THE DEVELOPING HUMAN

Clinically Oriented Embryology

8th Edition

Keith L. Moore, PhD, FIAC, FRSM
Professor Emeritus, Division of Anatomy, Department of Surgery, Faculty of Medicine, University of Toronto, Toronto, Ontario, Canada
Former Professor and Head, Department of Anatomy University of Manitoba, Winnipeg, Manitoba, Canada
Former Professor and Chairman, Department of Anatomy and Cell Biology, University of Toronto Toronto, Ontario, Canada

T.V.N. Persaud, MD, PhD, DSc, FRCPath (Lond.)
Professor Emeritus and Former Head
Department of Human Anatomy and Cell Science
Professor of Pediatrics and Child Health
Associate Professor of Obstetrics, Gynecology, and Reproductive Sciences
Faculty of Medicine, University of Manitoba, Winnipeg, Manitoba, Canada
Professor of Anatomy and Embryology, St. George's University, Grenada, West Indies

With the Collaboration of
Mark G. Torchia, MSc, PhD
Associate Professor and Director of Development
Department of Surgery, University of Manitoba
Director of Advanced Technologies
Winnipeg Regional Health Authority
Winnipeg, Manitoba, Canada

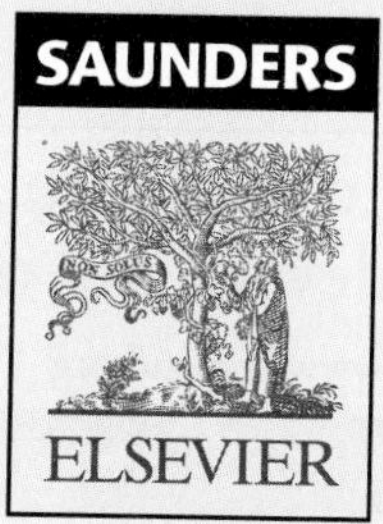

SAUNDERS
ELSEVIER

1600 John F. Kennedy Boulevard
Suite 1800
Philadelphia, PA 19103-2899

THE DEVELOPING HUMAN: CLINICALLY ORIENTED EMBRYOLOGY,
EIGHTH EDITION
ISBN: 978-1-4160-3706-4
International Edition: 978-0-8089-2387-9

Library of Congress Cataloging-in-Publication Data

Moore, Keith L.
The developing human : clinically oriented embryology / Keith L. Moore, T.V.N. Persaud; with the collaboration of Mark G. Torchia. —8th ed.
p. ; cm.
ISBN-13: 978-1-4160-3706-4
ISBN-10: 1-4160-3706-3
1. Embryology, Human. 2. Abnormalities, Human. I. Persaud, T. V. N. II. Torchia, Mark G. III. Title.
[DNLM: 1. Embryology. QS 604 M822d 2008]

QM601.M76 2008
612.6'4—dc22

2006039363

Acquisitions Editor: Inta Ozols/Madelene Hyde
Developmental Editor: Kathryn DeFrancesco
Project Manager: Bryan Hayward
Interior and Cover Designer: Steven Stave

Printed in China

Last digit is the print number: 9 8 7 6 5 4 3 2 1

In Memory of Marion Moore

Marion was my best friend, confidant, colleague, and wife for 57 years. She was the mother of our five children and grandmother of our nine grandchildren. Her assistance with the editing and preparation of earlier editions of this and other books was invaluable. Marion, you will always be in our thoughts and in our hearts. You will be surely missed but never forgotten.

Keith L. Moore

Contributors

Albert E. Chudley, MD, FRCPC, FCCMG
Professor of Pediatrics and Child Health, and Biochemistry and Metabolism
Program Director, Genetics and Metabolism
Health Sciences Centre and Winnipeg Regional Health Authority
Winnipeg, Manitoba, Canada

Jeffrey T. Wigle, PhD
Senior Scientist, Institute of Cardiovascular Sciences
St. Boniface General Hospital Research Centre
Assistant Professor, Department of Biochemistry and Medical Genetics
University of Manitoba, Winnipeg, Manitoba, Canada

David D. Eisenstat, MD, MA, FRCPC
Director, Neuro-Oncology, CancerCare Manitoba
Senior Investigator, Manitoba Institute of Cell Biology
Associate Professor, Departments of Pediatrics and Child Health, Human Anatomy and Cell Science, and Ophthalmology
University of Manitoba, Winnipeg, Manitoba, Canada

Preface

We are now entering an era of outstanding achievements in the fields of molecular biology and human embryology. The sequencing of the human genome has been achieved, and several mammalian species, including the human embryo, have been cloned. Scientists have isolated human embryonic stem cells, and suggestions for their use in treating certain intractable diseases continue to generate widespread debate. These remarkable scientific developments have already provided promising directions for research in human embryology, which will have an impact on medical practice in the future.

The eighth edition of *The Developing Human* has been thoroughly revised to reflect our current understanding of some of the molecular events that guide formation of the embryo. The book also contains more clinically oriented material than previous editions. These sections are highlighted in color to set them apart from the rest of the text. In addition to focusing on clinically relevant aspects of embryology, we have revised the clinically oriented problems with brief answers and added more case studies that emphasize that embryology is an important part of modern medical practice.

This edition includes numerous new color photographs of embryos (normal and abnormal). Many of the illustrations have been improved using three-dimensional renderings and more effective use of colors. There are also many new diagnostic images (ultrasound and MRI) of embryos and fetuses to illustrate three-dimensional aspects of embryos. An innovative set of animations that will help students to understand the complexities of embryological development now comes with this book.

The coverage of teratology has been increased because the study of abnormal development is helpful in understanding risk estimation, the causes of anomalies, and how malformations may be prevented. Recent advances in the molecular aspects of developmental biology have been highlighted throughout the book, especially in those areas that appear promising for clinical medicine or have the potential for making a significant impact on the direction of future research. With this is mind, we have added a chapter, contributed by Dr. Jeffrey T. Wigle and Dr. David D. Eisenstat, on some common signaling pathways during development.

We have continued our attempts to give an easy-to-read account of human development before birth. Each chapter has been thoroughly revised to reflect new findings in research and their clinical significance. The chapters are organized to present a systematic and logical approach that explains how embryos develop. The first chapter introduces the reader to the scope and importance of embryology, the historical background of the discipline, and the terms used to describe the stages of development. The next four chapters cover embryonic development, beginning with the formation of gametes and ending with the formation of basic organs and systems. The development of specific organs and systems is then described in a systematic manner, followed by chapters dealing with the highlights of the fetal period, the placenta and fetal membranes, and the causes of human congenital anomalies. At the end of each chapter there are references that contain both classic works and recent research publications.

Keith L. Moore
Vid Persaud

Acknowledgments

The Developing Human is widely used by medical, dental, and other students in the health sciences. The suggestions, criticisms, and comments we received from instructors and students around the world have helped us to improve this work. In a book such as this, the illustrations are an essential feature. Many colleagues have generously provided us with photographs of clinical cases from their practice.

We are indebted to the following colleagues (listed alphabetically) for critical reviewing of chapters, making suggestions for improvement of this book, or providing new figures: Dr. Judy Anderson, Department of Human Anatomy and Cell Science, University of Manitoba, Winnipeg, Manitoba; Dr. Stephen Ahing, Department of Dental Diagnostic and Surgical Sciences, Faculty of Dentistry, University of Manitoba, Winnipeg, Manitoba; Dr. Kunwar Batnagar, School of Medicine, University of Louisville, Louisville, Kentucky; Dr. David L. Bolender, Department of Cell Biology, Neurobiology, and Anatomy, Medical College of Wisconsin, Milwaukee, Wisconsin; Dr. Boris Kablar, Department of Anatomy and Neurobiology, Dalhousie University, Halifax, Nova Scotia; Dr. Albert Chudley, Departments of Pediatrics and Child Health, Biochemistry and Medical Genetics, University of Manitoba, Winnipeg, Manitoba; Dr. Blaine M. Cleghorn, Faculty of Dentistry, Dalhousie University, Halifax, Nova Scotia; Dr. Marc Del Bigio, Department of Pathology, University of Manitoba, Winnipeg, Manitoba; Dr. Stephen E. Dolgin, Division of Pediatric Surgery, Mount Sinai School of Medicine, New York, New York; Dr. Raymond Gasser, Department of Cell Biology and Anatomy, Louisiana State University School of Medicine, New Orleans, Louisiana; Dr. Barry Grayson, Institute of Reconstructive Plastic Surgery, New York University Medical Center, New York, New York; Dr. Byron Grove, Department of Anatomy and Cell Biology, University of North Dakota, Grand Forks, North Dakota; Dr. Brian K. Hall, Department of Biology, Dalhousie University, Halifax, Nova Scotia; Dr. Mark W. Hamrick, Department of Cellular Biology and Anatomy, Medical College of Georgia, Augusta, Georgia; Dr. Christopher Harman, Department of Obstetrics, Gynecology, and Reproductive Sciences, University of Maryland, Baltimore, Maryland; Dr. Dagmar Kalousek, Department of Pathology, University of British Columbia, Vancouver, British Columbia; Dr. Tom Klonisch, Department of Human Anatomy and Cell Science, University of Manitoba, Winnipeg, Manitoba; Dr. David J. Kozlowski, Department of Cellular Biology and Anatomy, Medical College of Georgia, Augusta, Georiga; Dr. Peeyush Lala, Faculty of Medicine, University of Western Ontario, London, Ontario; Dr. Deborah Levine, Beth Israel Deaconess Medical Center, Boston, Massachusetts; Dr. Edward A. Lyons, Department of Radiology, University of Manitoba, Winnipeg, Manitoba; Professor Bernard J. Moxham, Cardiff School of Biosciences, Cardiff University, Cardiff, Wales; Dr. John Mulliken, Department of Surgery and Craniofacial Center, Harvard Medical School, Boston, Massachusetts; Dr. Valerie Dean O'Loughlin, Department of Anatomy and Cell Biology, Indiana University, Bloomington, Indiana; Dr. Maria Patestas, Des Moines University, Des Moines, Iowa; Professor T.S. Ranganathan, Department of Anatomical Sciences, St. George's University, Grenada; Dr. Gregory Reid, Department of Obstetrics, Gynecology and Reproductive Sciences, University of Manitoba, Winnipeg, Manitoba; Dr. Norman Rosenblum, The Hospital for Sick Children and Department of Pediatrics, University of Toronto, Toronto, Ontario; Dr. J. Elliott Scott, Department of Oral Biology, Faculty of Dentistry, University of Manitoba, Winnipeg, Manitoba; Dr. Robert Semo, Department of Obstetrics and Gynecology, University of California, San Diego, California; Dr. Joseph Siebert, Research Associate Professor, Children's Hospital and Regional Medical Center, Seattle, Washington; Dr. Kohei Shiota, Department of Anatomy and Developmental Biology, Kyoto University, Kyoto, Japan; Dr. Gerald Smyser, Altru Health System, Grand Forks, North Dakota; Dr. Pierre Soucy, Division of Paediatric General Surgery, Children's Hospital of Eastern Ontario, University of Ottawa, Ottawa, Ontario; Dr. Richard Shane Tubbs, Children's Hospital, University of Alabama at Birmingham, Birmingham, Alabama; Professor Christoph Viebahn, Department of Anatomy and Embryology, Göttingen University, Göttingen, Germany; Christopher von Bartheld, Department of Physiology and Cell Biology, Medical School of Nevada, Reno, Nevada; Dr. Michael Wiley, Division of Anatomy, Department of Surgery, University of Toronto, Toronto, Ontario; and Dr. Donna L. Young, Department of Biology, University of Winnipeg, Winnipeg, Manitoba.

The new illustrations were prepared by Hans Neuhart, President of the Electronic Illustrators Group in Fountain Hills, Arizona. The stunning collection of animations was created by *Emantras*, and for skillfully reviewing them we thank Dr. David L. Bolender, Department of Cell Biology, Neurobiology, and Anatomy, Medical College of Wisconsin, Milwaukee, Wisconsin.

We are greatly indebted to Ms. Inta Ozols, Executive Medical Editor, and Ms. Madelene Hyde, Publisher, for their insight, encouragement, and many suggestions. We wish to thank Ms. Kathryn DeFrancesco, our Developmental Editor, for her specialist advice and skillful editing. For coordinating work relating to the animations, we would like to thank Ms. Carol Emery. Finally, our special thanks also go to the production staff, particularly Mr. Bryan Hayward, Project Manager, and Ms. Linnea Hermanson, Production Editor. This new edition of *The Developing Human* is largely the result of their professional dedication and technical expertise.

Keith L. Moore
Vid Persaud

Contents

1 Introduction to The Developing Human 1

Developmental Periods **2**
Embryologic Terminology **2**
Significance of Embryology **7**
Historical Gleanings **8**
  Ancient Views of Human Embryology **8**
  Embryology in the Middle Ages **8**
  The Renaissance **9**
Genetics and Human Development **11**
Molecular Biology of Human Development **11**
Descriptive Terms in Embryology **11**
Clinically Oriented Problems **13**

2 The Beginning of Human Development: First Week 14

Gametogenesis **15**
Meiosis **15**
Spermatogenesis **15**
Oogenesis **20**
  Prenatal Maturation of Oocytes **20**
  Postnatal Maturation of Oocytes **20**
Comparison of Gametes **20**
Uterus, Uterine Tubes, and Ovaries **21**
  Uterus **21**
  Uterine Tubes **21**
  Ovaries **23**
Female Reproductive Cycles **23**
Ovarian Cycle **23**
  Follicular Development **23**
  Ovulation **23**
  Corpus Luteum **25**
Menstrual Cycle **27**
  Phases of the Menstrual Cycle **27**
Transportation of Gametes **28**
  Oocyte Transport **28**
  Sperm Transport **28**
Maturation of Sperms **29**
Viability of Gametes **31**
Fertilization **31**
  Phases of Fertilization **31**
  Fertilization **33**
Cleavage of the Zygote **35**
Formation of the Blastocyst **36**
Summary of the First Week **39**
Clinically Oriented Problems **39**

3 Formation of the Bilaminar Embryonic Disc: Second Week 42

Completion of Implantation and Continuation of Embryonic Development **43**
Formation of the Amniotic Cavity, Embryonic Disc, and Umbilical Vesicle **44**
Development of the Chorionic Sac **45**
Implantation Sites of Blastocysts **45**
Summary of Implantation **48**
Summary of the Second Week **51**
Clinically Oriented Problems **53**

4 Formation of Germ Layers and Early Tissue and Organ Differentiation: Third Week 54

Gastrulation: Formation of Germ Layers **55**
Primitive Streak **57**
  Fate of the Primitive Streak **57**
Notochordal Process and Notochord **59**
The Allantois **62**
Neurulation: Formation of the Neural Tube **62**
  Neural Plate and Neural Tube **62**
  Neural Crest Formation **62**
Development of Somites **65**
Development of the Intraembryonic Coelom **65**
Early Development of the Cardiovascular System **65**
  Vasculogenesis and Angiogenesis **66**
  The Primordial Cardiovascular System **67**
Development of Chorionic Villi **68**
Summary of the Third Week **68**
Clinically Oriented Problems **70**

5 Organogenetic Period: Fourth to Eighth Weeks 72

Phases of Embryonic Development **73**
Folding of the Embryo **73**
  Folding of the Embryo in the Median Plane **73**
  Folding of the Embryo in the Horizontal Plane **73**
Germ Layer Derivatives **75**
Control of Embryonic Development **75**
Highlights of the Fourth to Eighth Weeks **79**
  Fourth Week **79**
  Fifth Week **79**
  Sixth Week **80**
  Seventh Week **80**
  Eighth Week **81**
Estimation of Embryonic Age **86**
Summary of the Fourth to Eighth Weeks **90**
Clinically Oriented Problems **91**

6 **The Fetal Period: Ninth Week to Birth 95**
Estimation of Fetal Age **96**
Trimesters of Pregnancy **97**
Measurements and Characteristics of Fetuses **98**
Highlights of the Fetal Period **98**
Nine to Twelve Weeks **98**
Thirteen to Sixteen Weeks **100**
Seventeen to Twenty Weeks **100**
Twenty-one to Twenty-five Weeks **101**
Twenty-six to Twenty-nine Weeks **102**
Thirty to Thirty-four Weeks **102**
Thirty-five to Thirty-eight Weeks **102**
Expected Date of Delivery **103**
Factors Influencing Fetal Growth **104**
Cigarette Smoking **104**
Multiple Pregnancy **104**
Alcohol and Illicit Drugs **104**
Impaired Uteroplacental and Fetoplacental Blood Flow **104**
Genetic Factors and Growth Retardation **104**
Procedures for Assessing Fetal Status **104**
Ultrasonography **105**
Diagnostic Amniocentesis **105**
Alpha-fetoprotein Assay **105**
Spectrophotometric Studies **105**
Chorionic Villus Sampling **106**
Sex Chromatin Patterns **106**
Cell Cultures and Chromosomal Analysis **106**
Fetal Transfusion **107**
Fetoscopy **107**
Percutaneous Umbilical Cord Blood Sampling **107**
Computed Tomography and Magnetic Resonance Imaging **107**
Fetal Monitoring **107**
Summary of the Fetal Period **107**
Clinically Oriented Problems **108**

7 **The Placenta and Fetal Membranes 110**
The Placenta **111**
The Decidua **111**
Development of the Placenta **111**
Placental Circulation **117**
The Placental Membrane **118**
Functions of the Placenta **118**
The Placenta as an Invasive Tumorlike Structure **122**
Uterine Growth during Pregnancy **122**
Parturition **123**
The Placenta and Fetal Membranes after Birth **123**
The Umbilical Cord **125**
The Umbilical Vesicle (Yolk Sac) **133**
Significance of the Umbilical Vesicle **134**
Fate of the Umbilical Vesicle (Yolk Sac) **134**
The Allantois **134**
Multiple Pregnancies **134**
Twins and Fetal Membranes **134**
Dizygotic Twins **137**
Monozygotic Twins **137**
Other Types of Multiple Births **140**
Summary of the Placenta and Fetal Membranes **140**
Clinically Oriented Problems **143**

8 **Body Cavities, Mesenteries, and Diaphragm 145**
The Embryonic Body Cavity **146**
Mesenteries **146**
Division of the Embryonic Body Cavity **146**
Development of the Diaphragm **150**
Septum Transversum **150**
Pleuroperitoneal Membranes **151**
Dorsal Mesentery of the Esophagus **151**
Muscular Ingrowth from Lateral Body Walls **152**
Positional Changes and Innervation of the Diaphragm **153**
Summary of the Development of the Body Cavities **157**
Clinically Oriented Problems **157**

9 **The Pharyngeal Apparatus 159**
Pharyngeal Arches **160**
Pharyngeal Arch Components **160**
Pharyngeal Pouches **166**
Derivatives of Pharyngeal Pouches **166**
Pharyngeal Grooves **169**
Pharyngeal Membranes **169**
Development of the Thyroid Gland **173**
Histogenesis of the Thyroid Gland **173**
Development of the Tongue **176**
Lingual Papillae and Taste Buds **176**
Nerve Supply of the Tongue **177**
Development of the Salivary Glands **179**
Development of the Face **179**
Summary of Facial Development **182**
Development of the Nasal Cavities **182**
Paranasal Sinuses **184**
Development of the Palate **185**
Primary Palate **185**
Secondary Palate **186**
Summary of the Pharyngeal Apparatus **195**
Clinically Oriented Problems **195**

10 **The Respiratory System 197**
Respiratory Primordium **198**
Development of the Larynx **198**
Development of the Trachea **198**
Development of the Bronchi and Lungs **202**
Maturation of the Lungs **203**
Summary of the Respiratory System **208**
Clinically Oriented Problems **209**

11 The Digestive System 211
Foregut 212
Development of the Esophagus 212
Development of the Stomach 213
Omental Bursa 216
Development of the Duodenum 216
Development of the Liver and Biliary Apparatus 218
Development of the Spleen 223
Midgut 224
Rotation of the Midgut Loop 224
The Cecum and Appendix 227
Hindgut 235
Cloaca 235
The Anal Canal 236
Summary of the Digestive System 241
Clinically Oriented Problems 241

12 The Urogenital System 243
Development of the Urinary System 244
Development of the Kidneys and Ureters 244
Development of the Urinary Bladder 256
Development of the Urethra 260
Development of the Suprarenal Glands 260
Development of the Genital System 262
Development of the Gonads 263
Development of the Genital Ducts 265
Development of the Male Genital Ducts and Glands 265
Development of the Female Genital Ducts and Glands 269
Development of the Uterus and Vagina 269
Development of the External Genitalia 271
Development of the Male External Genitalia 271
Development of the Female External Genitalia 273
Development of the Inguinal Canals 277
Relocation of the Testes and Ovaries 279
Descent of the Testes 279
Descent of the Ovaries 281
Summary of the Urogenital System 282
Clinically Oriented Problems 283

13 The Cardiovascular System 285
Early Development of the Heart and Blood Vessels 286
Development and Fate of Veins Associated with the Heart 286
Fate of the Vitelline and Umbilical Arteries 292
Later Development of the Heart 292
Circulation through the Primordial Heart 292
Partitioning of the Primordial Heart 292
Changes in the Sinus Venosus 297
Conducting System of the Heart 308
Anomalies of the Heart and Great Vessels 309
Derivatives of the Pharyngeal Arch Arteries 317
Derivatives of the First Pair of Pharyngeal Arch Arteries 318
Derivatives of the Second Pair of Pharyngeal Arch Arteries 318
Derivatives of the Third Pair of Pharyngeal Arch Arteries 318
Derivatives of the Fourth Pair of Pharyngeal Arch Arteries 319
Fate of the Fifth Pair of Pharyngeal Arch Arteries 319
Derivatives of the Sixth Pair of Pharyngeal Arch Arteries 319
Pharyngeal Arch Arterial Anomalies 319
Fetal and Neonatal Circulation 325
Fetal Circulation 325
Transitional Neonatal Circulation 327
Derivatives of Fetal Vascular Structures 330
Development of the Lymphatic System 333
Development of the Lymph Sacs and Lymphatic Ducts 333
Thoracic Duct 333
Development of the Lymph Nodes 333
Development of the Lymphocytes 333
Development of the Spleen and Tonsils 334
Summary of the Cardiovascular System 335
Clinically Oriented Problems 336

14 The Skeletal System 338
Development of Bone and Cartilage 339
Histogenesis of Cartilage 339
Histogenesis of Bone 339
Intramembranous Ossification 339
Endochondral Ossification 339
Development of Joints 342
Fibrous Joints 344
Cartilaginous Joints 344
Synovial Joints 344
Development of the Axial Skeleton 344
Development of the Vertebral Column 344
Development of the Ribs 346
Development of the Sternum 347
Development of the Cranium 347
Newborn Cranium 347
Postnatal Growth of the Cranium 348
Development of the Appendicular Skeleton 353
Summary of the Skeletal System 355
Clinically Oriented Problems 356

15 The Muscular System 357
Development of Skeletal Muscle 358
Myotomes 358
Pharyngeal Arch Muscles 358
Ocular Muscles 358
Tongue Muscles 359
Limb Muscles 359

Development of Smooth Muscle 360
Development of Cardiac Muscle 360
Summary of the Muscular System 362
Clinically Oriented Problems 363

16 **The Limbs** 364
Early Stages of Limb Development 365
Final Stages of Limb Development 366
Cutaneous Innervation of Limbs 368
Blood Supply to the Limbs 371
Anomalies of the Limbs 372
Summary of Limb Development 377
Clinically Oriented Problems 379

17 **The Nervous System** 380
Origin of the Nervous System 381
Development of the Spinal Cord 381
Development of the Spinal Ganglia 383
Development of the Spinal Meninges 384
Positional Changes of the Spinal Cord 384
Myelination of Nerve Fibers 386
Congenital Anomalies of the Spinal Cord 386
Development of the Brain 392
Brain Flexures 392
Hindbrain 393
Choroid Plexuses and Cerebrospinal Fluid (CSF) 398
Midbrain 398
Forebrain 399
Congenital Anomalies of the Brain 404
Development of the Peripheral Nervous System 413
Spinal Nerves 414
Cranial Nerves 414
Development of the Autonomic Nervous System 416
Sympathetic Nervous System 416
Parasympathetic Nervous System 416
Summary of the Nervous System 416
Clinically Oriented Problems 417

18 **The Eye and Ear** 419
Development of the Eye and Related Structures 420
Development of the Retina 420
Development of the Ciliary Body 425
Development of the Iris 425
Development of the Lens 427
Development of the Aqueous Chambers 428
Development of the Cornea 429
Development of the Choroid and Sclera 429
Development of the Eyelids 429
Development of the Lacrimal Glands 430
Development of the Ear 430
Development of the Internal Ear 431
Development of the Middle Ear 433
Development of the External Ear 433
Summary of the Development of the Eye 437
Summary of the Development of the Ear 437
Clinically Oriented Problems 437

19 **The Integumentary System** 439
Development of Skin and Skin Appendages 440
Epidermis 440
Dermis 441
Glands of the Skin 441
Development of Hairs 447
Development of Nails 448
Development of Teeth 448
Summary of the Integumentary System 455
Clinically Oriented Problems 456

20 **Congenital Anatomic Anomalies or Human Birth Defects** 457
Classification of Birth Defects 458
Teratology: The Study of Abnormal Development 458
Anomalies Caused by Genetic Factors 459
Numerical Chromosomal Abnormalities 459
Structural Chromosomal Abnormalities 466
Anomalies Caused by Mutant Genes 469
Developmental Signaling Pathways 471
Anomalies Caused by Environmental Factors 471
Principles in Teratogenesis 474
Human Teratogens 475
Anomalies Caused by Multifactorial Inheritance 484
Summary of Congential Anatomic Anomalies or Human Birth Defects 484
Clinically Oriented Problems 484

21 **Common Signaling Pathways Used during Development** 487
Morphogens 488
Retinoic Acid 488
Transforming Growth Factor β/Bone Morphogenetic Protein 489
Hedgehog 489
Wnt/β-Catenin Pathway 490
Notch-Delta Pathway 491
Transcription Factors 491
Hox/Homeobox Proteins 492
Pax Genes 493
Basic Helix-Loop-Helix Transcription Factors 493
Receptor Tyrosinase Kinases 493
Common Features 493
Regulation of Angiogenesis by Receptor Tyrosine Kinases 494
Summary of Common Signaling Pathways Used during Development 494

Appendix 496

Index 507

1

Introduction to the Developing Human

Developmental Periods 2

Embryologic Terminology 2

Significance of Embryology 7

Historical Gleanings 8

Ancient Views of Human Embryology 8

Embryology in the Middle Ages 8

The Renaissance 9

Genetics and Human Development 11

Molecular Biology of Human Development 11

Descriptive Terms in Embryology 11

Clinically Oriented Problems 13

Human development is a continuous process that begins when an **oocyte** (ovum) from a female is fertilized by a **sperm** (spermatozoon) from a male. Cell division, cell migration, programmed cell death, differentiation, growth, and cell rearrangement transform the fertilized oocyte, a highly specialized, totipotent cell, a **zygote**, into a multicellular human being. Although most developmental changes occur during the embryonic and fetal periods, important changes occur during later periods of development: infancy, childhood, adolescence, and early adulthood *Development does not stop at birth*. Important changes, in addition to growth, occur after birth (e.g., development of teeth and female breasts).

DEVELOPMENTAL PERIODS

It is customary to divide human development into *prenatal* (before birth) and *postnatal* (after birth) periods. The main developmental changes occurring before birth are illustrated in the *Timetable of Human Prenatal Development* (Figs. 1-1 and 1-2). Examination of the timetable reveals that the most visible advances occur during the third to eighth weeks of embryonic development. During the fetal period, differentiation and growth of tissues and organs occur. The rate of body growth increases during this period.

EMBRYOLOGIC TERMINOLOGY

The following terms are commonly used in discussions of developing humans; several of these terms are used in the *Timetable of Human Prenatal Development*. Most terms have Latin (L.) or Greek (Gr.) origins.

Oocyte (*L. ovum*, egg). The female germ or sex cells are produced in the *ovaries*. When mature, the oocytes are called secondary oocytes or mature oocytes.

Sperm (Gr. *sperma*, seed). The sperm, or spermatozoon, refers to the male germ cell produced in the testes (testicles). Numerous sperms (spermatozoa) are expelled from the male urethra during ejaculation.

Zygote. This cell results from the union of an oocyte and a sperm during fertilization. A zygote or embryo is the beginning of a new human being.

Gestational Age. It is difficult to determine exactly when fertilization (conception) occurs because the process cannot be observed in vivo (within the living body). Physicians calculate the age of the embryo or fetus from the presumed first day of the last normal menstrual period. This is the *gestational age*, which is approximately 2 weeks longer than the *fertilization age* because the oocyte is not fertilized until approximately 2 weeks after the preceding menstruation (see Fig. 1-1).

Cleavage. This is the *series of mitotic cell divisions of the zygote* that result in the formation of early embryonic cells, *blastomeres*. The size of the cleaving zygote remains unchanged because at each succeeding cleavage division, the blastomeres become smaller.

Morula (L. *morus*, mulberry). This solid mass of 12 to approximately 32 blastomeres is formed by cleavage of a zygote. The blastomeres change their shape and tightly align themselves against each other to form a compact ball of cells. This phenomenon, **compaction**, is probably mediated by cell surface adhesion glycoproteins. The morula stage occurs 3 to 4 days after fertilization, just as the early embryo enters the uterus.

Blastocyst (Gr. *blastos*, germ + *kystis*, bladder). After 2 to 3 days, the morula enters the uterus from the uterine tube (fallopian tube). Soon a fluid-filled cavity, the *blastocystic cavity*, develops inside it. This change converts the morula into a blastocyst. Its centrally located cells, the *inner cell mass* or *embryoblast*, is the embryonic part of the embryo.

Implantation. The process during which the blastocyst attaches to the *endometrium*, the mucous membrane or lining of uterus, and subsequently embeds in it. The preimplantation period of embryonic development is the time between fertilization and the beginning of implantation, a period of approximately 6 days.

Gastrula (Gr. *gaster*, stomach). During gastrulation (transformation of a blastocyst into a gastrula), a three-layered or trilaminar embryonic disc forms (third week). The three germ layers of the gastrula (ectoderm, mesoderm, and endoderm) subsequently differentiate into the tissues and organs of the embryo.

Neurula (Gr. *neuron*, nerve). The early embryo during the third and fourth weeks when the neural tube is developing from the neural plate (see Fig. 1-1). It is the first appearance of the nervous system and the next stage after the gastrula.

Embryo (Gr. *embryon*). The developing human during its early stages of development. The *embryonic period* extends to the end of the eighth week (56 days), by which time the beginnings of all major structures are present. The size of embryos is given as crown-rump length, which is measured from the vertex of the cranium (crown of head) to the rump (buttocks).

Stages of Prenatal Development. Early embryonic development is described in stages because of the variable period it takes for embryos to develop certain morphologic characteristics (see Fig. 1-1). *Stage 1* begins at fertilization and embryonic development ends at stage 23, which occurs on day 56. The *fetal period* begins on day 57 and ends when the fetus is completely outside the mother.

Conceptus (L. *conceptio*, derivatives of zygote). The embryo and its adnexa (L., appendages or adjunct parts) or associated membranes (i.e., the *products of conception*). The conceptus includes all structures that develop from the zygote, both embryonic and extraembryonic. Hence, it includes the embryo as well as the embryonic part of the placenta and its associated membranes: amnion, chorionic (gestational) sac, and umbilical vesicle or yolk sac (see Chapter 7).

Primordium (L. *primus*, first + *ordior*, to begin). The beginning or first discernible indication of an organ or structure. The terms *anlage* and rudiment have similar meanings. The primordium of the upper limb appears as a bud on day 26 (see Fig. 1-1).

Fetus (L., unborn offspring). After the embryonic period (8 weeks) and until birth, the developing human is called a fetus. During the *fetal period* (ninth week to birth), differentiation and growth of the tissues and organs formed during the embryonic period occur. These developmental changes are not dramatic.

Text continues on p. 7

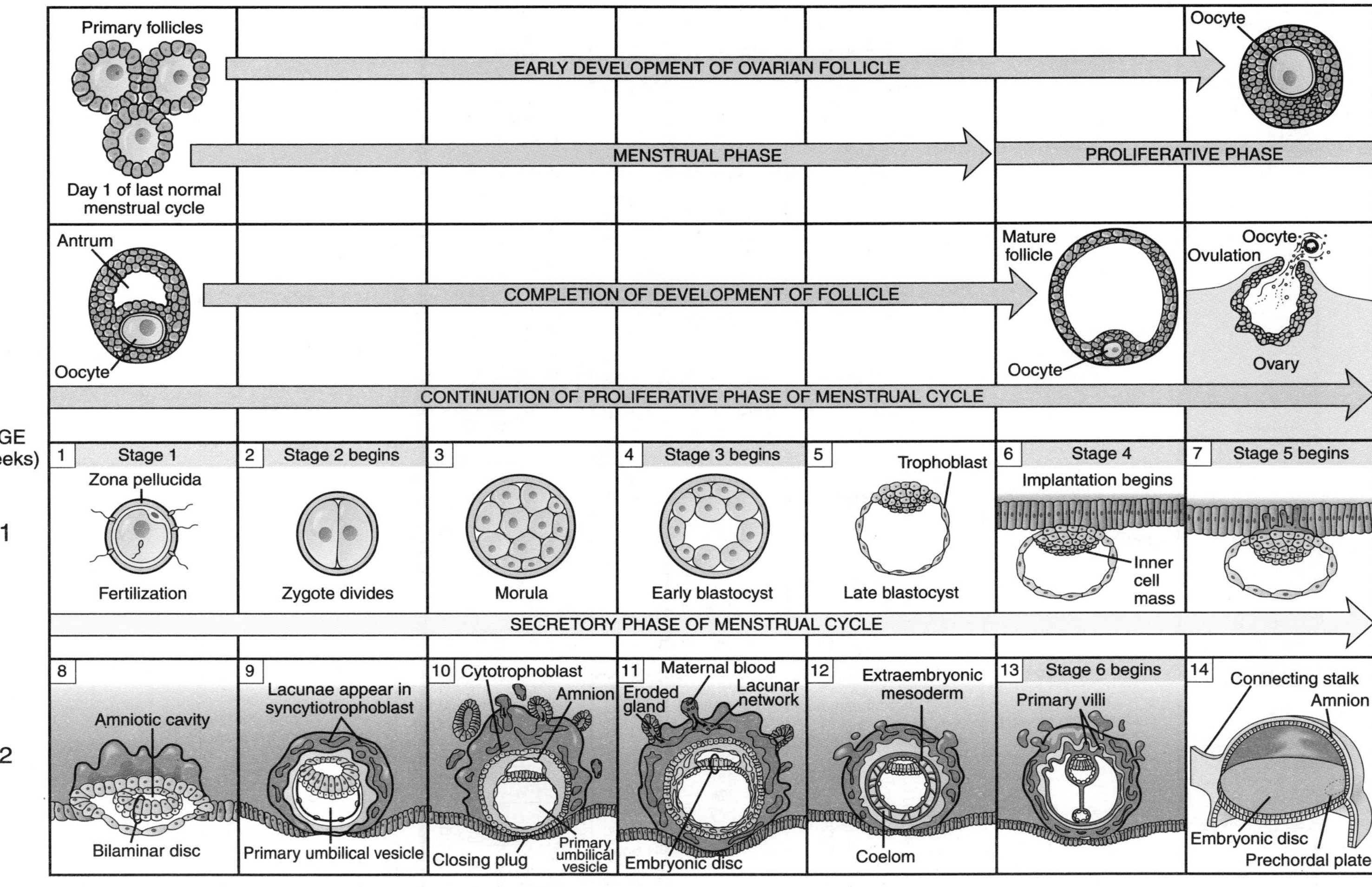

FIGURE 1-1. Early stages of development. Development of an ovarian follicle containing an oocyte, ovulation, and the phases of the menstrual cycle are illustrated. Human development begins at fertilization, approximately 14 days after the onset of the last normal menstrual period. Cleavage of the zygote in the uterine tube, implantation of the blastocyst in the endometrium (lining) of the uterus, and early development of the embryo are also shown. Beginning students should not attempt to memorize these tables or the stages (e.g., that stage 3 begins on day 4 and stage 5 on day 7). *Continued*

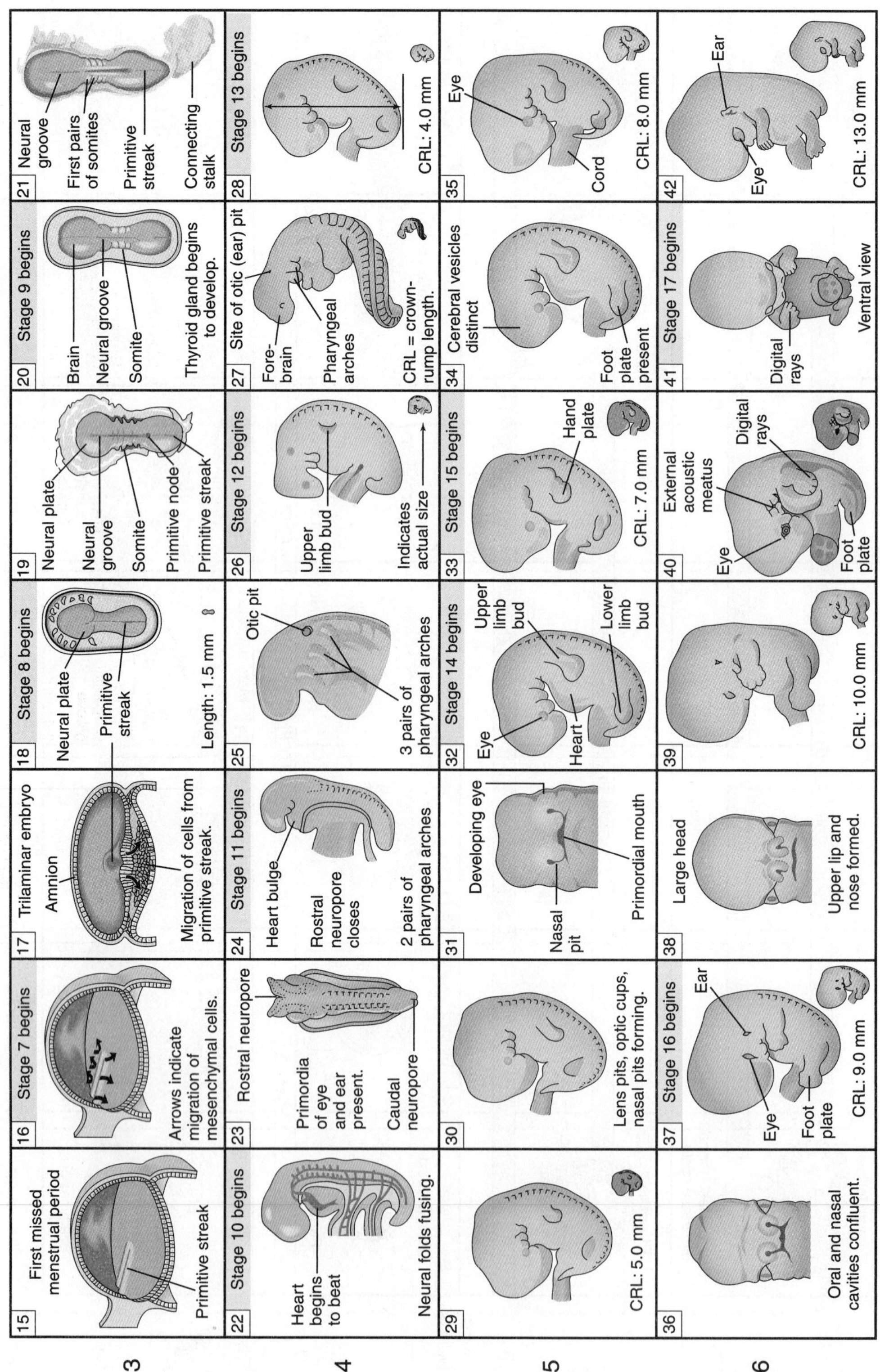

Figure 1-1. *Cont'd.*

TIMETABLE OF HUMAN PRENATAL DEVELOPMENT
7 to 38 weeks

AGE (weeks)							
7	43 Actual size CRL: 16 mm	44 Stage 18 begins Eyelids forming	45 Head large but chin poorly formed. Grooves between digital rays indicate fingers.	46 Wall of uterus Amniotic sac Uterine cavity Smooth chorion	47 Genital tubercle Urogenital membrane Anal membrane ♀ or ♂	48 Stage 19 begins Eyelid External ear Wrist, fingers fused	49 Actual size CRL: 18 mm
8	50 Stage 20 begins Upper limbs longer and bent at elbows. Fingers distinct but webbed.	51 Eye Ear Nose Fingers Toes	52 Stage 21 begins Large forehead	53 External genitalia have begun to differentiate.	54 Stage 22 begins Genital tubercle Urethral groove Anus ♀ or ♂	55 Eye Ear Wrist Knee Elbow Toes	56 Stage 23 CRL: 30 mm
9	57 Beginning of fetal period.	58 Eye Ear Wrist Knee Toes Elbow	59 Placenta	60 Genitalia Phallus Urogenital fold Labioscrotal fold Perineum ♀	61 CRL: 45 mm	62 Genitalia Phallus Urogenital fold Labioscrotal fold Perineum ♂	63 CRL: 50 mm
10	64 Face has human profile. Note growth of chin compared to day 44.	65	66 Ears still lower than normal.	67 Clitoris Labium minus Urogenital groove Labium majus ♀	68 Genitalia have ♀ or ♂ characteristics but still not fully formed.	69 Glans penis Urethral groove Scrotum ♂	70 CRL: 61 mm

FIGURE 1-1. *Cont'd.*

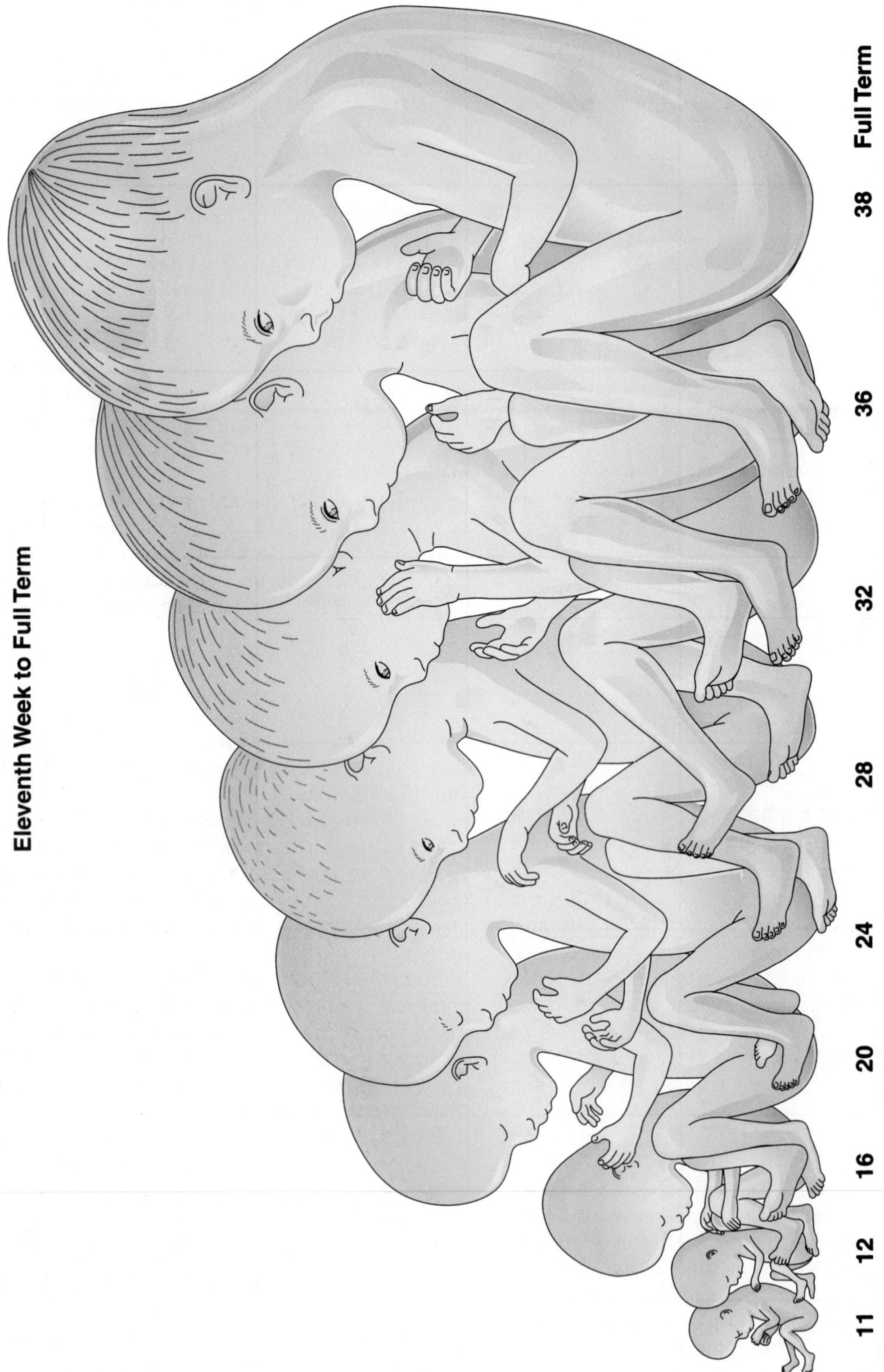

FIGURE 1-2. The embryonic period terminates at the end of the eighth week; by this time, the beginnings (primordia) of all essential structures are present. The fetal period, extending from 9 weeks to birth, is characterized by growth and elaboration of structures. Sex is clearly distinguishable by 12 weeks. Fetuses are viable 22 weeks after fertilization, but their chances of survival are not good until they are several weeks older. The 11- to 38-week fetuses shown are approximately half of their actual sizes. For more information, see Chapter 6.

Changes occurring during the embryonic period are very important because they make it possible for the tissues and organs to function. The rate of body growth is remarkable, especially during the third and fourth months (see Fig. 1-2), and weight gain is phenomenal during the terminal months.

Abortion (L. *aboriri*, to miscarry). A premature stoppage of development and expulsion of a conceptus from the uterus or expulsion of an embryo or fetus before it is viable—capable of living outside the uterus. An abortus is the products of an abortion (i.e., the embryo/fetus and its membranes). There are different types of abortion:

- *Threatened abortion* (bleeding with the possibility of abortion) is a complication in approximately 25% of clinically apparent pregnancies. Despite every effort to prevent an abortion, approximately half of these concepti ultimately abort.
- A *spontaneous abortion* is one that occurs naturally and is most common during the third week after fertilization. Approximately 15% of recognized pregnancies end in spontaneous abortion, usually during the first 12 weeks.
- A *habitual abortion* is the spontaneous expulsion of a dead or nonviable embryo or fetus in three or more consecutive pregnancies.
- An *induced abortion* is a birth that is medically induced before 20 weeks (i.e., before the fetus is viable). This type of abortion refers to the expulsion of an embryo or fetus induced intentionally by drugs or mechanical means
- A *complete abortion* is one in which all the products of conception are expelled from the uterus.
- A *missed abortion* is the retention of a conceptus in the uterus after death of the embryo or fetus.
- A *miscarriage* is the spontaneous abortion of a fetus and its membranes before the middle of the second trimester (approximately 135 days).

Trimester. A period of *three calendar months* during a pregnancy. Obstetricians commonly divide the 9-month period of gestation into three trimesters. The most critical stages of development occur during the first trimester (13 weeks) when embryonic and early fetal development is occurring.

Postnatal Period. The period occurring after birth. Explanations of frequently used developmental terms and periods follow.

Infancy refers to the earliest period of extrauterine life, roughly the *first year after birth*. An infant aged 1 month or younger is called a *newborn* or *neonate*. Transition from intrauterine to extrauterine existence requires many critical changes, especially in the cardiovascular and respiratory systems. If newborn infants survive the first crucial hours after birth, their chances of living are usually good. The body as a whole grows particularly rapidly during infancy; total length increases by approximately one half and weight is usually tripled. By 1 year of age, most children have six to eight teeth.

Childhood is the period from approximately 13 months until puberty. The primary (deciduous) teeth continue to appear and are later replaced by the secondary (permanent) teeth. During early childhood, there is active ossification (formation of bone), but as the child becomes older, the rate of body growth slows down. Just before puberty, however, growth accelerates—the *prepubertal growth spurt*.

Puberty occurs usually between the ages of 12 and 15 years in girls and 13 and 16 years in boys, during which *secondary sexual characteristics* develop and the capability of sexual reproduction is attained. The stages of pubertal development follow a consistent pattern and are defined by the appearance of secondary sexual characteristics (e.g., pubic hair development, breasts in females, and growth of external genitalia in males). Puberty ends in females with the first menstrual period or *menarche*, the beginning of the menstrual cycles or periods. Puberty ends in males when mature sperms are produced.

Adolescence is the period from approximately 11 to 19 years of age, which is characterized by rapid physical and sexual maturation. It extends from the earliest signs of sexual maturity—puberty—until the attainment of adult physical, mental, and emotional maturity. *The ability to reproduce is achieved during adolescence.* The general growth rate decelerates as this period terminates, but growth of some structures accelerates (e.g., female breasts and male genitalia).

Adulthood (L. *adultus*, grown up), attainment of full growth and maturity, is generally reached between the ages of 18 and 21 years. Ossification and growth are virtually completed during early adulthood (21 to 25 years). Thereafter, developmental changes occur very slowly.

SIGNIFICANCE OF EMBRYOLOGY

Literally, **embryology** means the study of embryos; however, the term generally refers to prenatal development of embryos and fetuses.

Developmental anatomy is the field of embryology concerned with the changes that cells, tissues, organs, and the body as a whole undergo from a germ cell of each parent to the resulting adult. Prenatal development is more rapid than postnatal development and results in more striking changes.

Teratology (Gr. *teratos*, monster) is the division of embryology and pathology that deals with abnormal development (birth defects). This branch of embryology is concerned with various genetic and/or environmental factors that disturb normal development and produce birth defects (see Chapter 20).

Embryology

- Bridges the gap between prenatal development and obstetrics, perinatal medicine, pediatrics, and clinical anatomy.
- Develops knowledge concerning the beginnings of human life and the changes occurring during prenatal development.
- Is of practical value in helping to understand the causes of variations in human structure.
- Illuminates gross anatomy and explains how normal and abnormal relations develop.

Knowledge that physicians have of normal development and of the causes of anomalies is necessary for giving the embryo and fetus the greatest possible chance of developing normally. Much of the modern practice of obstetrics involves **applied embryology**. Embryologic topics of special interest to obstetricians are ovulation, oocyte and sperm transport, fertilization, implantation, fetal-maternal relations, fetal circulation, critical periods of development, and causes of birth defects. In addition to caring for the mother, physicians guard the health of the embryo and fetus. The *significance of embryology* is readily apparent to pediatricians because some of their patients have birth defects resulting from maldevelopment, e.g., diaphragmatic hernia, spina bifida, and congenital heart disease.

Developmental anomalies cause most deaths during infancy. Knowledge of the development of structure and function is essential for understanding the physiologic changes that occur during the newborn period and for helping fetuses and babies in distress. Progress in surgery, especially in the fetal, perinatal, and pediatric age groups, has made knowledge of human development even more clinically significant. *Surgical treatment of the fetus is now possible.* The understanding and correction of most congenital anomalies depend on knowledge of normal development and of the deviations that may occur. An understanding of common congenital anomalies and their causes also enables physicians, dentists, and other health care providers to explain the developmental basis of abnormalities, often dispelling parental guilt feelings.

Physicians and other health care professionals who are aware of common anomalies and their embryologic bases approach unusual situations with confidence rather than surprise. For example, when it is realized that the renal artery represents only one of several vessels originally supplying the embryonic kidney, the frequent variations in number and arrangement of renal vessels are understandable and not unexpected.

HISTORICAL GLEANINGS

> If I have seen further, it is by standing on the shoulders of giants.
>
> — Sir Isaac Newton, English mathematician, 1643–1727

This statement, made more than 300 years ago, emphasizes that each new study of a problem rests on a base of knowledge established by earlier investigators. The theories of every age offer explanations based on the knowledge and experience of investigators of the period. Although we should not consider them final, we should appreciate rather than scorn their ideas. People have always been interested in knowing how they originated, developed, and were born, and why some people develop abnormally. Ancient people, filled with curiosity, developed many answers to these questions.

Ancient Views of Human Embryology

Egyptians of the Old Kingdom, approximately 3000 BC, knew of methods for incubating birds' eggs, but they left no records. *Akhnaton (Amenophis IV)* praised the sun god Aton as the creator of the germ in woman, maker of the seed in man, and giver of life to the son in the body of his mother. The ancient Egyptians believed that the soul entered the child at birth through the placenta.

A brief *Sanskrit treatise* on ancient Indian embryology is thought to have been written in 1416 BC. This scripture of the Hindus, called **Garbha Upanishad**, describes ancient ideas concerning the embryo. It states:

> From the conjugation of blood and semen the embryo comes into existence. During the period favorable for conception, after the sexual intercourse, (it) becomes a *Kalada* (one-day-old embryo). After remaining seven nights, it becomes a vesicle. After a fortnight it becomes a spherical mass. After a month it becomes a firm mass. After two months the head is formed. After three months the limb regions appear.

Greek scholars made many important contributions to the science of embryology. The first recorded embryologic studies are in the books of **Hippocrates of Cos**, the famous Greek physician (circa 460–377 BC), who is regarded as the *Father of Medicine*. In order to understand how the human embryo develops, he recommended:

> Take twenty or more eggs and let them be incubated by two or more hens. Then each day from the second to that of hatching, remove an egg, break it, and examine it. You will find exactly as I say, for the nature of the bird can be likened to that of man.

Aristotle of Stagira (circa 384–322 BC), a Greek philosopher and scientist, wrote a treatise on embryology in which he described development of the chick and other embryos. Aristotle is regarded as the *Founder of Embryology*, despite the fact that he promoted the idea that the embryo developed from a formless mass, which he described as a "less fully concocted seed with a nutritive soul and all bodily parts." This embryo, he thought, arose from menstrual blood after activation by male semen.

Claudius Galen (circa 130–201 AD), a Greek physician and medical scientist in Rome, wrote a book, *On the Formation of the Foetus*, in which he described the development and nutrition of fetuses and the structures that we now call the allantois, amnion, and placenta.

The **Talmud** contains references to the formation of the embryo. The Jewish physician Samuel-el-Yehudi, who lived during the second century AD, described six stages in the formation of the embryo from a "formless, rolled-up thing" to a "child whose months have been completed." Talmud scholars believed that the bones and tendons, the nails, the marrow in the head, and the white of the eye, were derived from the father, "who sows the white," but the skin, flesh, blood, hair from the mother, "who sows the red." These views were according to the teachings of both Aristotle and Galen (Needham, 1959).

Embryology in the Middle Ages

Growth of science was slow during the medieval period, and few high points of embryologic investigation undertaken during this time are known to us. It is cited in the **Quran** (seventh century AD), the Holy Book of the Muslims, that human beings are produced from a mixture of secretions from the male and female. Several references are made to the creation of a human being from a *nutfa* (small drop). It also states that the resulting organism settles in the womb like a seed, 6 days after its beginning. Reference is also made to the leechlike appearance of the early embryo. Later the embryo is said to resemble a "chewed substance."

Constantinus Africanus of Salerno (circa 1020–1087 AD) wrote a concise treatise entitled *De Humana Natura*. He gave the West many classical learnings in readable Latin through his many translations of Greek, Roman, and Arabic scholars. Africanus described the composition and sequential development of the embryo in relation to the planets and each month during pregnancy, a concept unknown in antiquity. Medieval scholars hardly deviated from the theory of Aristotle, which stated that the embryo was derived from menstrual blood and semen. Because of a lack of knowledge, drawings of the fetus in the uterus often showed a preformed fully developed infant frolicking in the womb (Fig. 1-3).

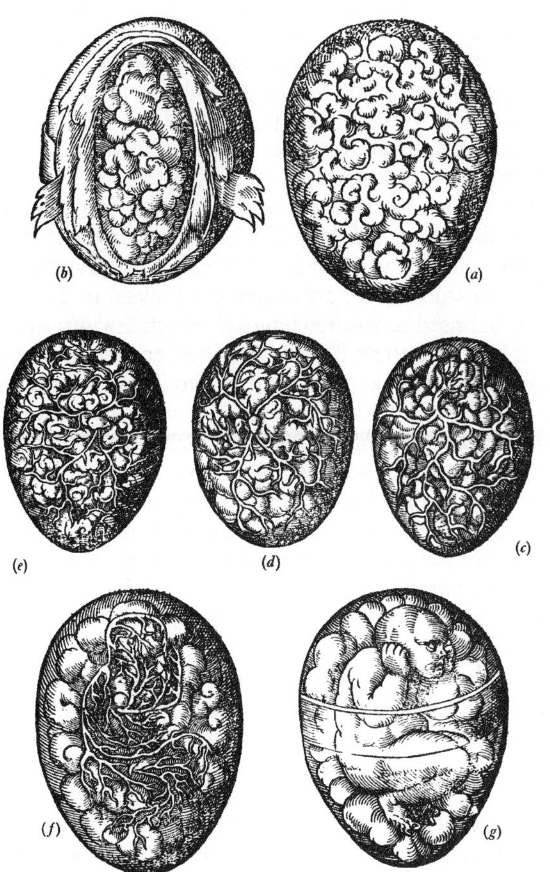

FIGURE 1-3. Illustrations from Jacob Rueff's *De Conceptu et Generatione Hominis* (1554) showing the fetus developing from a coagulum of blood and semen in the uterus. This theory was based on the teachings of Aristotle, and it survived until the late 18th century. (From Needham J: A History of Embryology. Cambridge, University Press, 1934; with permission of Cambridge University Press, England.)

The Renaissance

Leonardo da Vinci (1452–1519) made accurate drawings of dissections of pregnant uteri containing fetuses (Fig. 1-4). He introduced the quantitative approach to embryology by making measurements of prenatal growth.

It has been stated that the embryologic revolution began with the publication of **William Harvey's book**, *De Generatione Animalium*, in 1651. He believed that the male seed or sperm, after entering the womb or uterus, became metamorphosed into an egglike substance from which the embryo developed. Harvey (1578–1657) was greatly influenced by one of his professors at the University of Padua, **Fabricius of Aquapendente**, an Italian anatomist and embryologist who was the first to study embryos from different species of animals. Harvey examined chick embryos with simple lenses and made many new observations. He also studied the development of the fallow deer; however, when unable to observe early developmental stages, he concluded that embryos were secreted by the uterus. **Girolamo Fabricius** (1537–1619) wrote two major embryologic treatises, including one entitled *De Formato Foetu* (*The Formed Fetus*), which contained many illustrations of embryos and fetuses at different stages of development.

Early microscopes were simple but they opened an exciting new field of observation. In 1672, **Regnier de Graaf** observed small chambers in the rabbit's uterus and concluded that they could not have been secreted by the uterus. He stated that they must have come from organs that he called *ovaries*. Undoubtedly, the small chambers that de Graaf described were blastocysts (see Fig. 1-1). He also described vesicular ovarian follicles, which are still sometimes called *graafian follicles*.

Marcello Malpighi, studying what he believed were unfertilized hen's eggs in 1675, observed early embryos. As a result, he thought the egg contained a miniature chick.

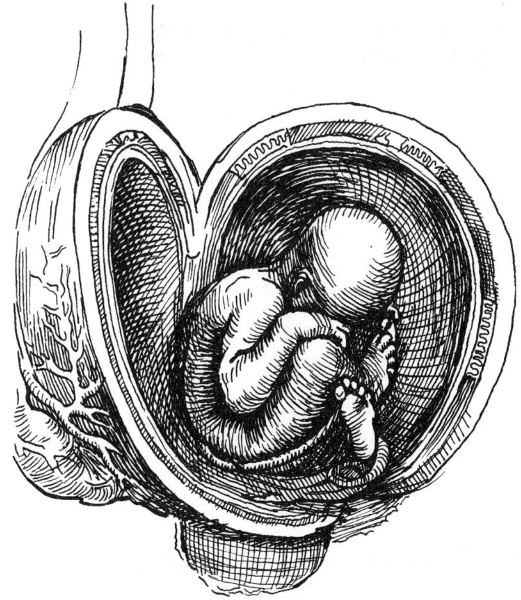

FIGURE 1-4. Reproduction of Leonardo da Vinci's drawing made in the 15th century AD showing a fetus in a uterus that has been incised and opened.

A young medical student in Leiden, **Johan Ham van Arnheim**, and his countryman **Anton van Leeuwenhoek** using an improved microscope in 1677 (Fig. 1-5), first observed a human sperm. However, they misunderstood the sperm's role in fertilization. They thought the sperm contained a miniature preformed human being that enlarged when it was deposited in the female genital tract (Fig. 1-6).

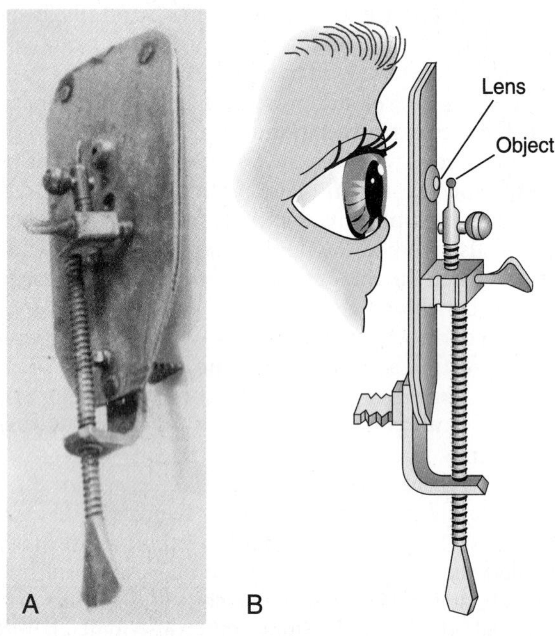

FIGURE 1-5. **A,** Photograph of a 1673 Leeuwenhoek microscope. **B,** Drawing of a lateral view illustrating the use of this primitive microscope. The object was held in front of the lens on the point of the short rod, and the screw arrangement was used to adjust the object under the lens.

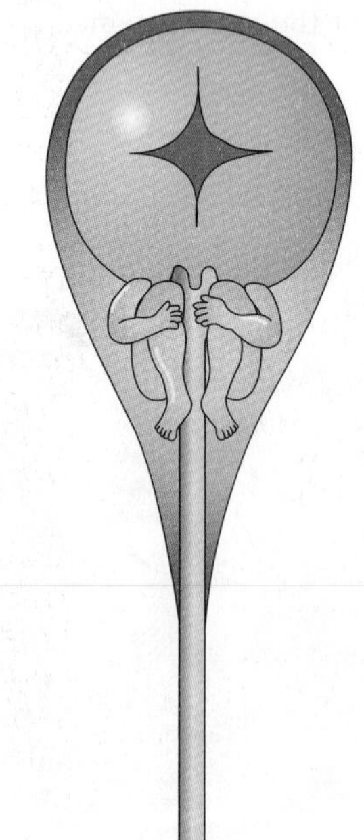

FIGURE 1-6. Copy of a 17th-century drawing of a sperm by Hartsoeker. The miniature human being within it was thought to enlarge after the sperm entered an ovum. Other embryologists at this time thought the oocyte contained a miniature human being that enlarged when it was stimulated by a sperm.

Caspar Friedrich Wolff refuted both versions of the *preformation theory* in 1759, after observing parts of the embryo develop from "globules" (small spherical bodies). He examined unincubated eggs but could not see the embryos described by Malpighi. He proposed the *layer concept*, whereby division of what we call the zygote produces layers of cells (now called the embryonic disc) from which the embryo develops. His ideas formed the basis of the *theory of epigenesis*, which states that development results from growth and differentiation of specialized cells. These important discoveries first appeared in Wolff's doctoral dissertation *Theoria Generationis*. He also observed embryonic masses of tissue that partly contribute to the development of the urinary and genital systems—Wolffian bodies and Wolffian ducts—now called the mesonephros and mesonephric ducts, respectively (see Chapter 12).

The preformation controversy ended in 1775 when **Lazaro Spallanzani** showed that both the oocyte and sperm were necessary for initiating the development of a new individual. From his experiments, including artificial insemination in dogs, he concluded that the sperm was the fertilizing agent that initiated the developmental processes. **Heinrich Christian Pander** discovered the three germ layers of the embryo, which he named the blastoderm. He reported this discovery in 1817 in his doctoral dissertation.

Etienne Saint Hilaire and his son, **Isidore Saint Hilaire**, made the first significant studies of abnormal development in 1818. They performed experiments in animals that were designed to produce developmental abnormalities, initiating what we now know as the *science of teratology*.

Karl Ernst von Baer described the oocyte in the ovarian follicle of a dog in 1827, approximately 150 years after the discovery of sperms. He also observed cleaving zygotes in the uterine tube and blastocysts in the uterus. He contributed new knowledge about the origin of tissues and organs from the layers described earlier by Malpighi and Pander. Von Baer formulated two important embryologic concepts: *corresponding stages of embryonic development and that general characteristics precede specific ones*. His significant and far-reaching contributions resulted in his being regarded as the *Father of Modern Embryology*.

Mattias Schleiden and **Theodor Schwann** were responsible for great advances being made in embryology when they formulated the *cell theory* in 1839. This concept stated that the body is composed of cells and cell products. The cell theory soon led to the realization that the embryo developed from a single cell, the zygote, which underwent many cell divisions as the tissues and organs formed.

Wilhelm His (1831–1904), a Swiss anatomist and embryologist, developed improved techniques for fixation, sectioning, and staining of tissues and for reconstruction of embryos. His method of graphic reconstruction paved the way for producing current three-dimensional, stereoscopic, and computer-generated images of embryos.

Franklin P. Mall (1862–1917), inspired by the work of His, began to collect human embryos for scientific study. Mall's collection forms a part of the *Carnegie Collection of embryos* that is known throughout the world. It is now in the National Museum of Health and Medicine in the Armed Forces Institute of Pathology in Washington, DC.

Wilhelm Roux (1850–1924) pioneered analytical experimental studies on the physiology of development in amphibia, which was pursued further by **Hans Spemann** (1869–1941). For his discovery of the phenomenon of primary induction—how one tissue determines the fate of another—Spemann received the Nobel Prize in 1935. Over the decades, scientists have been attempting to isolate the substances that are transmitted from one tissue to another, causing induction.

Robert G. Edwards and **Patrick Steptoe** pioneered one of the most revolutionary developments in the history of human reproduction: the technique of *in vitro fertilization*. These studies resulted in the birth of Louise Brown, the first "test tube baby," in 1978. Since then, more than one million couples throughout the world who were considered infertile have experienced the miracle of birth because of this new reproductive technology.

GENETICS AND HUMAN DEVELOPMENT

In 1859, **Charles Darwin** (1809–1882), an English biologist and evolutionist, published his book, *On the Origin of Species*, in which he emphasized the hereditary nature of variability among members of a species as an important factor in evolution. **Gregor Mendel**, an Austrian monk, developed the principles of heredity in 1865, but medical scientists and biologists did not understand the significance of these principles in the study of mammalian development for many years.

Walter Flemming observed chromosomes in 1878 and suggested their probable role in fertilization. In 1883, **Eduard von Beneden** observed that mature germ cells have a reduced number of chromosomes. He also described some features of meiosis, the process whereby the chromosome number is reduced in germ cells.

Walter Sutton (1877–1916) and **Theodor Boveri** (1862–1915) declared independently in 1902 that the behavior of chromosomes during germ cell formation and fertilization agreed with Mendel's principles of inheritance. In the same year, **Garrod** reported alcaptonuria (genetic disorder of phenylalanine-tyrosine metabolism) as the first example of mendelian inheritance in human beings. Many geneticists consider Sir Archibald Garrod (1857–1936) the *Father of Medical Genetics*. It was soon realized that the zygote contains all the genetic information necessary for directing the development of a new human being.

Felix von Winiwarter reported the first observations on human chromosomes in 1912, stating that there were 47 chromosomes in body cells. **Theophilus Shickel Painter** concluded in 1923 that 48 was the correct number, a conclusion that was widely accepted until 1956, when **Joe Hin Tjio** and **Albert Levan** reported finding only 46 chromosomes in embryonic cells.

James Watson and **Francis Crick** deciphered the molecular structure of DNA in 1953, and in 2000, the human genome was sequenced. The biochemical nature of the genes on the 46 human chromosomes has been decoded.

Chromosome studies were soon used in medicine in a number of ways, e.g., clinical diagnosis, chromosome mapping, and prenatal diagnosis. Once the normal chromosomal pattern was firmly established, it soon became evident that some persons with congenital anomalies had an abnormal number of chromosomes. A new era in medical genetics resulted from the demonstration by **Jérôme Jean Louis Marie Lejeune** and associates in 1959 that infants with mongolism (now known as *Down syndrome*) have 47 chromosomes instead of the usual 46 in their body cells. It is now known that chromosomal aberrations are a significant cause of congenital anomalies and embryonic death (see Chapter 20).

In 1941, **Sir Norman Gregg** reported an "unusual number of cases of cataracts" and other anomalies in infants whose mothers had contracted rubella in early pregnancy. For the first time, concrete evidence was presented showing that the development of the human embryo could be adversely affected by an environmental factor. Twenty years later, **Widukind Lenz** and **William McBride** reported rare limb deficiencies and other severe congenital abnormalities, induced by the sedative thalidomide, in the babies of infants of mothers who had ingested the drug. The thalidomide tragedy alerted the public and health care providers to the potential hazards of drugs, chemicals, and other environmental factors during pregnancy (see Chapter 20).

MOLECULAR BIOLOGY OF HUMAN DEVELOPMENT

Rapid advances in the field of *molecular biology* have led to the application of sophisticated techniques (e.g., *recombinant DNA technology*, *chimeric models*, transgenic mice, and *stem cell manipulation*). These techniques are now widely used in research laboratories to address such diverse problems as the genetic regulation of morphogenesis, the temporal and regional expression of specific genes, and how cells are committed to form the various parts of the embryo. For the first time, we are beginning to understand how, when, and where selected genes are activated and expressed in the embryo during normal and abnormal development (see Chapter 21).

The first mammal, **Dolly** the sheep, was cloned in 1997 by **Ian Wilmut** and his colleagues using the technique of somatic cell nuclear transfer. Since then, other animals have been successfully cloned from cultured differentiated adult cells. Interest in *human cloning* has generated considerable debate because of social, ethical, and legal implications. Moreover, there is concern that cloning may result in infants born with birth defects and serious diseases.

Human embryonic stem cells are pluripotential, capable of self-renewal, and are able to differentiate into specialized cell types. The isolation and programmed culture of human embryonic stem cells hold great potential for the treatment of degenerative, malignancy, and genetic diseases (see Lerou and associates, 2005).

DESCRIPTIVE TERMS IN EMBRYOLOGY

The English equivalents of the standard Latin forms of terms are given in some cases, e.g., sperm (spermatozoon).

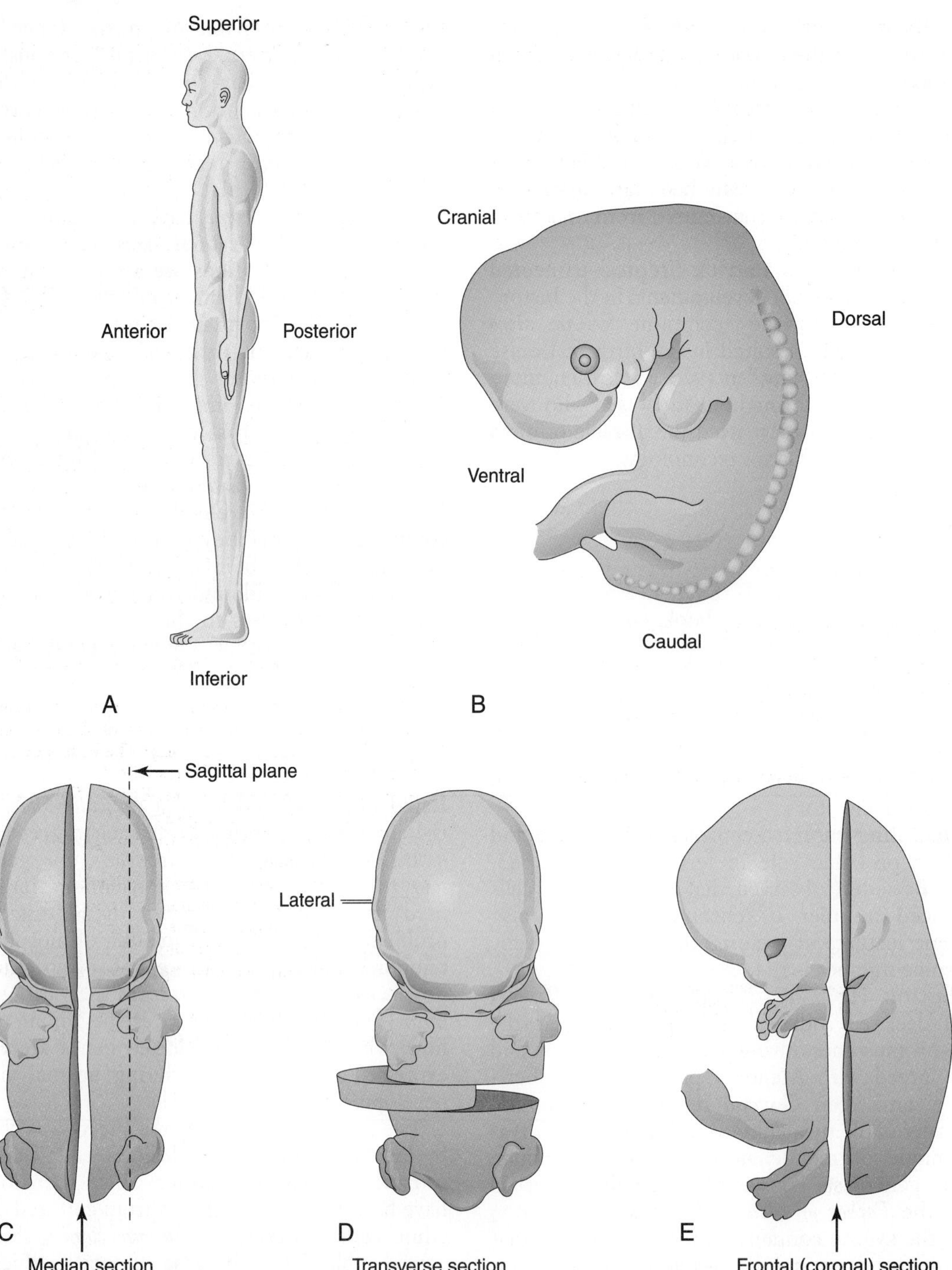

FIGURE 1-7. Drawings illustrating descriptive terms of position, direction, and planes of the body. **A,** Lateral view of an adult in the anatomical position. **B,** Lateral view of a 5-week embryo. **C** and **D,** Ventral views of 6-week embryo. **E,** Lateral view of a 7-week embryo. In describing development, it is necessary to use words denoting the position of one part to another or to the body as a whole. For example, the vertebral column (spine) develops in the dorsal part of the embryo, and the sternum (breast bone) in the ventral part of the embryo.

Eponyms commonly used clinically appear in parentheses, such as uterine tube (fallopian tube). In anatomy and embryology, several terms relating to position and direction are used, and reference is made to various planes of the body. All descriptions of the adult are based on the assumption that the body is erect, with the upper limbs by the sides and the palms directed anteriorly (Fig. 1-7*A*). This is the *anatomical position*. The terms anterior or ventral and posterior or dorsal are used to describe the front or back of the body or limbs and the relations of structures within the body to one another. When describing embryos, the terms dorsal and ventral are used (see Fig. 1-7*B*). Superior and inferior are used to indicate the relative levels of different structures (see Fig. 1-7*A*). For embryos, the terms cranial or rostral and caudal are used to denote relationships to the head and caudal eminence (tail), respectively (see Fig. 1-7*B*). Distances from the source or attachment of a structure are designated as proximal or distal. In the lower limb, for example, the knee is proximal to the ankle and the ankle is distal to the knee.

The *median plane* is an imaginary vertical plane of section that passes longitudinally through the body. Median sections divide the body into right and left halves (see Fig. 1-7*C*). The terms *lateral* and *medial* refer to structures that are, respectively, farther from or nearer to the median plane of the body. A *sagittal plane* is any vertical plane passing through the body that is parallel to the median plane (see Fig. 1-7*C*). A *transverse (axial) plane* refers to any plane that is at right angles to both the median and coronal planes (see Fig. 1-7*D*). A *frontal (coronal) plane* is any vertical plane that intersects the median plane at a right angle (see Fig. 1-7*E*) and divides the body into anterior or ventral and posterior or dorsal parts.

CLINICALLY ORIENTED PROBLEMS

1. What is the human embryo called at the beginning of its development?
2. How do the terms conceptus and abortus differ?
3. What sequence of events occurs during puberty? Are they the same in males and females? What are the respective ages of presumptive puberty in males and females?
4. How do the terms embryology and teratology differ?

Discussion of these problems appears at the back of the book.

References and Suggested Reading

Allen GE: Inducers and "organizers": Hans Spemann and experimental embryology. Pubbl Stn Zool Napoli 15:229, 1993.

Churchill FB: The rise of classical descriptive embryology. Dev Biol (NY) 7:1, 1991.

Dunstan GR (ed): The Human Embryo. Aristotle and the Arabic and European Traditions. Exeter, University of Exeter Press, 1990.

Gasser R: Atlas of Human Embryos. Hagerstown, Harper & Row, 1975.

Green RM: The Human Embryo Research Debates: Bioethics in the Vortex of Controversy. Oxford, Oxford University Press, 2001.

Hopwood N: Producing development: The anatomy of human embryos and the norms of Wilhelm His. Bull Hist Med 74:29, 2000.

Horder TJ, Witkowski JA, Wylie CC (eds): A History of Embryology. Cambridge, Cambridge University Press, 1986.

Kohl F: von Baer KE: 1792–1876. Zum 200. Geburtstag des "Vaters der Embryologie." Dtsch Med Wochenschr 117:1976, 1992.

Kuliev A, Rechitsky S, Tur-Kaspa I, Verlinsky Y: Preimplantation genetics: Improving access to stem cell therapy. Ann N Y Acad Sci 1054, 223, 2005.

Lerou PH, Daley GQ: Therapeutic potential of embryonic stem cells. Blood Rev 19:321, 2005.

Meyer AW: The Rise of Embryology. Stanford, CA, Stanford University Press, 1939.

Moore CA, Khoury MJ, Bradley LA: From genetics to genomics: Using gene-based medicine to prevent disease and promote health in children. Semin Perinatol 29:135, 2005.

Moore KL, Persaud TVN, Shiota K: Color Atlas of Clinical Embryology, 2nd ed. Philadelphia, WB Saunders, 2000.

Murillo-Gonzalés J: Evolution of embryology: A synthesis of classical, experimental, and molecular perspectives. Clin Anat 14:158, 2001.

Needham J: A History of Embryology, 2nd ed. Cambridge, Cambridge University Press, 1959.

O'Rahilly R: One hundred years of human embryology. In Kalter H (ed): Issues and Reviews in Teratology, vol 4. New York, Plenum Press, 1988.

O'Rahilly R, Müller F: Developmental Stages in Human Embryos. Washington, DC, Carnegie Institution of Washington, 1987.

Persaud TVN: A History of Anatomy: The Post-Vesalian Era. Springfield, IL, Charles C Thomas, 1997.

Pinto-Correia C: The Ovary of Eve: Egg and Sperm and Preformation. Chicago, University of Chicago Press, 1997.

Slack JMW: Essential Developmental Biology, 2nd ed. Oxford, Blackwell Publishing, 2006.

Streeter GL: Developmental horizons in human embryos. Description of age group XI, 13 to 20 somites, and age group XII, 21 to 29 somites. Contrib Embryol Carnegie Inst 30:211, 1942.

Turnpenny L, Cameron IT, Spalluto CM, et al: Human embryonic germ cells for future neuronal replacement therapy. Brain Res Bull 68:76, 2005.

Zavos PM: Stem cells and cellular therapy: Potential treatment for cardiovascular diseases. Int J Cardiol 107:1, 2006.

2 The Beginning of Human Development: First Week

He who sees things grow from the beginning will have the finest view of them. — Aristotle, 384–322 BC

Gametogenesis 15

Meiosis 15

Spermatogenesis 15

Oogenesis 20
- Prenatal Maturation of Oocytes 20
- Postnatal Maturation of Oocytes 20

Comparison of Gametes 20

Uterus, Uterine Tubes, and Ovaries 21
- Uterus 21
- Uterine Tubes 21
- Ovaries 23

Female Reproductive Cycles 23

Ovarian Cycle 23
- Follicular Development 23
- Ovulation 23
- Corpus Luteum 25

Menstrual Cycle 27
- Phases of the Menstrual Cycle 27

Transportation of Gametes 28
- Oocyte Transport 28
- Sperm Transport 28

Maturation of Sperms 29

Viability of Gametes 31

Fertilization 31
- Phases of Fertilization 31
- Fertilization 33

Cleavage of the Zygote 35

Formation of the Blastocyst 36

Summary of the First Week 39

Clinically Oriented Problems 39

Human development begins at fertilization when a male gamete or sperm unites with a female gamete or oocyte to form a single cell, a **zygote**. This highly specialized, totipotent cell marks the beginning of each of us as a unique individual. The zygote, just visible to the unaided eye, contains chromosomes and genes (units of genetic information) that are derived from the mother and father. The unicellular zygote divides many times and becomes progressively transformed into a multicellular human being through cell division, migration, growth, and differentiation.

Although development begins at fertilization, the stages and duration of pregnancy described in clinical medicine are calculated from the commencement of the mother's *last normal menstrual period*, which is approximately 14 days before conception occurs (see Fig. 1-1). Although referred to as the *gestational (menstrual) age*, this method overestimates the fertilization age by approximately 2 weeks. However, gestational age is widely used in clinical practice because the onset of the last normal menstrual period is usually easy to establish. Before describing the beginning of development, gametogenesis and the female reproductive system are reviewed.

GAMETOGENESIS

The sperm and oocyte, the male and female gametes, are highly specialized sex cells. Each of these cells contains half the number of chromosomes (haploid number) that are present in somatic (body) cells. The number of chromosomes is reduced during **meiosis**, a special type of cell division that occurs during gametogenesis. Gamete maturation is called **spermatogenesis** in males and **oogenesis** in females (Fig. 2-1). The sequence of gametogenesis is the same, but the timing of events during meiosis differs in the two sexes.

Gametogenesis (gamete formation) is the process of formation and development of specialized generative cells, **gametes**. This process, involving the chromosomes and cytoplasm of the gametes, prepares these sex cells for fertilization. During gametogenesis, the chromosome number is reduced by half and the shape of the cells is altered. A chromosome is defined by the presence of a *centromere*, the constricted part of a chromosome. Before DNA replication in the S phase of the cell cycle, chromosomes exist as single-chromatid chromosomes. A chromatid consists of parallel DNA strands. After DNA replication, chromosomes are double-chromatid chromosomes.

MEIOSIS

Meiosis is *a special type of cell division that involves two meiotic cell divisions*; it takes place in germ cells only (Fig. 2-2). Diploid germ cells give rise to haploid *gametes* (sperms and oocytes).

The **first meiotic division** is a *reduction division* because the chromosome number is reduced from diploid to haploid by pairing of homologous chromosomes in prophase and their segregation at anaphase. *Homologous chromosomes* (one from each parent) pair during prophase and separate during anaphase, with one representative of each pair randomly going to each pole of the meiotic spindle. The spindle connects to the chromosome at the centromere. At this stage, they are *double-chromatid chromosomes*. The X and Y chromosomes are not homologs, but they have homologous segments at the tips of their short arms. They pair in these regions only. By the end of the first meiotic division, each new cell formed (secondary spermatocyte or secondary oocyte) has the *haploid chromosome number* (double-chromatid chromosomes), i.e., half the number of chromosomes of the preceding cell (primary spermatocyte or primary oocyte). This separation or disjunction of paired homologous chromosomes is the *physical basis of segregation*, the separation of allelic genes during meiosis.

The **second meiotic division** follows the first division without a normal interphase (i.e., without an intervening step of DNA replication). Each chromosome divides and each half, or **chromatid**, is drawn to a different pole; thus, the haploid number of chromosomes (23) is retained and each daughter cell formed by meiosis has the reduced haploid number of chromosomes, with one representative of each chromosome pair (now a **single-chromatid chromosome**). The second meiotic division is similar to an ordinary mitosis except that the chromosome number of the cell entering the second meiotic division is haploid.

Meiosis

- Provides *constancy of the chromosome number* from generation to generation by reducing the chromosome number from diploid to haploid, thereby producing haploid gametes.
- Allows *random assortment of maternal and paternal chromosomes between the gametes.*
- Relocates segments of maternal and paternal chromosomes by *crossing over of chromosome segments*, which "shuffles" the genes and produces a *recombination of genetic material.*

ABNORMAL GAMETOGENESIS

Disturbances of meiosis during gametogenesis, e.g., nondisjunction (Fig. 2-3), result in the formation of chromosomally abnormal gametes. If involved in fertilization, these gametes with numerical chromosome abnormalities cause abnormal development such as occurs in infants with Down syndrome (see Chapter 20).

SPERMATOGENESIS

Spermatogenesis is the sequence of events by which *spermatogonia* are transformed into **mature sperms**. This maturation process begins at puberty. **Spermatogonia**, which have been dormant in the seminiferous tubules of the testes since the fetal period, begin to increase in number at puberty. After several mitotic divisions, the spermatogonia grow and undergo changes.

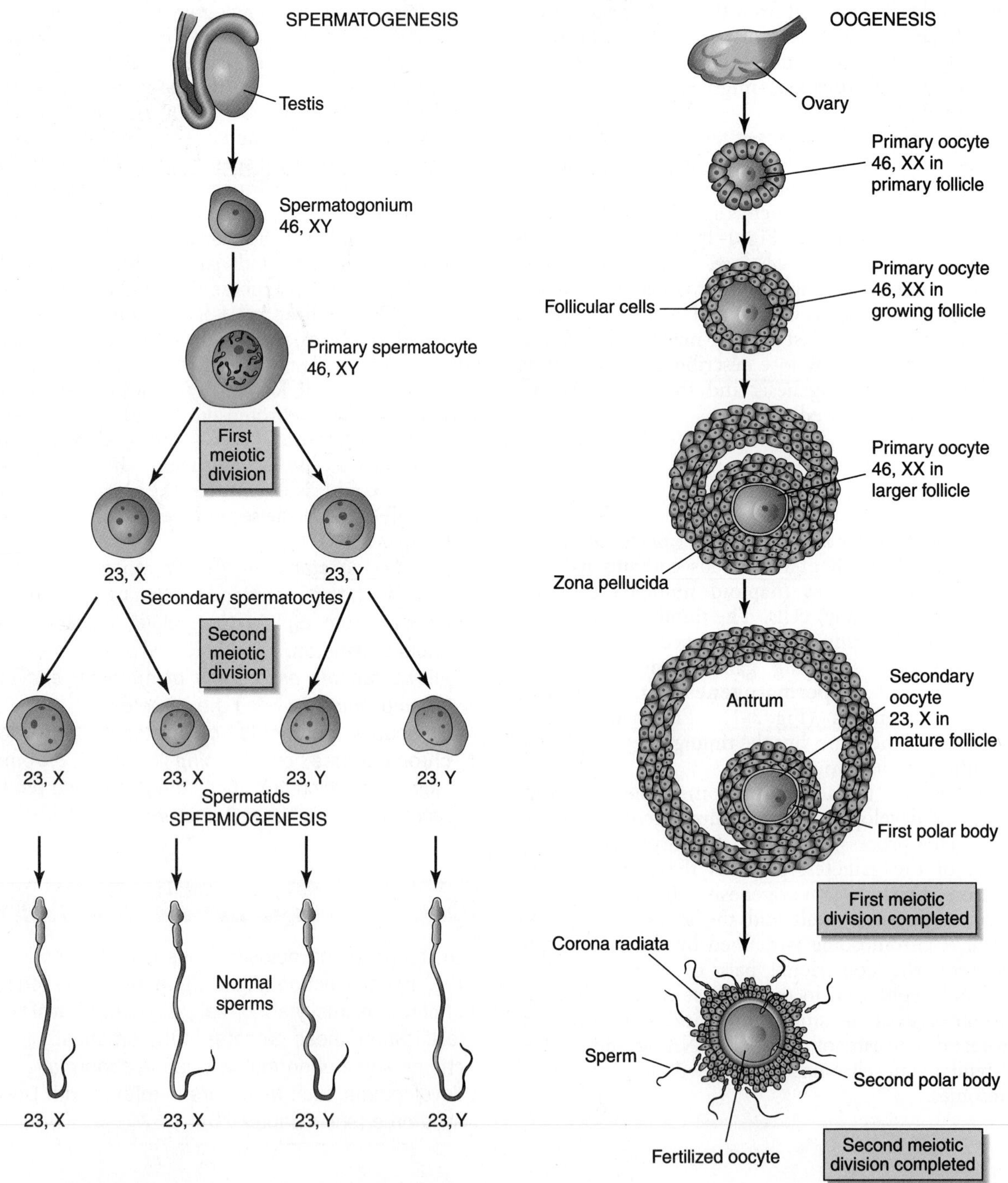

FIGURE 2-1. Normal gametogenesis: conversion of germ cells into gametes. The drawings compare spermatogenesis and oogenesis. Oogonia are not shown in this figure because they differentiate into primary oocytes before birth. The chromosome complement of the germ cells is shown at each stage. The number designates the total number of chromosomes, including the sex chromosome(s) shown after the comma. Note that (1) following the two meiotic divisions, the diploid number of chromosomes, 46, is reduced to the haploid number, 23; (2) four sperms form from one primary spermatocyte, whereas only one mature oocyte results from maturation of a primary oocyte; and (3) the cytoplasm is conserved during oogenesis to form one large cell, the mature oocyte. The polar bodies are small nonfunctional cells that eventually degenerate.

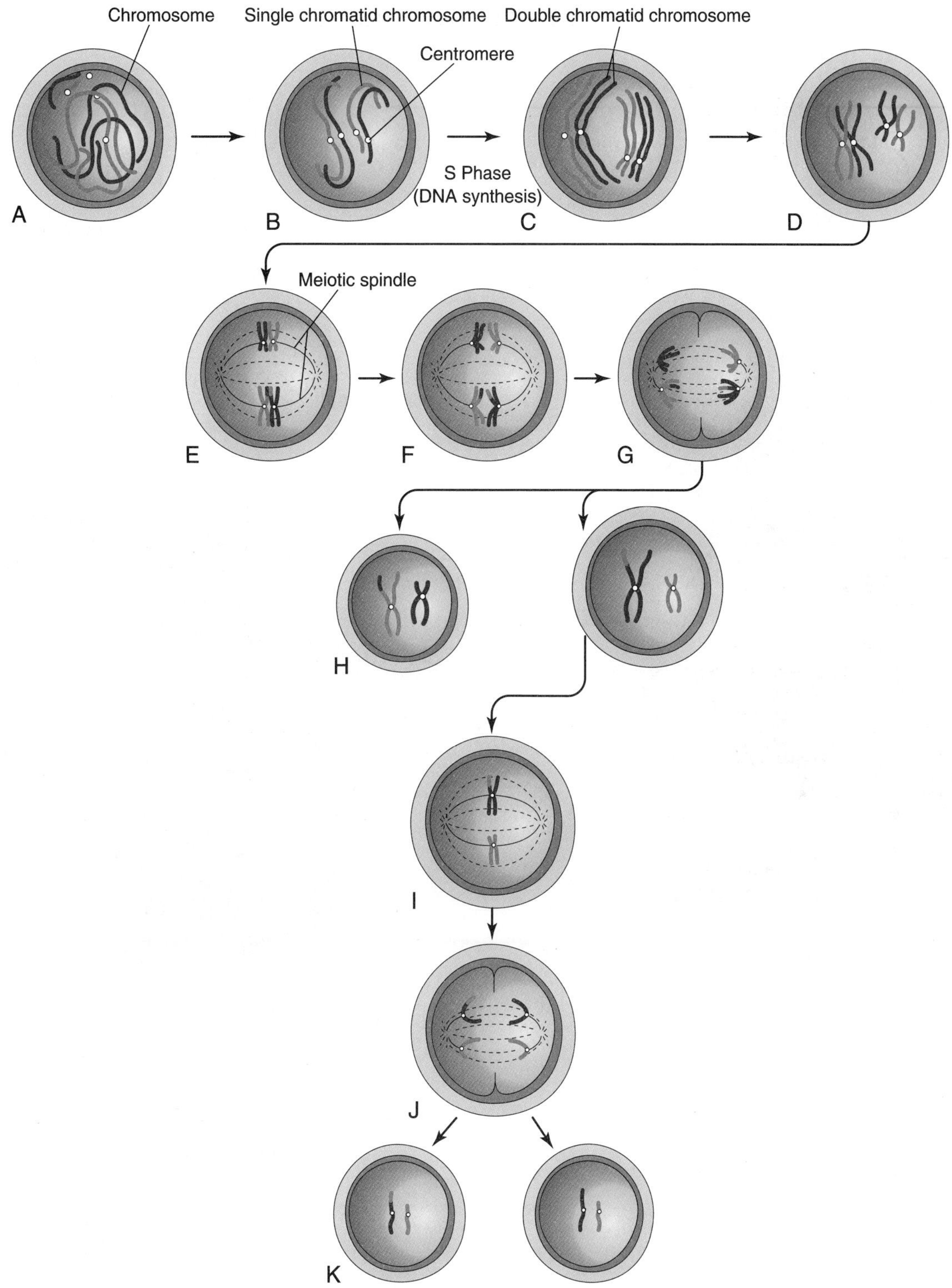

FIGURE 2-2. Diagrammatic representation of meiosis. Two chromosome pairs are shown. **A** to **D,** Stages of prophase of the first meiotic division. The homologous chromosomes approach each other and pair; each member of the pair consists of two chromatids. Observe the single crossover in one pair of chromosomes, resulting in the interchange of chromatid segments. **E,** Metaphase. The two members of each pair become oriented on the meiotic spindle. **F,** Anaphase. **G,** Telophase. The chromosomes migrate to opposite poles. **H,** Distribution of parental chromosome pairs at the end of the first meiotic division. **I** to **K,** Second meiotic division. It is similar to mitosis except that the cells are haploid.

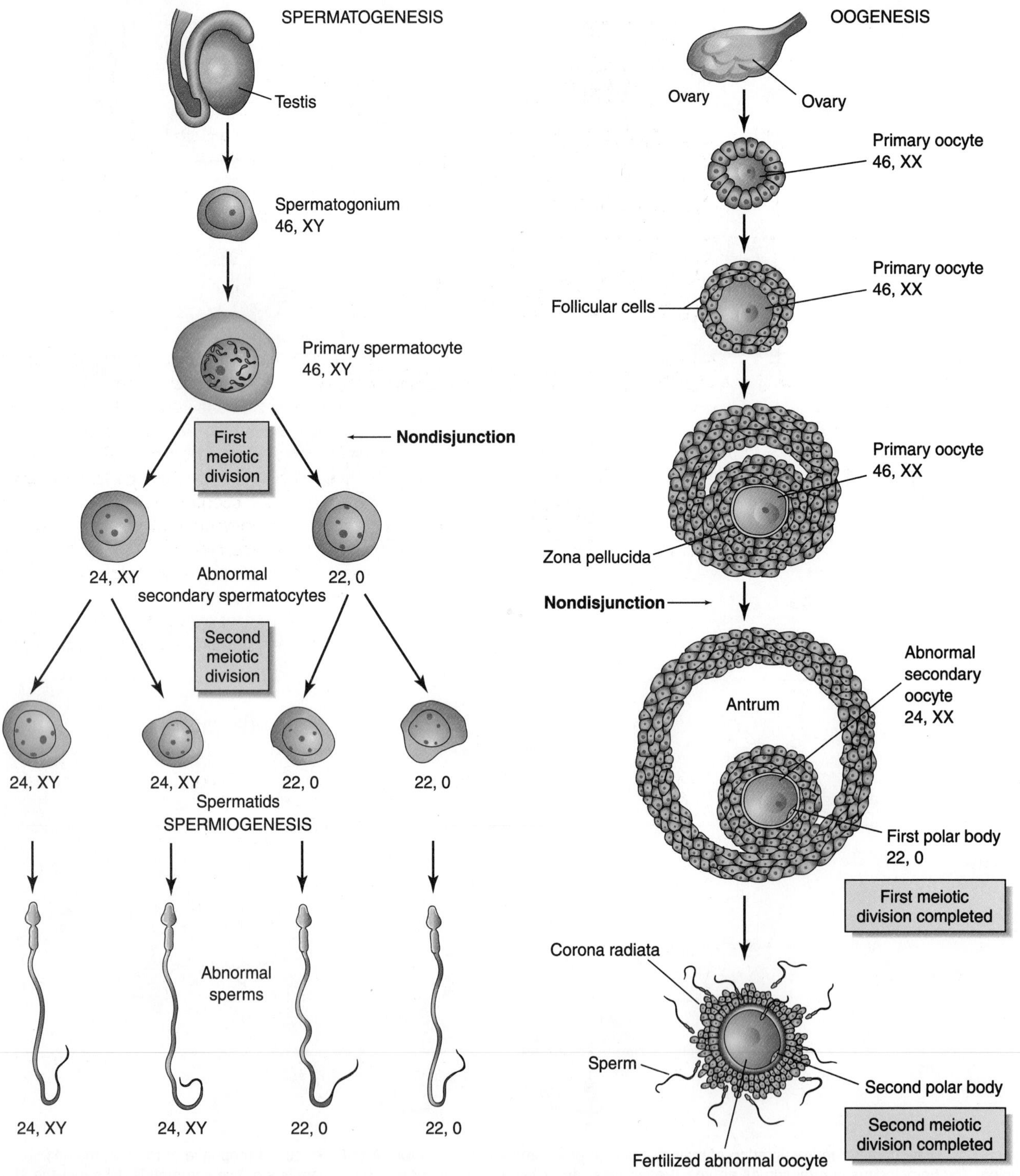

FIGURE 2-3. Abnormal gametogenesis. The drawings show how nondisjunction results in an abnormal chromosome distribution in gametes. Although nondisjunction of sex chromosomes is illustrated, a similar defect may occur in autosomes. When nondisjunction occurs during the first meiotic division of spermatogenesis, one secondary spermatocyte contains 22 autosomes plus an X and a Y chromosome, and the other one contains 22 autosomes and no sex chromosome. Similarly, nondisjunction during oogenesis may give rise to an oocyte with 22 autosomes and two X chromosomes (as shown) or may result in one with 22 autosomes and no sex chromosome.

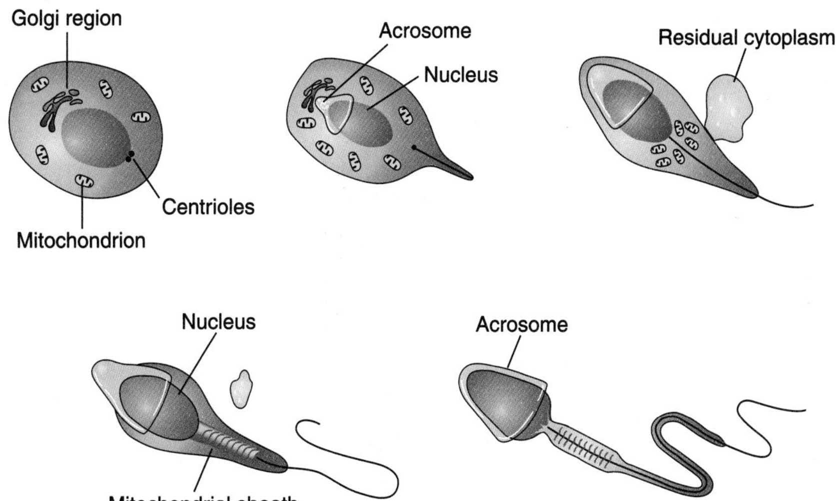

FIGURE 2-4. Illustrations of spermiogenesis, the last phase of spermatogenesis. During this process, the rounded spermatid is transformed into elongated sperm. Note the loss of cytoplasm, development of the tail, and formation of the acrosome. The acrosome, derived from the Golgi region of the spermatid, contains enzymes that are released at the beginning of fertilization to assist the sperm in penetrating the corona radiata and zona pellucida surrounding the secondary oocyte. The mitochondria arrange themselves end to end in the form of a tight helix, forming a collar-like mitochondrial sheath. Note that the residual cytoplasm is shed during spermiogenesis.

Spermatogonia are transformed into **primary spermatocytes**, the largest germ cells in the seminiferous tubules. Each primary spermatocyte subsequently undergoes a reduction division—the first meiotic division—to form two haploid **secondary spermatocytes**, which are approximately half the size of primary spermatocytes. Subsequently, the secondary spermatocytes undergo a second meiotic division to form four haploid spermatids, which are approximately half the size of secondary spermatocytes. The spermatids are gradually transformed into four mature sperm by a process known as **spermiogenesis** (Fig. 2-4). The entire process of spermatogenesis, which includes spermiogenesis, takes approximately 2 months. When spermiogenesis is complete, the sperms enter the lumina of the seminiferous tubules.

Sertoli cells lining the seminiferous tubules support and nurture the germ cells and may be involved in the regulation of spermatogenesis. Sperms are transported passively from the seminiferous tubules to the *epididymis*, where they are stored and become functionally mature. The epididymis is the elongated coiled duct along the posterior border of the testis (see Fig. 2-13). It is continuous with the *ductus deferens* (vas deferens), which transports the sperms to the urethra.

Mature sperms are free-swimming, actively motile cells consisting of a head and a tail (Fig. 2-5*A*). The **neck of the**

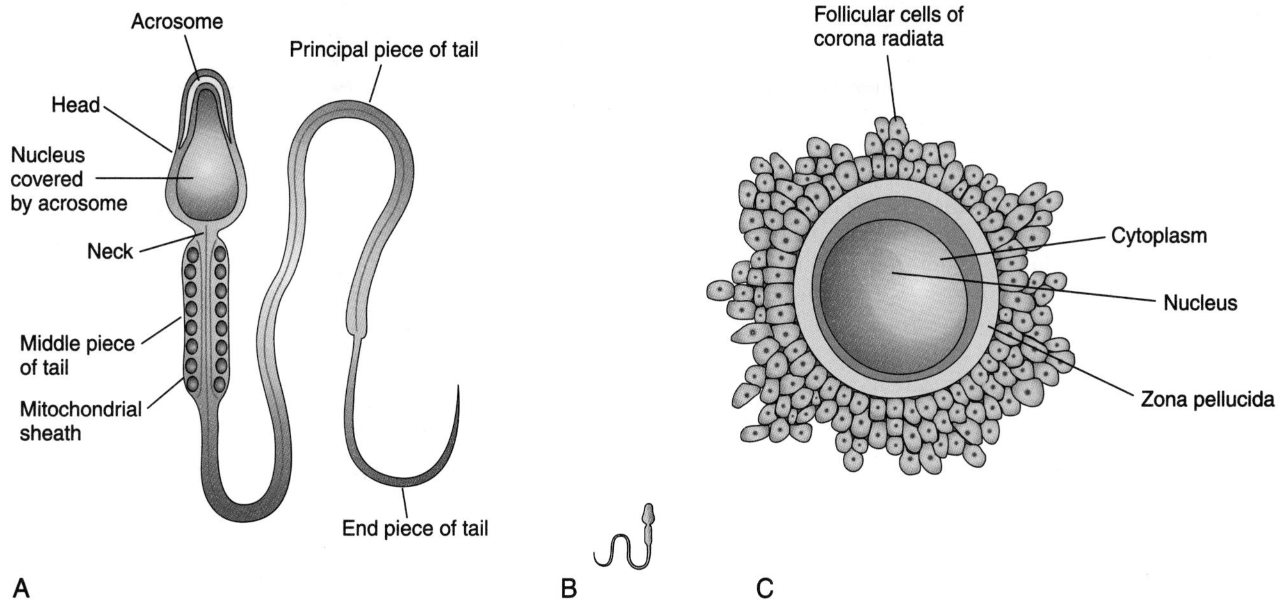

FIGURE 2-5. Male and female gametes. **A,** The main parts of a human sperm (×1250). The head, composed mostly of the nucleus, is partly covered by the caplike acrosome, an organelle containing enzymes. The tail of the sperm consists of three regions: the middle piece, principal piece, and end piece. **B,** A sperm drawn to approximately the same scale as the oocyte. **C,** A human secondary oocyte (×200), surrounded by the zone pellucida and corona radiata.

sperm is the junction between the head and tail. The **head of the sperm** forms most of the bulk of the sperm and contains the haploid nucleus. The anterior two thirds of the nucleus is covered by the **acrosome**, a caplike saccular organelle containing several enzymes. When released, these enzymes facilitate dispersion of the follicular cells of the corona radiata and sperm penetration of the zona pellucida during fertilization. The **tail of the sperm** consists of three segments: middle piece, principal piece, and end piece (see Fig. 2-5*A*). The tail provides the motility of the sperm that assists its transport to the site of fertilization. The **middle piece of the tail** contains mitochondria, which provide the adenosine triphosphate necessary for activity.

Many genes and molecular factors are implicated in spermatogenesis. For example, recent studies indicate that *proteins of the Bcl-2 family* are involved in the maturation of germ cells, as well as their survival at different stages. For normal spermatogenesis, the Y chromosome is essential; microdeletions result in defective spermatogenesis and infertility.

OOGENESIS

Oogenesis (ovogenesis) is the sequence of events by which oogonia are transformed into **mature oocytes**. This maturation process begins before birth and is completed after puberty. Oogenesis continues to *menopause*, which is permanent cessation of the *menses* (bleeding associated with the menstrual cycles).

Prenatal Maturation of Oocytes

During early fetal life, oogonia proliferate by mitosis. *Oogonia enlarge to form primary oocytes before birth*; for this reason, no oogonia are shown in Figures 2-1 and 2-3. As a **primary oocyte** forms, connective tissue cells surround it and form a single layer of flattened, follicular epithelial cells (see Fig. 2-8). The primary oocyte enclosed by this layer of cells constitutes a **primordial follicle** (see Fig. 2-9*A*). As the primary oocyte enlarges during puberty, the follicular epithelial cells become cuboidal in shape and then columnar, forming a **primary follicle** (see Fig. 2-1). The primary oocyte soon becomes surrounded by a covering of amorphous acellular glycoprotein material, the **zona pellucida** (see Figs. 2-8 and 2-9*B*). Scanning electron microscopy of the surface of the zona pellucida reveals a regular meshlike appearance with intricate fenestrations.

Primary oocytes begin the first meiotic division before birth, but completion of prophase does not occur until adolescence. The follicular cells surrounding the primary oocyte are believed to secrete a substance, *oocyte maturation inhibitor*, which keeps the meiotic process of the oocyte arrested.

Postnatal Maturation of Oocytes

Beginning during puberty, usually one follicle matures each month and ovulation occurs, except when oral contraceptives are used. The long duration of the first meiotic division (up to 45 years) may account in part for the relatively high frequency of meiotic errors, such as **nondisjunction** (failure of paired chromatids to dissociate), that occur with increasing maternal age. The primary oocytes in suspended prophase (dictyotene) are vulnerable to environmental agents such as radiation.

No primary oocytes form after birth in females, in contrast to the continuous production of primary spermatocytes in males. The primary oocytes remain dormant in the ovarian follicles until puberty. As a follicle matures, the **primary oocyte** increases in size and, shortly before ovulation, completes the first meiotic division to give rise to a secondary oocyte and the **first polar body.** Unlike the corresponding stage of spermatogenesis, however, the division of cytoplasm is unequal. The **secondary oocyte** receives almost all the cytoplasm (see Fig. 2-1), and the first polar body receives very little. The polar body is a small, nonfunctional cell that soon degenerates. At ovulation, the nucleus of the secondary oocyte begins the second meiotic division, but progresses only to metaphase, when division is arrested. If a sperm penetrates the secondary oocyte, the second meiotic division is completed, and most cytoplasm is again retained by one cell, the **fertilized oocyte** (see Fig. 2-1). The other cell, the **second polar body**, also a small nonfunctional cell, soon degenerates. As soon as the polar body is extruded, maturation of the oocyte is complete.

There are approximately two million primary oocytes in the ovaries of a newborn female, but most regress during childhood so that by adolescence no more than 40,000 remain. Of these, only approximately 400 become secondary oocytes and are expelled at ovulation during the reproductive period. Few of these oocytes, if any, are fertilized and become mature. The number of oocytes that ovulate is greatly reduced in women who take oral contraceptives because the hormones in them prevent ovulation from occurring.

COMPARISON OF GAMETES

The oocyte is a massive cell compared with the sperm and is immotile (see Fig. 2-5), whereas the microscopic sperm is highly motile. The oocyte is surrounded by the zona pellucida and a layer of follicular cells, *the corona radiata* (see Fig. 2-5*C*). The oocyte also has an abundance of cytoplasm containing yolk granules, which may provide nutrition to the dividing zygote during the first week of development.

With respect to sex chromosome constitution, there are *two kinds of normal sperm*: 23, X and 23, Y, whereas there is only *one kind of normal secondary oocyte*: 23, X (see Fig. 2-1). In the foregoing descriptions and illustrations, the number 23 is followed by a comma and an X or Y to indicate the sex chromosome constitution, e.g., 23, X indicates that there are 23 chromosomes in the complement, consisting of 22 autosomes and one sex chromosome (an X in this case). *The difference in the sex chromosome complement of sperms forms the basis of primary sex determination.*

ABNORMAL GAMETES

The ideal maternal age for reproduction is generally considered to be from 18 to 35 years. The likelihood of chromosomal abnormalities in the embryo increases after the mother is 35. In older mothers, there is an appreciable risk of Down syndrome or some other form of trisomy in the infant (see Chapter 20). The likelihood of a fresh gene mutation (change in DNA) also increases with age. The older the parents are at the time of conception, the more likely they are to have accumulated mutations that the embryo might inherit. For fathers of children with fresh mutations, such as the one causing achondroplasia, this age relationship has continually been demonstrated. This does not hold for all dominant mutations and is not an important consideration in older mothers.

During gametogenesis, homologous chromosomes sometimes fail to separate. As a result of this error of meiotic cell division—nondisjunction—some gametes have 24 chromosomes and others only 22 (see Fig. 2-3). If a gamete with 24 chromosomes unites with a normal one with 23 chromosomes during fertilization, a zygote with 47 chromosomes forms (see Fig. 20-2). This condition is called trisomy because of the presence of three representatives of a particular chromosome instead of the usual two. If a gamete with only 22 chromosomes unites with a normal one, a zygote with 45 chromosomes forms. This condition is known as monosomy because only one representative of the particular chromosome pair is present. For a description of the clinical conditions associated with numerical disorders of chromosomes, see Chapter 20.

As many as 10% of sperms in an ejaculate are grossly abnormal (e.g., with two heads), but it is generally believed that these abnormal sperms do not fertilize oocytes due to their lack of normal motility. Most morphologically abnormal sperms are unable to pass through the mucus in the cervical canal. Measurement of forward progression is a subjective assessment of the quality of sperm movement. Radiography, severe allergic reactions, and certain antispermatogenic agents have been reported to increase the percentage of abnormally shaped sperms. Such sperms are not believed to affect fertility unless their number exceeds 20%.

Although some oocytes have two or three nuclei, these cells die before they reach maturity. Similarly, some ovarian follicles contain two or more oocytes, but this phenomenon is infrequent. Although compound follicles could result in multiple births, it is believed that most of them never mature and expel the oocytes at ovulation.

UTERUS, UTERINE TUBES, AND OVARIES

A brief description of the structure of the uterus, uterine tubes, and ovaries is presented as a basis for understanding reproductive cycles and implantation of the blastocyst.

Uterus

The uterus (Latin [L.], womb) is a thick-walled, pear-shaped muscular organ averaging 7 to 8 cm in length, 5 to 7 cm in width at its superior part, and 2 to 3 cm in wall thickness. The uterus consists of two major parts (Fig. 2-6*A*):

- Body, the expanded superior two thirds
- Cervix, the cylindrical inferior one third

The **body of the uterus** narrows from the **fundus,** the rounded, superior part of the body, to the **isthmus**, the 1-cm-long constricted region between the body and cervix (L., neck). The **cervix of the uterus** is its tapered vaginal end that is nearly cylindrical in shape. The lumen of the cervix, the **cervical canal**, has a constricted opening at each end. The **internal os** communicates with the cavity of the uterine body and the **external os** communicates with the vagina. *The walls of the body of the uterus consist of three layers* (see Fig. 2-6*B*):

- Perimetrium, the thin external layer
- Myometrium, the thick smooth muscle layer
- Endometrium, the thin internal layer

The **perimetrium** is a peritoneal layer that is firmly attached to the myometrium. During the luteal (secretory) phase of the menstrual cycle, three layers of the endometrium can be distinguished microscopically (see Fig. 2-6*C*):

- A thin, **compact layer** consisting of densely packed, connective tissue around the necks of the uterine glands
- A thick, **spongy layer** composed of edematous connective tissue containing the dilated, tortuous bodies of the uterine glands
- A thin, **basal layer** containing the blind ends of the uterine glands

At the peak of its development, the endometrium is 4 to 5 mm thick. The basal layer of the endometrium has its own blood supply and is not sloughed off during menstruation. The compact and spongy layers, known collectively as the **functional layer**, disintegrate and are shed during menstruation and after parturition (delivery of a baby).

Uterine Tubes

The uterine tubes, approximately 10 cm long and 1 cm in diameter, extend laterally from the **horns** (L., *cornua*) **of the uterus** (see Fig. 2-6*A*). Each tube opens at its proximal end into the horn of the uterus and into the peritoneal cavity at its distal end. For descriptive purposes, *the uterine tube is divided into four parts*: the infundibulum, the ampulla, the isthmus, and the uterine part. The tubes carry oocytes from the ovaries and sperms entering from the uterus to reach the fertilization site in the **ampulla**

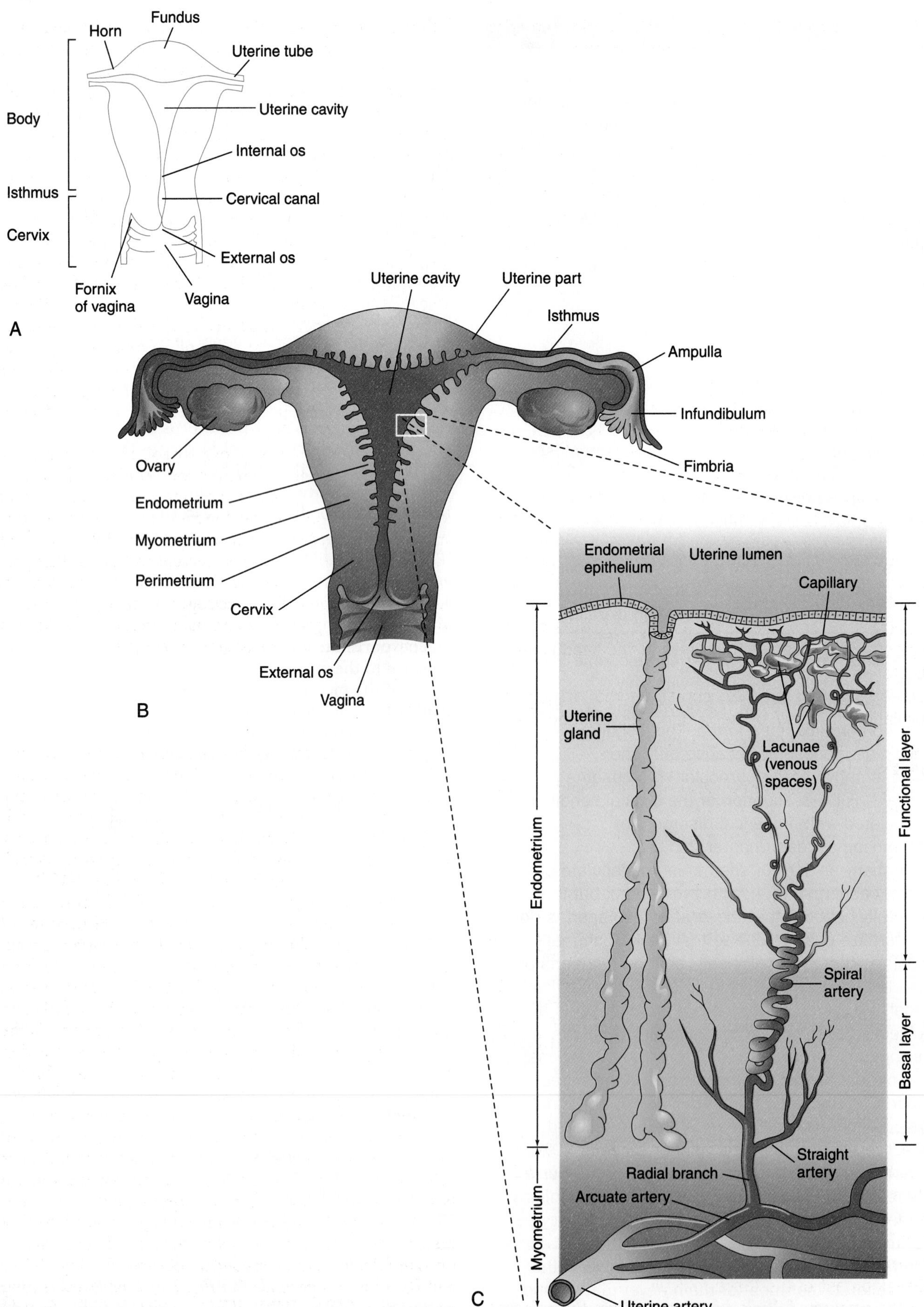

FIGURE 2-6. **A,** Parts of the uterus. **B,** Diagrammatic frontal section of the uterus, uterine tubes, and vagina. The ovaries are also shown. **C,** Enlargement of the area outlined in **B**. The functional layer of the endometrium is sloughed off during menstruation.

of the uterine tube (see Fig. 2-6*B*). The uterine tube also conveys the cleaving zygote to the uterine cavity.

Ovaries

The ovaries are almond-shaped reproductive glands located close to the lateral pelvic walls on each side of the uterus that produce oocytes (see Fig. 2-6*B*). The ovaries also produce estrogen and progesterone, the hormones responsible for the development of secondary sex characteristics and regulation of pregnancy.

FEMALE REPRODUCTIVE CYCLES

Commencing at puberty, females undergo reproductive cycles (sexual cycles), involving activities of the **hypothalamus** of the brain, **pituitary gland** (L., *hypophysis*), **ovaries, uterus, uterine tubes, vagina,** and **mammary glands** (Fig. 2-7). These monthly cycles prepare the reproductive system for pregnancy.

A *gonadotropin-releasing hormone* is synthesized by neurosecretory cells in the hypothalamus and is carried by the *hypophysial portal system* to the anterior lobe of the pituitary gland. Gonadotropin-releasing hormone stimulates the release of two hormones produced by this gland that act on the ovaries:

- *Follicle-stimulating hormone* (**FSH**) stimulates the development of ovarian follicles and the production of **estrogen** by the follicular cells.
- *Luteinizing hormone* (**LH**) serves as the "trigger" for ovulation (release of secondary oocyte) and stimulates the follicular cells and corpus luteum to produce **progesterone**.

These ovarian hormones also induce growth of the endometrium.

OVARIAN CYCLE

FSH and LH produce cyclic changes in the ovaries—the ovarian cycle (see Fig. 2-7)—development of follicles (Fig. 2-8), ovulation, and corpus luteum formation. During each cycle, FSH promotes growth of several *primordial follicles* into 5 to 12 primary follicles (Fig. 2-9*A*); however, only one primary follicle usually develops into a mature follicle and ruptures through the surface of the ovary, expelling its oocyte (Fig. 2-10).

Follicular Development

Development of an ovarian follicle (see Figs. 2-8 and 2-9) is characterized by:

- Growth and differentiation of primary oocyte
- Proliferation of follicular cells
- Formation of zona pellucida
- Development of the theca folliculi

As the **primary follicle** increases in size, the adjacent connective tissue organizes into a capsule, the **theca folliculi** (see Fig. 2-7). The theca soon differentiates into two layers, an internal vascular and glandular layer, the **theca interna**, and a capsule-like layer, the **theca externa.** Thecal cells are thought to produce an *angiogenesis factor* that promotes growth of blood vessels in the theca interna (see Fig. 2-9*B*), which provide nutritive support for follicular development. The follicular cells divide actively, producing a stratified layer around the oocyte (see Fig. 2-9*B*). The ovarian follicle soon becomes oval and the oocyte eccentric in position. Subsequently, fluid-filled spaces appear around the follicular cells, which coalesce to form a single large cavity, the **antrum**, which contains **follicular fluid** (see Figs. 2-8, and 2-9*B*). After the antrum forms, the ovarian follicle is called a vesicular or **secondary follicle.**

The primary oocyte is pushed to one side of the follicle, where it is surrounded by a mound of follicular cells, the **cumulus oophorus**, that projects into the antrum (see Figs. 2-9*B*). The follicle continues to enlarge until it reaches maturity and produces a swelling on the surface of the ovary (see Fig. 2-10*A*).

The early development of ovarian follicles is induced by FSH, but final stages of maturation require LH as well. Growing follicles produce **estrogen**, a hormone that regulates development and function of the reproductive organs. The vascular *theca interna* produces follicular fluid and some *estrogen*. Its cells also secrete androgens that pass to the follicular cells (see Fig. 2-8), which, in turn, convert them into estrogen. Some estrogen is also produced by widely scattered groups of stromal secretory cells, known collectively as the *interstitial gland of the ovary*.

Ovulation

Around midcycle, the ovarian follicle, under the influence of FSH and LH, undergoes a sudden *growth spurt*, producing a cystic swelling or bulge on the surface of the ovary. A small avascular spot, the **stigma**, soon appears on this swelling (see Fig. 2-10*A*). Before ovulation, the secondary oocyte and some cells of the cumulus oophorus detach from the interior of the distended follicle (Fig. 2-10*B*).

Ovulation is triggered by a surge of LH production (Fig. 2-11). Ovulation usually follows the LH peak by 12 to 24 hours. The **LH surge**, elicited by the high estrogen level in the blood, appears to cause the stigma to balloon out, forming a vesicle (see Fig. 2-10*A*). The stigma soon ruptures, expelling the secondary oocyte with the follicular fluid (see Fig. 2-10*B* to *D*). Expulsion of the oocyte is the result of intrafollicular pressure and possibly contraction of smooth muscle in the theca externa owing to stimulation by prostaglandins. *Enzymatic digestion of the follicular wall* seems to be one of the principal mechanisms leading to ovulation. The expelled secondary oocyte is surrounded by the zona pellucida and one or more layers of follicular cells, which are radially arranged as the **corona radiata** (see Fig. 2-10*C*), forming the oocyte-cumulus complex. The LH surge also seems to induce resumption of the first meiotic division of the primary oocyte. Hence, mature ovarian follicles contain secondary oocytes (see Fig. 2-10*A* and *B*). The *zona pellucida (see Fig. 2-8) is composed of three glycoproteins* (**ZPA, ZPB, ZPC**), which usually form a network of filaments with multiple pores. Binding of the

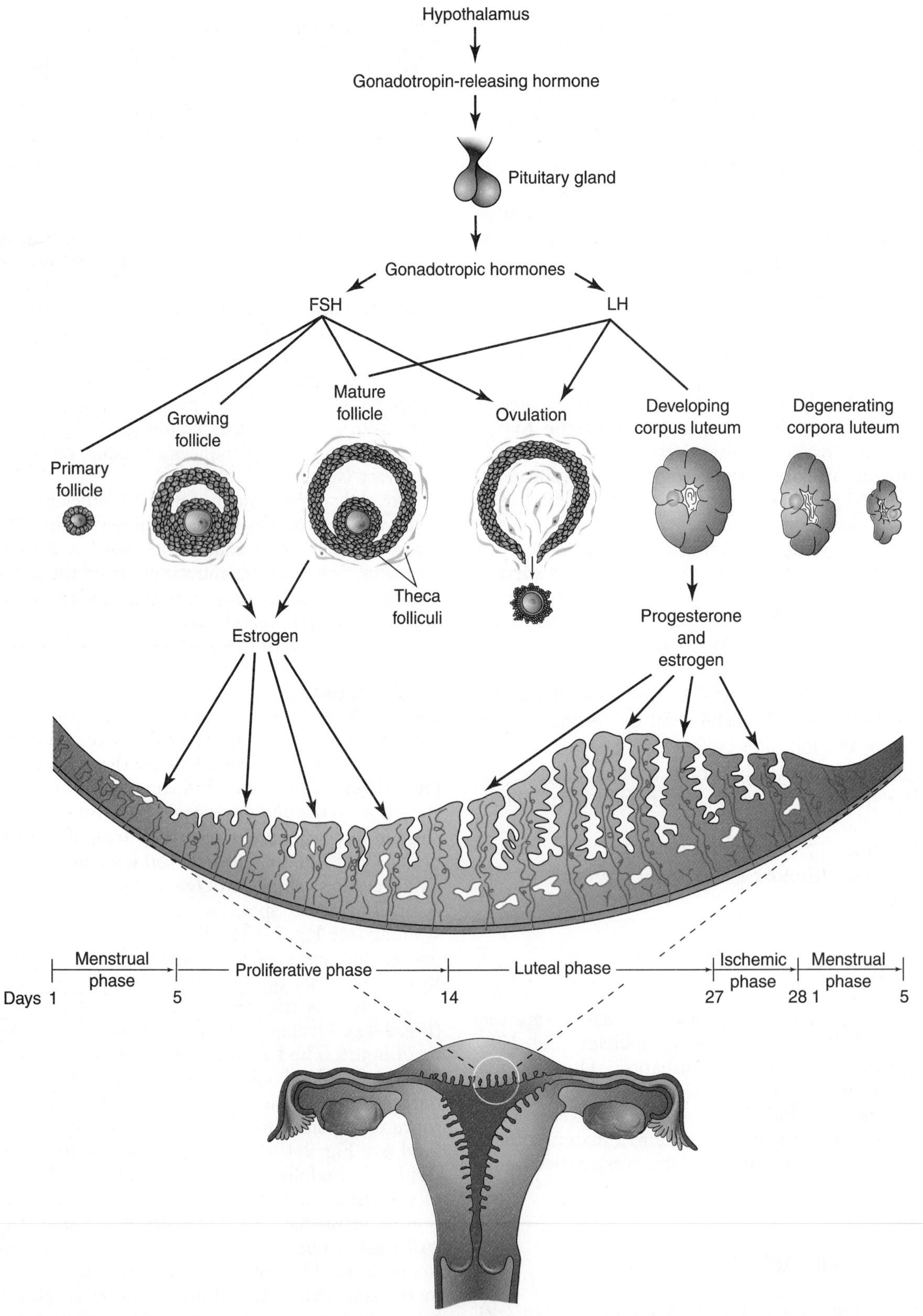

FIGURE 2-7. Schematic drawings illustrating the interrelations of the hypothalamus of the brain, pituitary gland, ovaries, and endometrium. One complete menstrual cycle and the beginning of another are shown. Changes in the ovaries, the ovarian cycle, are induced by the gonadotropic hormones (follicle-stimulating hormone and luteinizing hormone). Hormones from the ovaries (estrogens and progesterone) then promote cyclic changes in the structure and function of the endometrium, the menstrual cycle. Thus, the cyclical activity of the ovary is intimately linked with changes in the uterus. The ovarian cycles are under the rhythmic endocrine control of the pituitary gland, which in turn is controlled by gonadotropin-releasing hormone produced by neurosecretory cells in the hypothalamus.

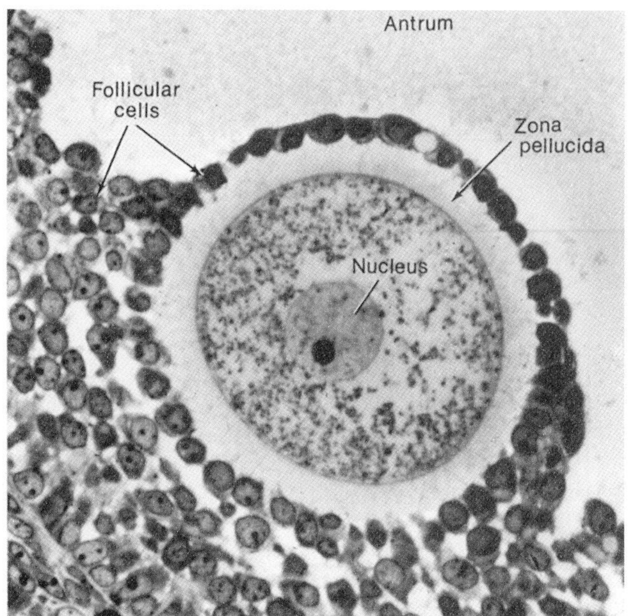

FIGURE 2-8. Photomicrograph of a human primary oocyte in a secondary follicle, surrounded by the zona pellucida and follicular cells. The mound of tissue, the cumulus oophorus, projects into the antrum. (From Bloom W, Fawcett DW: A Textbook of Histology, 10th ed. Philadelphia, WB Saunders, 1975. Courtesy of L. Zamboni.)

sperm to the zona pellucida (*sperm-oocyte interactions*) is a complex and critical event during fertilization.

MITTELSCHMERZ AND OVULATION

A variable amount of abdominal pain, mittelschmerz (German, *mittel*, mid + *schmerz*, pain), accompanies ovulation in some women. In these cases, ovulation results in slight bleeding into the peritoneal cavity, which results in sudden constant pain in the lower abdomen. Mittelschmerz may be used as a symptom of ovulation, but there are better symptoms, such as the slight drop in basal body temperature.

ANOVULATION

Some women do not ovulate (cessation of ovulation—anovulation) because of an inadequate release of gonadotropins. In some of these women, ovulation can be induced by the administration of gonadotropins or an ovulatory agent such as clomiphene citrate. This drug stimulates the release of pituitary gonadotropins (FSH and LH), resulting in maturation of several ovarian follicles and multiple ovulations. The incidence of multiple pregnancy increases as much as tenfold when ovulation is induced. Spontaneous abortions occur because there is no chance that more than seven embryos can survive.

Corpus Luteum

Shortly after ovulation, the walls of the ovarian follicle and theca folliculi collapse and are thrown into folds (see Fig. 2-10*D*). Under LH influence, they develop into a glandular structure, the **corpus luteum**, which secretes *progesterone* and some *estrogen*, causing the endometrial glands to secrete and prepare the endometrium for implantation of the blastocyst.

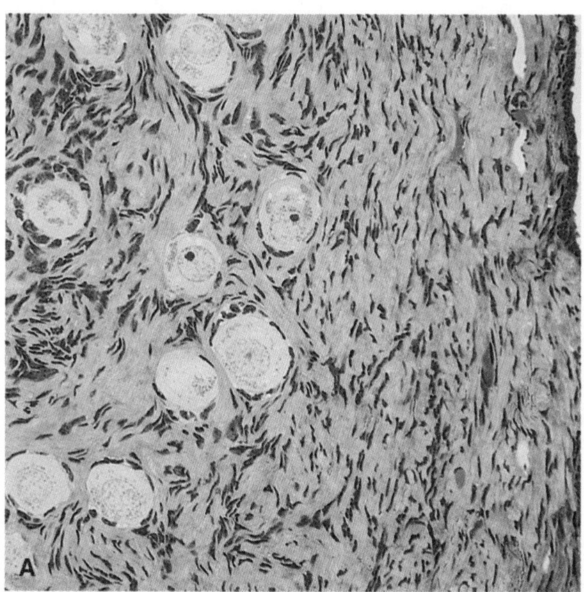

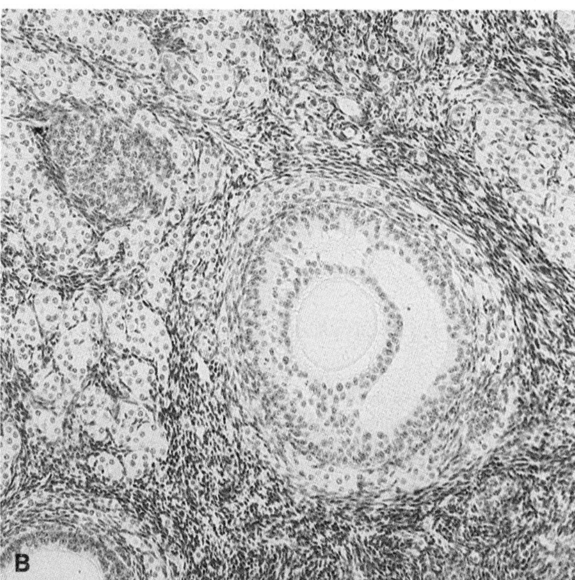

FIGURE 2-9. Micrographs of ovarian cortex. **A,** Several primordial follicles are visible (×270). Observe that the primary oocytes are surrounded by follicular cells. **B,** Secondary ovarian follicle. The oocyte is surrounded by granulosa cells of the cumulus oophorus (×132). (From Gartner LP, Hiatt JL: Color Textbook of Histology, 2nd ed. Philadelphia, WB Saunders, 2001.)

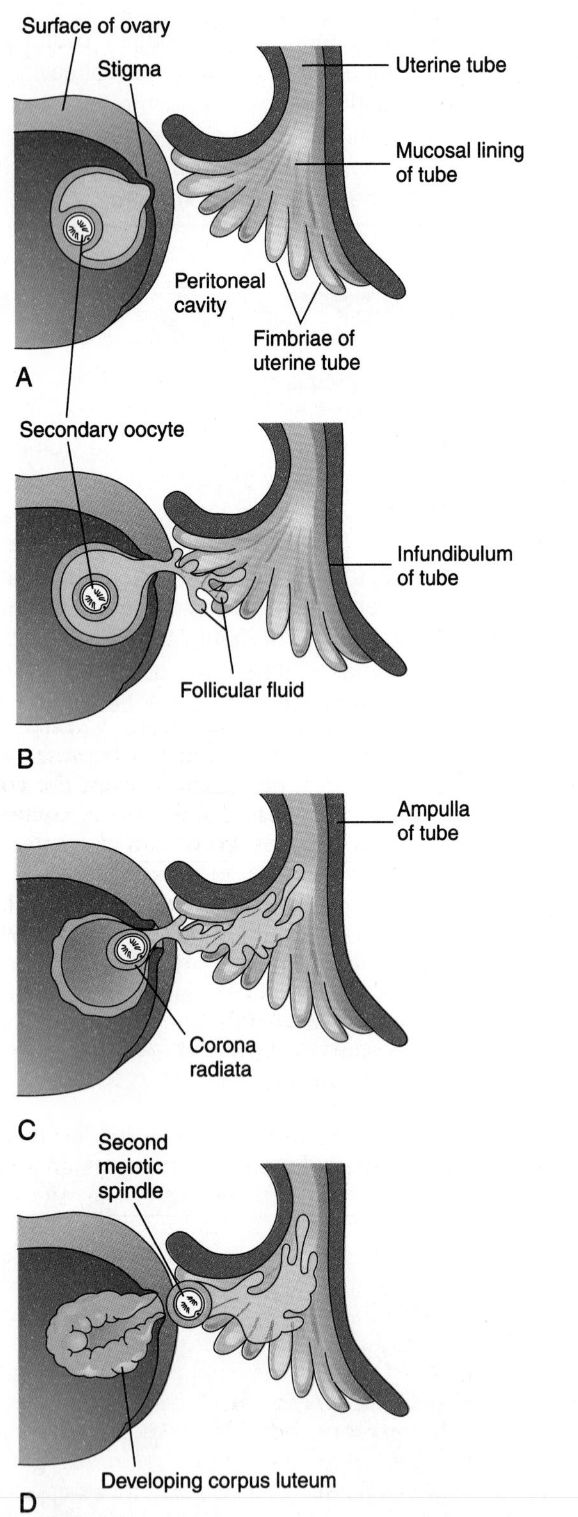

FIGURE 2-10. Illustrations of ovulation. When the stigma ruptures, the secondary oocyte is expelled from the ovarian follicle with the follicular fluid. After ovulation, the wall of the follicle collapses and is thrown into folds. The follicle is transformed into a glandular structure, the corpus luteum.

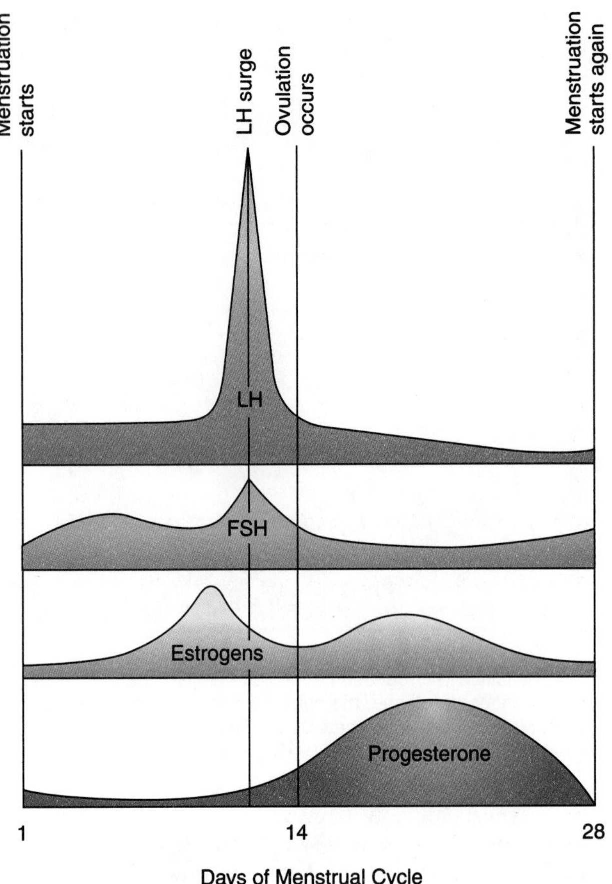

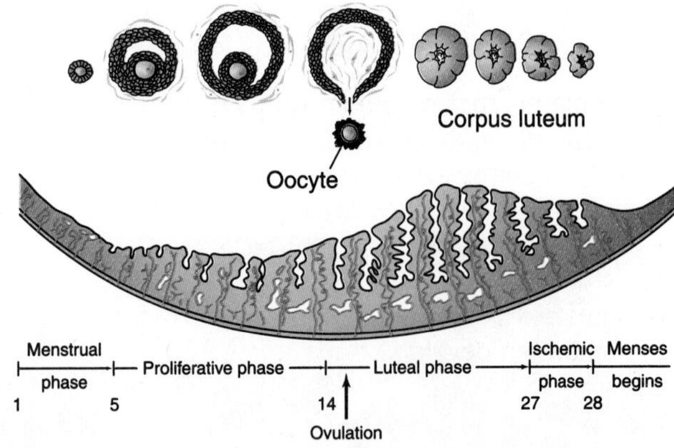

FIGURE 2-11. Illustration of the blood levels of various hormones during the menstrual cycle. Follicle-stimulating hormone (FSH) stimulates the ovarian follicles to develop and produce estrogens. The level of estrogens rises to a peak just before the luteinizing hormone (LH) surge. Ovulation normally occurs 24 to 36 hours after the LH surge. If fertilization does not occur, the blood levels of circulating estrogens and progesterone fall. This hormone withdrawal causes the endometrium to regress and menstruation to start again.

If the oocyte is fertilized, the corpus luteum enlarges to form a corpus luteum of pregnancy and increases its hormone production. Degeneration of the corpus luteum is prevented by *human chorionic gonadotropin*, a hormone secreted by the syncytiotrophoblast of the blastocyst (see Fig. 2-21*B*). The corpus luteum of pregnancy remains functionally active throughout the first 20 weeks of pregnancy. By this time, the placenta has assumed the production of the estrogen and progesterone that is necessary for the maintenance of pregnancy (see Chapter 7).

If the oocyte is not fertilized, the corpus luteum involutes and degenerates 10 to 12 days after ovulation. It is then called a *corpus luteum of menstruation*. The corpus luteum is subsequently transformed into white scar tissue in the ovary, a *corpus albicans*. Except during pregnancy, ovarian cycles normally persist throughout the reproductive life of women and terminate at **menopause**, the permanent cessation of menstruation, usually between the ages of 48 and 55. The endocrine, somatic (body), and psychological changes occurring at the termination of the reproductive period are called the **climacteric**.

MENSTRUAL CYCLE

The menstrual (endometrial) cycle is the time during which the oocyte matures, is ovulated, and enters the uterine tube. The hormones produced by the ovarian follicles and corpus luteum (estrogen and progesterone) produce cyclic changes in the endometrium (see Fig. 2-11). These monthly changes in the internal layer of the uterus constitute the **endometrial cycle**, commonly referred to as the **menstrual cycle** or period because menstruation (flow of blood from the uterus) is an obvious event.

The endometrium is a "mirror" of the ovarian cycle because it responds in a consistent manner to the fluctuating concentrations of gonadotropic and ovarian hormones (see Figs. 2-7 and 2-11). The average menstrual cycle is 28 days, with day 1 of the cycle designated as the day on which menstrual flow begins. Menstrual cycles normally vary in length by several days. In 90% of women, the length of the cycles ranges between 23 and 35 days. Almost all these variations result from alterations in the duration of the proliferative phase of the menstrual cycle.

ANOVULATORY MENSTRUAL CYCLES

The typical reproductive cycle illustrated in Figure 2-11 is not always realized because the ovary may not produce a mature follicle and ovulation does not occur. In *anovulatory cycles*, the endometrial changes are minimal; the proliferative endometrium develops as usual, but no ovulation occurs and no corpus luteum forms. Consequently, the endometrium does not progress to the luteal phase; it remains in the proliferative phase until menstruation begins. Anovulatory cycles may result from ovarian hypofunction. The estrogen, with or without progesterone, in oral contraceptives (birth control pills) acts on the hypothalamus and pituitary gland, resulting in inhibition of secretion of gonadotropin-releasing hormone and FSH and LH, the secretion of which is essential for ovulation to occur.

Phases of the Menstrual Cycle

Changes in the estrogen and progesterone levels cause cyclic changes in the structure of the female reproductive tract, notably the endometrium. Although the menstrual cycle is divided into three main phases for descriptive purposes (see Fig. 2-11), *the menstrual cycle is a continuous process; each phase gradually passes into the next one*.

Menstrual Phase. The functional layer of the uterine wall (see Fig. 2-6*C*) is sloughed off and discarded with the menstrual flow—menses (monthly bleeding), which usually lasts 4 to 5 days. The blood discharged through the vagina is combined with small pieces of endometrial tissue. After menstruation, the eroded endometrium is thin.

Proliferative Phase. The proliferative (follicular, estrogenic) phase, lasting approximately 9 days, coincides with growth of ovarian follicles and is controlled by estrogen secreted by these follicles. There is a two- to threefold increase in the thickness of the endometrium and in its water content during this phase of repair and proliferation. Early during this phase, the surface epithelium reforms and covers the endometrium. The glands increase in number and length, and the spiral arteries elongate.

Luteal Phase. The luteal (secretory, progesterone) phase, lasting approximately 13 days, coincides with the formation, functioning, and growth of the corpus luteum. The progesterone produced by the corpus luteum stimulates the glandular epithelium to secrete a glycogen-rich material. The glands become wide, tortuous, and saccular, and the endometrium thickens because of the influence of progesterone and estrogen from the corpus luteum and because of increased fluid in the connective tissue. As the **spiral arteries** grow into the superficial compact layer, they become increasingly coiled (see Fig. 2-6*C*). The venous network becomes complex and large *lacunae* (venous spaces) develop. *Direct arteriovenous anastomoses* are prominent features of this stage.

If fertilization does not occur:

- The corpus luteum degenerates.
- Estrogen and progesterone levels fall and the secretory endometrium enters an ischemic phase.
- Menstruation occurs.

Ischemic Phase. The ischemic phase occurs when the oocyte is not fertilized. *Ischemia* (reduced blood supply) occurs as the spiral arteries constrict, giving the endometrium a pale appearance. This constriction results from the decreasing secretion of hormones, primarily progesterone, by the degenerating corpus luteum. In addition to vascular changes, the hormone withdrawal results in the stoppage of glandular secretion, a loss of interstitial fluid, and a marked shrinking of the endometrium. Toward the end of the ischemic phase, the spiral arteries become constricted for longer periods. This results in *venous stasis* and patchy ischemic necrosis (death) in the superficial tissues. Eventually, rupture of damaged vessel walls follows and blood seeps into the surrounding connective tissue. Small pools of blood form and break through the endometrial surface, resulting in bleeding into the uterine lumen and from the vagina. As small pieces of the endometrium detach and pass into the uterine cavity, the torn ends of the arteries bleed into the uterine cavity, resulting in a loss of 20 to 80 mL of blood. Eventually, over 3 to 5 days, the entire compact layer and most of the spongy layer of the endometrium are discarded in the *menses*. Remnants of the spongy and basal layers remain to undergo regeneration during the subsequent proliferative phase of the endometrium. It is obvious from the previous descriptions that the cyclic hormonal activity of the ovary is intimately linked with cyclic histologic changes in the endometrium.

If fertilization occurs:

- Cleavage of the zygote and blastogenesis (formation of blastocyst) occur.
- The blastocyst begins to implant in the endometrium on approximately the sixth day of the luteal phase (day 20 of a 28-day cycle).
- Human chorionic gonadotropin, a hormone produced by the syncytiotrophoblast (see Fig. 2-21), keeps the corpus luteum secreting estrogens and progesterone.
- The luteal phase continues and menstruation does not occur.

Pregnancy Phase. *If pregnancy occurs, the menstrual cycles cease* and the endometrium passes into a pregnancy phase. With the termination of pregnancy, the ovarian and menstrual cycles resume after a variable period (usually 6 to 10 weeks if the woman is not breast-feeding her baby). *If pregnancy does not occur, the reproductive cycles normally continue* until menopause.

TRANSPORTATION OF GAMETES

Oocyte Transport

The secondary oocyte is expelled at ovulation from the ovarian follicle with the escaping follicular fluid (see Fig. 2-10*D*). During ovulation, the fimbriated end of the uterine tube becomes closely applied to the ovary. The fingerlike processes of the tube, *fimbriae*, move back and forth over the ovary (Fig. 2-12). The sweeping action of the fimbriae and fluid currents produced by the cilia of the mucosal cells of the fimbriae "sweep" the secondary oocyte into the funnel-shaped infundibulum of the uterine tube. The oocyte passes into the ampulla of the tube, mainly as the result of *peristalsis*—movements of the wall of the tube characterized by alternate contraction and relaxation—that pass toward the uterus.

Sperm Transport

From their storage site in the epididymis, mainly in its tail, the sperms are rapidly transported to the urethra by peristaltic contractions of the thick muscular coat of the ductus deferens (Fig. 2-13). The accessory sex glands—*seminal glands* (vesicles), *prostate*, and *bulbourethral glands*—produce secretions that are added to the sperm-containing fluid in the ductus deferens and urethra (see Fig. 2-13).

From 200 to 600 million sperms are deposited around the external os of the uterus and in the fornix of the vagina during sexual intercourse. The sperms pass slowly through the cervical canal by movements of their tails. The enzyme vesiculase, produced by the seminal glands, coagulates some of the semen or ejaculate and forms a vaginal plug that may prevent the backflow of semen into the vagina. When ovulation occurs, the cervical mucus increases in amount and becomes less viscid, making it more favorable for sperm transport.

The *reflex ejaculation of semen* may be divided into two phases:

- *Emission*: Semen is delivered to the prostatic part of the urethra through the ejaculatory ducts after peristalsis of the ductus deferens; emission is a sympathetic response.
- *Ejaculation*: Semen is expelled from the urethra through the external urethral orifice; this results from closure of the vesical sphincter at the neck of the bladder, contraction of urethral muscle, and contraction of the bulbospongiosus muscles.

Passage of sperms through the uterus and uterine tubes results mainly from muscular contractions of the walls of these organs. *Prostaglandins* in the semen are thought to stimulate uterine motility at the time of intercourse and assist in the movement of sperms to the site of fertilization in the ampulla of the tube. Fructose, secreted by the seminal glands, is an energy source for the sperms in the semen.

The volume of **sperm** or **ejaculate** (sperms suspended in secretions from accessory sex glands) averages 3.5 mL, with a range of 2 to 6 mL. The sperms move 2 to 3 mm

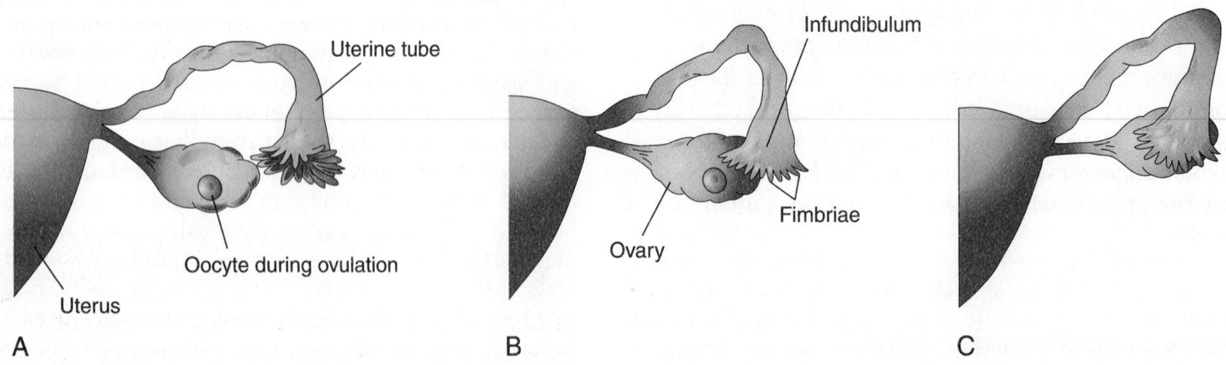

FIGURE 2-12. Illustrations of the movement of the uterine tube that occurs during ovulation. Note that the infundibulum of the tube becomes closely applied to the ovary. Its fingerlike fimbriae move back and forth over the ovary and "sweep" the secondary oocyte into the infundibulum as soon as it is expelled from the ovary during ovulation.

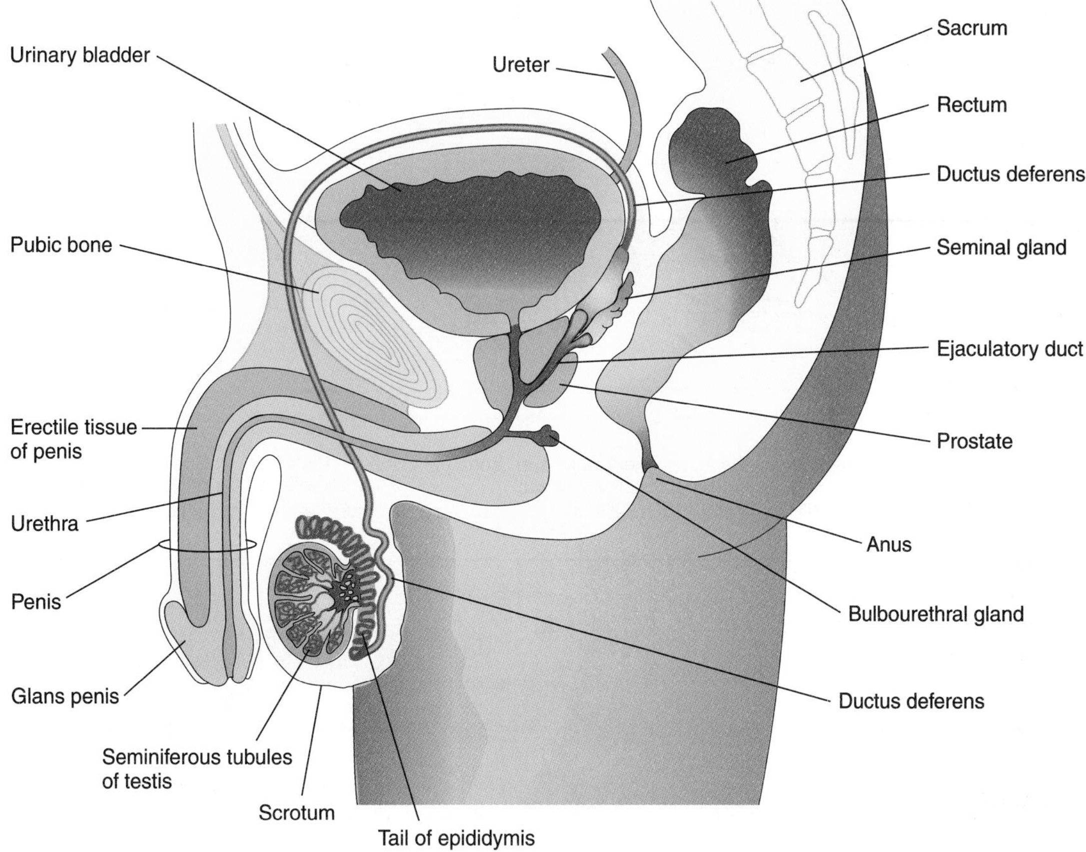

FIGURE 2-13. Sagittal section of male pelvis primarily to show the male reproductive system.

per minute, but the speed varies with the pH of the environment. They are nonmotile during storage in the epididymis, but become motile in the ejaculate. They move slowly in the acid environment of the vagina, but move more rapidly in the alkaline environment of the uterus. It is not known how long it takes sperms to reach the fertilization site, but the time of transport is probably short. Motile sperms have been recovered from the ampulla of the uterine tube 5 minutes after their deposition near the external uterine os. Some sperms, however, take as long as 45 minutes to complete the journey. Only approximately 200 sperms reach the fertilization site. Most sperms degenerate and are resorbed by the female genital tract.

MATURATION OF SPERMS

Freshly ejaculated sperms are unable to fertilize oocytes. *Sperms must undergo a period of conditioning*—**capacitation**—lasting approximately 7 hours. During this period, a glycoprotein coat and seminal proteins are removed from the surface of the sperm's acrosome. The membrane components of the sperms are extensively altered. Capacitated sperms show no morphologic changes, but they are more active. Sperms are usually capacitated in the uterus or uterine tubes by substances secreted by these parts of the female genital tract. During *in vitro fertilization*, a process whereby several oocytes are placed in an artificial medium to which sperms are added for fertilization (see Fig. 2-16), capacitation is induced by incubating the sperms in a defined medium for several hours. Completion of capacitation permits the acrosome reaction to occur.

The intact acrosome of the sperm binds to a *glycoprotein (ZP3)* on the zona pellucida. Studies have shown that the sperm plasma membrane, calcium ions, prostaglandins, and progesterone play a critical role in the acrosome reaction. The **acrosome reaction** of sperms must be completed before the sperm can fuse with the oocyte. When capacitated sperms come into contact with the corona radiata surrounding a secondary oocyte (Fig. 2-14), they undergo complex *molecular changes* that result in the development of perforations in the acrosome. Multiple point fusions of the plasma membrane of the sperm and the external acrosomal membrane occur. Breakdown of the membranes at these sites produces apertures. The changes induced by the acrosome reaction are associated with the release of enzymes, including *hyaluronidase* and *acrosin*, from the acrosome that facilitate fertilization.

SPERM COUNTS

During evaluation of male fertility, an analysis of semen is made. Sperms account for less than 10% of the semen. The remainder of the ejaculate consists of the secretions of the seminal glands,

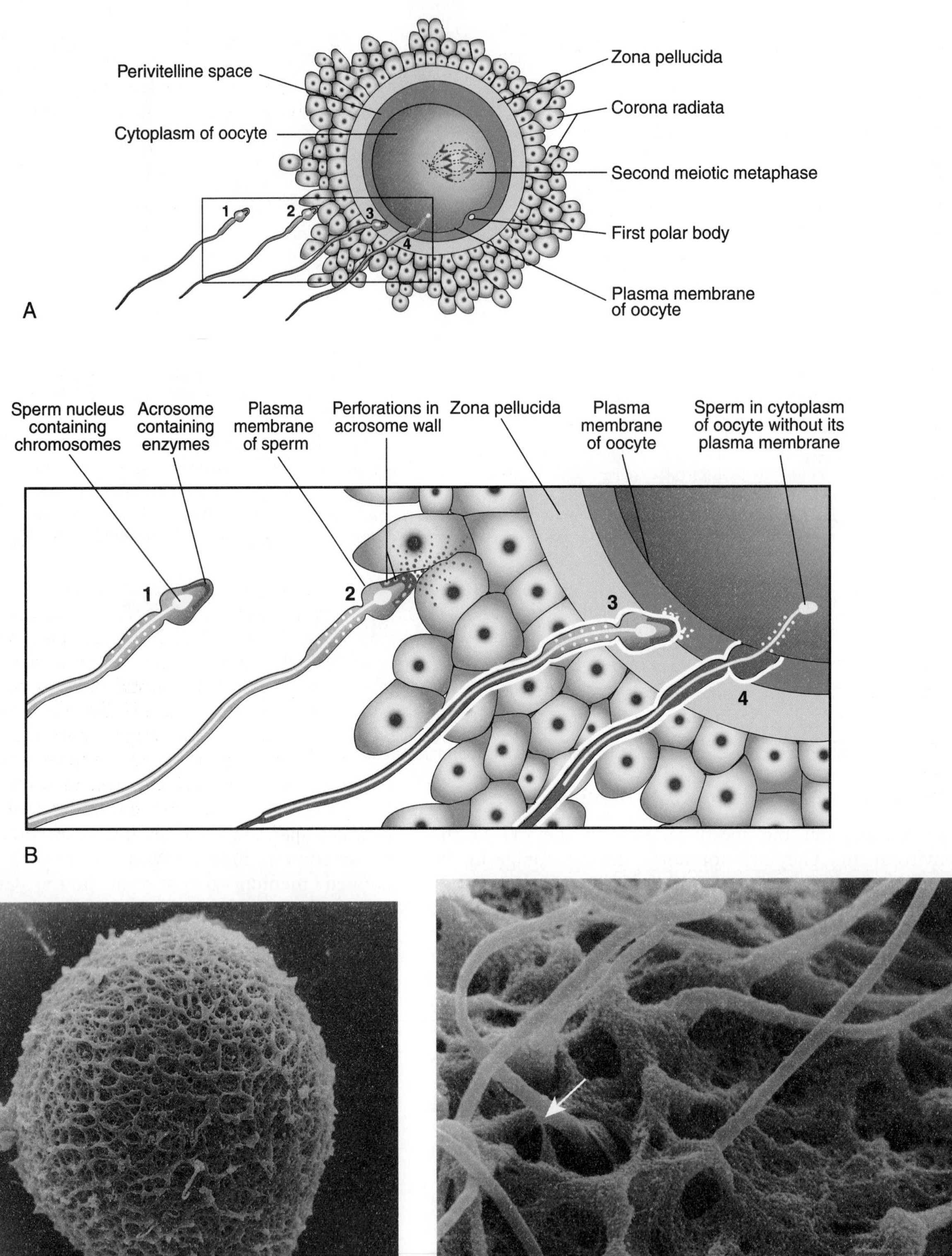

FIGURE 2-14. Acrosome reaction and a sperm penetrating an oocyte. The detail of the area outlined in **A** is given in **B**. 1, Sperm during capacitation, a period of conditioning that occurs in the female reproductive tract. 2, Sperm undergoing the acrosome reaction, during which perforations form in the acrosome. 3, Sperm digesting a path through the zona pellucida by the action of enzymes released from the acrosome. 4, Sperm after entering the cytoplasm of the oocyte. Note that the plasma membranes of the sperm and oocyte have fused and that the head and tail of the sperm enter the oocyte, leaving the sperm's plasma membrane attached to the oocyte's plasma membrane. **C,** Scanning electron microscopy of an unfertilized human oocyte shows relatively few sperms attached to the zona pellucida. **D,** Scanning electron microscopy of human oocyte shows penetration of the sperm (*arrow*) into the zona pellucida. (Courtesy of Professor P. Schwartz and Professor H.M. Michelmann, University of Goettingen, Goettingen, Germany.)

prostate, and bulbourethral glands. There are usually more than 100 million sperms per milliliter of semen in the ejaculate of normal males. Although there is much variation in individual cases, men whose semen contains 20 million sperms per milliliter, or 50 million in the total specimen, are probably fertile. A man with fewer than 10 million sperms per milliliter of semen is likely to be sterile, especially when the specimen contains immotile and abnormal sperms. For potential fertility, 50% of sperms should be motile after 2 hours and some should be motile after 24 hours. Male infertility may result from a low sperm count, poor sperm motility, medications and drugs, endocrine disorders, exposure to environmental pollutants, cigarette smoking, abnormal sperms, or obstruction of a genital duct such as in the ductus deferens (see Fig. 2-13) and represents approximately 30% to 50% of infertility in couples.

Vasectomy

The most effective method of permanent contraception in the male is vasectomy, or excision of a segment of each ductus (vas) deferens. This surgical procedure is reversible in more than 50% of cases. Following vasectomy, there are no sperms in the semen or ejaculate, but the volume is the same.

Dispermy and Triploidy

Although several sperms begin to penetrate the corona radiata and zona pellucida, usually only one sperm penetrates the oocyte and fertilizes it. Two sperms may participate in fertilization during an abnormal process known as dispermy, resulting in a zygote with an extra set of chromosomes. **Triploid conceptions** account for approximately 20% of chromosomally abnormal spontaneous abortions. **Triploid embryos** (69 chromosomes) may appear normal, but they nearly always abort. Aborted triploid fetuses have severe intrauterine growth retardation, disproportionately small trunks, and anomalies in the central nervous system. A few triploid infants have been born, but they all died shortly after birth.

VIABILITY OF GAMETES

Studies on early stages of development indicate that **human oocytes** are usually fertilized within 12 hours after ovulation. In vitro observations have shown that the oocyte cannot be fertilized after 24 hours and that it degenerates shortly thereafter. Most **human sperms** probably do not survive for more than 48 hours in the female genital tract. Some sperms are stored in folds of the mucosa of the cervix and are gradually released into the cervical canal and pass through the uterus into the uterine tubes. The short-term storage of sperms in the cervix provides a gradual release of sperms and thereby increases the chances of fertilization. Sperms and oocytes can be stored frozen for many years to be used in assisted reproduction.

FERTILIZATION

The usual site of fertilization is the ampulla of the uterine tube, its longest and widest part (see Fig. 2-6*B*). If the oocyte is not fertilized here, it slowly passes along the tube to the uterus, where it degenerates and is resorbed. Although fertilization may occur in other parts of the tube, it does not occur in the uterus. Chemical signals (*attractants*), secreted by the oocyte and surrounding follicular cells, guide the capacitated sperms (*sperm chemotaxis*) to the oocyte.

Fertilization is a complex sequence of coordinated molecular events that begins with contact between a sperm and an oocyte (see Fig. 2-14) and ends with the intermingling of maternal and paternal chromosomes at metaphase of the first mitotic division of the zygote, a unicellular embryo (Fig. 2-15). Defects at any stage in the sequence of these events might cause the zygote to die. The fertilization process takes approximately 24 hours. *Transgenic and gene knockout studies* in animals have shown that carbohydrate binding molecules and *gamete-specific proteins* on the surface of the sperms are involved in *sperm-egg recognition* and their union.

Phases of Fertilization

Fertilization is a sequence of coordinated events (see Figs. 2-14 and 2-15):

- **Passage of a sperm through the corona radiata.** Dispersal of the follicular cells of the corona radiata surrounding the oocyte and zona pellucida appears to result mainly from the action of the enzyme *hyaluronidase* released from the acrosome of the sperm, but the evidence of this is not unequivocal. *Tubal mucosal enzymes* also appear to assist the dispersal. Movements of the tail of the sperm are also important in its penetration of the corona radiata.
- **Penetration of the zona pellucida.** Passage of a sperm through the zona pellucida is the important phase in the initiation of fertilization. Formation of a pathway also results from the action of enzymes released from the acrosome. The enzymes *esterases*, *acrosin*, and *neuraminidase* appear to cause lysis of the zona pellucida, thereby forming a path for the sperm to follow to the oocyte. The most important of these enzymes is **acrosin,** a proteolytic enzyme. Once the sperm penetrates the zona pellucida, a **zona**

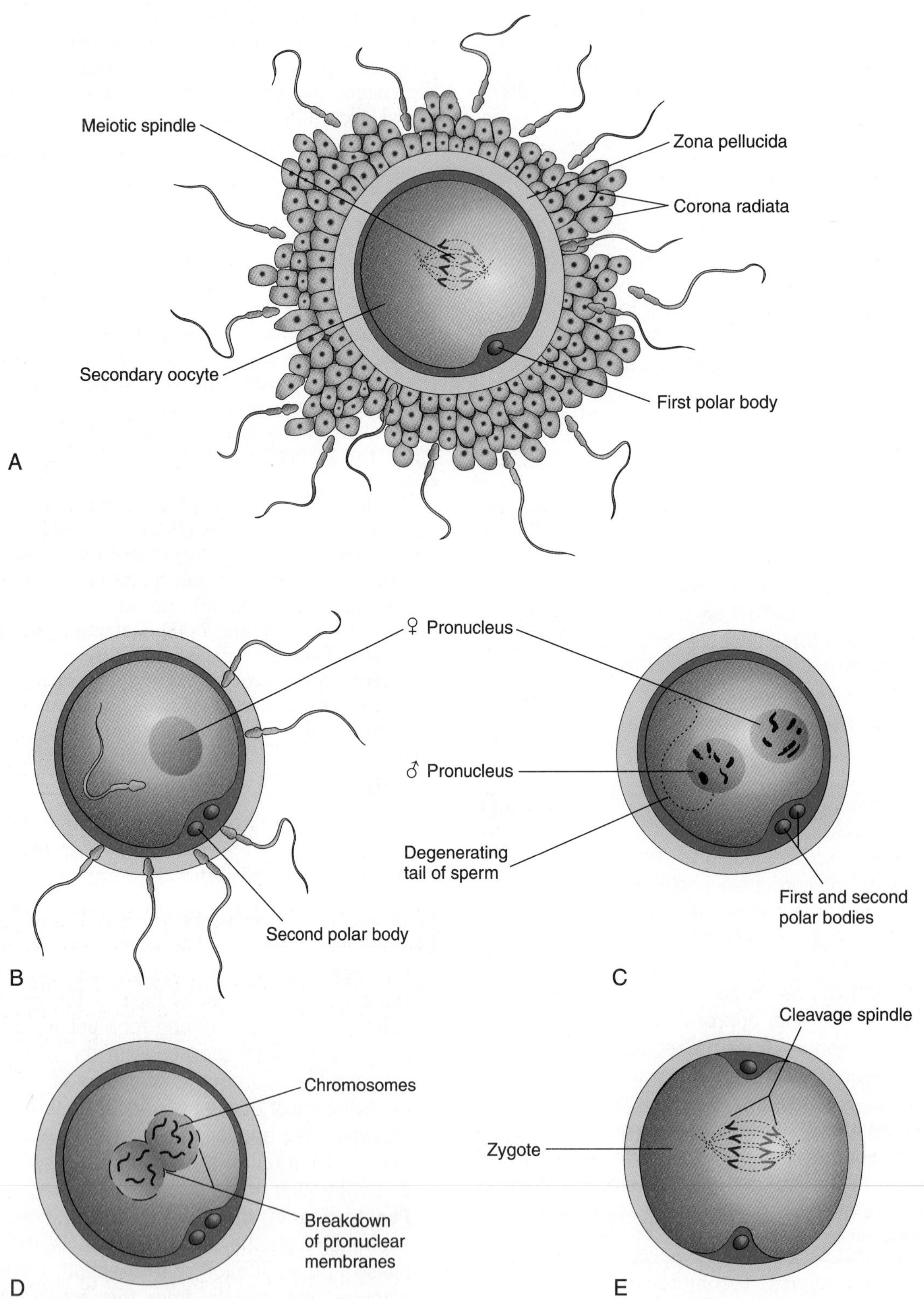

FIGURE 2-15. Illustrations of fertilization, the procession of events beginning when the sperm contacts the secondary oocyte's plasma membrane and ending with the intermingling of maternal and paternal chromosomes at metaphase of the first mitotic division of the zygote. **A,** Secondary oocyte surrounded by several sperms, two of which have penetrated the corona radiata. (Only four of the 23 chromosome pairs are shown.) **B,** The corona radiata has disappeared, a sperm has entered the oocyte, and the second meiotic division has occurred, forming a mature oocyte. The nucleus of the oocyte is now the female pronucleus. **C,** The sperm head has enlarged to form the male pronucleus. This cell, an ootid, contains the male and female pronuclei. **D,** The pronuclei are fusing. **E,** The zygote has formed; it contains 46 chromosomes, the diploid number.

reaction—a change in the properties of the zona pellucida—occurs that makes it impermeable to other sperms. The composition of this extracellular glycoprotein coat changes after fertilization. The zona reaction is believed to result from the action of lysosomal enzymes released by cortical granules near the plasma membrane of the oocyte. The contents of these granules, which are released into the perivitelline space (see Fig. 2-14*A*), also cause changes in the plasma membrane that make it impermeable to other sperms.

- **Fusion of plasma membranes of the oocyte and sperm.** The plasma or cell membranes of the oocyte and sperm fuse and break down at the area of fusion. The head and tail of the sperm enter the cytoplasm of the oocyte, but the sperm's plasma membrane remains behind (see Fig. 2-14*B*).
- **Completion of the second meiotic division of oocyte and formation of female pronucleus.** Penetration of the oocyte by a sperm activates the oocyte into completing the second meiotic division and forming a mature oocyte and a second polar body (see Fig. 2-15*B*). Following decondensation of the maternal chromosomes, the nucleus of the mature oocyte becomes the female pronucleus.
- **Formation of the male pronucleus.** Within the cytoplasm of the oocyte, the nucleus of the sperm enlarges to form the male pronucleus and the tail of the sperm degenerates (see Fig. 2-15*C*). *Morphologically, the male and female pronuclei are indistinguishable.* During growth of the pronuclei, they replicate their DNA-1 n (haploid), 2 c (two chromatids). The oocyte containing two haploid pronuclei is called an *ootid*.
- **As the pronuclei fuse into a single diploid aggregation of chromosomes, the ootid becomes a zygote.** The chromosomes in the zygote become arranged on a **cleavage spindle** (see Fig. 2-15*E*) in preparation for cleavage of the zygote (see Fig. 2-18).

Early pregnancy factor, an immunosuppressant protein, is secreted by the trophoblastic cells and appears in the maternal serum within 24 to 48 hours after fertilization. Early pregnancy factor forms the basis of a pregnancy test during the first 10 days of development.

The zygote is genetically unique because half of its chromosomes came from the mother and half from the father. The zygote contains a new combination of chromosomes that is different from that in the cells of either of the parents. This mechanism forms the basis of biparental inheritance and variation of the human species. Meiosis allows independent assortment of maternal and paternal chromosomes among the germ cells (see Fig. 2-2). Crossing over of chromosomes, by relocating segments of the maternal and paternal chromosomes, "shuffles" the genes, thereby producing a recombination of genetic material. The embryo's chromosomal sex is determined at fertilization by the kind of sperm (X or Y) that fertilizes the oocyte. Fertilization by an X-bearing sperm produces a 46, XX zygote, which normally develops into a female, whereas fertilization by a Y-bearing sperm produces a 46, XY zygote, which normally develops into a male.

Fertilization

- Stimulates the penetrated oocyte to complete the second meiotic division.
- Restores the normal diploid number of chromosomes (46) in the zygote.
- Results in variation of the human species through mingling of maternal and paternal chromosomes.
- Determines chromosomal sex of the embryo.
- Causes metabolic activation of the ootid and initiates cleavage (cell division) of the zygote.

Preselection of the Embryo's Sex

Because X and Y sperms are formed in equal numbers, the expectation is that the sex ratio at fertilization (primary sex ratio) would be 1.00 (100 boys per 100 girls). It is well known, however, that there are more male babies than female babies born in all countries. In North America, for example, the sex ratio at birth (secondary sex ratio) is approximately 1.05 (105 boys per 100 girls). Various microscopic techniques have been developed in an attempt to separate X and Y sperms (gender selection) using:

- The differential swimming abilities of the X and Y sperms
- Different speeds of migration of sperms in an electric field
- Differences in the appearance of X and Y sperms
- DNA difference between X (2.8% more DNA) and Y sperms

The use of a selected sperm sample in artificial insemination may produce the desired sex.

Assisted Reproductive Technologies

In Vitro Fertilization and Embryo Transfer

In vitro fertilization (IVF) of oocytes and transfer of the cleaving zygotes into the uterus have provided an opportunity for many women who are sterile (e.g., owing to tubal occlusion) to bear children. The first of these in vitro fertilization babies was born in 1978. Since then, *approximately* two million children have been born after an in vitro fertilization procedure. The steps involved during in vitro fertilization and embryo transfer are as follows (Figs. 2-16 and 2-17):

- Ovarian follicles are stimulated to grow and mature by the administration of clomiphene citrate or gonadotropin (superovulation).
- Several mature oocytes are aspirated from mature ovarian follicles during laparoscopy. Oocytes can also be removed by an ultrasonography-guided large-gauge needle

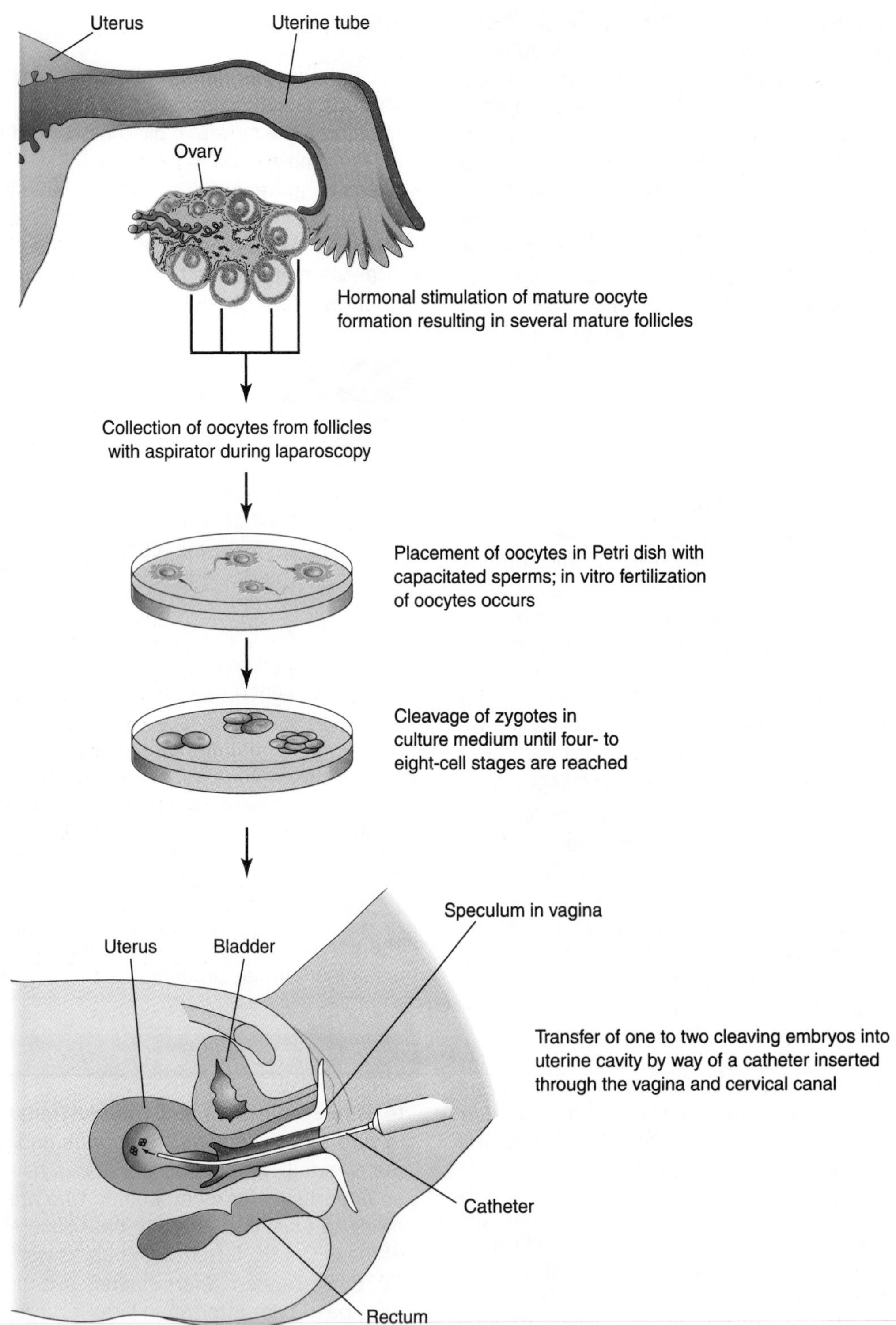

FIGURE 2-16. In vitro fertilization and embryo transfer procedures.

inserted through the vaginal wall into the ovarian follicles.

- The oocytes are placed in a Petri dish containing a special culture medium and capacitated sperms.
- Fertilization of the oocytes and cleavage of the zygotes are monitored microscopically for 3 to 5 days.
- One or two of the resulting embryos (four- to eight-cell stage or early blastocysts) are

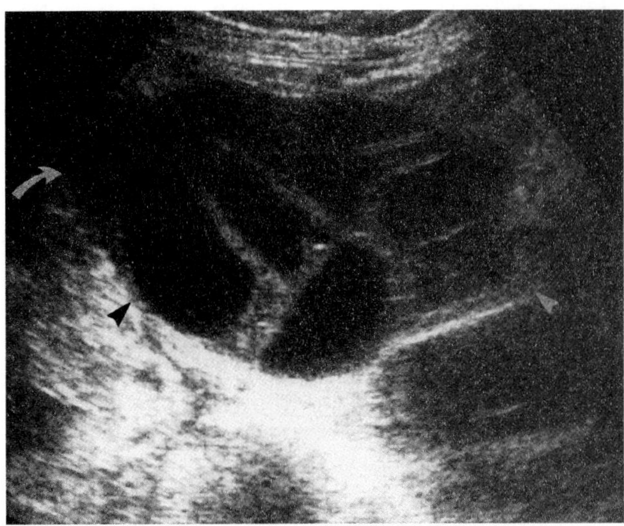

FIGURE 2-17. Ovarian hyperstimulation syndrome. Transabdominal scan demonstrating an enlarged multicystic ovary (*arrowheads*) and ascites (*curved arrow*) in a pregnant patient after assisted fertilization.

transferred by introducing a catheter through the vagina and cervical canal into the uterus. Any remaining embryos are stored in liquid nitrogen for later use.
- The patient lies supine (face upward) for several hours.

Obviously, the chances of multiple pregnancies are higher than when pregnancy results from normal ovulation, fertilization, and passage of the morula into the uterus via the uterine tube. The incidence of spontaneous abortion of transferred embryos is also higher than normal.

Cryopreservation of Embryos
Early embryos resulting from in vitro fertilization can be preserved for long periods by freezing them with a cryoprotectant (e.g., glycerol). Successful transfer of four- to eight-cell embryos and blastocysts to the uterus after thawing is now a common practice.

Intracytoplasmic Sperm Injection
A sperm can be injected directly into the cytoplasm of a mature oocyte. This technique has been successfully used for the treatment of couples for whom in vitro fertilization failed or in cases where there are too few sperms available for in vitro insemination.

Assisted In Vivo Fertilization
A technique enabling fertilization to occur in the uterine tube is called gamete intrafallopian transfer. It involves superovulation (similar to that used for in vitro fertilization), oocyte retrieval, sperm collection, and laparoscopic placement of several oocytes and sperms into the uterine tubes. Using this technique, fertilization occurs in the ampulla, its usual location.

Surrogate Mothers
Some women produce mature oocytes but are unable to become pregnant, for example, a woman who has had her uterus excised (hysterectomy). In these cases, in vitro fertilization may be performed and the embryos transferred to another woman's uterus for development and delivery.

CLEAVAGE OF THE ZYGOTE

Cleavage consists of repeated mitotic divisions of the zygote, resulting in a rapid increase in the number of cells. These embryonic cells—**blastomeres—**become smaller with each successive cleavage division (Figs. 2-18 and 2-19). Cleavage normally occurs as the zygote passes along the uterine tube toward the uterus (see Fig. 2-22). During cleavage, the zygote is within the rather thick zona pellucida. Division of the zygote into blastomeres begins approximately 30 hours after fertilization. Subsequent cleavage divisions follow one another, forming progressively smaller blastomeres (see Fig. 2-18). After the nine-cell stage, the blastomeres change their shape and tightly align themselves against each other to form a compact ball of cells. This phenomenon, **compaction,** is probably mediated by cell surface adhesion glycoproteins. Compaction permits greater cell-to-cell interaction and is a prerequisite for segregation of the internal cells that form the inner cell mass or *embryoblast* of the blastocyst (see Fig. 2-18*E* and *F*). When there are 12 to 32 blastomeres, the developing human is called a **morula** (L., *morus*, mulberry). Internal cells of the morula (*inner cell mass*) are surrounded by a layer of cells that form the outer cell layer. The spherical morula forms approximately 3 days after fertilization and enters the uterus.

NONDISJUNCTION OF CHROMOSOMES

If nondisjunction (failure of a chromosome pair to separate) occurs during an early cleavage division of a zygote, an embryo with two or more cell lines with different chromosome complements is produced. Individuals in whom numerical mosaicism is present are *mosaics*; for example, a zygote with an additional chromosome 21 might lose the extra chromosome during an early division of the zygote. Consequently, some cells of the embryo would have a normal chromosome complement and others would have an additional chromosome 21. In general, individuals who are mosaic for a given trisomy, such as mosaic Down syndrome, are less severely affected than those with the usual nonmosaic condition.

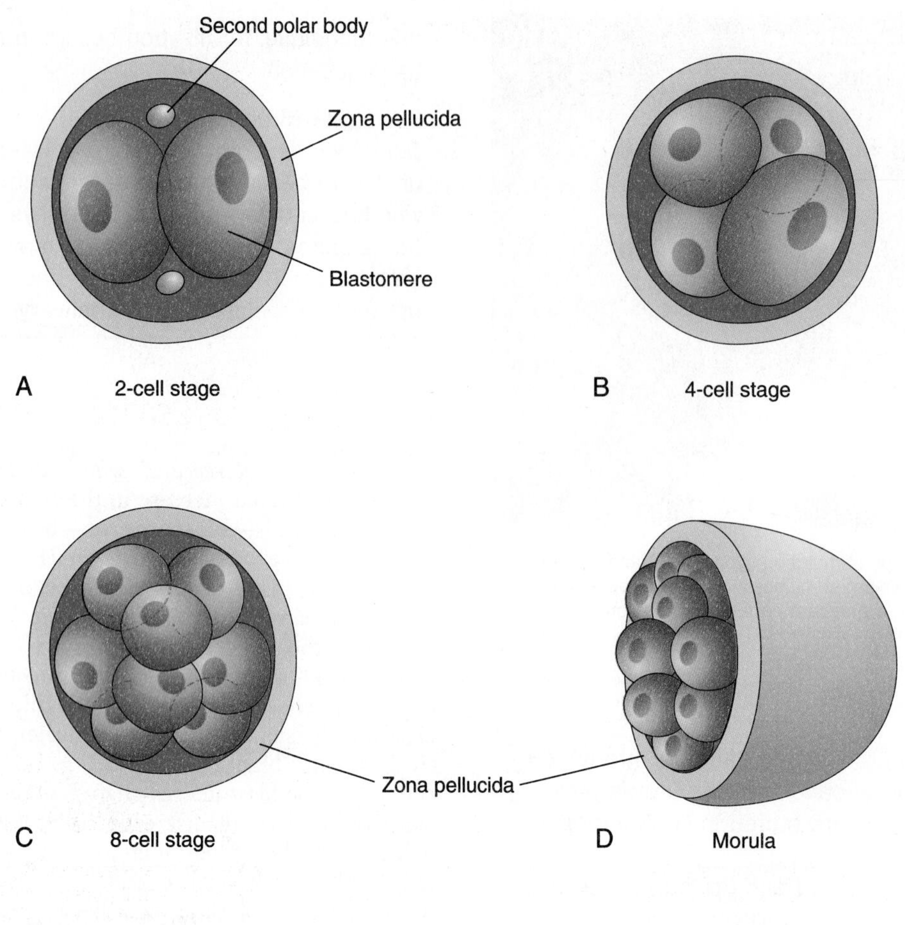

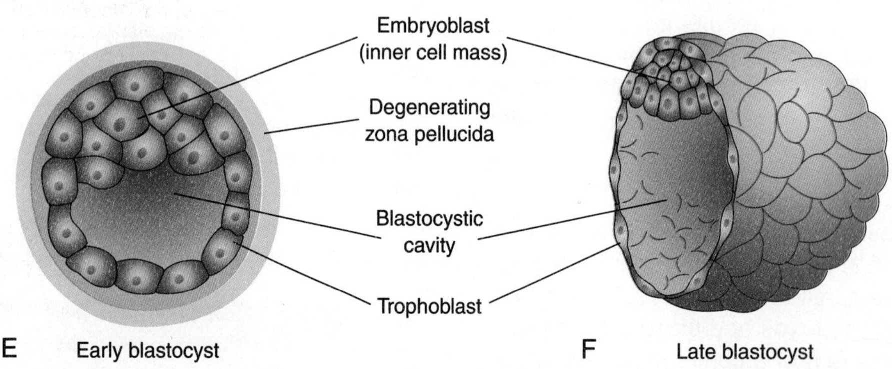

FIGURE 2-18. Illustrations of cleavage of the zygote and formation of the blastocyst. **A** to **D**, Various stages of cleavage. The period of the morula begins at the 12- to 16-cell stage and ends when the blastocyst forms. **E** and **F**, Sections of blastocysts. The zona pellucida has disappeared by the late blastocyst stage (5 days). The second polar bodies shown in **A** are small, nonfunctional cells that soon degenerate. Cleavage of the zygote and formation of the morula occur as the dividing zygote passes along the uterine tube. Blastocyst formation normally occurs in the uterus. Although cleavage increases the number of blastomeres, note that each of the daughter cells is smaller than the parent cells. As a result, there is no increase in the size of the developing embryo until the zona pellucida degenerates. The blastocyst then enlarges considerably.

FORMATION OF THE BLASTOCYST

Shortly after the morula enters the uterus (approximately 4 days after fertilization), a fluid-filled space called the **blastocystic cavity** appears inside the morula (see Fig. 2-18*E*). The fluid passes from the uterine cavity through the zona pellucida to form this space. As fluid increases in the blastocystic cavity, it separates the blastomeres into two parts:

- A thin, outer cell layer, the **trophoblast** (Greek, *trophe*, nutrition), which gives rise to the embryonic part of the placenta
- A group of centrally located blastomeres, the **inner cell mass,** which gives rise to the embryo; because it is the primordium of the embryo, the inner cell mass is called the **embryoblast**

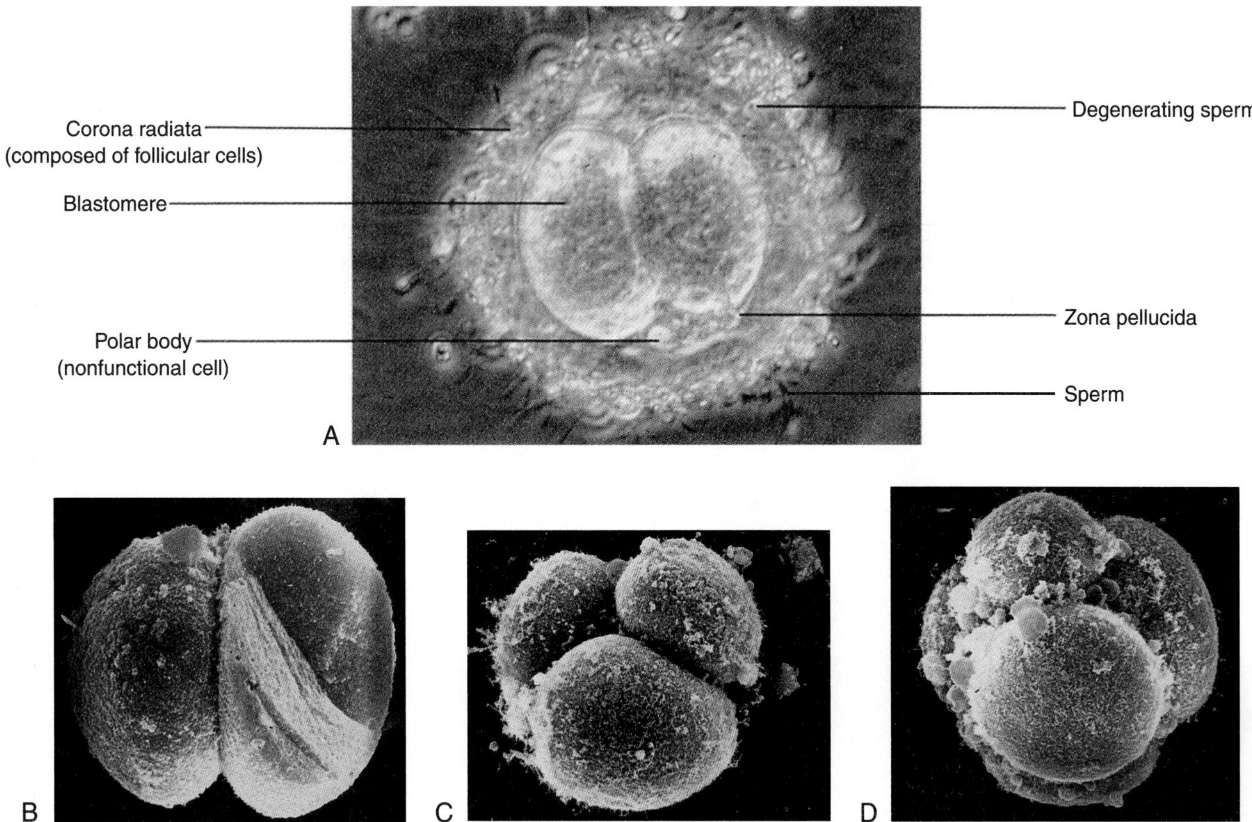

FIGURE 2-19. **A,** Two-cell stage of a cleaving zygote developing in vitro. Observe that it is surrounded by many sperms. **B,** In vitro fertilization, two-cell stage human embryo. The zona pellucida has been removed. A small rounded polar body (pink) is still present on the surface of a blastomere (artificially colored, scanning electron microscopy, ×1000). **C,** Three-cell stage human embryo, in vitro fertilization (scanning electron microscopy, ×1300). **D,** Eight-cell stage human embryo, in vitro fertilization (scanning electron microscopy, ×1100). Note the rounded large blastomeres with several spermatozoa attached. (**A,** Courtesy of Dr. M.T. Zenzes, In Vitro Fertilization Program, Toronto Hospital, Toronto, Ontario, Canada; **D,** From Makabe S, Naguro T, Motta PM: Three-dimensional features of human cleaving embryo by ODO method and field emission scanning electron microscopy. In Motta PM: Microscopy of Reproduction and Development: A Dynamic Approach. Rome, Antonio Delfino Editore, 1997.)

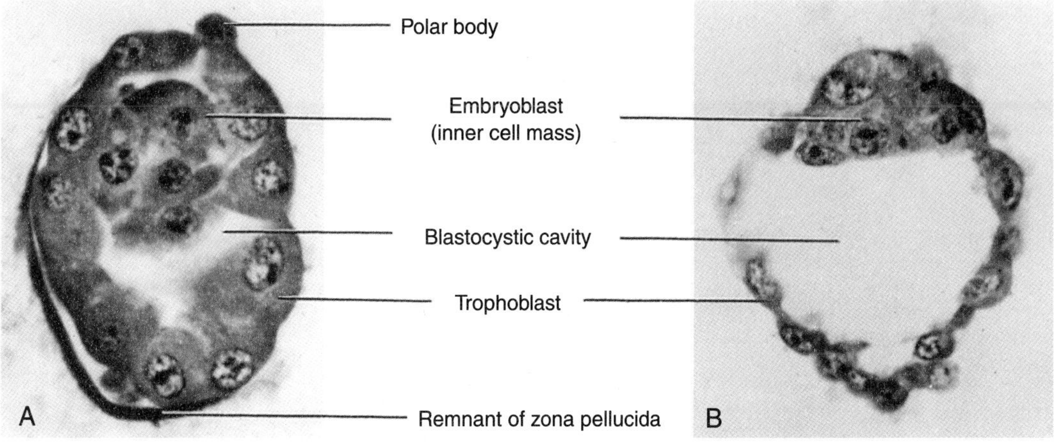

FIGURE 2-20. Photomicrographs of sections of human blastocysts recovered from the uterine cavity (×600). **A,** At 4 days: the blastocystic cavity is just beginning to form and the zona pellucida is deficient over part of the blastocyst. **B,** At $4^1/_2$ days; the blastocystic cavity has enlarged and the embryoblast and trophoblast are clearly defined. The zona pellucida has disappeared. (From Hertig AT, Rock J, Adams EC: Am J Anat 98:435, 1956. Courtesy of the Carnegie Institution of Washington.)

During this stage of development—**blastogenesis**—the conceptus is called a **blastocyst** (Fig. 2-20). The embryoblast now projects into the blastocystic cavity and the trophoblast forms the wall of the blastocyst. After the free blastocyst has floated in the uterine secretions for approximately 2 days, the zona pellucida gradually degenerates and disappears (see Figs. 2-18*F* and 2-20*A*). *Shedding of the zona pellucida and hatching of the blastocyst* have been observed in vitro. Shedding of the zona pellucida permits the hatched blastocyst to increase rapidly in size. While floating in the uterus, this early embryo derives nourishment from secretions of the uterine glands.

Approximately 6 days after fertilization (day 20 of a 28-day menstrual cycle), the blastocyst attaches to the endometrial epithelium, usually adjacent to the **embryonic pole** (Fig. 2-21*A*). As soon as it attaches to the endometrial epithelium, the trophoblast starts to proliferate rapidly and gradually differentiates into two layers (see Fig. 2-21*B*):

- An inner layer of **cytotrophoblast**
- An outer layer of **syncytiotrophoblast** consisting of a multinucleated protoplasmic mass in which no cell boundaries can be observed

Both intrinsic and extracellular matrix factors modulate, in carefully timed sequences, the differentiation of the trophoblast. *At approximately 6 days*, the fingerlike processes of syncytiotrophoblast extend through the endometrial epithelium and invade the connective tissue. By the end of the first week, the blastocyst is superficially implanted in the compact layer of the endometrium and is deriving its nourishment from the eroded maternal tissues (see Fig. 2-21*B*). The highly invasive syncytiotrophoblast expands quickly adjacent to the embryoblast, the area known as the **embryonic pole.** The syncytiotrophoblast produces enzymes that erode the maternal tissues, enabling the blastocyst to burrow into the endometrium. *At approximately 7 days*, a layer of cells, the **hypoblast** (primary endoderm), appears on the surface of the embryoblast facing the blastocystic cavity (see Fig. 2-21*B*). Comparative embryologic data suggest that the hypoblast arises by delamination of blastomeres from the embryoblast.

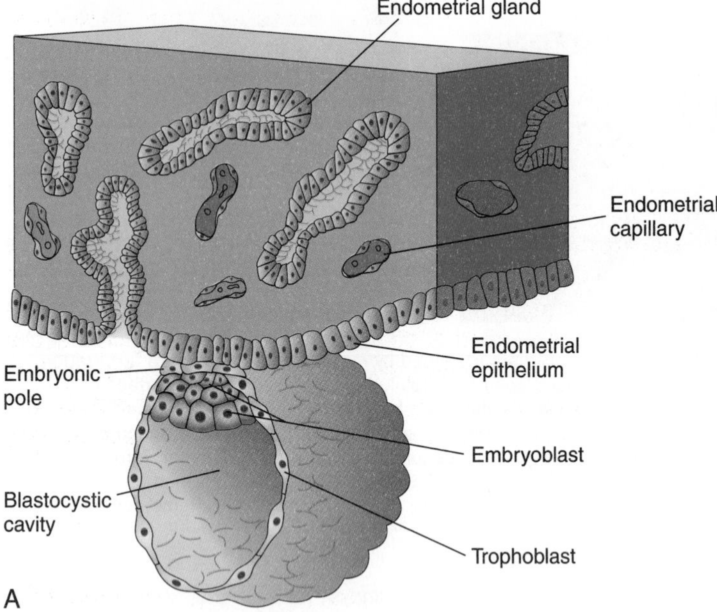

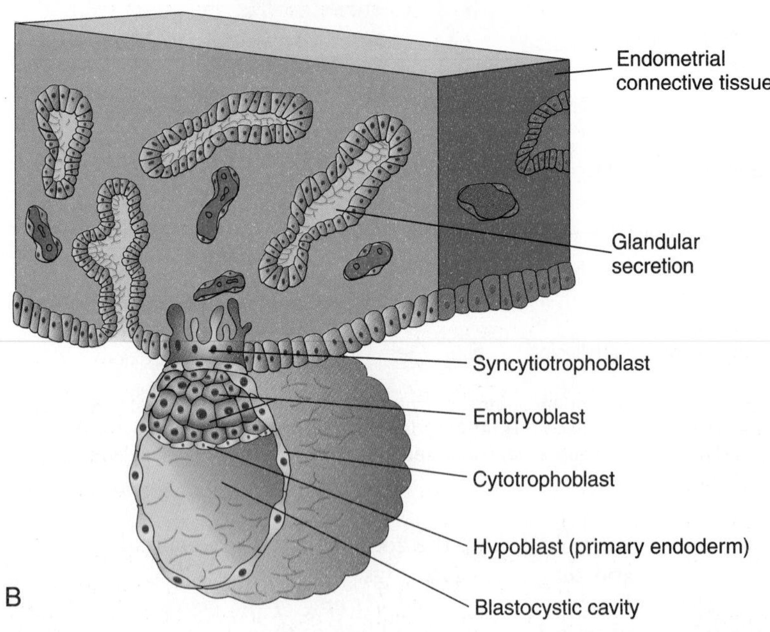

FIGURE 2-21. Attachment of the blastocyst to the endometrial epithelium during the early stages of its implantation. **A,** At 6 days: the trophoblast is attached to the endometrial epithelium at the embryonic pole of the blastocyst. **B,** At 7 days: the syncytiotrophoblast has penetrated the epithelium and has started to invade the endometrial connective tissue. Some students have difficulty interpreting illustrations such as these because in histologic studies, it is conventional to draw the endometrial epithelium upward, whereas in embryologic studies, the embryo is usually shown with its dorsal surface upward. Because the embryo implants on its future dorsal surface, it would appear upside down if the histologic convention were followed. In this book, the histologic convention is followed when the endometrium is the dominant consideration (e.g., Fig. 2-6C), and the embryologic convention is used when the embryo is the center of interest, as in the adjacent illustrations.

Preimplantation Genetic Diagnosis

Preimplantation genetic diagnosis can be carried out 3 to 5 days after in vitro fertilization of the oocyte. One or two cells (blastomeres) are removed from the embryo known to be at risk of a specific genetic disorder. These cells are then analyzed before transfer into the uterus. The sex of the embryo can also be determined from one blastomere taken from a six- to eight-cell dividing zygote and analyzed by DNA amplification of sequences from the Y chromosome. This procedure has been used to detect female embryos during in vitro fertilization in cases in which a male embryo would be at risk of a serious X-linked disorder.

Abnormal Embryos and Spontaneous Abortions

Many zygotes, morulae, and blastocysts abort spontaneously. Early implantation of the blastocyst is a critical period of development that may fail to occur owing to inadequate production of progesterone and estrogen by the corpus luteum. Clinicians occasionally see a patient who states that her last menstrual period was delayed by several days and that her last menstrual flow was unusually profuse. Very likely such patients have had early spontaneous abortions. The overall early spontaneous abortion rate is thought to be approximately 45%. Early spontaneous abortions occur *for a variety of reasons*, one being the presence of chromosomal abnormalities. More than half of all known spontaneous abortions occur because of these abnormalities. The early loss of embryos, once called pregnancy wastage, appears to represent a disposal of abnormal conceptuses that could not have developed normally, i.e., there is a natural screening of embryos. Without this screening, the incidence of infants born with congenital abnormalities would be far greater.

SUMMARY OF THE FIRST WEEK (Fig. 2-22)

- Oocytes are produced by the ovaries (oogenesis) and expelled from them during ovulation. The fimbriae of the uterine tube sweep the oocyte into the ampulla where it may be fertilized.
- Sperms are produced in the testes (spermatogenesis) and are stored in the epididymis. Ejaculation of semen during sexual intercourse results in the deposit of millions of sperms in the vagina. Several hundred sperms pass through the uterus and enter the uterine tubes.
- When an oocyte is contacted by a sperm, it completes the second meiotic division. As a result, a mature oocyte and a second polar body are formed. The nucleus of the mature oocyte constitutes the female pronucleus.
- After the sperm enters the oocyte, the head of the sperm separates from the tail and enlarges to become the male pronucleus. Fertilization is complete when the male and female pronuclei unite and the maternal and paternal chromosomes intermingle during metaphase of the first mitotic division of the zygote.
- As it passes along the uterine tube toward the uterus, the zygote undergoes cleavage (a series of mitotic cell divisions) into a number of smaller cells—blastomeres. Approximately 3 days after fertilization, a ball of 12 or more blastomeres—a morula—enters the uterus.
- A cavity forms in the morula, converting it into a blastocyst consisting of the embryoblast, a blastocystic cavity, and the trophoblast. The trophoblast encloses the embryoblast and blastocystic cavity and later forms extraembryonic structures and the embryonic part of the placenta.
- Four to 5 days after fertilization, the zona pellucida is shed and the trophoblast adjacent to the embryoblast attaches to the endometrial epithelium.
- The trophoblast at the embryonic pole differentiates into two layers, an outer syncytiotrophoblast and an inner cytotrophoblast. The syncytiotrophoblast invades the endometrial epithelium and underlying connective tissue. Concurrently, a cuboidal layer of hypoblast forms on the deep surface of the embryoblast. By the end of the first week, the blastocyst is superficially implanted in the endometrium.

CLINICALLY ORIENTED PROBLEMS

1. What is the main cause of numerical aberrations of chromosomes? Define this process. What is the usual result of this chromosomal abnormality?
2. During in vitro cleavage of a zygote, all blastomeres of a morula were found to have an extra set of chromosomes. Explain how this could happen. Can such a morula develop into a viable fetus?
3. In infertile couples, the inability to conceive is attributable to some factor in the woman or the man. What is a major cause of (a) female infertility and (b) male infertility?
4. Some people have a mixture of cells with 46 and 47 chromosomes (e.g., some persons with Down syndrome are *mosaics*). How do mosaics form? Would children with mosaicism and Down syndrome have the same stigmata as other infants with this syndrome? At what stage of development does mosaicism develop? Can this chromosomal abnormality be diagnosed before birth?
5. A young woman who feared that she might be pregnant asked you about the so-called morning-after pills (postcoital oral contraceptives). How would you explain to her the action of such medication?

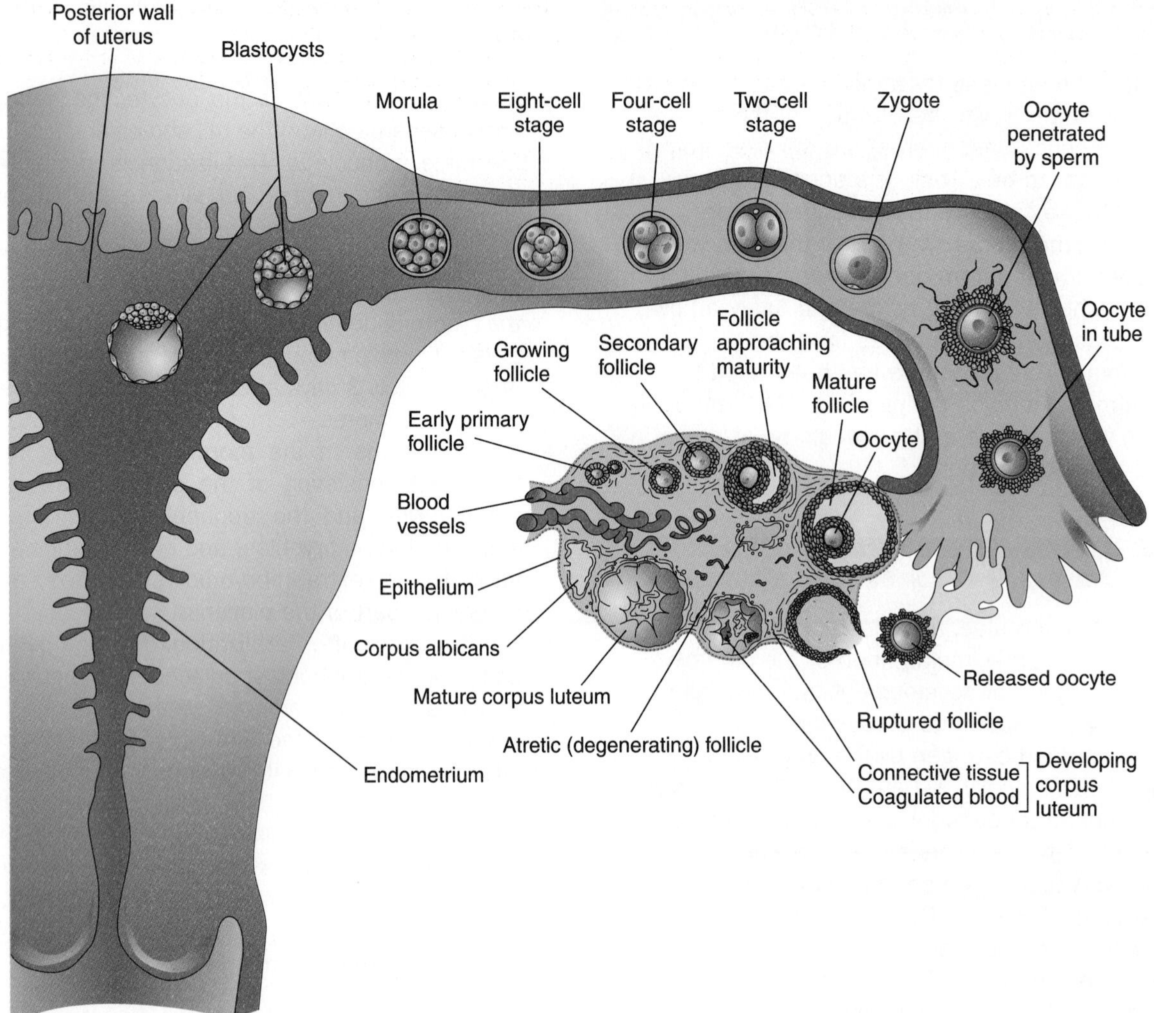

FIGURE 2-22. Summary of the ovarian cycle, fertilization, and human development during the first week. Stage 1 of development begins with fertilization in the uterine tube and ends when the zygote forms. Stage 2 (days 2 to 3) comprises the early stages of cleavage (from 2 to approximately 32 cells, the morula). Stage 3 (days 4 to 5) consists of the free (unattached) blastocyst. Stage 4 (days 5 to 6) is represented by the blastocyst attaching to the posterior wall of the uterus, the usual site of implantation. The blastocysts have been sectioned to show their internal structure.

6. What is the most common abnormality in early spontaneously aborted embryos?
7. Mary, 26 years old, is unable to conceive after 4 years of marriage. Her husband, Jerry, 32 years old, appears to be in good health. Mary and Jerry consulted their family physician who referred them to an infertility clinic. How common is infertility in couples who want to have a baby? What do you think is the likely problem in this couple? What investigation(s) would you recommend first?

Discussion of these problems appears at the back of the book.

References and Suggested Reading

Clermont Y, Trott M: Kinetics of spermatogenesis in mammals: Seminiferous epithelium cycle and spermatogonial renewal. Physiol Rev 52:198, 1972.

Cooke HJ, Hargreave T, Elliott DJ: Understanding the genes involved in spermatogenesis: A progress report. Fertil Steril 69:989, 1998.

Doody KJ: Advances in assisted reproduction. Semin Reprod Med 23:299, 2005.

Geber S, Winston RM, Handyside AH: Proliferation of blastomeres from biopsied cleavage stage human embryos in vitro: An alternative to blastocyst biopsy for preimplantation diagnosis. Hum Reprod 10:1492, 1995.

Guraya SS: Cellular and molecular biology of capacitation and acrosome reaction in spermatozoa. Int Rev Cytol 199:1, 2000.

Hampton T: Researchers discover a range of factors undermine sperm quality, male fertility. JAMA 294:2829, 2005.

Hansen M, Kurinczuk JJ, Bower C, et al: The risk of major birth defects after intracytoplasmic sperm injection and in vitro fertilization. N Engl J Med 346:725, 2002.

Hertig AT, Rock J, Adams EC, Menkin MC: Thirty-four fertilized human ova, good, bad, and indifferent, recovered from 210 women of known fertility. Pediatrics 23:202, 1959.

Hillier SG: Gonadotropic control of ovarian follicular growth and development. Mol Cell Endocrinol 179:39, 2001.

Horne AW, White JO, Lalani E: The endometrium and embryo implantation. BMJ 321:1301, 2000.

Kubiak JZ, Johnson M: Human infertility, reproductive cloning and nuclear transfer: A confusion of meanings. BioEssays 23:359, 2001.

Latham KE: Mechanisms and control of embryonic genome activation in mammalian embryos. Int Rev Cytol 193:71, 1999.

Magerkurth C, Topfer-Petersen E, Schwartz P, Michelmann HW: Scanning electron microscopy analysis of the human zona pellucida: Influence of maturity and fertilization on morphology and sperm binding pattern. Hum Reprod 14:1057, 1999.

Ngai SW, Fan S, Li S, et al: A randomized trial to compare 24 h versus 12 h double dose regimen of levonorgestrel for emergency contraception. Human Reprod 20:307, 2005.

Oehninger S, Hodgen GD: Hypothalamic-pituitary-ovary-uterine axis. In Copeland LJ, Jarrell J, McGregor J (eds): Textbook of Gynecology, 2nd ed. Philadelphia, WB Saunders, 2000.

Rock J, Hertig AT: The human conceptus during the first two weeks of gestation. Am J Obstet Gynecol 55:6, 1948.

Shevell T, Malone FD, Vidaver J, et al: Assisted reproductive technology and pregnancy outcome. Obstet Gynecol 106: 1039, 2005.

Sjoberg N-O, Hamberger L (eds): Blastocyst development and early implantation. Hum Reprod 15 (Suppl 6): 2000.

Steptoe PC, Edwards RG: Birth after implantation of a human embryo. Lancet 2:36, 1978.

Sutcliffe AG: Intracytoplasmic sperm injection and other aspects of new reproductive technologies. Arch Dis Child 83:48, 2000.

Swan SH, Elkin EP: Declining semen quality: Can the past inform the present? BioEssays 21:614, 1999.

Trounson A: Developments in infertility therapy. Diagnosis of genetic disease in embryos. Aust Fam Physician 34:123, 2005.

Veeck LL (ed): Atlas of Human Gametes and Early Conceptus. New York, Parthenon Publishing Group, 2000.

Weremowicz S, Sandstrom DJ, Morton CC, et al: Fluorescence in situ hybridization (FISH) for rapid detection of aneuploidy: Experience in 911 prenatal cases. Prenat Diagn 21:262, 2001.

Wilmut I, Schnieke AE, McWhir J, et al: Viable offspring derived from fetal and adult mammalian cells. Nature 385:810, 1997.

Wylie C: Germ cells. Curr Opin Genet Dev 10:410, 2000.

3

Formation of the Bilaminar Embryonic Disc: Second Week

Completion of Implantation and Continuation of Embryonic Development 43

Formation of the Amniotic Cavity, Embryonic Disc, and Umbilical Vesicle 44

Development of the Chorionic Sac 45

Implantation Sites of Blastocysts 45

Summary of Implantation 48

Summary of the Second Week 51

Clinically Oriented Problems 53

Implantation of the blastocyst is completed during the second week. As this process occurs, morphologic changes in the embryoblast produce a bilaminar embryonic disc composed of epiblast and hypoblast (Fig. 3-1*A*). The **embryonic disc** gives rise to the germ layers that form all the tissues and organs of the embryo. Extraembryonic structures forming during the second week are the amniotic cavity, amnion, umbilical vesicle (yolk sac), connecting stalk, and chorionic sac.

COMPLETION OF IMPLANTATION AND CONTINUATION OF EMBRYONIC DEVELOPMENT

Implantation of the blastocyst is completed by the end of the second week. It occurs during a restricted time period 6 to 10 days after ovulation. As the blastocyst implants (see Fig. 3-1), more trophoblast contacts the endometrium and differentiates into

- The cytotrophoblast, a layer of cells that is mitotically active and forms new cells that migrate into the increasing mass of syncytiotrophoblast, where they fuse and lose their cell membranes
- The syncytiotrophoblast, a rapidly expanding, multinucleated mass in which no cell boundaries are discernible

The erosive **syncytiotrophoblast** invades the endometrial connective tissue, and the blastocyst slowly embeds itself in the endometrium. Syncytiotrophoblastic cells displace endometrial cells at the implantation site. The endometrial cells undergo **apoptosis** (programmed cell death), which facilitates the invasion. The molecular mechanisms of implantation involve synchronization between the invading blastocyst and a receptive endometrium. The microvilli of endometrial cells (pinopodes), cell adhesion molecules, cytokines, prostaglandins, homeobox genes, growth factors, and matrix metalloproteins play a role in making the endometrium receptive. The connective tissue cells around the implantation site accumulate glycogen and lipids and assume a polyhedral appearance. Some of these cells—**decidual cells**—degenerate adjacent to the penetrating syncytiotrophoblast. The syncytiotrophoblast engulfs these degenerating cells, providing a rich source of embryonic nutrition.

The syncytiotrophoblast produces a hormone—*human chorionic gonadotrophin* (hCG), which enters the maternal blood via lacunae (Latin, hollow cavities) in the syncytiotrophoblast (see Fig. 3-1*C*). hCG maintains the hormonal activity of the corpus luteum in the ovary during preg-

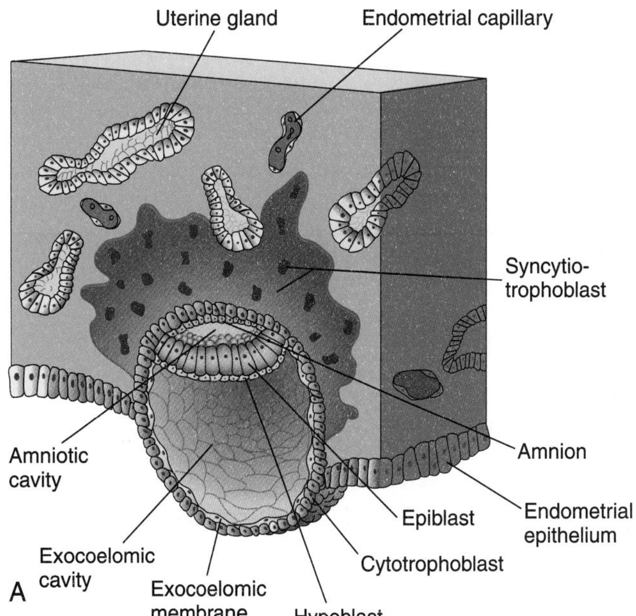

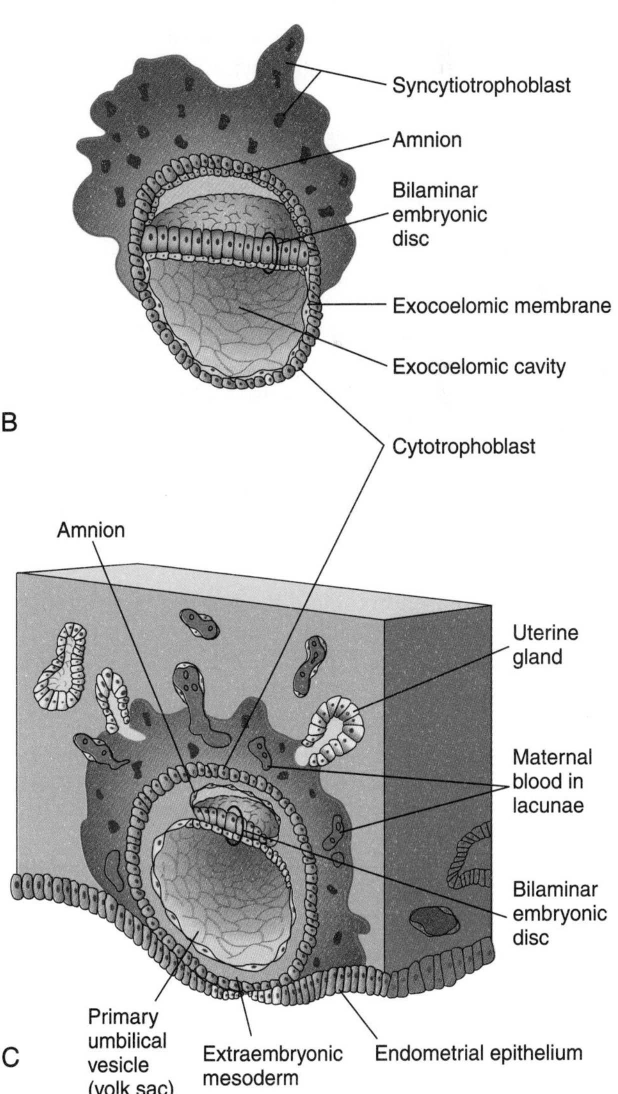

FIGURE 3-1. Implantation of a blastocyst in the endometrium. The actual size of the conceptus is 0.1 mm, approximately the size of the period at the end of this sentence. **A,** Drawing of a section through a blastocyst partially implanted in the endometrium (approximately 8 days). Note the slitlike amniotic cavity. **B,** An enlarged three-dimensional sketch of a slightly older blastocyst after removal from the endometrium. Note the extensive syncytiotrophoblast at the embryonic pole (side of the blastocyst containing the embryonic disc). **C,** Drawing of a section through a blastocyst of approximately 9 days implanted in the endometrium. Note the lacunae appearing in the syncytiotrophoblast. The term *yolk sac* is a misnomer because it contains no yolk.

nancy. The corpus luteum is an endocrine glandular structure that secretes estrogen and progesterone to maintain the pregnancy. Highly sensitive radioimmunoassays are available for detecting hCG and pregnancy and forms the basis for *pregnancy tests*. Enough hCG is produced by the syncytiotrophoblast at the end of the second week to give a positive pregnancy test, even though the woman is probably unaware that she is pregnant.

FORMATION OF THE AMNIOTIC CAVITY, EMBRYONIC DISC, AND UMBILICAL VESICLE

As implantation of the blastocyst progresses, a small space appears in the embryoblast. This space is the primordium of the **amniotic cavity** (see Fig. 3-1*A*). Soon amniogenic (amnion-forming) cells—*amnioblasts*—separate from the epiblast and form the **amnion**, which encloses the amniotic cavity (see Fig. 3-1*B* and *C*). Concurrently, morphologic changes occur in the embryoblast that result in the formation of a flat, almost circular bilaminar plate of cells, the **embryonic disc**, consisting of two layers (Fig. 3-2*A*):

- **Epiblast,** the thicker layer, consisting of high columnar cells related to the amniotic cavity
- **Hypoblast,** consisting of small cuboidal cells adjacent to the exocoelomic cavity

The epiblast forms the floor of the amniotic cavity and is continuous peripherally with the amnion. The hypoblast forms the roof of the **exocoelomic cavity** and is continuous with the thin exocoelomic **membrane** (see Fig. 3-1*B*). This membrane, together with the hypoblast, lines the **primary umbilical vesicle**. The embryonic disc now lies between the amniotic cavity and the umbilical vesicle (see Fig. 3-1*C*). Cells from the vesicle endoderm form a layer of connective tissue, the **extraembryonic mesoderm** (see Fig. 3-2*A*), which surrounds the amnion and umbilical vesicle. This mesoderm continues to form from cells that arise from the primitive streak (see Fig. 4-3). The umbilical vesicle and amniotic cavities make morphogenetic movements of the cells of the embryonic disc possible.

As the amnion, embryonic disc, and primary umbilical vesicle form, isolated cavities— **lacunae**—appear in the syncytiotrophoblast (see Figs. 3-1*C* and 3-2). The lacunae soon become filled with a mixture of maternal blood from ruptured endometrial capillaries and cellular debris from eroded uterine glands. The fluid in the lacunar spaces—*embryotroph* (Greek, *trophe*, nourishment)—passes to the embryonic disc by diffusion and provides nutritive material to the embryo.

The communication of the eroded endometrial capillaries with the lacunae establishes the **primordial uteroplacental circulation**. When maternal blood flows into the lacunae, oxygen and nutritive substances are available to the embryo. *Oxygenated blood* passes into the lacunae from the *spiral endometrial arteries*, and *poorly oxygenated blood* is removed from them through the endometrial veins.

The 10-day human conceptus (embryo and extraembryonic membranes) is completely embedded in the endometrium (see Fig. 3-2*A*). For approximately 2 days, there is a defect in the endometrial epithelium that is filled by a **closing plug**, a fibrinous coagulum of blood. By day 12, an almost completely regenerated uterine epithelium covers the closing plug (see Fig. 3-2*B*). As the conceptus implants, the endometrial connective tissue cells undergo a transformation, the **decidual reaction**. After the cells swell because of the accumulation of glycogen and lipid in their cytoplasm, they are known as **decidual cells**. The primary function of the decidual reaction is to provide nutrition for the early embryo and an immunologically privileged site for the conceptus.

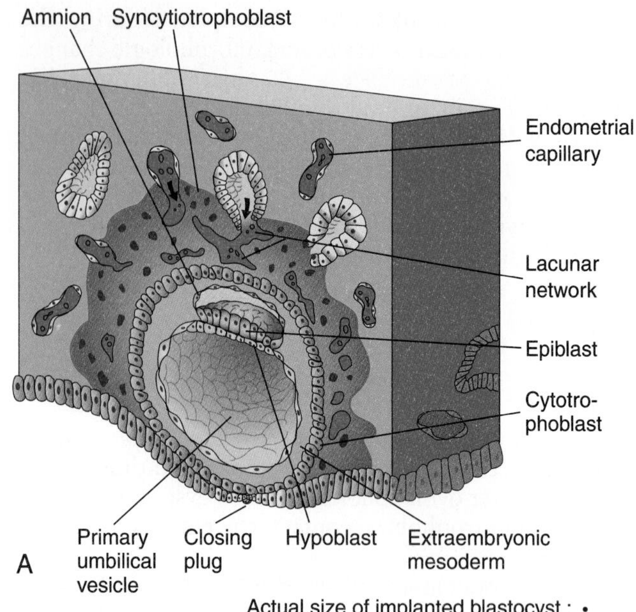

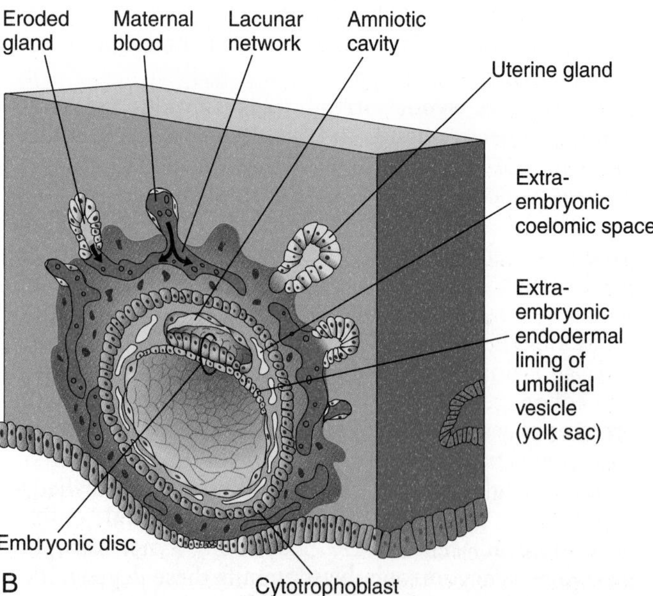

FIGURE 3-2. Implanted blastocysts. **A,** At 10 days; **B,** at 12 days. This stage of development is characterized by communication of the blood-filled lacunar networks. Note in **B** that coelomic spaces have appeared in the extraembryonic mesoderm, forming the beginning of the extraembryonic coelom.

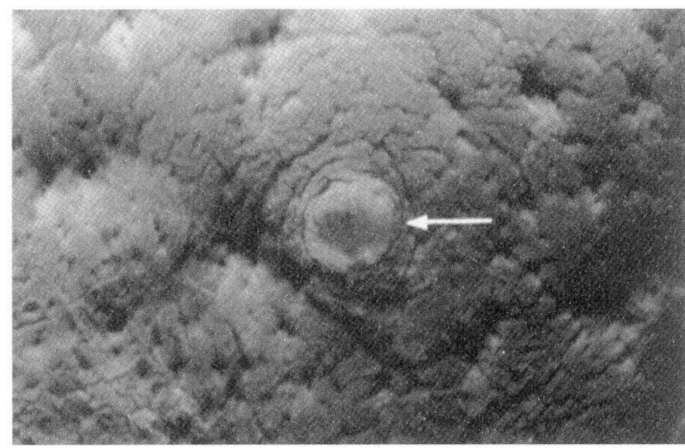

FIGURE 3-3. Photograph of the endometrial surface of the uterus, showing the implantation site of the 12-day embryo shown in Figure 3-4. The implanted conceptus produces a small elevation (*arrow*) (×8). (From Hertig AT, Rock J: Contrib Embryol Carnegie Inst 29:127, 1941. Courtesy of the Carnegie Institution of Washington.)

In a **12-day embryo**, adjacent syncytiotrophoblastic lacunae have fused to form **lacunar networks** (see Fig. 3-2*B*), giving the syncytiotrophoblast a spongelike appearance. The lacunar networks, particularly obvious around the embryonic pole, are the primordia of the intervillous spaces of the placenta (see Chapter 7). The endometrial capillaries around the implanted embryo become congested and dilated to form *sinusoids*, thin-walled terminal vessels that are larger than ordinary capillaries. The syncytiotrophoblast erodes the sinusoids, and maternal blood flows freely into the lacunar networks. The trophoblast absorbs nutritive fluid from the lacunar networks, which is transferred to the embryo. Growth of the bilaminar embryonic disc is slow compared with growth of the trophoblast (see Figs. 3-1 and 3-2). The implanted 12-day embryo produces a minute elevation on the endometrial surface that protrudes into the uterine lumen (Figs. 3-3 and 3-4).

As changes occur in the trophoblast and endometrium, the extraembryonic mesoderm increases and isolated **extraembryonic coelomic spaces** appear within it (see Figs. 3-2 and 3-4). These spaces rapidly fuse to form a large isolated cavity, the **extraembryonic coelom** (Fig. 3-5*A*). This fluid-filled cavity surrounds the amnion and umbilical vesicle, except where they are attached to the **chorion** by the **connecting stalk**. As the extraembryonic coelom forms, the primary umbilical vesicle decreases in size and a smaller **secondary umbilical vesicle** forms (see Fig. 3-5*B*). This smaller vesicle is formed by extraembryonic endodermal cells that migrate from the hypoblast inside the primary umbilical vesicle (Fig. 3-6). During formation of the secondary umbilical vesicle, a large part of the primary umbilical vesicle is pinched off (see Fig. 3-5*B*). *The umbilical vesicle contains no yolk*; however, it has important functions (e.g., it is the *site of origin of primordial germ cells* [see Chapter 12]). It may have a role in the selective transfer of nutrients to the embryo.

DEVELOPMENT OF THE CHORIONIC SAC

The end of the second week is characterized by the appearance of **primary chorionic villi** (Figs. 3-5 and 3-7). Proliferation of cytotrophoblastic cells produces cellular extensions that grow into the syncytiotrophoblast. The growth of these extensions is thought to be induced by the underlying **extraembryonic somatic mesoderm**. The cellular projections form primary chorionic villi, the first stage in the development of the chorionic villi of the placenta.

The extraembryonic coelom splits the extraembryonic mesoderm into two layers (see Fig. 3-5*A* and *B*):

- **Extraembryonic somatic mesoderm**, lining the trophoblast and covering the amnion
- **Extraembryonic splanchnic mesoderm**, surrounding the umbilical vesicle

The extraembryonic somatic mesoderm and the two layers of trophoblast form the **chorion** (see Fig. 3-7*B*). The *chorion forms the wall of the chorionic sac*, within which the embryo and its amniotic sac and umbilical vesicle are suspended by the connecting stalk. The extraembryonic coelom is now called the chorionic cavity. The amniotic sac and the umbilical vesicle can be thought of as two balloons pressed together (at the site of embryonic disc) and suspended by a cord (connecting stalk) from the inside of a larger balloon (chorionic sac). *Transvaginal ultrasonography* (endovaginal sonography) is used for measuring the chorionic (gestational) sac diameter (Fig. 3-8). This measurement is valuable for evaluating early embryonic development and pregnancy outcome.

The **14-day embryo** still has the form of a flat bilaminar embryonic disc (see Fig. 3-9), but the hypoblastic cells in a localized area are now columnar and form a thickened circular area—the **prechordal plate** (see Fig. 3-5*B* and *C*), which indicates the future site of the mouth and an important organizer of the head region.

IMPLANTATION SITES OF BLASTOCYSTS

Implantation of blastocysts usually occurs in the endometrium of the uterus, superior in the body of the uterus, slightly more often on the posterior than on the anterior wall. Implantation of a blastocyst can be detected by ultrasonography and highly sensitive radioimmunoassays of hCG as early as the end of the second week.

EXTRAUTERINE IMPLANTATION

Blastocysts may implant outside the uterus. These implantations result in **ectopic pregnancies**; 95% to 98% of ectopic implantations occur in the uterine tubes, *most often in the ampulla and isthmus* (Figs. 3-10 to 3-12). The incidence of ectopic pregnancy has increased in most countries, ranging from 1 in 80 to 1 in 250 pregnancies, depending on the socioeconomic level of the population. In the United States, the frequency of ectopic pregnancy is approximately 2% of all pregnancies, and it is the main cause of maternal deaths during the first trimester.

A woman with a **tubal pregnancy** has signs and symptoms of pregnancy (e.g., misses her menstrual period). She may also experience abdominal pain

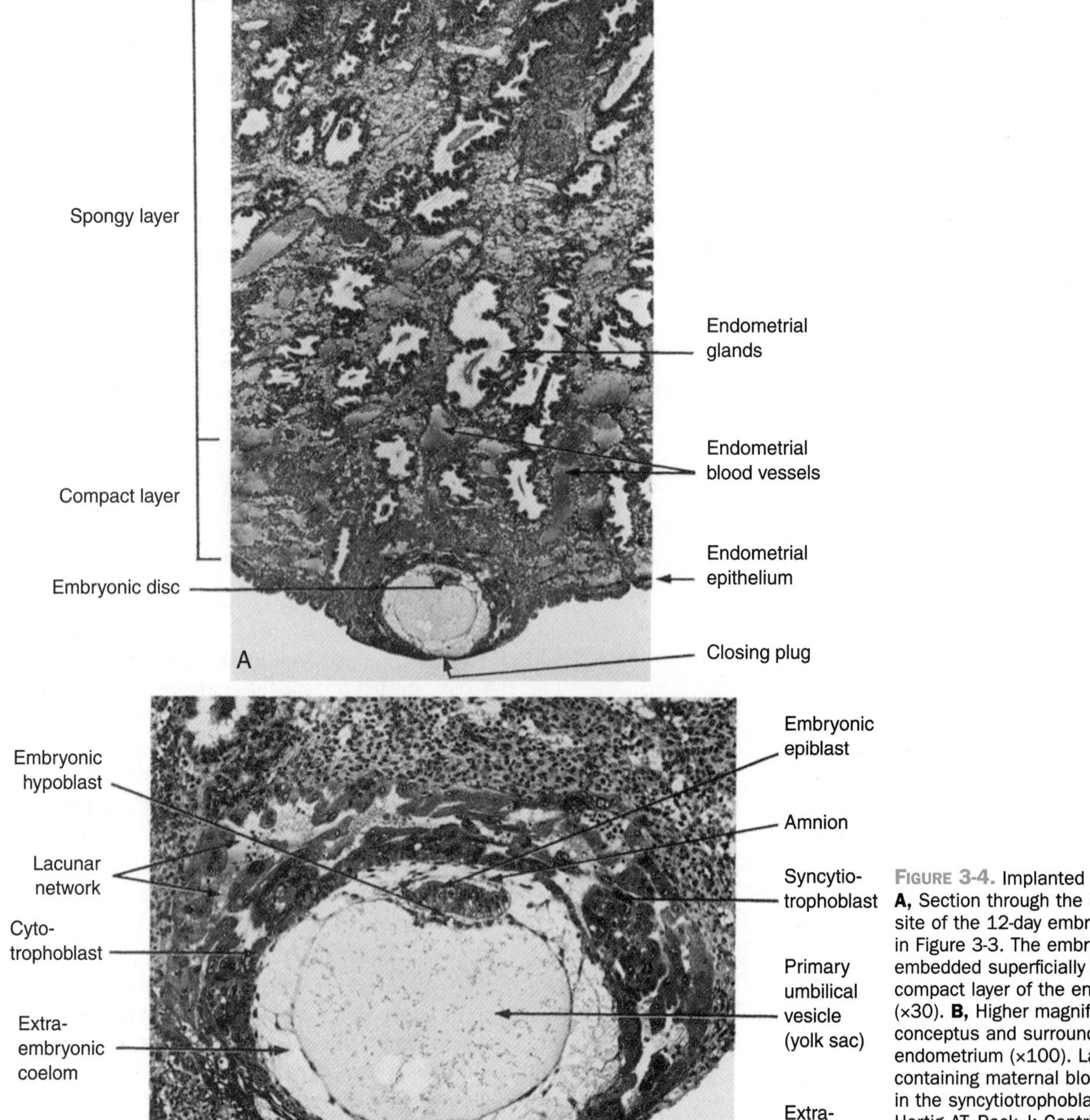

FIGURE 3-4. Implanted blastocyst. **A,** Section through the implantation site of the 12-day embryo described in Figure 3-3. The embryo is embedded superficially in the compact layer of the endometrium (×30). **B,** Higher magnification of the conceptus and surrounding endometrium (×100). Lacunae containing maternal blood are visible in the syncytiotrophoblast. (From Hertig AT, Rock J: Contrib Embryol Carnegie Inst 29:127, 1941. Courtesy of the Carnegie Institution of Washington.)

and tenderness because of distention of the uterine tube, abnormal bleeding, and irritation of the pelvic peritoneum (peritonitis). The pain may be confused with *appendicitis* if the pregnancy is in the right uterine tube. Ectopic pregnancies produce β-human chorionic gonadotropin at a slower rate than normal pregnancies; consequently β-human chorionic gonadotropin assays may give false-negative results if performed too early. *Transvaginal ultrasonography is very helpful in the early detection of ectopic tubal pregnancies.*

There are several causes of tubal pregnancy, but they are often related to factors that delay or prevent transport of the cleaving zygote to the uterus, for example, by mucosal adhesions in the uterine tube or from blockage of it that is caused by scarring resulting from *pelvic inflammatory disease*. Ectopic tubal pregnancies usually result in rupture of the uterine tube and hemorrhage into the peritoneal cavity during the first 8 weeks, followed by death of the embryo. Tubal rupture and hemorrhage constitute a threat to the mother's life. The affected tube and conceptus are usually surgically removed (see Fig. 3-12).

When blastocysts implant in the isthmus of the uterine tube (see Fig. 3-11*D*), the tube tends to

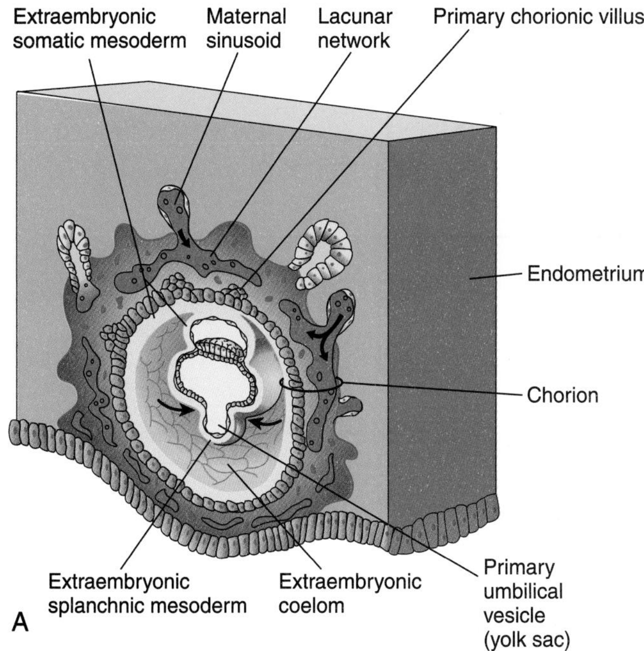

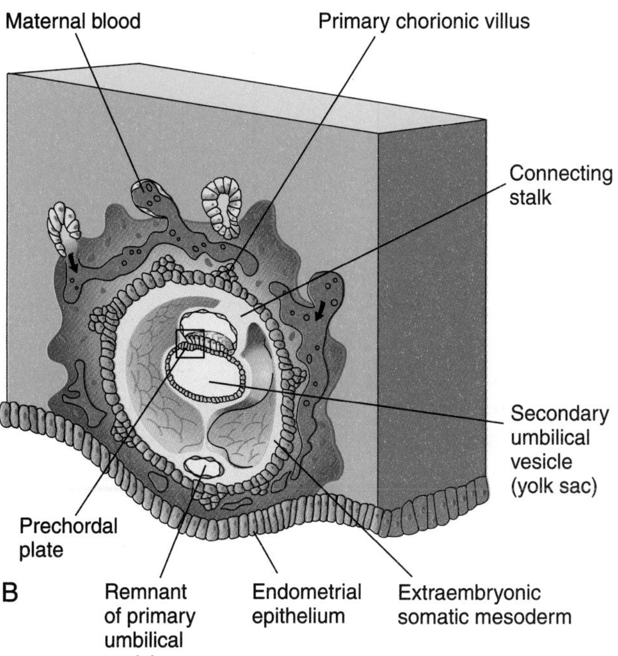

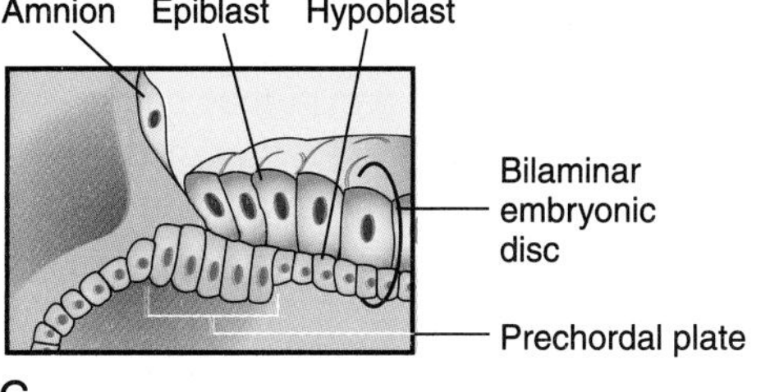

rupture early because this narrow part of the tube is relatively unexpandable, and often with extensive bleeding, probably because of the rich anastomoses between ovarian and uterine vessels in this area. When blastocysts implant in the uterine (intramural) part of the tube (see Fig. 3-11*E*), they may develop beyond 8 weeks before expulsion occurs. When a uterine tubal pregnancy ruptures, it usually bleeds profusely.

Blastocysts that implant in the ampulla or on fimbriae of the uterine tube may be expelled into the peritoneal cavity where they commonly implant in the rectouterine pouch. In exceptional cases, an **abdominal pregnancy** may continue to full term and the fetus may be delivered alive through an abdominal incision. Usually, however, the placenta attaches to abdominal organs (Fig. 3-11G) and causes considerable intraperitoneal bleeding. Abdominal pregnancy increases the risk of maternal death from hemorrhage by a factor of 90 when compared with intrauterine pregnancy, and seven times more than that for tubal pregnancy. In very unusual cases, an abdominal conceptus dies and is not detected; the fetus becomes calcified, forming a "stone fetus"—*lithopedion* (Greek, *lithos*, stone, + *paidion*, child).

Simultaneous intrauterine and extrauterine pregnancies are unusual, occurring approximately 1 in 7000. The ectopic pregnancy is masked initially by the presence of the uterine pregnancy. Usually the ectopic pregnancy can be terminated by surgical removal of the involved uterine tube without interfering with the intrauterine pregnancy (see Fig. 3-12). *Cervical implantations are unusual* (see Fig. 3-11); in some cases, the placenta becomes firmly attached to fibrous and muscular tissues of the cervix, often resulting in bleeding and requiring subsequent surgical intervention, such as *hysterectomy* (excision of uterus).

FIGURE 3-5. Drawings of sections through implanted human embryos, based mainly on Hertig and colleagues (1956). Observe that (1) the defect in the endometrial epithelium has disappeared; (2) a small secondary umbilical vesicle has formed; (3) a large cavity, the extraembryonic coelom, now surrounds the umbilical vesicle and amnion, except where the amnion is attached to the chorion by the connecting stalk; and (4) the extraembryonic coelom splits the extraembryonic mesoderm into two layers: extraembryonic somatic mesoderm lining the trophoblast and covering the amnion and the extraembryonic splanchnic mesoderm around the umbilical vesicle. **A,** At 13 days, illustrating the decrease in relative size of the primary umbilical vesicle and the early appearance of primary chorionic villi. **B,** At 14 days, showing the newly formed secondary umbilical vesicle and the location of the prechordal plate in its roof. **C,** Detail of the prechordal plate outlined in **B**.

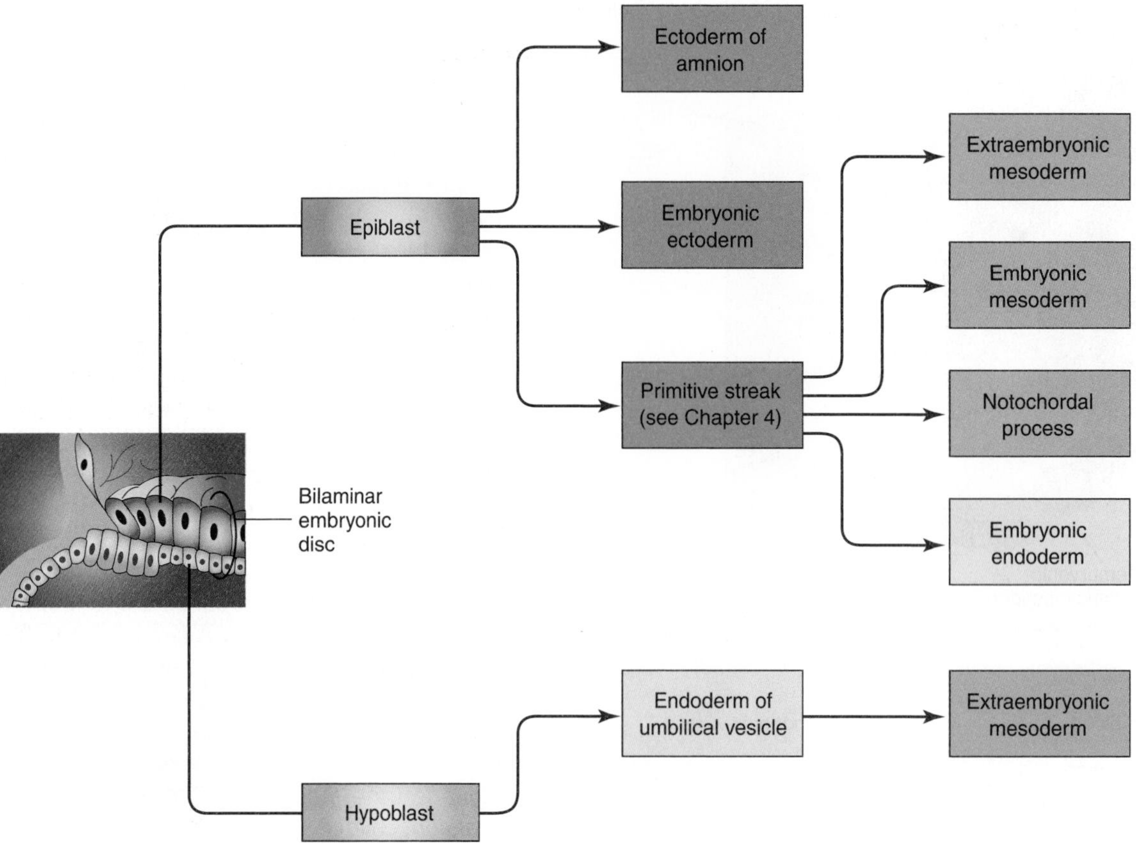

FIGURE 3-6. Origin of embryonic tissues. The colors in the boxes are used in drawings of sections of conceptuses.

SUMMARY OF IMPLANTATION

Implantation of the blastocyst begins at the end of the first week and is completed by the end of the second week. The cellular and molecular events relating to implantation are complex. It involves a receptive endometrium and hormonal factors, such as estrogen, progesterone, prolactin, as well as cell adhesion molecules, growth factors, and HOX genes, Implantation may be summarized as follows:

- The zona pellucida degenerates (*day 5*). Its disappearance results from enlargement of the blastocyst and degeneration caused by enzymatic lysis. The lytic enzymes are released from the acrosomes of the sperms that surround and partially penetrate the zona pellucida.
- The blastocyst adheres to the endometrial epithelium (*day 6*).
- The trophoblast differentiates into two layers: the syncytiotrophoblast and cytotrophoblast (*day 7*).
- The syncytiotrophoblast erodes endometrial tissues, and the blastocyst starts to embed in the endometrium (*day 8*).
- Blood-filled lacunae appear in the syncytiotrophoblast (*day 9*).
- The blastocyst sinks beneath the endometrial epithelium, and the defect is filled by a closing plug (*day 10*).
- Lacunar networks form by fusion of adjacent lacunae (*days 10 and 11*).
- The syncytiotrophoblast erodes endometrial blood vessels, allowing maternal blood to seep in and out of lacunar networks, thereby establishing a uteroplacental circulation (*days 11 and 12*).
- The defect in the endometrial epithelium is repaired (*days 12 and 13*).
- Primary chorionic villi develop (days 13 and 14).

PLACENTA PREVIA

Implantation of a blastocyst in the inferior segment of the uterus near the internal os results in placenta previa, a placenta that partially or completely covers the os (see Fig. 3-11). Placenta previa may cause bleeding because of premature separation of the placenta during pregnancy or at delivery of the fetus (see Chapter 7).

SPONTANEOUS ABORTION OF EMBRYOS

Most spontaneous abortions of embryos occur during the first 3 weeks. *Sporadic and recurrent*

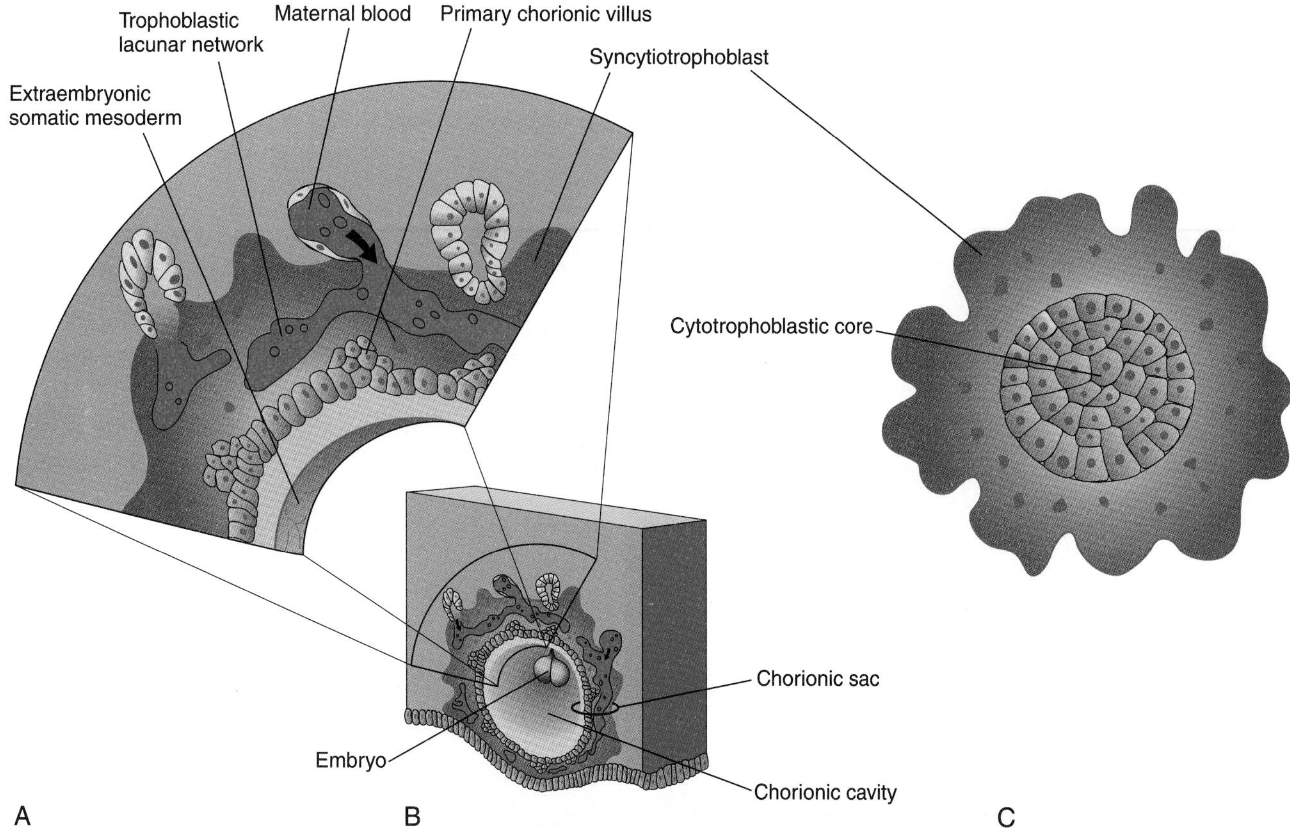

FIGURE 3-7. **A,** Detail of the section (outlined in **B**) of the wall of the chorionic sac. **B,** Sketch of a 14-day conceptus illustrating the chorionic sac and the shaggy appearance of it created by the primary chorionic villi. **C,** Drawing of a transverse section through a primary chorionic villus.

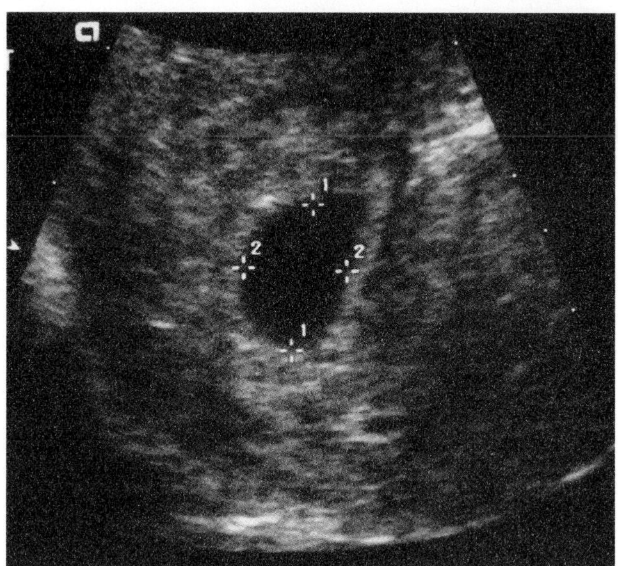

FIGURE 3-8. Endovaginal sonogram of an early chorionic (gestational) sac. The mean gestational sac diameter is determined by adding the three orthogonal dimensions (length, depth, and width) and dividing by 3. (From Laing FC, Frates MC: Ultrasound evaluation during the first trimester of pregnancy. In Callen PW [ed]: Ultrasonography in Obstetrics and Gynecology, 4th ed. Philadelphia, WB Saunders, 2000.)

spontaneous abortions are two of the most common gynecologic problems. The frequency of early abortions is difficult to establish because they often occur before a woman is aware that she is pregnant. An abortion occurring several days after the first missed period is very likely to be mistaken for a delayed menstruation. Detection of a conceptus in the menses (menstrual blood) is very difficult because of its small size.

Study of most early spontaneous abortions resulting from medical problems reveals abnormal conceptuses. More than 50% of all known spontaneous abortions result from chromosomal abnormalities. The higher incidence of early abortions in older women probably results from the increasing frequency of *nondisjunction* during oogenesis (see Chapter 2). It has been estimated that from 30% to 50% of all zygotes never develop into blastocysts and implant. Failure of blastocysts to implant may result from a poorly developed endometrium; however, in many cases, there are probably lethal chromosomal abnormalities in the embryo. There is a higher incidence of spontaneous abortion of fetuses with neural tube defects, cleft lip, and cleft palate.

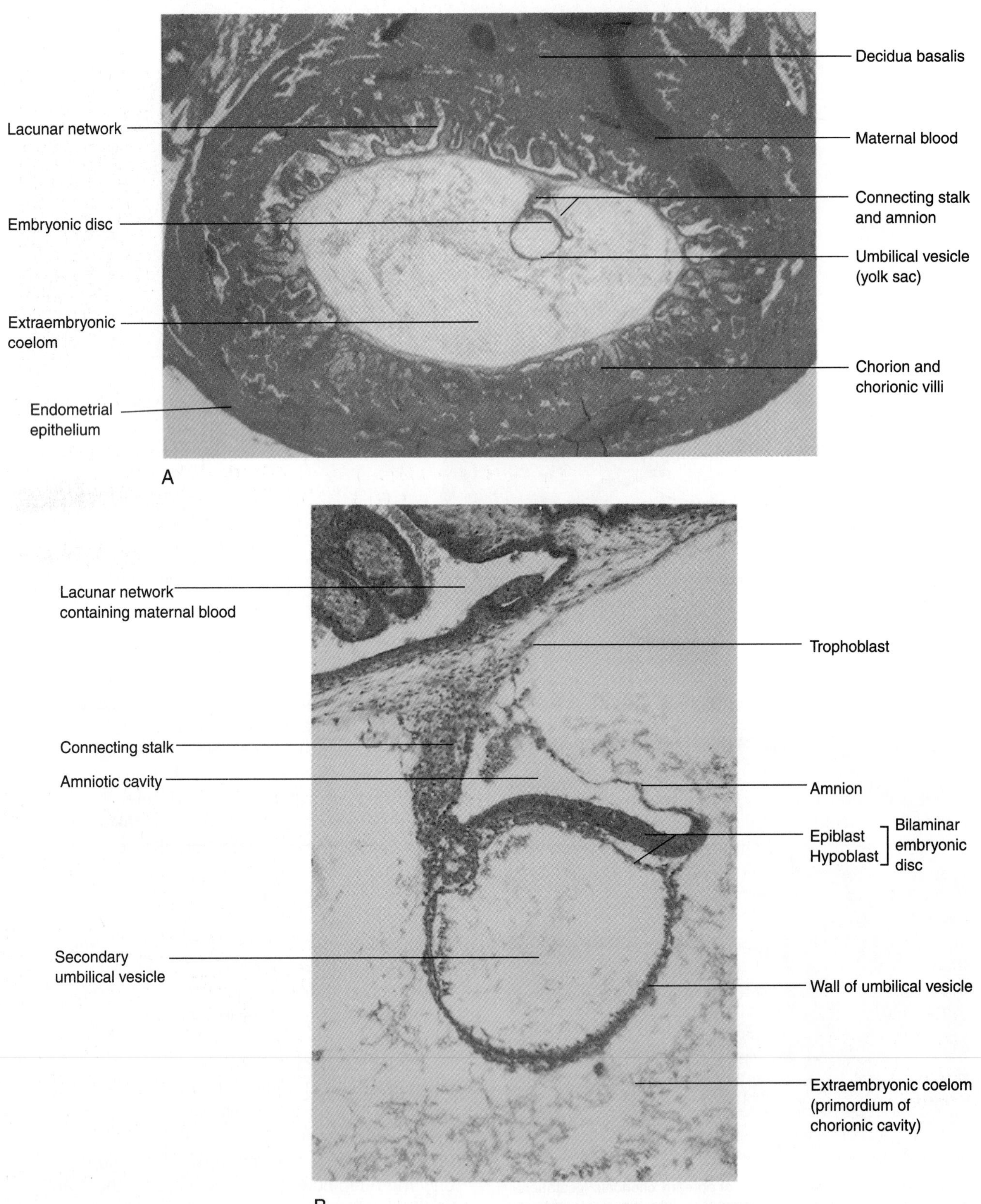

FIGURE 3-9. Photomicrographs of longitudinal sections of an implanted embryo at Carnegie stage 6, approximately 14 days. Note the large size of the extraembryonic coelom. **A,** Low-power view (×18). **B,** High-power view (×95). The embryo is represented by the bilaminar embryonic disc composed of epiblast and hypoblast. (From Nishimura H [ed]: Atlas of Human Prenatal Histology. Tokyo, Igaku-Shoin, 1983.)

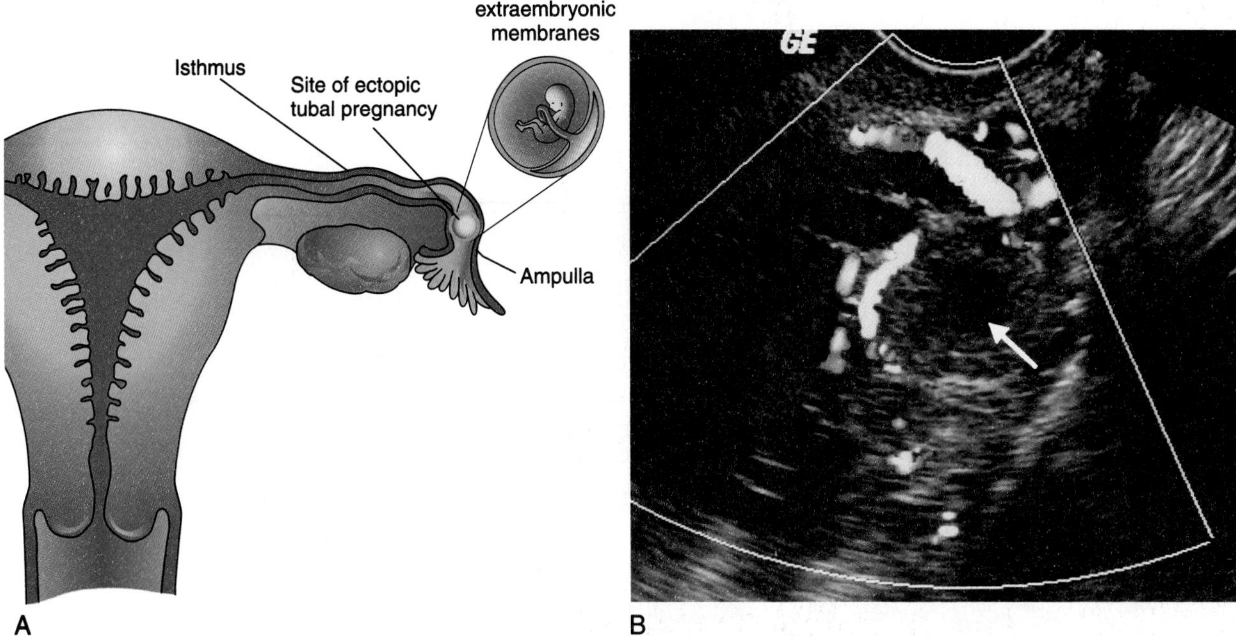

FIGURE 3-10. **A,** Frontal section of the uterus and left uterine tube, illustrating an ectopic pregnancy in the ampulla of the tube. **B,** Ectopic tubal pregnancy. This axial sonogram through the left adnexa (placenta and extraembryonic membranes) of a 6-week pregnant patient shows a small chorionic or gestational sac (*arrow*) in the left uterine tube with prominent vascularity in its periphery. This is characteristic of an ectopic tubal pregnancy. The incidence of tubal pregnancy ranges from 1 in 80 to 1 in 250 pregnancies. Most ectopic implantations (95% to 97%) occur in the uterine tube, usually in the isthmus or ampulla. (Courtesy of E.A. Lyons, MD, Professor of Radiology and Obstetrics and Gynecology, Health Sciences Centre, University of Manitoba, Winnipeg, Manitoba, Canada.)

INHIBITION OF IMPLANTATION

The administration of relatively large doses of progestins and/or estrogens ("morning-after pills") for several days, beginning shortly after unprotected sexual intercourse, usually does not prevent fertilization but often prevents implantation of the blastocyst. A high dose of *diethylstilbestrol*, given daily for 5 to 6 days, may also accelerate passage of the cleaving zygote along the uterine tube. Normally, the endometrium progresses to the secretory phase of the menstrual cycle as the zygote forms, undergoes cleavage, and enters the uterus. The large amount of estrogen disturbs the normal balance between estrogen and progesterone that is necessary for preparation of the endometrium for implantation.

An intrauterine device inserted into the uterus through the vagina and cervix usually interferes with implantation by causing a local inflammatory reaction. Some intrauterine devices contain progesterone that is slowly released and interferes with the development of the endometrium so that implantation does not usually occur.

SUMMARY OF THE SECOND WEEK

- Rapid proliferation and differentiation of the trophoblast occurs as the blastocyst completes its implantation in the endometrium.
- The endometrial changes resulting from the adaptation of these tissues in preparation for implantation are known as the **decidual reaction**.
- Concurrently, the *primary umbilical vesicle* (yolk sac) forms and **extraembryonic mesoderm** develops. The extraembryonic coelom forms from spaces that develop in the extraembryonic mesoderm. The coelom later becomes the **chorionic cavity**.
- The primary umbilical vesicle becomes smaller and gradually disappears as the **secondary umbilical vesicle** develops.
- The **amniotic cavity** appears as a space between the cytotrophoblast and the embryoblast.
- The **embryoblast** differentiates into a **bilaminar embryonic disc** consisting of *epiblast*, related to the amniotic cavity, and *hypoblast*, adjacent to the blastocyst cavity.
- The **prechordal plate** develops as a localized thickening of the hypoblast, which indicates the future

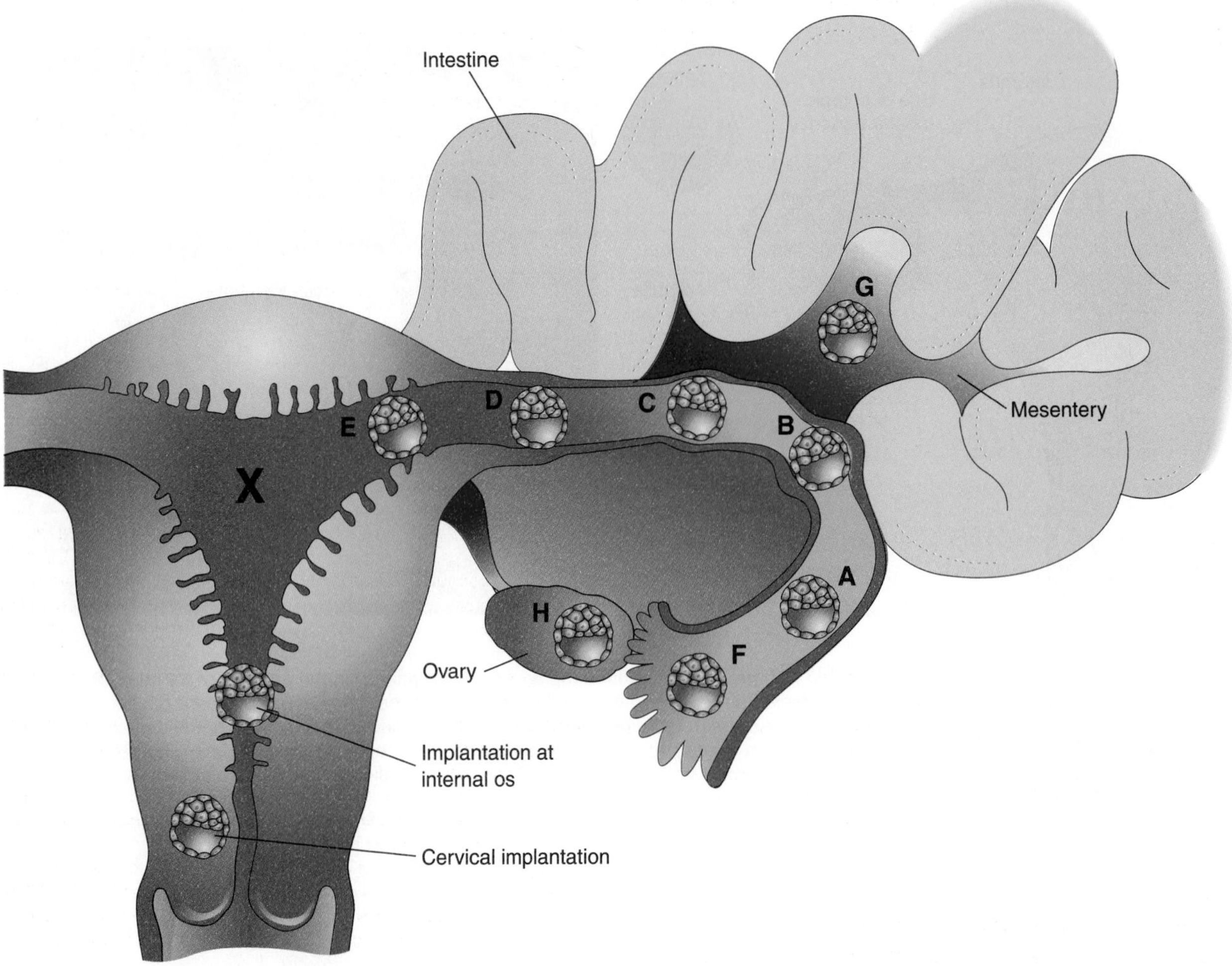

Intestine
G
Mesentery
E
D
C
B
X
A
H
F
Ovary
Implantation at internal os
Cervical implantation

FIGURE 3-11. Implantation sites of blastocysts. The usual site in the posterior wall of the uterus is indicated by an X. The approximate order of frequency of ectopic implantations is indicated alphabetically (A, most common, H, least common). **A** to **F**, tubal pregnancies; **G**, abdominal pregnancy; **H**, ovarian pregnancy. Tubal pregnancies are the most common type of ectopic pregnancy. Although appropriately included with uterine pregnancy sites, a cervical pregnancy is often considered to be an ectopic pregnancy.

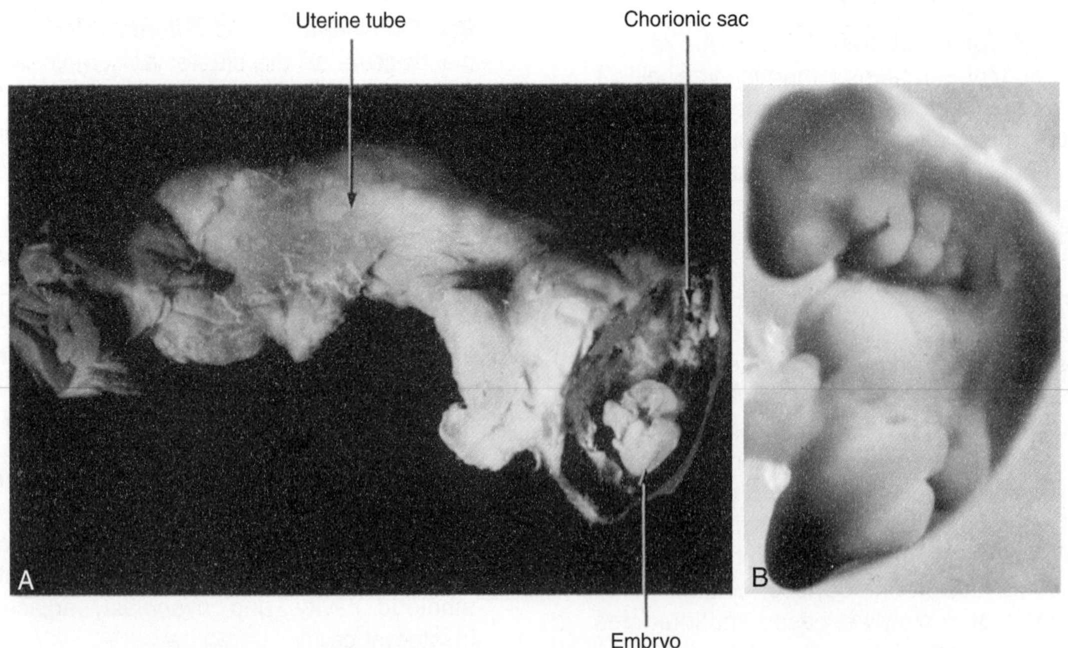

FIGURE 3-12. A tubal pregnancy. **A,** The uterine tube has been surgically removed and sectioned to show the conceptus implanted in the mucous membrane (×3). **B,** Enlarged photograph of the normal-appearing 4-week embryo (×13). (Courtesy of Professor Jean Hay [retired], Department of Anatomy and Cell Science, University of Manitoba, Winnipeg, Manitoba, Canada.)

cranial region of the embryo and the future site of the mouth; the prechordal plate is also an important organizer of the head region.

CLINICALLY ORIENTED PROBLEMS

CASE 3-1

A 22-year-old woman who complained of a severe "chest cold" was sent for a radiograph of her thorax.

- Is it advisable to examine a healthy female's chest radiographically during the last week of her menstrual cycle?
- Are birth defects likely to develop in her conceptus if she happens to be pregnant?

CASE 3-2

A woman who was sexually assaulted during her fertile period was given large doses of estrogen twice for 1 day to interrupt a possible pregnancy.

- If fertilization had occurred, what do you think would be the mechanism of action of this hormone?
- What do lay people call this type of medical treatment? Is this what the media refer to as the "abortion pill?" If not, explain the method of action of the hormone treatment.
- How early can a pregnancy be detected?

CASE 3-3

A 23-year-old woman consulted her physician about severe right lower abdominal pain. She said that she had missed two menstrual periods. A diagnosis of ectopic pregnancy was made.

- What techniques might be used to enable this diagnosis to be made?
- What is the most likely site of the extrauterine gestation?
- How do you think the physician would likely treat the condition?

CASE 3-4

A 30-year-old woman had an appendectomy toward the end of her menstrual cycle; 8½ months later, she had a child with a congenital anomaly of the brain.

- Could the surgery have produced this child's congenital anomaly?
- What is the basis for your views?

CASE 3-5

A 42-year-old woman finally became pregnant after many years of trying to conceive. She was concerned about the development of her baby.

- What would the physician likely tell her?
- Can women over 40 have normal babies?
- What tests and diagnostic techniques would likely be performed?

Discussion of these problems appears at the back of the book.

References and Suggested Reading

Attar E: Endocrinology of ectopic pregnancy. Obstet Gynecol Clin N Am 31:779, 2004.

Bianchi DW, Wilkins-Haug LE, Enders AC, Hay ED: Origin of extraembryonic mesoderm in experimental animals: relevance to chorionic mosaicism in humans. Am J Med Genet 46:542, 1993.

Bukulmez O, Arici A: Luteal phase defect: Myth or reality. Obstet Gynecol Clin N Am 31:727. 2004.

Cadkin AV, McAlpin J: The decidua-chorionic sac: A reliable sonographic indicator of intrauterine pregnancy prior to detection of a fetal pole. J Ultrasound Med 3:539, 1984.

Coulam CB, Faulk WP, McIntyre JA: Spontaneous and recurrent abortions. In Quilligan EJ, Zuspan FP (eds): Current Therapy in Obstetrics and Gynecology, Vol 3. Philadelphia, WB Saunders, 1990.

Dickey RP, Gasser R, Olar TT, et al: Relationship of initial chorionic sac diameter to abortion and abortus karyotype based on new growth curves for the 16 to 49 post-ovulation day. Hum Reprod 9:559, 1994.

Enders AC, King BF: Formation and differentiation of extraembryonic mesoderm in the rhesus monkey. Am J Anat 181:327, 1988.

Hertig AT, Rock J: Two human ova of the pre-villous stage, having a development age of about seven and nine days respectively. Contrib Embryol Carnegie Inst 31:65, 1945.

Hertig AT, Rock J: Two human ova of the pre-villous stage, having a developmental age of about eight and nine days, respectively. Contrib Embryol Carnegie Inst 33:169, 1949.

Hertig AT, Rock J, Adams EC: A description of 34 human ova within the first seventeen days of development. Am J Anat 98:435, 1956.

Hertig AT, Rock J, Adams EC, Menkin MC: Thirty-four fertilized human ova, good, bad, and indifferent, recovered from 210 women of known fertility. Pediatrics 23:202, 1959.

Kodaman PH, Taylor HS: Hormonal regulation of implantation. Obstet Gynecol Clin N Am 31:745, 2004.

Lessey BA: The role of the endometrium during embryo implantation. Human Reprod 15(Suppl 6):39, 2000.

Levine D: Ectopic pregnancy. In Callen PW (ed): Ultrasonography in Obstetrics and Gynecology, 4th ed. Philadelphia, WB Saunders, 2000.

Lindsay DJ, Lovett IS, Lyons EA, et al: Endovaginal sonography: Yolk sac diameter and shape as a predictor of pregnancy outcome in the first trimester. Radiology 183:115, 1992.

Lipscomb GH: Ectopic pregnancy. In Copeland LJ, Jarrell JF (eds): Textbook of Gynecology, 4th ed. Philadelphia, WB Saunders, 2000.

Luckett WP: The origin of extraembryonic mesoderm in the early human and rhesus monkey embryos. Anat Rec 169:369, 1971.

Luckett WP: Origin and differentiation of the yolk sac and extraembryonic mesoderm in presomite human and rhesus monkey embryos. Am J Anat 152:59, 1978.

Nogales FF (ed): The Human Yolk Sac and Yolk Sac Tumors. New York, Springer-Verlag, 1993.

Sen C, Yayla M: Chromosomal abnormalities of the embryo. In Kurjak A, Chervenak FA, Carrera JM (eds): The Embryo as a Patient. New York, Parthenon Publishing Group, 2001.

Streeter GL: Developmental horizons in human embryos. Description of age group XI, 13 to 20 somites, and age group XII, 21 to 29 somites. Contrib Embryol Carnegie Inst 30:211, 1942.

4

Formation of Germ Layers and Early Tissue and Organ Differentiation: Third Week

Gastrulation: Formation of Germ Layers 55

Primitive Streak 57

Fate of the Primitive Streak 57

Notochordal Process and Notochord 59

The Allantois 62

Neurulation: Formation of the Neural Tube 62

Neural Plate and Neural Tube 62

Neural Crest Formation 62

Development of Somites 65

Development of the Intraembryonic Coelom 65

Early Development of the Cardiovascular System 65

Vasculogenesis and Angiogenesis 66

The Primordial Cardiovascular System 67

Development of Chorionic Villi 68

Summary of the Third Week 68

Clinically Oriented Problems 70

Rapid development of the embryo from the embryonic disc during the third week is characterized by

- Appearance of primitive streak
- Development of notochord
- Differentiation of three germ layers

The third week of embryonic development coincides with the week following the first missed menstrual period; that is, 5 weeks after the first day of the last normal menstrual period. *Cessation of menstruation is often the first indication that a woman may be pregnant.* Approximately 3 weeks after conception, approximately 5 weeks after the last normal menstrual period (Fig. 4-1), a normal pregnancy can be detected with ultrasonography.

PREGNANCY SYMPTOMS

Frequent symptoms of pregnancy are nausea and vomiting, which may occur by the end of the third week; however, the time of onset of these symptoms varies. Vaginal bleeding at the expected time of menstruation does not rule out pregnancy because there may be a slight loss of blood from the implantation site of the blastocyst. Implantation bleeding results from leakage of blood into the uterine cavity from disrupted lacunar networks in the implanted blastocyst (see Fig. 3-7). When this bleeding is interpreted as menstruation, an error occurs in determining the expected date of confinement and delivery date of the baby.

GASTRULATION: FORMATION OF GERM LAYERS

Gastrulation is the formative process by which the three germ layers, which are precursors of all embryonic tissues, and axial orientation are established in embryos. During gastrulation, the bilaminar embryonic disc is converted into a trilaminar embryonic disc. Extensive cell shape changes, rearrangement, movement, and changes in adhesive properties contribute to the process of gastrulation. Gastrulation is the beginning of **morphogenesis** (development of body form) and is the significant event occurring during the third week. *Bone morphogenetic proteins* and other signaling molecules such as *FGFs* and *Wnts* play an essential role in this process. The first morphologic sign of gastrulation begins with formation of the *primitive streak* on the surface of the epiblast of the embryonic disc (Fig. 4-2*B*). During this period, the embryo may be referred to as a gastrula. Each of the three germ layers (ectoderm, mesoderm, and endoderm) gives rise to specific tissues and organs:

- **Embryonic ectoderm** gives rise to the epidermis, central and peripheral nervous systems, the eye, and inner ear, and, as neural crest cells, to many connective tissues of the head (see Chapter 5).
- **Embryonic endoderm** is the source of the epithelial linings of the respiratory and alimentary (digestive) tracts, including the glands opening into the gastrointestinal tract and the glandular cells of associated organs such as the liver and pancreas.
- **Embryonic mesoderm** gives rise to all skeletal muscles, blood cells and the lining of blood vessels, all visceral smooth muscular coats, the serosal

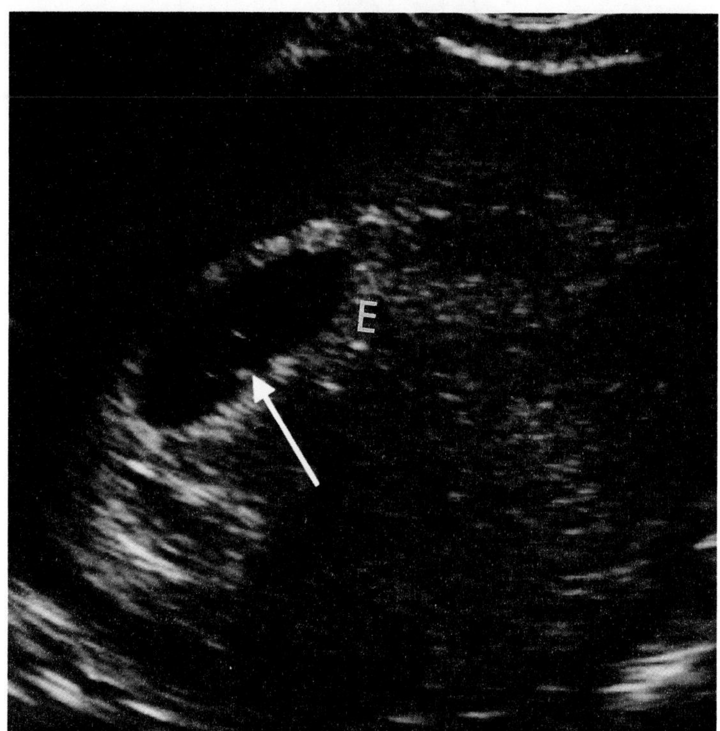

FIGURE 4-1. Ultrasonograph sonogram of a 3.5-week conceptus. Note the surrounding endometrium (E) and secondary umbilical vesicle (yolk sac) (*arrow*). (Courtesy of E.A. Lyons, MD, Professor of Radiology and Obstetrics and Gynecology, Health Sciences Centre, University of Manitoba, Winnipeg, Manitoba, Canada.)

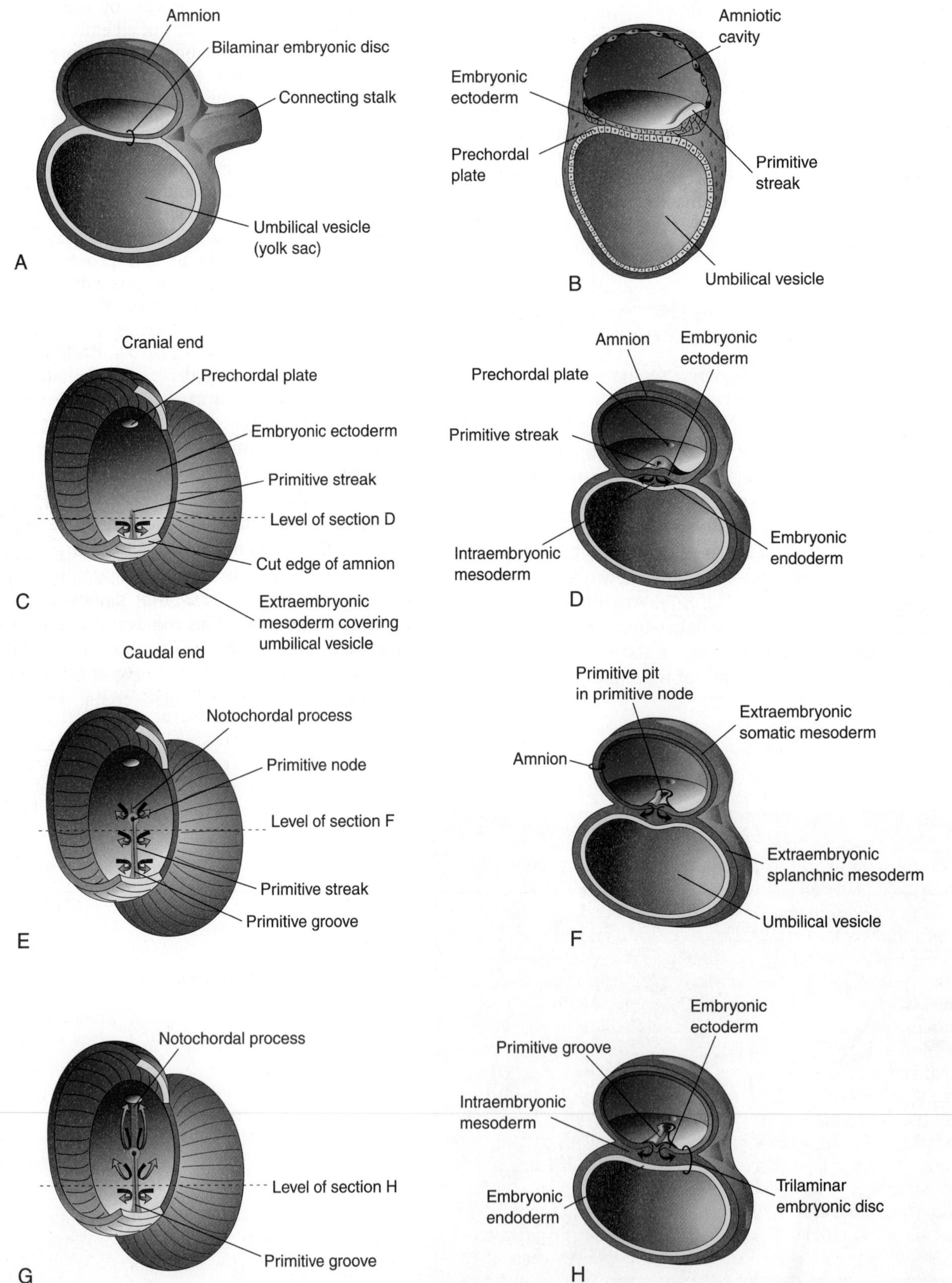

FIGURE 4-2. Illustrations of the formation of the trilaminar embryonic disc (days 15 to 16). The *arrows* indicate invagination and migration of mesenchymal cells from the primitive streak between the ectoderm and endoderm. **C, E,** and **G,** Dorsal views of the embryonic disc early in the third week, exposed by removal of the amnion. **A, B, D, F,** and **H,** Transverse sections through the embryonic disc. The levels of the sections are indicated in **C, E,** and **G.** The prechordal plate, indicating the head region in **C,** is indicated by a light blue oval because this thickening of endoderm cannot be seen from the dorsal surface.

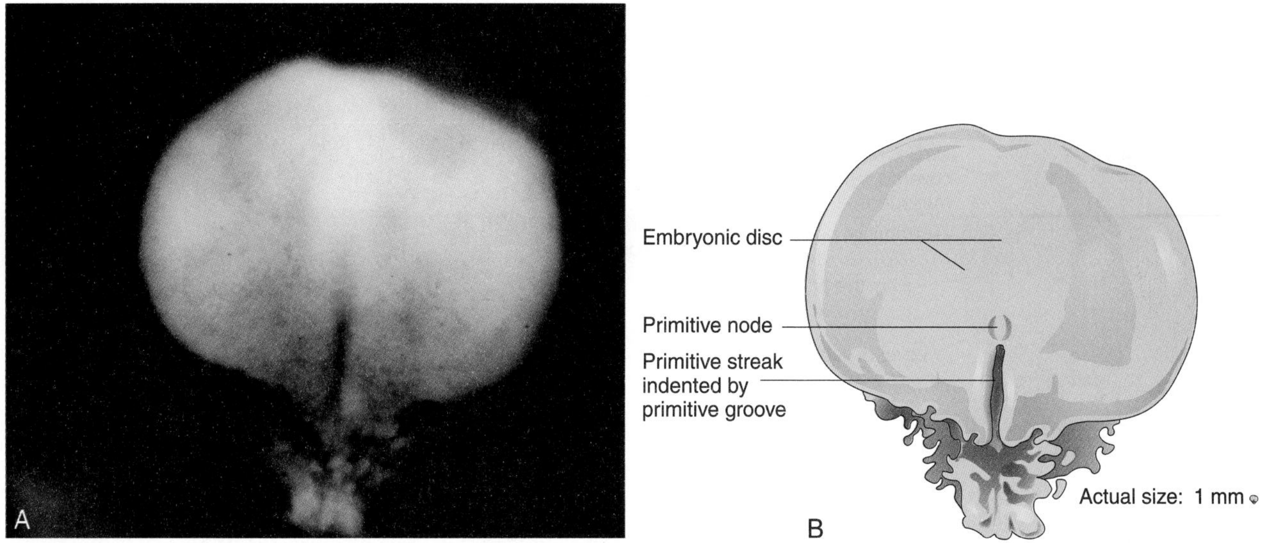

FIGURE 4-3. **A,** Dorsal view of an embryo approximately 16 days old. **B,** Illustration of structures shown in **A**. (**A,** From Moore KL, Persaud TVN, Shiota K: Color Atlas of Clinical Embryology, 2nd ed. Philadelphia, WB Saunders, 2000.)

linings of all body cavities, the ducts and organs of the reproductive and excretory systems, and most of the cardiovascular system. In the trunk, it is the source of all connective tissues, including cartilage, bones, tendons, ligaments, dermis, and stroma of internal organs.

PRIMITIVE STREAK

The first sign of gastrulation is the appearance of the primitive streak (see Fig. 4-2*B*). At the beginning of the third week, an opacity formed by a thickened linear band of epiblast—the **primitive streak**—appears caudally in the median plane of the dorsal aspect of the embryonic disc (Figs. 4-2*C* and 4-3). The primitive streak results from the proliferation and movement of cells of the epiblast to the median plane of the embryonic disc. As the streak elongates by addition of cells to its caudal end, its cranial end proliferates to form a **primitive node** (see Figs. 4-2*F* and 4-3). Concurrently, a narrow groove—**primitive groove**—develops in the primitive streak that is continuous with a small depression in the primitive node—the **primitive pit**. As soon as the primitive streak appears, it is possible to identify the embryo's craniocaudal axis, its cranial and caudal ends, its dorsal and ventral surfaces, and its right and left sides. The primitive groove and pit result from the invagination (inward movement) of epiblastic cells, which is indicated by arrows in Figure 4-2*E*.

Shortly after the primitive streak appears, cells leave its deep surface and form **mesenchyme**, a tissue consisting of loosely arranged cells suspended in a gelatinous matrix. **Mesenchymal cells** are ameboid and actively phagocytic (Fig. 4-4*B*). Mesenchyme forms the supporting tissues of the embryo, such as most of the connective tissues of the body and the connective tissue framework of glands. Some mesenchyme forms **mesoblast** (undifferentiated mesoderm), which forms the intraembryonic, or embryonic, mesoderm (see Fig. 4-2*D*). Cells from the epiblast as well as from the primitive node and other parts of the primitive streak displace the hypoblast, forming the **embryonic endoderm** in the roof of the umbilical vesicle. The cells remaining in the epiblast form the **embryonic ectoderm**. Research data suggest that *signaling molecules* (*nodal factors*) of the *transforming growth factor* β superfamily induce formation of mesoderm. The concerted action of other signaling molecules (e.g., *FGFs*) also participates in specifying germ cell layer fates. Moreover, transforming growth factor β (*nodal*), a *T-box* transcription factor (*veg T*), and the *Wnt* signaling pathway appear to be involved in specification of the endoderm. Mesenchymal cells derived from the primitive streak migrate widely. These pluripotential cells have the potential to proliferate and differentiate into diverse types of cells, such as fibroblasts, chondroblasts, and osteoblasts (see Chapter 5). In summary, cells of the epiblast, through the process of gastrulation, give rise to all three germ layers in the embryo, the primordia of all its tissues and organs.

Fate of the Primitive Streak

The primitive streak actively forms mesoderm by the ingression of cells until the early part of the fourth week; thereafter, production of mesoderm slows down. The primitive streak diminishes in relative size and becomes an insignificant structure in the sacrococcygeal region of the embryo (Fig. 4-5*D*). Normally the primitive streak undergoes degenerative changes and disappears by the end of the fourth week.

SACROCOCCYGEAL TERATOMA

Remnants of the primitive streak may persist and give rise to a **sacrococcygeal teratoma** (Fig. 4-6). Because they are derived from pluripotent primitive

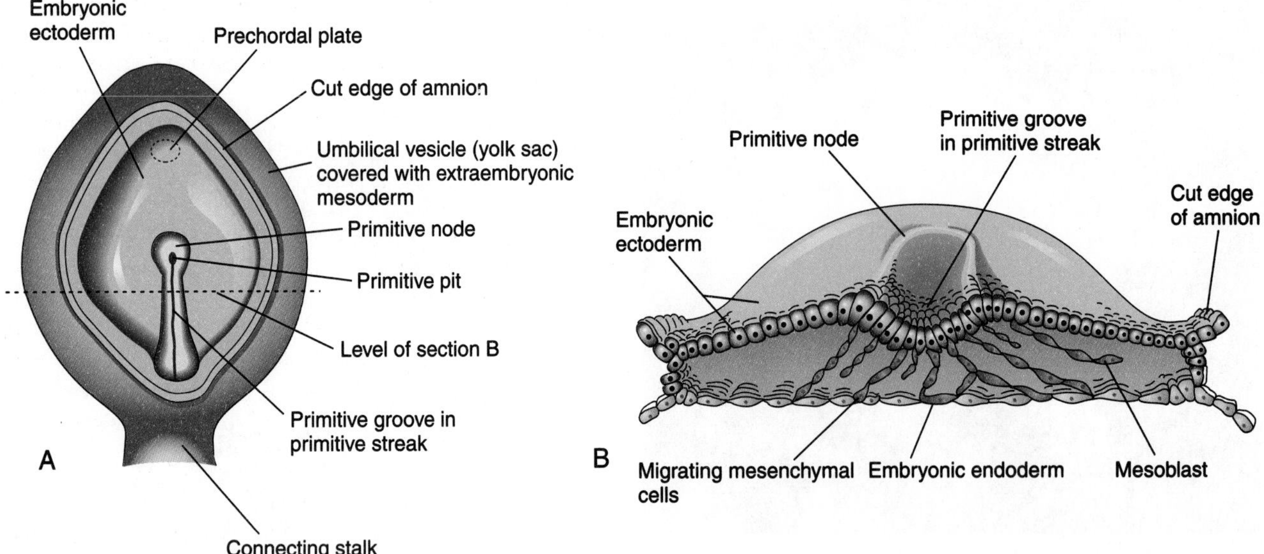

FIGURE 4-4. **A,** Drawing of a dorsal view of a 16-day embryo. The amnion has been removed to expose the embryonic disc. **B,** Drawing of the cranial half of the embryonic disc. The disc has been cut transversely to show the migration of mesenchymal cells from the primitive streak to form mesoblast that soon organizes to form the intraembryonic mesoderm. This illustration also shows that most of the embryonic endoderm also arises from the epiblast. Most of the hypoblastic cells are displaced to extraembryonic regions such as the wall of the umbilical vesicle.

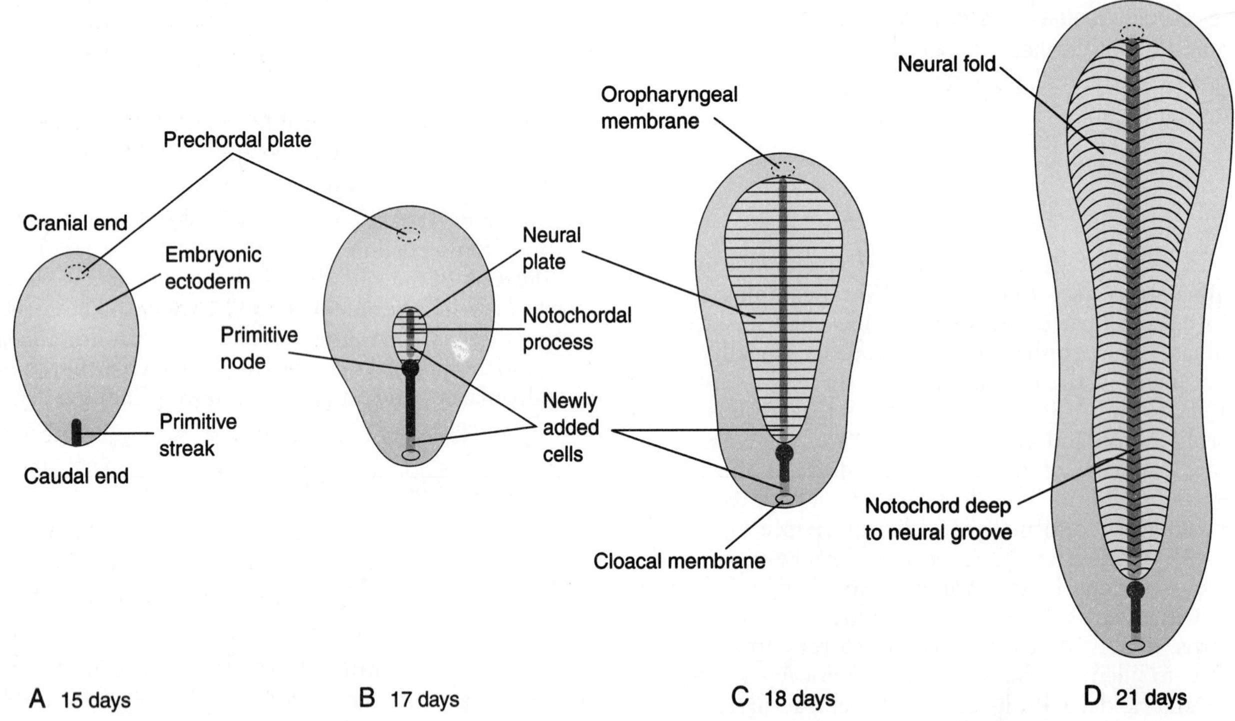

FIGURE 4-5. Diagrammatic sketches of dorsal views of the embryonic disc showing how it lengthens and changes shape during the third week. The primitive streak lengthens by addition of cells at its caudal end, and the notochordal process lengthens by migration of cells from the primitive node. The notochordal process and adjacent mesoderm induce the overlying embryonic ectoderm to form the neural plate, the primordium of the central nervous system. Observe that as the notochordal process elongates, the primitive streak shortens. At the end of the third week, the notochordal process is transformed into the notochord.

streak cells, these tumors contain tissues derived from all three germ layers in incomplete stages of differentiation. Sacrococcygeal teratomas are the most common tumor in newborns and have an incidence of approximately one in 35,000; most affected infants (80%) are female. Sacrococcygeal teratomas are usually diagnosed on routine antenatal ultrasonography, and most tumors are benign. These tumors are usually surgically excised promptly, and the prognosis is good.

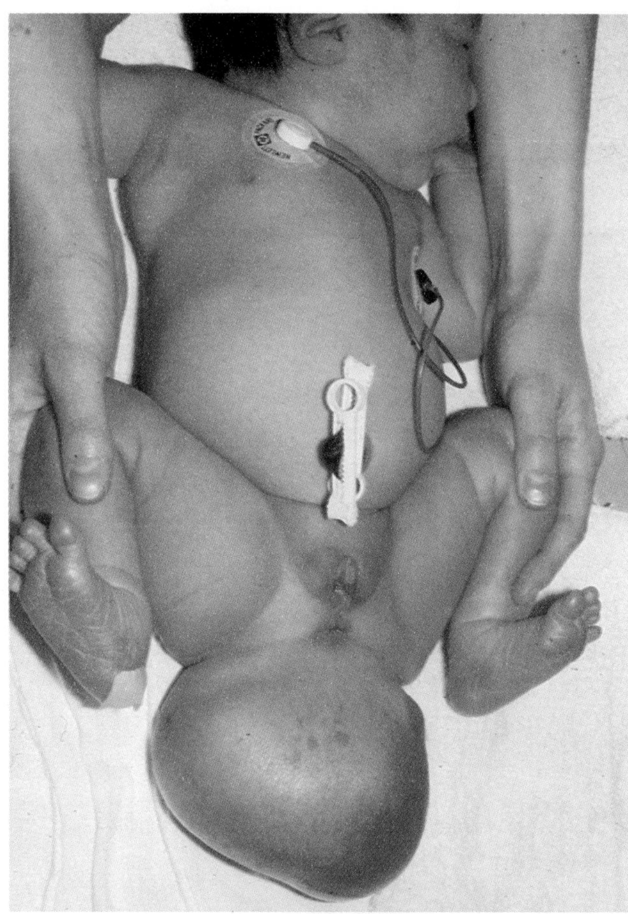

FIGURE 4-6. Female infant with a large sacrococcygeal teratoma that developed from remnants of the primitive streak. The tumor, a neoplasm made up of several different types of tissue, was surgically removed. (Courtesy of A.E. Chudley, MD, Section of Genetics and Metabolism, Department of Pediatrics and Child Health, Children's Hospital and University of Manitoba, Winnipeg, Manitoba, Canada.)

NOTOCHORDAL PROCESS AND NOTOCHORD

Some mesenchymal cells that have ingressed through the streak and, as a consequence, acquired mesodermal cell fates migrate cranially from the primitive node and pit, forming a median cellular cord, the **notochordal process** (Fig. 4-7*C*). This process soon acquires a lumen, the **notochordal canal**. The notochordal process grows cranially between the ectoderm and endoderm until it reaches the **prechordal plate**, a small circular area of columnar endodermal cells where the ectoderm and endoderm are in contact. Prechordal mesoderm is a mesenchymal population rostral to the notochord and essential in forebrain and eye induction. The prechordal plate is the primordium of the **oropharyngeal membrane**, located at the future site of the oral cavity (Fig. 4-8*C*) and may also have a role as a signaling center for controlling development of cranial structures.

Mesenchymal cells from the primitive streak and notochordal process migrate laterally and cranially, among other mesodermal cells, between the ectoderm and endoderm until they reach the margins of the embryonic disc. These cells are continuous with the extraembryonic mesoderm covering the amnion and umbilical vesicle (see Fig. 4-2*C* and *D*). Some mesenchymal cells from the primitive streak that have mesodermal fates migrate cranially on each side of the notochordal process and around the prechordal plate. Here they meet cranially to form cardiogenic mesoderm in the **cardiogenic area** where the **heart primordium** begins to develop at the end of the third week (see Fig. 4-11*B*).

Caudal to the primitive streak there is a circular area—the **cloacal membrane**, which indicates the future site of the anus (see Fig. 4-7*E*). The embryonic disc remains bilaminar here and at the **oropharyngeal membrane** because the embryonic ectoderm and endoderm are fused at these sites, thereby preventing migration of mesenchymal cells between them (see Fig. 4-8*C*). By the middle of the third week, intraembryonic mesoderm separates the ectoderm and endoderm everywhere except

- At the oropharyngeal membrane cranially
- In the median plane cranial to the primitive node, where the notochordal process is located
- At the cloacal membrane caudally

Instructive signals from the primitive streak region induce notochordal precursor cells to form the **notochord**, a cellular rodlike structure. The molecular mechanism that induces these cells involves (at least) Shh signaling from the floor plate of the neural tube. The notochord

- Defines the primordial longitudinal axis of the embryo and gives it some rigidity
- Provides signals that are necessary for the development of axial musculoskeletal structures and the central nervous system
- Contributes to the intervertebral discs

The notochord develops as follows:

- The **notochordal process** elongates by invagination of cells from the primitive pit.
- The primitive pit extends into the notochordal process, forming a **notochordal canal** (see Fig. 4-7*C*).
- The notochordal process is now a cellular tube that extends cranially from the primitive node to the prechordal plate.
- The floor of the notochordal process fuses with the underlying embryonic endoderm (see Fig. 4-7*E*).
- The fused layers gradually undergo degeneration, resulting in the formation of openings in the floor of the notochordal process, which brings the notochordal canal into communication with the umbilical vesicle (see Fig. 4-8*B*).
- The openings rapidly become confluent and the floor of the notochordal canal disappears (see Fig. 4-8*C*); the remains of the notochordal process form a flattened, grooved **notochordal plate** (see Fig. 4-8*D*).
- Beginning at the cranial end of the embryo, the notochordal cells proliferate and the notochordal plate infolds to form the **notochord** (see Fig. 4-8*F* and *G*).
- The proximal part of the notochordal canal persists temporarily as the *neurenteric canal* (see Fig. 4-8*C* and *E*), which forms a transitory communication between the amniotic and umbilical vesicle cavities. When

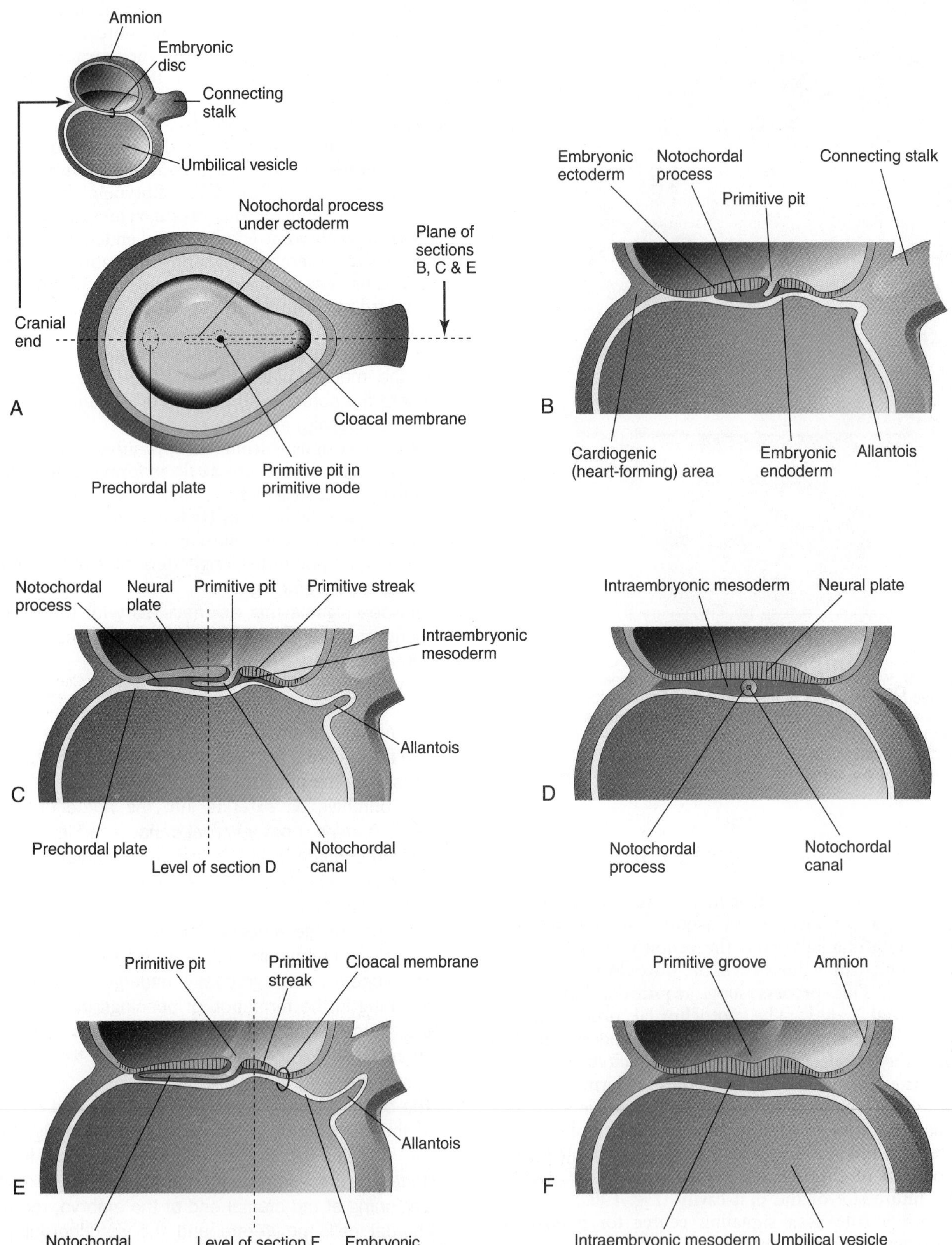

FIGURE 4-7. Illustrations of the development of the notochordal process. The small sketch at the upper left is for orientation. **A,** Dorsal view of the embryonic disc (approximately 16 days) exposed by removal of the amnion. The notochordal process is shown as if it were visible through the embryonic ectoderm. **B, C,** and **E,** Median sections at the plane shown in **A**, illustrating successive stages in the development of the notochordal process and canal. The stages shown in **C** and **E** occur at approximately 18 days. **D** and **F**, Transverse sections through the embryonic disc at the levels shown in **C** and **E**.

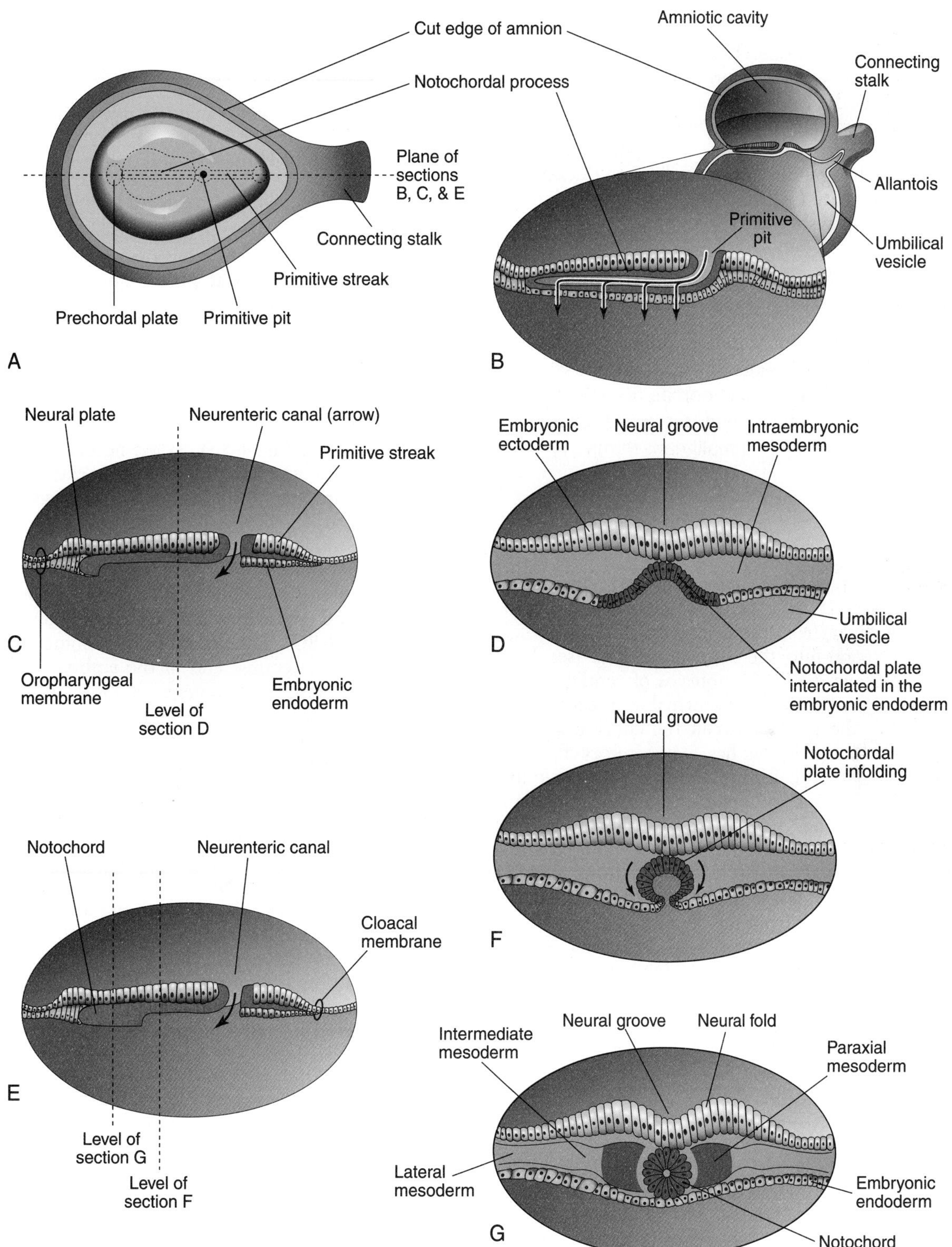

FIGURE 4-8. Illustrations of the further development of the notochord by transformation of the notochordal process. **A,** Dorsal view of the embryonic disc (approximately 18 days), exposed by removing the amnion. **B,** Three-dimensional median section of the embryo. **C** and **E,** Similar sections of slightly older embryos. **D, F,** and **G,** Transverse sections of the trilaminar embryonic disc at the levels shown in **C** and **E**.

development of the notochord is complete, the neurenteric canal normally obliterates.

- The notochord becomes detached from the endoderm of the umbilical vesicle, which again becomes a continuous layer (see Fig. 4-8G).

The notochord extends from the oropharyngeal membrane to the primitive node. The notochord degenerates as the bodies of the vertebrae form, but small portions of it persist as the *nucleus pulposus* of each intervertebral disc.

The notochord functions as the primary inductor (signaling center) in the early embryo. The developing notochord induces the overlying embryonic ectoderm to thicken and form the **neural plate** (see Fig. 4-8*C*), the primordium of the central nervous system (CNS).

REMNANTS OF NOTOCHORDAL TISSUE

Both benign and malignant tumors (**chordomas**) may form from vestigial remnants of notochordal tissue. Approximately one third of chordomas occur at the base of the cranium and extend to the nasopharynx. Chordomas grow slowly and malignant forms infiltrate bone.

THE ALLANTOIS

The allantois (Greek [Gr.] *allas*, sausage) appears on approximately day 16 as a small, sausage-shaped diverticulum (outpouching) from the caudal wall of the umbilical vesicle that extends into the connecting stalk (see Figs. 4-7*B*, *C*, and *E* and 4-8*B*). In embryos of reptiles, birds, and most mammals, this endodermal sac expands to occupy most of the space between the chorion and the amnion. In those species, it has a respiratory function and/or acts as a reservoir for urine during embryonic life. In humans, the allantoic sac remains very small, but allantoic mesoderm expands beneath the chorion and forms blood vessels that will serve the placenta. The proximal part of the original allantoic diverticulum persists throughout much of development as a stalk called the **urachus**, which extends from the bladder to the umbilical region. The urachus is represented in adults by the **median umbilical ligament**. The blood vessels of the allantoic stalk become the umbilical arteries (see Fig. 4-12). The intraembryonic part of the umbilical veins has a separate origin.

ALLANTOIC CYSTS

Allantoic cysts, remnants of the extraembryonic portion of the allantois, are usually found between the fetal umbilical vessels and can be detected by ultrasonography. They are most commonly detected in the proximal part of the umbilical cord, near its attachment to the anterior abdominal wall. The cysts are generally asymptomatic until childhood or adolescence, when they may present with infection and inflammation.

NEURULATION: FORMATION OF THE NEURAL TUBE

The processes involved in the formation of the neural plate and neural folds and closure of the folds to form the neural tube constitute **neurulation.** These processes are completed by the end of the fourth week, when closure of the caudal **neuropore** occurs (see Chapter 5). During neurulation, the embryo may be referred to as a **neurula.**

Neural Plate and Neural Tube

As the notochord develops, it induces the overlying embryonic ectoderm located at or adjacent to the midline to thicken and form an elongated plate of thickened epithelial cells, the **neural plate.** The ectoderm of the neural plate (neuroectoderm) gives rise to the **CNS**—the brain and spinal cord. **Neuroectoderm** also gives rise to various other structures, for example, the retina. At first, the elongated neural plate corresponds in length to the underlying notochord. It appears rostral to the primitive node and dorsal to the notochord and the mesoderm adjacent to it (see Fig. 4-5*B*). As the notochord elongates, the neural plate broadens and eventually extends cranially as far as the oropharyngeal membrane (see Figs. 4-5*C* and 4-8*C*). Eventually the neural plate extends beyond the notochord.

On approximately the 18th day, the neural plate invaginates along its central axis to form a longitudinal median **neural groove**, which has neural folds on each side (see Fig. 4-8*G*). The **neural folds** become particularly prominent at the cranial end of the embryo and are the first signs of brain development. By the end of the third week, the neural folds have begun to move together and fuse, converting the neural plate into a **neural tube**, the primordium of the CNS (Figs. 4-9 and 4-10). The neural tube soon separates from the surface ectoderm as the neural folds meet. Neural crest cells undergo an epithelial to mesenchymal transition and migrate away as the neural folds meet and the free edges of the surface ectoderm (non-neural ectoderm) fuse so that this layer becomes continuous over the neural tube and the back of the embryo (see Fig. 4-10*E* and *F*). Subsequently, the surface ectoderm differentiates into the epidermis. Neurulation is completed during the fourth week. Neural tube formation is a complex cellular and multifactorial process involving a cascade of *molecular mechanisms* and extrinsic factors (see Chapter 17).

Neural Crest Formation

As the neural folds fuse to form the neural tube, some neuroectodermal cells lying along the inner margin of each neural fold lose their epithelial affinities and attachments to neighboring cells (see Fig. 4-10). As the neural tube separates from the surface ectoderm, **neural crest cells** form a flattened irregular mass, the **neural crest**, between the neural tube and the overlying surface ectoderm (see Fig. 4-10*E*). The neural crest soon separates into right and left parts that shift to the dorsolateral

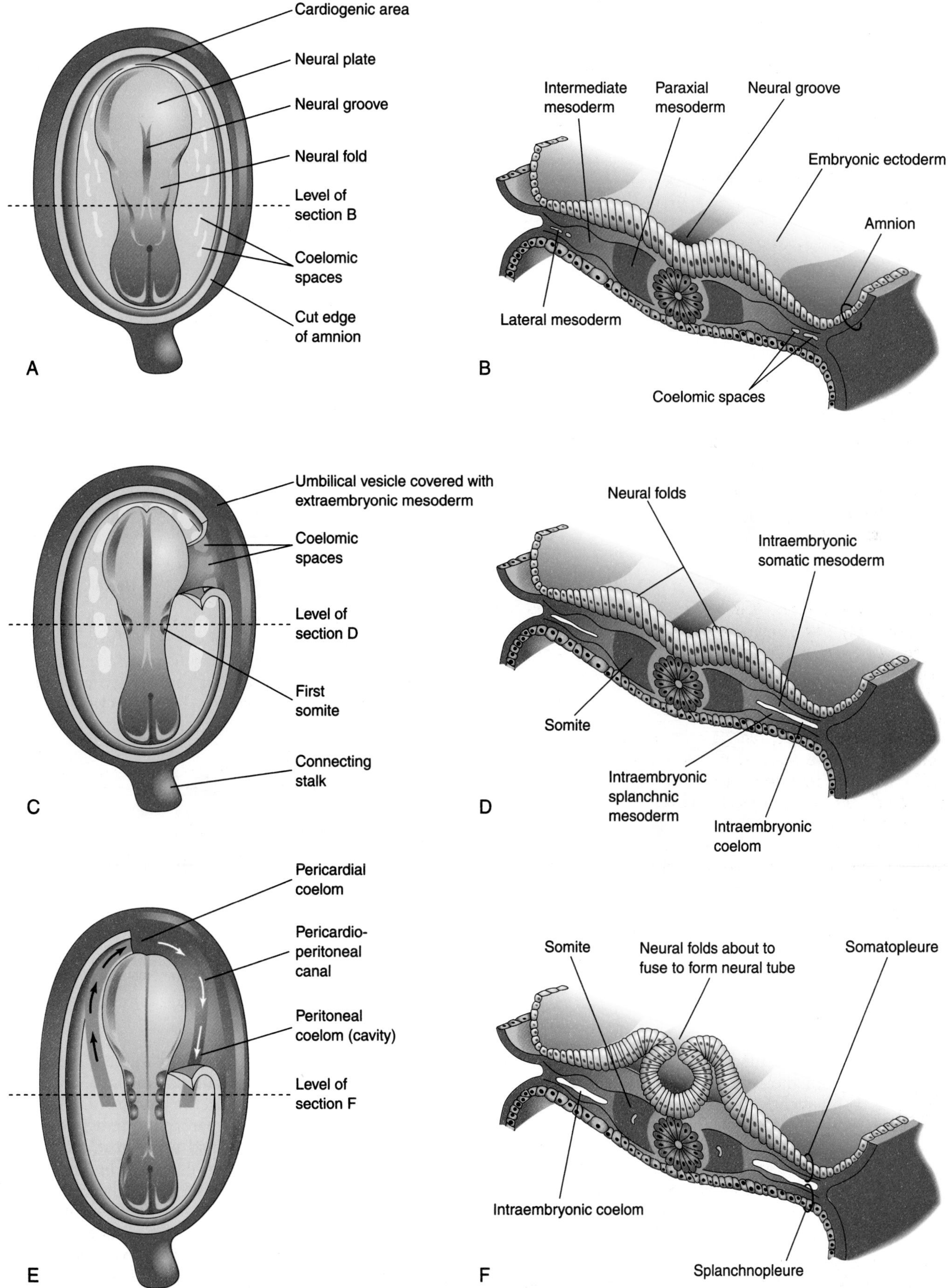

FIGURE 4-9. Drawings of embryos of 19 to 21 days illustrating development of the somites and intraembryonic coelom. **A, C,** and **E,** Dorsal views of the embryo, exposed by removal of the amnion. **B, D,** and **F,** Transverse sections through the embryonic disc at the levels shown. **A,** Presomite embryo of approximately 18 days. **C,** An embryo of approximately 20 days showing the first pair of somites. Part of the somatopleure on the right has been removed to show the coelomic spaces in the lateral mesoderm. **E,** A three-somite embryo (approximately 21 days) showing the horseshoe-shaped intraembryonic coelom, exposed on the right by removal of part of the somatopleure.

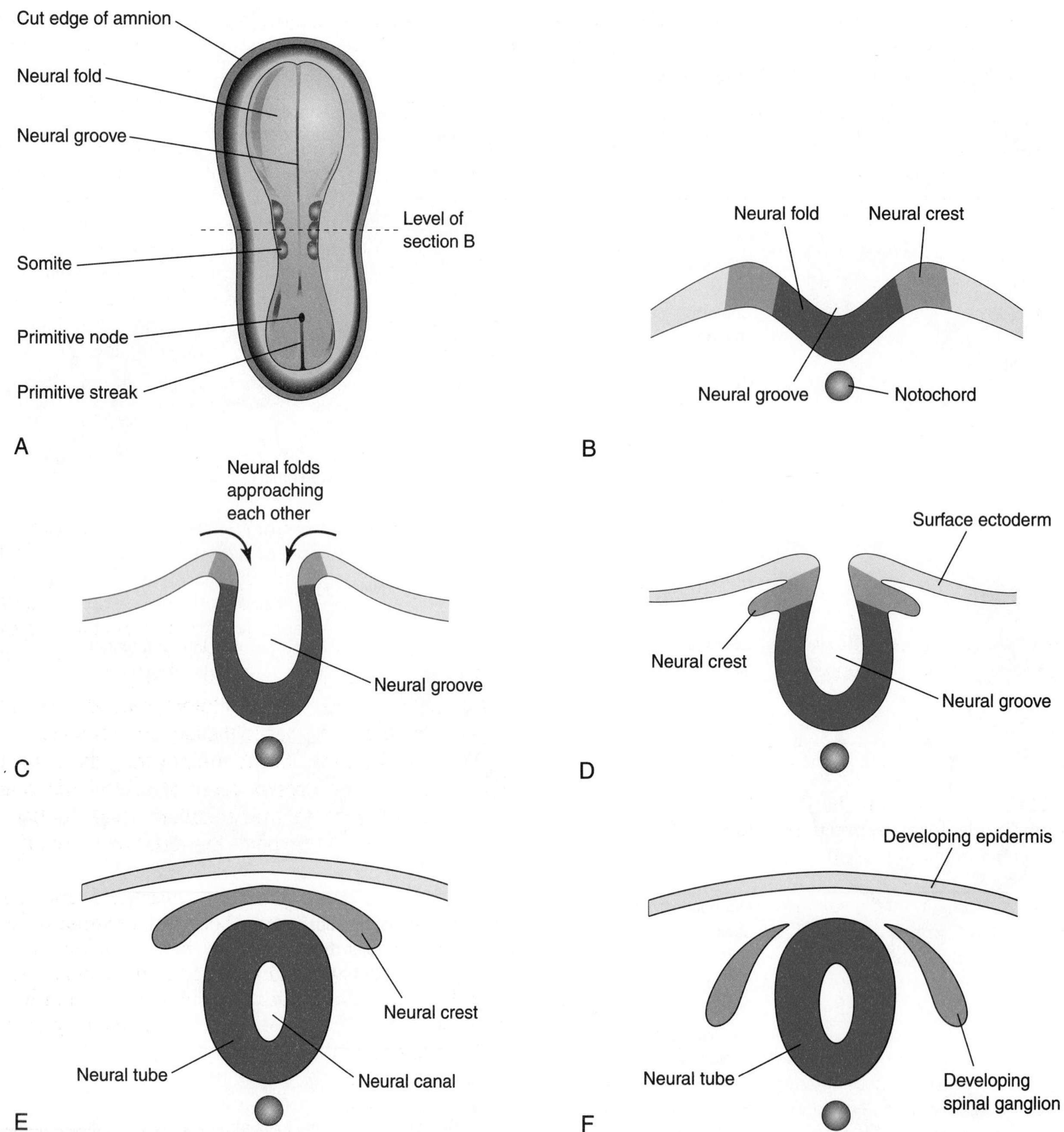

FIGURE 4-10. Diagrammatic transverse sections through progressively older embryos illustrating formation of the neural groove, neural folds, neural tube, and neural crest.

aspects of the neural tube; here they give rise to the sensory ganglia of the spinal and cranial nerves. Neural crest cells subsequently move both into and over the surface of somites. Although these cells are difficult to identify, special tracer techniques have revealed that neural crest cells disseminate widely but usually along predefined pathways. Neural crest cells give rise to the spinal ganglia (dorsal root ganglia) and the ganglia of the autonomic nervous system. The ganglia of cranial nerves V, VII, IX, and X are also partly derived from neural crest cells. In addition to forming ganglion cells, neural crest cells form the neurolemma sheaths of peripheral nerves and contribute to the formation of the leptomeninges (see Chapter 17). **Neural crest cells** also contribute to the formation of pigment cells, the suprarenal (adrenal) medulla, and many connective tissue components in the head (see Chapter 9). Laboratory studies indicate that cell interactions both within the surface epithelium and between it and underlying mesoderm are required to establish the boundaries of the neural plate and specify the sites where *epithelial-mesenchymal transformation* will occur. These are mediated by bone morphogenetic proteins, *Wnt*, *Notch*, and *FGF signaling systems*. Also, molecules such as *ephrins* are important in guiding specific streams of migrating neural crest cells. Many human diseases result from defective migration and/or differentiation of neural crest cells.

Congenital Anomalies Resulting from Abnormal Neurulation

Because the neural plate, the primordium of the CNS, appears during the third week and gives rise to the neural folds and the beginning of the neural tube, disturbance of neurulation may result in severe abnormalities of the brain and spinal cord (see Chapter 17). **Neural tube defects** are among the most common congenital anomalies. Meroencephaly (partial absence of the brain) is the most severe neural tube defect and is also the most common anomaly affecting the CNS. Although the term anencephaly (Gr. *an*, without + *enkephalos*, brain) is commonly used, it is a misnomer because a remnant of the brain is present. Available evidence suggests that the primary disturbance (e.g., a teratogenic drug; see Chapter 20) affects cell fates, cell adhesion, and the mechanism of neural tube closure. This results in failure of the neural folds to fuse and form the neural tube. Neural tube defects may also be secondary to or linked to lesions affecting the degree of flexion imposed on the neural plate during folding of the embryo.

DEVELOPMENT OF SOMITES

In addition to the notochord, cells derived from the primitive node form **paraxial mesoderm**. Close to the node, this population appears as a thick, longitudinal column of cells (see Figs. 4-8*G* and 4-9*B*). Each column is continuous laterally with the **intermediate mesoderm**, which gradually thins into a layer of lateral mesoderm. The **lateral mesoderm** is continuous with the extraembryonic mesoderm covering the umbilical vesicle and amnion. Toward the end of the third week, the **paraxial mesoderm** differentiates, condenses, and begins to divide into paired cuboidal bodies, the **somites** (Gr. *soma*, body), which form in a craniocaudal sequence. These blocks of mesoderm are located on each side of the developing neural tube (see Fig. 4-9*C* to *F*). About 38 pairs of somites form during the *somite period of human development* (days 20 to 30). By the end of the fifth week, 42 to 44 pairs of somites are present. The somites form distinct surface elevations on the embryo and are somewhat triangular in transverse section (see Fig. 4-9*C* to *F*). Because the somites are so prominent during the fourth and fifth weeks, they are used as one of several criteria for determining an embryo's age (see Chapter 5, Table 5-1).

Somites first appear in the future occipital region of the embryo. They soon develop craniocaudally and give rise to most of the *axial skeleton* and associated musculature as well as to the adjacent dermis of the skin. The first pair of somites appears at the end of the third week (see Fig. 4-9*C*) a short distance caudal to the site at which the otic placode forms. Subsequent pairs form in a craniocaudal sequence. Cranial somites are the oldest and caudal somites are the youngest. The ordered progression of segmentation involves a clock mechanism (oscillator) of gene expression, in particular Notch. Also, motor axons from the spinal cord innervate muscle cells in the somites, a process that requires the correct guidance of axons from the spinal cord to the appropriate target cells.

Experimental studies indicate that formation of somites from the paraxial mesoderm involves the expression of *Notch pathway genes* (Notch signaling), *Hox genes*, and other signaling factors. Moreover, *somite formation from paraxial mesoderm is preceded by expression of the forkhead transcription factors Fox C1 and C2 and the craniocaudal segmental pattern of the somites is regulated by the Delta-Notch signaling system.* A hypothetical molecular oscillator or clock has been proposed as the mechanism responsible for the orderly sequencing of somites.

DEVELOPMENT OF THE INTRAEMBRYONIC COELOM

The primordium of the intraembryonic coelom (embryonic body cavity) appears as isolated *coelomic spaces* in the lateral mesoderm and cardiogenic (heart-forming) mesoderm (see Fig. 4-9*A*). These spaces soon coalesce to form a single horseshoe-shaped cavity, the **intraembryonic coelom** (see Fig. 4-9*E*), which divides the lateral mesoderm into two layers (see Fig. 4-9*D*):

- A somatic or *parietal layer* of lateral mesoderm located beneath the ectodermal epithelium and continuous with the extraembryonic mesoderm covering the amnion
- A splanchnic or *visceral layer* of lateral mesoderm located adjacent to the endoderm and continuous with the extraembryonic mesoderm covering the umbilical vesicle

The somatic mesoderm and overlying embryonic ectoderm form the embryonic body wall or **somatopleure** (see Fig. 4-9*F*), whereas the splanchnic mesoderm and underlying embryonic endoderm form the embryonic gut or **splanchnopleure**. During the second month, the intraembryonic coelom is divided into three body cavities:

- Pericardial cavity
- Pleural cavities
- Peritoneal cavity

For a description of these divisions of the intraembryonic coelom, see Chapter 8.

EARLY DEVELOPMENT OF THE CARDIOVASCULAR SYSTEM

At the end of the second week, embryonic nutrition is obtained from the maternal blood by diffusion through the extraembryonic coelom and umbilical vesicle. At the beginning of the third week, *vasculogenesis* and *angiogenesis* (Gr. *angeion*, vessel + *genesis*, production), or blood vessel formation, begins in the extraembryonic mesoderm of the umbilical vesicle, connecting stalk, and chorion (Fig. 4-11). Embryonic blood vessels begin to develop approximately 2 days later. The early formation of the cardiovascular system is correlated with the urgent need for blood vessels to bring oxygen and nourishment to the embryo from

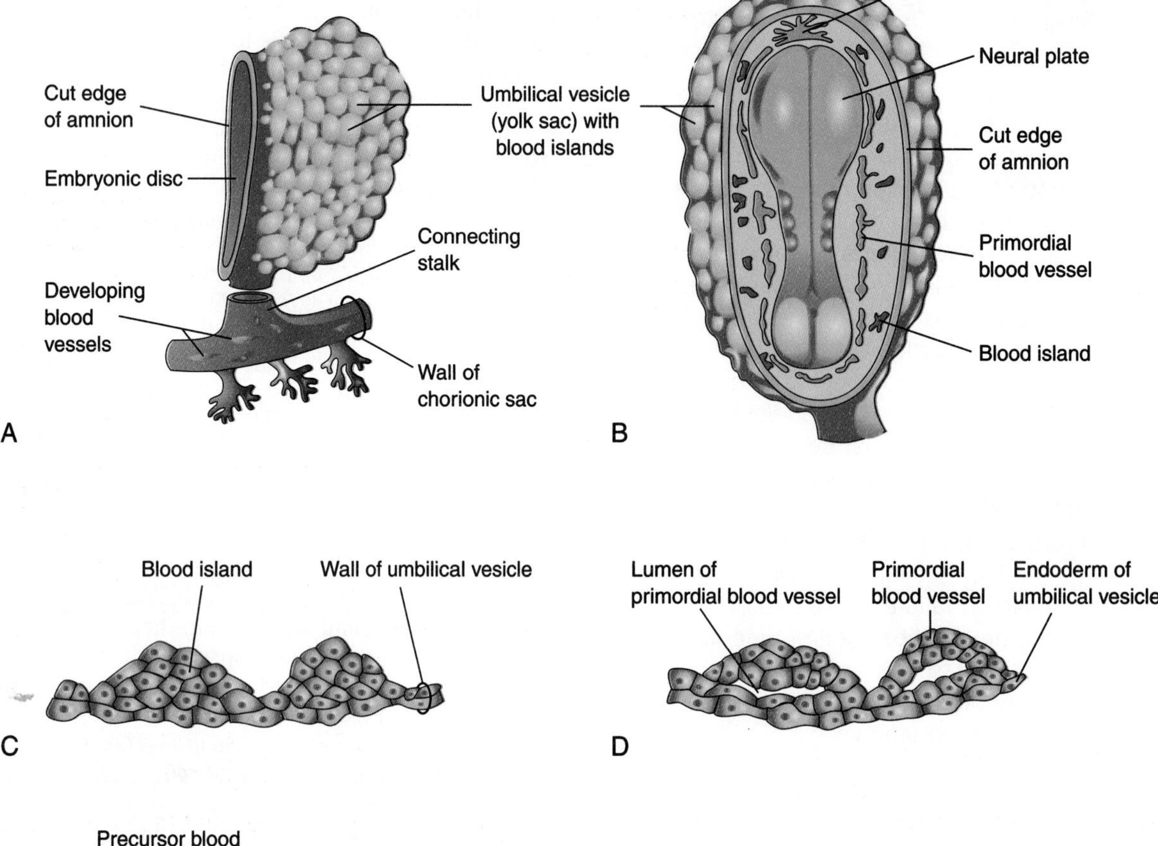

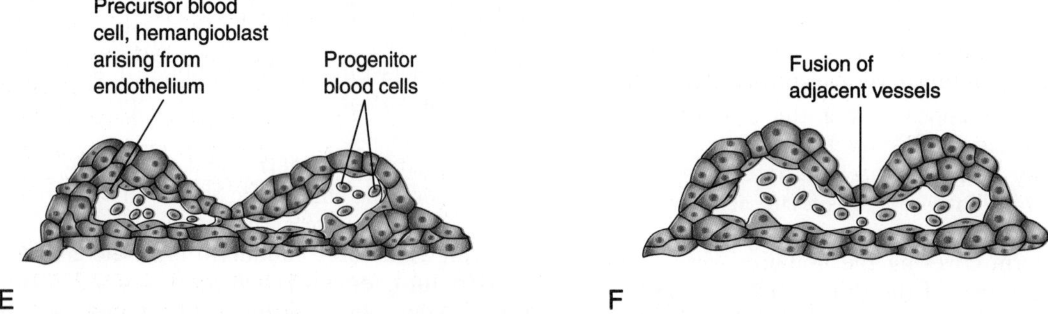

FIGURE 4-11. Successive stages in the development of blood and blood vessels. **A,** Lateral view of the umbilical vesicle and part of the chorionic sac (approximately 18 days). **B,** Dorsal view of the embryo exposed by removing the amnion. **C** to **F,** Sections of blood islands showing progressive stages in the development of blood and blood vessels.

the maternal circulation through the placenta. During the third week, a primordial uteroplacental circulation develops (Fig. 4-12).

Vasculogenesis and Angiogenesis

The formation of the embryonic vascular system involves two processes: *vasculogenesis* and *angiogenesis*. **Vasculogenesis** is the formation of new vascular channels by assembly of individual cell precursors called angioblasts. **Angiogenesis** is the formation of new vessels by budding and branching from preexisting vessels. Blood vessel formation (*vasculogenesis*) in the embryo and extraembryonic membranes during the third week may be summarized as follows (see Fig. 4-11):

- Mesenchymal cells (mesoderm derived) differentiate into endothelial cell precursors—**angioblasts** (vessel-forming cells), which aggregate to form isolated angiogenic cell clusters called **blood islands**, which are associated with the umbilical vesicle or endothelial cords within the embryo.
- Small cavities appear within the blood islands and endothelial cords by confluence of intercellular clefts.
- Angioblasts flatten to form endothelial cells that arrange themselves around the cavities in the blood island to form the endothelium.

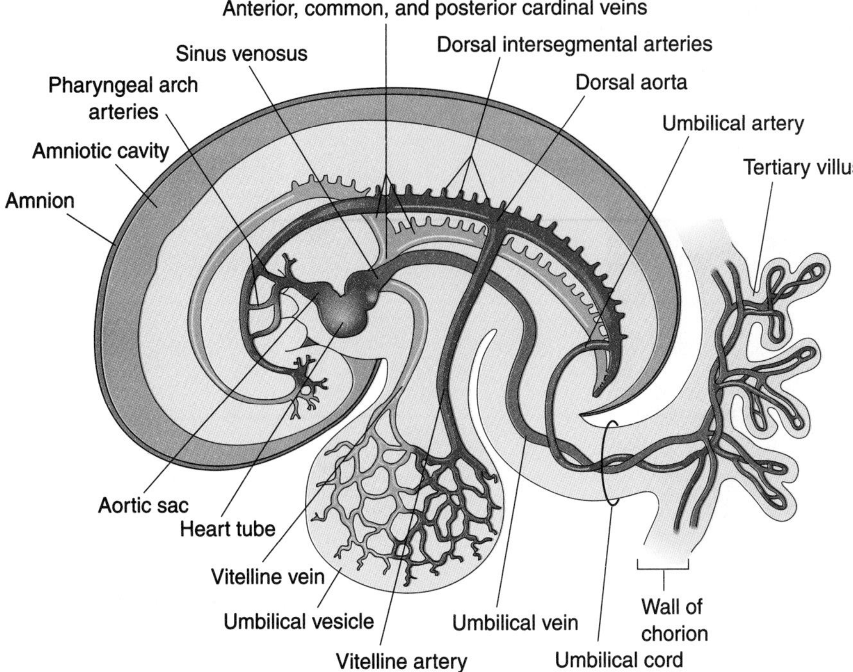

FIGURE 4-12. Diagram of the primordial cardiovascular system in an embryo of approximately 21 days, viewed from the left side. Observe the transitory stage of paired symmetrical vessels. Each heart tube continues dorsally into a dorsal aorta that passes caudally. Branches of the aortae are (1) umbilical arteries establishing connections with vessels in the chorion, (2) vitelline arteries to the umbilical vesicle, and (3) dorsal intersegmental arteries to the body of the embryo. Vessels on the umbilical vesicle form a vascular plexus that is connected to the heart tubes by vitelline veins. The cardinal veins return blood from the body of the embryo. The umbilical vein carries oxygenated blood and nutrients from the chorion. The arteries carry poorly oxygenated blood and waste products to the chorionic villi for transfer to the mother's blood.

- These endothelium-lined cavities soon fuse to form networks of endothelial channels (vasculogenesis).
- Vessels sprout into adjacent areas by endothelial budding and fuse with other vessels.

Blood cells develop from the endothelial cells of vessels as they develop on the umbilical vesicle and allantois at the end of the third week (see Fig. 4-11*E* and *F*) and later in specialized sites along the dorsal aorta. Blood formation (**hematogenesis**) does not begin in the embryo until the fifth week. It occurs first along the aorta and then in various parts of the embryonic mesenchyme, mainly, the liver, and later in the spleen, bone marrow, and lymph nodes. Fetal and adult erythrocytes are derived from different hematopoietic progenitor cells (*hemangioblasts*). The mesenchymal cells surrounding the primordial endothelial blood vessels differentiate into the muscular and connective tissue elements of the vessels.

The Primordial Cardiovascular System

The **heart and great vessels** form from mesenchymal cells in the cardiogenic area (see Fig. 4-11*B*). Paired, longitudinal endothelial-lined channels—the **endocardial heart tubes**—develop during the third week and fuse to form a primordial **heart tube**. The tubular heart joins with blood vessels in the embryo, connecting stalk, chorion, and umbilical vesicle to form a primordial cardiovascular system (see Fig. 4-12). By the end of the third week, the blood is circulating and the heart begins to beat on the 21st or 22nd day. *The cardiovascular system is the first organ system to reach a functional state.* The embryonic heartbeat can be detected using Doppler ultrasonography during the fifth week, approximately 7 weeks after the last normal menstrual period (Fig. 4-13).

ABNORMAL GROWTH OF TROPHOBLAST

Sometimes the embryo dies and the chorionic villi do not complete their development; that is, they do not become vascularized to form tertiary villi. These degenerating villi form cystic swellings—**hydatidiform moles**—which resemble a bunch of grapes. The moles exhibit variable degrees of trophoblastic proliferation and produce excessive amounts of human chorionic gonadotropin. Complete hydatidiform moles are of paternal origin. Three percent to 5% of moles develop into malignant trophoblastic lesions—**choriocarcinomas**. Some moles develop after spontaneous abortions, and others occur after normal deliveries. Choriocarcinomas invariably metastasize (spread) through the bloodstream to various sites, such as the lungs, vagina, liver, bone, intestine, and brain.

The main mechanisms for development of **complete hydatidiform** moles are

- Fertilization of an empty oocyte by a sperm, followed by duplication (monospermic mole)
- Fertilization of an empty oocyte by two sperms (dispermic mole)

A complete (monospermic) hydatidiform mole results from fertilization of an oocyte in which the female pronucleus is absent or inactive—an empty oocyte. A partial (dispermic) hydatidiform mole usually results from fertilization of an oocyte by two sperms (dispermy). Most complete hydatidiform moles are monospermic. For both types, the genetic origin of the nuclear DNA is paternal.

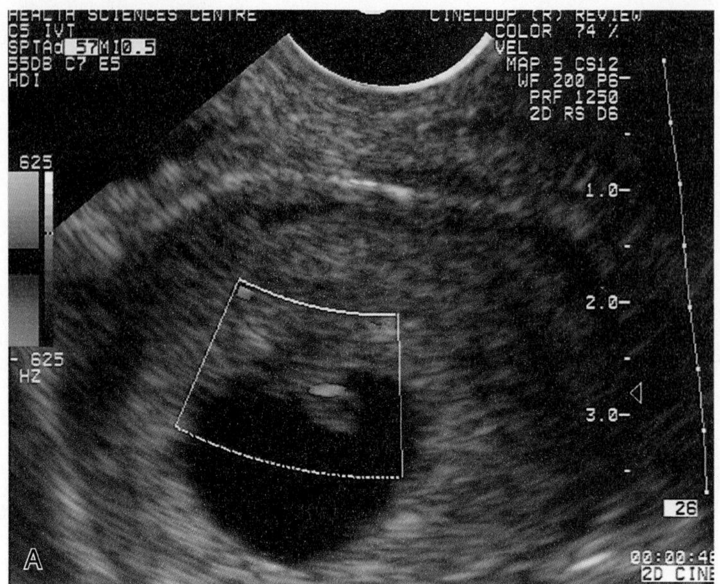

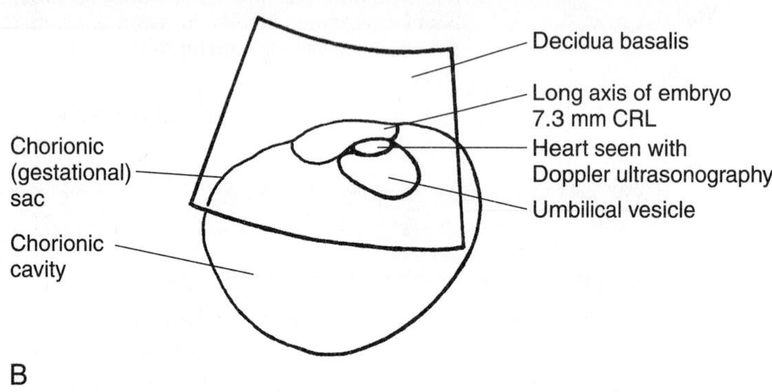

FIGURE 4-13. **A,** Ultrasonogram (sonogram) of a 5-week embryo and its attached umbilical vesicle within its chorionic (gestational) sac. The pulsating heart (red) of the embryo was visualized using Doppler ultrasonography. **B,** Sketch of the ultrasonogram for orientation and identification of structures. (Courtesy of E.A. Lyons, MD, Professor of Radiology and Obstetrics and Gynecology, Health Sciences Centre, University of Manitoba, Winnipeg, Manitoba, Canada.)

DEVELOPMENT OF CHORIONIC VILLI

Shortly after **primary chorionic villi** appear at the end of the second week, they begin to branch. Early in the third week, mesenchyme grows into these primary villi, forming a core of mesenchymal tissue. The villi at this stage—**secondary chorionic villi**—cover the entire surface of the chorionic sac (Fig. 4-14*A* and *B*). Some mesenchymal cells in the villi soon differentiate into capillaries and blood cells (see Fig. 4-14*C* and *D*). They are called **tertiary chorionic villi** when blood vessels are visible in them. The capillaries in the chorionic villi fuse to form **arteriocapillary networks,** which soon become connected with the embryonic heart through vessels that differentiate in the mesenchyme of the chorion and connecting stalk (see Fig. 4-12). By the end of the third week, embryonic blood begins to flow slowly through the capillaries in the chorionic villi. Oxygen and nutrients in the maternal blood in the intervillous space diffuse through the walls of the villi and enter the embryo's blood (see Fig. 4-14*C* and *D*). Carbon dioxide and waste products diffuse from blood in the fetal capillaries through the wall of the chorionic villi into the maternal blood. Concurrently, cytotrophoblastic cells of the chorionic villi proliferate and extend through the syncytiotrophoblast to form a **cytotrophoblastic shell** (see Fig. 4-14*C*), which gradually surrounds the chorionic sac and attaches it to the endometrium. Villi that attach to the maternal tissues through the cytotrophoblastic shell are **stem chorionic villi** (anchoring villi). The villi that grow from the sides of the stem villi are **branch chorionic villi** (terminal villi). It is through the walls of the branch villi that the main exchange of material between the blood of the mother and the embryo takes place. The branch villi are bathed in continually changing maternal blood in the intervillous space.

SUMMARY OF THE THIRD WEEK

- The *bilaminar embryonic disc* is converted into a *trilaminar embryonic disc* during **gastrulation**. These changes begin with the appearance of the *primitive streak*, which appears at the beginning of the third week as a thickening of the epiblast at the caudal end of the embryonic disc.
- The **primitive streak** results from migration of epiblastic cells to the median plane of the disc. Invagination of epiblastic cells from the primitive streak gives rise to mesenchymal cells that migrate ventrally, laterally, and cranially between the **epiblast and hypoblast**.

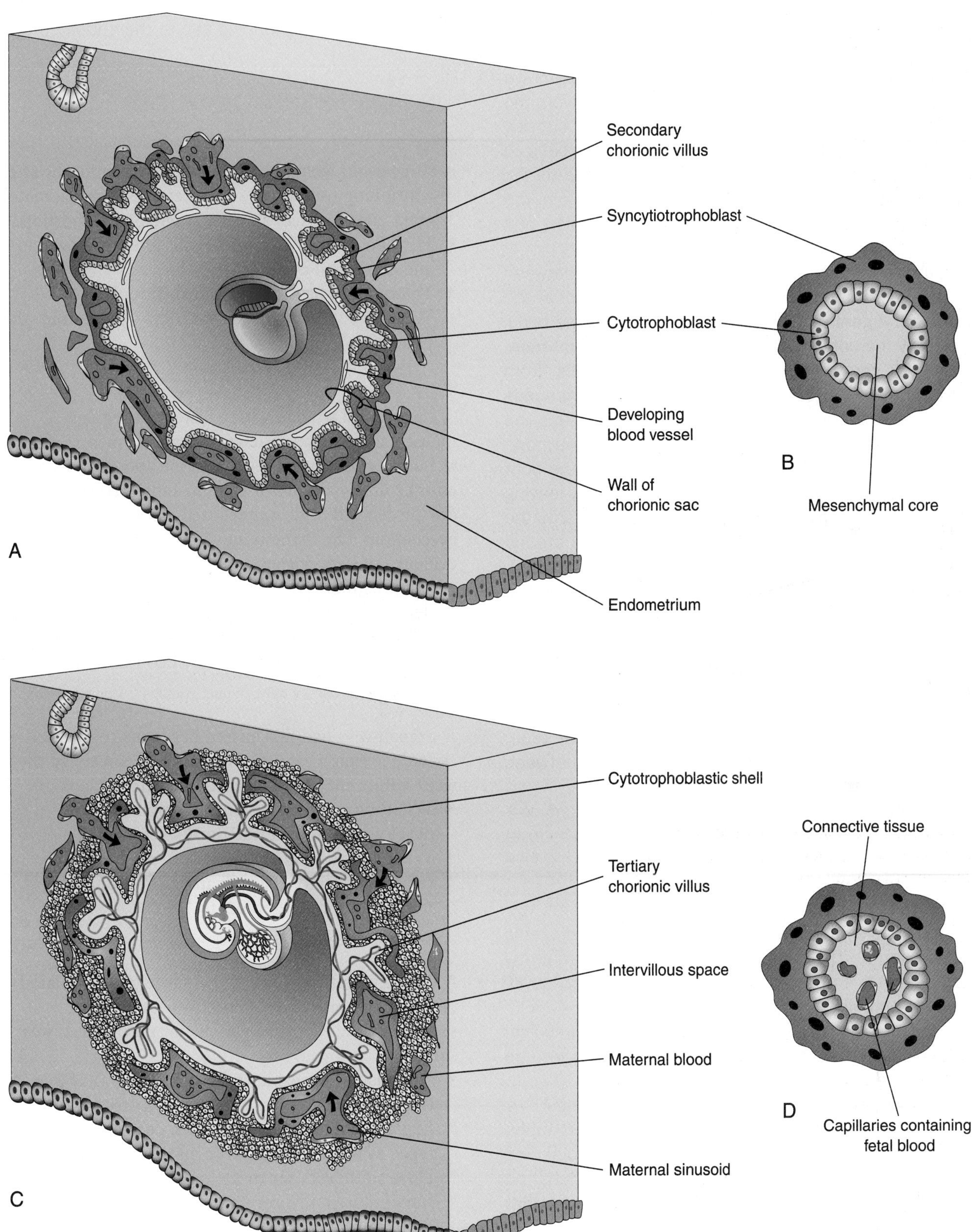

FIGURE 4-14. Diagrams illustrating development of secondary chorionic villi into tertiary chorionic villi. Early formation of the placenta is also shown. **A,** Sagittal section of an embryo (approximately 16 days). **B,** Section of a secondary chorionic villus. **C,** Section of an implanted embryo (approximately 21 days). **D,** Section of a tertiary chorionic villus. The fetal blood in the capillaries is separated from the maternal blood surrounding the villus by the endothelium of the capillary, embryonic connective tissue, cytotrophoblast, and syncytiotrophoblast.

- As soon as the primitive streak begins to produce mesenchymal cells, the epiblast is known as **embryonic ectoderm**. Some cells of the epiblast displace the hypoblast and form **embryonic endoderm**. Mesenchymal cells produced by the primitive streak soon organize into a third germ layer, the **intraembryonic or embryonic mesoderm**, occupying the area between the former hypoblast and cells in the epiblast. Cells of the mesoderm migrate to the edges of the embryonic disc, where they join the extraembryonic mesoderm covering the amnion and umbilical vesicle.
- By the end of the third week, mesoderm exists between the ectoderm and endoderm everywhere except at the **oropharyngeal membrane**, in the median plane occupied by the notochord, and at the **cloacal membrane**.
- Early in the third week, mesenchymal cells from the primitive streak form the **notochordal process** between the embryonic ectoderm and endoderm. The *notochordal process* extends from the primitive node to the *prechordal plate*. Openings develop in the floor of the *notochordal canal* and soon coalesce, leaving a notochordal plate. This plate infolds to form the **notochord**, the primordial axis of the embryo around which the axial skeleton forms (e.g., vertebral column).
- The **neural plate** appears as a thickening of the embryonic ectoderm, induced by the developing notochord. A longitudinal neural groove develops in the neural plate, which is flanked by **neural folds**. Fusion of the folds forms the **neural tube**, the primordium of the central nervous system.
- As the neural folds fuse to form the neural tube, neuroectodermal cells form a **neural crest** between the surface ectoderm and the neural tube.
- The mesoderm on each side of the notochord condenses to form longitudinal columns of paraxial mesoderm, which, by the end of the third week, give rise to **somites**.
- The **coelom** (cavity) within the embryo arises as isolated spaces in the lateral mesoderm and cardiogenic mesoderm. The coelomic vesicles subsequently coalesce to form a single, horseshoe-shaped cavity that eventually gives rise to the *body cavities*.
- **Blood vessels** first appear in the wall of the umbilical vesicle (yolk sac), allantois, and chorion. They develop within the embryo shortly thereafter.
- The **heart** is represented by *paired endocardial heart tubes*. By the end of the third week, the heart tubes have fused to form a *tubular heart* that is joined to vessels in the embryo, umbilical vesicle, chorion, and connecting stalk to form a **primordial cardiovascular system**. Fetal and adult erythrocytes develop from different hematopoietic precursors.
- **Primary chorionic villi** become **secondary chorionic villi** as they acquire mesenchymal cores. Before the end of the third week, capillaries develop in the secondary chorionic villi, transforming them into **tertiary chorionic villi**. Cytotrophoblastic extensions from these stem villi join to form a **cytotrophoblastic shell** that anchors the chorionic sac to the endometrium.

CLINICALLY ORIENTED PROBLEMS

Case 4-1

A 30-year-old woman became pregnant 2 months after discontinuing use of oral contraceptives. Approximately 3 weeks later, she had an early spontaneous abortion.

- How do hormones in these pills affect the ovarian and menstrual cycles?
- What might have caused the abortion?
- What would the physician likely have told this patient?

Case 4-2

A 25-year-old woman with a history of regular menstrual cycles was 5 days overdue on menses. Owing to her mental distress related to the abnormal bleeding and the undesirability of a possible pregnancy, the doctor decided to do a menstrual extraction or uterine evacuation. The tissue removed was examined for evidence of a pregnancy.

- Would a highly sensitive radioimmune assay have detected pregnancy at this early stage?
- What findings would indicate an early pregnancy?
- How old would the products of conception be?

Case 4-3

A woman who had just missed her menstrual period was concerned that a glass of wine she had consumed the week before may have harmed her embryo.

- What major organ systems undergo early development during the third week?
- What severe congenital anomaly might result from teratologic factors (see Chapter 20) acting during this period of development?

Case 4-4

A female infant was born with a large tumor situated between her anus and sacrum. A diagnosis of sacrococcygeal teratoma was made and the mass was surgically removed.

- What is the probable embryologic origin of this tumor?
- Explain why these tumors often contain various types of tissue derived from all three germ layers.
- Does an infant's sex make him or her more susceptible to the development of one of these tumors?

Case 4-5

A woman with a history of early spontaneous abortions had an ultrasound examination to determine whether her embryo was still implanted.

- Is ultrasonography of any value in assessing pregnancy during the third week?
- What structures might be recognizable?
- If a pregnancy test is negative, is it safe to assume that the woman is not pregnant?
- Could an extrauterine gestation be present?

Discussion of these problems appears at the back of the book.

References and Suggested Reading

Aulehla A, Herrmann BG: Segmentation in vertebrates: Clock and gradient finally joined. Genes Dev 18:2060–2067, 2004.

Aybar MJ, Glavic A, Mayor R: Extracellular signals, cell interactions and transcription factors involved in the induction of the neural crest cells. Biol Res 35:267–275, 2002.

Barembaum M, Bronner-Fraser M: Early steps in neural crest specification. Semin Cell Dev Biol 16:642–646, 2005.

Bianchi DW, Wilkins-Haug LE, Enders AC, Hay ED: Origin of extraembryonic mesoderm in experimental animals: Relevance to chorionic mosaicism in humans. Am J Med Genet 46:542, 1993.

Dale KJ, Pourquié O: A clock-work somite. BioEssays 22:72, 2000.

Djonov V, Baum O, Burri PH: Vascular remodeling by intussusceptive angiogenesis. Cell Tissue Res 314:107–117, 2003.

Drake CJ: Embryonic and adult vasculogenesis. Birth Defects Res C Embryo Today 69:73–82, 2003.

Dubrulle J, Pourquie O: Coupling segmentation to axis formation. Development 131:5783–5793, 2004.

Flake AW: The fetus with sacrococcygeal teratoma. In Harrison MR, Evans MI, Adzick NS, Holzgrev W (eds): The Unborn Patient: The Art and Science of Fetal Therapy, 3rd ed. Philadelphia, WB Saunders, 2001.

Gasser RF: Evidence that some events of mammalian embryogenesis can result from differential growth, making migration unnecessary. Anat Rec B New Anat 289B:53, 2006.

Hall BK: Bones and Cartilage: Developmental Skeletal Biology. Philadelphia, Elsevier, 2005.

Hardin J, Walston T: Models of morphogenesis: the mechanisms and mechanics of cell rearrangement. Curr Opin Genet Dev 14:399, 2004.

Harvey NL, Oliver G: Choose your fate: artery, vein or lymphatic vessel? Curr Opin Genet Dev 14:499, 2004.

Hollway G, Currie P: Vertebrate myotome development. Birth Defects Res C Embryo Today. 75:172–179, 2005.

Kalcheim C, Ben-Yair R: Cell rearrangements during development of the somite and its derivatives. Curr Opin Genet Dev 15:371, 2005.

Lerou PH, Daley GQ: Therapeutic potential of embryonic stem cells. Blood Rev 19:321, 2005.

Levine D: Ectopic pregnancy. In Callen PW (ed): Ultrasonography in Obstetrics and Gynecology, 4th ed. Philadelphia, WB Saunders, 2000.

Monsoro-Burq AH: Sclerotome development and morphogenesis: When experimental embryology meets genetics. Int J Dev Biol 49:301–308, 2005.

Morales AV, Barbas JA, Nieto MA: How to become neural crest: From segregation to delamination. Semin Cell Dev Biol 16:655–662, 2005.

Ohls RK, Christensen RD: Development of the hematopoietic system. In Behrman RE, Kliegman Jenson HB (eds): Nelson Textbook of Pediatrics, 17th ed. Philadelphia, Elsevier/Saunders, 2004.

Passegue E, Wagers AJ, Giuriato S, et al: Global analysis of proliferation and cell cycle gene expression in the regulation of hematopoietic stem and progenitor cell fates. J Exp Med 202:1599, 2005.

Pourquié O: Vertebrate segmentation: Is cycling the rule? Curr Opin Cell Biol 12:747, 2000.

Robb L, Tam PP: Gastrula organiser and embryonic patterning in the mouse. Semin Cell Dev Biol 15:543–554, 2004.

Roman BL, Weinstein BM: Building the vertebrate vasculature: Research is going swimmingly. BioEssays 22:882, 2000.

Sebire NJ, Foskett M, Fisher RA, et al: Risk of partial and complete hydatidiform molar pregnancy in relation to maternal age. Br J Obstet Gynaecol 109:99, 2002.

Seckl MJ, Fisher RA, Salerno G, et al: Choriocarcinoma and partial hydatidiform moles. Lancet 356:36, 2000.

Slack JMW: Essential Developmental Biology, 2nd ed. Oxford, Blackwell Publishing, 2006.

Smith JL, Schoenwolf GC: Neurulation: Coming to closure. Trends Neurosci 20:510, 1997.

Tam PPL, Kanai-Azuma M, Kanai Y: Early endoderm development in vertebrates: Lineage differentiation and morphogenetic function. Curr Opin Genet Dev 13:393, 2003.

5

Organogenetic Period: Fourth to Eighth Weeks

Phases of Embryonic Development 73

Folding of the Embryo 73
- Folding of the Embryo in the Median Plane 73
- Folding of the Embryo in the Horizontal Plane 73

Germ Layer Derivatives 75

Control of Embryonic Development 75

Highlights of the Fourth to Eighth Weeks 79
- Fourth Week 79
- Fifth Week 79
- Sixth Week 80
- Seventh Week 80
- Eighth Week 81

Estimation of Embryonic Age 86

Summary of the Fourth to Eighth Weeks 90

Clinically Oriented Problems 91

All major external and internal structures are established during the fourth to eighth weeks. By the end of this period, the main organ systems have begun to develop; however, the function of most of them is minimal except for the cardiovascular system. As the tissues and organs form, the shape of the embryo changes, and by the eighth week, it has a distinctly human appearance. Because the tissues and organs are differentiating rapidly during the fourth to eighth weeks, exposure of embryos to teratogens during this period may cause major congenital anomalies. **Teratogens** are agents such as drugs and viruses that produce or increase the incidence of congenital anomalies (see Chapter 20).

PHASES OF EMBRYONIC DEVELOPMENT

Human development may be divided into three phases, which to some extent are interrelated:

- The first phase is **growth**, which involves cell division and the elaboration of cell products.
- The second phase is **morphogenesis** (development of shape, size, or other features of a particular organ or part or the whole of the body). Morphogenesis is an elaborate process during which many complex interactions occur in an orderly sequence. The movement of cells allows them to interact with each other during the formation of tissues and organs.
- The third phase is **differentiation** (maturation of physiologic processes). Completion of differentiation results in the formation of tissues and organs that are capable of performing specialized functions.

FOLDING OF THE EMBRYO

A significant event in the establishment of body form is folding of the flat trilaminar embryonic disc into a somewhat cylindrical embryo (Fig. 5-1). Folding occurs in both the median and horizontal planes and results from rapid growth of the embryo. The growth rate at the sides of the embryonic disc fails to keep pace with the rate of growth in the long axis as the embryo increases rapidly in length. Folding at the cranial and caudal ends and sides of the embryo occurs simultaneously. Concurrently, there is relative constriction at the junction of the embryo and umbilical vesicle (yolk sac).

Folding of the Embryo in the Median Plane

Folding of the ends of the embryo ventrally produces head and tail folds that result in the cranial and caudal regions moving ventrally as the embryo elongates cranially and caudally (see Fig. 5-1A_2 to D_2).

Head Fold

By the beginning of the fourth week, the neural folds in the cranial region have thickened to form the primordium of the brain. Initially, the developing brain projects dorsally into the amniotic cavity. Later, the developing forebrain grows cranially beyond the oropharyngeal membrane and overhangs the developing heart. Concomitantly, the **septum transversum** (transverse septum), primordial heart, pericardial coelom, and oropharyngeal membrane move onto the ventral surface of the embryo (Fig. 5-2). During folding, part of the endoderm of the umbilical vesicle is incorporated into the embryo as the **foregut** (primordium of pharynx, esophagus, etc.; see Chapter 11). The foregut lies between the brain and heart, and the **oropharyngeal membrane** separates the foregut from the **stomodeum** (see Fig. 5-2*C*). After folding, the septum transversum lies caudal to the heart where it subsequently develops into the central tendon of the diaphragm (see Chapter 8). The head fold also affects the arrangement of the embryonic coelom (primordium of body cavities). Before folding, the coelom consists of a flattened, horseshoe-shaped cavity (see Fig. 5-1A_1). After folding, the pericardial coelom lies ventral to the heart and cranial to the septum transversum (see Fig. 5-2*C*). At this stage, the intraembryonic coelom communicates widely on each side with the extraembryonic coelom (Figs. 5-1A_3 and 5-3).

Tail Fold

Folding of the caudal end of the embryo results primarily from growth of the distal part of the neural tube—the primordium of the spinal cord (Fig. 5-4). As the embryo grows, the **caudal eminence** (tail region) projects over the **cloacal membrane** (future site of anus). During folding, part of the endodermal germ layer is incorporated into the embryo as the **hindgut** (primordium of descending colon). The terminal part of the hindgut soon dilates slightly to form the **cloaca** (primordium of urinary bladder and rectum; see Chapters 11 and 12). Before folding, the **primitive streak** lies cranial to the cloacal membrane (see Fig. 5-4*B*); after folding, it lies caudal to it (see Fig. 5-4*C*). The **connecting stalk** (primordium of umbilical cord) is now attached to the ventral surface of the embryo, and the **allantois**—a diverticulum of the umbilical vesicle—is partially incorporated into the embryo.

Folding of the Embryo in the Horizontal Plane

Folding of the sides of the embryo produces right and left **lateral folds** (see Fig. 5-1A_3 to D_3). Lateral folding is produced by the rapidly growing spinal cord and somites. The primordia of the ventrolateral wall fold toward the median plane, rolling the edges of the embryonic disc ventrally and forming a roughly cylindrical embryo. As the abdominal walls form, part of the endoderm germ layer is incorporated into the embryo as the **midgut** (primordium of small intestine, etc.; see Chapter 11). Initially, there is a wide connection between the midgut and umbilical vesicle (see Fig. 5-1A_2), however; after lateral folding, the connection is reduced to an **omphaloenteric duct** (Fig. 5-1C_2). The region of attachment of the amnion to the ventral surface of the embryo is also reduced to a relatively narrow umbilical region (Fig. 5-1D_2 and D_3). As the umbilical cord forms from the connecting stalk,

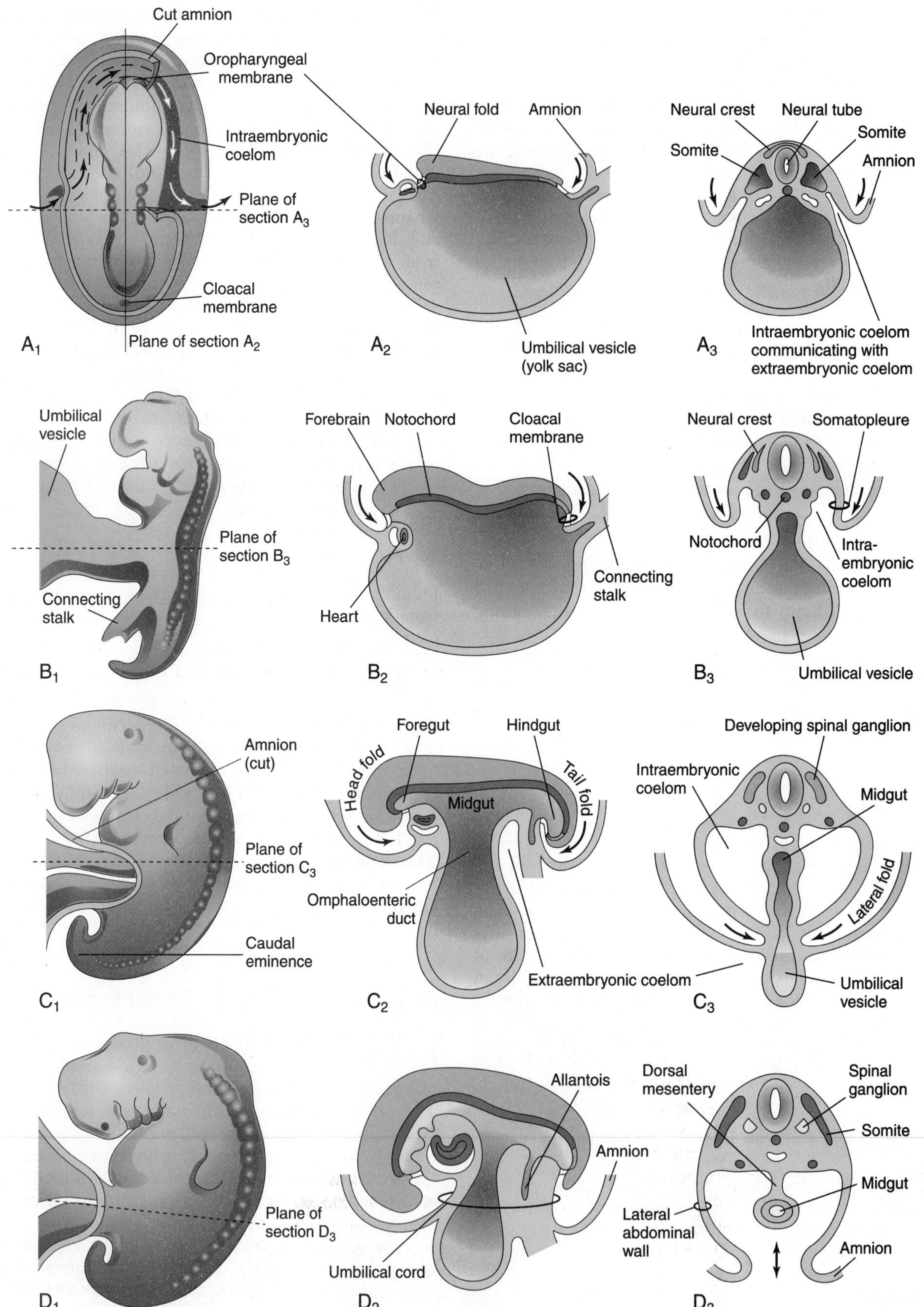

FIGURE 5-1. Illustrations of folding of embryos during the fourth week. **A_1**, Dorsal view of an embryo early in the fourth week. Three pairs of somites are visible. The continuity of the intraembryonic coelom and extraembryonic coelom is illustrated on the right side by removal of a part of the embryonic ectoderm and mesoderm. **B_1**, **C_1**, and **D_1**, Lateral views of embryos at 22, 26, and 28 days, respectively. **A_2** to **D_2**, Sagittal sections at the plane shown in **A_1**. **A_3** to **D_3**, Transverse sections at the levels indicated in **A_1** to **D_1**.

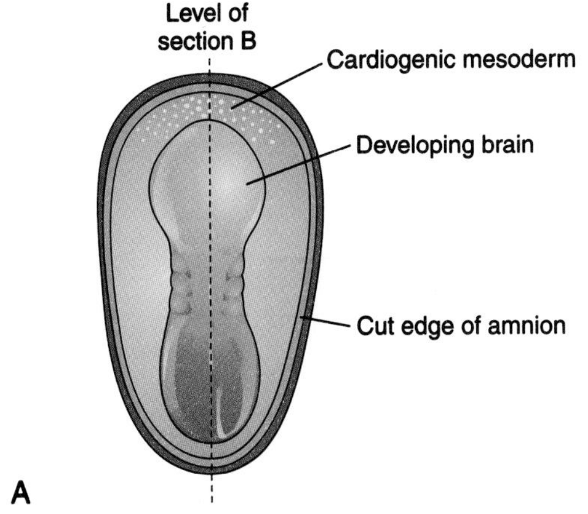

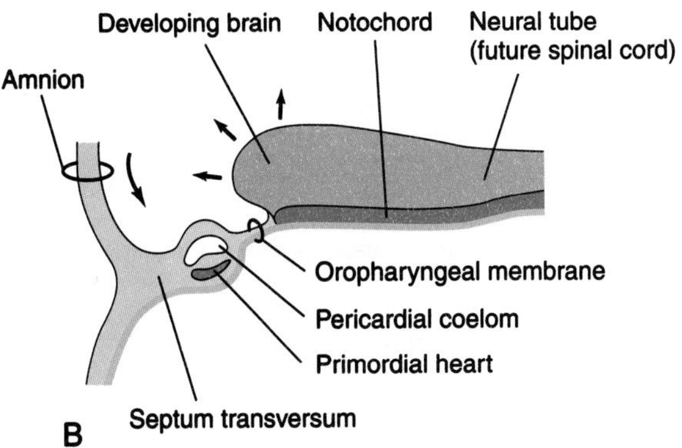

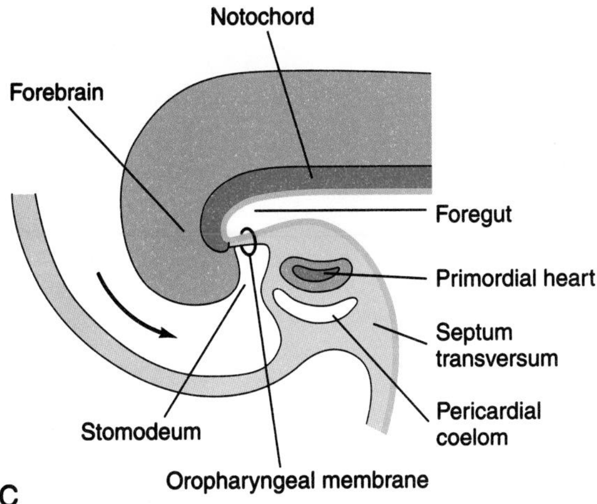

FIGURE 5-2. Folding of cranial end of embryo. **A,** Dorsal view of embryo at 21 days. **B,** Sagittal section of cranial part of the embryo at the plane shown in **A**. Observe the ventral movement of the heart. **C,** Sagittal section of an embryo at 26 days. Note that the septum transversum, primordial heart, pericardial coelom, and oropharyngeal membrane have moved onto the ventral surface of the embryo. Observe also that part of the umbilical vesicle is incorporated into the embryo as the foregut.

ventral fusion of the lateral folds reduces the region of communication between the intraembryonic and extraembryonic coelomic cavities to a narrow communication (see Fig. 5-1C_2). As the amniotic cavity expands and obliterates most of the extraembryonic coelom, the amnion forms the epithelial covering of the umbilical cord (see Fig. 5-1D_2).

GERM LAYER DERIVATIVES

The three germ layers (ectoderm, mesoderm, and endoderm) formed during gastrulation (see Chapter 4) give rise to the primordia of all the tissues and organs. The specificity of the germ layers, however, is not rigidly fixed. The cells of each germ layer divide, migrate, aggregate, and differentiate in rather precise patterns as they form the various organ systems. The main germ layer derivatives are as follows (Fig. 5-5):

- **Ectoderm** gives rise to the central nervous system, peripheral nervous system; sensory epithelia of the eye, ear, and nose; epidermis and its appendages (hair and nails); mammary glands; pituitary gland; subcutaneous glands; and enamel of teeth. **Neural crest cells**, derived from neuroectoderm, give rise to the cells of the spinal, cranial (cranial nerves V, VII, IX, and X), and autonomic ganglia; ensheathing cells of the peripheral nervous system; pigment cells of the dermis; muscle, connective tissues, and bone of pharyngeal arch origin; suprarenal medulla; and meninges (coverings) of the brain and spinal cord.
- **Mesoderm** gives rise to connective tissue; cartilage; bone; striated and smooth muscles; heart, blood, and lymphatic vessels; kidneys; ovaries; testes; genital ducts; serous membranes lining the body cavities (pericardial, pleural, and peritoneal); spleen; and cortex of suprarenal glands.
- **Endoderm** gives rise to the epithelial lining of the gastrointestinal and respiratory tracts, parenchyma of the tonsils, thyroid and parathyroid glands, thymus, liver, and pancreas, epithelial lining of the urinary bladder and most of the urethra, and the epithelial lining of the tympanic cavity, tympanic antrum, and pharyngotympanic (auditory) tube.

CONTROL OF EMBRYONIC DEVELOPMENT

Development results from genetic plans in the chromosomes. Knowledge of the genes that control human development is increasing. Most information about developmental processes has come from studies in other organisms, especially *Drosophila* (fruit fly) and mice because of ethical problems associated with the use of human embryos for laboratory studies. Most developmental processes depend on a precisely coordinated interaction of genetic and environmental factors. Several control mechanisms guide differentiation and ensure synchronized development, such as tissue interactions,

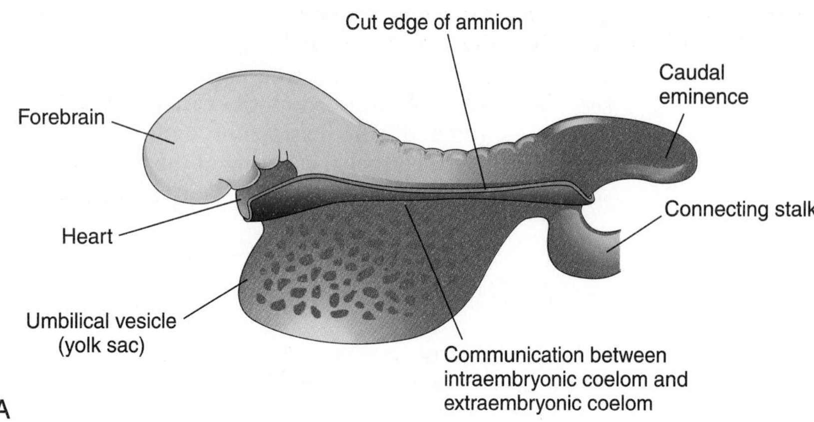

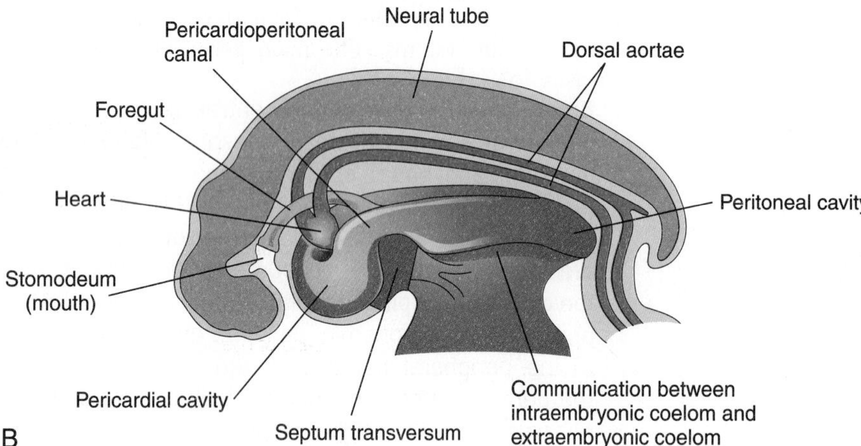

FIGURE 5-3. Illustrations of the effect of the head fold on the intraembryonic coelom. **A,** Lateral view of an embryo (24 to 25 days) during folding, showing the large forebrain, ventral position of the heart, and communication between the intraembryonic and extraembryonic parts of the coelom. **B,** Schematic drawing of an embryo (26 to 27 days) after folding, showing the pericardial cavity ventrally, the pericardioperitoneal canals running dorsally on each side of the foregut, and the intraembryonic coelom in communication with the extraembryonic coelom.

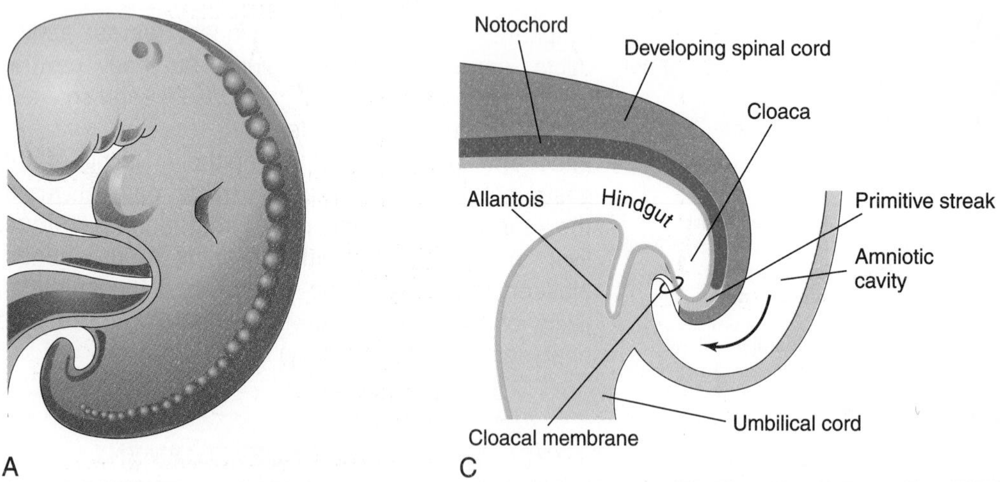

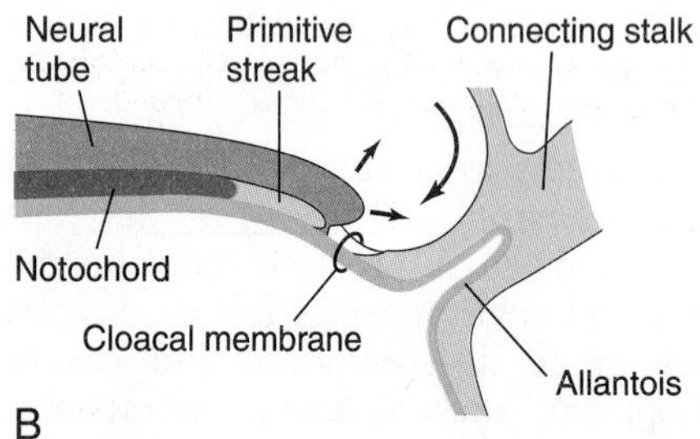

FIGURE 5-4. Folding of caudal end of the embryo. **A,** Lateral view of a 4-week embryo. **B,** Sagittal section of caudal part of the embryo at the beginning of the fourth week. **C,** Similar section at the end of the fourth week. Note that part of the umbilical vesicle is incorporated into the embryo as the hindgut and that the terminal part of the hindgut has dilated to form the cloaca. Observe also the change in position of the primitive streak, allantois, cloacal membrane, and connecting stalk.

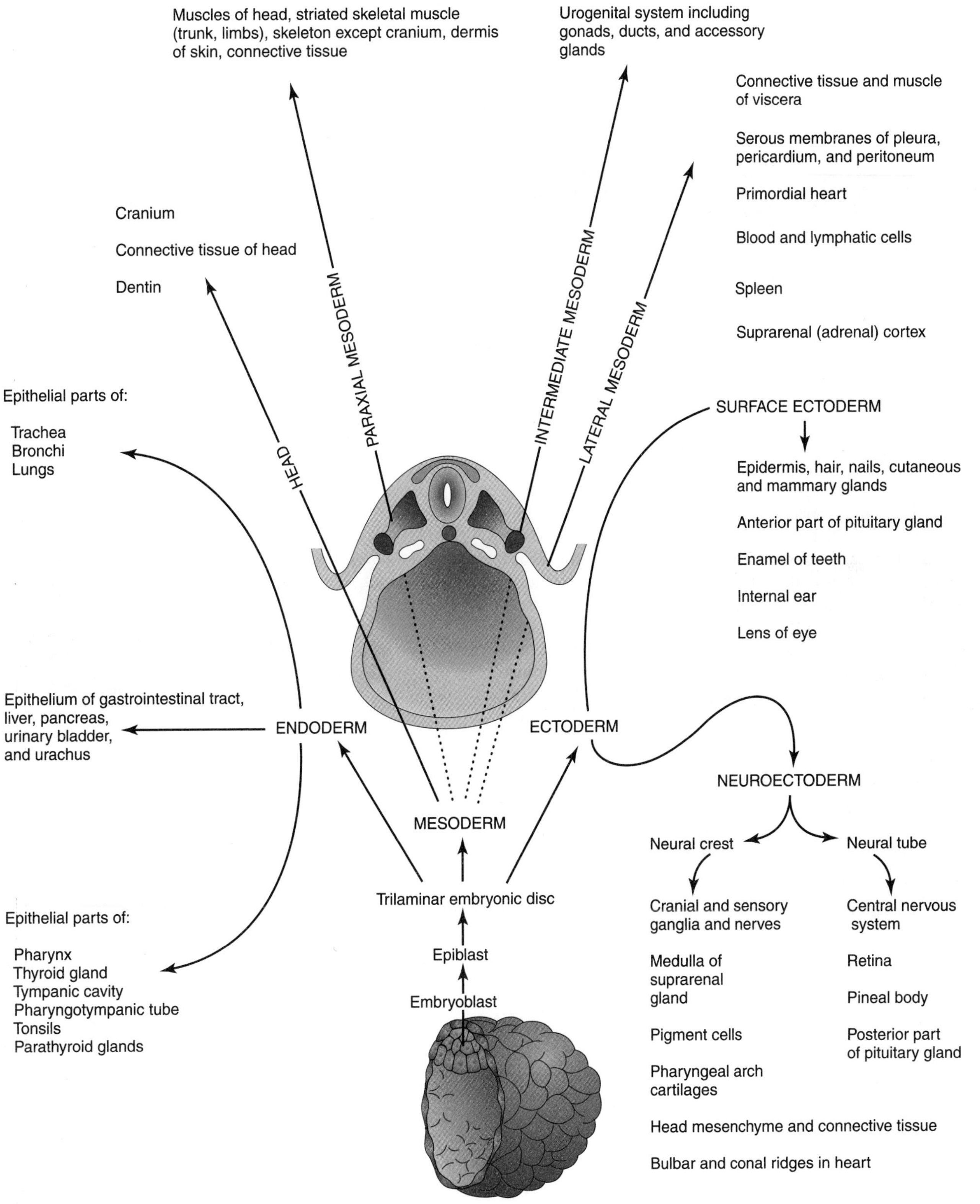

FIGURE 5-5. Schematic drawing of derivatives of the three germ layers: ectoderm, endoderm, and mesoderm. Cells from these layers contribute to the formation of different tissues and organs, e.g., the endoderm forms the epithelial lining of the gastrointestinal tract and the mesoderm gives rise to connective tissues and muscles.

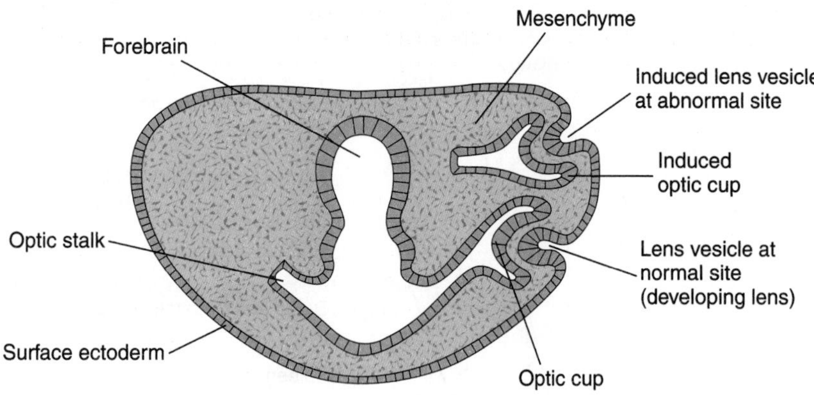

FIGURE 5-6. Schematic transverse section through the head of an embryo in the region of the developing eyes to illustrate inductive tissue interaction. At the normal site (*lower right*), observe that the optic stalk, the precursor of the optic cup, has acted on the surface ectoderm of the head to induce formation of a lens vesicle, the primordium of the lens. On the opposite side, the optic stalk was cut and the optic vesicle removed. As a result, no lens placode (first indication of a lens) developed. At the abnormal site (*upper right*), the optic vesicle removed from the right side was inserted deep to the skin. Here, it acted on the surface ectoderm to induce the formation of a lens vesicle that has induced the formation of an optic cup (primordium of eyeball).

regulated migration of cells and cell colonies, controlled proliferation, and programmed cell death. Each system of the body has its own developmental pattern.

Embryonic development is essentially a process of growth and increasing complexity of structure and function. Growth is achieved by mitosis together with the production of extracellular matrices, whereas complexity is achieved through morphogenesis and differentiation. The cells that make up the tissues of very early embryos are pluripotential, which under different circumstances are able to follow more than one pathway of development. This broad developmental potential becomes progressively restricted as tissues acquire the specialized features necessary for increasing their sophistication of structure and function. Such restriction presumes that choices must be made to achieve tissue diversification. At present, most evidence indicates that these choices are determined, not as a consequence of cell lineage, but rather in response to cues from the immediate surroundings, including the adjacent tissues. As a result, the architectural precision and coordination that are often required for the normal function of an organ appear to be achieved by the interaction of its constituent parts during development.

The interaction of tissues during development is a recurring theme in embryology. The interactions that lead to a change in the course of development of at least one of the interactants are called **inductions**. Numerous examples of such inductive interactions can be found in the literature; for example, during *development of the eye*, the optic vesicle induces the development of the lens from the surface ectoderm of the head. When the optic vesicle is absent, the eye fails to develop. Moreover, if the optic vesicle is removed and placed in association with surface ectoderm that is not usually involved in eye development, lens formation can be induced (Fig. 5-6). Clearly then, development of a lens is dependent on the ectoderm acquiring an association with a second tissue. In the presence of the neuroectoderm of the optic vesicle, the surface ectoderm of the head adopts a pathway of development that it would not otherwise have taken. In a similar fashion, many of the morphogenetic tissue movements that play such important roles in shaping the embryo also provide for the changing tissue associations that are fundamental to inductive *tissue interactions*.

The fact that one tissue can influence the *developmental pathway* adopted by another tissue presumes that a signal passes between the two interactants. Analysis of the molecular defects in mutant strains that show abnormal tissue interactions during embryonic development, and studies of the development of embryos with targeted gene mutations have begun to reveal the *molecular mechanisms of induction*. The mechanism of signal transfer appears to vary with the specific tissues involved. In some cases, the signal appears to take the form of a diffusible molecule, such as

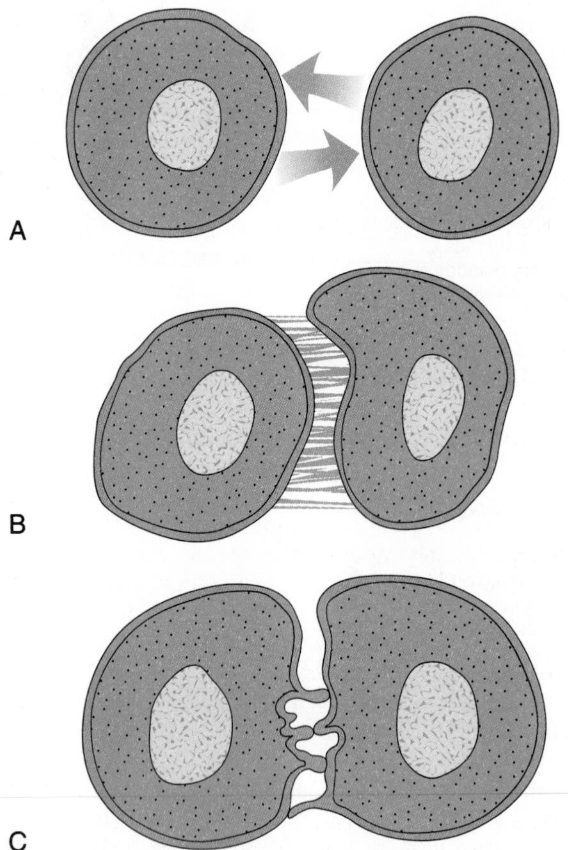

FIGURE 5-7. Sketches of three possible methods of transmission of signal substances in inductive cell interactions. **A,** Diffusion of signal substances. The signal appears to take the form of a diffusible molecule that passes from the inductor to the reacting tissue. **B,** Matrix-mediated interaction. The signal is mediated through a nondiffusible extracellular matrix, secreted by the inductor, with which the reacting tissue comes in contact. **C,** Cell contact–mediated interaction. The signal requires physical contact between the inducing and responding tissues. (Modified from Grobstein C: Adv Cancer Res 4:187, 1956; and Saxen L: In Tarin D [ed]: Tissue Interactions in Carcinogenesis. London, Academic Press, 1972.)

sonic hedgehog, that passes from the inductor to the reacting tissue (Fig. 5-7*A*). In others, the message appears to be mediated through a nondiffusible extracellular matrix that is secreted by the inductor and with which the reacting tissue comes into contact (see Fig. 5-7*B*). In still other cases, the signal appears to require that physical contacts occur between the inducing and responding tissues (see Fig. 5-7*C*). Regardless of the mechanism of intercellular transfer involved, the signal is translated into an intracellular message that influences the genetic activity of the responding cells.

Laboratory studies have established that the signal can be relatively nonspecific in some interactions. Under experimental conditions, the role of the natural inductor in a variety of interactions has been shown to be mimicked by a number of heterologous tissue sources and, in some instances, even by a variety of cell-free preparations. These studies suggest that the specificity of a given induction is a property of the reacting tissue rather than that of the inductor. Inductions should not be thought of as isolated phenomena. Often they occur in a sequential fashion that results in the orderly development of a complex structure; for example, following induction of the lens by the optic vesicle, the lens induces the development of the cornea from the surface ectoderm and adjacent mesenchyme. This ensures the formation of component parts that are appropriate in size and relationship for the function of the organ. In other systems, there is evidence that the interactions between tissues are reciprocal. During *development of the kidney*, for instance, the metanephric diverticulum (ureteric bud) induces the formation of tubules in the metanephric mesoderm (see Chapter 12). This mesoderm, in turn, induces branching of the diverticulum that results in the development of the collecting tubules and calices of the kidney.

To be competent to respond to an inducing stimulus, the cells of the reacting system must express the appropriate receptor for the specific inducing signal molecule, the components of the particular *intracellular signal transduction pathway*, and the *transcription factors* that will mediate the particular response. Experimental evidence suggests that the acquisition of competence by the responding tissue is often dependent on its previous interactions with other tissues. For example, the lens-forming response of head ectoderm to the stimulus provided by the optic vesicle appears to be dependent on a previous association of the head ectoderm with the anterior neural plate.

The ability of the reacting system to respond to an inducing stimulus is not unlimited. Most inducible tissues appear to pass through a transient, but more or less sharply delimited physiologic state in which they are competent to respond to an inductive signal from the neighboring tissue. Because this state of receptiveness is limited in time, a delay in the development of one or more components in an interacting system may lead to failure of an inductive interaction. Regardless of the signal mechanism employed, inductive systems seem to have the common feature of close proximity between the interacting tissues. Experimental evidence has demonstrated that interactions may fail if the interactants are too widely separated. Consequently, inductive processes appear to be limited in space as well as by time. Because tissue induction plays such a fundamental role in ensuring the orderly formation of precise structure, failed interactions can be expected to have drastic developmental consequences (e.g., congenital anomalies such as absence of the lens).

HIGHLIGHTS OF THE FOURTH TO EIGHTH WEEKS

The following descriptions summarize the main developmental events and changes in external form of the embryo during the fourth to eighth weeks. The main criteria for estimating developmental stages in human embryos are listed in Table 5-1.

Fourth Week

Major changes in body form occur during the fourth week. At the beginning, the embryo is almost straight and has four to 12 somites that produce conspicuous surface elevations (Fig. 5-8*A*). The **neural tube** is formed opposite the somites, but it is widely open at the rostral and caudal **neuropores** (Figs. 5-8*B* and 5-9). By 24 days, the first two pharyngeal arches are visible. The first (mandibular arch) and the second (hyoid arch) are distinct (Figs. 5-8*C* and 5-10). The major part of the first arch gives rise to the mandible (lower jaw), and a rostral extension of the arch, the maxillary prominence, contributes to the maxilla (upper jaw). The embryo is now slightly curved because of the head and tail folds. The heart produces a large ventral prominence and pumps blood.

Three pairs of **pharyngeal arches** are visible by 26 days (Figs. 5-8*D* and 5-11), and the rostral neuropore is closed. The **forebrain** produces a prominent elevation of the head, and folding of the embryo has given the embryo a C-shaped curvature. **Upper limb buds** are recognizable by day 26 or 27 as small swellings on the ventrolateral body walls (see Figs. 5-8*D* and *E*). The **otic pits**, the primordia of the internal ears, are also visible. Ectodermal thickenings (**lens placodes**) indicating the future lenses of the eyes are visible on the sides of the head. The fourth pair of pharyngeal arches and the lower limb buds are visible by the end of the fourth week (see Fig. 5-8*E*). Toward the end of the fourth week, a long tail-like **caudal eminence** is a characteristic feature (Figs. 5-11, 5-12, and 5-13). Rudiments of many of the organ systems, especially the *cardiovascular system*, are established (Fig. 5-14). *By the end of the fourth week, the caudal neuropore is usually closed.*

Fifth Week

Changes in body form are minor during the fifth week compared with those that occurred during the fourth week, but growth of the head exceeds that of other regions (Figs. 5-15 and 5-16). Enlargement of the head is caused mainly by the rapid development of the brain and facial prominences. The face soon contacts the heart prominence. The rapidly growing second pharyngeal arch overgrows the third and fourth arches, forming a lateral ectodermal depression on each side—the **cervical sinus**.

Table 5-1. Criteria for Estimating Developmental Stages in Human Embryos

AGE (DAYS)	FIGURE REFERENCE	CARNEGIE STAGE	NO. OF SOMITES	LENGTH (MM)*	MAIN EXTERNAL CHARACTERISTICS†
20–21	5–1A_1	9	1–3	1.5–3.0	*Flat embryonic disc. Deep neural groove and prominent neural folds. One to three pairs of somites present.* Head fold evident.
22–23	5–8*A* 5–9*A,B*	10	4–12	1.0–3.5	*Embryo straight or slightly curved.* Neural tube forming or formed opposite somites, but widely open at rostral and caudal neuropores. First and second pairs of pharyngeal arches visible.
24–25	5–8*C* 5–10	11	13–20	2.5–4.5	*Embryo curved owing to head and tail folds.* Rostral neuropore closing. Otic placodes present. Optic vesicles formed.
26–27	5–8*D* 5–11	12	21–29	3.0–5.0	*Upper limb buds appear.* Rostral neuropore closed. Caudal neuropore closing. Three pairs of pharyngeal arches visible. Heart prominence distinct. Otic pits present.
28–30	5–8*E* 5–12	13	30–35	4.0–6.0	*Embryo has C-shaped curve.* Caudal neuropore closed. Upper limb buds are flipper-like. Four pairs of pharyngeal arches visible. Lower limb buds appear. Otic vesicles present. Lens placodes distinct. *Tail-like caudal eminence* present.
31–32	5–15 5–16	14	‡	5.0–7.0	*Upper limbs are paddle shaped.* Lens pits and nasal pits visible. Optic cups present.
33–36		15		7.0–9.0	*Handplates formed; digital rays visible.* Lens vesicles present. Nasal pits prominent. *Lower limbs are paddle shaped.* Cervical sinuses visible.
37–40		16		8.0–11.0	*Footplates formed.* Pigment visible in retina. Auricular hillocks developing.
41–43	5–17	17		11.0–14.0	*Digital rays clearly visible in handplates.* Auricular hillocks outline future auricle of external ear. Trunk beginning to straighten. Cerebral vesicles prominent.
44–46		18		13.0–17.0	*Digital rays clearly visible in footplates.* Elbow region visible. Eyelids forming. Notches between the digital rays in the hands. Nipples visible.
47–48	5–18	19		16.0–18.0	*Limbs extend ventrally.* Trunk elongating and straightening. Midgut herniation prominent.
49–51	5–19*C*	20		18.0–22.0	*Upper limbs longer and bent at elbows. Fingers distinct but webbed.* Notches between the digital rays in the feet. Scalp vascular plexus appears.
52–53	5–19	21		22.0–24.0	*Hands and feet approach each other. Fingers are free and longer. Toes distinct but webbed.*
54–55		22		23.0–28.0	*Toes free and longer.* Eyelids and auricles of external ears more developed.
56	5–20 5–21	23		27.0–31.0	*Head more rounded and shows human characteristics.* External genitalia still have sexless appearance. Distinct bulge still present in umbilical cord, caused by herniation of intestines. *Caudal eminence ("tail") has disappeared.*

*The embryonic lengths indicate the usual range. In stages 9 and 10, the measurement is greatest length; in subsequent stages, crown-rump measurements are given (see Fig. 5-23).

†Based on Nishimura et al (1974), O'Rahilly and Müller (1987), Shiota (1991), and Gasser (2004).

‡At this and subsequent stages, the number of somites is difficult to determine and so is not a useful criterion.

Mesonephric ridges indicate the site of the mesonephric kidneys, which are interim excretory organs in humans.

Sixth Week

By the sixth week, embryos show reflex response to touch. The upper limbs begin to show regional differentiation as the elbows and large **handplates** develop (Fig. 5-17). The primordia of the digits (fingers), called **digital rays**, begin to develop in the handplates, which indicate the formation of digits. Embryos in the sixth week show spontaneous movements, such as twitching of the trunk and limbs. Development of the lower limbs occurs 4 to 5 days later than that of the upper limbs. Several small swellings—**auricular hillocks**—develop around the pharyngeal groove or cleft between the first two pharyngeal arches. This groove becomes the **external acoustic meatus** (external auditory canal). The auricular hillocks contribute to the formation of the auricle, the shell-shaped part of the external ear. Largely because retinal pigment has formed, the eye is now obvious. The head is now much larger relative to the trunk and is bent over the **heart prominence**. This head position results from bending in the cervical (neck) region. The trunk and neck have begun to straighten. The intestines enter the extraembryonic coelom in the proximal part of the umbilical cord. This umbilical herniation is a normal event in the embryo. The herniation occurs because the abdominal cavity is too small at this age to accommodate the rapidly growing intestine.

Seventh Week

The limbs undergo considerable change during the seventh week. Notches appear between the digital rays in the handplates, clearly indicating the future digits

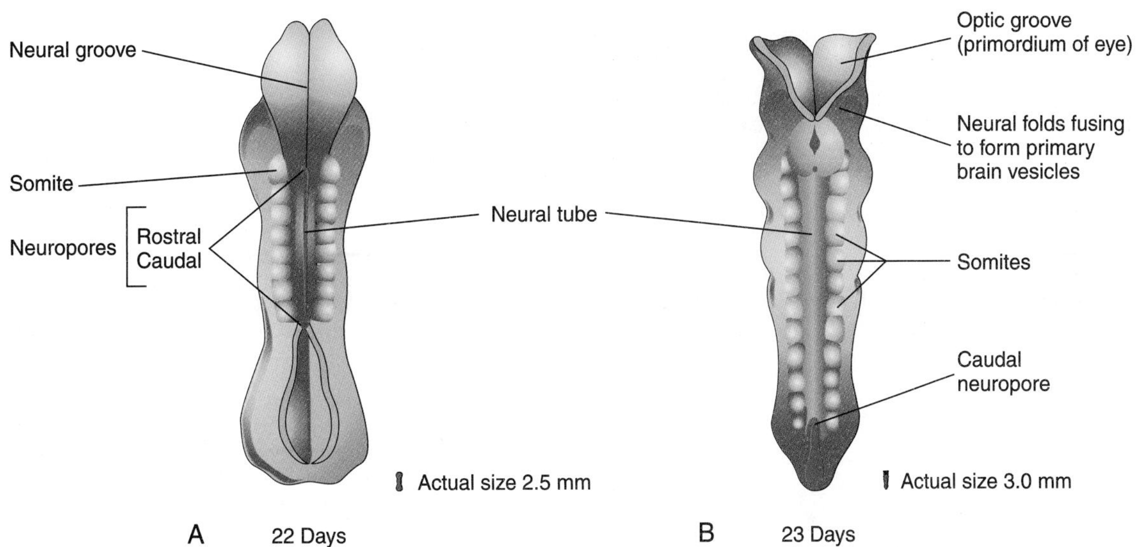

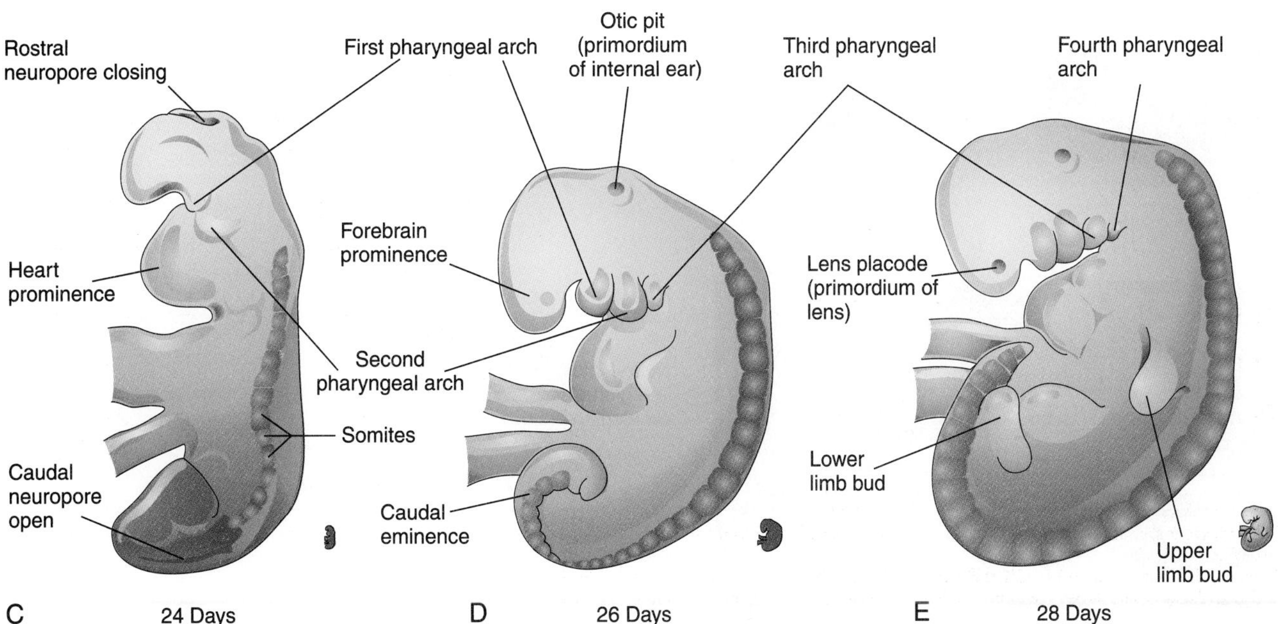

FIGURE 5-8. A and **B,** Drawings of dorsal views of embryos early in the fourth week showing 8 and 12 pairs of somites, respectively. **C, D,** and **E,** Lateral views of older embryos showing 16, 27, and 33 pairs of somites, respectively. The rostral neuropore is normally closed by 25 to 26 days, and the caudal neuropore is usually closed by the end of the fourth week.

(Fig. 5-18). Communication between the primordial gut and umbilical vesicle is now reduced to a relatively slender duct, the omphaloenteric duct. By the end of the seventh week, ossification of the bones of the upper limbs has begun.

Eighth Week

At the beginning of this final week of the embryonic period, the digits of the hand are separated but noticeably webbed (Fig. 5-19). Notches are now clearly visible between the digital rays of the feet. The caudal eminence is still present but stubby. The **scalp vascular plexus** has appeared and forms a characteristic band around the head. By the end of the eighth week, all regions of the limbs are apparent, the digits have lengthened and are completely separated (Fig. 5-20). Purposeful limb movements first occur during this week. Ossification begins in the femur. All evidence of the caudal eminence has disappeared by the end of the eighth week. Both hands and feet approach each other ventrally. At the end of the eighth week, the embryo has distinct human characteristics (Fig. 5-21); however, the head is still disproportionately large, constituting almost half of the embryo. The neck region is established, and the eyelids are more obvious. The eyelids are closing, and by the end of the eighth week, they begin to unite by epithelial fusion. The intestines are still in the proximal portion of the umbilical cord. The auricles of the external ears begin to assume their final shape. Although there are

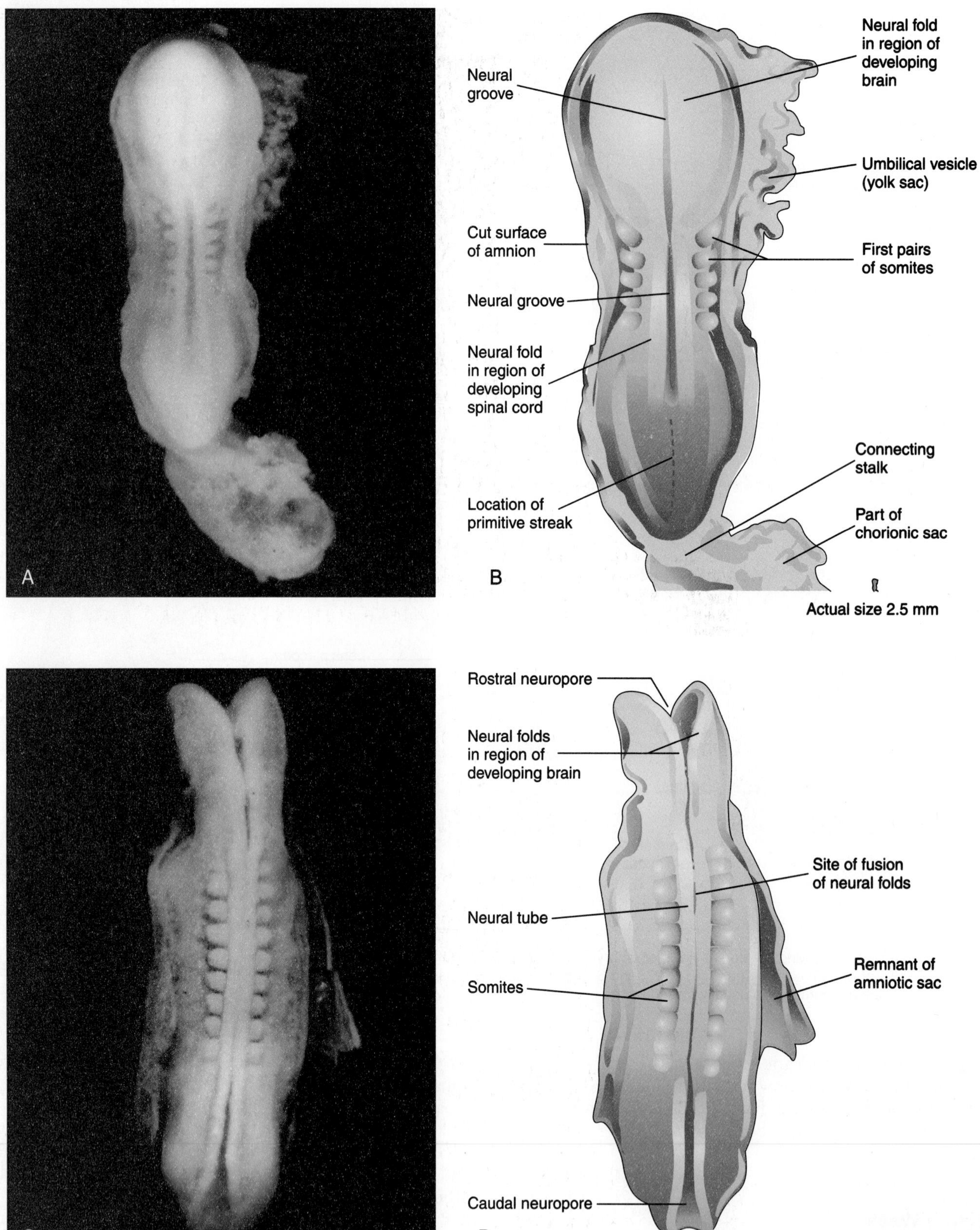

FIGURE 5-9. **A,** Dorsal view of a five-somite embryo at Carnegie stage 10, approximately 22 days. Observe the neural folds and deep neural groove. The neural folds in the cranial region have thickened to form the primordium of the brain. **B,** Illustration of the structures shown in **A**. Most of the amniotic and chorionic sacs have been cut away to expose the embryo. **C,** Dorsal view of an older eight-somite embryo at Carnegie stage 10. The neural tube is in open communication with the amniotic cavity at the cranial and caudal ends through the rostral and caudal neuropores, respectively. **D,** Diagram of the structures shown in **C**. The neural folds have fused opposite the somites to form the neural tube (primordium of spinal cord in this region). (**A** and **C,** From Moore KL, Persaud TVN, Shiota K: Color Atlas of Clinical Embryology, 2nd ed. Philadelphia, WB Saunders, 2000.)

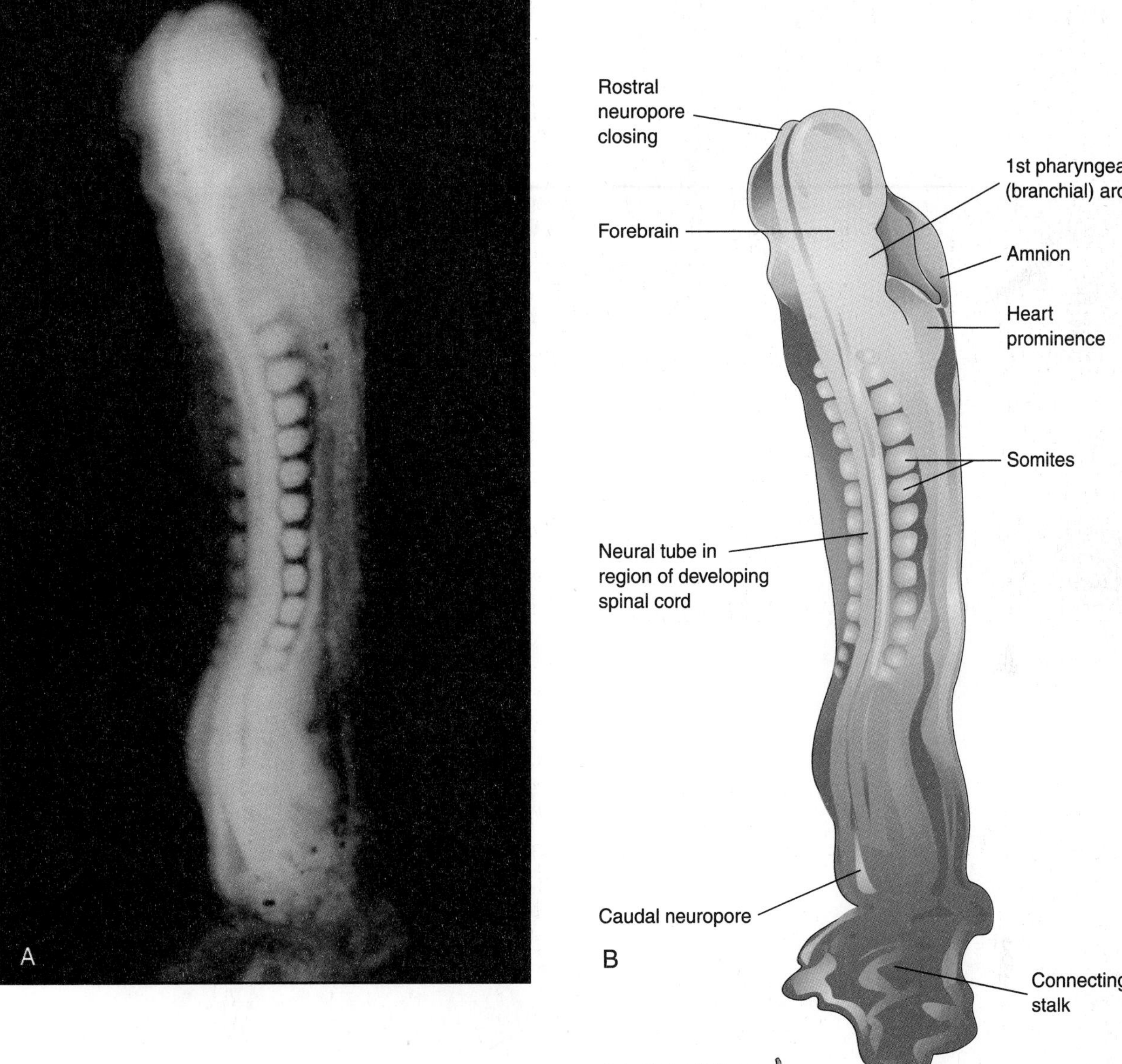

FIGURE 5-10. **A,** Dorsal view of a 13-somite embryo at Carnegie stage 11, approximately 24 days. The rostral neuropore is closing, but the caudal neuropore is wide open. **B,** Illustration of the structures shown in **A**. The embryo is lightly curved because of folding at the cranial and caudal ends. (**A,** From Moore KL, Persaud TVN, Shiota K: Color Atlas of Clinical Embryology, 2nd ed. Philadelphia, WB Saunders, 2000.)

sex differences in the appearance of the external genitalia, they are not distinctive enough to permit accurate sexual identification (see Chapter 12).

ESTIMATION OF GESTATIONAL AND EMBRYONIC AGE

By convention, obstetricians date pregnancy from the first day of the LNMP. This is the gestational age. Embryonic age begins at fertilization, approximately 2 weeks after the LNMP. Fertilization age is used in patients who have undergone in vitro fertilization or artificial insemination (see Chapter 2).

Knowledge of embryonic age is important because it affects clinical management, especially when invasive procedures such as chorionic villus sampling and amniocentesis are necessary (see Chapter 6). In some women, estimation of gestational age from the menstrual history alone may be unreliable. The probability of error in establishing the LNMP is highest in women who become pregnant after cessation of oral contraception because the interval between discontinuance of hormones and the onset of ovulation is highly variable. In others, slight uterine bleeding ("spotting"), which sometimes occurs

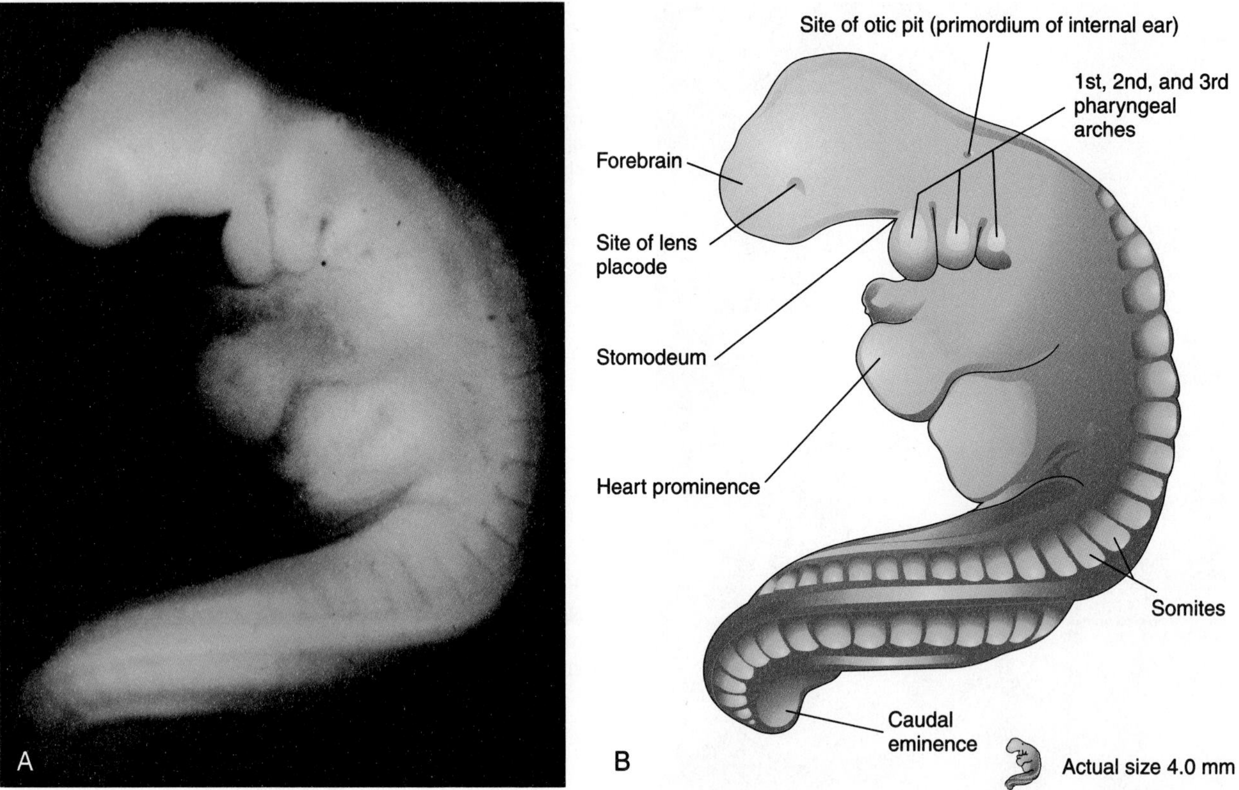

FIGURE 5-11. **A,** Lateral view of a 27-somite embryo at Carnegie stage 12, approximately 26 days. The embryo is curved, especially its tail-like caudal eminence. Observe the lens placode (primordium of lens of eye) and the otic pit indicating early development of internal ear. **B,** Illustration of the structures shown in **A**. The rostral neuropore is closed, and three pairs of pharyngeal arches are present. (**A,** From Nishimura H, Semba R, Tanimura T, Tanaka O: Prenatal Development of the Human with Special Reference to Craniofacial Structures: An Atlas. Washington, DC, National Institutes of Health, 1977.)

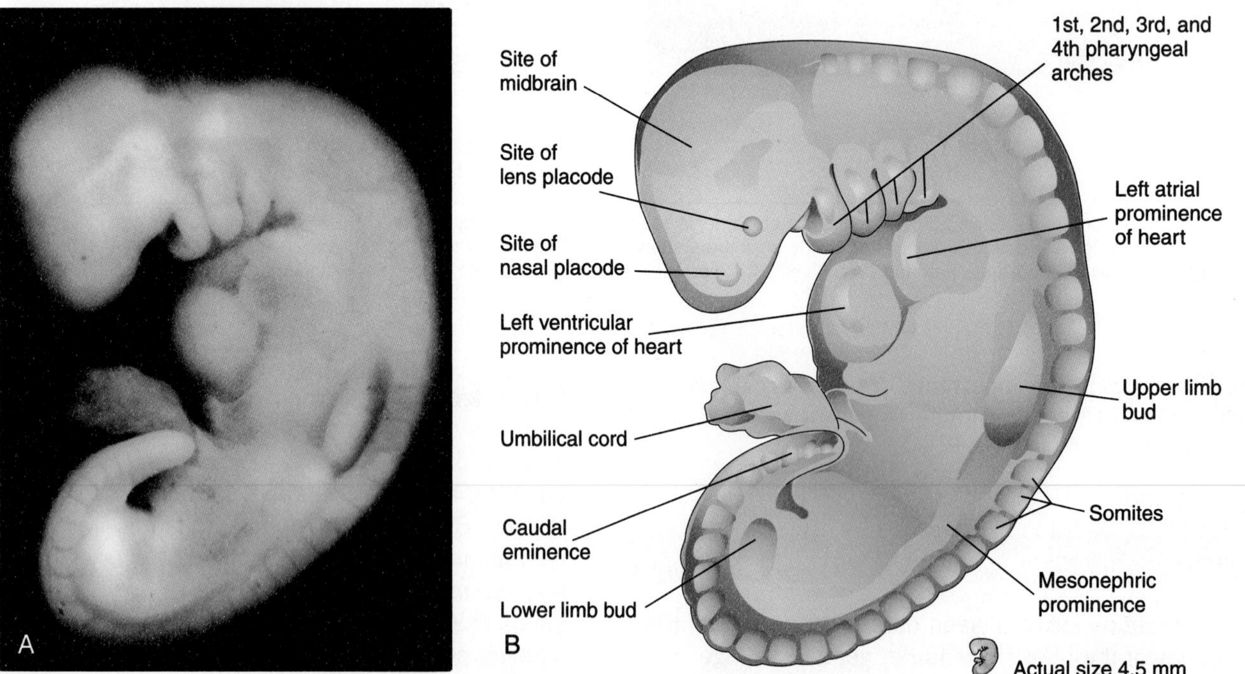

FIGURE 5-12. **A,** Lateral view of an embryo at Carnegie stage 13, approximately 28 days. The primordial heart is large, and its division into a primordial atrium and ventricle is visible. The rostral and caudal neuropores are closed. **B,** Drawing indicating the structures shown in **A**. The embryo has a characteristic C-shaped curvature, four pharyngeal arches, and upper and lower limb buds. (**A,** From Nishimura H, Semba R, Tanimura T, Tanaka O: Prenatal Development of the Human with Special Reference to Craniofacial Structures: An Atlas. Washington, DC, National Institutes of Health, 1977.)

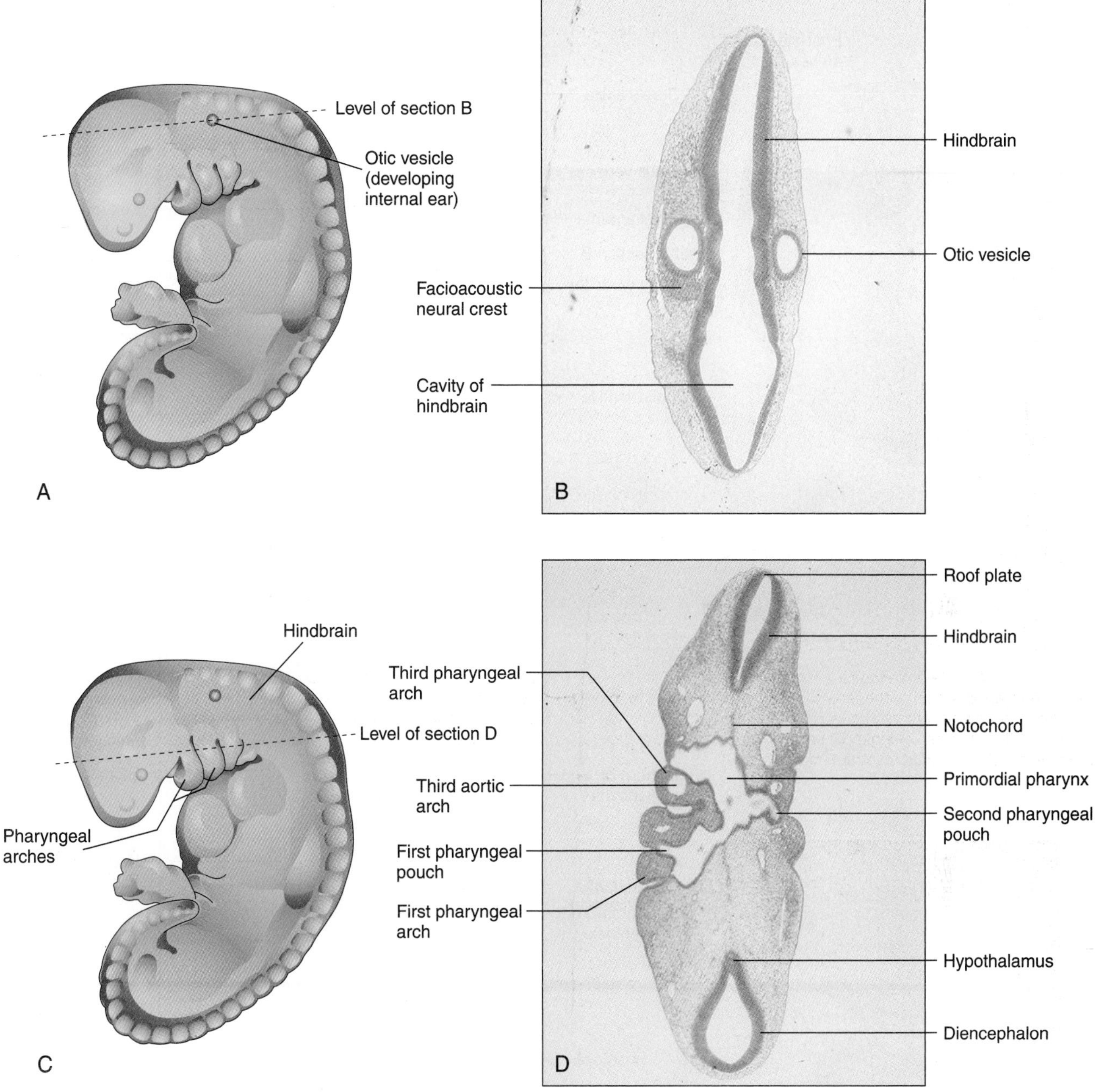

FIGURE 5-13. **A,** Drawing of an embryo at Carnegie stage 13, approximately 28 days. **B,** Photomicrograph of a section of the embryo at the level shown in **A**. Observe the hindbrain and otic vesicle (primordium of internal ear). **C,** Drawing of same embryo showing the level of the section in **D**. Observe the primordial pharynx and pharyngeal arches. (**B** and **D,** From Moore KL, Persaud TVN, Shiota K: Color Atlas of Clinical Embryology, 2nd ed. Philadelphia, WB Saunders, 2000.)

during implantation of the blastocyst, may be incorrectly regarded by a woman as light menstruation. Other contributing factors to LNMP unreliability may include oligomenorrhea (scanty menstruation), pregnancy in the postpartum period (i.e., several weeks after childbirth), and use of intrauterine devices. Despite possible sources of error, the LNMP is a reliable criterion in most cases. Ultrasound assessment of the size of the chorionic (gestational) cavity and its embryonic contents (see Fig. 5-22) enables clinicians to obtain an accurate estimate of the date of conception.

The day on which fertilization occurs is the most accurate reference point for estimating age; this is commonly calculated from the estimated time of ovulation because the oocyte is usually fertilized within 12 hours after ovulation. All statements about age should indicate the reference point used, that is, days after the LNMP or after the estimated time of fertilization.

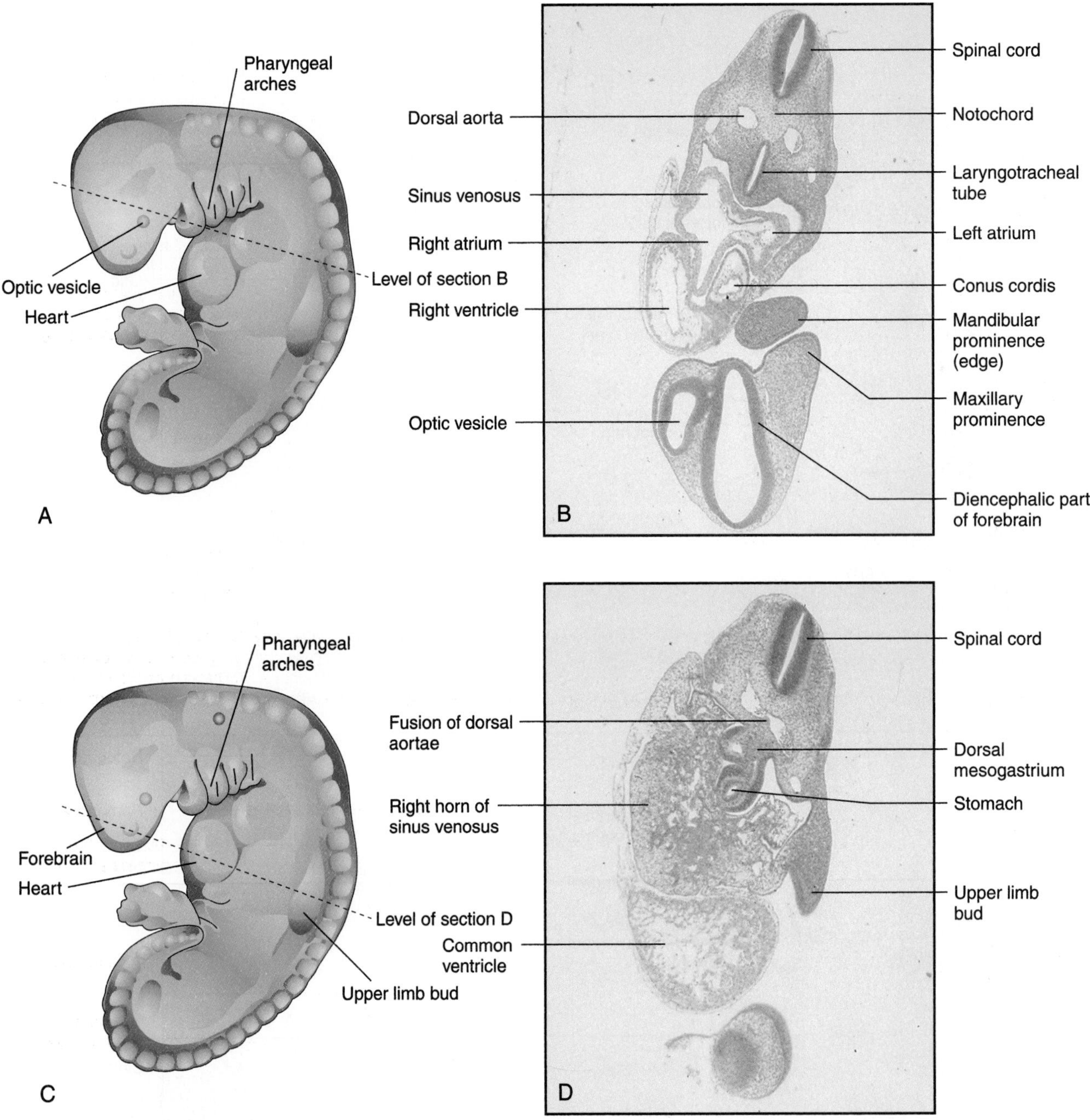

FIGURE 5-14. **A,** Drawing of an embryo at Carnegie stage 13, approximately 28 days. **B,** Photomicrograph of a section of the embryo at the level shown in **A**. Observe the parts of the primordial heart. **C,** Drawing of the same embryo showing the level of section in **D**. Observe the primordial heart and stomach. (**B** and **D,** From Moore KL, Persaud TVN, Shiota K: Color Atlas of Clinical Embryology, 2nd ed. Philadelphia, WB Saunders, 2000.)

ESTIMATION OF EMBRYONIC AGE

Estimates of the age of embryos recovered after a spontaneous abortion, for example, are determined from their external characteristics and measurements of their length (Figs. 5-22 and 5-23; see Table 5-1). Size alone may be an unreliable criterion because some embryos undergo a progressively slower rate of growth before death. The appearance of the developing limbs is a helpful criterion for estimating embryonic age. Because embryos of the third and early fourth weeks are straight (see Fig. 5-23*A*), measurements indicate the greatest length. The crown-rump length is most frequently used for older embryos (see Fig. 5-23*B*). Because no anatomic marker clearly indicates the crown or rump, one assumes that the longest crown-rump length is the most accurate. Standing height, or crown-heel length, is sometimes measured for 8-week embryos. The length of an embryo is only one criterion for establishing age (see Table 5-1). The Carnegie Embryonic Staging System is used internationally (see Table 5-1); its use enables comparisons to be made between the findings of one person and those of another.

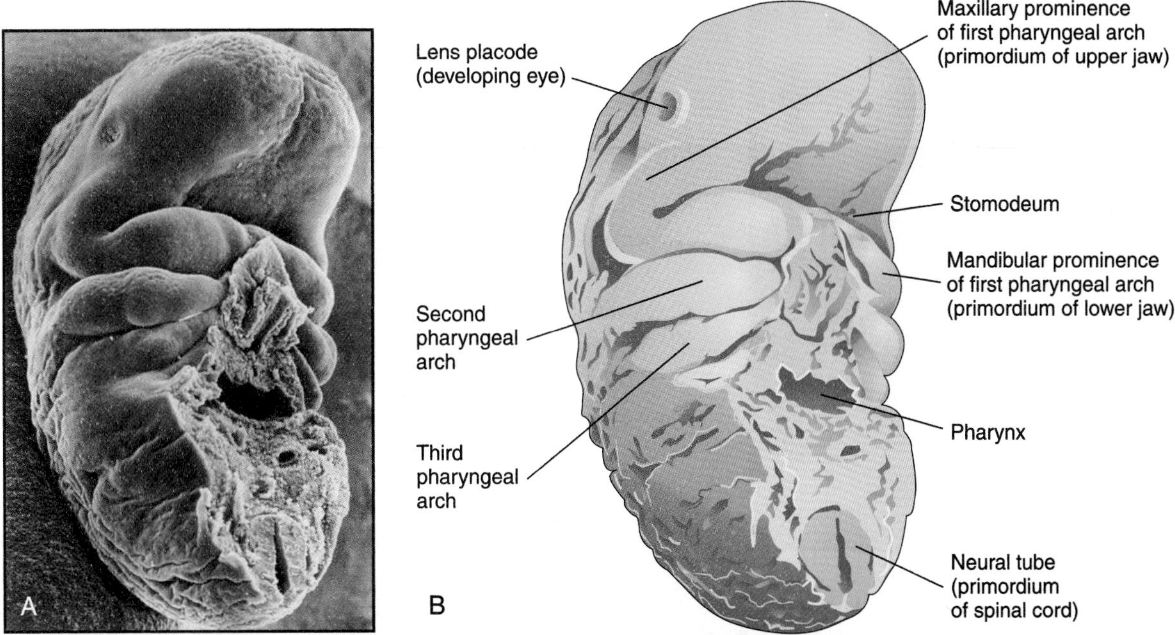

FIGURE 5-15. **A,** Scanning electron micrograph of the craniofacial region of a human embryo of approximately 32 days (Carnegie stage 14, 6.8 mm). Three pairs of pharyngeal arches are present. The maxillary and mandibular prominences of the first arch are clearly delineated. Observe the large mouth located between the maxillary prominences and the fused mandibular prominences. **B,** Drawing of the scanning electron micrograph illustrating the structures shown in **A**. (**A,** Courtesy of the late Professor K. Hinrichsen, Ruhr-Universität Bochum, Bochum, Germany.)

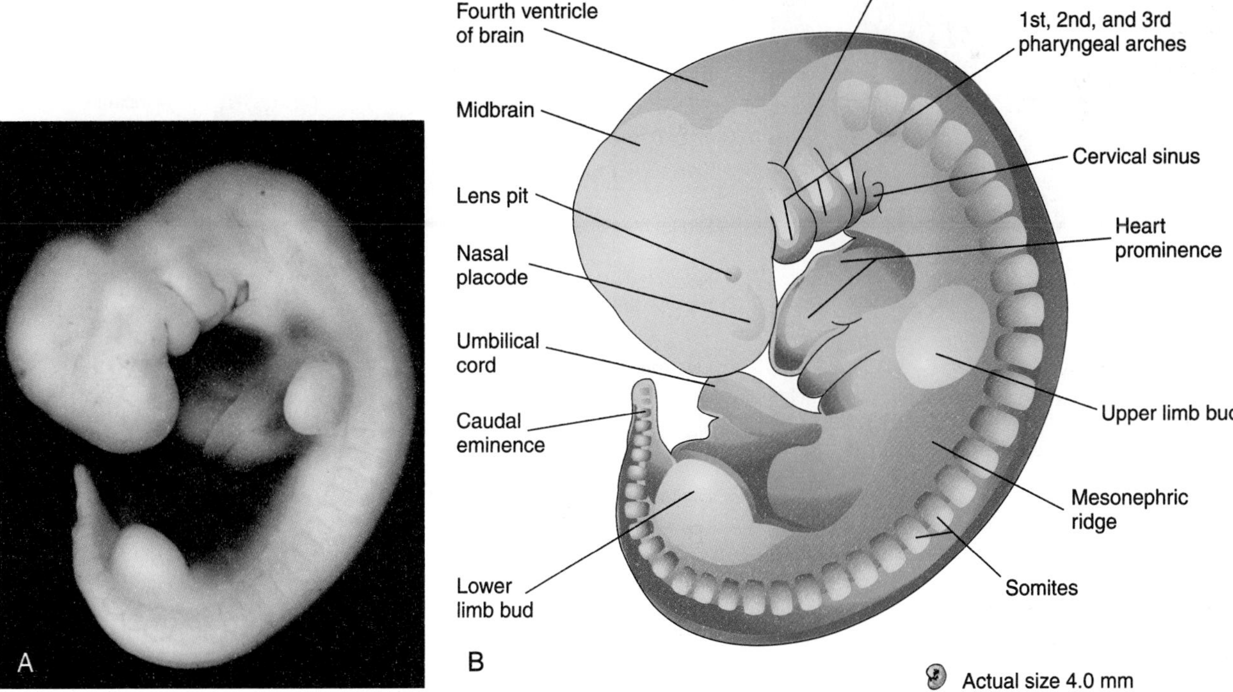

FIGURE 5-16. **A,** Lateral view of an embryo at Carnegie stage 14, approximately 32 days. The second pharyngeal arch has overgrown the third arch, forming a depression known as the cervical sinus. The mesonephric ridge indicates the site of the mesonephric kidney, an interim kidney (see Chapter 12). **B,** Illustration of the structures shown in **A**. The upper limb buds are paddle shaped and the lower limb buds are flipper-like. (**A,** From Nishimura H, Semba R, Tanimura T, Tanaka O: Prenatal Development of the Human with Special Reference to Craniofacial Structures: An Atlas. Washington, DC, National Institutes of Health, 1977.)

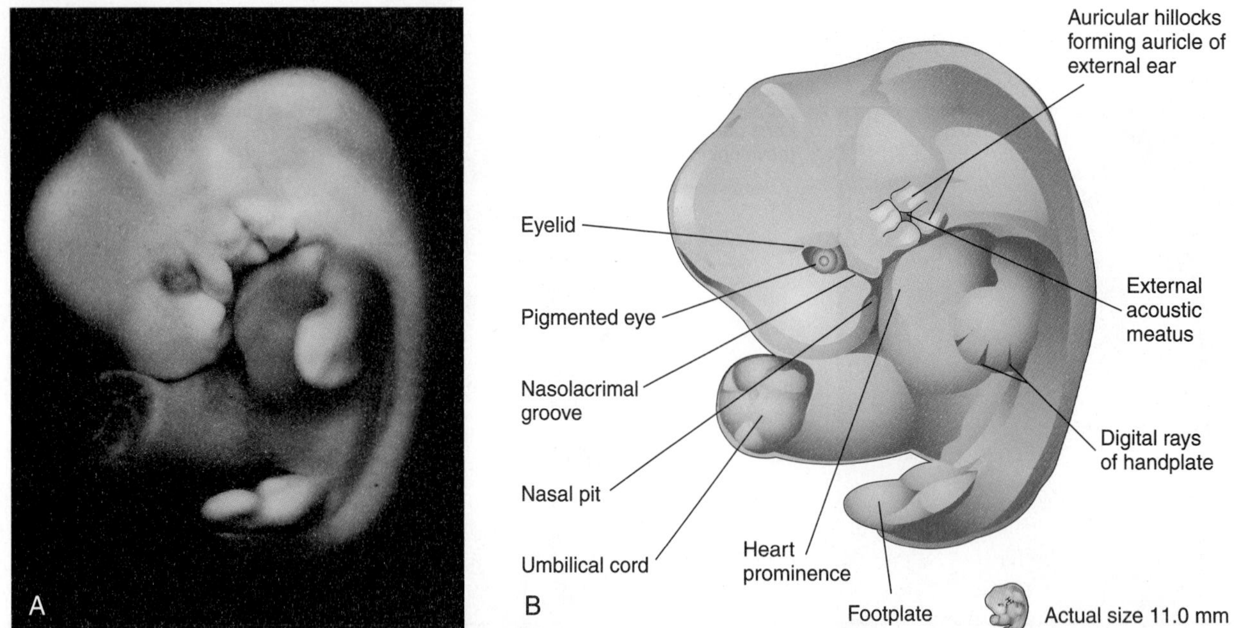

FIGURE 5-17. **A,** Lateral view of an embryo at Carnegie stage 17, approximately 42 days. Digital rays are visible in the handplate, indicating the future site of the digits. **B,** Drawing illustrating the structures shown in **A**. The eye, auricular hillocks, and external acoustic meatus are now obvious. (**A,** From Moore KL, Persaud TVN, Shiota K: Color Atlas of Clinical Embryology, 2nd ed. Philadelphia, WB Saunders, 2000.)

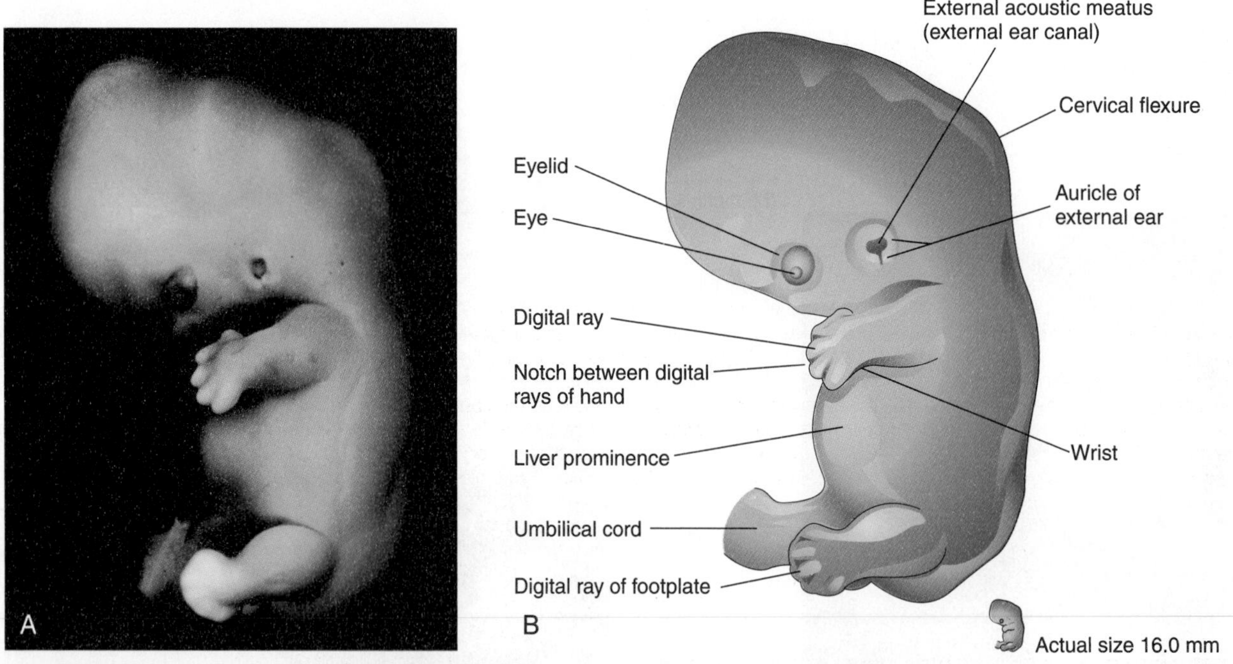

FIGURE 5-18. **A,** Lateral view of an embryo at Carnegie stage 19, about 48 days. The auricle and external acoustic meatus are now clearly visible. Note the relatively low position of the ear at this stage. Digital rays are now visible in the footplate. The prominence of the abdomen is caused mainly by the large size of the liver. **B,** Drawing indicating the structures shown in **A**. Observe the large hand and the notches between the digital rays, which clearly indicate the developing digits or fingers. (**A,** From Moore KL, Persaud TVN, Shiota K: Color Atlas of Clinical Embryology, 2nd ed. Philadelphia, WB Saunders, 2000.)

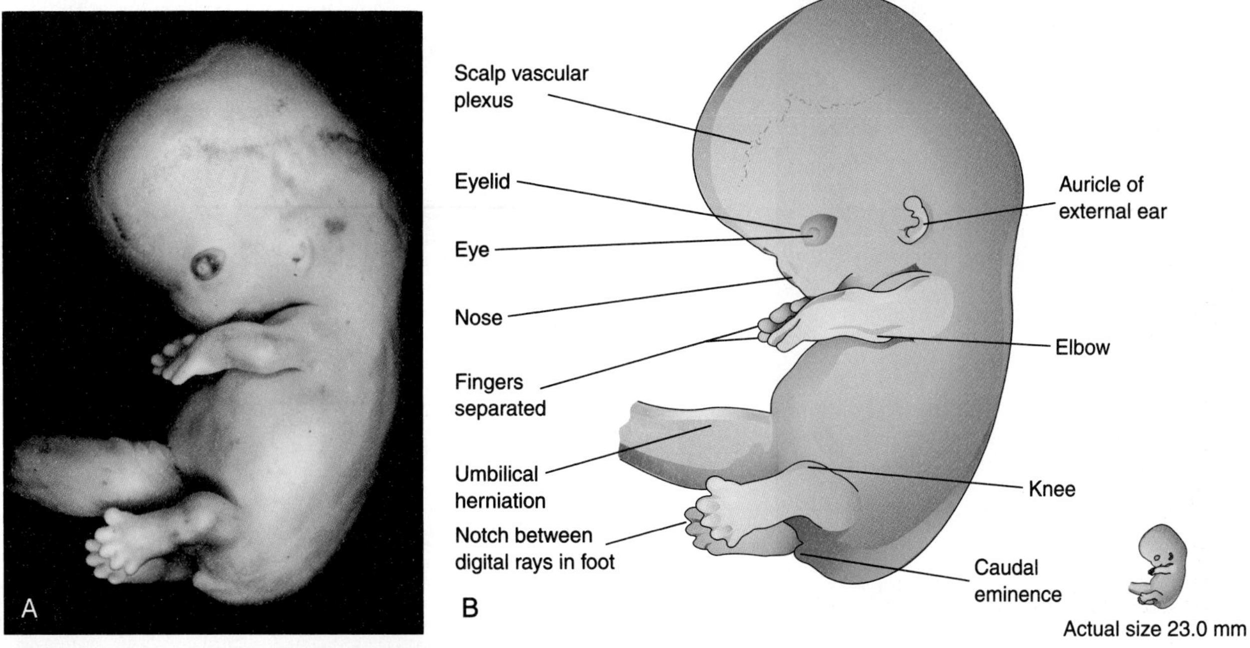

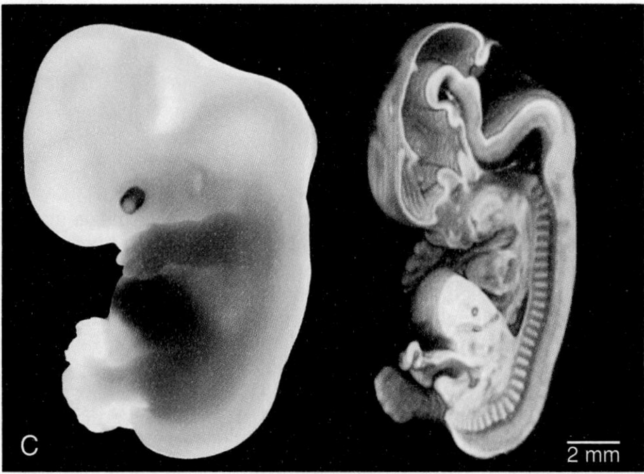

FIGURE 5-19. **A,** Lateral view of an embryo at Carnegie stage 21, approximately 52 days. Note that the feet are fan shaped. The scalp vascular plexus now forms a characteristic band across the head. The nose is stubby and the eye is heavily pigmented. **B,** Illustration of the structures shown in **A**. The fingers are separated and the toes are beginning to separate. **C,** A Carnegie stage 20 human embryo, approximately 50 days after ovulation, imaged with optical microscopy (*left*) and magnetic resonance microscopy (*right*). The three-dimensional data set from magnetic resonance microscopy has been edited to reveal anatomic detail from a mid-sagittal plane. (**A,** From Nishimura H, Semba R, Tanimura T, Tanaka O: Prenatal Development of the Human with Special Reference to Craniofacial Structures: An Atlas. Washington, DC, National Institutes of Health, 1977; **B,** From Moore KL, Persaud TVN, Shiota K: Color Atlas of Clinical Embryology, 2nd ed. Philadelphia, WB Saunders 2000; **C,** Courtesy of Dr. Bradley R. Smith, Center for In Vivo Microscopy, Duke University Medical Center, Durham, NC.)

ULTRASOUND EXAMINATION OF EMBRYOS

Most women seeking obstetric care have at least one ultrasound examination during their pregnancy for one or more of the following reasons:

- Estimation of gestational age for confirmation of clinical dating
- Evaluation of embryonic growth when intrauterine growth retardation is suspected
- Guidance during chorionic villus or amniotic fluid sampling (see Chapter 6)
- Examination of a clinically detected pelvic mass
- Suspected ectopic pregnancy (see Chapter 3)
- Possible uterine abnormality
- Detection of congenital anomalies

Current data indicate that there are no confirmed biologic effects of ultrasonography on embryos or fetuses from the use of diagnostic ultrasound evaluation.

The size of an embryo in a pregnant woman can be estimated using ultrasound measurements. Transvaginal endovaginal/sonography permits an

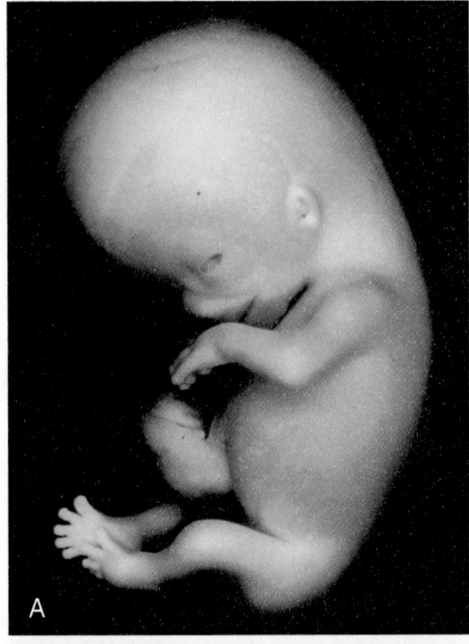

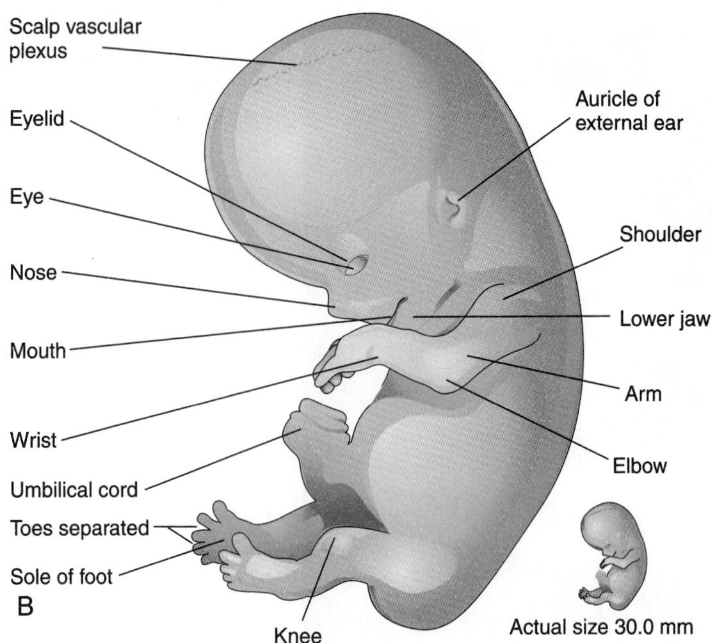

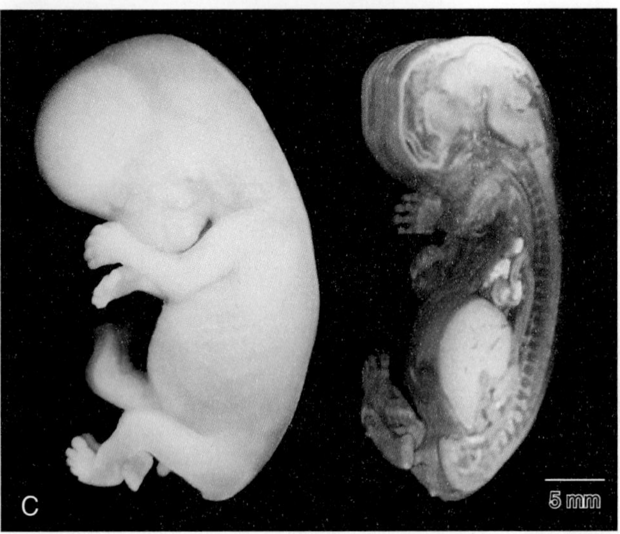

FIGURE 5-20. **A,** Lateral view of an embryo at Carnegie stage 23, approximately 56 days. The embryo has a distinct human appearance. **B,** Illustration of the structures shown in **A**. **C,** A Carnegie stage 23 embryo, approximately 56 days after ovulation, imaged with optical microscopy (*left*) and magnetic resonance microscopy (*right*). (**A,** From Nishimura H, Semba R, Tanimura T, Tanaka O: Prenatal Development of the Human with Special Reference to Craniofacial Structures: An Atlas. Washington, DC, National Institutes of Health, 1977; **B,** From Moore KL, Persaud TVN, Shiota K: Color Atlas of Clinical Embryology, 2nd ed. Philadelphia, WB Saunders, 2000; **C,** Courtesy of Dr. Bradley R. Smith, Center for In Vivo Microscopy, Duke University Medical Center, Durham, NC.)

earlier and more accurate measurement of CRL in early pregnancy. Early in the fifth week, the embryo is 4 to 7 mm long (see Figs. 5-16 and 5-22*A*). During the sixth and seventh weeks, discrete embryonic structures can be visualized (e.g., parts of limbs), and crown-rump measurements are predictive of embryonic age with an accuracy of 1 to 4 days. Furthermore, after the sixth week, dimensions of the head and trunk can be obtained and used for assessment of embryonic age. There is, however, considerable variability in early embryonic growth and development. Differences are greatest before the end of the first 4 weeks of development, but less so by the end of the embryonic period.

SUMMARY OF THE FOURTH TO EIGHTH WEEKS

- At the beginning of the fourth week, *folding in the median and horizontal planes* converts the flat trilaminar embryonic disc into a C-shaped, cylindrical embryo. The formation of the head, caudal eminence, and lateral folds is a continuous sequence of events that results in a constriction between the embryo and the umbilical vesicle (yolk sac).
- As the head folds ventrally, part of the endodermal layer is incorporated into the developing embryonic head region as the *foregut*. Folding of the head region also results in the *oropharyngeal membrane and heart being carried ventrally*, and the developing brain becoming the most cranial part of the embryo.
- As the caudal eminence folds ventrally, part of the endodermal germ layer is incorporated into the caudal

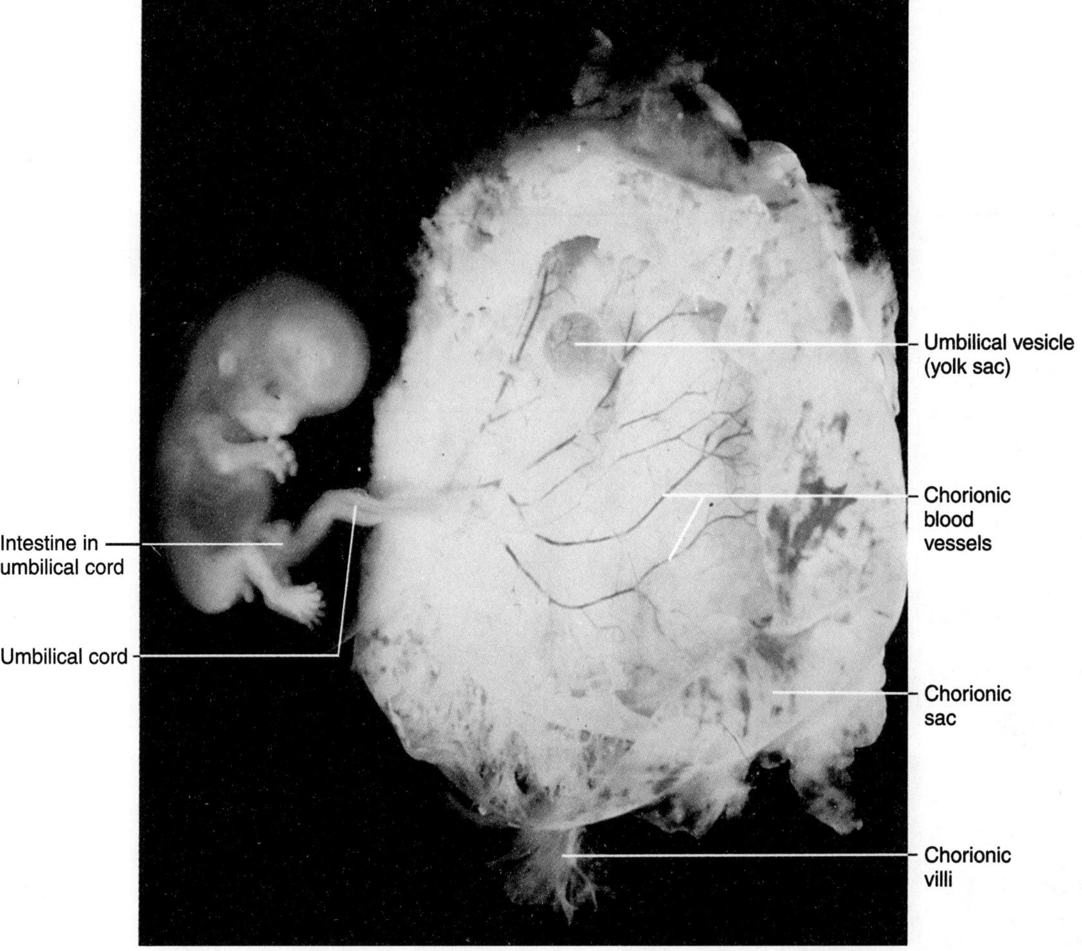

FIGURE 5-21. Lateral view of an embryo and its chorionic sac at Carnegie stage 23, approximately 56 days. Observe the human appearance of the embryo. (From Nishimura H, Semba R, Tanimura T, Tanaka O: Prenatal Development of the Human with Special Reference to Craniofacial Structures: An Atlas. Washington, DC, National Institutes of Health, 1977.)

end of the embryo as the *hindgut*. The terminal part of the hindgut expands to form the *cloaca*. Folding of the caudal region also results in the cloacal membrane, allantois, and connecting stalk being carried to the ventral surface of the embryo.

- Folding of the embryo in the horizontal plane incorporates part of the endoderm into the embryo as the *midgut*.
- The umbilical vesicle remains attached to the midgut by a narrow omphaloenteric duct (yolk stalk). During folding of the embryo in the horizontal plane, the *primordia of the lateral and ventral body walls are formed*. As the amnion expands, it envelops the connecting stalk, omphaloenteric duct, and allantois, thereby forming an epithelial covering for the umbilical cord.
- The *three germ layers differentiate into various tissues and organs* so that by the end of the embryonic period, the beginnings of all the main organ systems have been established.
- The external appearance of the embryo is greatly affected by the formation of the brain, heart, liver, somites, limbs, ears, nose, and eyes. As these structures develop, the appearance of the embryo changes so that *it has unquestionably human characteristics at the end of the eighth week*.
- Because the beginnings of most essential external and internal structures are formed during the fourth to eighth weeks, *this is the most critical period of development*. Developmental disturbances during this period may give rise to major congenital anomalies of the embryo.
- Reasonable estimates of the age of embryos can be determined from the day of onset of the last normal menstrual period (LNMP), the estimated time of fertilization, ultrasound measurements of the chorionic sac and embryo, and examination of external characteristics of the embryo.

CLINICALLY ORIENTED PROBLEMS

CASE 5-1

A 28-year-old woman who has been a heavy cigarette smoker since her teens was informed that she was in the second month of pregnancy.

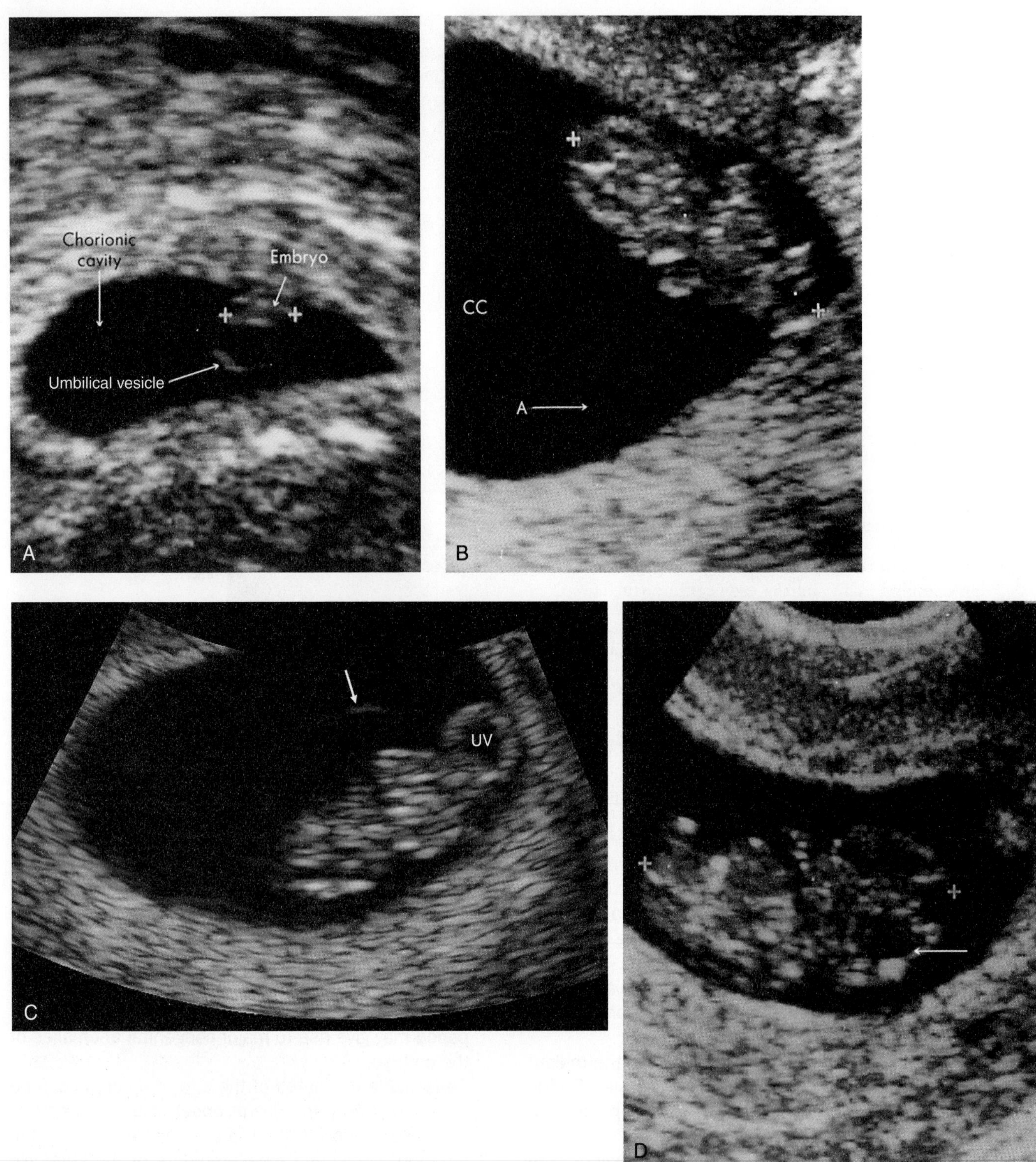

FIGURE 5-22. Ultrasound images of embryos. **A,** Crown-rump length is 4.8 mm. The 4.5-week embryo is indicated by the measurement cursors (+). Ventral to the embryo is the umbilical vesicle. The chorionic cavity appears black. **B,** Coronal scan of 5-week embryo (crown-rump length, 2.09 cm). The upper limbs are clearly shown. The embryo is surrounded by a thin amnion (A), which is difficult to see. The fluid in the chorionic cavity (CC) is more particulate than the amniotic fluid. **C,** Ultrasound image of a 6-week embryo (8 weeks gestational age) Observe the umbilical vesicle (UV) and the amnion (*arrow*). **D,** Sagittal scan of a 7-week embryo (CRL of 2.14 cm) demonstrating the eye, limbs, and the developing fourth ventricle (arrow) of the brain. (**A, B,** and **D,** Courtesy of E.A. Lyons, MD, Professor of Radiology and Obstetrics and Gynecology, Health Sciences Centre, University of Manitoba, Winnipeg, Manitoba, Canada. **C,** Courtesy of Dr. G. J. Reid, Department of Obstetrics, Gynecology, and Reproductive Sciences, University of Manitoba, Women's Hospital, Winnipeg, Manitoba, Canada.)

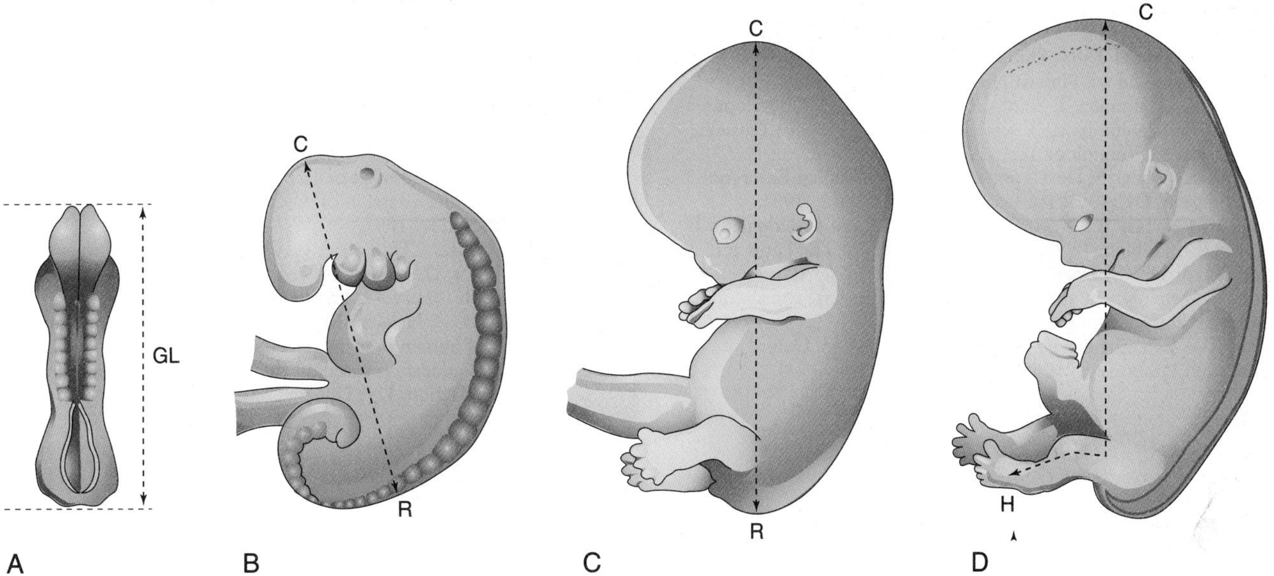

FIGURE 5-23. Illustrations of methods used to measure the length of embryos. **A,** Greatest length (GL). **B** and **C,** Crown (C)-rump (R) length. **D,** Crown (C)-heel (H) length.

- What would the doctor likely tell the patient about her smoking habit and the use of other drugs (e.g., alcohol)?

CASE 5-2

Physicians usually discuss the critical period of development with their patients.

- Why is the embryonic period such a critical stage of development?

CASE 5-3

- A patient was concerned about what she had read in the newspaper about recent effects of drugs on laboratory animals.
- Can one predict the possible harmful effects of drugs on the human embryo from studies performed in experimental animals?
- Discuss germ layer formation and organogenesis.

CASE 5-4

A 30-year-old woman was unsure when her LNMP was. She stated that her periods were irregular.

- Why may information about the starting date of a pregnancy provided by a patient be unreliable?
- What clinical techniques are now available for evaluating embryonic age?

CASE 5-5

A woman who had just become pregnant told her doctor that she had accidentally taken a sleeping pill given to her by a friend. She wondered whether it could harm the development of her baby's limbs.

- Would a drug known to cause severe limb defects be likely to cause these abnormalities if it was administered during the eighth week?
- Discuss the mechanism of the action of these teratogens (see Chapter 20).

Discussion of these problems appears at the back of the book.

References and Suggested Reading

Ashe HL, Briscoe J: The interpretation of morphogen gradients. Development 133:385, 2006.

Barnea ER, Hustin J, Jauniaux E (eds): The First Twelve Weeks of Gestation. Berlin, Springer-Verlag, 1992.

Bhalla US: Models of cell signaling pathways. Curr Opin Genet Dev 14:375, 2004.

Cooke J: Vertebrate left and right: Finally a cascade, but first a flow? BioEssays 21:537, 1999.

Dickey RP, Gasser RF: Computer analysis of the human embryo growth curve: Differences between published ultrasound findings on living embryos in utero and data on fixed specimens. Anat Rec 237:400, 1993.

Dickey RP, Gasser RF: Ultrasound evidence for variability in the size and development of normal human embryos before the tenth post-insemination week after assisted reproductive technologies. Hum Reprod 8:331, 1993.

Filly RA, Hadlock FP: Sonographic determination of menstrual age. In Callen PW (ed): Ultrasonography in Obstetrics and Gynecology, 4th ed. Philadelphia, WB Saunders, 2000.

Gasser, RF: Digitally reproduced embryonic morphology DVD. Computer Imaging Laboratory, Cell Biology and Anatomy, LSU Health Sciences Center, New Orleans, LA, 2004.

Gilbert SF: Developmental Biology, 7th ed. Sunderland, Sinauer, 2003.

Hardin J, Walston T: Models of morphogenesis: The mechanisms and mechanics of cell rearrangement. Curr Opin Genet Dev 14: 399, 2004.

Iffy L, Shepard TH, Jakobovits A, et al: The rate of growth in young human embryos of Streeter's horizons XIII and XXIII. Acta Anat 66:178, 1967.

Jirásek JE: An Atlas of Human Prenatal Developmental Mechanics. Anatomy and Staging. London and New York, Taylor & Francis, 2004.

Kalousek DK, Fitch N, Paradice BA: Pathology of the Human Embryo and Previable Fetus: An Atlas. New York, Springer-Verlag, 1990.

Laing FC, Frates MC: Ultrasound evaluation during the first trimester of pregnancy. In Callen PW (ed): Ultrasonography in Obstetrics and Gynecology, 4th ed. Philadelphia, WB Saunders, 2000.

Lerner JP: Fetal growth and well-being. Obstet Gynecol Clin N Am 31:159, 2004.
Moore KL, Persaud TVN, Shiota K: Color Atlas of Clinical Embryology, 2nd ed. Philadelphia, WB Saunders, 2000.
Nishimura H, Tanimura T, Semba R, Uwabe C: Normal development of early human embryos: Observation of 90 specimens at Carnegie stages 7 to 13. Teratology 10:1, 1974.
O'Rahilly R, Müller F: Developmental Stages in Human Embryos. Washington, DC: Carnegie Institute of Washington, 1987.
Persaud TVN, Hay JC: Normal embryonic and fetal development. In Reece EA, Hobbins JC (eds): Clinical Obstetrics: The Fetus and Mother, 3rd ed. Blackwell Publishing, UK, 2006, pp 19–32.
Shiota K: Development and intrauterine fate of normal and abnormal human conceptuses. Congen Anom 31:67, 1991.
Slack JMW: Essential Developmental Biology, 2nd ed. Oxford, Blackwell Publishing, 2006.
Streeter GL: Developmental horizons in human embryos: Description of age groups XV, XVI, XVII, and XVIII. Contrib Embryol Carnegie Inst 32:133, 1948.
Streeter GL: Developmental horizons in human embryos: Description of age group XI, 13 to 20 somites, and age group XII, 21 to 29 somites. Contrib Embryol Carnegie Inst 30:211, 1942.
Streeter GL: Developmental horizons in human embryos: Description of age group XIII, embryos of 4 or 5 millimeters long, and age group XIV, period of identification of the lens vesicle. Contrib Embryol Carnegie Inst 31:27, 1945.
Streeter GL, Heuser CH, Corner GW: Developmental horizons in human embryos: Description of age groups XIX, XX, XXI, XXII, and XXIII. Contrib Embryol Carnegie Inst 34:165, 1951.
Yamada S, Uwabe C, Nakatsu-Komatsu T, et al: Graphic and movie illustrations of human prenatal development and their application to embryological education based on the human embryo specimens in the Kyoto Collection. Dev Dynam 235:468, 2006.

6 The Fetal Period: Ninth Week to Birth

Estimation of Fetal Age 96
Trimesters of Pregnancy 97
Measurements and Characteristics of Fetuses 98
Highlights of the Fetal Period 98
Nine to Twelve Weeks 98
Thirteen to Sixteen Weeks 100
Seventeen to Twenty Weeks 100
Twenty-one to Twenty-five Weeks 101
Twenty-six to Twenty-nine Weeks 102
Thirty to Thirty-four Weeks 102
Thirty-five to Thirty-eight Weeks 102
Expected Date of Delivery 103
Factors Influencing Fetal Growth 104
Cigarette Smoking 104
Multiple Pregnancy 104
Alcohol and Illicit Drugs 104
Impaired Uteroplacental and Fetoplacental Blood Flow 104
Genetic Factors and Growth Retardation 104
Procedures for Assessing Fetal Status 104
Ultrasonography 105
Diagnostic Amniocentesis 105
Alpha-fetoprotein Assay 105
Spectrophotometric Studies 105
Chorionic Villus Sampling 106
Sex Chromatin Patterns 106
Cell Cultures and Chromosomal Analysis 106
Fetal Transfusion 107
Fetoscopy 107
Percutaneous Umbilical Cord Blood Sampling 107
Computed Tomography and Magnetic Resonance Imaging 107
Fetal Monitoring 107
Summary of the Fetal Period 107
Clinically Oriented Problems 108

The transformation of an embryo to a fetus is gradual, but the name change is meaningful because it signifies that the embryo has developed into a recognizable human being and that the primordia of all major systems have formed. Development during the fetal period is primarily concerned with rapid body growth and differentiation of tissues, organs, and systems. A notable change occurring during the fetal period is the relative slowdown in the growth of the head compared with the rest of the body. The rate of body growth during the fetal period is very rapid (Table 6-1, Fig. 6-1), and fetal weight gain is phenomenal during the terminal weeks. Periods of normal continuous growth alternate with prolonged intervals of absent growth.

Viability of Fetuses

Viability is defined as the ability of fetuses to survive in the extrauterine environment (i.e., after a premature birth). Fetuses weighing less than 500 g at birth usually do not survive. Many full-term, low birth weight babies result from intrauterine growth restriction (IUGR). Consequently, if given expert postnatal care, some fetuses weighing less than 500 g may survive; they are referred to as extremely low birth weight or immature infants. Most fetuses weighing between 1500 and 2500 g survive, but complications may occur; they are premature infants. Prematurity is one of the most common causes of morbidity and perinatal death.

ESTIMATION OF FETAL AGE

Ultrasound measurements of the crown-rump length (CRL) are taken to determine the size and probable age of the fetus and to provide a prediction of the *expected date of delivery*. Fetal head measurements and femur length are also used to evaluate age. *Gestational age* is commonly used clinically, and it may be confusing because the term seems to imply the actual age of the fetus from fertilization. In fact, this term is most often meant to be synonymous with last normal menstrual period (LNMP). It is important that the person ordering the ultrasound examination and the ultrasonographer use the same terminology.

The intrauterine period may be divided into days, weeks, or months (Table 6-2), but confusion arises if it is not stated whether the age is calculated from the onset of the LNMP or the estimated day of fertilization. Most uncertainty about age arises when months are used, particularly when it is not stated whether calendar months (28–31 days) or lunar months (28 days) are meant. Unless otherwise stated, fetal age in this book is calculated from the estimated time of fertilization.

Table 6–1. Criteria for Estimating Fertilization Age during the Fetal Period

AGE (WEEKS)	CR LENGTH (MM)*	FOOT LENGTH (MM)*	FETAL WEIGHT (G)†	MAIN EXTERNAL CHARACTERISTICS
Previable Fetuses				
9	50	7	8	*Eyelids closing or closed.* Head large and more rounded. External genitalia still not distinguishable as male or female. Intestines in proximal part of umbilical cord. Ears are low-set.
10	61	9	14	*Intestines in abdomen.* Early fingernail development.
12	87	14	45	*Sex distinguishable externally.* Well-defined neck.
14	120	20	110	*Head erect.* Eyes face anteriorly. Ears are close to their definitive position. Lower limbs well developed. Early toenail development.
16	140	27	200	*External ears stand out from head.*
18	160	33	320	*Vernix caseosa covers skin.* Quickening (first movements) felt by mother.
20	190	39	460	*Head and body hair (lanugo) visible.*
Viable Fetuses‡				
22	210	45	630	*Skin wrinkled, translucent, and pink to red.*
24	230	50	820	*Fingernails present.* Lean body.
26	250	55	1000	*Eyelids partially open.* Eyelashes present.
28	270	59	1300	*Eyes wide open.* Good head of hair often present. Skin slightly wrinkled.
30	280	63	1700	*Toenails present.* Body filling out. Testes descending.
32	300	68	2100	*Fingernails reach fingertips.* Skin smooth.
36	340	79	2900	*Body usually plump.* Lanugo (hairs) almost absent. Toenails reach toe-tips. Flexed limbs; firm grasp.
38	360	83	3400	*Prominent chest; breasts protrude.* Testes in scrotum or palpable in inguinal canals. Fingernails extend beyond fingertips.

*These measurements are averages and so may not apply to specific cases; dimensional variations increase with age.

†These weights refer to fetuses that have been fixed for approximately 2 weeks in 10% formalin. Fresh specimens usually weigh approximately 5% less.

‡There is no sharp limit of development, age, or weight at which a fetus automatically becomes viable or beyond which survival is ensured, but experience has shown that it is rare for a baby to survive whose weight is less than 500 g or whose fertilization age is less than 22 weeks. Even fetuses born between 26 and 28 weeks have difficulty surviving, mainly because the respiratory system and the central nervous system are not completely differentiated.

CR, crown-rump.

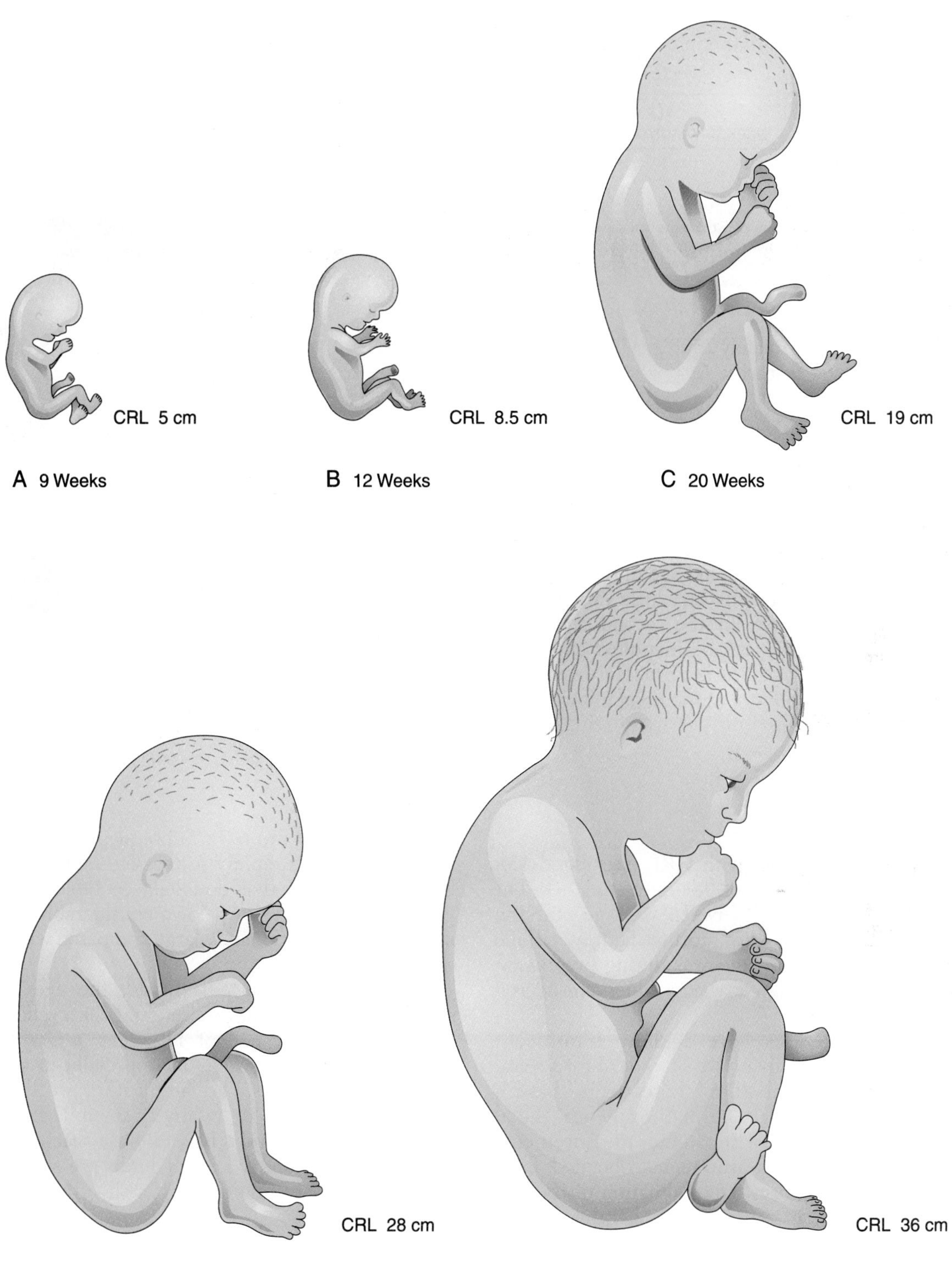

FIGURE 6-1. Drawings of fetuses at various stages of development. Head hair usually begins to appear at 20 weeks and eyebrows and eyelashes are usually recognizable by 24 weeks. The eyes open at approximately 26 weeks. CRL, crown-rump length.

Trimesters of Pregnancy

Clinically, the gestational period is divided into three trimesters, each lasting 3 months. At the end of the first trimester, all major systems are developed (see Fig. 6-1*B*). In the second trimester, the fetus grows sufficiently in size so that good anatomic detail can be visualized during ultrasonography. During this period, most major fetal anomalies can be detected using high-resolution real-time ultrasonography. By the beginning of the third trimester, the fetus may survive if born prematurely. The fetus reaches a major developmental landmark at 35 weeks of

Table 6-2. Comparison of Gestational Time Units and Date of Birth

REFERENCE POINT	DAYS	WEEKS	CALENDAR MONTHS	LUNAR MONTHS
Fertilization*	266	38	$8^3/_4$	$9^1/_2$
LNMP	280	40	$9^1/_4$	10

*The date of birth is calculated as 266 days after the estimated day of fertilizaton or 280 days after the onset of the last normal menstrual period (LNMP). From fertilization to the end of the embryonic period (8 weeks), age is best expressed in days; thereafter, age is often given in weeks.

gestation. It weighs approximately 2500 g, which is used to define the level of fetal maturity. At this stage, the fetus usually survives if born prematurely.

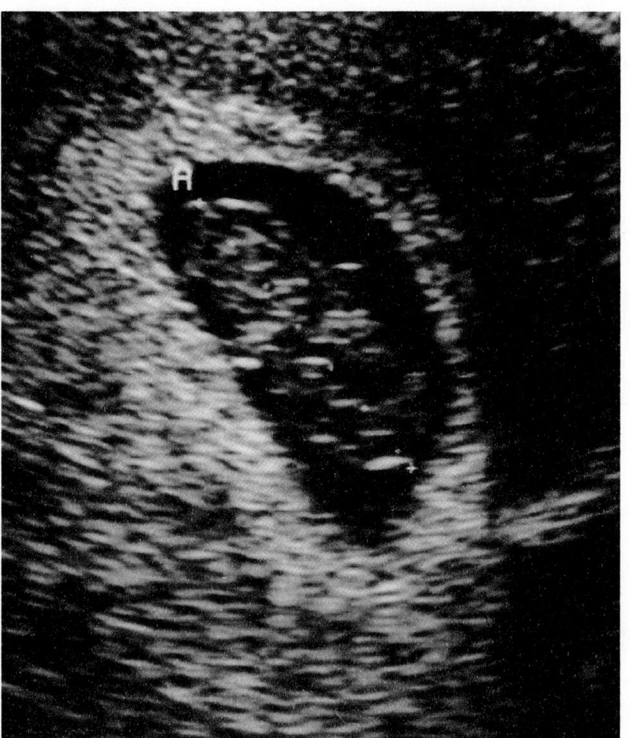

FIGURE 6-2. Ultrasound image of 9-week fetus (11 weeks gestational age). Note the amnion, umbilical cord, amniotic cavity (A), and chorionic cavity. (Courtesy of E.A. Lyons, MD, Professor of Radiology and Obstetrics and Gynecology, Health Sciences Centre, University of Manitoba, Winnipeg, Manitoba, Canada.)

Measurements and Characteristics of Fetuses

Various measurements and external characteristics are useful for estimating fetal age (see Table 6-1). CRL is the method of choice for estimating fetal age until the end of the first trimester because there is very little variability in fetal size during this period. In the second and third trimesters, several structures can be identified and measured ultrasonographically, but the basic measurements are

- Biparietal diameter (diameter of the head between the two parietal eminences)
- Head circumference
- Abdominal circumference
- Femur length
- Foot length

Foot length correlates well with CRL (see Fig. 6-12). Weight is often a useful criterion for estimating age, but there may be a discrepancy between the age and the weight, particularly when the mother had metabolic disturbances such as diabetes mellitus during pregnancy. In these cases, weight often exceeds values considered normal for CRL.

Freshly expelled fetuses have a shiny translucent appearance, whereas those that have been dead for several days before spontaneous abortion (miscarriage) have a tanned appearance and lack normal resilience. Fetal dimensions obtained from ultrasound measurements closely approximate CRL measurements obtained from spontaneously aborted fetuses. Determination of the size of a fetus, especially of its head, is helpful to the obstetrician for management of patients.

HIGHLIGHTS OF THE FETAL PERIOD

There is no formal staging system for the fetal period; however, it is helpful to consider the changes that occur in periods of 4 to 5 weeks.

Nine to Twelve Weeks

At the beginning of the ninth week, the head constitutes approximately half the crown-heel length of the fetus (Figs. 6-1*A*, 6-2, and 6-3). Subsequently, growth in body length accelerates rapidly so that by the end of 12 weeks, the CRL has more than doubled (see Table 6-1). Although growth of the head slows down considerably by this time, it is still disproportionately large compared with the rest of the body.

At 9 weeks, the face is broad, the eyes are widely separated, the ears are low set, and the eyelids are fused (Fig. 6-4*B*). By the end of 12 weeks, *primary ossification centers* appear in the skeleton, especially in the cranium (skull) and long bones. Early in the ninth week, the legs are short and the thighs are relatively small. By the end of 12 weeks, the upper limbs have almost reached their final relative lengths, but the lower limbs are still not so well developed and are slightly shorter than their final relative lengths.

The external genitalia of males and females appear similar until the end of the ninth week. Their mature fetal form is not established until the 12th week. Intestinal coils are clearly visible in the proximal end of the umbilical cord until the middle of the tenth week (see Fig. 6-4*B*). By the 11th week, the intestines have returned to the abdomen (Fig. 6-5).

At 9 weeks, the liver is the major site of *erythropoiesis* (formation of red blood cells). By the end of 12 weeks, this activity has decreased in the liver and has begun in the spleen. *Urine formation* begins between the 9th and 12th weeks, and urine is discharged through the urethra into the amniotic fluid. The fetus reabsorbs some amniotic fluid after swallowing it. Fetal waste products are

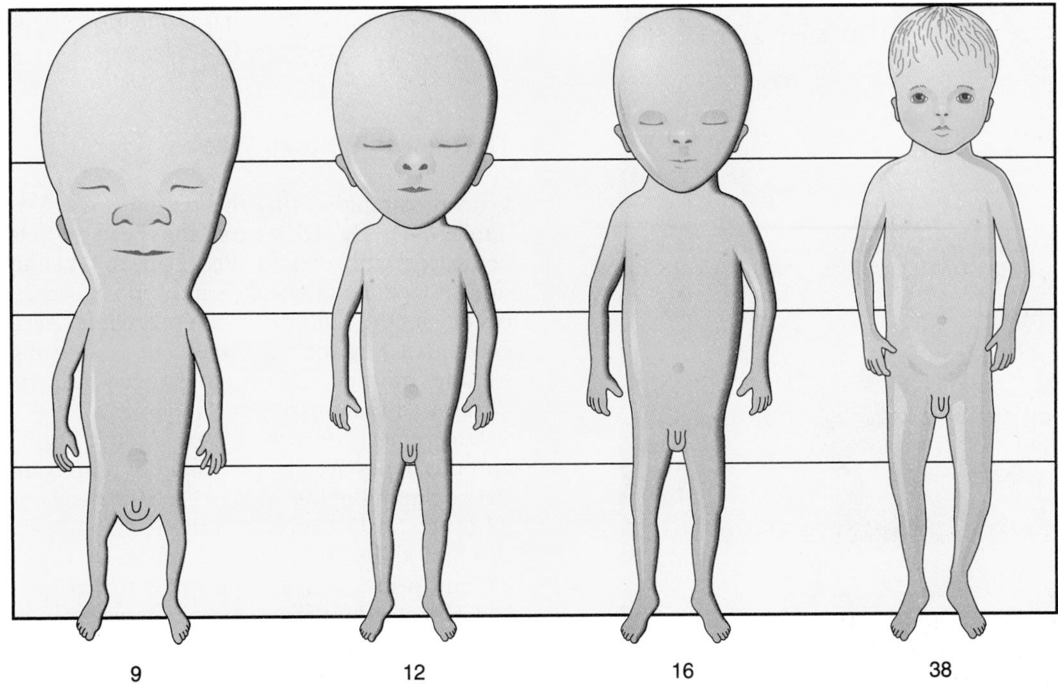

FIGURE 6-3. Diagram illustrating the changing proportions of the body during the fetal period. At 9 weeks, the head is approximately half the crown-heel length of the fetus. By 36 weeks, the circumferences of the head and the abdomen are approximately equal. After this (38 weeks), the circumference of the abdomen may be greater. All stages are drawn to the same total height.

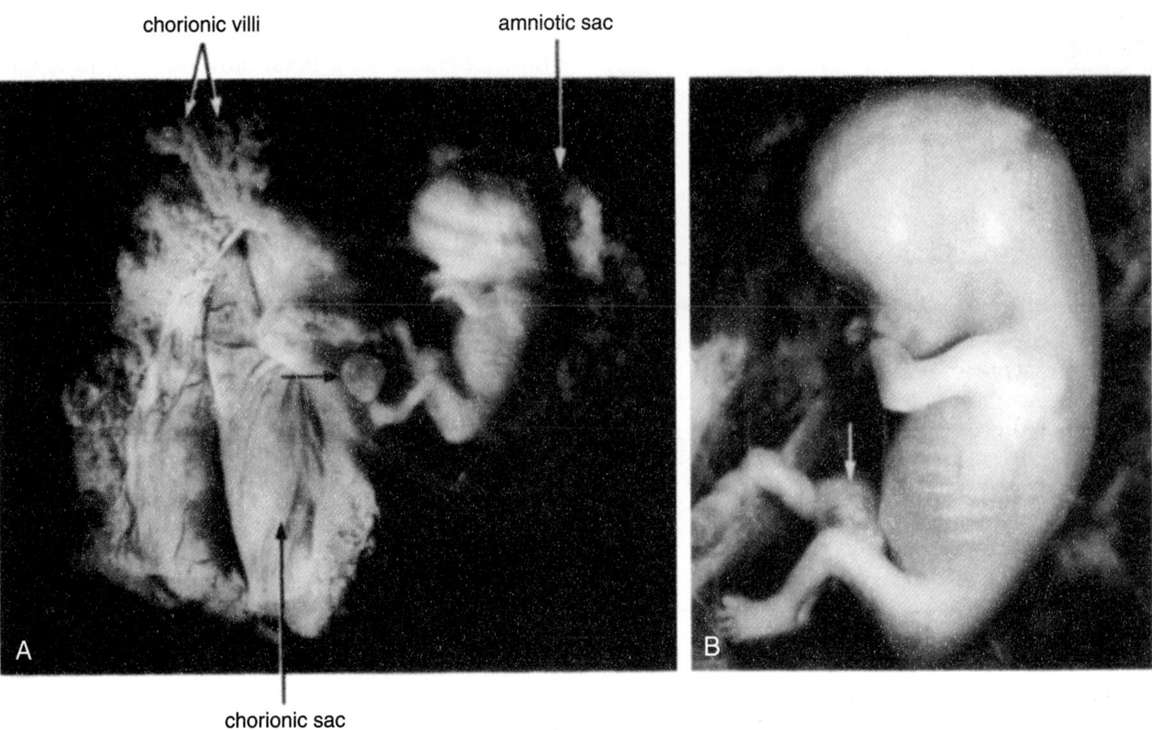

FIGURE 6-4. A 9-week fetus in the amniotic sac exposed by removal from the chorionic sac. **A,** Actual size. The remnant of the umbilical vesicle is indicated by an *arrow*. **B,** Enlarged photograph of the fetus (×2). Note the following features: large head, fused eyelids, cartilaginous ribs, and intestines in umbilical cord (*arrow*). (Courtesy of Professor Jean Hay [retired], Department of Human Anatomy and Cell Science, University of Manitoba, Winnipeg, Manitoba, Canada.)

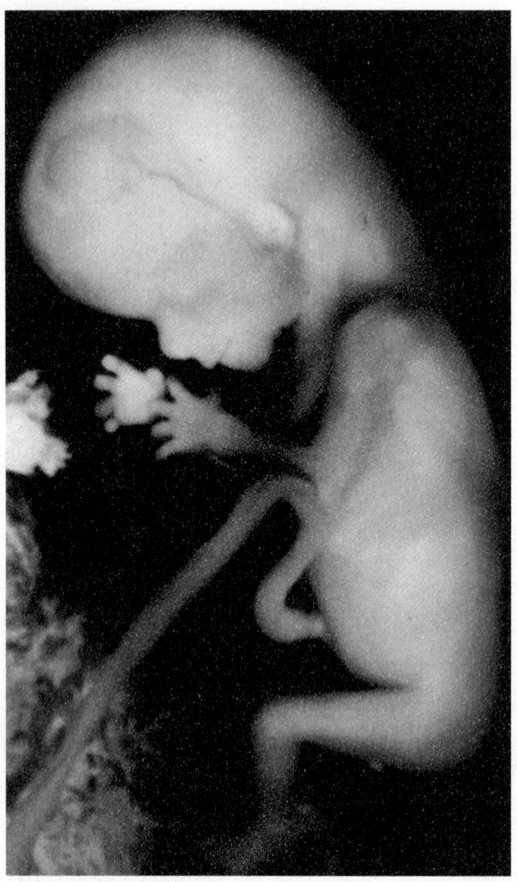

FIGURE 6-5. An 11-week fetus exposed by removal from its chorionic and amniotic sacs (×1.5). Note its relatively large head and that the intestines are no longer in the umbilical cord. (Courtesy of Professor Jean Hay [retired], Department of Human Anatomy and Cell Science, University of Manitoba, Winnipeg, Manitoba, Canada.)

transferred to the maternal circulation by passing across the placental membrane (see Chapter 7).

Thirteen to Sixteen Weeks

Growth is rapid during this period (Figs. 6-6 and 6-7; see Table 6-1). By 16 weeks, the head is relatively small compared with that of the 12-week fetus and the lower limbs have lengthened. Limb movements, which first occur at the end of the embryonic period, become coordinated by the 14th week but are too slight to be felt by the mother. Limb movements are visible during ultrasound examinations.

Ossification of the fetal skeleton is active during this period, and the bones are clearly visible on ultrasound images by the beginning of the 16th week. *Slow eye movements occur at 14 weeks.* Scalp hair patterning is also determined during this period. By 16 weeks, the ovaries are differentiated and contain primordial ovarian follicles that contain oogonia (see Chapter 12). The sex of the fetuses can be recognized by 12 to 14 weeks. By 16 weeks, the eyes face anteriorly rather than anterolaterally. In addition, the external ears are close to their definitive position on the sides of the head.

Seventeen to Twenty Weeks

Growth slows down during this period, but the fetus still increases its CRL by approximately 50 mm (Figs. 6-6 and 6-8; see Table 6-1). Fetal movements—**quickening**—are commonly felt by the mother. The skin is now covered with a greasy, cheeselike material—**vernix caseosa**. It consists of a mixture of dead epidermal cells and a fatty substance (secretion) from the fetal sebaceous glands. The

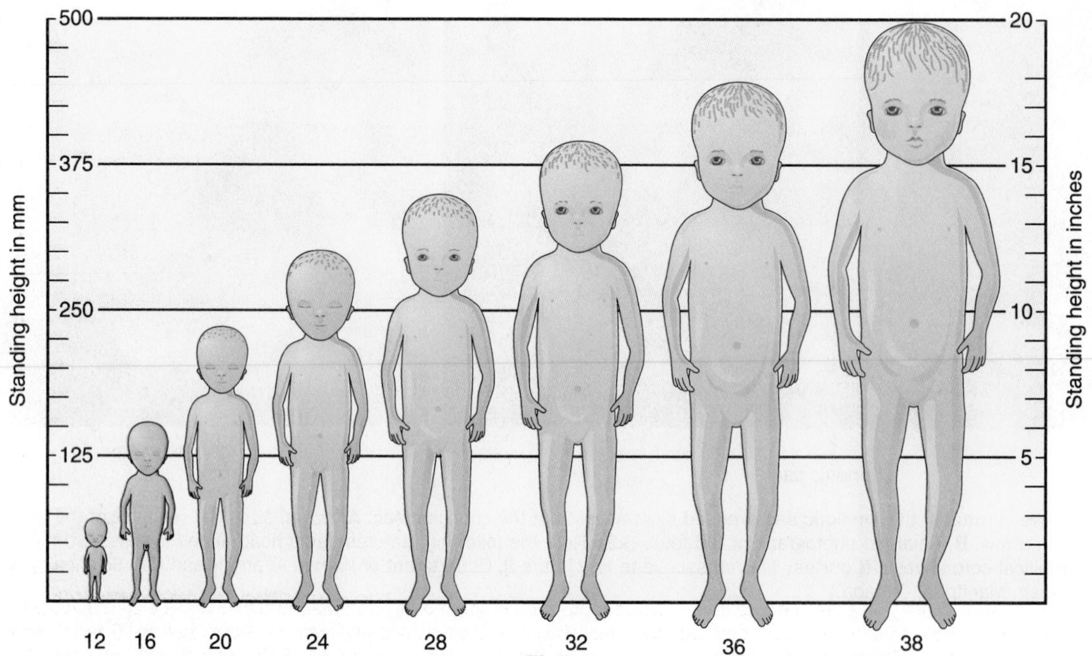

FIGURE 6-6. Diagram, drawn to scale, illustrating the changes in the size of the human fetus.

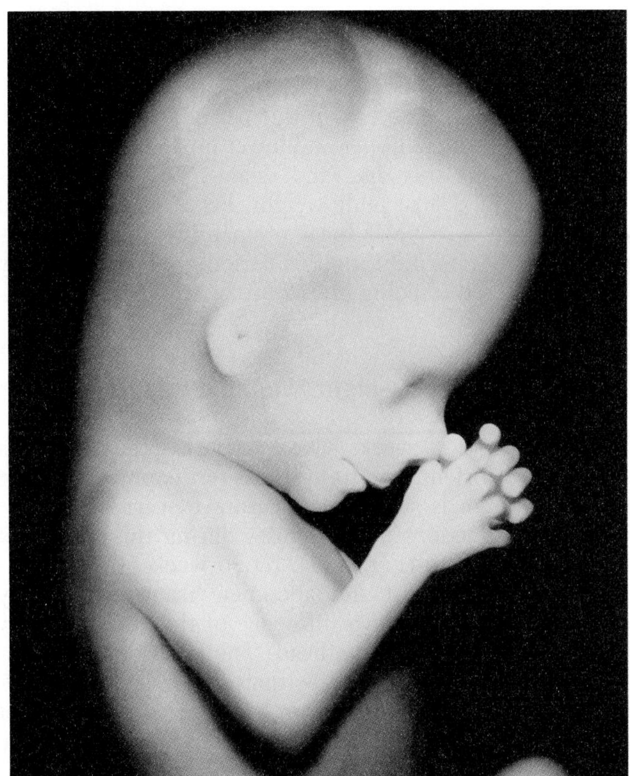

FIGURE 6-7. Enlarged photograph of the head and shoulders of a 13-week fetus. (Courtesy of Professor Jean Hay [retired], Department of Human Anatomy and Cell Science, University of Manitoba, Winnipeg, Manitoba, Canada.)

vernix caseosa protects the delicate fetal skin from abrasions, chapping, and hardening that result from exposure to the amniotic fluid.

Eyebrows and head hair are visible at 20 weeks. The fetuses are usually completely covered with fine downy hair—**lanugo**—that helps to hold the vernix caseosa on the skin. Brown fat forms during this period and is the site of heat production, particularly in the newborn infant. This specialized adipose tissue produces heat by oxidizing fatty acids. Brown fat is chiefly found at the root of the neck, posterior to the sternum, and in the perirenal area. By 18 weeks, the uterus is formed and canalization of the vagina has begun. By this time, many primordial ovarian follicles containing oogonia are visible. By 20 weeks, the testes have begun to descend, but they are still located on the posterior abdominal wall, as are the ovaries in female fetuses.

Twenty-one to Twenty-five Weeks

There is a substantial weight gain during this period, and the fetus is better proportioned (Fig. 6-9). The skin is usually wrinkled and more translucent, particularly during the early part of this period. The skin is pink to red in fresh specimens because blood is visible in the capillaries. At 21 weeks, rapid eye movements begin and blink-startle responses have been reported at 22 to 23 weeks. By 24 weeks, the secretory epithelial cells (type II pneumocytes) in the interalveolar walls of the lung have begun to secrete **surfactant**, a surface-active lipid that maintains the patency of the developing alveoli of the lungs (see Chapter 10). Fingernails are present by 24 weeks. Although a 22- to 25-week fetus born prematurely may survive if given intensive care (Fig. 6-9), it may die because its respiratory system is still immature.

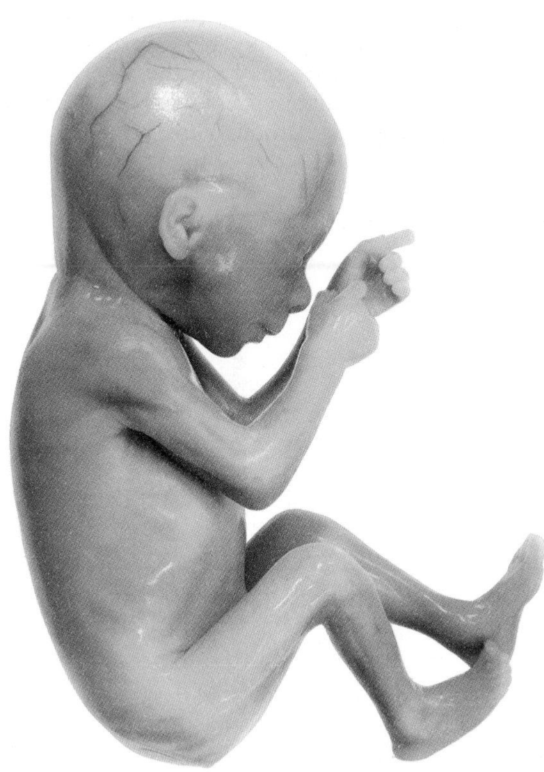

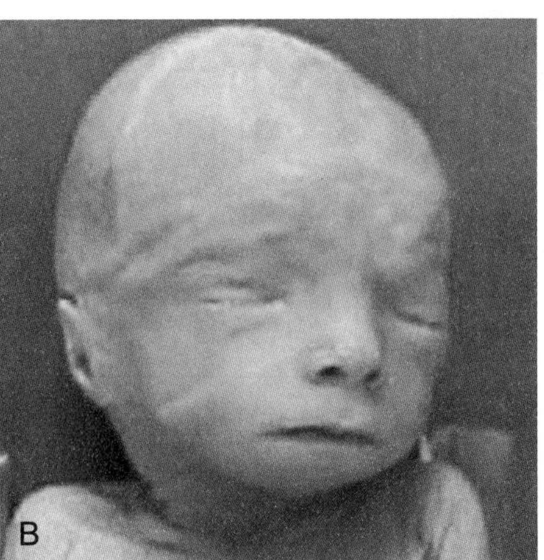

FIGURE 6-8. **A,** A 17-week fetus. Because there is little subcutaneous tissue and the skin is thin, the blood vessels of the scalp are visible. Fetuses at this age are unable to survive if born prematurely, mainly because their respiratory systems are immature. **B,** A 17-week fetus, frontal view. (**A,** From Moore KL, Persaud TVN, Shiota K: Color Atlas of Clinical Embryology, 2nd ed. Philadelphia, WB Saunders, 2000; **B,** Courtesy of Dr. Robert Jordan, St. Georges University Medical School, Grenada.)

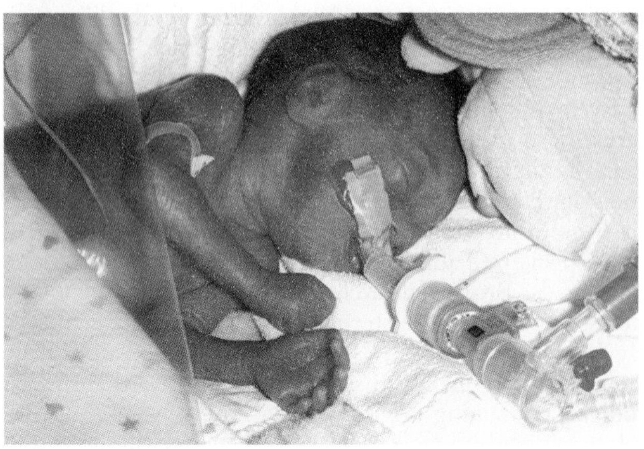

FIGURE 6-9. A 25-week-old normal female newborn weighing 725 g. (Courtesy of Dean Barringer and Marnie Danzinger.)

Twenty-six to Twenty-nine Weeks

At this age, a fetus often survives if born prematurely and given intensive care. The *lungs and pulmonary vasculature* have developed sufficiently to provide adequate gas exchange. In addition, the central nervous system has matured to the stage where it can direct rhythmic breathing movements and control body temperature. The highest neonatal mortality occurs in infants of low (≤2500 g) and very low (≤1500 g) birth weight.

The *eyelids are open* at 26 weeks, and lanugo and head hair are well developed. Toenails become visible, and considerable subcutaneous fat is now present under the skin, smoothing out many of the wrinkles. During this period, the quantity of white fat increases to approximately 3.5% of body weight. The fetal spleen has been an important site of erythropoiesis. This ends by 28 weeks, by which time bone marrow has become the major site of this process. MRIs produce clear images (Fig. 6-10).

Thirty to Thirty-four Weeks

The *pupillary light reflex* of the eyes can be elicited at 30 weeks. Usually by the end of this period, the skin is pink and smooth and the upper and lower limbs have a chubby appearance. At this age, the quantity of white fat is approximately 8% of body weight. Fetuses 32 weeks and older usually survive if born prematurely. If a normal-weight fetus is born during this period, it is premature by date as opposed to being premature by weight.

Thirty-five to Thirty-eight Weeks

Fetuses born at 35 weeks have a firm grasp and exhibit a spontaneous orientation to light. As term approaches, the nervous system is sufficiently mature to carry out some integrative functions. Most fetuses during this "finishing period" are plump (Fig. 6-11). By 36 weeks, the circumferences of the head and abdomen are approximately equal. After this, the circumference of the abdomen may be greater than that of the head. The fetal foot measurement is usually slightly larger than femoral length at 37 weeks and is an alternative parameter for confirmation of fetal age (Fig. 6-12). There is a slowing of growth as the time of birth approaches (Fig. 6-13).

By full term, most fetuses usually reach a CRL of 360 mm and weigh approximately 3400 g. The amount of white fat is approximately 16% of body weight. A fetus adds approximately 14 g of fat per day during these last weeks of gestation. In general, male fetuses are longer and weigh more at birth than females. The thorax (chest) is prominent, and the breasts often protrude slightly in both sexes. The testes are usually in the scrotum in full-term male infants; premature male infants commonly have undescended testes. Although the head is smaller at full term in relation to the rest of the body than it was earlier in fetal life, it still is one of the largest regions of the fetus.

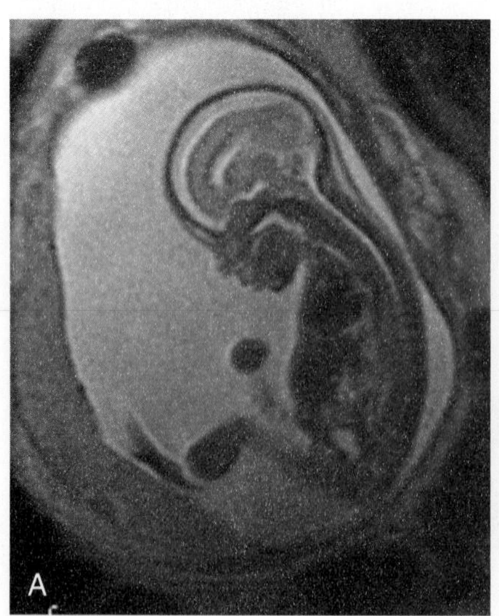

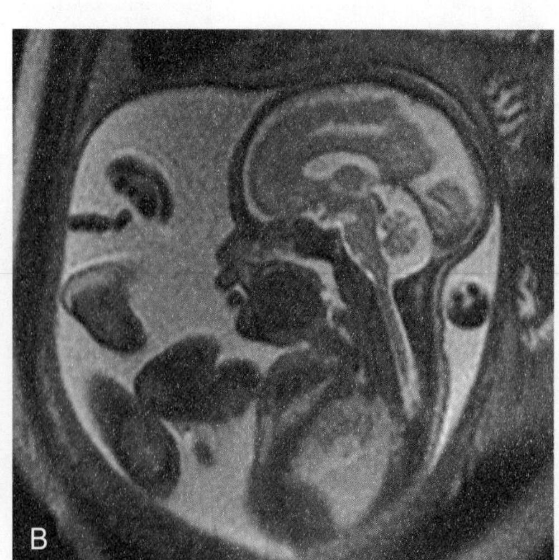

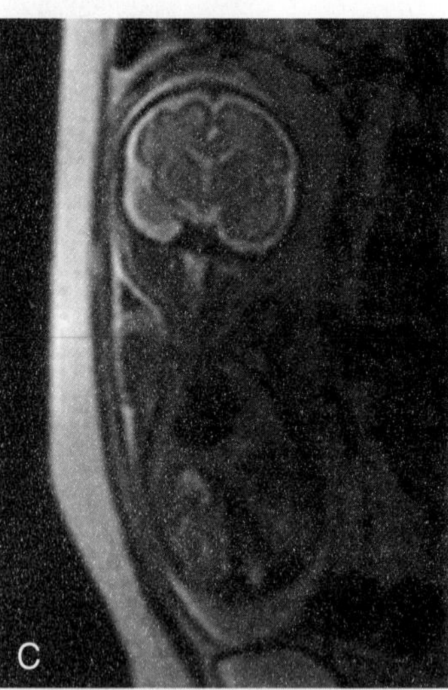

FIGURE 6-10. Magnetic resonance images (MRIs) of normal fetuses. **A,** At 18 weeks (20-week gestational age). **B,** At 26 weeks. **C,** At 28 weeks. (Courtesy of Deborah Levine, MD, Director of Obstetric and Gynecologic Ultrasound, Beth Israel Deaconess Medical Center, Boston, MA.)

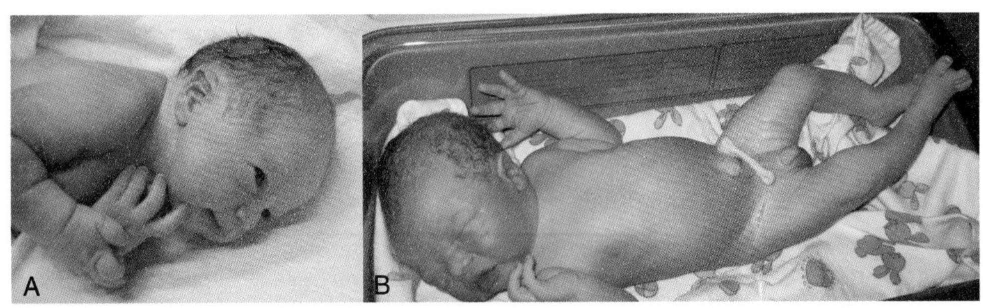

FIGURE 6-11. Healthy newborns. **A,** At 34 weeks (36-week gestational age). **B,** At 38 weeks (40-week gestational age). (**A,** Courtesy of Michael and Michele Rice; **B,** Courtesy of Dr. and Mrs. Don Jackson.)

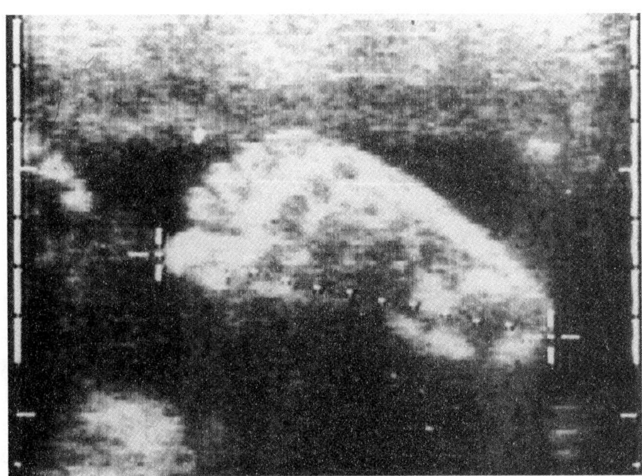

FIGURE 6-12. Ultrasound scan of the foot of a fetus at 37 weeks' gestation. (Courtesy of Dr. C.R. Harman, Department of Obstetrics, Gynecology and Reproductive Sciences, University of Maryland, Baltimore, MD.)

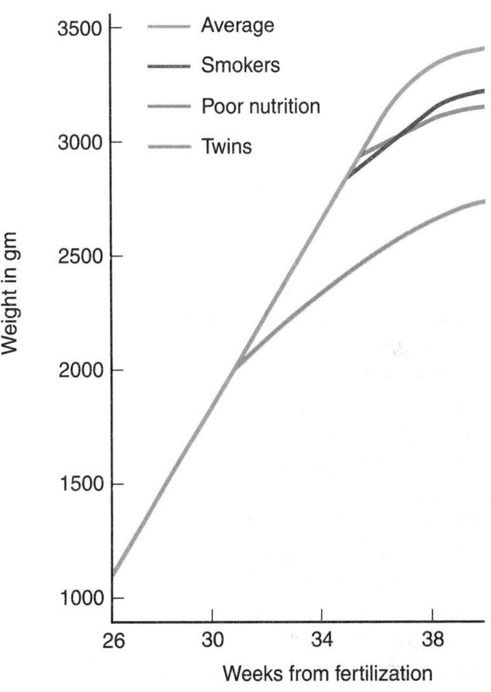

FIGURE 6-13. Graph showing the rate of fetal growth during the last trimester. Average refers to babies born in the United States. After 36 weeks, the growth rate deviates from the straight line. The decline, particularly after full term (38 weeks), probably reflects inadequate fetal nutrition caused by placental changes. (Adapted from Gruenwald P: Growth of the human fetus. I. Normal growth and its variation. Am J Obstet Gynecol 94:1112–1119, 1966.)

LOW BIRTH WEIGHT

Not all low birth weight babies are premature. Approximately one third of those with a birth weight of 2500 g or less are actually small for gestational age. These "small for dates" infants may be underweight because of placental insufficiency (see Chapter 7). The placentas are often small or poorly attached and/or have undergone degenerative changes that progressively reduce the oxygen supply and nourishment to the fetus.

It is important to distinguish between full-term infants who have a low birth weight because of IUGR and preterm infants who are underweight because of a shortened gestation (i.e., premature by date). IUGR may be caused by placental insufficiency, multiple gestations (e.g., triplets), infectious diseases, cardiovascular anomalies, inadequate maternal nutrition, and maternal and fetal hormones. Teratogens (drugs, chemicals, and viruses) and genetic factors are also known to cause IUGR (see Chapter 20). Infants with IUGR show a characteristic lack of subcutaneous fat and their skin is wrinkled, suggesting that white fat has actually been lost.

EXPECTED DATE OF DELIVERY

The expected date of delivery of a fetus is 266 days or 38 weeks after fertilization, that is, 280 days or 40 weeks after LNMP (see Table 6-2). Approximately 12% of babies are born 1 to 2 weeks after the expected time of birth. The common delivery date rule (Nägele's rule) for estimating the expected date of delivery is to count back 3 months from the first day of the LNMP and add a year and 7 days.

POSTMATURITY SYNDROME

Prolongation of pregnancy for 3 or more weeks beyond the expected date of delivery occurs in 5% to 6% of women. Some infants in such pregnancies develop the postmaturity syndrome and have an increased risk of mortality. Because of this, labor is often induced (see Chapter 7). These fetuses have dry, parchment-like skin, are often overweight, and have no lanugo, decreased or absent vernix caseosa, long nails, and increased alertness.

FACTORS INFLUENCING FETAL GROWTH

The fetus requires substrates for growth and production of energy. Gases and nutrients pass freely to the fetus from the mother through the placental membrane (see Chapter 7). **Glucose** is a primary source of energy for fetal metabolism and growth; *amino acids* are also required. These substances pass from the mother's blood to the fetus through the placental membrane. Insulin required for the metabolism of glucose is secreted by the fetal pancreas; no significant quantities of maternal insulin reach the fetus because the placental membrane is relatively impermeable to this hormone. Insulin, insulin-like growth factors, human growth hormone, and some small polypeptides (such as somatomedin C) are believed to stimulate fetal growth.

Many factors may affect prenatal growth: maternal, fetal, and environmental. Some factors operating throughout pregnancy, such as maternal vascular disease, intrauterine infection, cigarette smoking, and consumption of alcohol, tend to produce *intrauterine growth restriction (IUGR) infants* or *small for gestational age (SGA) infants*, whereas factors operating during the last trimester, such as maternal malnutrition, usually produce underweight infants with normal length and head size. The terms IUGR and SGA are related, but they are not synonymous. IUGR refers to a process that causes a reduction in the expected pattern of fetal growth as well as fetal growth potential. SGA refers to an infant whose birth weight is lower than a predetermined cutoff value for a particular gestational age (<2 SDs below the mean or less than the third percentile). Severe maternal malnutrition resulting from a poor-quality diet is known to cause reduced fetal growth (see Fig. 6-13).

Cigarette Smoking

Smoking is a well-established cause of IUGR. The growth rate for fetuses of mothers who smoke cigarettes is less than normal during the last 6 to 8 weeks of pregnancy (see Fig. 6-13). On average, the birth weight of infants whose mothers smoke heavily during pregnancy is 200 g less than normal, and *perinatal morbidity* is increased when adequate medical care is unavailable. The effect of maternal smoking is greater on fetuses whose mothers also receive inadequate nutrition. Presumably, there is an additive effect of heavy smoking and poor-quality diet.

Multiple Pregnancy

Individuals of multiple births usually weigh considerably less than infants resulting from a single pregnancy (see Fig. 6-13). It is evident that the total metabolic requirements of two or more fetuses exceed the nutritional supply available from the placenta during the third trimester.

Alcohol and Illicit Drugs

Infants born to alcoholic mothers often exhibit IUGR as part of the *fetal alcohol syndrome* (see Chapter 20). Similarly, the use of marijuana and other illicit drugs (e.g., cocaine) can cause IUGR and other obstetric complications.

Impaired Uteroplacental and Fetoplacental Blood Flow

Maternal placental circulation may be reduced by conditions that decrease uterine blood flow (e.g., small chorionic vessels, severe maternal hypotension, and renal disease). Chronic reduction of uterine blood flow can cause fetal starvation resulting in IUGR. Placental dysfunction or defects (e.g., infarction; see Chapter 7) can also cause IUGR. The net effect of these placental abnormalities is a reduction of the total area for exchange of nutrients between the fetal and maternal blood streams. It is very difficult to separate the effect of these placental changes from the effect of reduced maternal blood flow to the placenta. In some instances of chronic maternal disease, the maternal vascular changes in the uterus are primary and the placental defects are secondary.

Genetic Factors and Growth Retardation

It is well established that genetic factors can cause IUGR. Repeated cases of this condition in one family indicate that recessive genes may be the cause of the abnormal growth. In recent years, structural and numerical chromosomal aberrations have also been shown to be associated with cases of retarded fetal growth. IUGR is pronounced in infants with Down syndrome and is very characteristic of fetuses with trisomy 18 syndrome (see Chapter 20).

PROCEDURES FOR ASSESSING FETAL STATUS

> By accepting the shelter of the uterus, the fetus also takes the risk of maternal disease or malnutrition and of biochemical, immunological and hormonal adjustment.
>
> — George W. Corner, Renowned American Embryologist, 1888–1981

Perinatology is the branch of medicine that is concerned with the well-being of the fetus and newborn infant, generally covering the period from approximately 26 weeks after fertilization to 4 weeks after birth. This subspecialty of medicine combines aspects of obstetrics and pediatrics. A third-trimester fetus is regarded as an unborn patient.

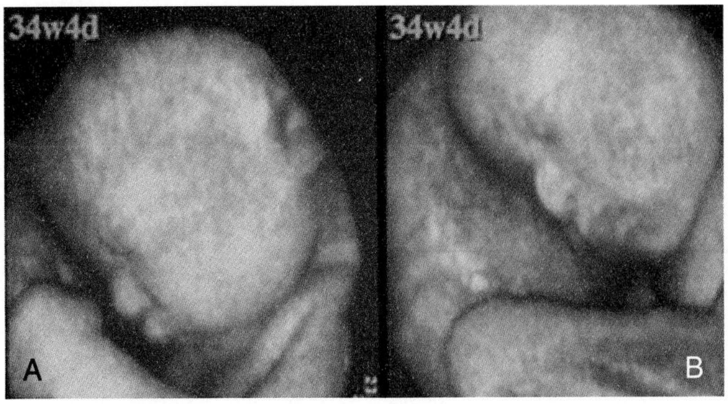

FIGURE 6-14. **A** and **B,** Three-dimensional ultrasonograms (sonograms) of a third-trimester fetus showing the normal face. The surface features are clearly recognizable. (Courtesy of Dr. Toshiyuki Hata, Department of Perinatology, Kagawa Medical University, Japan.)

Ultrasonography

Ultrasonography is the primary imaging modality in the evaluation of the fetus because of its wide availability, low cost, and lack of known adverse effects. The chorionic sac and its contents may be visualized by ultrasonography during the embryonic and fetal periods. Placental and fetal size, multiple births, abnormalities of placental shape, and abnormal presentations can also be determined. Ultrasound scans give accurate measurements of the biparietal diameter of the fetal cranium, from which close estimates of fetal age and length can be made. Figures 6-12 and 6-14 illustrate how details of the fetus can be observed in ultrasound scans. Ultrasound examinations are also helpful for diagnosing abnormal pregnancies at a very early stage. Rapid advances in ultrasonography have made this technique a major tool for prenatal diagnosis of fetal abnormalities.

Diagnostic Amniocentesis

This is a common invasive prenatal diagnostic procedure, usually performed between 15 and 18 weeks gestation. Amniotic fluid is sampled by inserting a 22-gauge needle through the mother's anterior abdominal and uterine walls into the amniotic cavity by piercing the chorion and amnion (Fig. 6-15*A*). A syringe is attached and amniotic fluid is withdrawn. Because there is relatively little amniotic fluid before the 14th week (LNMP), amniocentesis is difficult to perform before this time. The amniotic fluid volume is approximately 200 mL, and 15 to 20 mL can be safely withdrawn. Amniocentesis is relatively devoid of risk, especially when the procedure is performed by an experienced physician who is guided by real-time ultrasonography for outlining the position of the fetus and placenta.

TRANSABDOMINAL AMNIOCENTESIS

Amniocentesis is a common technique for detecting genetic disorders (e.g., Down syndrome). The common indications for amniocentesis are

- Advanced maternal age (38 years or older)
- Previous birth of a trisomic child (e.g., Down syndrome)
- Chromosome abnormality in either parent (e.g., a chromosome translocation; see Chapter 20)
- Women who are carriers of X-linked recessive disorders (e.g., hemophilia)
- History of neural tube defects in the family (e.g., spina bifida cystica; see Chapter 20)
- Carriers of inborn errors of metabolism

Alpha-fetoprotein Assay

Alpha fetoprotein (AFP) is a glycoprotein that is synthesized in the fetal liver, umbilical vesicle, and gut. AFP is found in high concentration in fetal serum, peaking 14 weeks after the LNMP. Small amounts of AFP normally enter the amniotic fluid.

ALPHA-FETOPROTEIN AND FETAL ANOMALIES

The concentration of AFP in the amniotic fluid surrounding fetuses with severe anomalies of the central nervous system and ventral abdominal wall is high. Amniotic fluid AFP concentration is measured by immunoassay, and, when used with ultrasonographic scanning, approximately 99% of fetuses with these severe defects can be diagnosed prenatally. When a fetus has an open neural tube defect, the concentration of AFP is also likely to be higher than normal in the maternal serum. Maternal serum AFP concentration is low when the fetus has Down syndrome (trisomy 21), trisomy 18, or other chromosome defects.

Spectrophotometric Studies

Examination of amniotic fluid by this method may be used for assessing the degree of erythroblastosis fetalis, also called hemolytic disease of newborn. This disease results from destruction of fetal red blood cells by maternal antibodies (see Chapter 7).

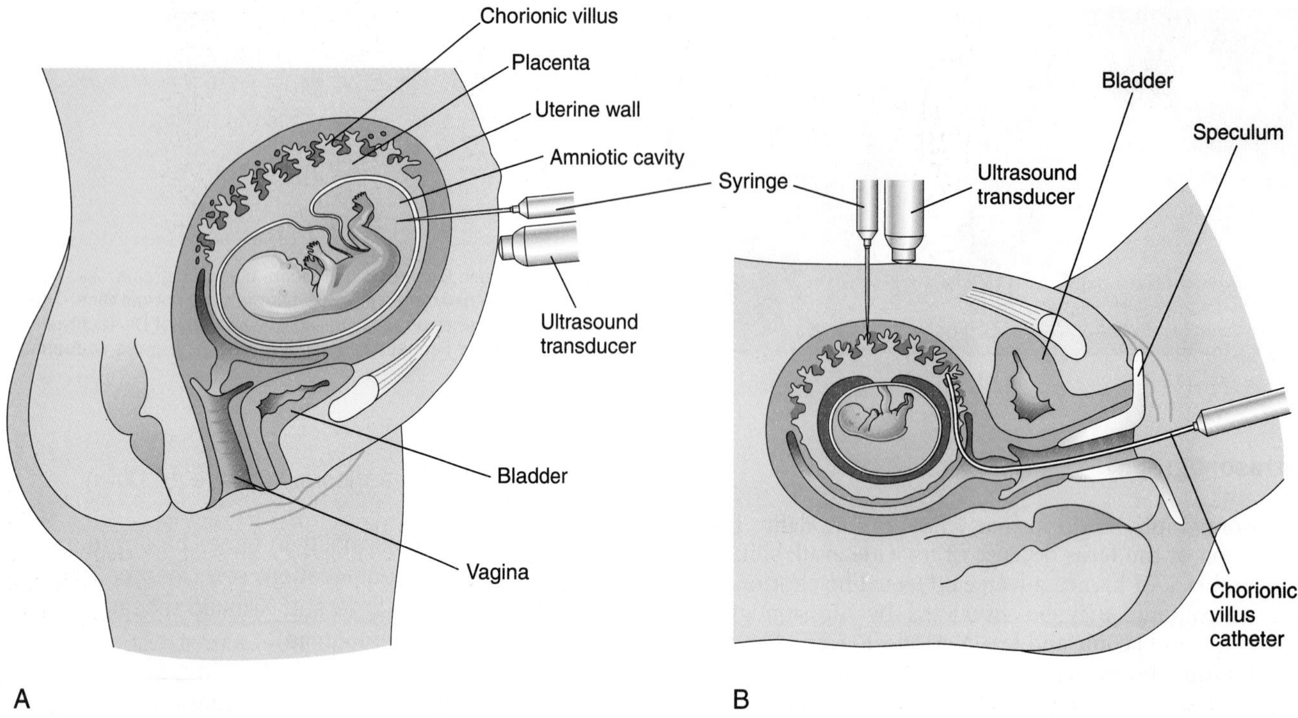

FIGURE 6-15. **A,** Illustration of amniocentesis. A needle is inserted through the lower abdominal and uterine walls into the amniotic cavity. A syringe is attached and amniotic fluid is withdrawn for diagnostic purposes. **B,** Drawing illustrating chorionic villus sampling. Two sampling approaches are illustrated: through the maternal anterior abdominal wall with a needle and through the vagina and cervical canal using a malleable catheter.

Chorionic Villus Sampling

Biopsies of trophoblastic tissue (5–20 mg) may be obtained by inserting a needle, guided by ultrasonography, through the mother's abdominal and uterine walls (transabdominal) into the uterine cavity (see Fig. 6-15*B*). Chorionic villus sampling (CVS) is also performed transcervically by passing a polyethylene catheter through the cervix and guided by real-time ultrasonography. For assessing the condition of a fetus at risk, the fetal karyotype can be obtained and a diagnosis made weeks earlier when CVS is performed, compared with amniocentesis. The risk of miscarriage with CVS is approximately 1%, more than with amniocentesis.

DIAGNOSTIC VALUE OF CHORIONIC VILLUS SAMPLING

Biopsies of chorionic villi are used for detecting chromosomal abnormalities, inborn errors of metabolism, and X-linked disorders. CVS can be performed between 10 and 12 weeks of gestation. The rate of fetal loss is approximately 1%, slightly more than the risk from amniocentesis. Reports regarding an increased risk of limb defects after CVS are conflicting. The major advantage of CVS over amniocentesis is that it allows the results of chromosomal analysis to be performed several weeks earlier than when performed by amniocentesis.

Sex Chromatin Patterns

Fetal sex can be determined by noting the presence or absence of sex chromatin in the nuclei of cells recovered from amniotic fluid. These tests were developed after it was discovered that sex chromatin was visible in nuclei of normal female cells but not in normal male cells (Fig. 6-16*A* and *B*). Females with three X chromosomes (46, XXX) have two masses of sex chromatin (see Fig. 6-16*C*). By use of a special staining technique, the Y chromosome can also be identified in cells recovered from the amniotic fluid surrounding male fetuses (see Fig. 6-16*D*). Knowledge of *fetal sex* can be useful in diagnosing the presence of severe sex-linked hereditary diseases, such as hemophilia and muscular dystrophy.

Cell Cultures and Chromosomal Analysis

The prevalence of chromosomal disorders is approximately one in 120 live-born infants. Fetal sex and chromosomal aberrations can be determined by studying the sex chromosomes in cultured fetal cells obtained during amniocentesis. These cultures are commonly done when an autosomal abnormality, such as occurs in *Down syndrome*, is suspected. Moreover, microdeletions and microduplications, as well as subtelomeric rearrangements, can now be detected with fluorescence in situ hybridization technology. *Inborn errors of metabolism* in fetuses can also be detected by studying cell cultures. Enzyme deficiencies can be determined by incubating cells recovered from amniotic fluid and then detecting the specific enzyme deficiency in the cells (see Chapter 20).

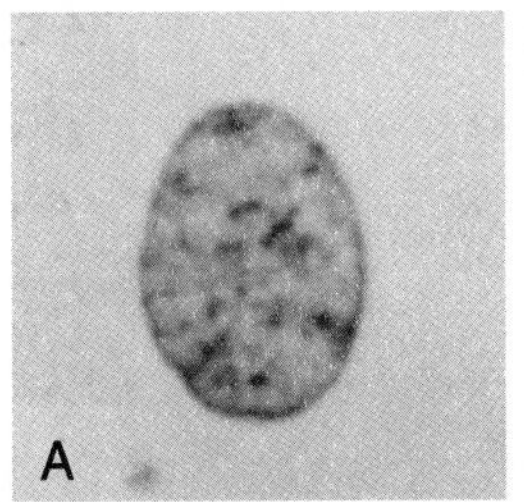

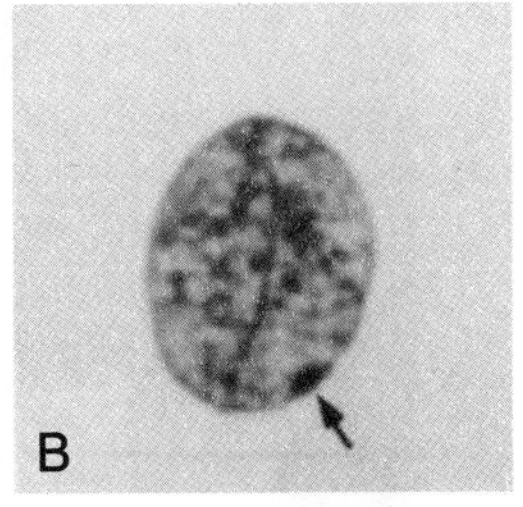

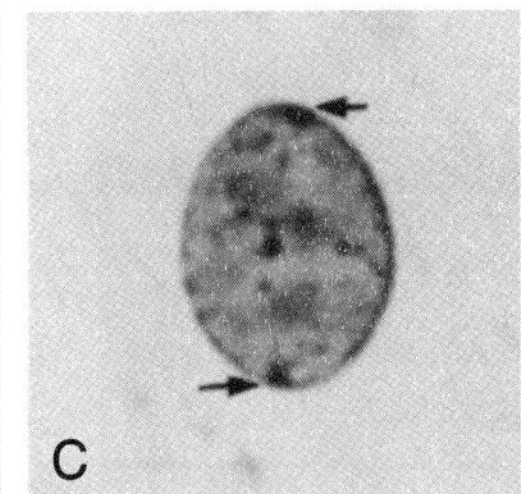

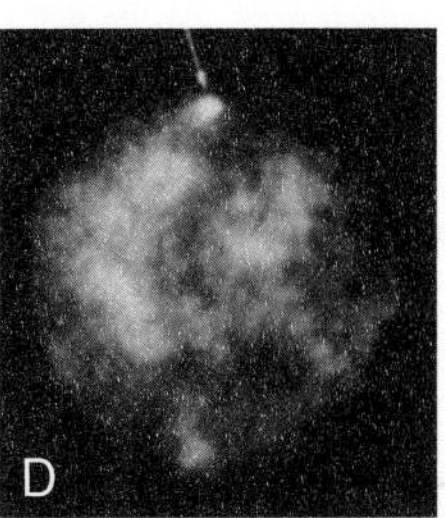

FIGURE 6-16. Oral epithelial nuclei stained with cresylecht violet (**A**, **B**, and **C**) and quinacrine mustard (**D**) (×2000). **A**, From normal male. No sex chromatin is visible (chromatin negative). **B**, From normal female. The *arrow* indicates a typical mass of sex chromatin (chromatin positive). **C**, From female with XXX trisomy. The *arrows* indicate two masses of sex chromatin. **D**, From normal male. The *arrow* indicates a mass of Y chromatin as an intensely fluorescent body. (**A** and **B**, From Moore KL, Barr ML: Smears from the oral mucosa in the detection of chromosomal sex. Lancet 2:57, 1955.)

Fetal Transfusion

Fetuses with *hemolytic disease of the newborn* (HDN) can be treated by intrauterine blood transfusions. The blood is injected through a needle inserted into the fetal peritoneal cavity. With recent advances in percutaneous umbilical cord blood sampling (PUBS), blood and packed red blood cells are transfused directly into the umbilical vein for the treatment of fetal anemia due to isoimmunization. The need for fetal blood transfusions is reduced nowadays owing to the treatment of Rh-negative mothers of Rh-positive fetuses with anti-Rh immunoglobulin. *HDN is relatively uncommon now* because Rh immunoglobulin usually prevents development of this disease of the Rh system. Fetal transfusion of platelets directly into the umbilical cord vein is carried out for the treatment of alloimmune thrombocytopenia. Also, fetal transfusion of drugs in a similar manner for the treatment of a few medical conditions in the fetus has been reported.

Fetoscopy

Using fiberoptic lighting instruments, parts of the fetal body may be directly observed. It is possible to scan the entire fetus looking for congenital anomalies such as cleft lip and limb defects. The fetoscope is usually introduced through the anterior abdominal and uterine walls into the amniotic cavity, similarly to the way in which the needle is inserted during amniocentesis. Fetoscopy is usually carried out at 17 to 20 weeks of gestation, but with new approaches such as *transabdominal thin-gauge embryo-fetoscopy*, it is possible to detect certain anomalies in the embryo or fetus during the first trimester. Because of the risk to the fetus compared with other prenatal diagnostic procedures, fetoscopy now has few indications for routine prenatal diagnosis or treatment of the fetus. Biopsy of fetal tissues, such as skin, liver, kidney, and muscle, can be performed with ultrasound guidance.

Percutaneous Umbilical Cord Blood Sampling

Fetal blood samples may be obtained directly from the umbilical vein by PUBS or cordocentesis for the diagnosis of many fetal conditions, including aneuploidy, fetal growth restriction, fetal infection, and fetal anemia. PUBS is usually performed after 18 weeks of gestation under continuous direct ultrasound guidance, which is used to locate the umbilical cord and its vessels. Moreover, the procedure permits treating the fetus directly, including the transfusion of packed red blood cells for the management of fetal anemia resulting from isoimmunization.

Computed Tomography and Magnetic Resonance Imaging

When planning fetal treatment, computed tomography (CT) and magnetic resonance imaging (MRI) may be used to provide more information about an abnormality that has been detected in ultrasonic images. Important advantages of magnetic resonance imaging are that it does not use ionizing radiation and that it has high soft-tissue contrast and resolution (Fig. 6-17).

Fetal Monitoring

Continuous fetal heart rate monitoring in high-risk pregnancies is routine and provides information about the oxygenation of the fetus. There are various causes of prenatal fetal distress such as maternal diseases that reduce oxygen transport to the fetus (e.g., cyanotic heart disease). Fetal distress (e.g., indicated by an abnormal heart rate or rhythm) suggests that the fetus is in jeopardy. A noninvasive method of monitoring uses transducers placed on the mother's abdomen.

SUMMARY OF THE FETAL PERIOD

- The fetal period begins 9 weeks after fertilization (11 weeks after the LNMP) and ends at birth. It is characterized by *rapid body growth and differentiation of tissues and organ systems*. An obvious change in the fetal period is the relative slowing of head growth compared with that of the rest of the body.
- By the beginning of the *20th week*, lanugo and head hair appear, and the skin is coated with vernix caseosa. The eyelids are closed during most of the

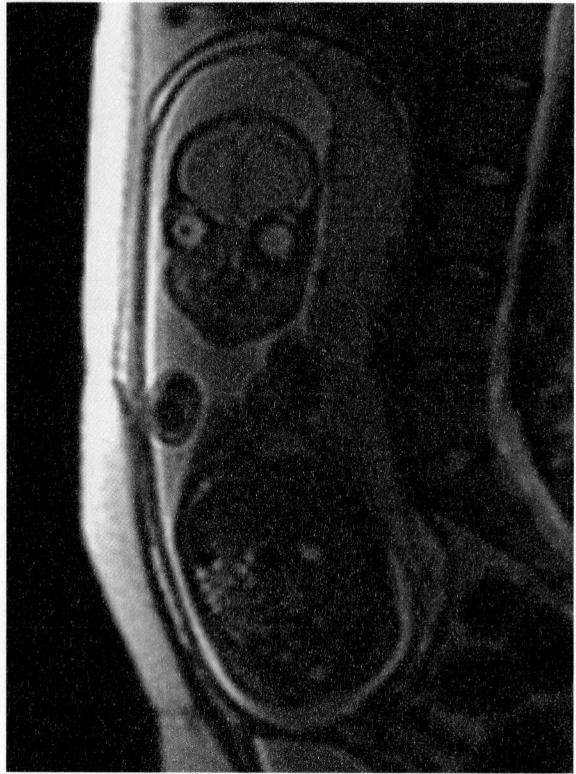

FIGURE 6-17. Sagittal magnetic resonance image of the pelvis of a pregnant woman. The fetus is in the breech presentation. Note the brain, eyes, and liver (below the diaphragm). (Courtesy of Deborah Levine, MD, Director of Obstetric and Gynecologic Ultrasound, Beth Israel Deaconess Medical Center, Boston, MA.)

fetal period but begin to reopen at approximately *26 weeks*. At this time, the fetus is usually capable of extrauterine existence, mainly because of the maturity of its respiratory system.

- Until approximately *30 weeks*, the fetus appears reddish and wizened because of the thinness of its skin and the relative absence of subcutaneous fat. Fat usually develops rapidly during the last 6 to 8 weeks, giving the fetus a smooth, plump appearance.
- The fetus is less vulnerable to the teratogenic effects of drugs, viruses, and radiation, but these agents may interfere with growth and normal functional development, especially of the brain and eyes.
- The physician can now determine whether a fetus has a particular disease or a congenital anomaly by using various diagnostic techniques, e.g., amniocentesis, CVS, ultrasonography, and magnetic resonance imaging. Prenatal diagnosis can be made early enough to allow early termination of the pregnancy if elected, e.g., when severe anomalies incompatible with postnatal life are diagnosed, such as absence of most of the brain.
- In selected cases, treatments can be given to the fetus, e.g., the administration of drugs to correct cardiac arrhythmia or thyroid disorders. Surgical correction of some congenital anomalies in utero (Fig. 6-18) is also possible (e.g., fetuses that have ureters that do not open into the bladder).

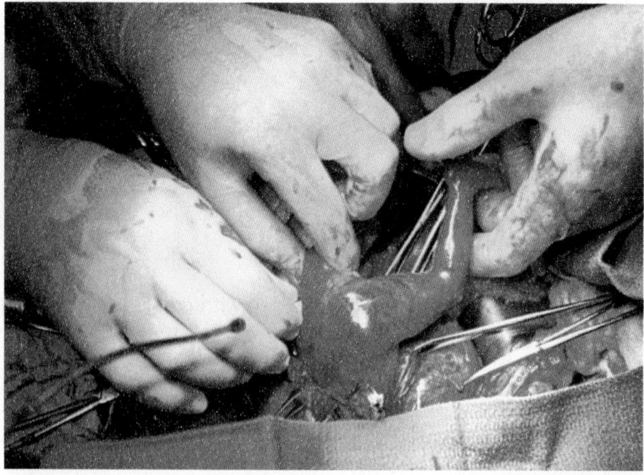

FIGURE 6-18. Fetus at 21 weeks undergoing bilateral ureterostomies, the establishment of openings of the ureters into the bladder. (From Harrison MR, Globus MS, Filly RA [eds]: The Unborn Patient. Prenatal Diagnosis and Treatment, 2nd ed. Philadelphia, WB Saunders, 1994.)

CLINICALLY ORIENTED PROBLEMS

CASE 6-1

A woman in the 20th week of a high-risk pregnancy was scheduled for a repeat cesarean section. Her physician wanted to establish an expected date of delivery.

- How would an expected date of delivery be established?
- When would labor likely be induced?
- How could this be accomplished?

CASE 6-2

A 44-year-old pregnant woman was worried that she might be carrying a fetus with major congenital anomalies.

- How could the status of her fetus be determined?
- What chromosomal abnormality would most likely be found?
- What other chromosomal aberrations might be detected?
- If this was of clinical interest, how could the sex of the fetus be determined in a family known to have hemophilia or muscular dystrophy?

CASE 6-3

A 19-year-old woman in the second trimester of pregnancy asked a physician whether her fetus was vulnerable to over-the-counter drugs and street drugs. She also wondered about the effect of her heavy drinking and cigarette smoking on her fetus.

- What would the physician likely tell her?

CASE 6-4

An ultrasound examination of a pregnant woman revealed IUGR of the fetus.

- What factors may cause IUGR? Discuss them.
- Which factors can the mother eliminate?

CASE 6-5

A woman in the first trimester of pregnancy who was to undergo amniocentesis expressed concerns about a miscarriage and the possibility of injury to her fetus.

- What are the risks of these complications?
- What procedures are used to minimize these risks?
- What other technique might be used for obtaining cells for chromosomal study?
- What does the acronym PUBS stand for?
- Describe how this technique is performed and how it is used to assess the status of a fetus.

CASE 6-6

A pregnant woman is told that she is going to have an AFP test to determine whether there are any fetal anomalies.

- What types of fetal anomalies can be detected by an AFP assay of maternal serum? Explain.
- What is the significance of high and low levels of AFP?

Discussion of these problems appears at the back of the book.

References and Suggested Reading

Anderson MS, Hay WW: Intrauterine growth restriction and the small-for-gestational-age infant. In MacDonald MG, Seshia MMK, Mullett MD (eds): Avery's Neonatology. Pathophysiology & Management of the Newborn, 6th ed. Philadelphia, Lippincott Williams & Wilkins, 2005.

Blickstein I: Growth aberration in multiple pregnancy. Obstet Gynecol Clin N Am 32:39, 2005.

Bulas DI: Fetal imaging: ultrasound and magnetic resonance imaging. In MacDonald MG, Seshia MMK, Mullett MD (eds): Avery's Neonatology. Pathophysiology & Management of the Newborn, 6th ed. Philadelphia, Lippincott Williams & Wilkins, 2005.

Canick JA, MacRae AR: Second trimester serum markers. Semin Perinatol 29:203, 2005.

Das UG, Sysyn GD: Abnormal fetal growth: Intrauterine growth retardation, small for gestational age, large for gestational age. Pediatr Clin N Am 51:639, 2004.

Doubilet PM, Benson CB, Callen PW: Ultrasound evaluation of normal fetal anatomy. In Callen PW (ed): Ultrasonography in Obstetrics and Gynecology, 4th ed. Philadelphia, WB Saunders, 2000.

Drugan A, Isada NB, Evans MI: Prenatal diagnosis in the molecular age—indications, procedures, and laboratory techniques. In MacDonald MG, Seshia MMK, Mullett MD (eds): Avery's Neonatology, Pathophysiology & Management of the Newborn, 6th ed. Philadelphia, Lippincott Williams & Wilkins, 2005.

Evans MI, Johnson MP, Flake AW, et al: Fetal therapy. In MacDonald MG, Seshia MMK, Mullett MD (eds): Avery's Neonatology. Pathophysiology & Management of the Newborn, 6th ed. Philadelphia, Lippincott Williams & Wilkins, 2005.

Evans MI, Wapner RJ: Invasive prenatal diagnostic procedures 2005. Semin Perinatol 29: 215, 2005.

Filly RA: Sonographic anatomy of the normal fetus. In Harrison MR, Evans MI, Adzick NS, et al (eds): The Unborn Patient. Prenatal Diagnosis and Treatment, 3rd ed. Philadelphia, WB Saunders, 2001.

Hinrichsen KV (ed): Humanembryologie. Berlin, Springer-Verlag, 1990.

Jirásel JE: An Atlas of Human Prenatal Developmental Mechanics. Anatomy and Staging, London and New York, Taylor & Francis, 2004.

Kalousek DK, Fitch N, Paradice BA: Pathology of the Human Embryo and Previable Fetus. An Atlas. New York, Springer-Verlag, 1990.

Kliegman RM: Intrauterine growth restriction. In Martin RJ, Fanaroff AA, Walsh MC (eds): Fanaroff and Martin's Neonatal-Perinatal Medicine. Diseases of the Fetus and Infant, 8th ed. Philadelphia, Mosby, 2006.

Leung KY, Ngai CS, Chan BC, et al: Three-dimensional extended imaging: A new display modality for three-dimensional ultrasound examination. Ultrasound Obstet Gynecol 26:244, 2005.

Lyons EA, Levi CS: Ultrasound of the normal first trimester of pregnancy. Syllabus: Special Course Ultrasound. Radiological Society of North America, 1991.

Moore CA, Khoury MJ, Bradley LA: From genetics to genomics: Using gene-based medicine to prevent disease and promote health in children. Semin Perinatol 29:135, 2005.

Needlman RD: Fetal growth and development. In Behrman RE, Kliegman RM, Jenson HB (eds): Nelson Textbook of Pediatrics, 17th ed. Philadelphia, Elsevier/Saunders, 2004.

Nicolaides KH: First-trimester screening for chromosomal abnormalities. Semin Perinatol 29:190, 2005.

O'Rahilly R, Müller F: Development Stages in Human Embryos. Publication 637. Washington, DC: Carnegie Institution of Washington, 1987.

Persaud TVN, Hay JC: Normal embryonic and fetal development. In Reece EA, et al. (eds): Clinical Obstetrics: The Fetus and Mother, 3rd ed. Malden, MA, Blackwell Publishing, 2006, pp 19–32.

Reed MD, Blumer JL: Pharmacologic treatment of the fetus. In Martin RJ, Fanaroff AA, Walsh MC (eds): Fanaroff and Martin's Neonatal-Perinatal Medicine. Diseases of the Fetus and Infant, 8th ed. Philadelphia, Mosby, 2006.

Sheridan C: Intrauterine growth restriction. Aust Fam Physician 34:717, 2005.

Streeter GL: Weight, sitting height, head size, foot length and menstrual age of the human embryo. Contrib Embryol Carnegie Inst 11:143, 1920.

Wilton L: Preimplantation genetic diagnosis for aneuploidy screening in early human embryo: A review. Prenat Diagn 22:512, 2002.

7

The Placenta and Fetal Membranes

The Placenta 111
- The Decidua 111
- Development of the Placenta 111
- Placental Circulation 117
- The Placental Membrane 118
- Functions of the Placenta 118
- Placental Metabolism 118
- The Placenta as an Invasive Tumorlike Structure 122
- Uterine Growth during Pregnancy 122

Parturition 123
- The Placenta and Fetal Membranes after Birth 123
- The Umbilical Cord 125

The Umbilical Vesicle (Yolk Sac) 133
- Significance of the Umbilical Vesicle 134
- Fate of the Umbilical Vesicle 134

The Allantois 134

Multiple Pregnancies 134
- Twins and Fetal Membranes 134
- Dizygotic Twins 137
- Monozygotic Twins 137
- Other Types of Multiple Births 140

Summary of the Placenta and Fetal Membranes 140

Clinically Oriented Problems 143

The placenta and fetal membranes separate the fetus from the **endometrium**—the mucous membrane of the inner layer of the uterine wall. An interchange of substances, such as nutrients and oxygen, occurs between the maternal and fetal bloodstreams through the placenta. The vessels in the umbilical cord connect the placental circulation with the fetal circulation. The chorion, amnion, umbilical vesicle, and allantois constitute the fetal membranes.

THE PLACENTA

The placenta is the primary site of nutrient and gas exchange between the mother and fetus. The placenta is a fetomaternal organ that has two components:

- A fetal part that develops from the chorionic sac
- A maternal part that is derived from the endometrium

The placenta and umbilical cord form a transport system for substances passing between the mother and fetus. Nutrients and oxygen pass from the maternal blood through the placenta to the fetal blood, and waste materials and carbon dioxide pass from the fetal blood through the placenta to the maternal blood. The placenta and fetal membranes perform the following functions and activities: protection, nutrition, respiration, excretion, and hormone production. Shortly after birth, the placenta and fetal membranes are expelled from the uterus as the afterbirth.

The Decidua

Decidua refers to the **gravid endometrium,** the functional layer of the endometrium in a pregnant woman that separates from the remainder of the uterus after parturition (childbirth). The three regions of the decidua are named according to their relation to the implantation site (Fig. 7-1):

- The decidua basalis is the part of the decidua deep to the conceptus that forms the maternal part of the placenta.
- The decidua capsularis is the superficial part of the decidua overlying the conceptus.
- The decidua parietalis is all the remaining parts of the decidua.

In response to increasing progesterone levels in the maternal blood, the connective tissue cells of the decidua enlarge to form pale-staining **decidual cells**. These cells enlarge as glycogen and lipid accumulate in their cytoplasm. The cellular and vascular changes occurring in the endometrium as the blastocyst implants constitute the **decidual reaction**. Many decidual cells degenerate near the chorionic sac in the region of the syncytiotrophoblast and, together with maternal blood and uterine secretions, provide a rich source of nutrition for the embryo. The full significance of decidual cells is not understood, but it has also been suggested that they protect the maternal tissue against uncontrolled invasion by the syncytiotrophoblast and that they may be involved in hormone production. Decidual regions, clearly recognizable during ultrasonography, are important in diagnosing early pregnancy.

Development of the Placenta

Early placental development is characterized by the rapid proliferation of the trophoblast and development of the chorionic sac and chorionic villi (see Chapters 3 and 4). By the end of the third week, the anatomic arrangements necessary for physiologic exchanges between the mother and her embryo are established. A complex vascular network is established in the placenta by the end of the fourth week, which facilitates maternal-embryonic exchanges of gases, nutrients, and metabolic waste products.

Chorionic villi cover the entire chorionic sac until the beginning of the eighth week (Figs. 7-1*C*, 7-2, and 7-3). As this sac grows, the villi associated with the decidua capsularis are compressed, reducing the blood supply to them. These villi soon degenerate (see Figs. 7-1*D* and 7-3*B*), producing a relatively avascular bare area, the **smooth chorion**. As these villi disappear, those associated with the decidua basalis rapidly increase in number, branch profusely, and enlarge. This bushy area of the chorionic sac is the **villous chorion** (Fig. 7-4).

Ultrasonography of Chorionic Sac

The size of the chorionic (gestational) sac is useful in determining gestational age of embryos in patients with uncertain menstrual histories. Growth of the chorionic sac is extremely rapid between weeks 5 and 10. Modern ultrasound equipment, especially instruments equipped with intravaginal transducers, enables ultrasonographers to detect the chorionic sac, or gestational sac, when it has a median sac diameter of 2 to 3 mm (Fig. 7-5). Chorionic sacs with this diameter indicate that the gestational age is 4 weeks and 3 to 4 days, that is, approximately 18 days after fertilization.

The uterus, chorionic sac, and placenta enlarge as the embryo and later the fetus grow. Growth in the size and thickness of the placenta continues rapidly until the fetus is approximately 18 weeks old (20 weeks' gestation). The fully developed placenta covers 15% to 30% of the decidua and weighs approximately one sixth that of the fetus. The placenta has two parts (Figs. 7-1*E* and *F* and 7-6):

- **The fetal part of the placenta** is formed by the villous chorion. The chorionic villi that arise from it project into the intervillous space containing maternal blood.
- **The maternal part of the placenta** is formed by the decidua basalis, the part of the decidua related to the fetal component of the placenta. By the end of the fourth month, the decidua basalis is almost entirely replaced by the fetal part of the placenta.

The fetal part of the placenta (villous chorion) is attached to the maternal part of the placenta (decidua basalis) by the **cytotrophoblastic shell**, the external layer of trophoblastic cells on the maternal surface of the

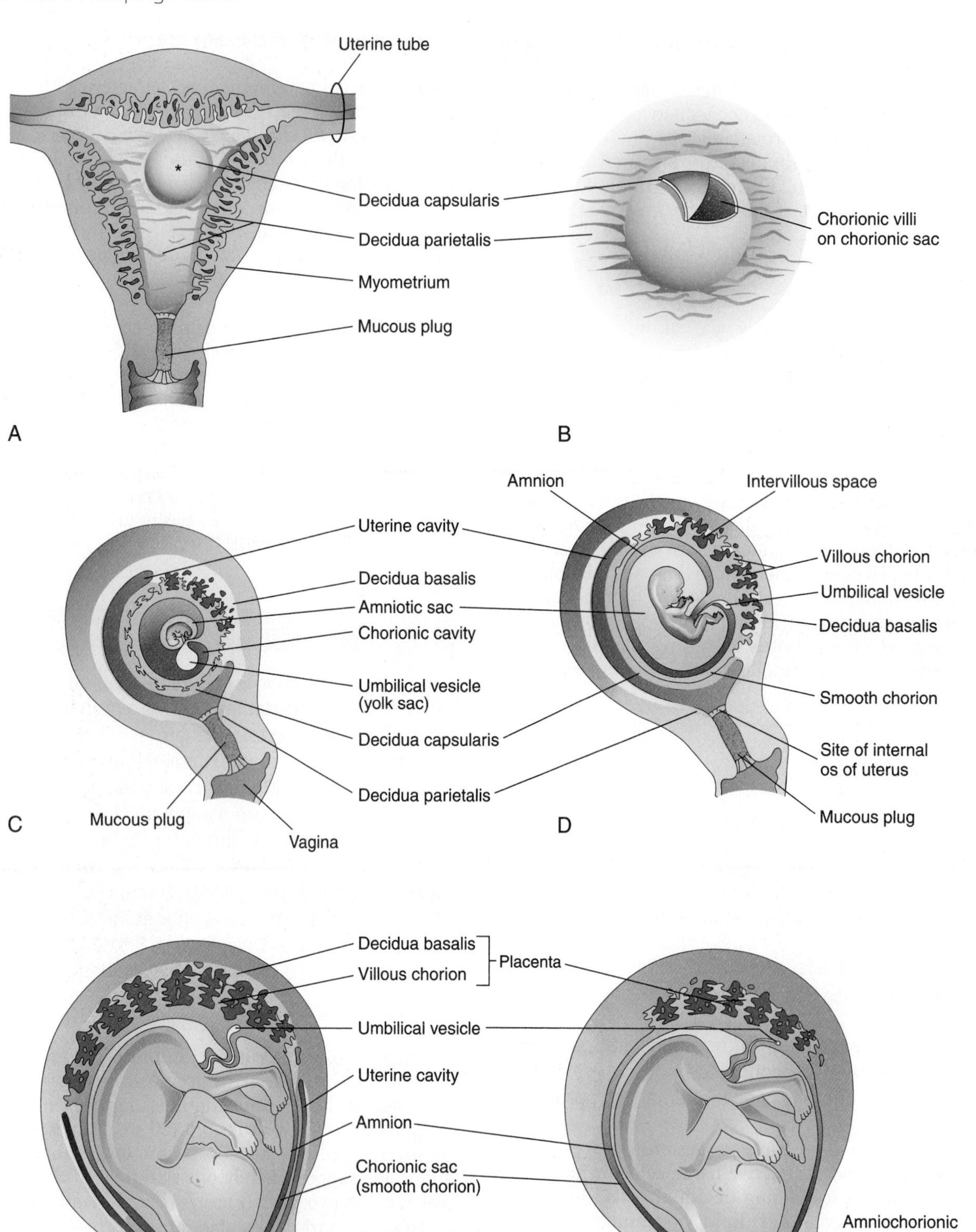

FIGURE 7-1. Development of the placenta and fetal membranes. **A,** Frontal section of the uterus showing elevation of the decidua capsularis by the expanding chorionic sac of a 4-week embryo implanted in the endometrium on the posterior wall (*). **B,** Enlarged drawing of the implantation site. The chorionic villi were exposed by cutting an opening in the decidua capsularis. **C** to **F,** Sagittal sections of the gravid uterus from weeks 5 to 22 showing the changing relations of the fetal membranes to the decidua. In **F,** the amnion and chorion are fused with each other and the decidua parietalis, thereby obliterating the uterine cavity. Note in **D** to **F** that the chorionic villi persist only where the chorion is associated with the decidua basalis.

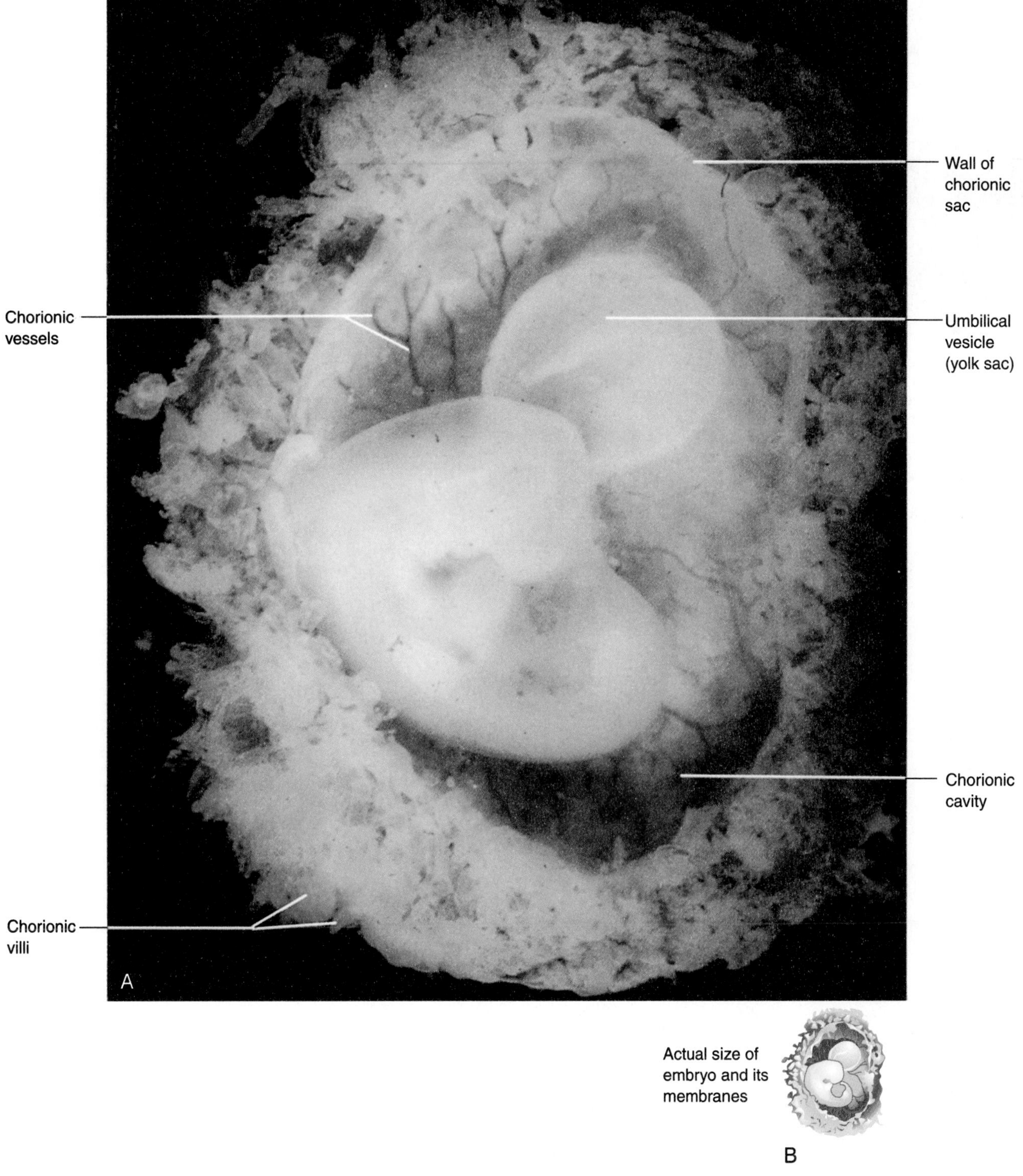

FIGURE 7-2. **A,** Lateral view of a spontaneously aborted embryo at Carnegie stage 14, approximately 32 days. The chorionic and amniotic sacs have been opened to show the embryo. Note the large size of the umbilical vesicle at this stage. **B,** The sketch shows the actual size of the embryo and its membranes. (**A,** From Moore KL, Persaud TVN, Shiota K: Color Atlas of Clinical Embryology, 2nd ed. Philadelphia, WB Saunders, 2000.)

placenta (Fig. 7-7). The chorionic villi attach firmly to the decidua basalis through the cytotrophoblastic shell and anchor the chorionic sac to the decidua basalis. Endometrial arteries and veins pass freely through gaps in the **cytotrophoblastic shell** and open into the intervillous space.

The shape of the placenta is determined by the persistent area of chorionic villi (see Fig. 7-1*F*). Usually this is a circular area, giving the placenta a discoid shape. As the chorionic villi invade the decidua basalis, decidual tissue is eroded to enlarge the intervillous space. This erosion produces several wedge-shaped areas of decidua,

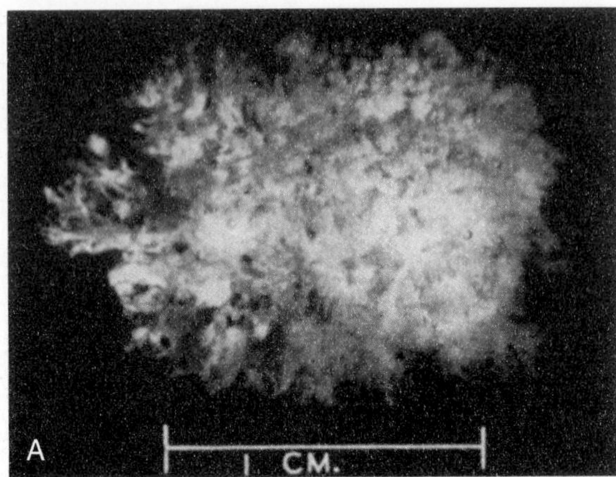

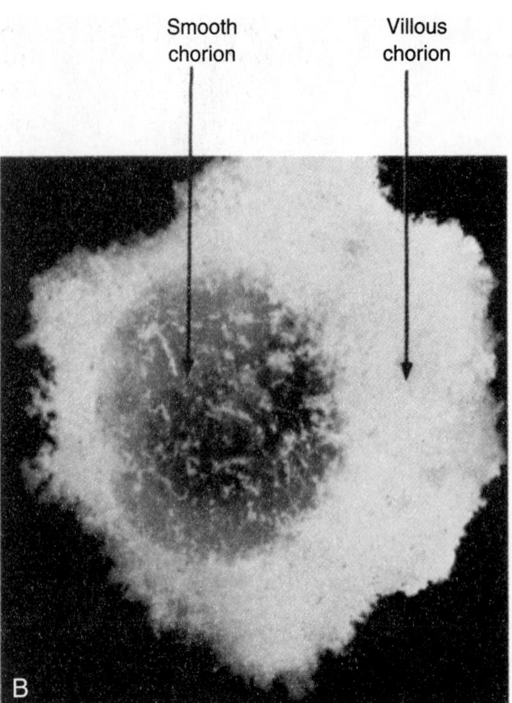

FIGURE 7-3. Spontaneously aborted human chorionic sacs. **A,** At 21 days. The entire sac is covered with chorionic villi (×4). **B,** At 8 weeks. Actual size. As the decidua capsularis becomes stretched and thin, the chorionic villi on the corresponding part of the chorionic sac gradually degenerate and disappear, leaving a smooth chorion. The remaining villous chorion forms the fetal part of the placenta. (From Potter EL, Craig JM: Pathology of the Fetus and the Infant, 3rd ed. Copyright 1975 by Year Book Medical Publishers, Chicago.)

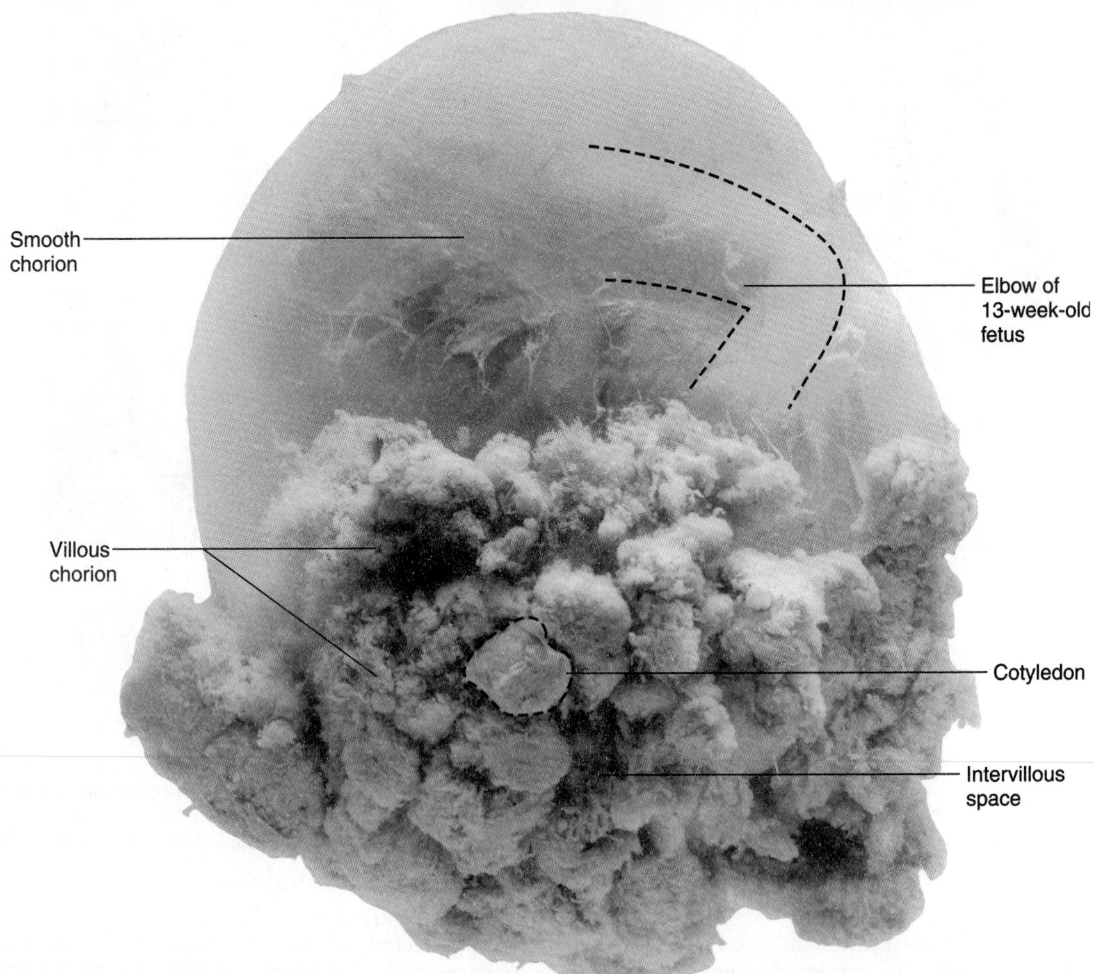

FIGURE 7-4. Spontaneously aborted human chorionic sac containing a 13-week fetus. The smooth chorion formed when the chorionic villi degenerated and disappeared from this area of the chorionic sac. The villous chorion is where chorionic villi persist and form the fetal part of the placenta. In situ, the cotyledons were attached to the decidua basalis and the intervillous space was filled with maternal blood. (From Moore KL, Persaud TVN, Shiota K: Color Atlas of Clinical Embryology, 2nd ed. Philadelphia, WB Saunders, 2000.)

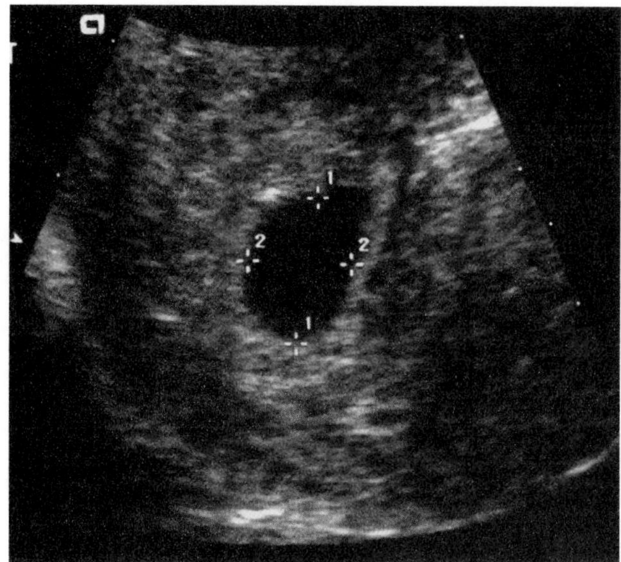

FIGURE 7-5. Sonogram of an early chorionic (gestational) sac showing how the mean sac diameter is measured. The mean sac diameter is determined by adding the three orthogonal dimensions of the chorionic sac and dividing by 3. (From Laing FC, Frates MC: Ultrasound evaluation during the first trimester of pregnancy. In Callen PW [ed]: Ultrasonography in Obstetrics and Gynecology, 4th ed. Philadelphia, WB Saunders, 2000.)

placental septa, that project toward the chorionic plate, the part of the chorionic wall related to the placenta (see Fig. 7-7). The placental septa divide the fetal part of the placenta into irregular convex areas—**cotyledons** (see Fig. 7-4). Each cotyledon consists of two or more stem villi and their many branch villi (Fig. 7-8*A*). By the end of the fourth month, the decidua basalis is almost entirely replaced by the cotyledons. Expression of the transcription factor Gcm1 (glial cells missing-1) in trophoblast stem cells regulates the branching process of the stem villi to form the vascular network in the placenta.

The **decidua capsularis**, the layer of decidua overlying the implanted chorionic sac, forms a capsule over the external surface of the sac (see Fig. 7-1*A* to *D*). As the conceptus enlarges, the decidua capsularis bulges into the uterine cavity and becomes greatly attenuated. Eventually the decidua capsularis contacts and fuses with the decidua parietalis, thereby slowly obliterating the uterine cavity (see Fig. 7-1*E* and *F*). By 22 to 24 weeks, the reduced blood supply to the decidua capsularis causes it to degenerate and disappear. After disappearance of the decidua capsularis, the smooth part of the chorionic sac fuses with the decidua parietalis. This fusion can be separated and usually occurs when blood escapes from the intervillous space (see Fig. 7-6). The collection of blood (hematoma) pushes the chorionic membrane away from the decidua parietalis, thereby reestablishing the potential space of the uterine cavity.

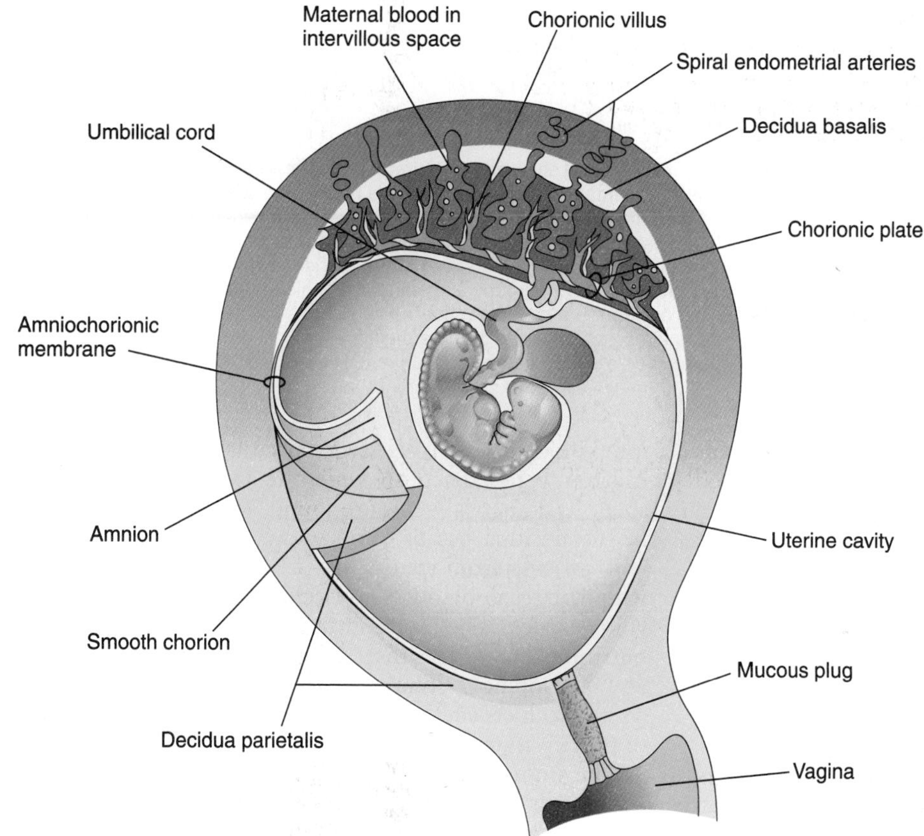

FIGURE 7-6. Drawing of a sagittal section of a gravid uterus at 4 weeks shows the relation of the fetal membranes to each other and to the decidua and embryo. The amnion and smooth chorion have been cut and reflected to show their relationship to each other and the decidua parietalis.

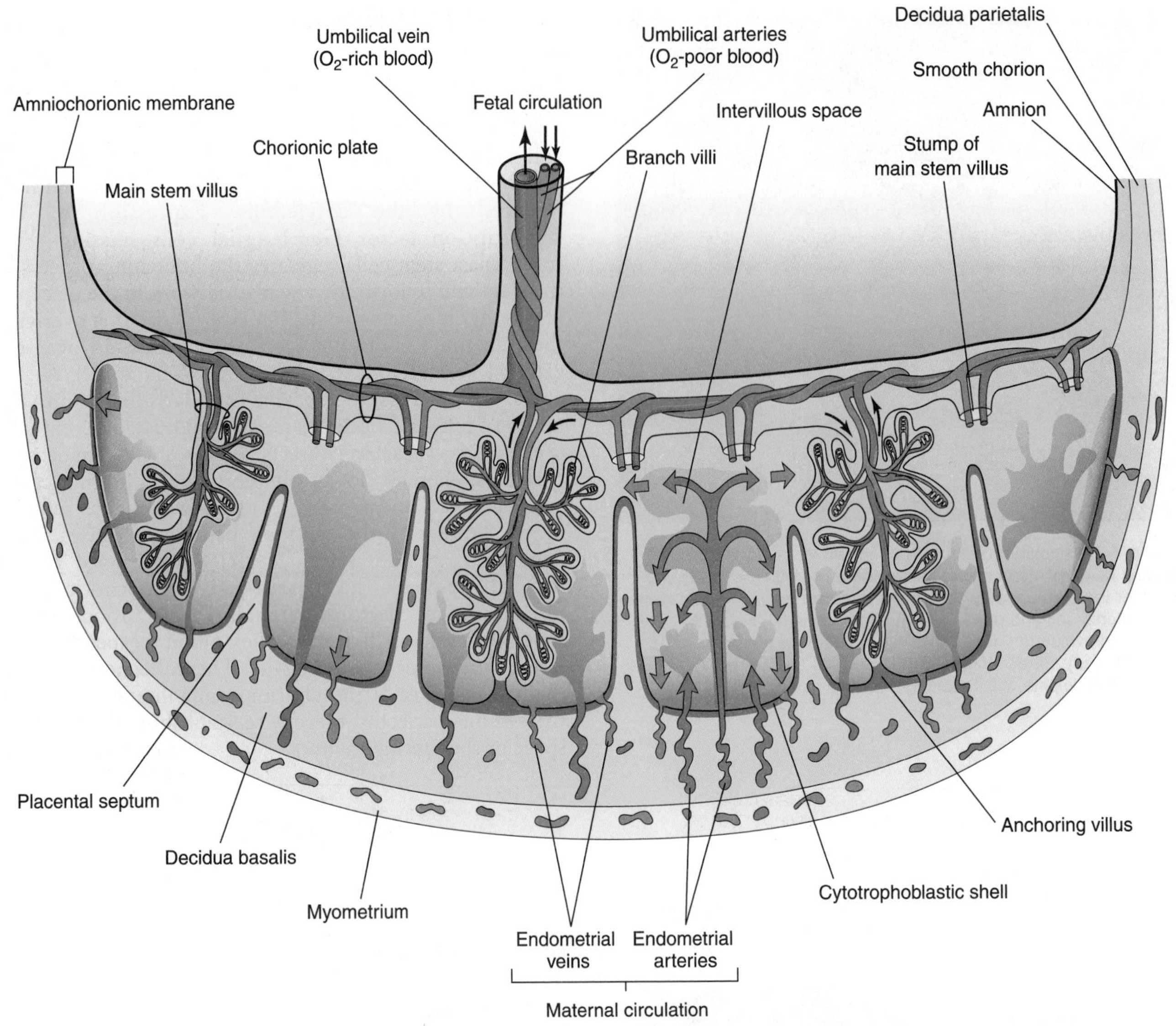

FIGURE 7-7. Schematic drawing of a transverse section through a full-term placenta, showing (1) the relation of the villous chorion (fetal part of placenta) to the decidua basalis (maternal part of placenta), (2) the fetal placental circulation, and (3) the maternal placental circulation. Maternal blood flows into the intervillous space in funnel-shaped spurts from the spiral endometrial arteries, and exchanges occur with the fetal blood as the maternal blood flows around the branch villi. It is through these villi that the main exchange of material between the mother and embryo/fetus occurs. The inflowing arterial blood pushes venous blood out of the intervillous space into the endometrial veins, which are scattered over the surface of the decidua basalis. Note that the umbilical arteries carry poorly oxygenated fetal blood (shown in blue) to the placenta and that the umbilical vein carries oxygenated blood (shown in red) to the fetus. Note that the cotyledons are separated from each other by placental septa, projections of the decidua basalis. Each cotyledon consists of two or more main stem villi and many branch villi. In this drawing, only one stem villus is shown in each cotyledon, but the stumps of those that have been removed are indicated.

The **intervillous space** of the placenta, which contains maternal blood, is derived from the lacunae that developed in the syncytiotrophoblast during the second week of development (see Chapter 3). This large blood-filled space results from the coalescence and enlargement of the lacunar networks. The intervillous space of the placenta is divided into compartments by the **placental septa**; however, there is free communication between the compartments because the septa do not reach the chorionic plate (see Fig. 7-7).

Maternal blood enters the intervillous space from the **spiral endometrial arteries** in the decidua basalis (see Figs. 7-6 and 7-7). The spiral arteries pass through gaps in the cytotrophoblastic shell and discharge blood into the intervillous space. This large space is drained by **endometrial veins** that also penetrate the cytotrophoblastic shell. Endometrial veins are found over the entire surface of the decidua basalis. The numerous branch chorionic villi—arising from stem villi—are continuously showered with maternal blood that circulates through the intervillous space. The blood in this space carries oxygen and nutritional materials that are necessary for fetal growth and development. The maternal blood also contains fetal waste products such as carbon dioxide, salts, and products of protein metabolism.

The amniotic sac enlarges faster than the chorionic sac. As a result, the amnion and smooth chorion soon fuse to form the **amniochorionic membrane** (see Figs. 7-6 and

7-7). This composite membrane fuses with the decidua capsularis and, after disappearance of this capsular part of the decidua, adheres to the decidua parietalis (see Fig. 7-1*F*). It is the amniochorionic membrane that ruptures during labor (the expulsion of the fetus and placenta from the uterus). Preterm rupture of this membrane is the most common event leading to premature labor. When the membrane ruptures, amniotic fluid escapes through the cervix and vagina to the exterior.

Placental Circulation

The branch chorionic villi of the placenta provide a large surface area where materials may be exchanged across the very thin placental membrane ("barrier") interposed between the fetal and maternal circulations (see Figs. 7-7 and 7-8). It is through the numerous branch villi that arise from the stem villi that the main exchange of material between the mother and fetus takes place. The circulations of the fetus and the mother are separated by the placental membrane consisting of extrafetal tissues (see Fig. 7-8*B* and *C*).

Fetal Placental Circulation

Poorly oxygenated blood leaves the fetus and passes through the umbilical arteries to the placenta. At the site of attachment of the umbilical cord to the placenta, these arteries divide into several radially disposed chorionic arteries that branch freely in the chorionic plate before entering the chorionic villi (see Fig. 7-7). The blood vessels form an extensive arteriocapillary-venous system within the chorionic villi (see Fig. 7-8*A*), which brings the fetal blood extremely close to the maternal blood. This system provides a very large surface area for the exchange of metabolic and gaseous products between the maternal and fetal bloodstreams. There is normally no intermingling of fetal and maternal blood; however, very small amounts of fetal blood may enter the maternal circulation when minute defects develop in the placental membrane. The well-oxygenated fetal blood in the fetal capillaries passes into thin-walled veins that follow the chorionic arteries to the site of attachment of the umbilical cord. They converge here to form the umbilical vein. This large vessel carries oxygen-rich blood to the fetus (see Fig. 7-7).

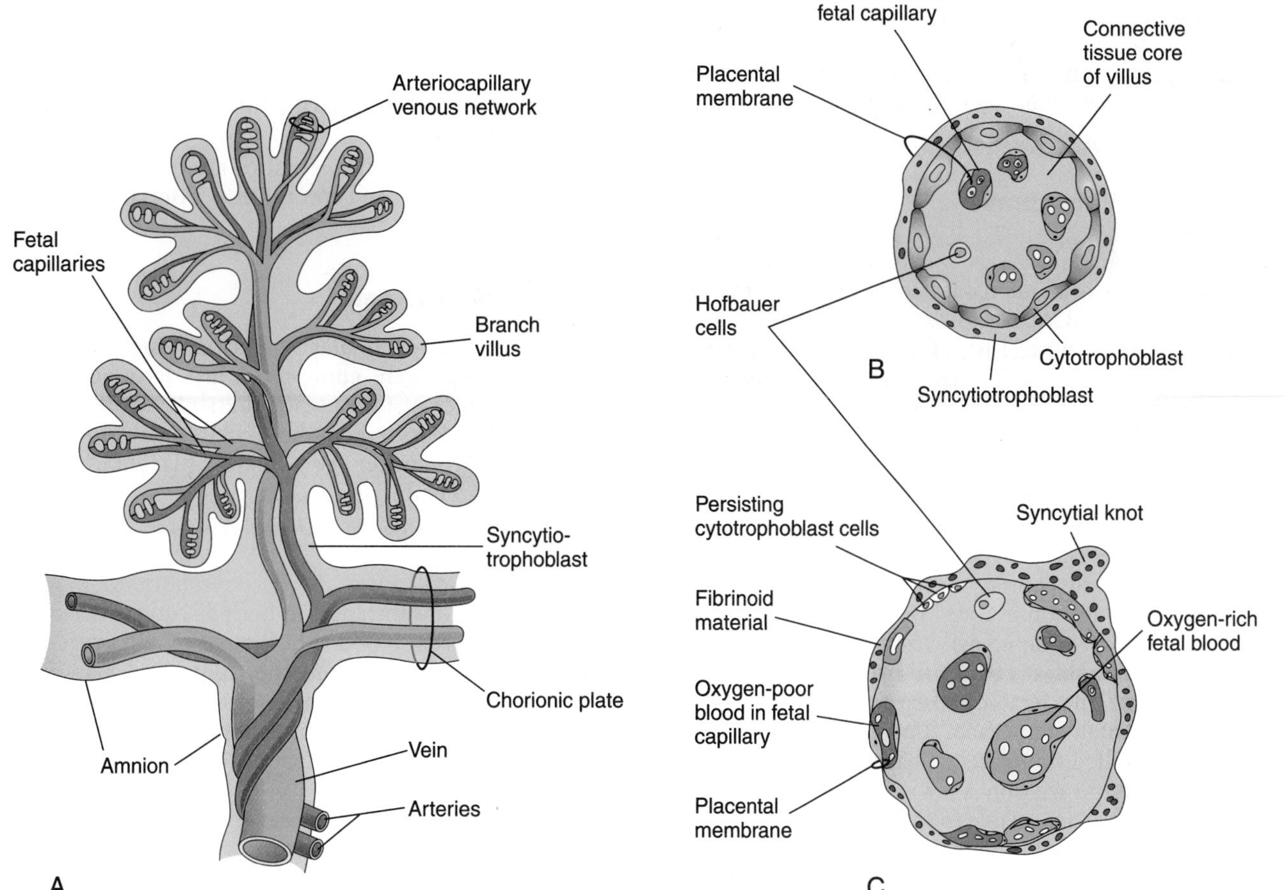

FIGURE 7-8. **A,** Drawing of a stem chorionic villus showing its arteriocapillary-venous system. The arteries carry poorly oxygenated fetal blood and waste products from the fetus, whereas the vein carries oxygenated blood and nutrients to the fetus. **B** and **C,** Drawings of sections through a branch villus at 10 weeks and full term, respectively. The placental membrane, composed of extrafetal tissues, separates the maternal blood in the intervillous space from the fetal blood in the capillaries in the villi. Note that the placental membrane becomes very thin at full term. Hofbauer cells are thought to be phagocytic cells.

Maternal Placental Circulation

The maternal blood in the intervillous space is temporarily outside the maternal circulatory system. It enters the intervillous space through 80 to 100 spiral endometrial arteries in the decidua basalis. These vessels discharge into the intervillous space through gaps in the cytotrophoblastic shell. The blood flow from the **spiral arteries** is pulsatile and is propelled in jetlike fountains by the maternal blood pressure (see Fig. 7-7). The entering blood is at a considerably higher pressure than that in the intervillous space and spurts toward the **chorionic plate** forming the "roof" of the intervillous space. As the pressure dissipates, the blood flows slowly over the branch villi, allowing an exchange of metabolic and gaseous products with the fetal blood. The blood eventually returns through the endometrial veins to the maternal circulation.

The welfare of the embryo and fetus depends more on the adequate bathing of the branch villi with maternal blood than on any other factor. Reductions of uteroplacental circulation result in **fetal hypoxia** and intrauterine growth restriction (IUGR). Severe reductions of uteroplacental circulation may result in fetal death. The intervillous space of the mature placenta contains approximately 150 mL of blood that is replenished three or four times per minute. The intermittent contractions of the uterus during pregnancy decrease uteroplacental blood flow slightly; however, they do not force significant amounts of blood out of the intervillous space. Consequently, oxygen transfer to the fetus is decreased during uterine contractions, but does not stop.

The Placental Membrane

The placental membrane is a composite structure that consists of the extrafetal tissues separating the maternal and fetal blood. Until approximately 20 weeks, the **placental membrane** consists of four layers (Figs. 7-8 and 7-9): syncytiotrophoblast, cytotrophoblast, connective tissue of villus, and endothelium of fetal capillaries.

After the 20th week, histologic changes occur in the branch villi that result in the cytotrophoblast in many of the villi becoming attenuated. Eventually cytotrophoblastic cells disappear over large areas of the villi, leaving only thin patches of syncytiotrophoblast. As a result, the placental membrane consists of three layers in most places (see Fig. 7-8*C*). In some areas, the placental membrane becomes markedly thinned and attenuated. At these sites, the syncytiotrophoblast comes in direct contact with the endothelium of the fetal capillaries to form a vasculosyncytial placental membrane. The placental membrane was formerly called the placental barrier, an inappropriate term because there are only a few substances, endogenous or exogenous, that are unable to pass through the placental membrane in detectable amounts. The placental membrane acts as a barrier only when the molecule is of a certain size, configuration, and charge such as heparin and bacteria. Some metabolites, toxins, and hormones, although present in the maternal circulation, do not pass through the placental membrane in sufficient concentrations to affect the embryo/fetus.

Most drugs and other substances in the maternal plasma pass through the placental membrane and enter the fetal plasma (see Fig. 7-9). Electron micrographs of the syncytiotrophoblast show that its free surface has many microvilli, more than 1 billion/cm^2 at term, that increase the surface area for exchange between the maternal and fetal circulations. As pregnancy advances, the placental membrane becomes progressively thinner so that blood in many fetal capillaries is extremely close to the maternal blood in the intervillous space (see Fig. 7-8*C*).

During the third trimester, numerous nuclei in the syncytiotrophoblast aggregate to form multinucleated protrusions called nuclear aggregations or **syncytial knots**. These aggregations continually break off and are carried from the intervillous space into the maternal circulation. Some knots lodge in capillaries of the maternal lung where they are rapidly destroyed by local enzyme action. Toward the end of pregnancy, fibrinoid material forms on the surfaces of villi. This material consists of fibrin and other unidentified substances that stain intensely with eosin. Fibrinoid material results mainly from aging and appears to reduce placental transfer.

Functions of the Placenta

The placenta has three main functions:

- Metabolism (e.g., synthesis of glycogen)
- Transport of gases and nutrients
- Endocrine secretion (e.g., human chorionic gonadotropin [hCG])

These comprehensive activities are essential for maintaining pregnancy and promoting normal fetal development.

Placental Metabolism

The placenta, particularly during early pregnancy, synthesizes glycogen, cholesterol, and fatty acids, which serve as sources of nutrients and energy for the embryo/fetus. Many of its metabolic activities are undoubtedly critical for its other two major placental activities (transport and endocrine secretion).

Placental Transfer

The transport of substances in both directions between the fetal and maternal blood is facilitated by the great surface area of the placental membrane. Almost all materials are transported across the placental membrane by one of the following four main transport mechanisms: simple diffusion, facilitated diffusion, active transport, and pinocytosis.

Passive transport by **simple diffusion** is usually characteristic of substances moving from areas of higher to lower concentration until equilibrium is established. In **facilitated diffusion**, there is transport through electrical gradients. **Active transport** against a concentration gradient requires energy. Such systems may involve carrier molecules that temporarily combine with the substances to be transported. **Pinocytosis** is a form of endocytosis in

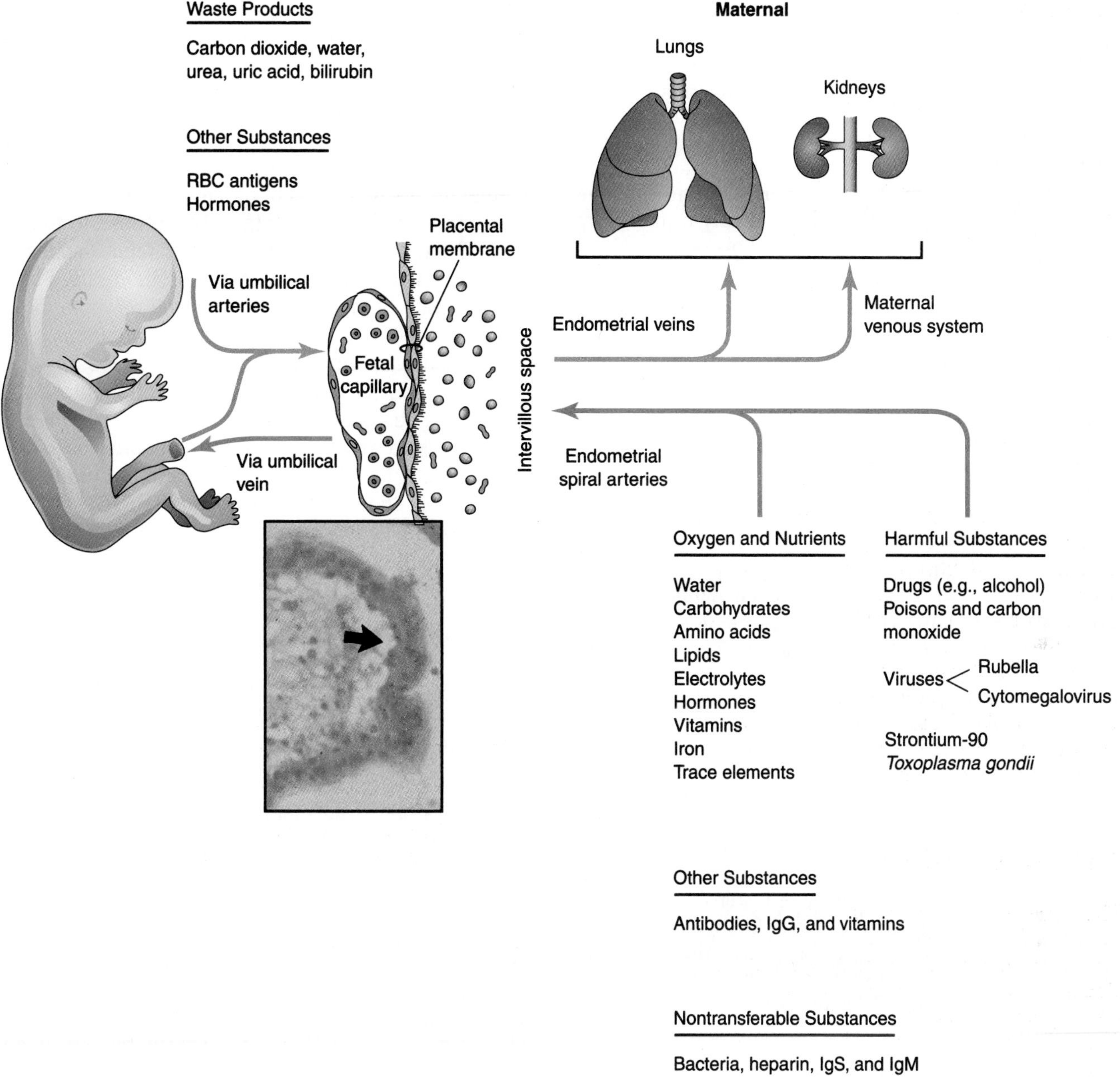

FIGURE 7-9. Diagrammatic illustration of transfer across the placental membrane (barrier). The extrafetal tissues, across which transport of substances between the mother and fetus occurs, collectively constitute the placental membrane. *Inset*, Light micrograph of chorionic villus showing a fetal capillary (*arrow*) and the placental membrane.

which the material being engulfed is a small amount of extracellular fluid. This method of transport is usually reserved for large molecules. Some proteins are transferred very slowly through the placenta by pinocytosis.

OTHER PLACENTAL TRANSPORT MECHANISMS

There are three other methods of transfer across the placental membrane. In the first, fetal red blood cells pass into the maternal circulation, particularly during parturition, through microscopic breaks in the placental membrane. Labeled maternal red blood cells have also been found in the fetal circulation. Consequently, red blood cells may pass in either direction through very small defects in the placental membrane. In the second method of transport, cells cross the placental membrane under their own power, e.g., maternal leukocytes and *Treponema pallidum*, the organism that causes syphilis. In the third method of transport, some bacteria and protozoa such as *Toxoplasma gondii* infect the placenta by creating lesions and then cross the placental membrane through the defects that are created.

Transfer of Gases

Oxygen, carbon dioxide, and carbon monoxide cross the placental membrane by simple diffusion. Interruption of oxygen transport for several minutes endangers survival of the embryo or fetus. The placental membrane approaches the efficiency of the lungs for gas exchange. The quantity of oxygen reaching the fetus is primarily flow limited rather than diffusion limited; hence, fetal hypoxia (decreased levels of oxygen) results primarily from factors that diminish either the uterine blood flow or fetal blood flow.

Nutritional Substances

Nutrients constitute the bulk of substances transferred from the mother to the embryo/fetus. Water is rapidly exchanged by simple diffusion and in increasing amounts as pregnancy advances. Glucose produced by the mother and placenta is quickly transferred to the embryo/fetus by facilitated diffusion. There is little or no transfer of maternal cholesterol, triglycerides, or phospholipids. Although there is transport of free fatty acids, the amount transferred appears to be relatively small. Amino acids are actively transported across the placental membrane and are essential for fetal growth. For most amino acids, the plasma concentrations in the fetus are higher than in the mother. Vitamins cross the placental membrane and are essential for normal development. Water-soluble vitamins cross the placental membrane more quickly than fat-soluble ones.

Hormones

Protein hormones do not reach the embryo or fetus in significant amounts, except for a slow transfer of thyroxine and triiodothyronine. Unconjugated steroid hormones cross the placental membrane rather freely. Testosterone and certain synthetic progestins cross the placental membrane and may cause masculinization of female fetuses in some cases (see Chapter 20).

Electrolytes

These compounds are freely exchanged across the placental membrane in significant quantities, each at its own rate. When a mother receives intravenous fluids with electrolytes, they also pass to the fetus and affect its water and electrolyte status.

Maternal Antibodies

The fetus produces only small amounts of antibodies because of its immature immune system. Some passive immunity is conferred on the fetus by the placental transfer of maternal antibodies. IgG gamma globulins are readily transported to the fetus by transcytosis. Maternal antibodies confer fetal immunity to some diseases such as diphtheria, smallpox, and measles; however, no immunity is acquired to pertussis (whooping cough) or varicella (chickenpox). A maternal protein, transferrin, crosses the placental membrane and carries iron to the embryo or fetus. The placental surface contains special receptors for this protein.

Hemolytic Disease of the Newborn

Small amounts of fetal blood may pass to the maternal blood through microscopic breaks in the placental membrane. If the fetus is Rh positive and the mother Rh negative, the fetal blood cells may stimulate the formation of anti-Rh antibodies by the immune system of the mother. These pass to the fetal blood and causes hemolysis of fetal Rh-positive blood cells, jaundice, and anemia in the fetus. Some fetuses with hemolytic disease of the newborn, or fetal erythroblastosis, fail to make a satisfactory intrauterine adjustment. They may die unless delivered early or given intrauterine, intraperitoneal, or intravenous transfusions of packed Rh-negative blood cells to maintain the fetus until after birth (see Chapter 6). Hemolytic disease of the newborn is relatively uncommon now because Rh (D) immunoglobulin given to the mother usually prevents development of this disease in the fetus.

Waste Products

Urea and uric acid pass through the placental membrane by simple diffusion. Conjugated bilirubin (which is fat soluble) is easily transported by the placenta for rapid clearance.

Drugs and Drug Metabolites

Most drugs and drug metabolites cross the placenta by simple diffusion, the exception being those with a structural similarity to amino acids, such as methyldopa and antimetabolites. Some drugs cause major congenital anomalies (see Chapter 20). Fetal drug addiction may occur after maternal use of drugs such as heroin and 50% to 75% of these newborns experience withdrawal symptoms. Because psychic dependence on these drugs is not developed during the fetal period, no liability to subsequent narcotic addiction exists in the infant after withdrawal is complete.

Most drugs used for the management of labor readily cross the placental membrane. Depending on the dose and its timing in relation to delivery, these drugs may cause respiratory depression of the newborn infant. All sedatives and analgesics affect the fetus to some degree. Neuromuscular blocking agents that may be used during operative obstetrics cross the placenta in only small amounts. Drugs taken by the mother can affect the embryo/fetus directly or indirectly by interfering with maternal or placental metabolism. Inhaled anesthetics can also cross the placental membrane and affect fetal breathing if used during parturition. The amount of drug or metabolite reaching the placenta is controlled by the maternal blood level and blood flow through the placenta.

Infectious Agents

Cytomegalovirus, rubella, and coxsackie viruses, and viruses associated with variola, varicella, measles, and poliomyelitis may pass through the placental membrane and cause fetal infection. In some cases, such as the rubella virus, congenital anomalies, such as cataracts, may be produced (see Chapter 20). Microorganisms such as *Treponema pallidum*, which causes syphilis, and *Toxoplasma gondii*, which produces destructive changes in the brain and eyes, also cross the placental membrane, often causing congenital anomalies and/or death of the embryo or fetus.

Placental Endocrine Synthesis and Secretion

Using precursors derived from the fetus and/or the mother, the syncytiotrophoblast of the placenta synthesizes protein and steroid hormones. The protein hormones synthesized by the placenta are

- hCG
- Human chorionic somatomammotropin or human placental lactogen
- Human chorionic thyrotropin
- Human chorionic corticotropin

The glycoprotein hCG, similar to luteinizing hormone, is first secreted by the syncytiotrophoblast during the second week; hCG maintains the corpus luteum, preventing the onset of menstrual periods. The concentration of hCG in the maternal blood and urine increases to a maximum by the eighth week and then declines. The steroid hormones synthesized by the placenta are progesterone and estrogens. Progesterone can be obtained from the placenta at all stages of gestation, indicating that it is essential for the maintenance of pregnancy. The placenta forms progesterone from maternal cholesterol or pregnenolone. The ovaries of a pregnant woman can be removed after the first trimester without causing an abortion because the placenta takes over the production of progesterone from the corpus luteum. Estrogens are also produced in large quantities by the syncytiotrophoblast.

The Placenta as an Allograft*

The placenta can be regarded as an **allograft** with respect to the mother. The fetal part of the placenta is a derivative of the conceptus, which inherits both paternal and maternal genes. What protects the placenta from rejection by the mother's immune system? This question remains a major biologic enigma in nature. The syncytiotrophoblast of the chorionic villi, although exposed to maternal immune cells within the blood sinusoids, lacks major histocompatibility (MHC) antigens and thus does not evoke rejection responses. However, extravillous trophoblast (EVT) cells, which invade the uterine decidua and its vasculature (spiral arteries), express class I MHC antigens. These antigens include HLA-G, which, being nonpolymorphic (class Ib), is poorly recognizable by T lymphocytes as an alloantigen, as well as HLA-C, which, being polymorphic (class Ia), is recognizable by T cells. In addition to averting T cells, EVT cells must also shield themselves from potential attack by natural killer (NK) lymphocytes and injury inflicted by activation of complement. Multiple mechanisms appear to be in place to guard the placenta:

1. Expression of HLA-G is restricted to a few tissues including placental EVT cells. Its strategic location in the placenta is believed to provide a dual immunoprotective role: evasion of T-cell recognition owing to its nonpolymorphic nature, and a recognition by the "killer-inhibitory receptors" on NK cells, thus turning off their killer function. Inadequacy of this hypothesis is suggested by several observations: (a) healthy individuals showing biallelic loss of HLA-G1 have been identified, indicating that HLA-G is not essential for fetoplacental survival; (b) human EVT cells were found to be vulnerable to NK cell–mediated killing; and (c) it does not explain why HLA-C, a polymorphic antigen, also expressed by EVT cells, does not evoke a rejection response in situ. Because both HLA-G and HLA-C were shown to have the unique ability to resist human cytomegalovirus-mediated MHC class I degradation, it is speculated that a selective location of these two antigens at the fetomaternal interface may help to withstand viral assault.
2. Immunoprotection is provided locally by certain immunosuppressor molecules, e.g., prostaglandin E_2, transforming growth factor (TGF) β and interleukin-10. Decidua-derived prostaglandin E_2 was shown to block activation of maternal T cells as well as NK cells in situ. Indeed, immunoregulatory function of decidual cells is consistent with their genealogy. It was shown that uterine endometrial stromal cells, which differentiate into decidual cells during pregnancy, are derived from progenitor (stem) cells that migrate from hemopoietic organs such as the fetal liver and the bone marrow during ontogeny.
3. Transient tolerance of maternal T-cell repertoire to fetal MHC antigens may serve as a backup mechanism for placental immunoprotection. A similar B-cell tolerance has also been reported.
4. A trafficking of activated maternal leukocytes into the placenta or the fetus is prevented by deletion of these cells triggered by apoptosis-inducing ligands present on the trophoblast.
5. Based on genetic manipulation in mice, it was shown that the presence of complement regulatory proteins (Crry in the mouse, membrane cofactor protein or CD46 in the human), which can block activation of the third component of complement (C3) in the complement cascade, protects the placenta from complement-mediated destruction, which may happen otherwise because of residual C3 activation remaining after defending against pathogens. Crry gene knockout mice died in utero because of complement-mediated placental damage, which could be averted by additional knockout of the C3 gene.
6. Experiments in mice revealed that the presence of the enzyme indoleamine 2,3-deoxygenase in trophoblastic cells was critical for immunoprotection of the allogeneic conceptus by suppressing T cell–driven local inflammatory responses including complement activation. Treatment of pregnant mice with an indoleamine 2,3-deoxygenase inhibitor, 1-methyl tryptophan, caused selective death of allogeneic (but not syngeneic) conceptuses due to massive deposition of complement and hemorrhagic necrosis at the placental sites.

*The authors are grateful to Dr. Peeyush Lala, Professor Emeritus, Department of Anatomy and Cell Biology, Faculty of Medicine, University of Western Ontario, London, Ontario, Canada, for preparing these sections.

The Placenta as an Invasive Tumorlike Structure

The placenta in many species, including human, is a highly invasive tumor-like structure that invades the uterus to tap on its blood supply to establish an adequate exchange of key molecules between the mother and the fetus. What protects the uterus from placental overinvasion? Following the development of chorionic villi, the invasive function of the placenta is provided by the subset of cytotrophoblastic cells, EVT cells, which are divided by proliferation and differentiation of stem cells located in the cytotrophoblast layer of certain chorionic villi (anchoring villi). They break out of the villous confines and migrate as cell columns to invade the decidua where they reorganize as distinct subsets: a nearly continuous cell layer (cytotrophoblastic shell) separating the decidua from maternal blood sinusoids; cells dispersed within the decidua (interstitial trophoblast); multinucleate placental bed giant cells produced by EVT cell fusion; and endovascular trophoblast, which invade and remodel the uteroplacental (spiral) arteries within the endometrium and a part of the myometrium. Optimal arterial remodeling (loss of tunica media and replacement of the endothelium by the EVT cells) allows steady placental perfusion with maternal blood unhindered by the presence of vasoactive molecules. Inadequate EVT cell invasion leading to poor placental perfusion underlies the pathogenesis of preeclampsia (a major pregnancy-associated hypertensive disorder in the mother) and certain forms of IUGR of the fetus, whereas excessive invasion is a hallmark of gestational trophoblastic neoplasias and choriocarcinomas.

Trophoblastic stem cells have been successfully propagated from the murine but not from the human placenta. However, normal human EVT cells have been successfully propagated from first-trimester human placentas. Using these cells for functional assays in vitro, it was shown that molecular mechanisms responsible for their invasiveness are identical to those of cancer cells, whereas their proliferation, migration, and invasiveness are stringently regulated in situ by a variety of locally produced molecules: growth factors, growth factor–binding proteins, proteoglycans, and components of the extracellular matrix. Numerous growth factors, e.g., epidermal growth factor, TGF-α, amphiregulin, colony-stimulating factor 1, vascular endothelial growth factor, and placental growth factor, all were shown to stimulate EVT cell proliferation without affecting migration or invasiveness, whereas insulin-like growth factor II and an insulin-like growth factor–binding protein, IGFBP-1, were shown to stimulate EVT cell migration and invasiveness without affecting proliferation. TGF-β, primarily produced by the decidua, was shown to provide the key control of EVT cell proliferation, migration, and invasiveness, whereas trophoblastic cancer (choriocarcinoma) cells were shown to be resistant to the inhibitory signals of TGF-β. Thus, it appears that the decidua plays a dual role in uteroplacental homeostasis by immunoprotection of the placenta and protection of the uterus from placental overinvasion.

Uterine Growth during Pregnancy

The uterus of a nonpregnant woman lies in the pelvis. To accommodate the growing conceptus, the uterus increases in size (Fig. 7-10*A*). It also increases in weight, and its walls become thinner (see Fig. 7-10*B* and *C*). During the first trimester, the uterus moves out of the pelvis and by 20 weeks reaches the level of the umbilicus. By 28 to 30 weeks, the uterus reaches the epigastric region, the area between the xiphoid process of the sternum and the umbilicus. The increase in size of the uterus largely results from hypertrophy of preexisting smooth muscular fibers and partly from the development of new fibers.

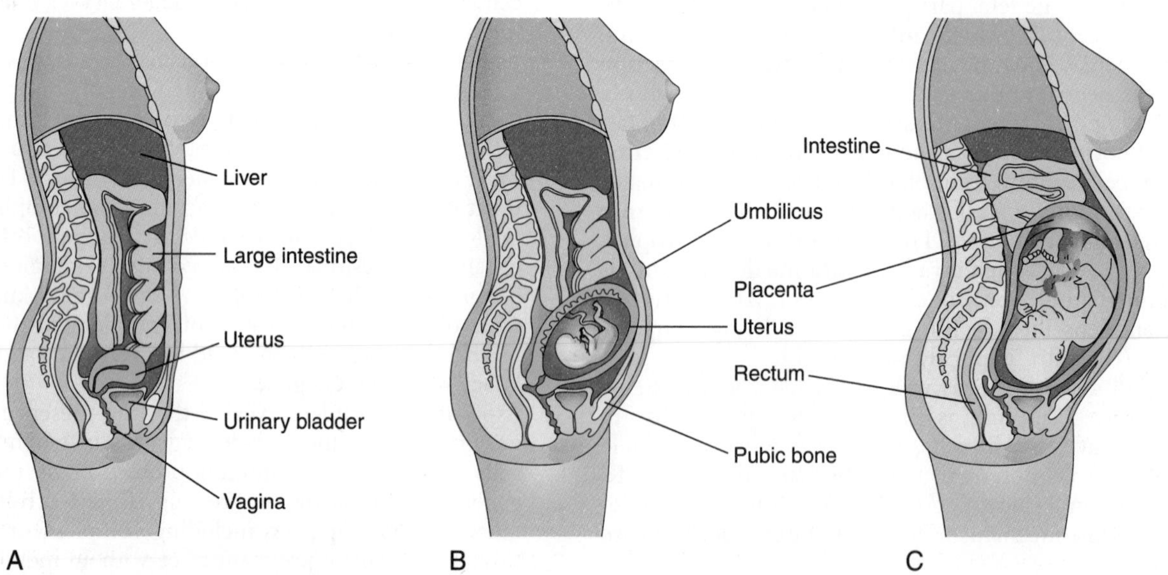

FIGURE 7-10. Drawings of median sections of a woman's body. **A,** Not pregnant. **B,** Twenty weeks pregnant. **C,** Thirty weeks pregnant. Note that as the conceptus enlarges, the uterus increases in size to accommodate the rapidly growing fetus. By 20 weeks, the uterus and fetus reach the level of the umbilicus, and by 30 weeks, they reach the epigastric region. The mother's abdominal viscera are displaced and compressed, and the skin and muscles of her anterior abdominal wall are stretched.

PARTURITION

Parturition (childbirth) is the process during which the fetus, placenta, and fetal membranes are expelled from the mother's reproductive tract (Fig. 7-11). **Labor** is the sequence of involuntary uterine contractions that result in dilation of the uterine cervix and expulsion of the fetus and placenta from the uterus. The factors that trigger labor are not completely understood, but several hormones are related to the initiation of contractions. The fetal hypothalamus secretes corticotropin-releasing hormone, which stimulates the anterior hypophysis (pituitary) to produce **adrenocorticotropin**. Adrenocorticotropin causes the secretion of **corticol** from the suprarenal (adrenal) cortex. Corticol is involved in the synthesis of estrogens. These steroids stimulate uterine contraction.

Peristaltic contractions of uterine smooth muscle are elicited by **oxytocin**, which is released by the neurohypophysis of the pituitary gland. This hormone is administered clinically when it is necessary to induce labor. Oxytocin also stimulates release of **prostaglandins** from the decidua that stimulate myometrial contractility by sensitizing the myometrial cells to oxytocin. **Estrogens** also increase myometrial contractile activity and stimulate the release of oxytocin and prostaglandins. From studies carried out in sheep and nonhuman primates, it seems that the duration of pregnancy and the process of birth are under the direct control of the fetus.

Labor is a continuous process; however, for clinical purposes, it is usually divided into three stages:

- **Dilation** begins with progressive dilation of the cervix (see Fig. 7-11*A* and *B*) and ends when the cervix is completely dilated. During this phase, regular painful contractions of the uterus occur less than 10 minutes apart. The average duration is approximately 12 hours for first pregnancies (primigravidas) and approximately 7 hours for women who have had a child previously (multigravidas).
- **Expulsion** begins when the cervix is fully dilated and ends with delivery of the baby (Figs. 7-11*C* to *E* and 7-12). During the second stage of labor, the fetus descends through the cervix and vagina. As soon as the fetus is outside the mother, it is called a newborn infant or neonate. The average duration of the second stage is 50 minutes for primigravidas and 20 minutes for multigravidas.
- **The placental stage** begins as soon as the baby is born and ends with the expulsion of the placenta and membranes. The duration of the third stage of labor is 15 minutes in approximately 90% of pregnancies. A retained placenta is one that has not been expelled within 60 minutes of delivery of the baby.

Retraction of the uterus reduces the area of placental attachment (see Fig. 7-11*G*). A hematoma, a localized mass of extravasated blood, soon forms deep to the placenta and separates it from the uterine wall. The placenta and fetal membranes are expelled through the vaginal canal. The placenta separates through the spongy layer of the decidua basalis (see Chapter 2). After delivery of the baby, the uterus continues to contract (see Fig. 7-11*H*). The myometrial contractions constrict the spiral arteries that supplied blood to the intervillous space. These contractions prevent excessive uterine bleeding.

The Placenta and Fetal Membranes after Birth

The placenta and fetal membranes are extruded from the uterus after birth. The **placenta** commonly has a discoid shape, with a diameter of 15 to 20 cm and a thickness of 2 to 3 cm (Fig. 7-13). It weighs 500 to 600 g, which is approximately one sixth the weight of the average fetus. The margins of the placenta are continuous with the ruptured amniotic and chorionic sacs. As the placenta develops, chorionic villi usually persist only where the villous chorion is in contact with the decidua basalis. This usually produces a discoid placenta (see Fig. 7-13). When villi persist on the entire surface of the chorionic sac (an uncommon occurrence), a thin layer of placenta attaches to a large area of the uterus. This type of placenta is a membranous placenta—placenta membranacea. When villi persist elsewhere, several variations in placental shape occur: accessory placenta (Fig. 7-14), bidiscoid placenta, and horseshoe placenta. Although there are variations in the size and shape of the placenta, most of them are of little physiologic or clinical significance.

GESTATIONAL CHORIOCARCINOMA

Abnormal proliferation of the trophoblast results in gestational trophoblastic disease, a spectrum of lesions including highly malignant tumors. The cells invade the decidua basalis, penetrate its blood vessels and lymphatics, and may metastasize to the maternal lungs, bone marrow, liver, and other organs. Gestational choriocarcinomas are highly sensitive to chemotherapy, and cures are usually achieved.

Maternal Surface of the Placenta

The characteristic cobblestone appearance of the maternal surface is produced by slightly bulging villous areas—**cotyledons**—that are separated by grooves that were formerly occupied by placental septa (see Figs. 7-7 and 7-13*A*). The surface of the cotyledons is covered by thin grayish shreds of decidua basalis that separated from the uterine wall when the placenta was extruded. These shreds of tissue are recognizable in sections of the placenta that are examined under a microscope. Most of the decidua is temporarily retained in the uterus and is shed with the uterine bleeding.

Examination of the placenta prenatally by ultrasonography or magnetic resonance imaging (Fig. 7-15) or postnatally by gross and microscopic study may provide clinical information about the causes of IUGR, placental dysfunction, fetal distress and death, and neonatal illness.

Placental studies can also determine whether the placenta is complete. Retention of a cotyledon or an

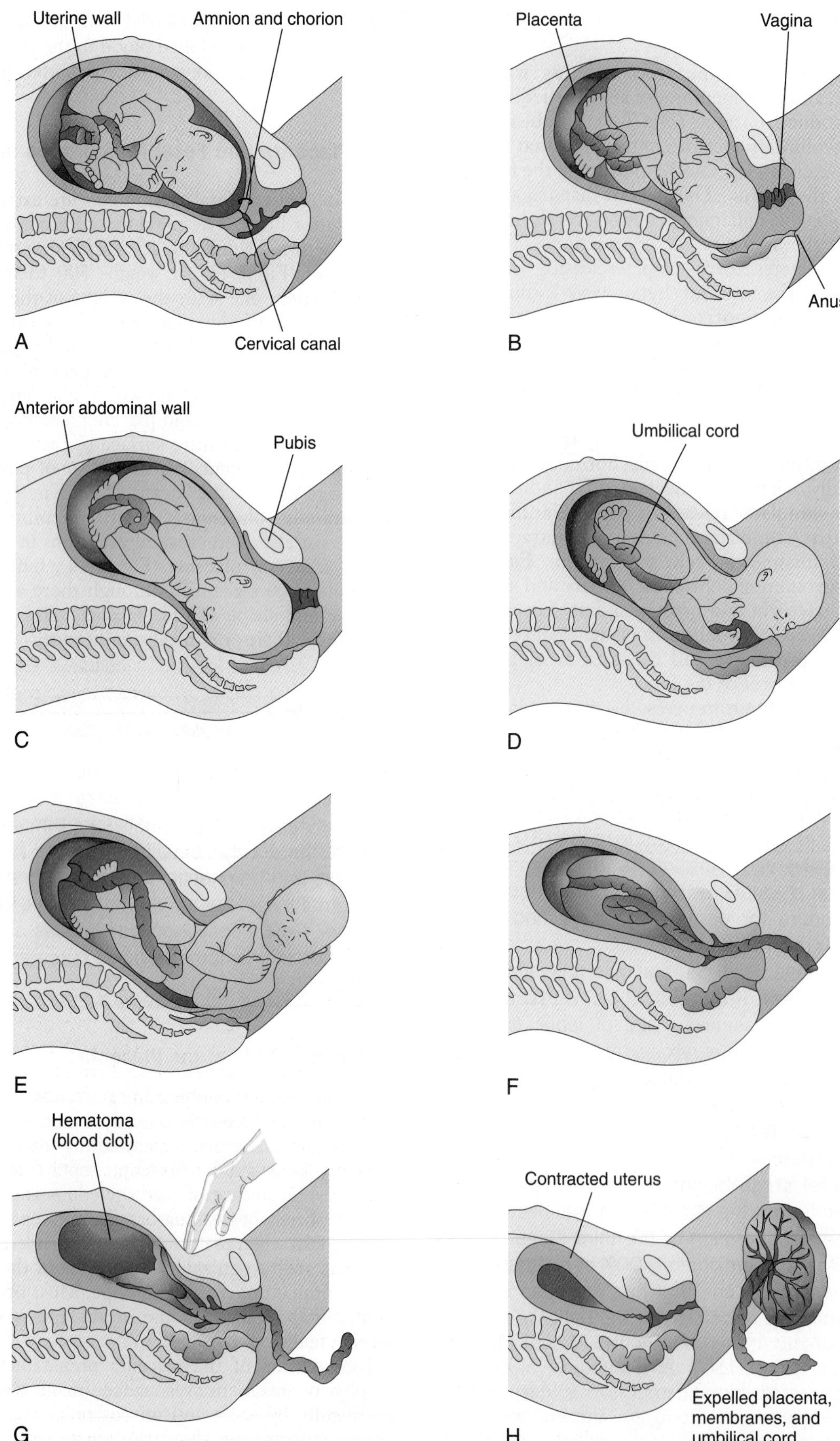

FIGURE 7-11. Drawings illustrating parturition (childbirth). **A** and **B,** The cervix is dilating during the first stage of labor. **C** to **E,** The fetus is passing through the cervix and vagina during the second stage of labor. **F** and **G,** As the uterus contracts during the third stage of labor, the placenta folds and pulls away from the uterine wall. Separation of the placenta results in bleeding and formation of a large hematoma (mass of blood). Pressure on the abdomen facilitates placental separation. **H,** The placenta is expelled and the uterus contracts.

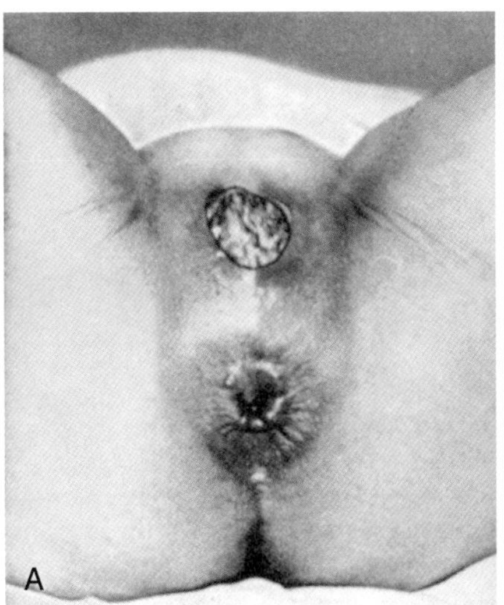

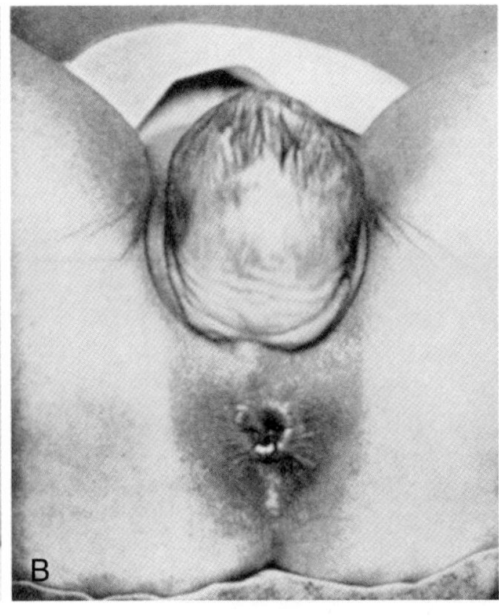

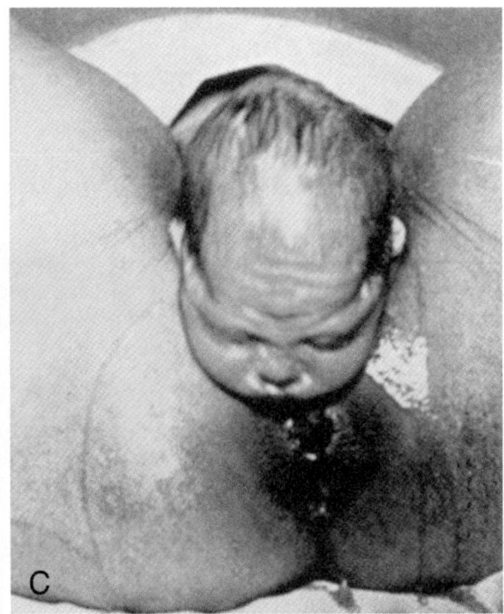

FIGURE 7-12. Delivery of the baby's head during the second stage of labor is shown. **A,** The crown of the head distends the mother's perineum. **B,** The perineum slips over the head and face. **C,** The head is delivered; subsequently, the body of the fetus is expelled. Episiotomy, surgical incision of the perineum to facilitate birth, may be performed as the fetal head distends the perineum. (From Greenhill JB, Friedman EA: Biological Principles and Modern Practice of Obstetrics. Philadelphia, WB Saunders, 1974.)

accessory placenta (see Fig. 7-14) in the uterus may cause severe uterine hemorrhage.

Fetal Surface of Placenta

The umbilical cord usually attaches to the fetal surface of the placenta, and its epithelium is continuous with the amnion adhering to the fetal surface (see Figs. 7-7 and 7-13*B* and *C*). The fetal surface of a freshly delivered placenta is smooth and shiny because it is covered by the amnion. The chorionic vessels radiating to and from the umbilical cord are clearly visible through the transparent amnion. The umbilical vessels branch on the fetal surface to form chorionic vessels, which enter the chorionic villi and form the arteriocapillary-venous system (see Fig. 7-8*A*).

Placental Abnormalities

Abnormal adherence of chorionic villi to the myometrium is called **placenta accreta** (Fig. 7-16). When chorionic villi penetrate the full thickness of the myometrium to or through the perimetrium (peritoneal covering), the abnormality is called **placenta percreta**. Third-trimester bleeding is the common presenting sign of these placental abnormalities. Most patients with placenta accreta have normal pregnancies and labors. After birth, the placenta fails to separate from the uterine wall, and attempts to remove it may cause hemorrhage that is difficult to control.

When the blastocyst implants close to or overlying the internal os of the uterus, the abnormality is called **placenta previa**. Late pregnancy bleeding may result from this placental abnormality. The fetus has to be delivered by cesarean section when the placenta completely obstructs the internal uterine os.

The Umbilical Cord

The attachment of the umbilical cord to the placenta is usually near the center of the fetal surface of this organ (see Fig. 7-13*B*), but it may attach at any point. For example, insertion of it at the placental margin produces a battledore placenta (see Fig. 7-13*D*), and its attachment to the fetal membranes is a velamentous insertion of the cord (Fig. 7-17).

Color flow Doppler ultrasonography may be used for the prenatal diagnosis of the position and structural abnormalities of the umbilical cord and its vessels. The umbilical cord is usually 1 to 2 cm in diameter and 30 to 90 cm in length (average, 55 cm). Excessively long or short cords are uncommon. Long cords have a tendency to prolapse and/or to coil around the fetus (see Fig. 7-21). Prompt recognition of prolapse of the umbilical cord is important because the cord may be compressed between the presenting body part of the fetus and the mother's bony pelvis, causing fetal hypoxia or anoxia. If the deficiency of oxygen persists for more than 5 minutes, the baby's brain may be damaged, producing mental retardation. A very short cord may cause premature separation of the placenta from the wall of the uterus during delivery.

The umbilical cord usually has two arteries and one vein that are surrounded by mucoid connective tissue (Wharton jelly). Because the umbilical vessels are longer than the cord, twisting and bending of the vessels are common. They frequently form loops, producing false knots that are of no significance; however, in approximately 1% of pregnancies, true knots form in the cord,

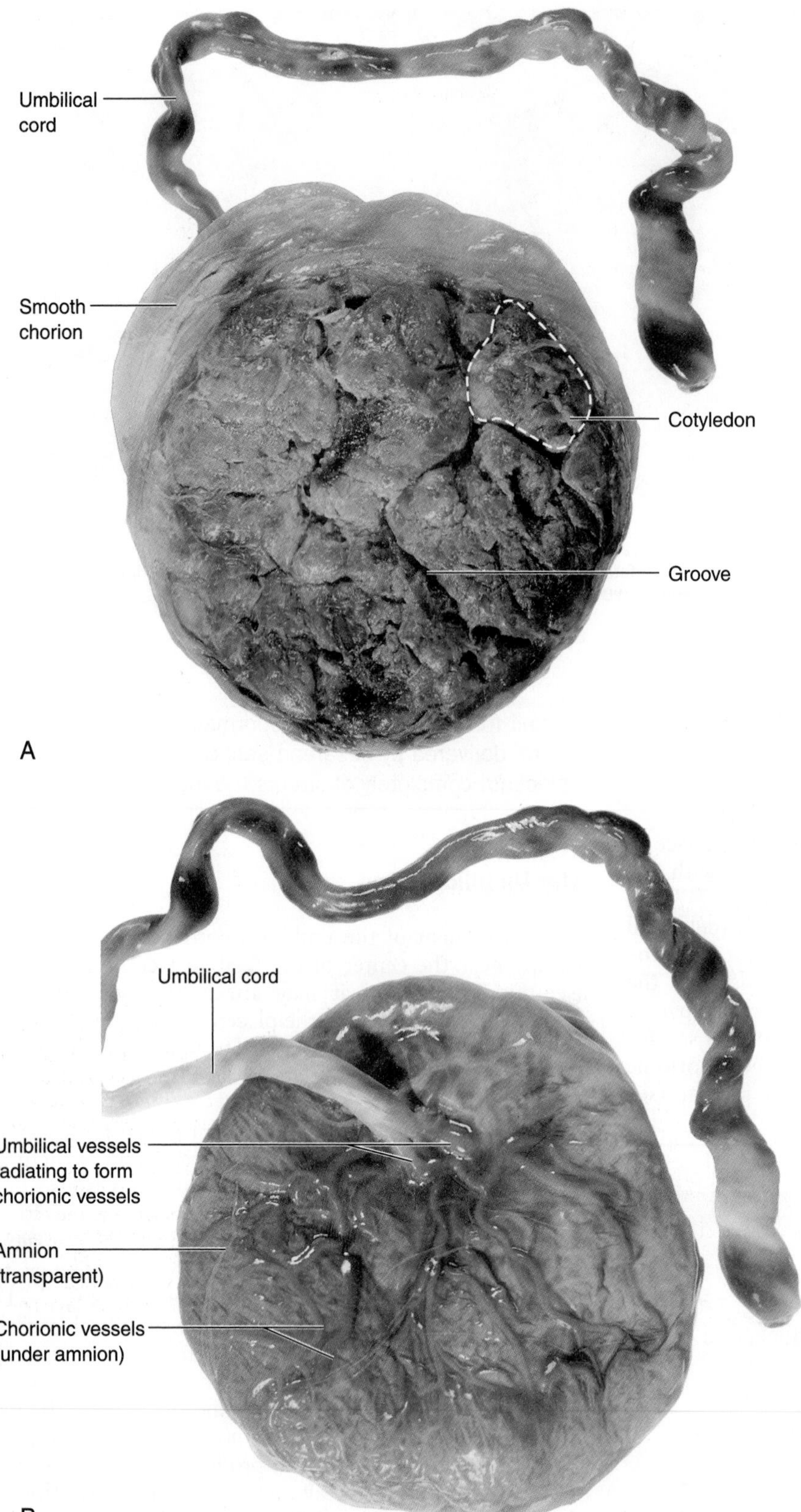

FIGURE 7-13. Placentas and fetal membranes after birth, approximately one third actual size. **A,** Maternal surface showing cotyledons and the grooves around them. Each cotyledon consists of a number of main stem villi with their many branch villi. The grooves were occupied by the placental septa when the maternal and fetal parts of the placenta were together (see Fig. 7-7). **B,** Fetal surface showing blood vessels running in the chorionic plate deep to the amnion and converging to form the umbilical vessels at the attachment of the umbilical cord.

Continued

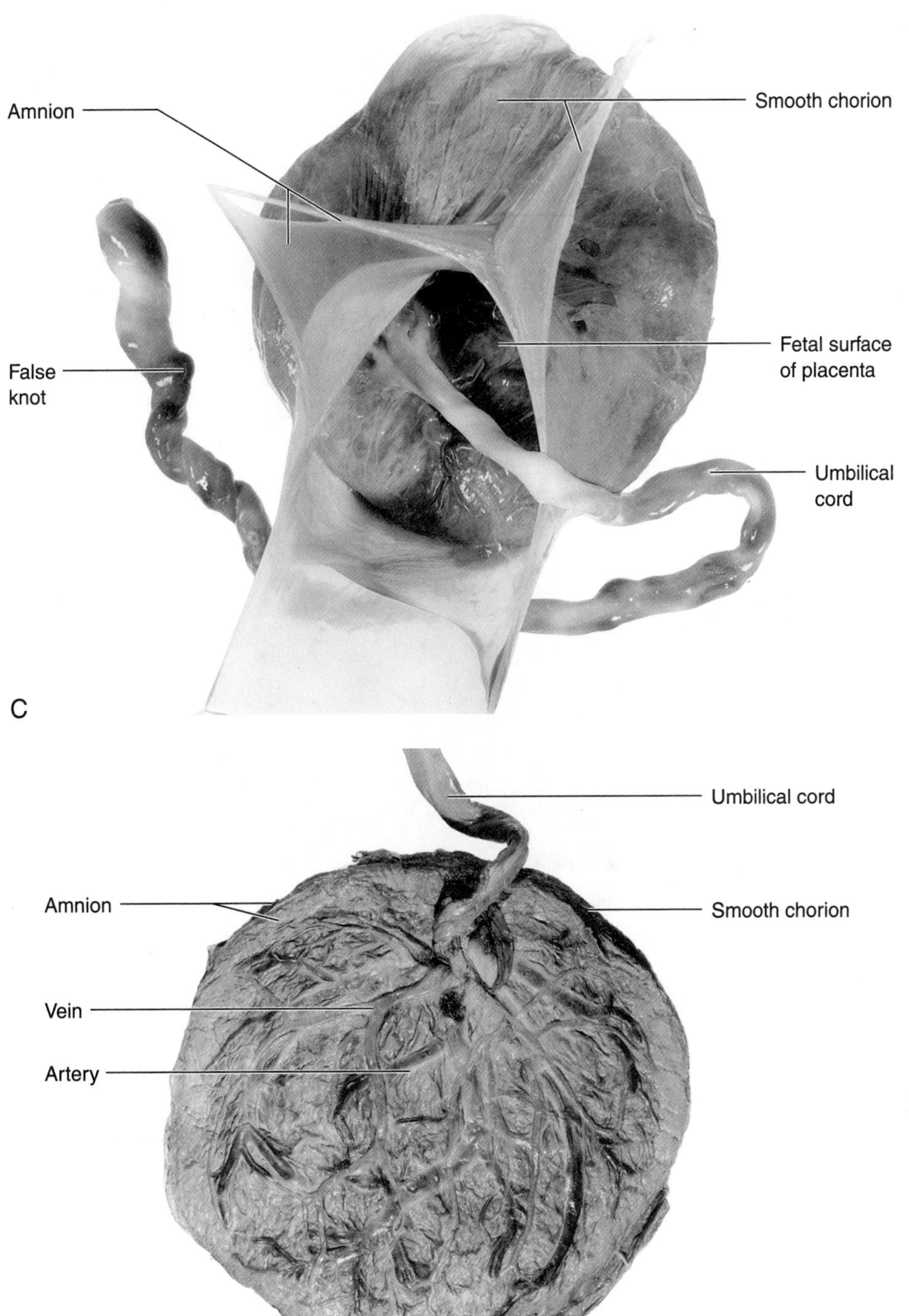

FIGURE 7-13, CONT'D. Placentas and fetal membranes after birth, approximately one third actual size. **C,** The amnion and smooth chorion are arranged to show that they are fused and continuous with the margins of the placenta. **D,** Placenta with a marginal attachment of the cord, often called a battledore placenta because of its resemblance to the bat used in the medieval game of battledore and shuttlecock. (From Moore KL, Persaud TVN, Shiota K: Color Atlas of Clinical Embryology, 2nd ed. Philadelphia, WB Saunders, 2000.)

which may tighten and cause fetal death resulting from fetal anoxia (Fig. 7-18). In most cases, the knots form during labor as a result of the fetus passing through a loop of the cord. Simple looping of the cord around the fetus occasionally occurs (see Fig. 7-21*B*). In approximately one fifth of deliveries, the cord is loosely looped around the neck without increased fetal risk.

UMBILICAL ARTERY DOPPLER VELOCIMETRY

As gestation and trophoblastic invasion of the decidua basalis progress, there is a progressive increase in the diastolic flow velocity in the umbilical

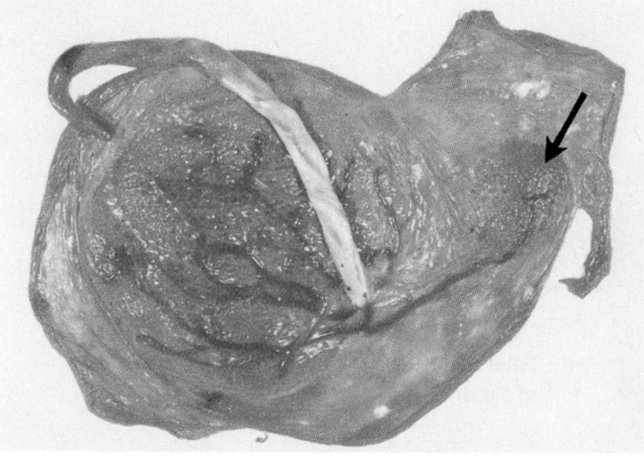

FIGURE 7-14. A full-term placenta and an accessory placenta (*arrow*). The accessory placenta developed from a patch of chorionic villi that persisted a short distance from the main placenta.

arteries. Doppler velocimetry of the uteroplacental and fetoplacental circulation is used to investigate complications of pregnancy such as IUGR and fetal distress resulting from fetal hypoxia and asphyxia (Fig. 7-19). For example, there is a statistically significant association between IUGR and abnormally increased resistance in an umbilical artery.

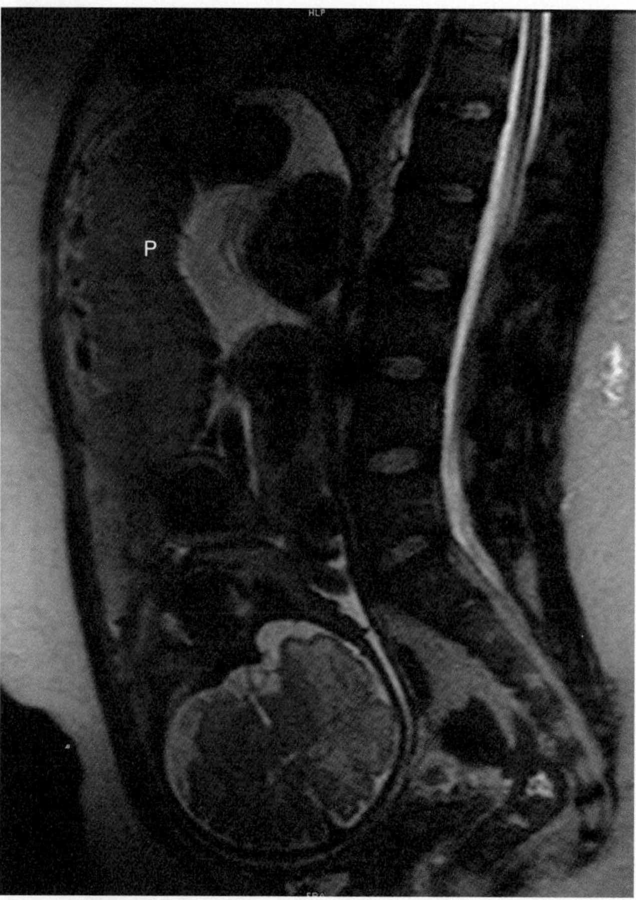

FIGURE 7-15. Sagittal magnetic resonance image of the pelvis of a pregnant woman. The vertebral column and pelvis of the mother are visible, as are the fetal brain and limbs and the placenta (P). (Courtesy of Stuart C. Morrison, Section of Pediatric Radiology, The Children's Hospital, Cleveland Clinic, Cleveland, OH.)

ABSENCE OF AN UMBILICAL ARTERY

In approximately one in 100 newborns, only one umbilical artery is present (Fig. 7-20), a condition that may be associated with chromosomal and fetal abnormalities. Absence of an umbilical artery is accompanied by a 15% to 20% incidence of cardiovascular anomalies in the fetus. Absence of an artery results from either agenesis or degeneration of one of the two umbilical arteries. A single umbilical artery and the anatomic defects associated with it can be detected before birth by ultrasonography.

Amnion and Amniotic Fluid

The thin but tough amnion forms a fluid-filled, membranous amniotic sac that surrounds the embryo and fetus (Fig. 7-21). Because the amnion is attached to the margins of the embryonic disc, its junction with the embryo (future umbilicus) is located on the ventral surface after embryonic folding (Fig. 7-22*B*). As the amnion enlarges, it gradually obliterates the chorionic cavity and forms the epithelial covering of the umbilical cord (see Fig. 7-22*C* and *D*).

AMNIOTIC FLUID

Amniotic fluid plays a major role in fetal growth and development. Initially, some amniotic fluid is secreted by amniotic cells; most is derived from maternal tissue and interstitial fluid by diffusion across the amniochorionic membrane from the decidua parietalis (see Fig. 7-7). Later there is diffusion of fluid through the chorionic plate from blood in the intervillous space of the placenta. Before keratinization of the skin occurs, a major pathway for passage of water and solutes in tissue fluid from the fetus to the amniotic cavity is through the skin; thus, amniotic fluid is similar to fetal tissue fluid. Fluid is also secreted by the fetal respiratory and gastrointestinal tracts and enters the amniotic cavity. The daily rate of contribution of fluid to the amniotic cavity from the respiratory tract is 300 to 400 mL. Beginning in the 11th week, the fetus contributes to the amniotic fluid by excreting urine into the amniotic cavity. By late pregnancy, approximately 500 mL of urine is added daily. The volume of amniotic fluid normally increases slowly, reaching approximately 30 mL at 10 weeks, 350 mL at 20 weeks, and 700 to 1000 mL by 37 weeks.

CIRCULATION OF AMNIOTIC FLUID

The water content of amniotic fluid changes every 3 hours. Large amounts of water pass through the amniochorionic membrane into the maternal tissue fluid and enter the uterine capillaries. An exchange of fluid with fetal blood also occurs through the umbilical cord and where the amnion adheres to the chorionic plate on the

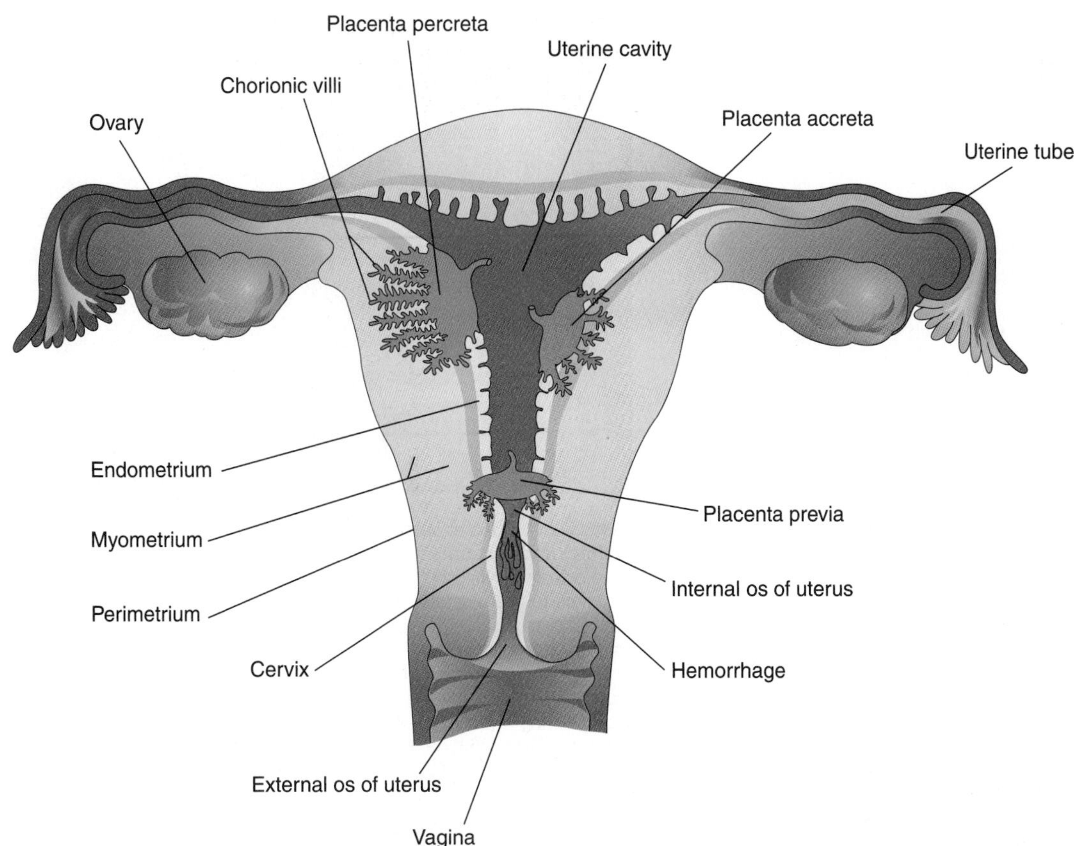

FIGURE 7-16. Placental abnormalities. In placenta accreta, there is abnormal adherence of the placenta to the myometrium. In placenta percreta, the placenta has penetrated the full thickness of the myometrium. In this example of placenta previa, the placenta overlies the internal os of the uterus and blocks the cervical canal.

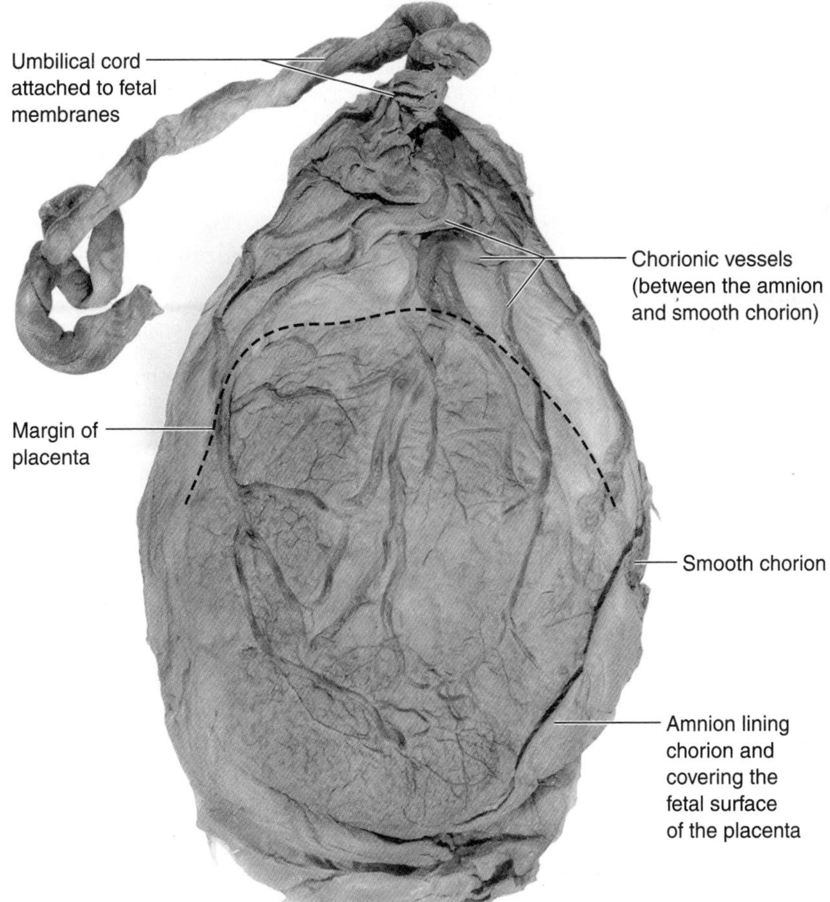

FIGURE 7-17. A placenta with a velamentous insertion of the umbilical cord. The cord is attached to the membranes (amnion and chorion), not to the placenta. The umbilical vessels leave the cord and run between the amnion and chorion before spreading over the placenta. The vessels are easily torn in this location, especially when they cross over the inferior uterine segment; the latter condition is known as vasa previa. If the vessels rupture before birth, the fetus loses blood and could be near exsanguination when born. (From Moore KL, Persaud TVN, Shiota K: Color Atlas of Clinical Embryology, 2nd ed. Philadelphia, WB Saunders, 2000.)

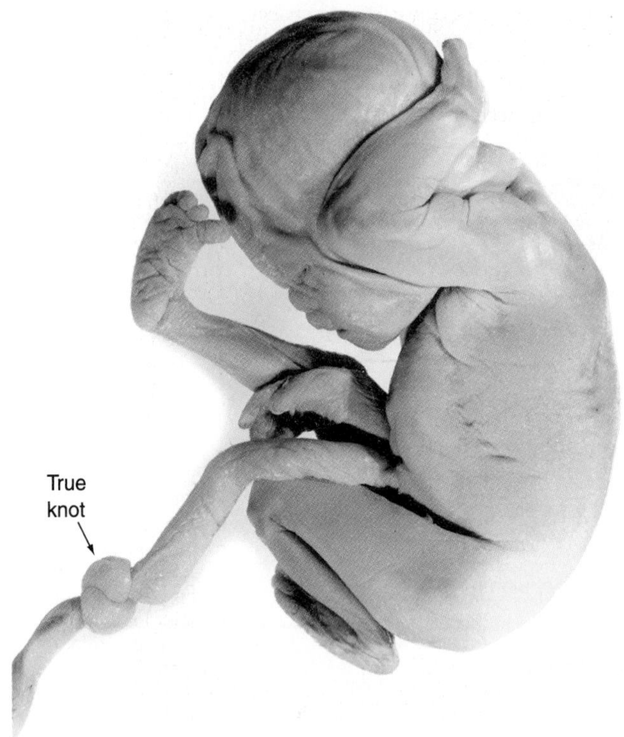

FIGURE 7-18. A 20-week fetus with a true knot (*arrow*) in its umbilical cord. Half actual size. The diameter of the cord is greater in the part closest to the fetus, indicating that there was an obstruction of blood flow from the fetus in the umbilical arteries and compression of the umbilical vein. Undoubtedly, this knot caused severe anoxia (decreased oxygen in the fetal tissues and organs) and was a major cause of the fetus's death. (From Moore KL, Persaud TVN, Shiota K: Color Atlas of Clinical Embryology, 2nd ed. Philadelphia, WB Saunders, 2000.)

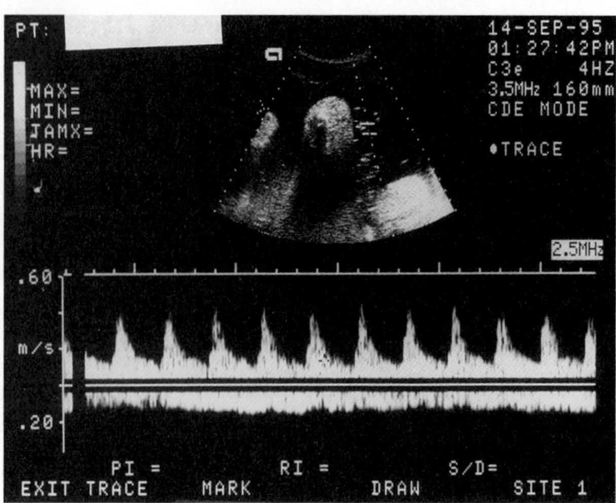

FIGURE 7-19. Doppler velocimetry of the umbilical cord. The arterial waveform (*top*) illustrates pulsatile forward flow, with high peaks and low velocities during diastole. This combination suggests high resistance in the placenta to placental blood flow. Because this index changes over gestation, it is important to know that the pregnancy was 18 weeks' gestation. For this period, the flow pattern is normal. The nonpulsatile flow in the opposite, negative direction represents venous return from the placenta. Both waveforms are normal for this gestational age. (Courtesy of Dr. C.R. Harman, Department of Obstetrics, Gynecology and Reproductive Sciences, University of Maryland, Baltimore, MD.)

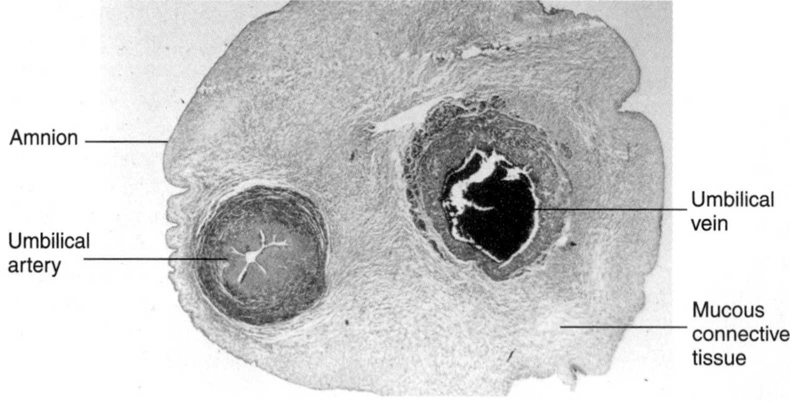

FIGURE 7-20. Transverse section of an umbilical cord. Observe that the cord is covered by epithelium derived from the enveloping amnion. It has a core of mucous connective tissue (Wharton jelly). Observe also that the cord has one umbilical artery and one vein. Usually there are two umbilical arteries. The vein, which carries oxygenated blood from the placenta, is unusual in that its wall, unlike that of most veins, consists principally of a tunica media. (Courtesy of Professor V. Becker, Pathologisches Institut der Universität, Erlangen, Germany.)

fetal surface of the placenta (see Figs. 7-7 and 7-13*B*); thus, amniotic fluid is in balance with the fetal circulation.

Amniotic fluid is swallowed by the fetus and absorbed by the fetus's respiratory and digestive tracts. It has been estimated that during the final stages of pregnancy, the fetus swallows up to 400 mL of amniotic fluid per day. The fluid passes into the fetal bloodstream and the waste products in it cross the placental membrane and enter the maternal blood in the intervillous space. Excess water in the fetal blood is excreted by the fetal kidneys and returned to the amniotic sac through the fetal urinary tract.

DISORDERS OF AMNIOTIC FLUID VOLUME

Low volumes of amniotic fluid for any particular gestational age—**oligohydramnios**—result in many cases from placental insufficiency with diminished placental blood flow. Preterm rupture of the amniochorionic membrane occurs in approximately 10% of pregnancies and is the most common cause of oligohydramnios. When there is **renal agenesis**

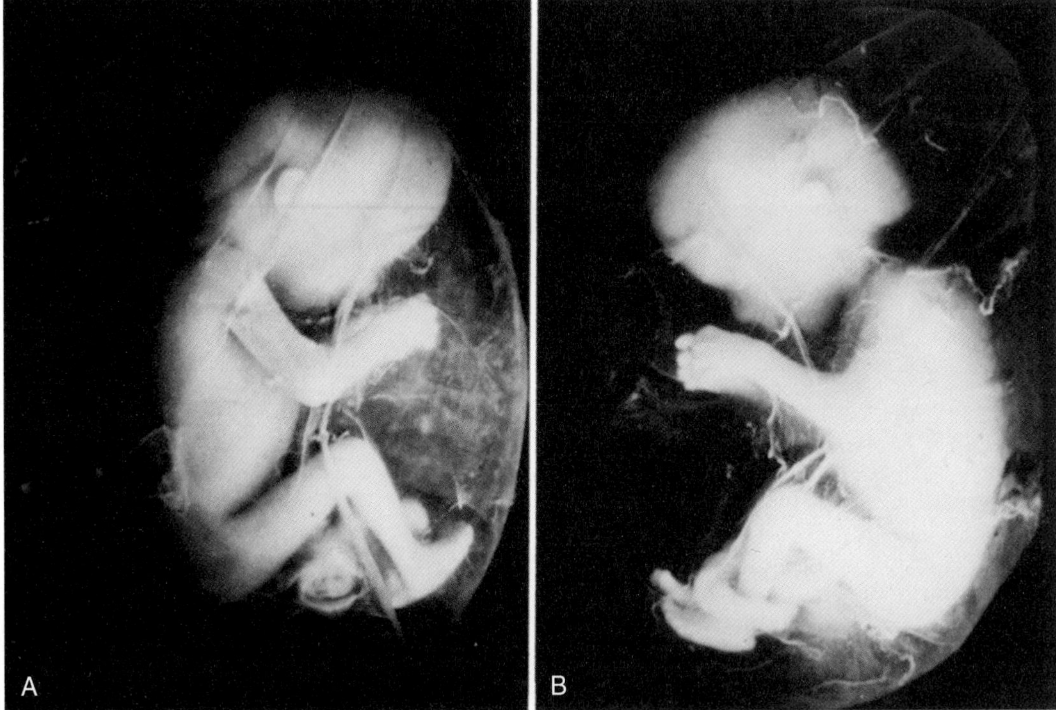

FIGURE 7-21. **A,** 12-week fetus within its amniotic sac. The fetus and its membranes aborted spontaneously. It was removed from its chorionic sac with its amniotic sac intact. Actual size. **B,** Note that the umbilical cord is looped around the left ankle of the fetus. Coiling of the cord around parts of the fetus affects their development when the coils are so tight that the circulation to the parts is affected.

(failure of kidney formation), the absence of fetal urine contribution to the amniotic fluid is the main cause of oligohydramnios. A similar decrease in fluid occurs when there is **obstructive uropathy** (urinary tract obstruction). Complications of oligohydramnios include fetal abnormalities (pulmonary hypoplasia, facial defects, and limb defects) that are caused by fetal compression by the uterine wall. Compression of the umbilical cord is also a potential complication of severe oligohydramnios.

High volumes of amniotic fluid—**polyhydramnios**—result when the fetus does not swallow the usual amount of amniotic fluid. Most cases of polyhydramnios (60%) are idiopathic (unknown cause), 20% are caused by maternal factors, and 20% are fetal in origin. Polyhydramnios may be associated with severe anomalies of the central nervous system, such as meroencephaly (anencephaly). When there are other anomalies, esophageal atresia (blockage), for example, amniotic fluid accumulates because it is unable to pass to the fetal stomach and intestines for absorption. Ultrasonography has become the technique of choice for diagnosing oligo- and polyhydramnios.

Composition of Amniotic Fluid

Amniotic fluid is an aqueous solution in which undissolved material (desquamated fetal epithelial cells) is suspended. Amniotic fluid contains approximately equal portions of organic and inorganic salts. Half of the organic constituents are protein; the other half consists of carbohydrates, fats, enzymes, hormones, and pigments. As pregnancy advances, the composition of the amniotic fluid changes as fetal excreta (meconium [fetal feces] and urine) are added. Because fetal urine enters the amniotic fluid, studies of fetal enzyme systems, amino acids, hormones, and other substances can be conducted on fluid removed by amniocentesis (see Chapter 6). Studies of cells in the amniotic fluid permit diagnosis of chromosomal abnormalities such as trisomy 21 (Down syndrome). Moreover, fluorescent in situ hybridization analyses are often carried out on fetal cells if there is a family history or clinical indication of certain genetic disorders. High levels of alpha fetoprotein usually indicate the presence of a severe neural tube defect. Low levels of alpha fetoprotein may indicate chromosomal aberrations such as trisomy 21 (see Chapter 20).

Significance of Amniotic Fluid

The embryo, suspended in amniotic fluid by the umbilical cord, floats freely. Amniotic fluid has critical functions in the normal development of the fetus. The buoyant amniotic fluid

- Permits symmetric external growth of the embryo and fetus
- Acts as a barrier to infection
- Permits normal fetal lung development
- Prevents adherence of the amnion to the embryo and fetus

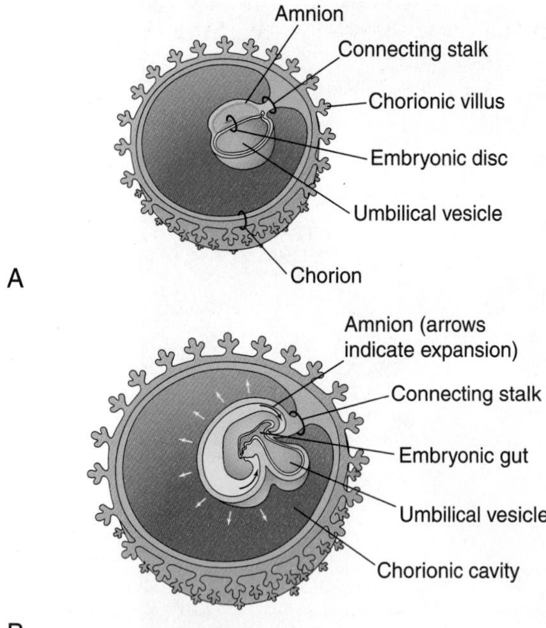

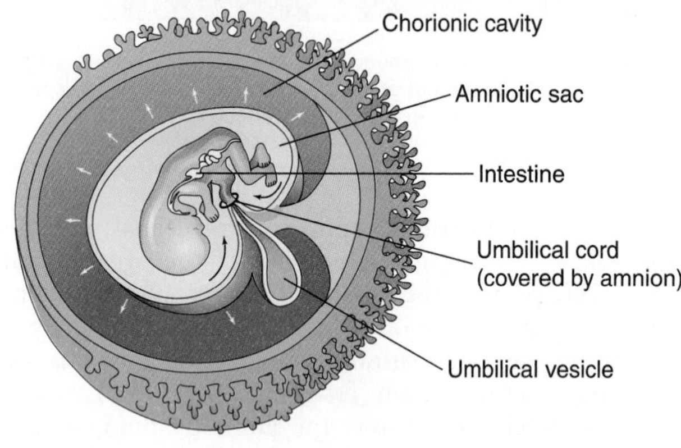

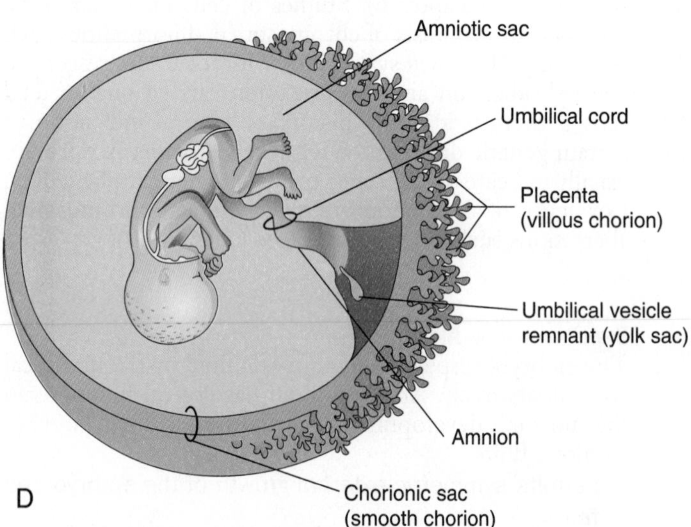

FIGURE 7-22. Illustrations showing how the amnion enlarges, obliterates the chorionic cavity, and envelops the umbilical cord. Observe that part of the umbilical vesicle is incorporated into the embryo as the primordial gut. Formation of the fetal part of the placenta and degeneration of chorionic villi are also shown. **A,** At 3 weeks; **B,** at 4 weeks; **C,** at 10 weeks; **D,** at 20 weeks.

- Cushions the embryo and fetus against injuries by distributing impacts the mother receives
- Helps control the embryo's body temperature by maintaining a relatively constant temperature
- Enables the fetus to move freely, thereby aiding muscular development in the limbs, for example
- Assists in maintaining homeostasis of fluid and electrolytes

PREMATURE RUPTURE OF FETAL MEMBRANES

Rupture of the amniochorionic membrane is the most common event leading to premature labor and delivery and the most common complication resulting in oligohydramnios. Loss of amniotic fluid removes the major protection that the fetus has against infection. **Rupture of the amnion** may cause various fetal anomalies that constitute the **amniotic band syndrome** (ABS), or the amniotic band disruption complex. The incidence of the ABS is approximately one in every 1200 live births. Prenatal ultrasound diagnosis of ABS is now possible. The malformations caused by ABS vary from digital constriction to major scalp, craniofacial, and visceral defects. The cause of these anomalies is probably related to constriction by encircling amniotic bands (Fig. 7-23). Other heterogeneous factors may be involved.

THE UMBILICAL VESICLE (YOLK SAC)

The umbilical vesicle (yolk sac) can be observed sonographically early in the fifth week (see Chapter 5). Early development of the umbilical vesicle was described in Chapters 3 and 5. At 32 days, the umbilical vesicle is large (see Fig. 7-2). By 10 weeks, the umbilical vesicle has shrunk to a pear-shaped remnant approximately 5 mm in diameter (see Fig. 7-22*C*) and is connected to the midgut by a narrow omphaloenteric duct (yolk stalk). By 20 weeks,

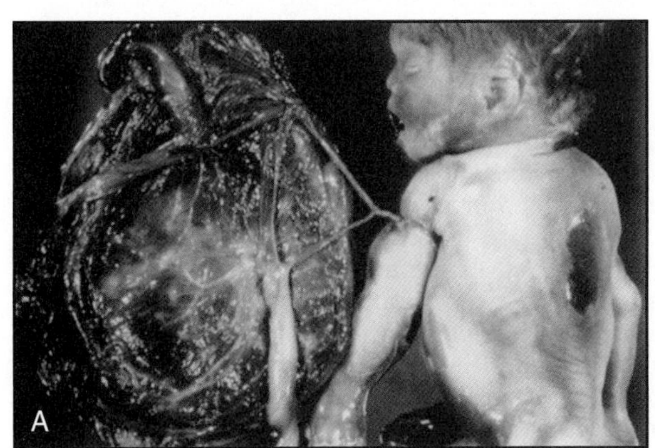

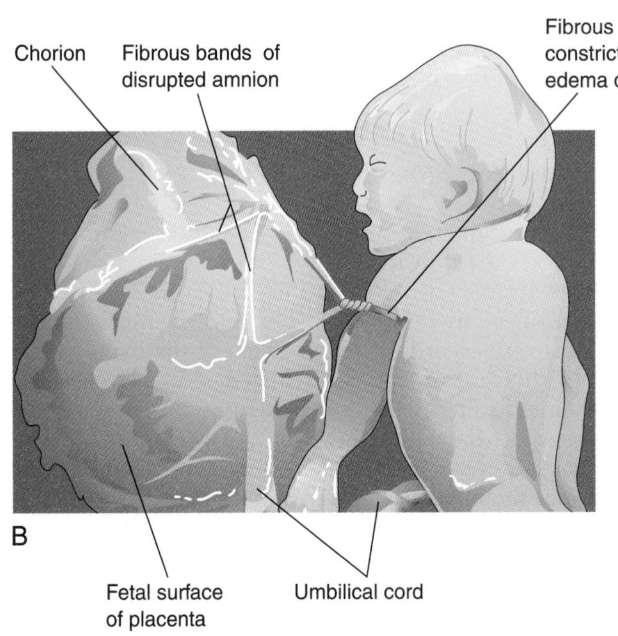

FIGURE 7-23. **A,** A fetus with the amniotic band syndrome showing amniotic bands constricting the left arm. **B,** Drawing indicating the structures shown in **A**. (**A,** Courtesy of Professor V. Becker, Pathologisches Institut der Universität, Erlangen, Germany.)

the umbilical vesicle is very small (see Fig. 7-22*D*); thereafter, it is usually not visible. The presence of the amniotic sac and umbilical vesicle enables early recognition and measurement of the embryo. The umbilical vesicle is recognizable in ultrasound examinations until the end of the first trimester.

Significance of the Umbilical Vesicle

Although the umbilical vesicle is nonfunctional as far as yolk storage is concerned (hence the name change), its presence is essential for several reasons:

- It has a role in the transfer of nutrients to the embryo during the second and third weeks when the uteroplacental circulation is being established.
- Blood development first occurs in the well-vascularized extraembryonic mesoderm covering the wall of the umbilical vesicle beginning in the third week (see Chapter 4) and continues to form there until hemopoietic activity begins in the liver during the sixth week.
- During the fourth week, the endoderm of the umbilical vesicle is incorporated into the embryo as the primordial gut (see Fig. 5-1). Its endoderm, derived from epiblast, gives rise to the epithelium of the trachea, bronchi, lungs, and digestive tract.
- Primordial germ cells appear in the endodermal lining of the wall of the umbilical vesicle in the third week and subsequently migrate to the developing gonads (see Chapter 12). They differentiate into spermatogonia in males and oogonia in females.

Fate of the Umbilical Vesicle

At 10 weeks, the small umbilical vesicle lies in the chorionic cavity between the amniotic and chorionic sacs (see Fig. 7-22*C*). It atrophies as pregnancy advances, eventually becoming very small (see Fig. 7-22*D*). In very unusual cases, the umbilical vesicle persists throughout pregnancy and appears under the amnion as a small structure on the fetal surface of the placenta near the attachment of the umbilical cord. Persistence of the umbilical vesicle is of no significance. The omphaloenteric duct usually detaches from the midgut loop by the end of the sixth week. In approximately 2% of adults, the proximal intra-abdominal part of the omphaloenteric duct persists as an ileal diverticulum (Meckel diverticulum [see Chapter 11]).

THE ALLANTOIS

Early development of the allantois is described in Chapter 4. In the third week, it appears as a sausage-like diverticulum from the caudal wall of the umbilical vesicle that extends into the connecting stalk (Fig. 7-24*A*). During the second month, the extraembryonic part of the allantois degenerates (see Fig. 7-24*B*). Although the allantois is not functional in human embryos, it is important for three reasons:

- Blood formation occurs in its wall during the third to fifth weeks.
- Its blood vessels persist as the umbilical vein and arteries.
- The intraembryonic part of the allantois runs from the umbilicus to the urinary bladder, with which it is continuous. As the bladder enlarges, the allantois involutes to form a thick tube, the urachus. After birth, the urachus becomes a fibrous cord, the median umbilical ligament, that extends from the apex of the urinary bladder to the umbilicus.

Allantoic Cysts

A cystic mass in the umbilical cord may represent the remains of the extraembryonic part of the allantois (Fig. 7-25). These cysts usually resolve but may be associated with omphalocele—congenital herniation of viscera into the proximal part of the umbilical cord (see Chapter 11).

MULTIPLE PREGNANCIES

The risks of chromosomal anomalies and fetal morbidity and mortality are higher in multiple gestations than in single gestations. As the number of fetuses increases, the risks are progressively greater. In most countries, multiple births are more common now because of greater access to fertility therapies, including induction of ovulation that occurs when exogenous gonadotropins are administered to women with ovulatory failure and to those being treated for infertility by assisted reproductive technologies. In North America, twins normally occur approximately once in every 85 pregnancies, triplets approximately once in 90^2 pregnancies, quadruplets once in 90^3 pregnancies, and quintuplets approximately once in every 90^4 pregnancies.

Twins and Fetal Membranes

Twins that originate from two zygotes are dizygotic (DZ) twins or fraternal twins (Fig. 7-26), whereas twins that originate from one zygote are monozygotic (MZ) twins or identical twins (Fig. 7-27). The fetal membranes and placentas vary according to the origin of the twins (Table 7-1). In the case of MZ twins, the type of placenta and membranes formed depends on when the twinning process occurs. Approximately two thirds of twins are DZ. The frequency of DZ twinning shows marked racial differences, but the incidence of MZ twinning is approximately the same in all populations. In addition, the rate of MZ twinning shows little variation with the mother's age, whereas the rate of DZ twinning increases with maternal age.

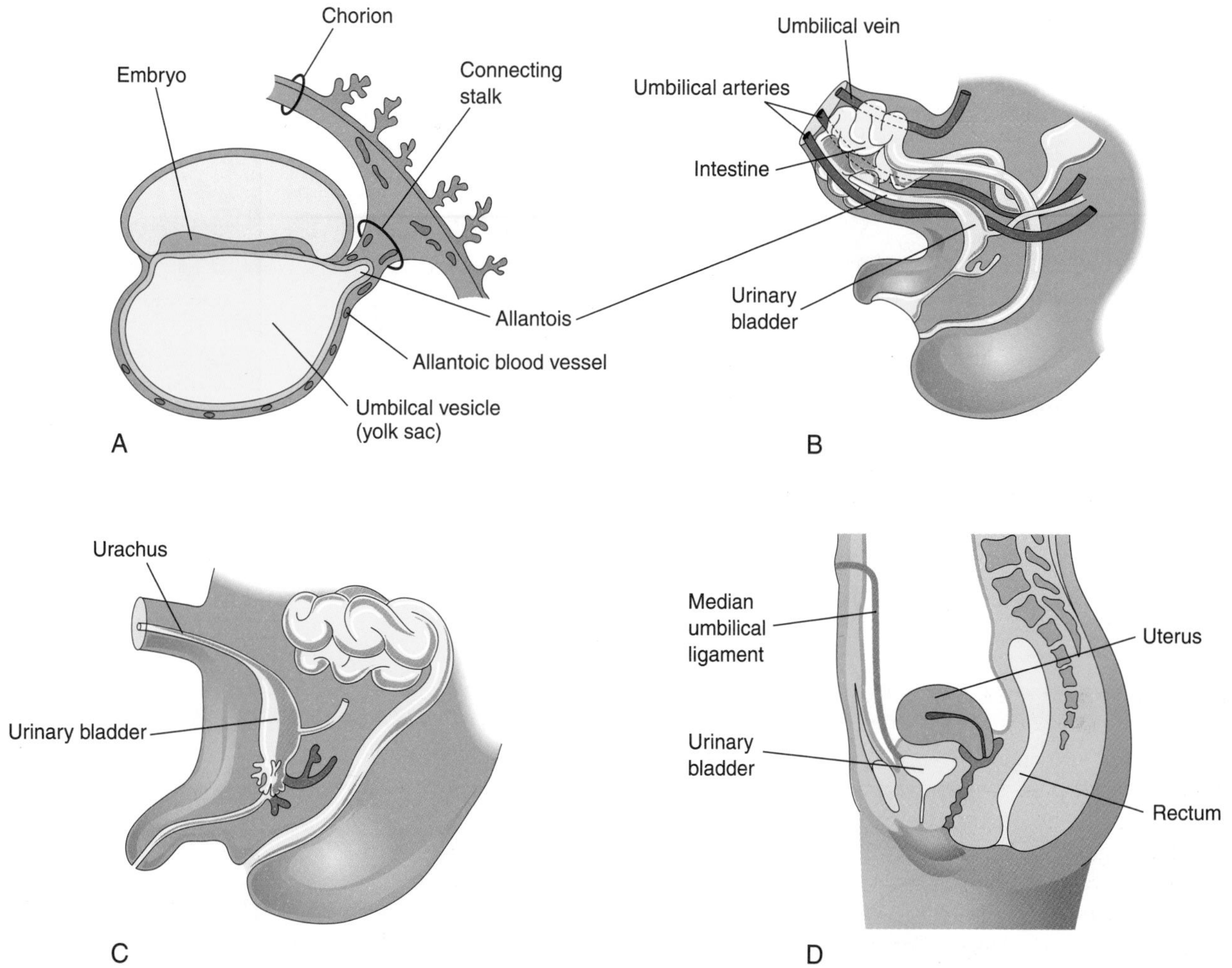

FIGURE 7-24. Illustrations of the development and usual fate of the allantois. **A,** A 3-week embryo. **B,** A 9-week fetus. **C,** A 3-month male fetus. **D,** Adult female. The nonfunctional allantois forms the urachus in the fetus and the median umbilical ligament in the adult.

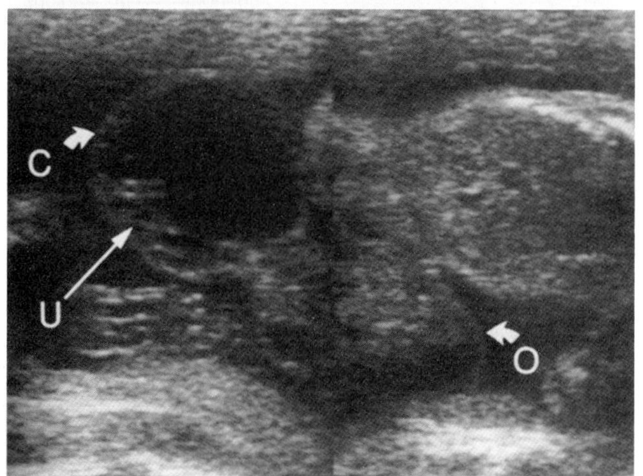

FIGURE 7-25. Sonogram of the umbilical cord (U) of a fetus exhibiting an allantoic cyst (C), which is associated with an omphalocele (O)—herniation of viscera into the proximal part of the umbilical cord. (From Townsend RR: Ultrasound evaluation of the placenta and umbilical cord. In Callen PW [ed]: Ultrasonography in Obstetrics and Gynecology, 3rd ed. Philadelphia, WB Saunders, 1994.)

The study of twins is important in human genetics because it is useful for comparing the effects of genes and environment on development. If an abnormal condition does not show a simple genetic pattern, comparison of its incidence in MZ and DZ twins may reveal that heredity is involved. The tendency for DZ, but not MZ, twins to repeat in families is evidence of hereditary influence. Studies in a Mormon population showed that the genotype of the mother affects the frequency of DZ twins, but the genotype of the father has no effect. It has also been observed that if the firstborn are twins, a repetition of twinning or some other form of multiple birth is approximately five times more likely to occur with the next pregnancy than in the general population.

ANASTOMOSIS OF PLACENTAL BLOOD VESSELS

Anastomoses between blood vessels of fused placentas of DZ twins may result in **erythrocyte mosaicism**. The members of these DZ twins have red blood cells of two different types because red

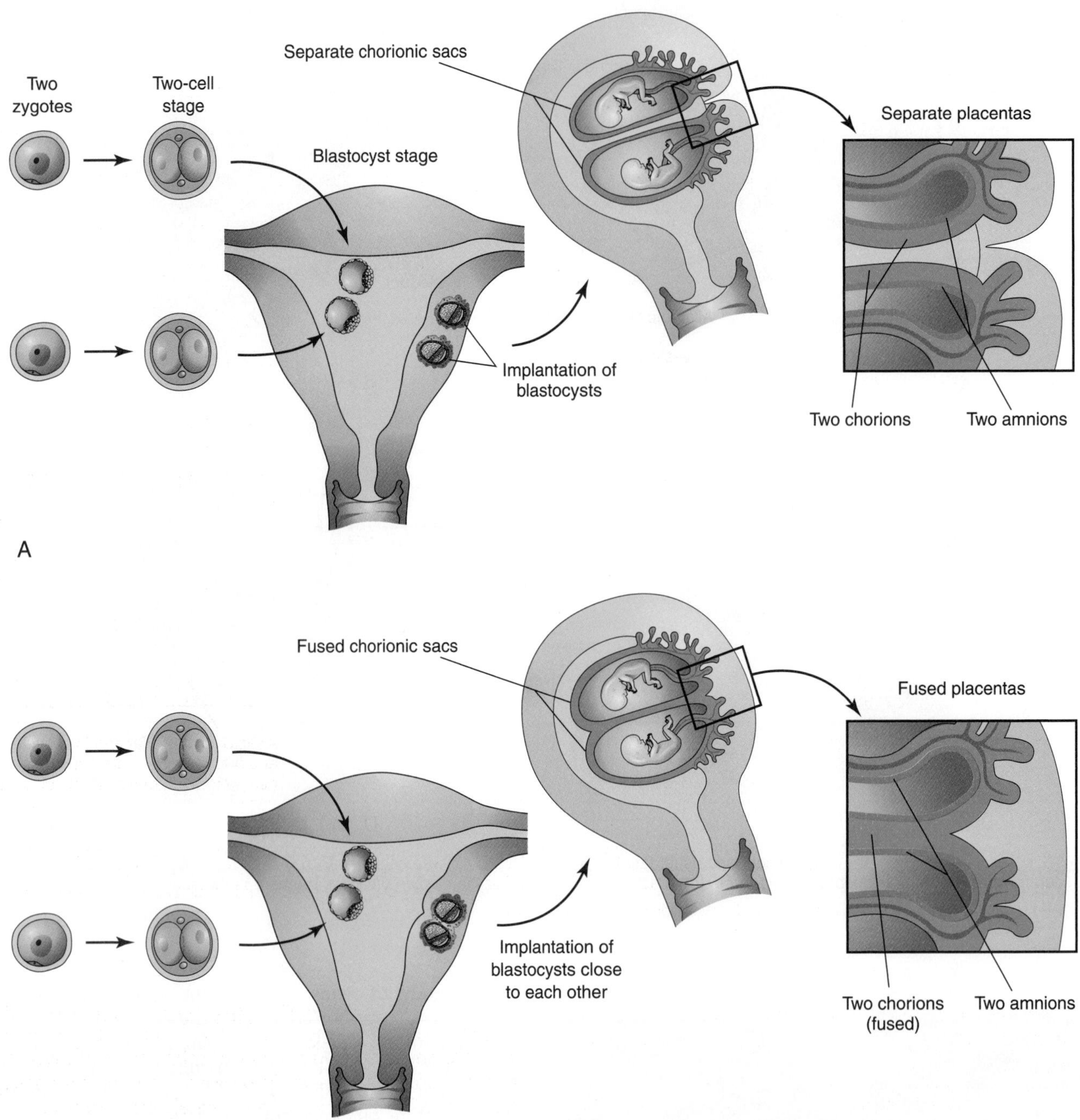

FIGURE 7-26. Diagrams illustrating how dizygotic twins develop from two zygotes. The relationships of the fetal membranes and placentas are shown for instances in which the blastocysts implant separately (**A**) and the blastocysts implant close together (**B**). In both cases, there are two amnions and two chorions. The placentas are usually fused when they implant close together.

cells were exchanged between the circulations of the twins. In cases in which one fetus is a male and the other is female, masculinization of the female fetus does not occur.

Twin Transfusion Syndrome

This syndrome occurs in as many as 30% of monochorionic-diamniotic MZ twins. There is shunting of arterial blood from one twin through arteriovenous anastomoses into the venous circulation of the other twin. The donor twin is small, pale, and anemic (Fig. 7-28), whereas the recipient twin is large and polycythemic, an increase above the normal in the number of red blood cells. The placenta shows similar abnormalities; the part of the placenta supplying the anemic twin is pale, whereas the part supplying the polycythemic twin is dark red. In lethal cases, death results from anemia in the donor twin and congestive heart failure in the recipient twin.

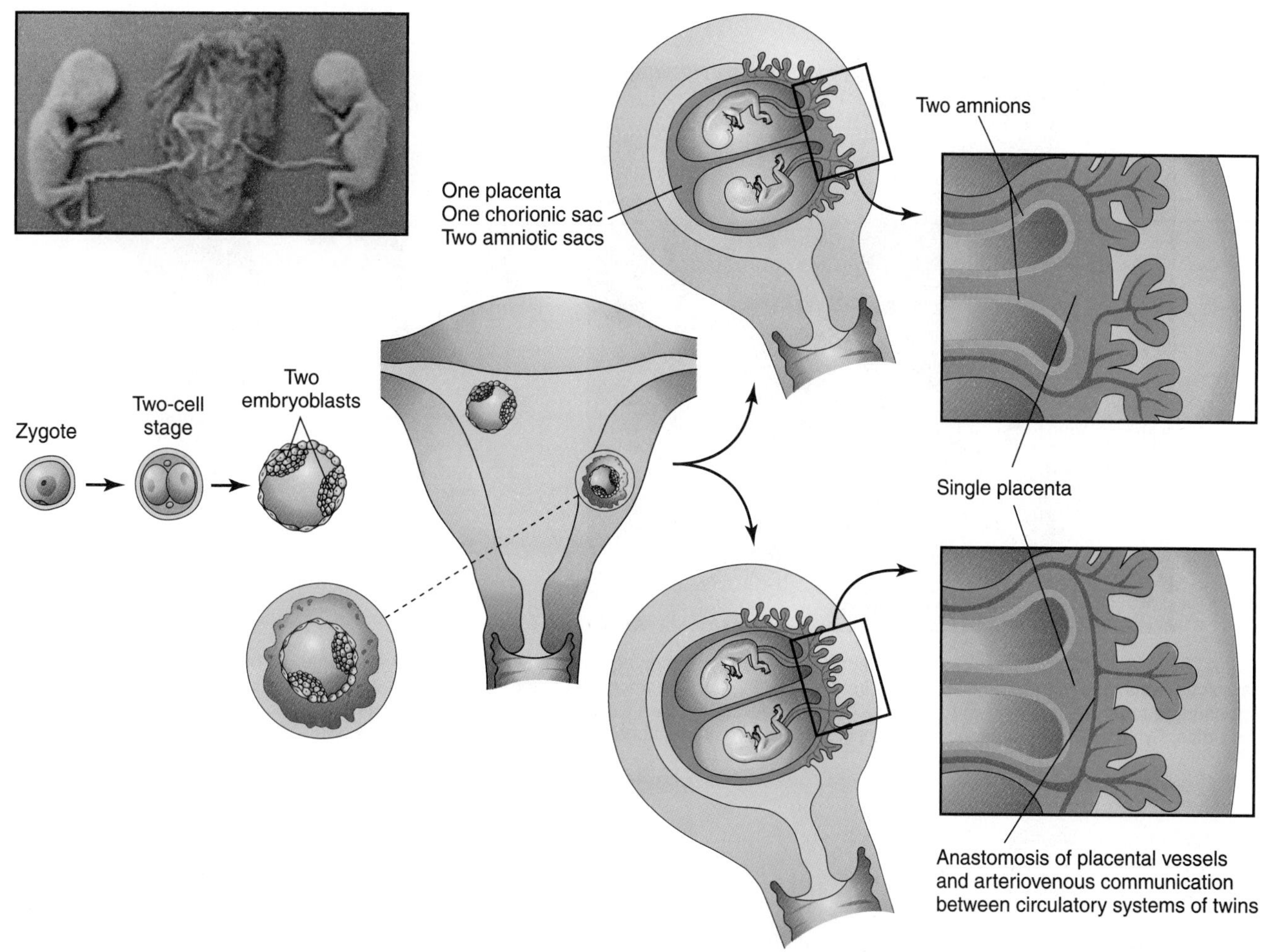

FIGURE 7-27. Diagrams illustrating how approximately 65% of monozygotic twins develop from one zygote by division of the embryoblast (inner cell mass) of the blastocyst. These twins always have separate amnions, a single chorionic sac, and a common placenta. If there is anastomosis of the placental vessels, one twin may receive most of the nutrition from the placenta. *Inset*, Monozygotic twins, 17 weeks' gestation. (Courtesy of Dr. Robert Jordan, St. Georges University Medical School, Grenada.)

TABLE 7–1. Frequency of Types of Placentas and Fetal Membranes in Monozygotic (MZ) and Dizygotic (DZ) Twins

	SINGLE CHORION		TWO CHORIONS	
ZYGOSITY	SINGLE AMNION	TWO AMNIONS	FUSED PLACENTAS*	TWO PLACENTAS
MZ	Very rare	65%	25%	10%
DZ	—	—	40%†	60%

Modified from Thompson MW, McInnes RR, Willard HF: Thompson & Thompson Genetics in Medicine, 5th ed. Philadelphia, WB Saunders, 1991.
*Results from secondary fusion.
†Dizygotic twins, the most common type, have their own amniotic and chorionic sacs, but the placentas may be fused (see Fig. 7-26*B*).

Dizygotic Twins

Because they result from fertilization of two oocytes, DZ twins develop from two zygotes and may be of the same sex or different sexes (see Fig. 7-26). For the same reason, they are no more alike genetically than brothers or sisters born at different times. The only thing they have in common is that they were in their mother's uterus at the same time (i.e., "womb mates"). DZ twins always have two amnions and two chorions, but the chorions and placentas may be fused. DZ twinning shows a hereditary tendency. Recurrence in families is approximately three times that of the general population. The incidence of DZ twinning shows considerable variation, being approximately 1 in 500 in Asians, 1 in 125 in whites, and as high as 1 in 20 in some African populations.

Monozygotic Twins

Because they result from the fertilization of one oocyte and develop from one zygote (see Fig. 7-27), MZ twins are of the same sex, genetically identical, and very similar in physical appearance. Physical differences between MZ twins are environmentally induced, e.g., because of anastomosis of placental vessels (Fig. 7-28). MZ twinning usually begins in the blastocyst stage, approximately at the end of the first week, and results from division of the embryoblast into two embryonic primordia. Subsequently,

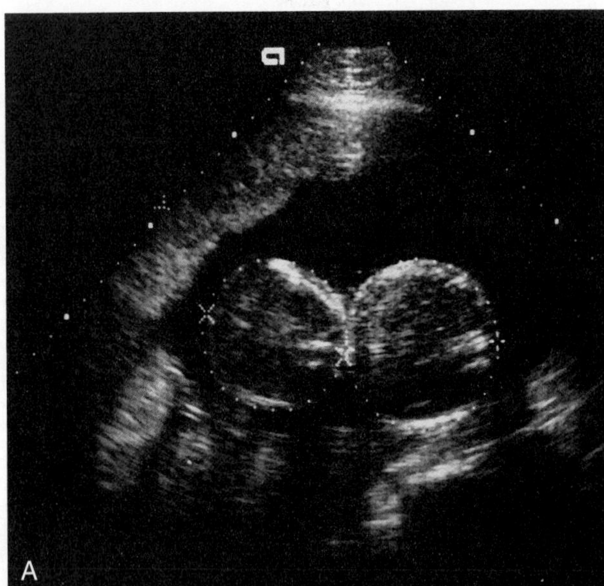

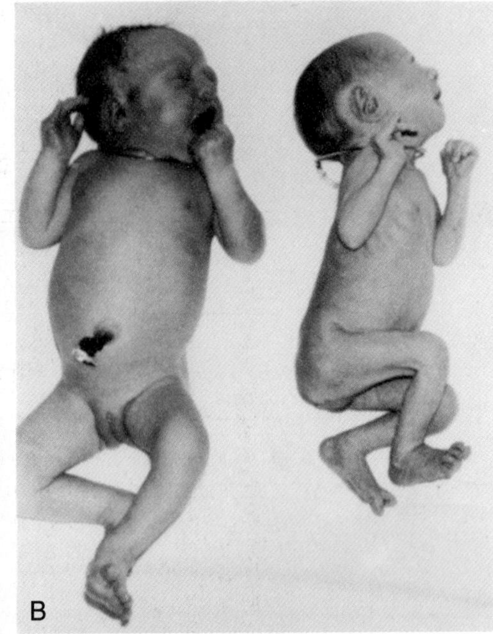

FIGURE 7-28. **A,** Ultrasound image of discordant (MZ) twins (24 weeks' gestation), twin transfusion syndrome. **B,** Monozygotic, monochorionic, diamniotic twins showing a wide discrepancy in size resulting from an uncompensated arteriovenous anastomosis of placental vessels. Blood was shunted from the smaller twin to the larger one, producing the twin transfusion syndrome. (**A,** Courtesy of Dr. G.J. Reid, Department of Obstetrics, Gynecology, and Reproductive Sciences, University of Manitoba, Women's Hospital, Winnipeg, Manitoba, Canada.)

two embryos, each in its own amniotic sac, develop within the same chorionic sac and share a common placenta—a monochorionic—diamniotic twin placenta. Uncommonly, early separation of embryonic blastomeres (e.g., during the two- to eight-cell stages) results in MZ twins with two amnions, two chorions, and two placentas that may or may not be fused (Fig. 7-29). In such cases, it is impossible to determine from the membranes alone whether the twins are MZ or DZ.

ESTABLISHING THE ZYGOSITY OF TWINS

Establishing the zygosity of twins is important in tissue and organ transplantation (e.g., bone marrow transplantations). The determination of twin zygosity is now done by molecular diagnosis because any two people who are not MZ twins are virtually certain to show differences in some of the large number of DNA markers that can be studied.

Approximately 35% of MZ twins result from early separation of the embryonic blastomeres, i.e., during the first 3 days of development (Fig. 7-29). The other 65% of MZ twins originate at the end of the first week of development (see Fig. 7-27). Late division of early embryonic cells, such as division of the embryonic disc during the second week, results in MZ twins that are in one amniotic sac and one chorionic sac (Fig. 7-30*A*). A monochorionic-monoamniotic twin placenta is associated with a fetal mortality rate approaching 50%. These MZ twins are rarely delivered alive because the umbilical cords are frequently so entangled that circulation of blood through their vessels ceases and one or both fetuses die. Sonography plays an important role in the diagnosis and management of twin pregnancies (Figs. 7-28*A* and 7-31). Ultrasound evaluation is necessary to identify various conditions that may complicate MZ twinning such as IUGR, fetal distress, and premature labor.

MZ twins may be discordant for a variety of birth defects and genetic disorders, despite their origin from the same zygote. In addition to environmental differences and chance variation, the following have been implicated:

- Mechanisms of embryologic development, such as vascular abnormalities, that can lead to discordance for anomalies
- Postzygotic changes, such as somatic mutation leading to discordance for cancer, or somatic rearrangement of immunoglobulin or T cell–receptor genes
- Chromosome aberrations originating in one blastocyst after the twinning event

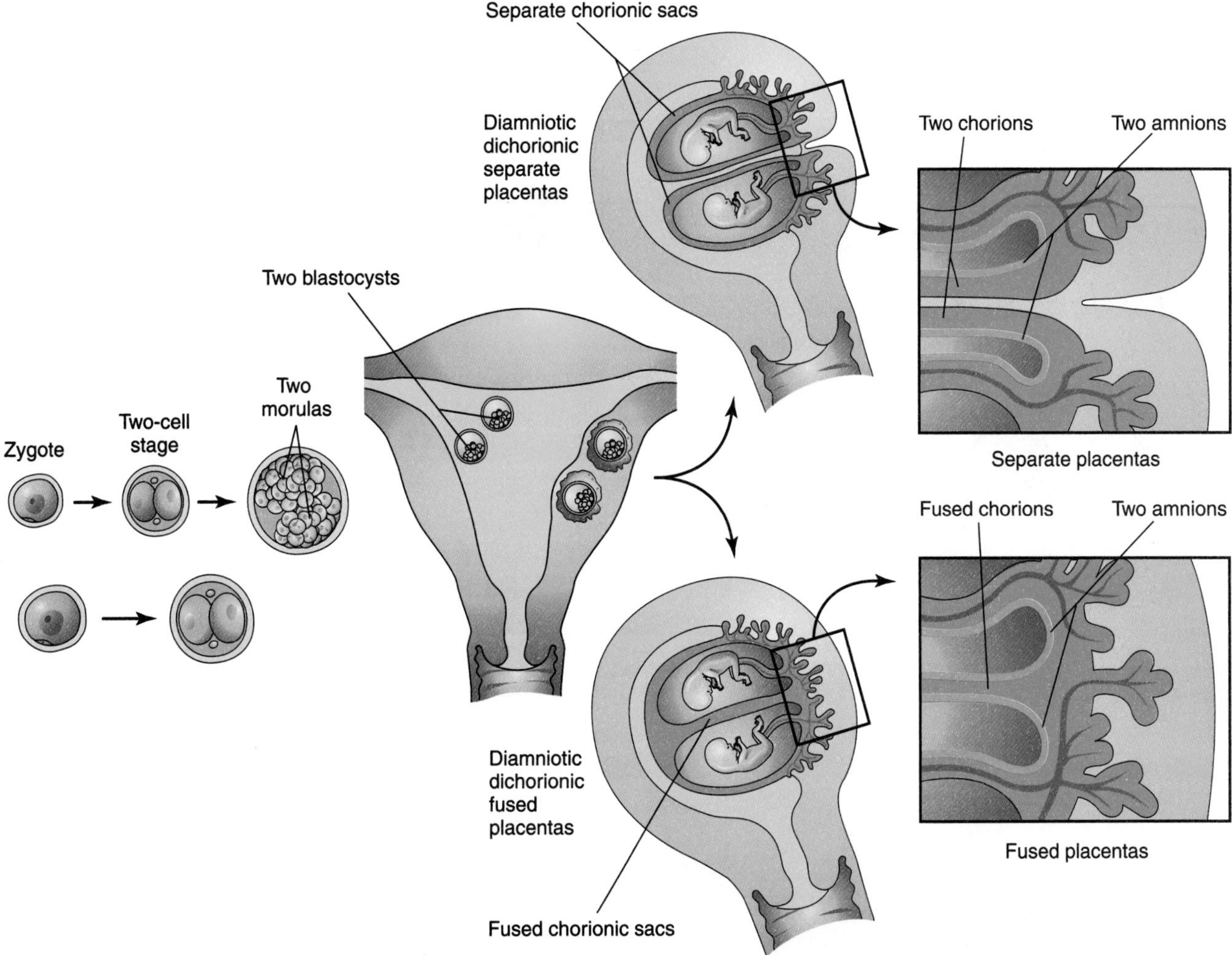

FIGURE 7-29. Diagrams illustrating how approximately 35% of monozygotic twins develop from one zygote. Separation of the blastomeres may occur anywhere from the two-cell stage to the morula stage, producing two identical blastocysts. Each embryo subsequently develops its own amniotic and chorionic sacs. The placentas may be separate or fused. In 25% of cases, there is a single placenta resulting from secondary fusion, and in 10% of cases, there are two placentas. In the latter cases, examination of the placenta would suggest that they were dizygotic twins. This explains why some monozygotic twins are wrongly stated to be dizygotic twins at birth.

- Uneven X chromosome inactivation between female MZ twins, with the result that one twin preferentially expresses the paternal X and the other the maternal X.

EARLY DEATH OF A TWIN

Because ultrasonographic studies are a common part of prenatal care, it is known that early death and resorption of one member of a twin pair is fairly common. Awareness of this possibility must be considered when discrepancies occur between prenatal cytogenetic findings and the karyotype of an infant. Errors in prenatal cytogenetic diagnosis may arise if extraembryonic tissues (e.g., part of a chorionic villus) from the resorbed twin are examined.

CONJOINED MONOZYGOTIC TWINS

If the embryonic disc does not divide completely, or adjacent embryonic discs fuse, various types of conjoined MZ twins may form (Figs. 7-30*B* and *C*, 7-32, 7-33, and 7-34). These attached (Greek, *pagos*, fixed) twins are named according to the regions that are attached, e.g., thoracopagus indicates that there is anterior union of the thoracic regions. It has been estimated that the incidence of conjoined twins is 1 in 50,000 to 100,000 births. In some cases, the twins are connected to each other by skin only or by cutaneous and other tissues, e.g., fused livers (see Fig. 7-33). Some conjoined twins can be successfully separated by surgical procedures (see Fig. 7-32*B*); however, the anatomic relations in most conjoined twins do not permit surgical separation with sustained viability (see Fig. 7-34).

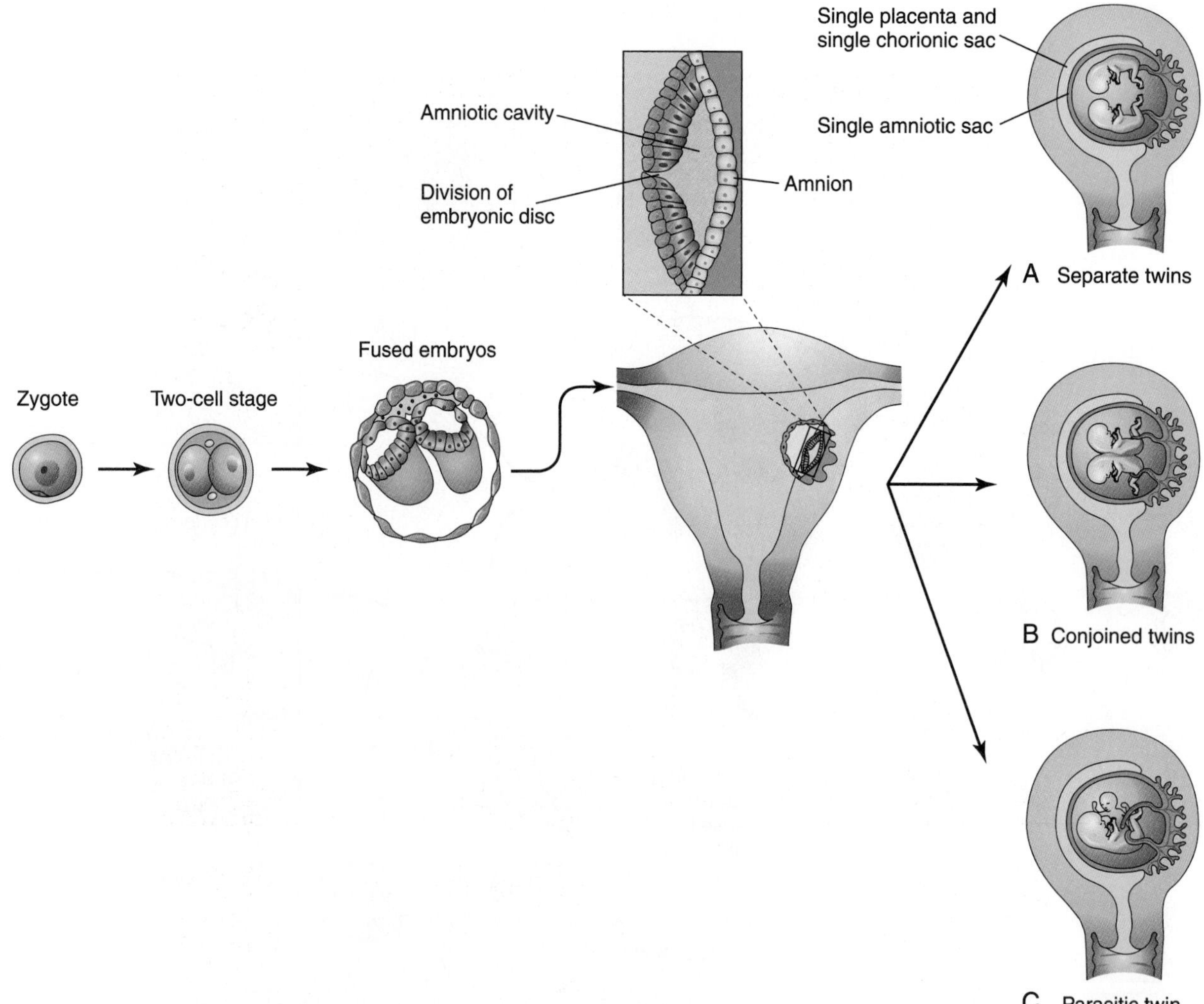

FIGURE 7-30. Diagrams illustrating how some monozygotic twins develop. This method of development is very uncommon. Division of the embryonic disc results in two embryos within one amniotic sac. **A,** Complete division of the embryonic disc gives rise to twins. Such twins rarely survive because their umbilical cords are often so entangled that interruption of the blood supply to the fetuses occurs. **B** and **C,** Incomplete division of the disc results in various types of conjoined twins.

SUPERFECUNDATION

Superfecundation is the fertilization of two or more oocytes at different times. In humans, the presence of two fetuses in the uterus caused by fertilization at different times (superfetation) is rare. DZ human twins with different fathers have been confirmed by genetic markers.

Other Types of Multiple Births

Triplets may be derived from:

- One zygote and be identical
- Two zygotes and consist of identical twins and a singleton
- Three zygotes and be of the same sex or of different sexes

In the last case, the infants are no more similar than infants from three separate pregnancies. Similar combinations occur in quadruplets, quintuplets, sextuplets, and septuplets.

SUMMARY OF THE PLACENTA AND FETAL MEMBRANES

- The placenta consists of two parts: a larger fetal part derived from the villous chorion and a smaller maternal part developed from the decidua basalis. The two parts are held together by stem chorionic villi that attach to the cytotrophoblastic shell surrounding the chorionic sac, which attaches the sac to the decidua basalis.
- The principal activities of the placenta are metabolism (synthesis of glycogen, cholesterol, and fatty acids), respiratory gas exchange (oxygen, carbon

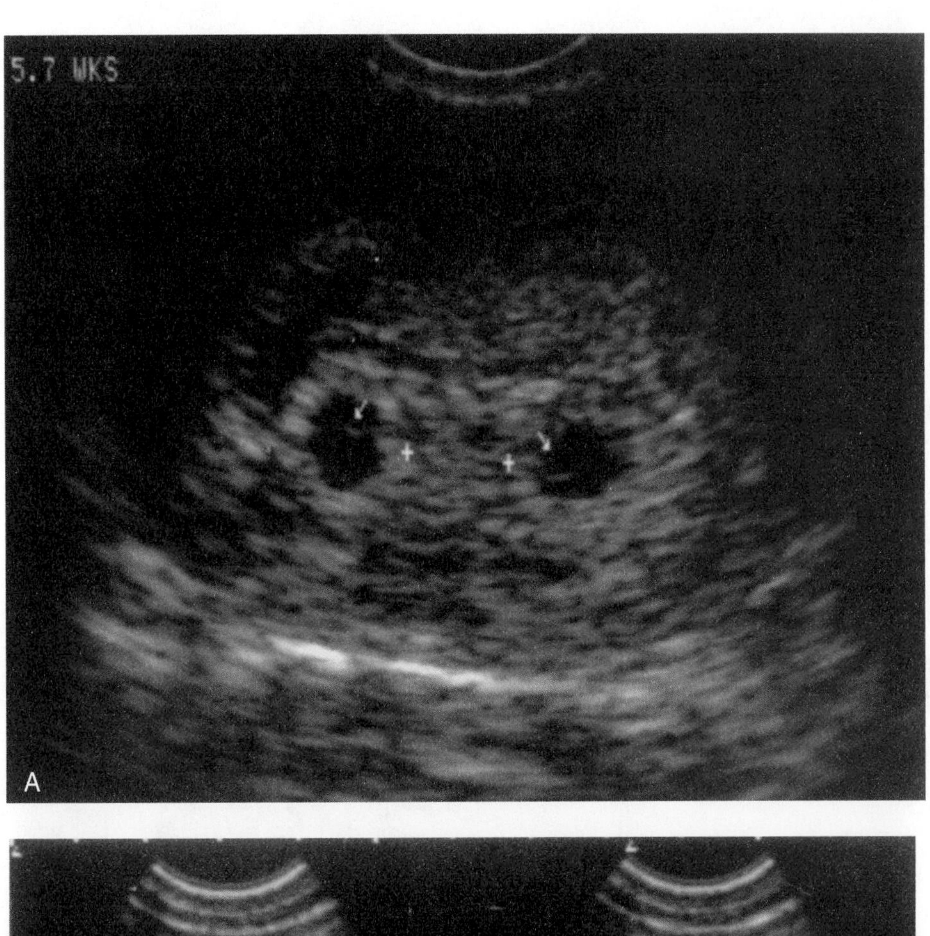

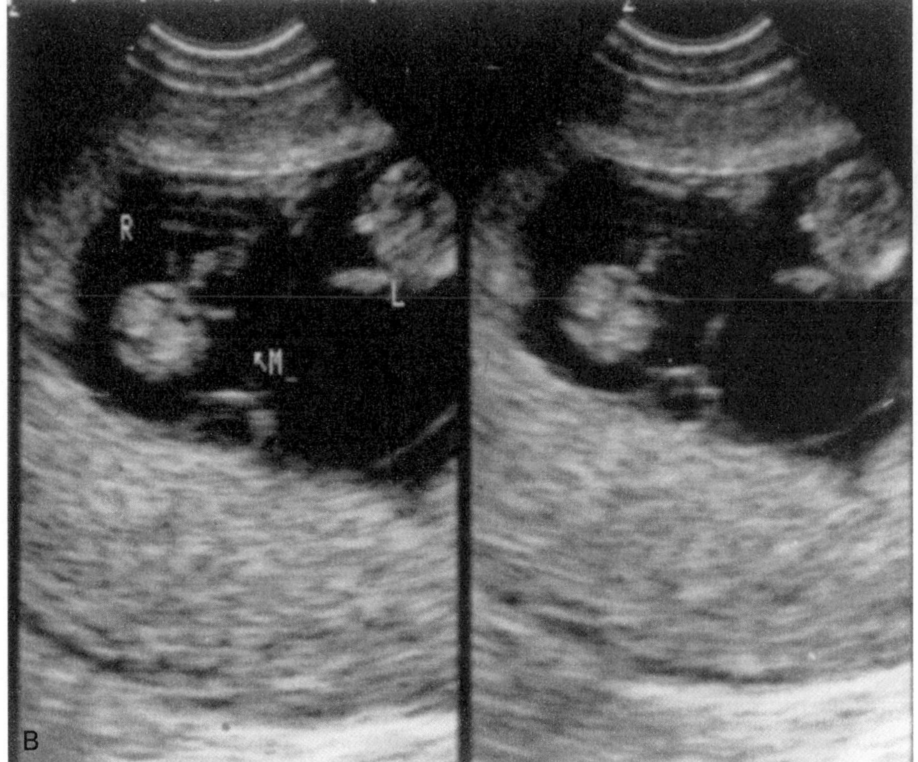

FIGURE 7-31. Ultrasound scans of pregnant women. **A,** Diamniotic/dichorionic twin gestation at 5.7 weeks, 3.7 weeks after fertilization. The *arrows* indicate the umbilical vesicles of the dizygotic twins in their chorionic sacs. **B,** Diamniotic/monochorionic twin gestation at 11 weeks, 9 weeks after fertilization. The fused amnions (M) separate the monozygotic fetuses (R and L). (Courtesy of Dr. Lyndon M. Hill, Department of Obstetrics and Gynecology, Division of Maternal-Fetal Medicine, University of Pittsburgh, Pittsburgh, PA.)

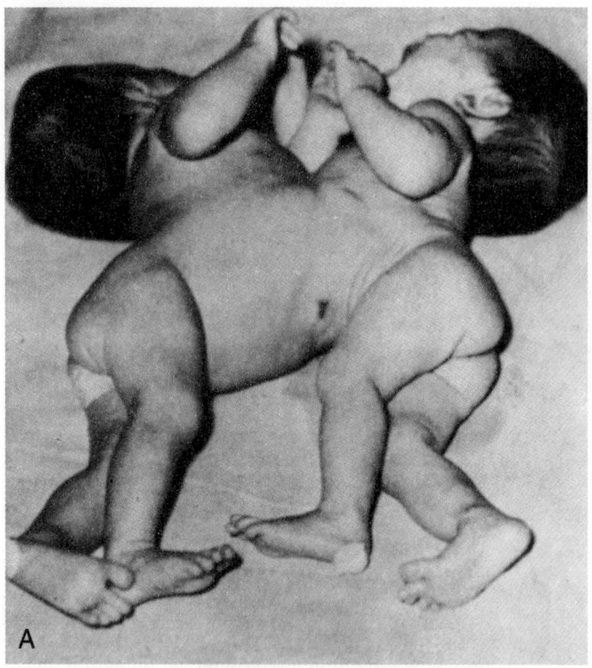

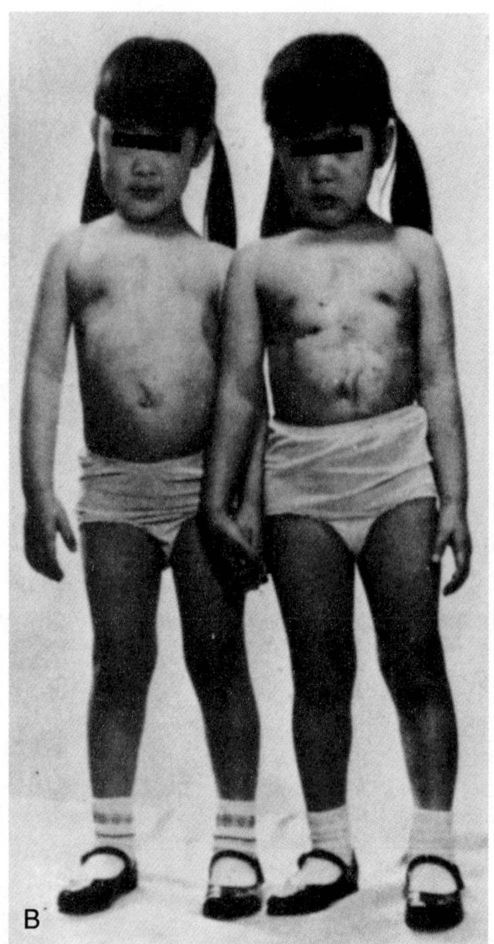

FIGURE 7-32. **A,** Newborn monozygotic conjoined twins showing union in the thoracic regions (thoracopagus). **B,** The twins approximately 4 years after separation. (From deVries PA: Case history—the San Francisco twins. In Bergsma D [ed]: Conjoined Twins. New York, Alan R. Liss for the National Foundation–March of Dimes, DBOAS III, [1], 141–142, 1967, with permission of the copyright holder.)

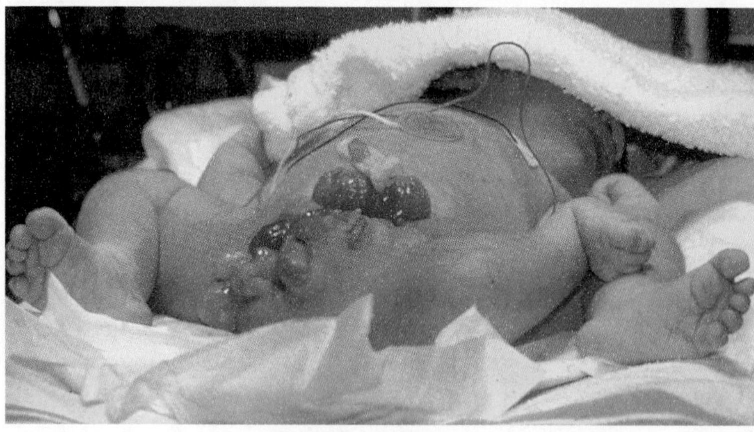

FIGURE 7-33. Parasitic twins, anterior view. Note normal tone and posture of fully developed host twin with meconium staining, exstrophy of the bladder in both host and parasitic twins, exposed small bowel in parasitic twin, and fully formed right lower limb with normal tone and flexion in the parasitic twin. (Courtesy of Dr. Linda J. Juretschke, The Ronald McDonald Children's Hospital of Loyola University Medical Center, Maywood, IL.)

dioxide, and carbon monoxide), transfer of nutrients (vitamins, hormones, and antibodies; elimination of waste products), and endocrine secretion (e.g., hCG) for maintenance of pregnancy

- The fetal circulation is separated from the maternal circulation by a thin layer of extrafetal tissues—the placental membrane. It is a permeable membrane that allows water, oxygen, nutritive substances, hormones, and noxious agents to pass from the mother to the embryo or fetus. Excretory products pass through the placental membrane from the fetus to the mother.
- The fetal membranes and placenta(s) in multiple pregnancies vary considerably, depending on the derivation of the embryos and the time when division of embryonic cells occurs. The common type of twins is DZ twins, with two amnions, two chorions, and two placentas that may or may not be fused.

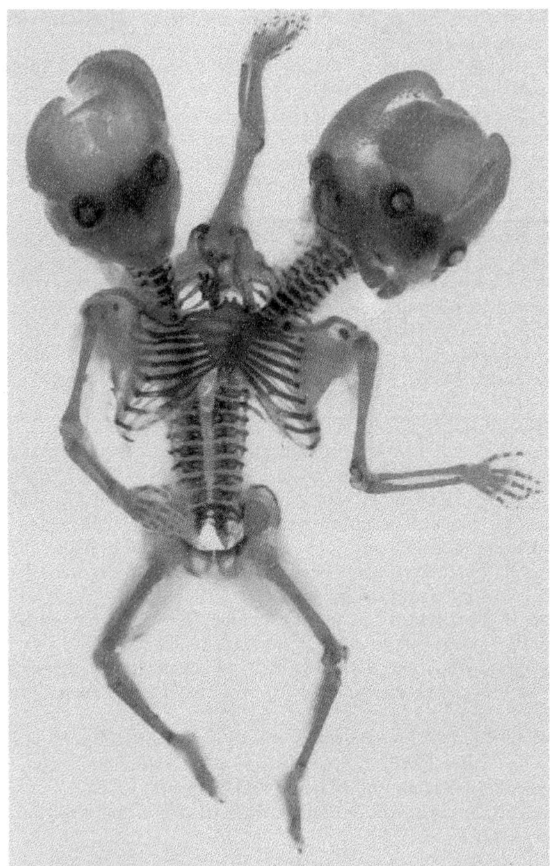

FIGURE 7-34. Dicephalic (two heads) conjoined twins, alizarin stained, showing bone (red) and cartilage (blue). Note the two clavicles supporting the midline upper limb, fused thoracic cage, and parallel vertebral columns. (Courtesy of Dr. Joseph R. Siebert, Children's Hospital and Regional Center, Seattle, WA.)

- MZ twins, the less common type, represent approximately one third of all twins; they are derived from one zygote. MZ twins commonly have one chorion, two amnions, and one placenta. Twins with one amnion, one chorion, and one placenta are always monozygotic, and their umbilical cords are often entangled. Other types of multiple birth (triplets, etc.) may be derived from one or more zygotes.
- The umbilical vesicle and allantois are vestigial structures; however, their presence is essential to normal embryonic development. Both are early sites of blood formation and both are partly incorporated into the embryo. Primordial germ cells also originate in the wall of the umbilical vesicle (yolk sac).
- The amnion forms an amniotic sac for amniotic fluid and provides a covering for the umbilical cord. The amniotic fluid has three main functions: to provide a protective buffer for the embryo or fetus, to allow room for fetal movements, and to assist in the regulation of fetal body temperature.

CLINICALLY ORIENTED PROBLEMS

CASE 7-1

A physician is concerned about the effects of a drug on the embryo of one of his patients.

- How is the estimated date of confinement or estimated delivery date of a baby determined?
- How could the estimated delivery date be confirmed in a high-risk obstetric patient?

CASE 7-2

A physician told a pregnant woman that she had polyhydramnios.

- If you were asked to explain the meaning of this clinical condition, what would be your answer?
- What conditions are often associated with polyhydramnios?
- Explain why polyhydramnios occurs.

CASE 7-3

A physician was asked, "Does twinning run in families?"

- Is maternal age a factor?
- If uncertainty exists about the origin of twins, how would you determine whether they were MZ or DZ?

CASE 7-4

A pathologist asked you to examine a section of an umbilical cord. You observed that there was only one umbilical artery.

- How often does this anomaly occur?
- What kind of fetal abnormalities might be associated with this condition?

CASE 7-5

An ultrasonound examination revealed a twin pregnancy with a single placenta. Chorionic villus sampling and chromosome analysis revealed that the twins were likely female. At birth, the twins were of different sexes.

- How could this error have occurred?

CASE 7-6

An ultrasound examination of a pregnant woman during the second trimester revealed multiple amniotic bands associated with the fetus.

- What produces these bands?
- What congenital defects may result from them?
- What is the syndrome called?

Discussion of these problems appears at the back of the book.

References and Suggested Reading

Alexander GR, Wingate MS, Salihu H, et al: Fetal and neonatal mortality risks of multiple births. Obstet Gynecol Clin N Am 32:1, 2005.

American College of Obstetrics and Gynecology. Intrauterine growth restriction. Washington, DC, The American College of Obstetricians and Gynecologists. Practice Bulletin No. 12, 2000.

Annas GJ: Conjoined twins—the limits of law at the limits of life. N Engl J Med 344:1104, 2001.

Battaglia FC: Fetoplacental perfusion and transfer of nutrients. In Reece EA, Hobbins JC (eds): Medicine of the Fetus and Mother, 2nd ed. Philadelphia, Lippincott-Raven, 1999.

Benirschke K, Kaufmann P: Pathology of the Human Placenta, 4th ed. New York, Springer-Verlag, 2000.

Brace RA: Amniotic fluid dynamics. In Creasy RK, Resnik R (eds): Maternal-Fetal Medicine, 5th ed. Philadelphia, WB Saunders, 2004.

Bronsan PG: The hypothalamic pituitary axis in the fetus and newborn. Semin Perinatol 25:371, 2001.

Collins JH: Umbilical cord accidents: Human studies. Semin Perinatol 26:79, 2002.

Cross JC: Formation of the placenta and extraembryonic membranes. Ann N Y Acad Sci 857:23, 1998.

Cunningham FG, Leveno KJ, Bloom SL, et al: Williams Obstetrics, 22nd ed. New York, McGraw-Hill, 2005.

Egan JF, Borgida AF: Multiple gestations: the importance of ultrasound. Obstet Gynecol Clin N Am 31:141, 2004.

Enders AC: Structural responses of the primate endometrium to implantation. Placenta 12:309, 1991.

Filly RA: Ultrasound evaluation during the first trimester. In Callen PW (ed): Ultrasonography in Obstetrics and Gynecology, 4th ed. Philadelphia, WB Saunders, 2000.

Foidart J-M, Hustin J, Dubois M, Schaaps J-P: The human placenta becomes haemochorial at the 13th week of pregnancy. Int J Dev Biol 36:451, 1992.

Harman CR, Baschatt AA: Comprehensive assessment of fetal well being: Which Doppler tests should be performed? Curr Opin Obstet Gynecol 15:147, 2003.

Jirásel JE: An Atlas of Human Prenatal Developmental Mechanics. Anatomy and Staging. London and New York, Taylor & Francis, 2004.

Kodaman PH, Taylor HS: Hormonal regulation of implantation. Obstet Gynecol Clin N Am 31:745, 2004.

Liao JB, Buhimschi CS, Norwitz ER: Normal labor: Mechanism and duration. Obstet Gynecol Clin N Am 32: 145, 2005.

Lockwood CJ: The initiation of parturition at term. Obstet Gynecol Clin N Am 31:935, 2004.

Ma GT, Soloveva V, Tzeng S-J, et al: Nodal regulates trophoblast differentiation and placental development. Dev Biol 236:124, 2001.

Marino T: Ultrasound abnormalities of the amniotic fluid, membranes, umbilical cord, and placenta. Obstet Gynecol Clin N Am 31:177, 2004.

Moore KL, Dalley AD: Clinically Oriented Anatomy, 5th ed. Baltimore, Williams & Wilkins, 2006.

Mundy CA: Intravenous immunoglobulin in the management of hemolytic disease of the newborn. Neonat Netwk 24:17, 2005.

Pridjian G: Fetomaternal interactions: Placental physiology, the in utero environment, and fetal determinants of adult disease. In MacDonald MG, Seshia MMK, Mullett MD (eds): Avery's Neonatology. Pathophysiology & Management of the Newborn, 6th ed. Philadelphia, Lippincott Williams & Wilkins, 2005.

Ralston SJ, Craigo SD: Ultrasound-guided procedures for prenatal diagnosis and therapy. Obstet Gynecol Clin N Am 31:101, 2004.

Redline RW: Placental pathology. In Martin RJ, Fanaroff AA, Walsh MC (eds): Fanaroff and Martin's Neonatal-Perinatal Medicine. Diseases of the Fetus and Infant, 8th ed. Philadelphia, Mosby, 2006.

Spencer R: Theoretical and analytical embryology of conjoined twins: Part I: Embryogenesis. Clin Anat 13:36, 2000.

Spencer R: Theoretical and analytical embryology of conjoined twins: Part II: Adjustments to union. Clin Anat 13:97, 2000.

Tongsong T, Wanapirak C, Kunavikatikul C, et al: Cordocentesis at 16–24 weeks of gestation: Experience of 1320 cases. Prenat Diagn 20:224, 2000.

Townsend RR: Ultrasound evaluation of the placenta and umbilical cord. In Callen PW (ed): Ultrasonography in Obstetrics and Gynecology, 4th ed. Philadelphia, WB Saunders, 2000.

Wachtel SS, Shulman LP, Sammons D: Fetal cells in maternal blood. Clin Genet 59:74, 2001.

8

Body Cavities, Mesenteries, and Diaphragm

The Embryonic Body Cavity 146
Mesenteries 146
Division of the Embryonic Body Cavity 146
Development of the Diaphragm 150
Septum Transversum 150
Pleuroperitoneal Membranes 151
Dorsal Mesentery of the Esophagus 151
Muscular Ingrowth from Lateral Body Walls 152
Positional Changes and Innervation of the Diaphragm 153
Summary of the Development of the Body Cavities 157
Clinically Oriented Problems 157

Early in the fourth week, the **intraembryonic coelom** appears as a horseshoe-shaped cavity (Fig. 8-1*A*). The curve or bend in this cavity at the cranial end of the embryo represents the future *pericardial cavity*, and its limbs (lateral extensions) indicate the future *pleural* and *peritoneal cavities*. The distal part of each limb of the intraembryonic coelom is continuous with the **extraembryonic coelom** at the lateral edges of the embryonic disc (see Fig. 8-1*B*). This communication is important because most of the midgut normally herniates through this communication into the umbilical cord, where it develops into most of the small intestine and part of the large intestine (see Chapter 11). The intraembryonic coelom provides room for the organs to develop and move. During embryonic folding in the horizontal plane, the limbs of the coelom are brought together on the ventral aspect of the embryo (Fig. 8-2). The ventral mesentery degenerates in the region of the future peritoneal cavity (see Fig. 8-2*F*), resulting in a large embryonic **peritoneal cavity** extending from the heart to the pelvic region.

THE EMBRYONIC BODY CAVITY

The intraembryonic coelom becomes the embryonic body cavity, which is divided into three well-defined cavities during the fourth week (Figs. 8-2 and 8-3):

- A pericardial cavity
- Two pericardioperitoneal canals
- A peritoneal cavity

These body cavities have a parietal wall lined by mesothelium (future parietal layer of peritoneum) derived from somatic mesoderm and a visceral wall covered by mesothelium (future visceral layer of peritoneum) derived from splanchnic mesoderm (see Fig. 8-3*E*). The peritoneal cavity (the major part of intraembryonic coelom) is connected with the extraembryonic coelom at the umbilicus (Fig. 8-4*C* and *D*). The peritoneal cavity loses its connection with the extraembryonic coelom during the 10th week as the intestines return to the abdomen from the umbilical cord (see Chapter 11).

During formation of the head fold, the heart and pericardial cavity are relocated ventrocaudally, anterior to the foregut (see Fig. 8-2*B*). As a result, the pericardial cavity opens into pericardioperitoneal canals, which pass dorsal to the foregut (see Fig. 8-4*B* and *D*). After embryonic folding, the caudal part of the foregut, the midgut, and the hindgut are suspended in the peritoneal cavity from the dorsal abdominal wall by the dorsal mesentery (see Figs. 8-2*F* and 8-3*C* to *E*).

Mesenteries

A mesentery is a double layer of peritoneum that begins as an extension of the visceral peritoneum covering an organ. The mesentery connects the organ to the body wall and conveys vessels and nerves to it. Transiently, the dorsal and ventral mesenteries divide the peritoneal cavity into right and left halves (see Fig. 8-3*C*). The ventral mesentery soon disappears (see Fig. 8-3*E*), except where it is attached to the caudal part of the foregut (primordium of stomach and proximal part of duodenum). The peritoneal cavity then becomes a continuous space (see Fig. 8-4*D*). The arteries supplying the primordial gut—celiac arterial trunk (foregut), superior mesenteric artery (midgut), and inferior mesenteric artery (hindgut)—pass between the layers of the dorsal mesentery (see Fig. 8-3*C*).

Division of the Embryonic Body Cavity

Each pericardioperitoneal canal lies lateral to the proximal part of the foregut (future esophagus) and dorsal to the **septum transversum**—a thick plate of mesodermal tissue that occupies the space between the thoracic cavity and

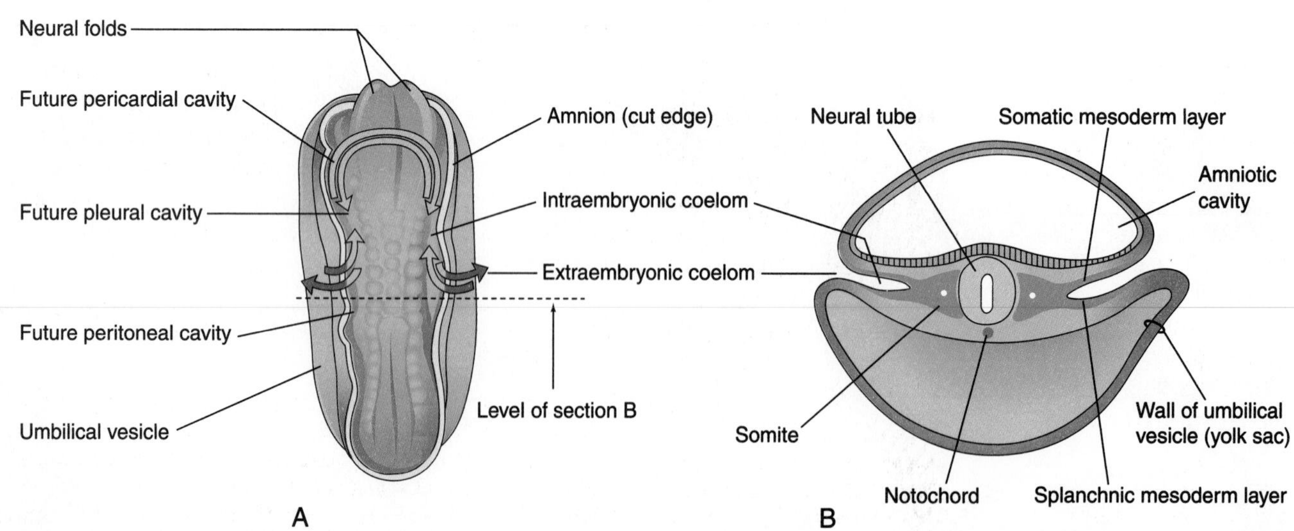

FIGURE 8-1. **A,** Drawing of a dorsal view of a 22-day embryo showing the outline of the horseshoe-shaped intraembryonic coelom. The amnion has been removed, and the coelom is shown as if the embryo were translucent. The continuity of the intraembryonic coelom, as well as the communication of its right and left limbs with the extraembryonic coelom, is indicated by arrows. **B,** Transverse section through the embryo at the level shown in **A**.

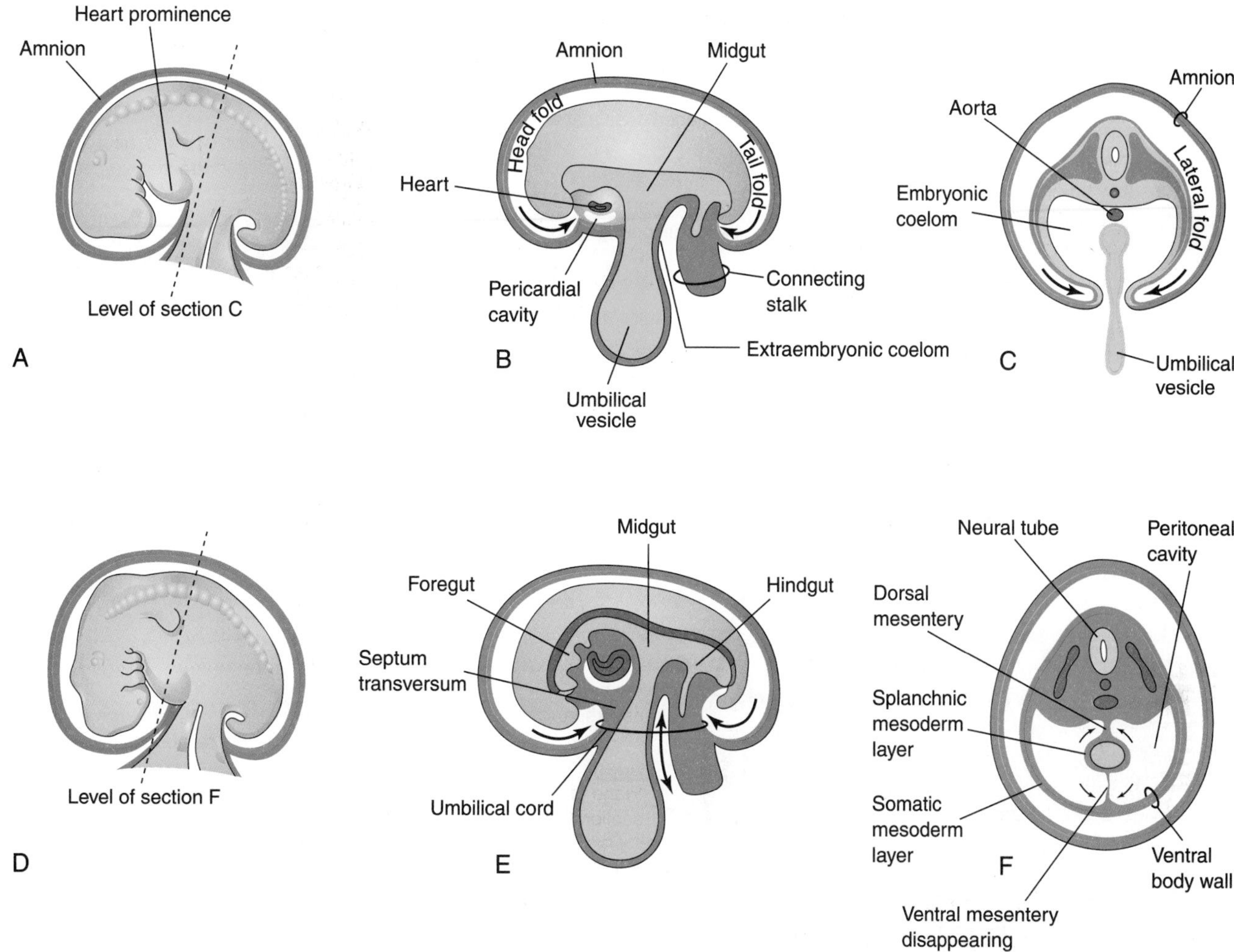

FIGURE 8-2. Illustrations of embryonic folding and its effects on the intraembryonic coelom and other structures. **A,** Lateral view of an embryo (approximately 26 days). **B,** Schematic sagittal section of this embryo showing the head and tail folds. **C,** Transverse section at the level shown in **A,** indicating how fusion of the lateral folds gives the embryo a cylindrical form. **D,** Lateral view of an embryo (approximately 28 days). **E,** Schematic sagittal section of this embryo showing the reduced communication between the intraembryonic and extraembryonic coeloms (*double-headed arrow*). **F,** Transverse section as indicated in **D,** illustrating formation of the ventral body wall and disappearance of the ventral mesentery. The *arrows* indicate the junction of the somatic and splanchnic layers of mesoderm. The somatic mesoderm will become the parietal peritoneum lining the abdominal wall, and the splanchnic mesoderm will become the visceral peritoneum covering the organs (e.g., the stomach).

omphaloenteric duct (see Fig. 8-4*A* and *B*). The septum transversum is the primordium of the central tendon of the diaphragm. Partitions form in each pericardioperitoneal canal that separate the pericardial cavity from the pleural cavities and the pleural cavities from the peritoneal cavity. Because of the growth of the **bronchial buds** (primordia of bronchi and lungs) into the pericardioperitoneal canals (Fig. 8-5*A*), a pair of membranous ridges is produced in the lateral wall of each canal:

- The cranial ridges—*pleuropericardial folds*—are located superior to the developing lungs.
- The caudal ridges—*pleuroperitoneal folds*—are located inferior to the lungs.

Congenital Pericardial Defects

Defective formation and/or fusion of the pleuropericardial membranes separating the pericardial and pleural cavities is uncommon. This anomaly results in a congenital defect of the pericardium, usually on the left side. Consequently, the pericardial cavity communicates with the pleural cavity. In very unusual cases, part of the left atrium of the heart herniates into the pleural cavity at each heartbeat.

Pleuropericardial Membranes

As the pleuropericardial folds enlarge, they form partitions that separate the pericardial cavity from the pleural cavities. These partitions—**pleuropericardial membranes**—contain the common cardinal veins (see Figs. 8-4*C* and 8-5*A*), which drain the venous system into the sinus venosus of the heart (see Chapter 13). Initially the bronchial buds are small relative to the heart and pericardial cavity (see Fig. 8-5*A*). They soon grow laterally from the caudal end of the trachea into the pericardio-

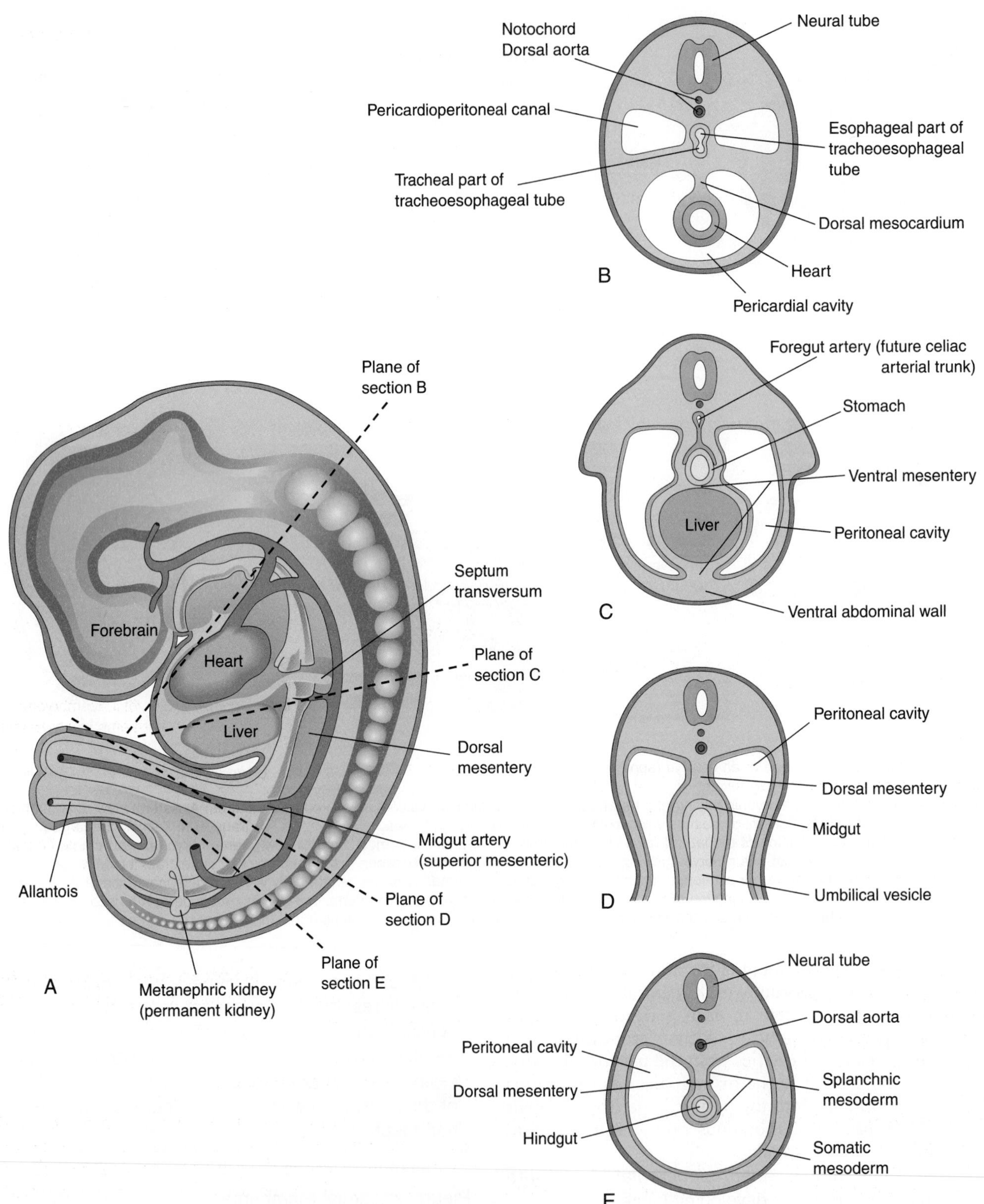

FIGURE 8-3. Illustrations of the mesenteries and body cavities at the beginning of the fifth week. **A,** Schematic sagittal section. Note that the dorsal mesentery serves as a pathway for the arteries supplying the developing gut. Nerves and lymphatics also pass between the layers of this mesentery. **B** to **E,** Transverse sections through the embryo at the levels indicated in **A**. The ventral mesentery disappears, except in the region of the terminal esophagus, stomach, and first part of the duodenum. Note that the right and left parts of the peritoneal cavity, separate in **C,** are continuous in **E**.

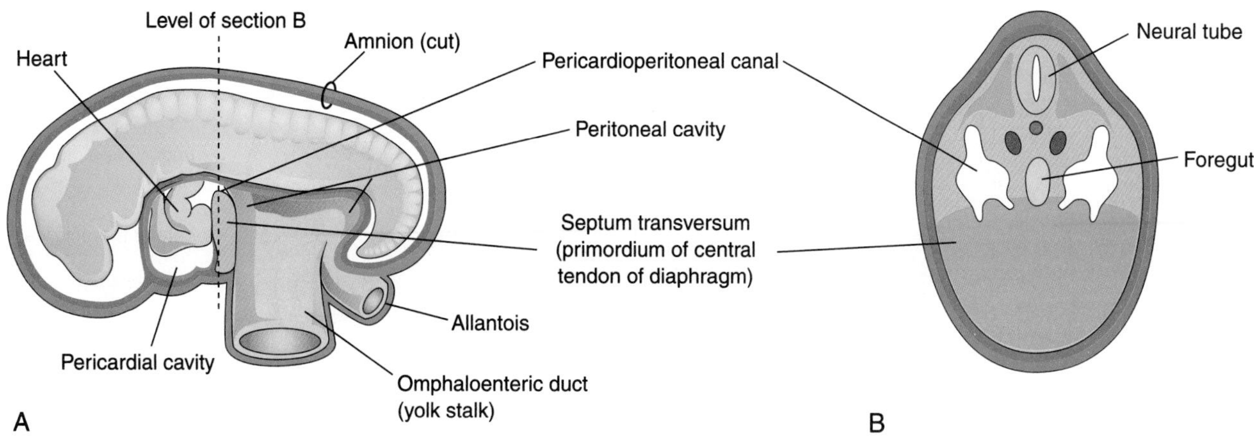

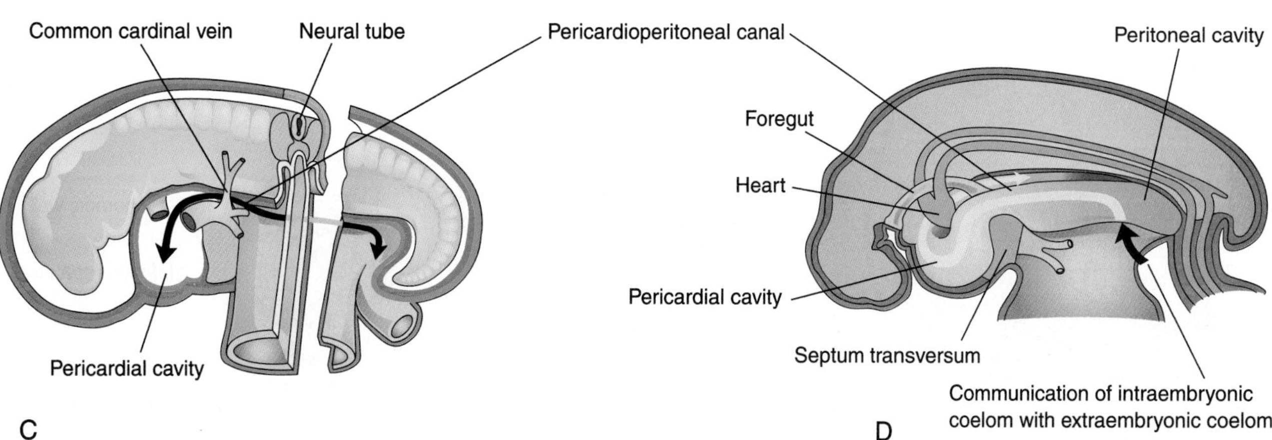

FIGURE 8-4. Schematic drawings of an embryo (approximately 24 days). **A,** The lateral wall of the pericardial cavity has been removed to show the primordial heart. **B,** Transverse section of the embryo illustrates the relationship of the pericardioperitoneal canals to the septum transversum (primordium of central tendon of diaphragm) and the foregut. **C,** Lateral view of the embryo with the heart removed. The embryo has also been sectioned transversely to show the continuity of the intraembryonic and extraembryonic coeloms (*arrow*). **D,** Sketch showing the pericardioperitoneal canals arising from the dorsal wall of the pericardial cavity and passing on each side of the foregut to join the peritoneal cavity. The *arrow* shows the communication of the extraembryonic coelom with the intraembryonic coelom and the continuity of the intraembryonic coelom at this stage.

peritoneal canals (future pleural canals). As the primordial pleural cavities expand ventrally around the heart, they extend into the body wall, splitting the mesenchyme into:

- An outer layer that becomes the thoracic wall
- An inner layer (pleuropericardial membrane) that becomes the fibrous pericardium, the outer layer of the pericardial sac enclosing the heart (see Fig. 8-5*C* and *D*)

The pleuropericardial membranes project into the cranial ends of the pericardioperitoneal canals (see Fig. 8-5*B*). With subsequent growth of the common cardinal veins, positional displacement of the heart, and expansion of the pleural cavities, the pleuropericardial membranes become mesentery-like folds extending from the lateral thoracic wall. By the seventh week, the pleuropericardial membranes fuse with the mesenchyme ventral to the esophagus, separating the pericardial cavity from the pleural cavities (see Fig. 8-5*C*). This **primordial mediastinum** consists of a mass of mesenchyme that extends from the sternum to the vertebral column, separating the developing lungs (see Fig. 8-5*D*). The right pleuropericardial opening closes slightly earlier than the left one and produces a larger pleuropericardial membrane.

Pleuroperitoneal Membranes

As the pleuroperitoneal folds enlarge, they project into the pericardioperitoneal canals. Gradually the folds become membranous, forming the **pleuroperitoneal membranes** (Figs. 8-6 and 8-7). Eventually these membranes separate the pleural cavities from the peritoneal cavity. The pleuroperitoneal membranes are produced as the developing lungs and pleural cavities expand and invade the body wall. They are attached dorsolaterally to the abdominal wall and initially their crescentic free edges project into the caudal ends of the **pericardioperitoneal canals**. During the sixth week, the pleuroperitoneal membranes extend ventromedially until their free edges fuse with the dorsal mesentery of the esophagus and septum transversum (see Fig. 8-7*C*). This separates the pleural cavities from the

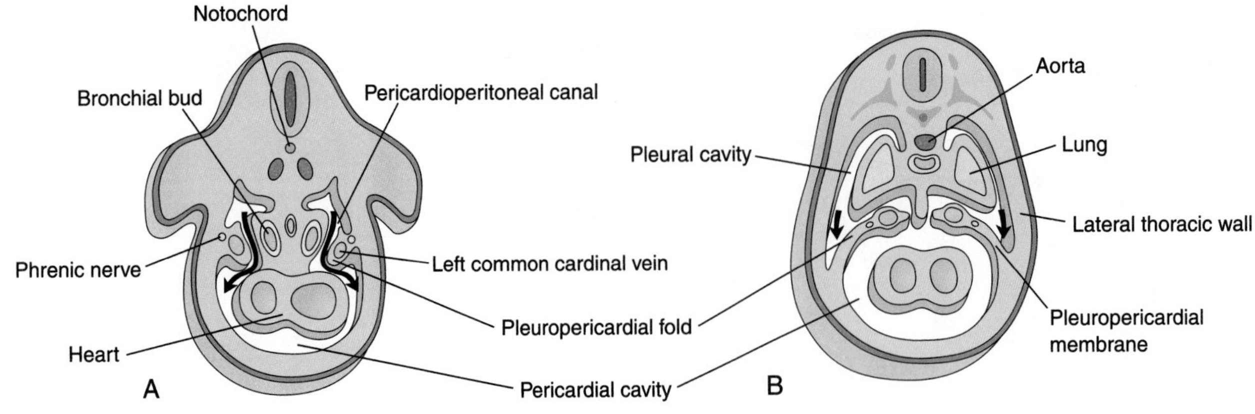

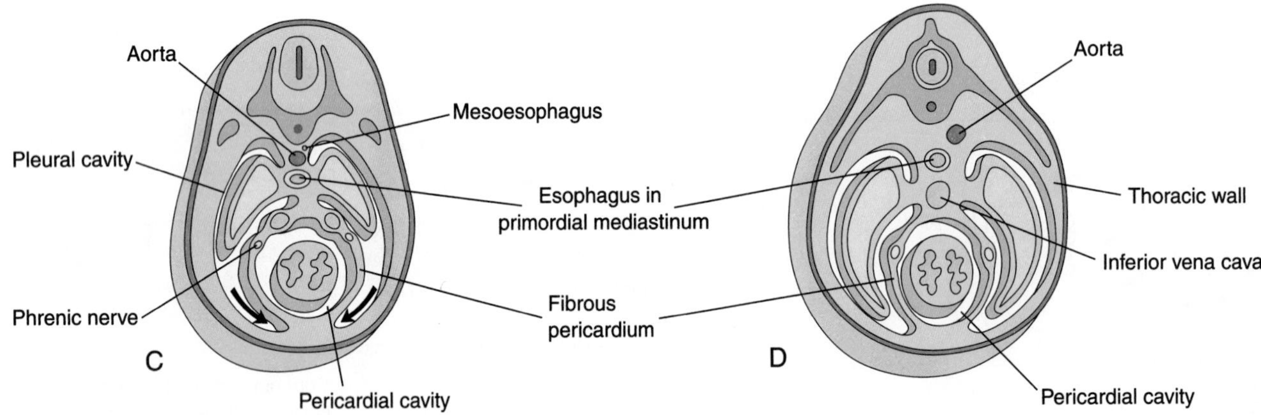

FIGURE 8-5. Schematic drawings of transverse sections through embryos cranial to the septum transversum, illustrating successive stages in the separation of the pleural cavities from the pericardial cavity. Growth and development of the lungs, expansion of the pleural cavities, and formation of the fibrous pericardium are also shown. **A,** At 5 weeks. The *arrows* indicate the communications between the pericardioperitoneal canals and the pericardial cavity. **B,** At 6 weeks. The *arrows* indicate development of the pleural cavities as they expand into the body wall. **C,** At 7 weeks. Expansion of the pleural cavities ventrally around the heart is shown. The pleuropericardial membranes are now fused in the median plane with each other and with the mesoderm ventral to the esophagus. **D,** At 8 weeks. Continued expansion of the lungs and pleural cavities and formation of the fibrous pericardium and thoracic wall are illustrated.

peritoneal cavity. Closure of the pleuroperitoneal openings is assisted by the migration of myoblasts (primordial muscle cells) into the pleuroperitoneal membranes (see Fig. 8-7*E*). The pleuroperitoneal opening on the right side closes slightly before the left one. The reason for this is uncertain, but it may be related to the relatively large size of the right lobe of the liver at this stage of development.

DEVELOPMENT OF THE DIAPHRAGM

The diaphragm is a dome-shaped, musculotendinous partition that separates the thoracic and abdominal cavities. It is a composite structure that develops from four embryonic components (see Fig. 8-7):

- Septum transversum
- Pleuroperitoneal membranes
- Dorsal mesentery of esophagus
- Muscular ingrowth from lateral body walls

Recent studies indicate that several candidate genes on the long arm of chromosome 15 (15q) play a critical role in the development of the diaphragm.

Septum Transversum

This transverse septum, composed of mesodermal tissue, is the primordium of the **central tendon of the diaphragm** (see Fig. 8-7*D* and *E*). The septum transversum grows dorsally from the ventrolateral body wall and forms a semicircular shelf, which separates the heart from the liver (see Fig. 8-6). The septum transversum is first identifiable at the end of the third week as a mass of mesodermal tissue cranial to the pericardial cavity (see Chapter 5). After the head folds ventrally during the fourth week, the septum transversum forms a thick incomplete partition between the pericardial and abdominal cavities (see Fig. 8-4). The septum transversum does not separate the thoracic and abdominal cavities completely. During its early development, a large part of the liver is embedded in the septum transversum. There are large openings, the **pericardioperitoneal canals,** along the sides of the esophagus (see Fig. 8-7*B*). The septum transversum expands and fuses with the dorsal mesentery of the esophagus and the pleuroperitoneal membranes (see Fig. 8-7*C*).

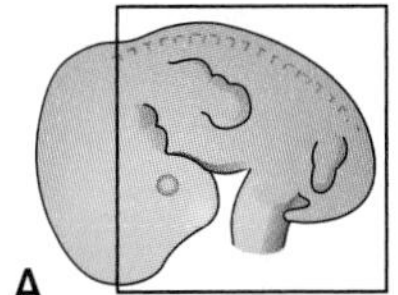

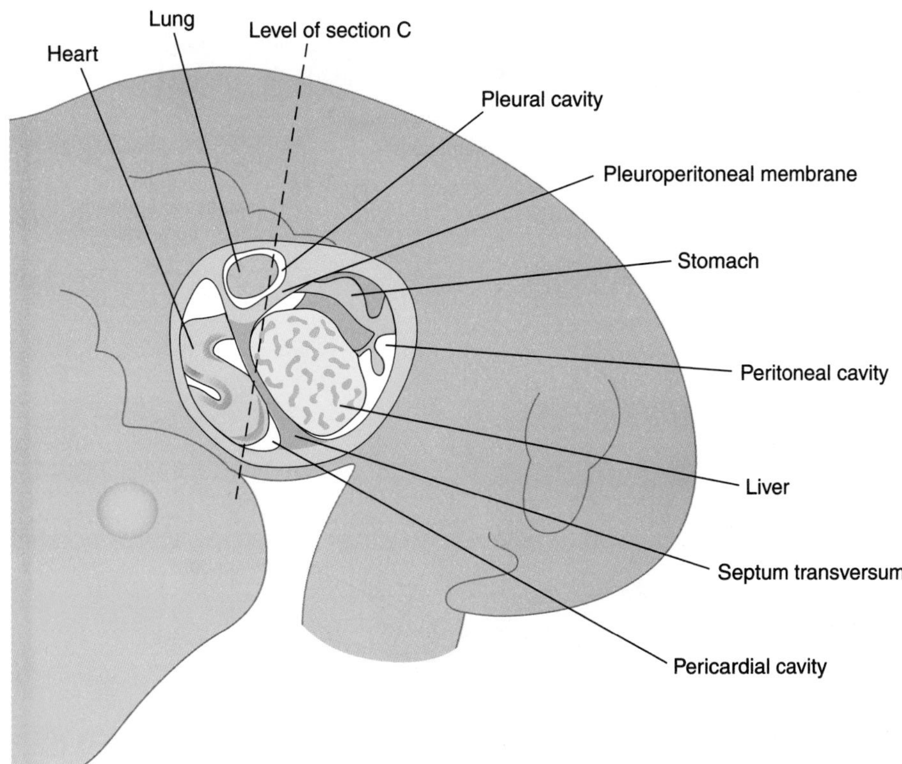

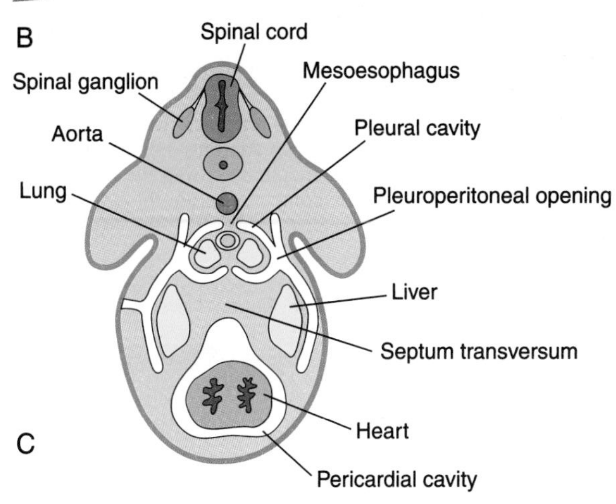

FIGURE 8-6. **A,** Sketch of a lateral view of an embryo (approximately 33 days). The rectangle indicates the area enlarged in **B**. The primordial body cavities are viewed from the left side after removal of the lateral body wall. **C,** Transverse section through the embryo at the level shown in **B**.

Pleuroperitoneal Membranes

These membranes fuse with the dorsal mesentery of the esophagus and the septum transversum (see Fig. 8-7*C*). This completes the partition between the thoracic and abdominal cavities and forms the **primordial diaphragm**. Although the pleuroperitoneal membranes form large portions of the early fetal diaphragm, they represent relatively small portions of the newborn's diaphragm (see Fig. 8-7*E*).

Dorsal Mesentery of the Esophagus

As previously described, the septum transversum and pleuroperitoneal membranes fuse with the dorsal mesentery of the esophagus (mesoesophagus). This mesentery constitutes the median portion of the diaphragm. The **crura of the diaphragm**, a leglike pair of diverging muscle bundles that cross in the median plane anterior to the aorta (see Fig. 8-7*E*), develop from myoblasts that grow into the dorsal mesentery of the esophagus.

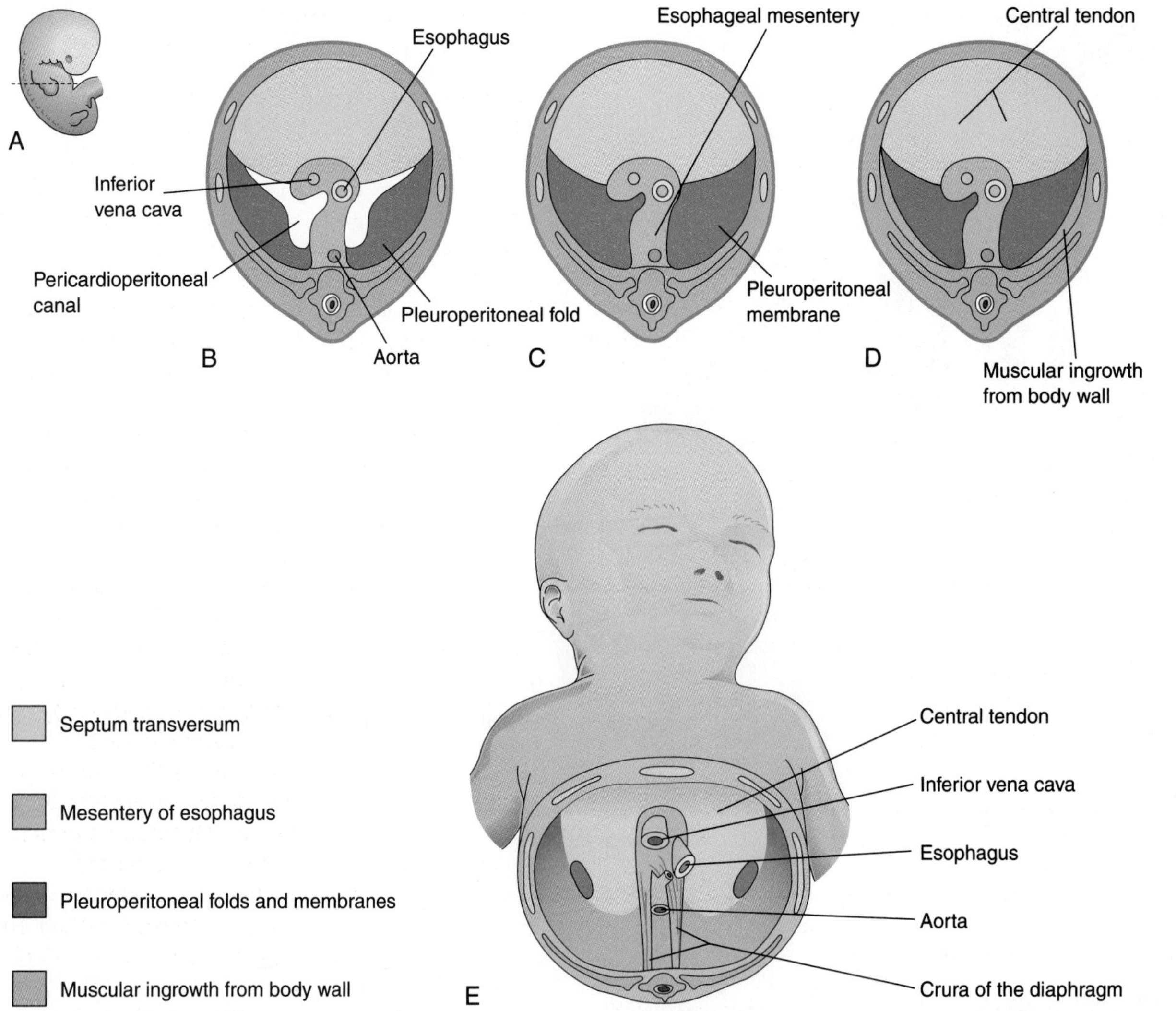

A

Esophagus

Inferior vena cava

Pericardioperitoneal canal

Pleuroperitoneal fold

Aorta

B

Esophageal mesentery

Pleuroperitoneal membrane

C

Central tendon

Muscular ingrowth from body wall

D

Septum transversum

Mesentery of esophagus

Pleuroperitoneal folds and membranes

Muscular ingrowth from body wall

Central tendon

Inferior vena cava

Esophagus

Aorta

Crura of the diaphragm

E

FIGURE 8-7. Illustrations of development of the diaphragm. **A,** Sketch of a lateral view of an embryo at the end of the fifth week (actual size) indicating the level of sections in **B** to **D**. **B** to **E,** The developing diaphragm as viewed inferiorly. **B,** Transverse section showing the unfused pleuroperitoneal membranes. **C,** Similar section at the end of the sixth week after fusion of the pleuroperitoneal membranes with the other two diaphragmatic components. **D,** Transverse section of a 12-week fetus after ingrowth of the fourth diaphragmatic component from the body wall. **E,** Inferior view of the diaphragm of a newborn indicating the embryologic origin of its components.

Muscular Ingrowth from Lateral Body Walls

During the 9th to 12th weeks, the lungs and pleural cavities enlarge, "burrowing" into the lateral body walls (see Fig. 8-5). During this process, the body-wall tissue is split into two layers:

- An external layer that becomes part of the definitive abdominal wall
- An internal layer that contributes to peripheral parts of the diaphragm, external to the parts derived from the pleuroperitoneal membranes (see Fig. 8-7*D* and *E*)

Further extension of the developing pleural cavities into the lateral body walls forms the right and left **costodiaphragmatic recesses** (Fig. 8-8), establishing the characteristic dome-shaped configuration of the diaphragm. After birth, the costodiaphragmatic recesses become alternately smaller and larger as the lungs move in and out of them during inspiration and expiration.

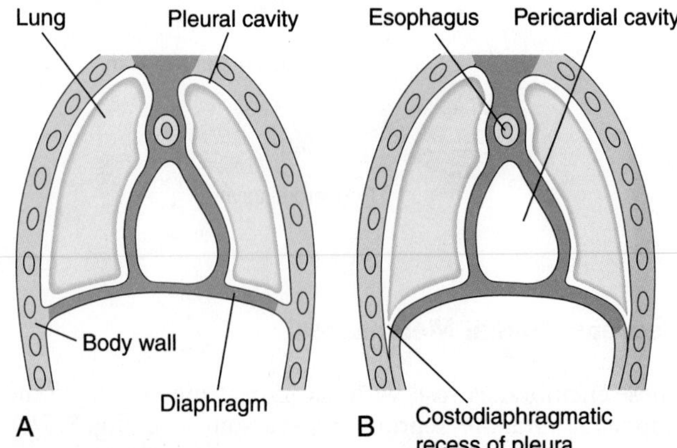

FIGURE 8-8. Illustrations of extension of the pleural cavities into the body walls to form peripheral parts of the diaphragm, the costodiaphragmatic recesses, and the establishment of the characteristic dome-shaped configuration of the diaphragm. Note that body wall tissue is added peripherally to the diaphragm as the lungs and pleural cavities enlarge.

Positional Changes and Innervation of the Diaphragm

During the fourth week, the septum transversum, before relocation of the heart, lies opposite the third to fifth cervical somites (Fig. 8-9*A*). During the fifth week, myoblasts from these somites migrate into the developing diaphragm, bringing their nerve fibers with them. Consequently, the **phrenic nerves** that supply motor innervation to the diaphragm arise from the ventral primary rami of the third, fourth, and fifth cervical spinal nerves. The three twigs on each side join together to form a phrenic nerve. The phrenic nerves also supply sensory fibers to the superior and inferior surfaces of the right and left domes of the diaphragm.

Rapid growth of the dorsal part of the embryo's body results in an apparent descent of the diaphragm. By the sixth week, the developing diaphragm is at the level of the thoracic somites (see Fig. 8-9*B*). The phrenic nerves now have a descending course. As the diaphragm appears relatively farther caudally in the body, the nerves are correspondingly lengthened. By the beginning of the eighth week, the dorsal part of the diaphragm lies at the level of the first lumbar vertebra (see Fig. 8-9*C*). Because of the cervical origin of the phrenic nerves, they are approximately 30 cm long in adults. The phrenic nerves in the embryo enter the diaphragm by passing through the pleuropericardial membranes. This explains why the phrenic nerves subsequently lie on the fibrous pericardium, the adult derivative of the pleuropericardial membranes (see Fig. 8-5*C* and *D*).

As the four parts of the diaphragm fuse (see Fig. 8-7), mesenchyme in the septum transversum extends into the other three parts. It forms myoblasts that differentiate into the skeletal muscle of the diaphragm. The costal border receives sensory fibers from the lower intercostal nerves because of the origin of the peripheral part of the diaphragm from the lateral body walls (see Fig. 8-7*D* and *E*).

POSTEROLATERAL DEFECTS OF DIAPHRAGM

Posterolateral defect of the diaphragm is the only relatively common congenital anomaly of the diaphragm (Figs. 8-10*A* and *B* and 8-11). This diaphragmatic defect occurs about once in 2200 newborn infants and is associated with **congenital diaphragmatic hernia**—(CDH, herniation of abdominal contents into the thoracic cavity). Life-threatening breathing difficulties may be associated with CDH because of inhibition of development and inflation of lungs (Fig. 8-12). The candidate region for CDH was reported to be chromosome 15q26. Moreover, fetal lung maturation may be delayed. *CDH is the most common cause of pulmonary hypoplasia.* **Polyhydramnios** (excess amniotic fluid) may also be present. CDH, usually unilateral, results from defective formation and/or fusion of the pleuroperitoneal membrane with the other three parts of the diaphragm (see Fig. 8-7). This results in a large opening in the posterolateral region of the diaphragm. As a result, the peritoneal and pleural cavities are continuous with one another along the posterior body wall. This congenital defect, sometimes referred to clinically as the *foramen of Bochdalek*, occurs on the left side in 85% to 90% of cases. The preponderance of left-sided defects may be related to the earlier closure of the right pleuroperitoneal opening. Prenatal diagnosis of CDH (Fig. 8-13) depends on ultrasound examination and magnetic resonance imaging of abdominal organs in the thorax.

The pleuroperitoneal membranes normally fuse with the other three diaphragmatic components by

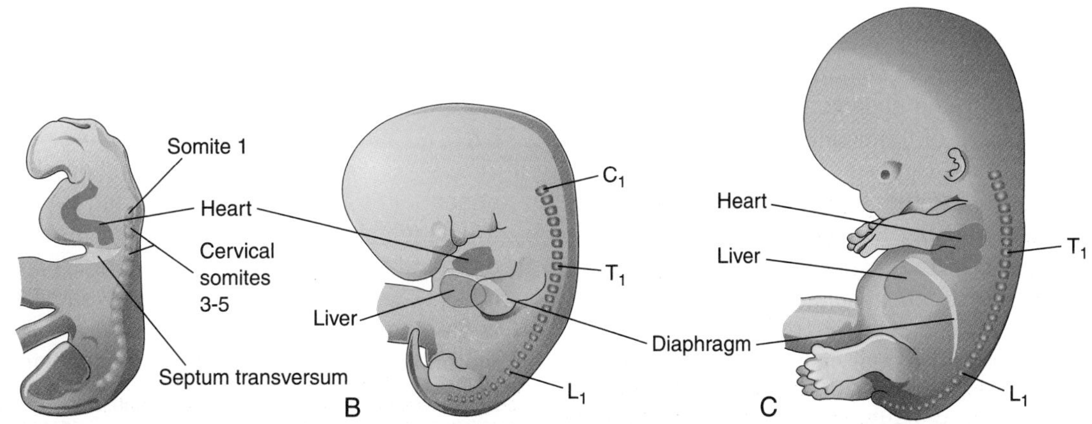

FIGURE 8-9. Illustrations of positional changes of the developing diaphragm. **A,** Approximately 24 days. The septum transversum is at the level of the third, fourth, and fifth cervical segments. **B,** Approximately 41 days. **C,** Approximately 52 days.

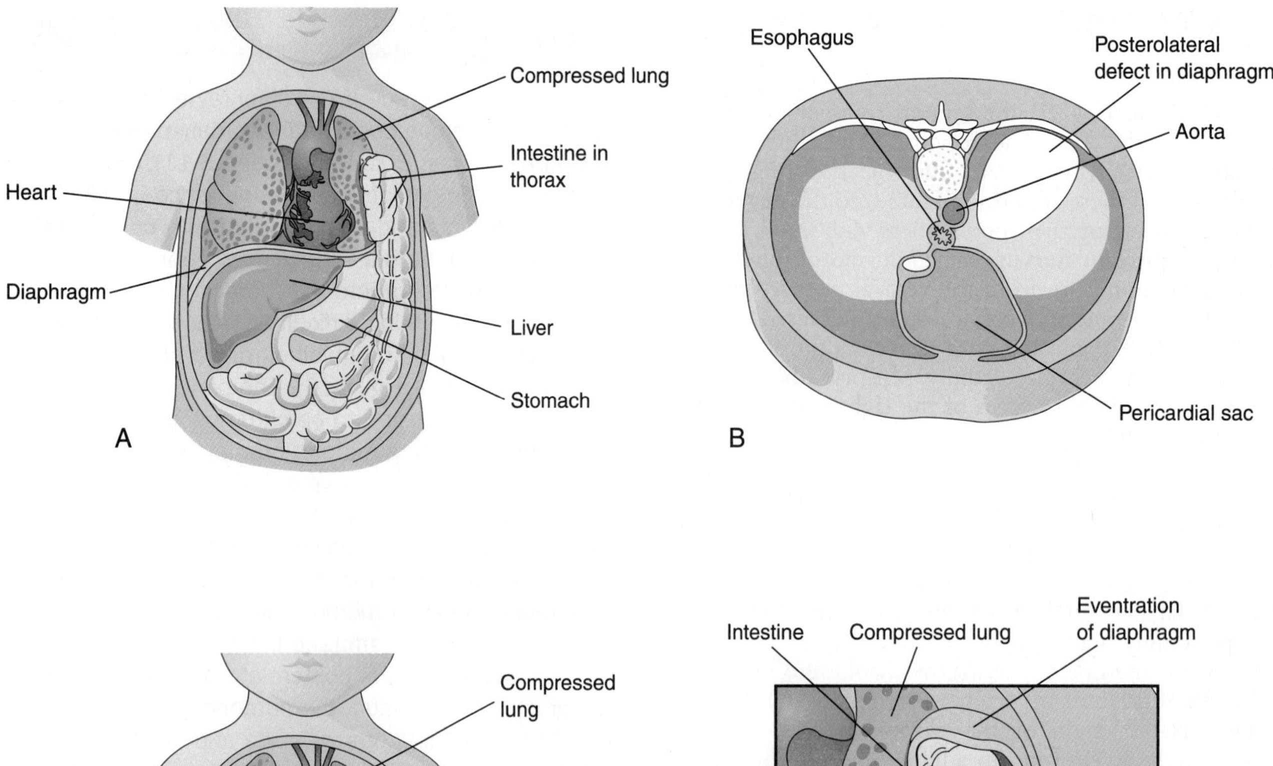

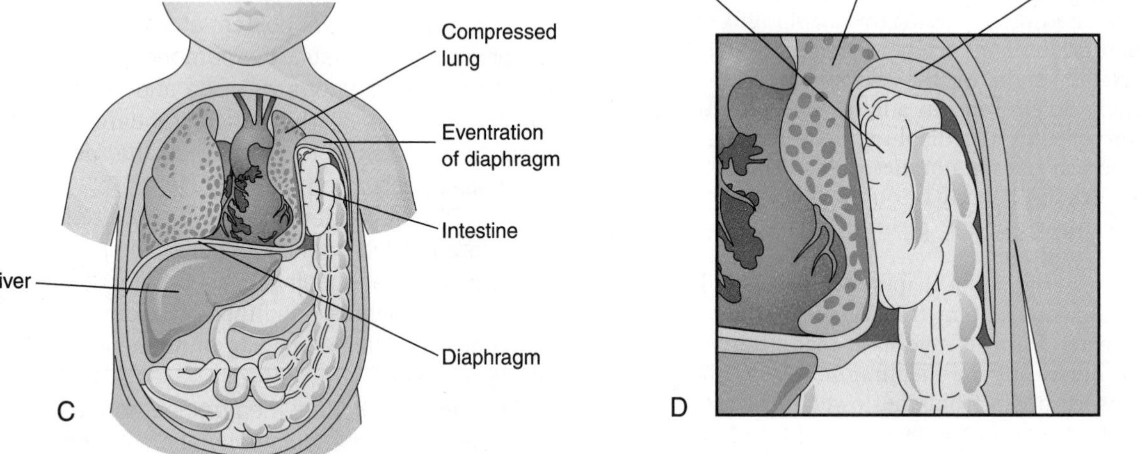

FIGURE 8-10. **A,** A "window" has been drawn on the thorax and abdomen to show the herniation of the intestine into the thorax through a posterolateral defect in the left side of the diaphragm. Note that the left lung is compressed and hypoplastic. **B,** Drawing of a diaphragm with a large posterolateral defect on the left side due to abnormal formation and/or fusion of the pleuroperitoneal membrane on the left side with the mesoesophagus and septum transversum. **C** and **D,** Eventration of the diaphragm resulting from defective muscular development of the diaphragm. The abdominal viscera are displaced into the thorax within a pouch of diaphragmatic tissue.

the end of the sixth week (see Fig. 8-7C). If a pleuroperitoneal canal is still open when the intestines return to the abdomen from the physiological hernia of the umbilical cord in the 10th week (see Chapter 11), some intestine and other viscera may pass into the thorax. The presence of abdominal viscera in the thorax pushes the lungs and heart anteriorly and compression of the lungs occurs. Often the stomach, spleen, and most of the intestines herniate (see Figs. 8-12 and 8-13). The abdominal viscera can usually move freely through the defect; consequently, they may be in the thoracic cavity when the infant is lying down and in the abdominal cavity when the infant is upright. Most babies born with CDH die not because there is simply a defect in the diaphragm or abdominal viscera in the chest, but because the lungs are hypoplastic due to compression during development. The severity of pulmonary developmental abnormalities depends on when and to what extent the abdominal viscera herniate into the thorax, i.e., on the timing and degree of compression of the fetal lungs. The effect on the ipsilateral (same side) lung is greater, but the contralateral lung also shows morphologic changes. If the abdominal viscera are in the thoracic cavity at birth, the initiation of respiration is likely to be impaired. The intestines dilate with swallowed air and compromise the

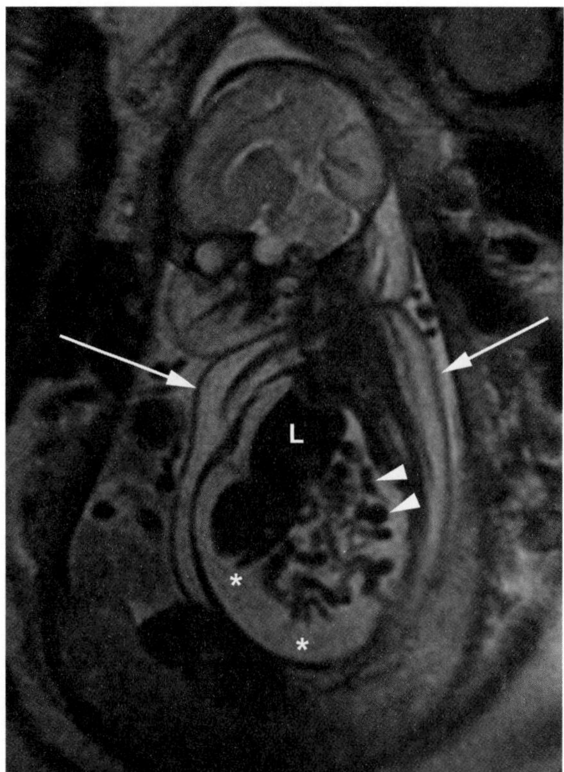

FIGURE 8-11. Coronal magnetic resonance image of a fetus with right-sided congenital diaphragmatic hernia. Note the liver (L) in the thoracic cavity and loops of small bowel (*arrowheads*). There are ascites (*), with fluid extending up into the chest, and skin thickening (*arrows*). (Courtesy of Deborah Levine, MD, Director of Obstetric and Gynecologic Ultrasound, Beth Israel Deaconess Medical Center, Boston, MA.)

functioning of the heart and lungs. Because the abdominal organs are most often in the left side of the thorax, the heart and mediastinum are usually displaced to the right.

The lungs in infants with CDH are often hypoplastic and greatly reduced in size. The growth retardation of the lungs results from the lack of room for them to develop normally. The lungs are often aerated and achieve their normal size after reduction (repositioning) of the herniated viscera and repair of the defect in the diaphragm; however, the mortality rate is high. Prenatal detection of CDH occurs in about 50% of cases. The role of fetal surgery in the treatment of these patients is at present not clear.

EVENTRATION OF DIAPHRAGM

In this uncommon condition, half the diaphragm has defective musculature and balloons into the thoracic cavity as an aponeurotic (membranous) sheet, forming a diaphragmatic pouch (see Fig. 8-10*C* and *D*). Consequently, there is superior displacement of abdominal viscera into the pocket-like outpouching of the diaphragm. This congenital anomaly results mainly from failure of muscular tissue from the body wall to extend into the pleuroperitoneal membrane on the affected side. Eventration of the diaphragm is not a true diaphragmatic herniation; it is a superior displacement of viscera into a saclike part of the diaphragm. However, the clinical manifestations of diaphragmatic eventration may simulate CDH. During surgical repair, a muscular flap (e.g., from a back muscle such as the latissimus dorsi) or a prosthetic patch is used to strengthen the diaphragm.

GASTROSCHISIS AND CONGENITAL EPIGASTRIC HERNIA

This uncommon hernia occurs in the median plane between the xiphoid process and umbilicus. These defects are similar to umbilical hernias (see Chapter 11) except for their location. Gastroschisis and epigastric hernias result from failure of the lateral body folds to fuse completely when forming the anterior abdominal wall during folding in the fourth week (see Fig. 8-2*C* and *F*). The small intestine herniates into the amniotic cavity, which can be detected prenatally by ultrasonography.

CONGENITAL HIATAL HERNIA

There may be herniation of part of the fetal stomach through an excessively large **esophageal hiatus**—the opening in the diaphragm through which the esophagus and vagus nerves pass; however, this is an uncommon congenital defect. Although **hiatal hernia** is usually an acquired lesion occurring during adult life, a congenitally enlarged esophageal hiatus may be the predisposing factor in some cases.

RETROSTERNAL (PARASTERNAL) HERNIA

Herniations through the sternocostal hiatus (foramen of Morgagni)—the opening for the superior epigastric vessels in the retrosternal area may occur; however, they are uncommon. This hiatus is located between the sternal and costal parts of the diaphragm. Herniation of intestine into the pericardial sac may occur or conversely, part of the heart may descend into the peritoneal cavity in the epigastric region. Large defects are commonly associated with body wall defects in the umbilical region (e.g., omphalocele; see Chapter 11). Radiologists and pathologists often observe fatty herniations through the sternocostal hiatus; however, they are usually of no clinical significance.

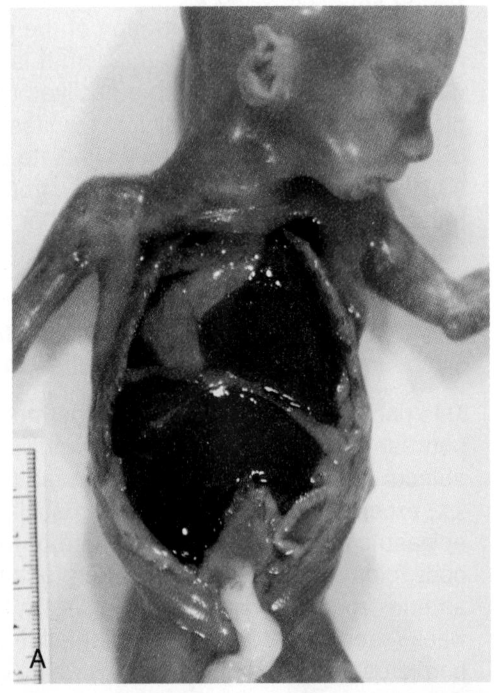

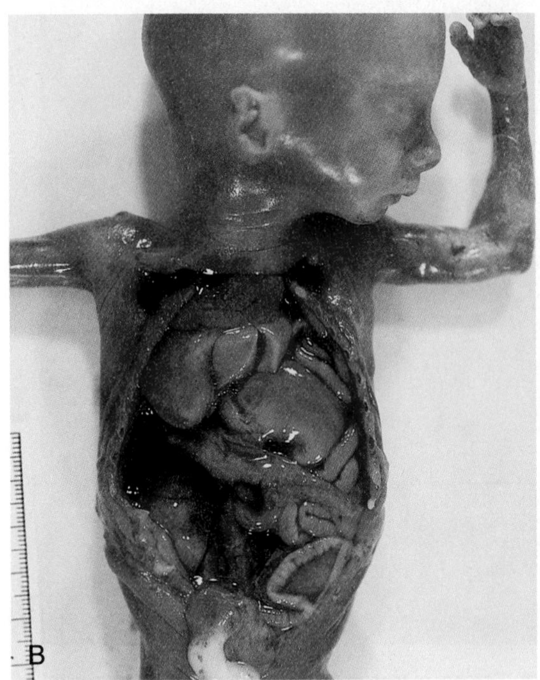

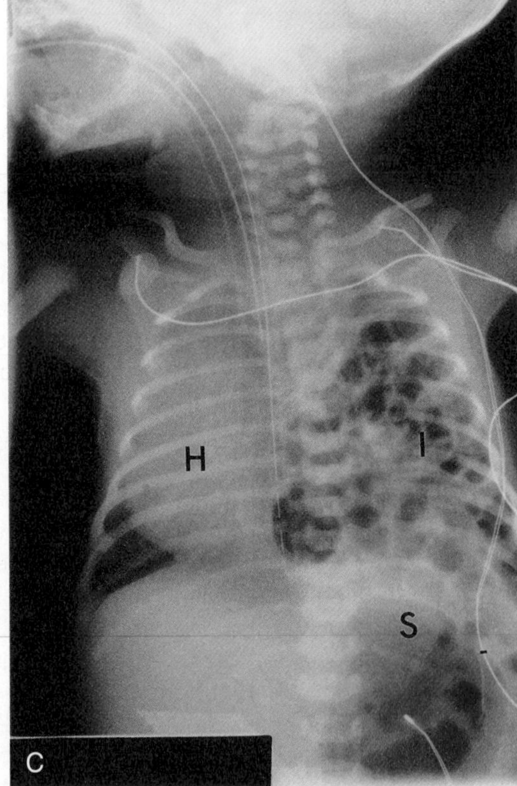

FIGURE 8-12. Diaphragmatic hernia on left side showing herniation of liver (**A**), stomach, and bowel (**B**), underneath the liver into left chest cavity. Note pulmonary hypoplasia visible after liver removal (female fetus at 19 to 20 weeks developmental age). **C,** Diaphragmatic hernia (posterolateral defect). Chest radiograph of a newborn infant showing herniation of intestinal loops (I) into the left side of the chest. Note that the heart (H) is displaced to the right and that the stomach (S) is on the left side of the upper abdominal cavity. (**A** and **B,** Courtesy of Dr. D.K. Kalousek, Department of Pathology, University of British Columbia, Children's Hospital, Vancouver, British Columbia, Canada; **C,** Courtesy of Dr. Prem S. Sahni, formerly of the Department of Radiology, Children's Hospital, Winnipeg, Manitoba, Canada.)

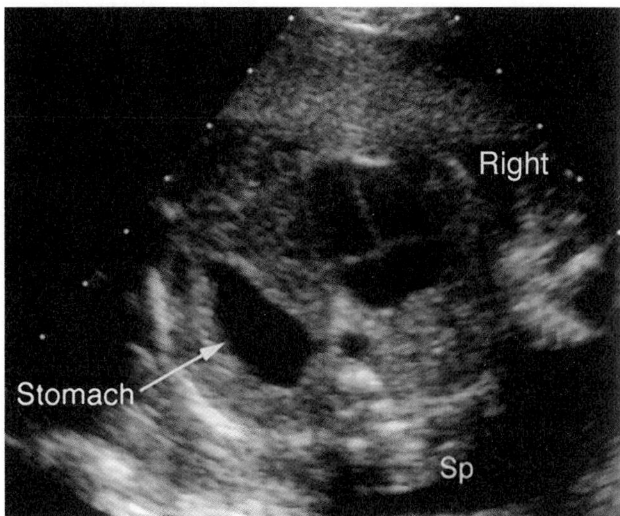

FIGURE 8-13. Ultrasound scan of the thorax showing the heart shifted to the right and the stomach on the left. The diaphragmatic hernia was detected at 23.4 weeks' gestation. The stomach herniated through a posterolateral defect in the diaphragm (congenital diaphragmatic hernia). Sp, vertebral column/spine. (Courtesy of Dr. Wesley Lee, Division of Fetal Imaging, William Beaumont Hospital, Royal Oak, MI.)

ACCESSORY DIAPHRAGM

More than 30 cases of this rare anomaly have been reported. It is most often on the right side and associated with lung hypoplasia and other respiratory complications. An accessory diaphragm can be diagnosed by magnetic resonance imaging and computed tomography and is treated by surgical excision.

SUMMARY OF THE DEVELOPMENT OF THE BODY CAVITIES

- The intraembryonic coelom begins to develop near the end of the third week. By the fourth week, it appears as a horseshoe-shaped cavity in the cardiogenic and lateral mesoderm. The curve of the cavity represents the future pericardial cavity and its lateral extensions represent the future pleural and peritoneal cavities.
- During folding of the embryonic disc in the fourth week, lateral parts of the intraembryonic coelom move together on the ventral aspect of the embryo. When the caudal part of the ventral mesentery disappears, the right and left parts of the intraembryonic coelom merge to form the peritoneal cavity.
- As peritoneal parts of the intraembryonic coelom come together, the splanchnic layer of mesoderm encloses the primordial gut and suspends it from the dorsal body wall by a double-layered peritoneal membrane, the dorsal mesentery.
- The parietal layer of mesoderm lining the peritoneal, pleural, and pericardial cavities becomes the parietal peritoneum, parietal pleura, and serous pericardium, respectively.
- Until the seventh week, the embryonic pericardial cavity communicates with the peritoneal cavity through paired pericardioperitoneal canals. During the fifth and sixth weeks, folds (later membranes) form near the cranial and caudal ends of these canals.
- Fusion of the cranial pleuropericardial membranes with mesoderm ventral to the esophagus separates the pericardial cavity from the pleural cavities. Fusion of the caudal pleuroperitoneal membranes during formation of the diaphragm separates the pleural cavities from the peritoneal cavity.

CLINICALLY ORIENTED PROBLEMS

CASE 8-1

A newborn infant suffers from severe respiratory distress. The abdomen is unusually flat and intestinal peristaltic movements are heard over the left side of the thorax.

- What congenital anomaly would you suspect?
- Explain the basis of the signs described above.
- How would the diagnosis likely be established?

CASE 8-2

An ultrasound scan of an infant's thorax revealed intestine in the pericardial sac.

- What congenital anomaly could result in herniation of intestine into the pericardial cavity?
- What is the embryologic basis of this defect?

CASE 8-3

A CDH was diagnosed prenatally during an ultrasound examination.

- How common is posterolateral defect of the diaphragm?
- How do you think a newborn infant in whom this diagnosis is suspected should be positioned?
- Why would this positional treatment be given?
- Briefly describe surgical repair of a CDH.
- Why do most newborns with CDH die?

CASE 8-4

A baby was born with a hernia in the median plane, between the xiphoid process and umbilicus.

- Name this type of hernia.
- Is it common?
- What is the embryologic basis of this congenital anomaly?

Discussion of these problems appears at the back of the book.

References and Suggested Reading

Becmeur F, Horta P, Donata L, et al: Accessory diaphragm: Review of 31 cases in the literature. Eur J Pediatr Surg 5:43, 1995.

Cass DL: Fetal surgery for congenital diaphragmatic hernia: The North American Experience. Semin Perinatol 29:104, 2005.

The Congenital Diaphragmatic Hernia Study Group: Estimating disease severity of congenital diaphragmatic hernia in the first five minutes of life. J Pediatr Surg 36:141, 2001.

Deprest J, Jani J, Gratacos E, et al: Fetal intervention for congenital diaphragmatic hernia: The European experience. Semin Perinatol 29:94, 2005.

Goldstein RB: Ultrasound evaluation of the fetal abdomen. In Callen PW (ed): Ultrasonography in Obstetrics and Gynecology, 4th ed. Philadelphia, WB Saunders, 2000.

Goldstein RB: Ultrasound evaluation of the fetal thorax. In Callen PW (ed): Ultrasonography in Obstetrics and Gynecology, 4th ed. Philadelphia, WB Saunders, 2000.

Graham G, Devine PC: Antenatal diagnosis of congenital diaphragmatic hernia. Sem Perinatol 29:69, 2005.

Harrison MR: The fetus with a diaphragmatic hernia: In Harrison MR, Evans MI, Adzick NS, Holzgreve W (eds): The Unborn Patient: The Art and Science of Fetal Therapy, 3rd ed. Philadelphia, WB Saunders, 2001.

Kays DW: Congenital diaphragmatic hernia and neonatal lung lesions. Surg Clin N Am 86:329, 2006.

Moore KL, Dalley AF: Clinically Oriented Anatomy, 5th ed. Baltimore, Williams & Wilkins, 2005.

Moya FR, Lally KP: Evidence-based management of infants with congenital diaphragmatic hernia. Semin Perinatol 29:112, 2005.

Rottier R, Tibboel D: Fetal lung and diaphragm development in congenital diaphragmatic hernia. Semin Perinatol 29:86, 2005.

Schlembach D, Zenker M, Trautmann U, et al: Deletion 15q24-26 in prenatally detected diaphragmatic hernia: Increasing evidence of a candidate region for diaphragmatic development. Prenat Diagn 21:289, 2001.

Skandalakis JE, Colborn GL, Weidman TA, Symbas P N: Diaphragm. In Skandalakis JE (ed): Surgical Anatomy. The Embryological and Anatomic Basis of Modern Surgery. Athens, Greece, Paschalidid Medical Publications, 2004.

Slavotinek AM: The genetics of congenital diaphragmatic hernia. Semin Perinatol 29:77, 2005.

Wells LJ: Development of the human diaphragm and pleural sacs. Contr Embryol Carnegie Inst 35:107, 1954.

Yang W, Carmichael SL, Harris JA, Shaw GM: Epidemiologic characteristics of congenital diaphragmatic hernia among 2.5 million California births, 1899–1997. Birth Defects Res (Part A) 76:170, 2006.

9

The Pharyngeal Apparatus

Pharyngeal Arches	160
Pharyngeal Arch Components	160
Pharyngeal Pouches	166
Derivatives of the Pharyngeal Pouches	166
Pharyngeal Grooves	169
Pharyngeal Membranes	169
Development of the Thyroid Gland	173
Histogenesis of the Thyroid Gland	173
Development of the Tongue	176
Lingual Papillae and Taste Buds	176
Nerve Supply of the Tongue	177
Development of the Salivary Glands	179
Development of the Face	179
Summary of Facial Development	182
Development of the Nasal Cavities	182
Paranasal Sinuses	184
Development of the Palate	185
Primary Palate	185
Secondary Palate	186
Summary of the Pharyngeal Apparatus	195
Clinically Oriented Problems	195

The head and neck regions of a 4-week human embryo somewhat resemble these regions of a fish embryo at a comparable stage of development. This explains the former use of the designation *branchial apparatus*; the adjective *branchial* is derived from the Greek word *branchia*, gill. A primordial pharyngeal (branchial) apparatus develops in human embryos; however, no gills form. Consequently, the term pharyngeal arch is now used instead of branchial arch when describing the development of the head and neck regions of human embryos. By the end of the embryonic period, these structures have either become rearranged and adapted to new functions or disappeared. The pharyngeal apparatus (Fig. 9-1) consists of pharyngeal arches, pouches, grooves, and membranes. These embryonic structures contribute to the formation of the lateral and ventral regions of the head and neck. Most congenital anomalies, often characterized as branchial anomalies, in these regions originate during transformation of the pharyngeal apparatus into its adult derivatives.

PHARYNGEAL ARCHES

The pharyngeal arches begin to develop early in the fourth week as **neural crest cells** migrate into the future head and neck regions (see Chapter 5). The first pair of pharyngeal arches, the primordium of the jaws, appears as surface elevations lateral to the developing pharynx (see Fig. 9-1*A* and *B*). Soon other arches appear as obliquely disposed, rounded ridges on each side of the future head and neck regions (see Fig. 9-1*C* and *D*). By the end of the fourth week, four pairs of pharyngeal arches are visible externally (Fig. 9-1*D*). The fifth and sixth arches are rudimentary and are not visible on the surface of the embryo. The pharyngeal arches are separated from each other by the pharyngeal grooves. Like the pharyngeal arches, the grooves are numbered in a craniocaudal sequence.

The first pharyngeal arch (mandibular arch) separates into two prominences (see Figs. 9-1*E* and 9-2):

- The maxillary prominence gives rise to the maxilla, zygomatic bone, and a portion of the vomer.
- The mandibular prominence forms the mandible. The proximal mandibular prominence also forms the squamous temporal bone.

The second pharyngeal arch (hyoid arch) contributes, along with parts of the third and fourth arches, to the formation of the hyoid bone.

The pharyngeal arches support the lateral walls of the primordial pharynx, which is derived from the cranial part of the foregut. The stomodeum (primordial mouth) initially appears as a slight depression of the surface ectoderm (see Fig. 9-1*D* and *E*). It is separated from the cavity of the primordial pharynx by a bilaminar membrane—the oropharyngeal membrane, which is composed of ectoderm externally and endoderm internally. The oropharyngeal membrane ruptures at approximately 26 days, bringing the pharynx and foregut into communication with the amniotic cavity (see Fig. 9-1*F* and *G*).

Pharyngeal Arch Components

Each pharyngeal arch consists of a core of mesenchyme (embryonic connective tissue) and is covered externally by ectoderm and internally by endoderm (see Fig. 9-1*H* and *I*). Originally, this mesenchyme is derived from mesoderm in the third week. During the fourth week, most of the mesenchyme is derived from neural crest cells that migrate into the pharyngeal arches. It is the migration of neural crest cells into the arches and their differentiation into mesenchyme that produces the maxillary and mandibular prominences (see Fig. 9-2), in addition to all connective tissue including the dermis and smooth muscle. Coincident with immigration of neural crest cells, myogenic mesoderm from paraxial regions moves into each pharyngeal arch, forming a central core of muscle primordium. Endothelial cells in the arches are derived from both the lateral mesoderm and the invasive angioblasts that move into the arches.

A typical pharyngeal arch contains

- A pharyngeal arch artery that arises from the truncus arteriosus of the primordial heart (Fig. 9-3*B*) and passes around the primordial pharynx to enter the dorsal aorta
- A cartilaginous rod that forms the skeleton of the arch
- A muscular component that differentiates into muscles in the head and neck
- Sensory and motor nerves that supply the mucosa and muscles derived from the arch

The nerves that grow into the arches are derived from neuroectoderm of the primordial brain.

Fate of the Pharyngeal Arches

The pharyngeal arches contribute extensively to the formation of the face, nasal cavities, mouth, larynx, pharynx, and neck (Figs. 9-3 and 9-4). During the fifth week, the second pharyngeal arch enlarges and overgrows the third and fourth arches, forming an ectodermal depression—the **cervical sinus** (see Figs. 9-2 and 9-4*A* to *D*). By the end of the seventh week, the second to fourth pharyngeal grooves and the cervical sinus have disappeared, giving the neck a smooth contour.

Derivatives of the Pharyngeal Arch Cartilages

The dorsal end of the **first pharyngeal arch cartilage** (Meckel cartilage) is closely related to the developing ear. Early in development, small nodules break away from the proximal part of this cartilage and form two of the middle ear bones, the **malleus** and **incus** (Fig. 9-5, Table 9-1). The middle part of the cartilage regresses, but its perichondrium forms *the anterior ligament of malleus* and the *sphenomandibular ligament*. Ventral parts of the first arch cartilages form the horseshoe-shaped primordium of the mandible and, by keeping pace with its growth, guide its early morphogenesis. Each half of the mandible forms lateral to and in close association with its cartilage. The cartilage disappears as the mandible develops around it by *intramembranous ossification* (see Fig. 9-5*B*).

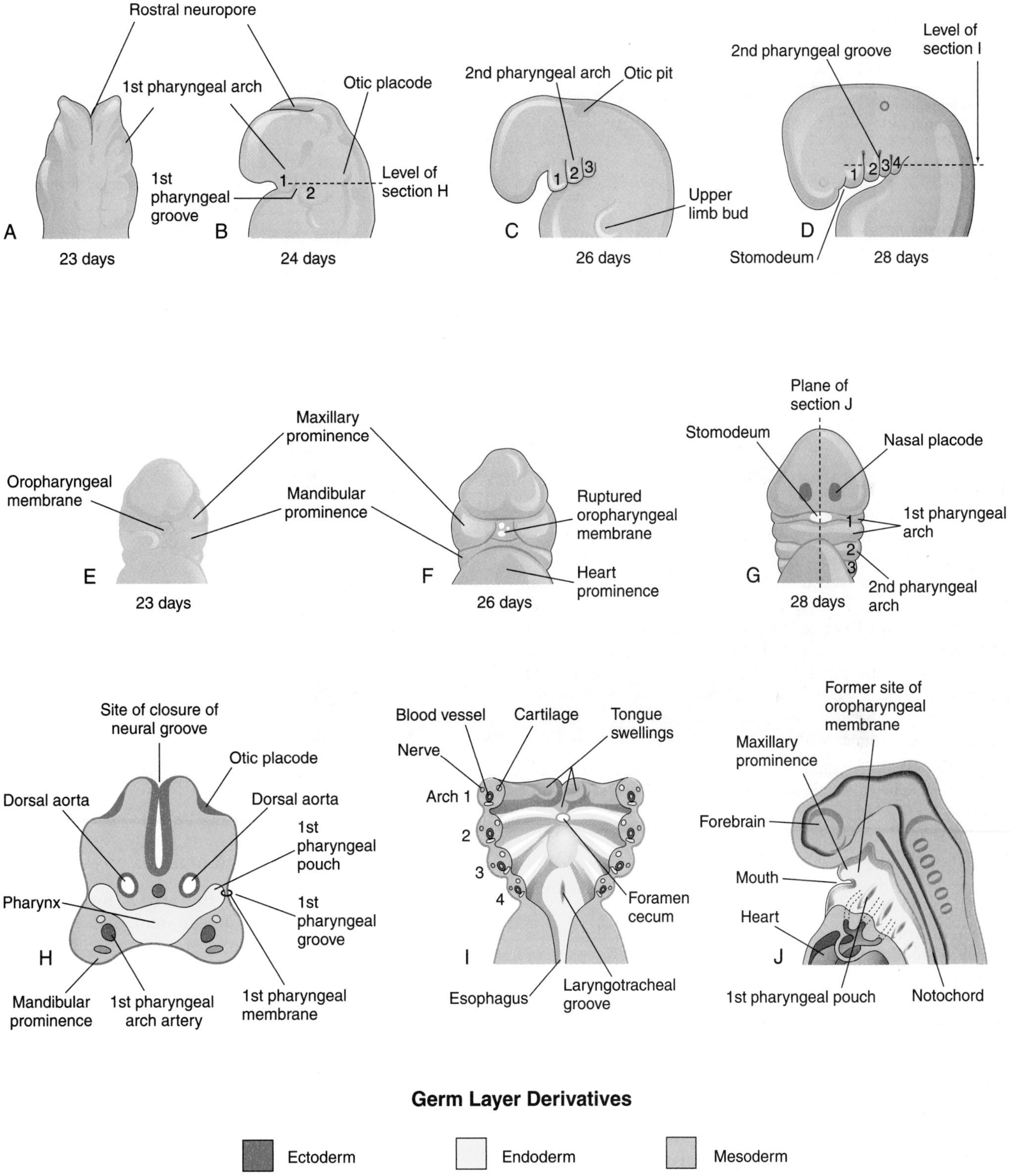

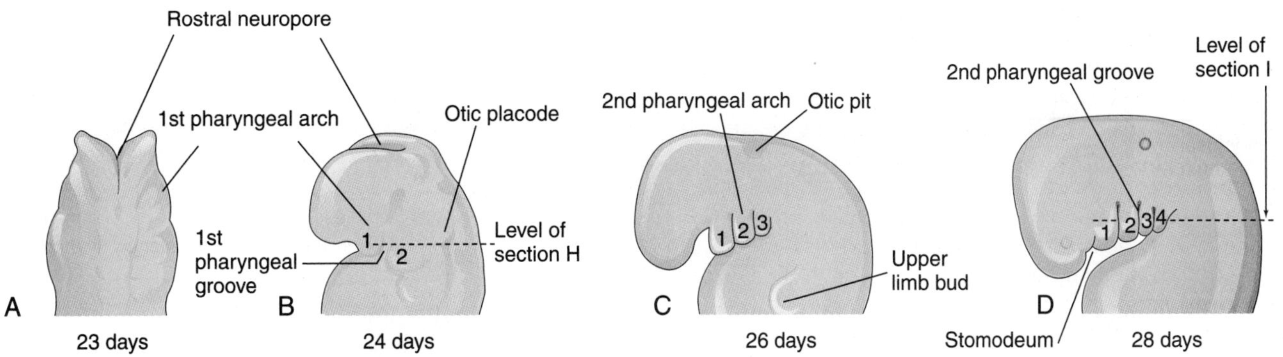

Germ Layer Derivatives

FIGURE 9-1. Illustrations of the human pharyngeal apparatus. **A,** Dorsal view of the cranial part of an early embryo. **B** to **D,** Lateral views showing later development of the pharyngeal arches. **E** to **G,** Ventral or facial views illustrating the relationship of the first pharyngeal arch to the stomodeum. **H,** Horizontal section through the cranial region of an embryo. **I,** Similar section illustrating the arch components and floor of the primordial pharynx. **J,** Sagittal section of the cranial region of an embryo, illustrating the openings of the pharyngeal pouches in the lateral wall of the primordial pharynx.

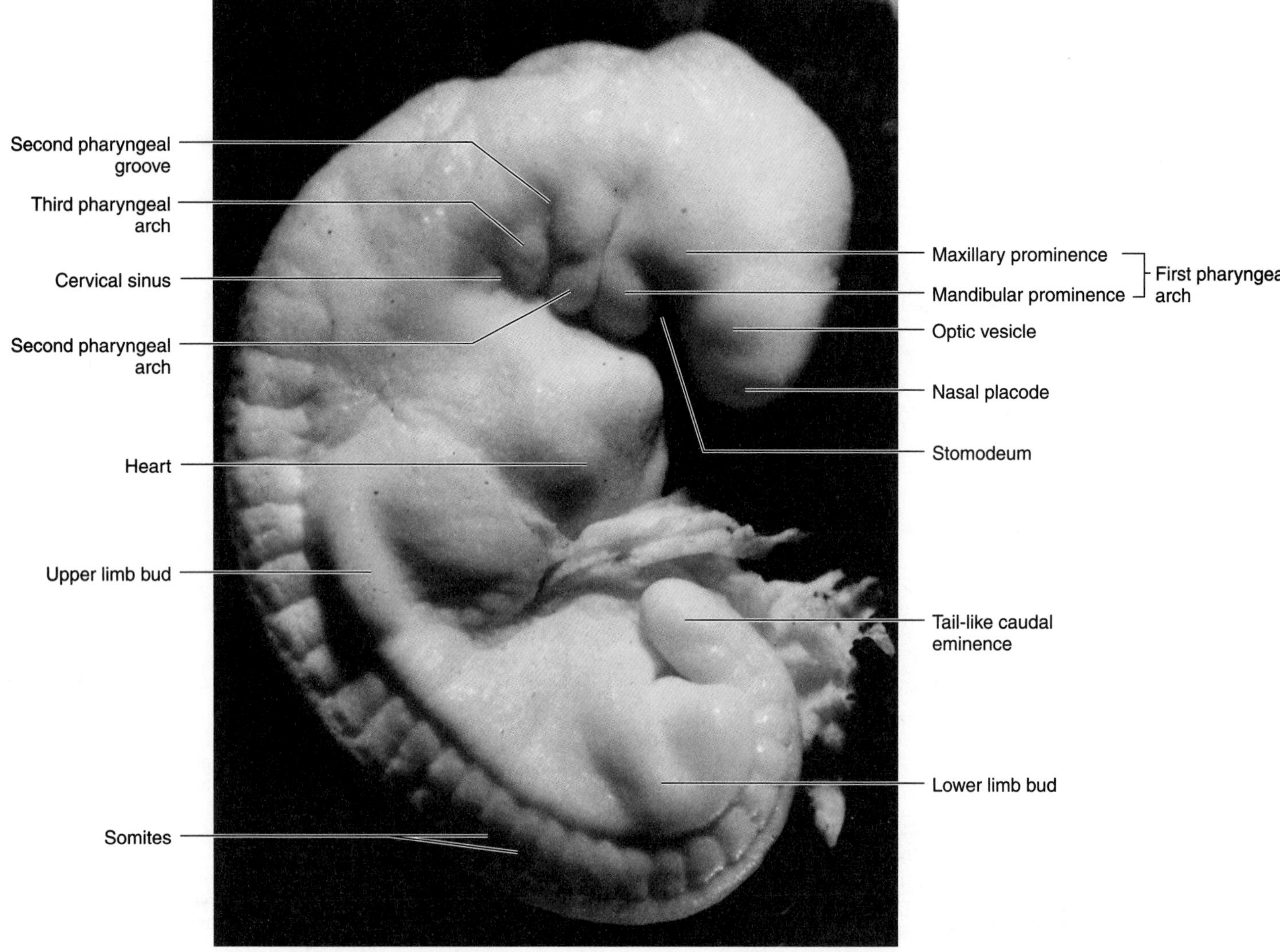

FIGURE 9-2. Macrophotograph of a stage 13, 4 1/2-week human embryo. (Courtesy of the late Professor Emeritus Dr. K.V. Hinrichsen, Medizinische Fakultät, Institut für Anatomie, Ruhr-Universität Bochum, Bochum, Germany.)

An independent cartilage anlage near the dorsal end of the **second pharyngeal arch cartilage** (Reichert cartilage), also closely related to the developing ear, ossifies to form the *stapes of the middle ear* and the *styloid process of the temporal bone* (see Fig. 9-5*B*). The part of cartilage between the styloid process and hyoid bone regresses; its perichondrium forms the *stylohyoid ligament*. The ventral end of the second arch cartilage ossifies to form the lesser cornu (Latin, horn) and the superior part of the body of the hyoid bone (see Fig. 9-5*B*).

The **third pharyngeal arch cartilage**, located in the ventral part of the arch, ossifies to form the greater cornu and the inferior part of the body of the hyoid bone.

The **fourth and sixth pharyngeal arch cartilages** fuse to form the laryngeal cartilages (see Fig. 9-5*B*, Table 9-1), except for the epiglottis. The cartilage of the epiglottis develops from mesenchyme in the *hypopharyngeal eminence* (see Fig. 9-24*A*), a prominence in the floor of the embryonic pharynx that is derived from the third and fourth pharyngeal arches. The fifth pharyngeal arch is rudimentary (if present) and has no derivatives.

Derivatives of Pharyngeal Arch Muscles

The muscular components of the arches form various muscles in the head and neck. The musculature of the *first pharyngeal arch* forms the **muscles of mastication** and other muscles (Fig. 9-6, Table 9-1). The musculature of the *second pharyngeal arch* forms the **stapedius**, stylohyoid, posterior belly of digastric, auricular, and **muscles of facial expression**. The musculature of the third pharyngeal arch forms the **stylopharyngeus**. The musculature of the *fourth pharyngeal arch* forms the **cricothyroid**, levator veli palatini, and constrictors of the pharynx. The musculature of the *sixth pharyngeal arch* forms the intrinsic muscles of the larynx.

Derivatives of the Pharyngeal Arch Nerves

Each arch is supplied by its own cranial nerve (CN). The special visceral efferent (branchial) components of the CNs supply muscles derived from the pharyngeal arches (Fig. 9-7, Table 9-1). Because mesenchyme from the

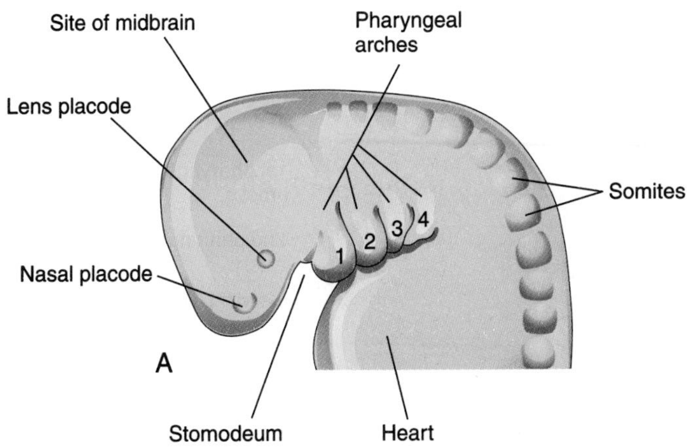

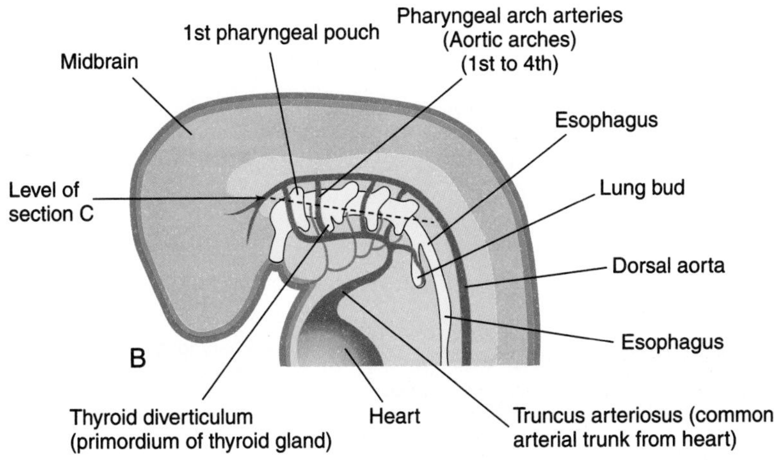

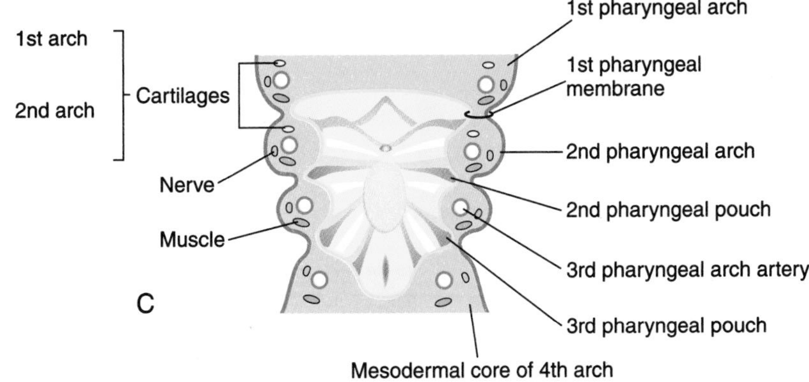

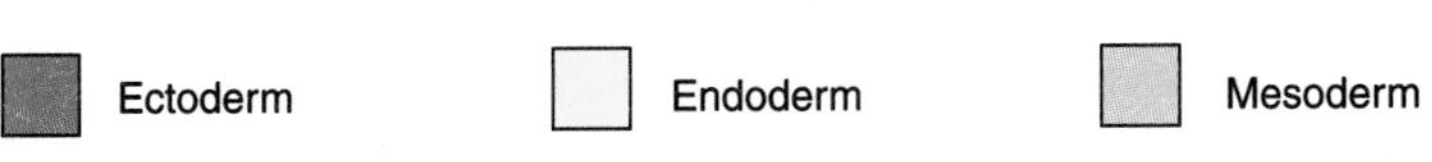

FIGURE 9-3. **A,** Drawing of the head, neck, and thoracic regions of a human embryo (approximately 28 days), illustrating the pharyngeal apparatus. **B,** Schematic drawing showing the pharyngeal pouches and pharyngeal arch arteries. **C,** Horizontal section through the embryo showing the floor of the primordial pharynx and illustrating the germ layer of origin of the pharyngeal arch components.

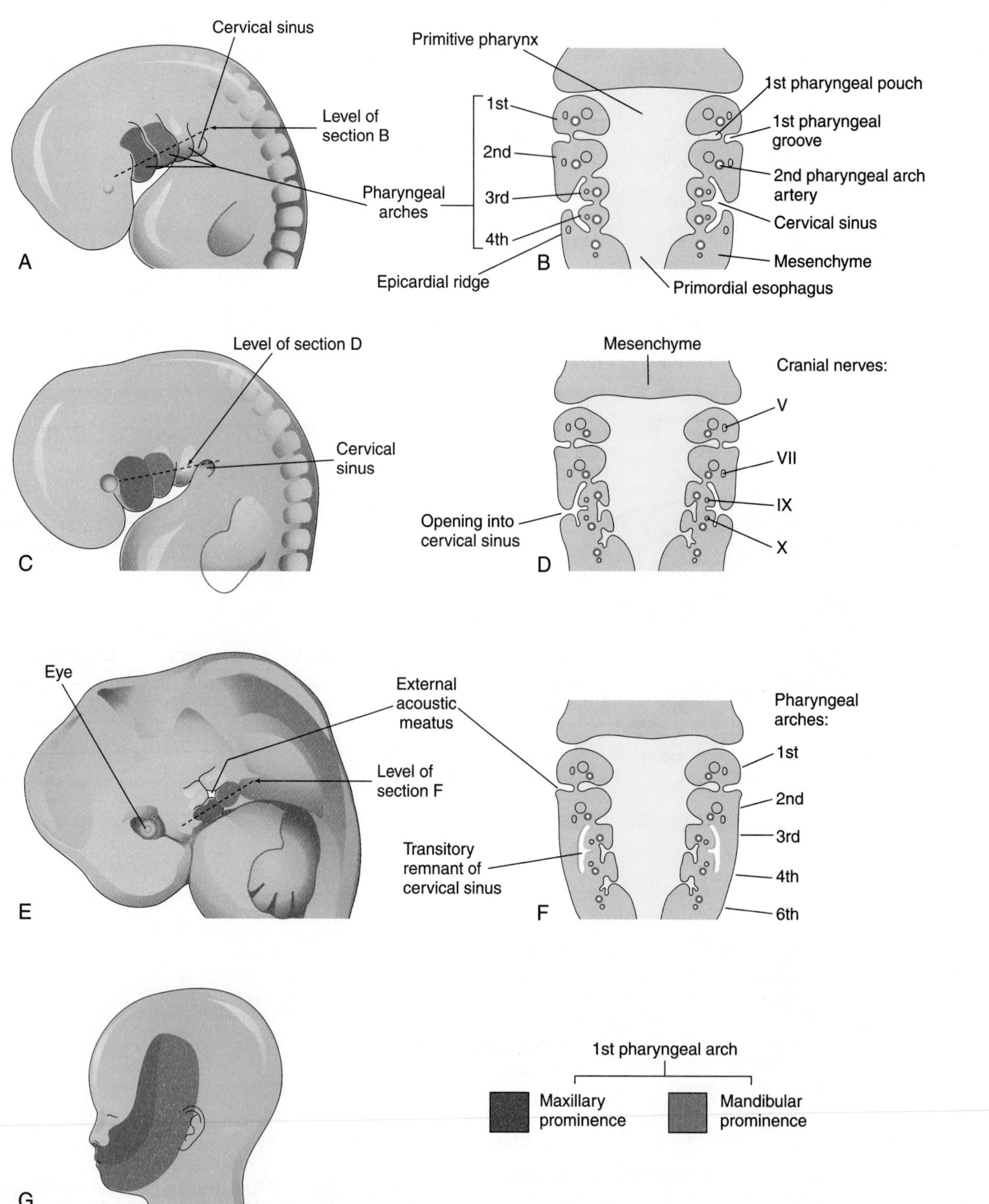

FIGURE 9-4. **A,** Lateral view of the head, neck, and thoracic regions of an embryo (approximately 32 days), showing the pharyngeal arches and cervical sinus. **B,** Diagrammatic section through the embryo at the level shown in **A**, illustrating growth of the second arch over the third and fourth arches. **C,** An embryo of approximately 33 days. **D,** Section of the embryo at the level shown in **C**, illustrating early closure of the cervical sinus. **E,** An embryo of approximately 41 days. **F,** Section of the embryo at the level shown in **E**, showing the transitory cystic remnant of the cervical sinus. **G,** Drawing of a 20-week fetus illustrating the area of the face derived from the first pair of pharyngeal arches.

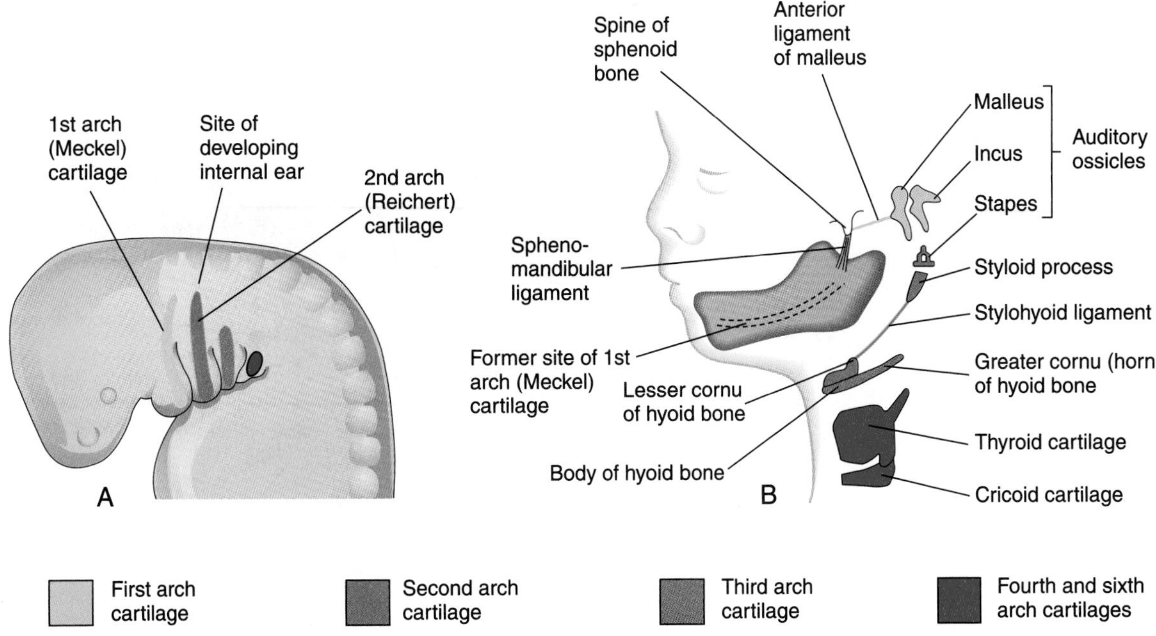

FIGURE 9-5. **A,** Schematic lateral view of the head, neck, and thoracic regions of a 4-week embryo illustrating the location of the cartilages in the pharyngeal arches. **B,** Similar view of a 24-week fetus illustrating the adult derivatives of the arch cartilages. Note that the mandible is formed by intramembranous ossification of mesenchymal tissue surrounding the first arch cartilage. This cartilage acts as a template for development of the mandible, but does not contribute directly to the formation of it. Occasionally ossification of the second arch cartilage may extend from the styloid process along the stylohyoid ligament. When this occurs, it may cause pain in the region of the palatine tonsil.

TABLE 9–1. Structures Derived from Pharyngeal Arch Components*

ARCH	NERVE	MUSCLES	SKELETAL STRUCTURES	LIGAMENTS
First (mandibular)	Trigeminal† (CN V)	Muscles of mastication‡ Mylohyoid and anterior belly of digastric Tensor tympani Tensor veli palatini	Malleus Incus	Anterior ligament of malleus Sphenomandibular ligament
Second (hyoid)	Facial (CN VII)	Muscles of facial expression§ Stapedius Stylohyoid Posterior belly of digastric	Stapes Styloid process Lesser cornu of hyoid bone Upper part of body of hyoid bone	Stylohyoid ligament
Third	Glossopharyngeal (CN IX)	Stylopharyngeus	Greater cornu of hyoid bone Lower part of body of hyoid bone	
Fourth and sixth¶	Superior laryngeal branch of vagus (CN X) Recurrent laryngeal branch of vagus (CN X)	Cricothyroid Levator veli palatini Constrictors of pharynx Intrinsic muscles of larynx Striated muscles of esophagus	Thyroid cartilage Cricoid cartilage Arytenoid cartilage Corniculate cartilage Cuneiform cartilage	

*The derivatives of the aortic arch arteries are described in Chapter 13.
†The ophthalmic division fifth cranial nerve (CN V) does not supply any pharyngeal arch components.
‡Temporalis, masseter, medial, and lateral pterygoids.
§Buccinator, auricularis, frontalis, platysma, orbicularis oris, and orbicularis oculi.
¶The fifth pharyngeal arch is often absent. When present, it is rudimentary and usually has no recognizable cartilage bar. The cartilaginous components of the fourth and sixth arches fuse to form the cartilages of the larynx.

pharyngeal arches contributes to the dermis and mucous membranes of the head and neck, these areas are supplied with special visceral afferent nerves.

The facial skin is supplied by the CN V—the **trigeminal nerve**. However, only its caudal two branches (maxillary and mandibular) supply derivatives of the first pharyngeal arch (see Fig. 9-7*B*). CN V is the principal sensory nerve of the head and neck and is the motor nerve for the muscles of mastication (see Table 9-1). Its sensory branches innervate the face, teeth, and mucous membranes of the nasal cavities, palate, mouth, and tongue (see Fig. 9-7*C*).

CN VII—the **facial nerve**, CN IX—the **glossopharyngeal nerve**, and CN X—the **vagus nerve**—supply the second, third, and caudal (fourth to sixth) arches, respectively. The fourth arch is supplied by the superior laryngeal branch of the vagus (CN X) and by its recurrent laryngeal branch. The nerves of the second to sixth

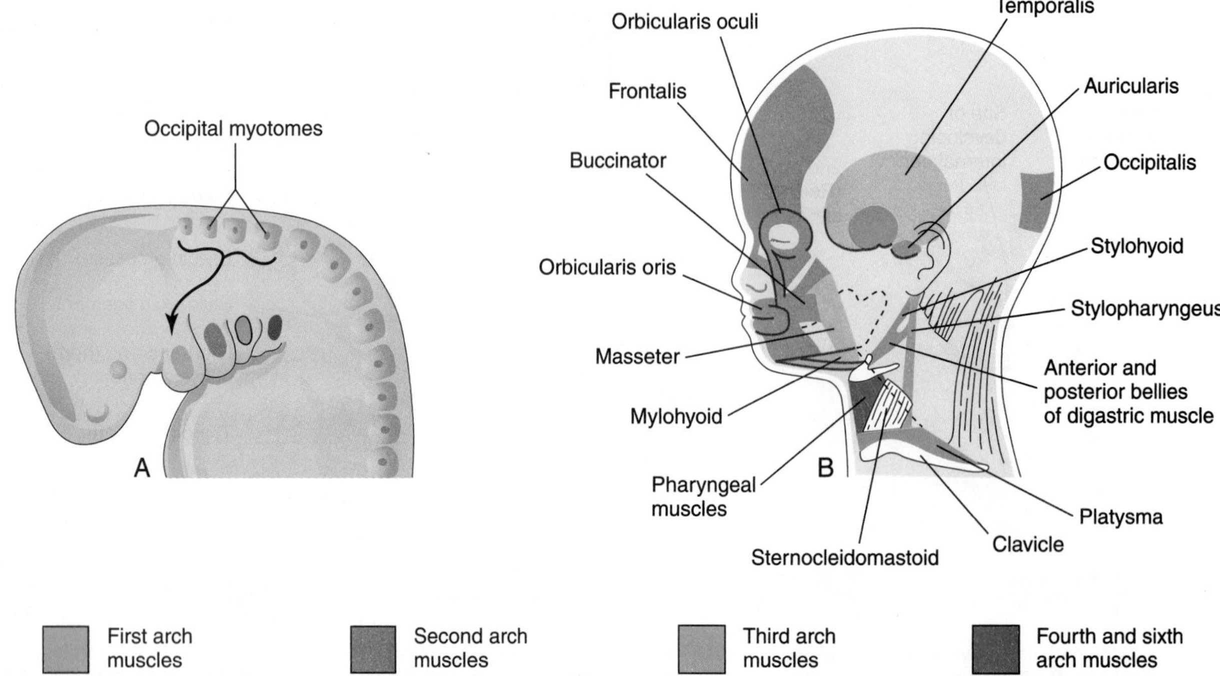

FIGURE 9-6. **A,** Lateral view of the head, neck, and thoracic regions of a 4-week embryo showing the muscles derived from the pharyngeal arches. The *arrow* shows the pathway taken by myoblasts from the occipital myotomes to form the tongue musculature. **B,** Sketch of the head and neck regions of a 20-week fetus, dissected to show the muscles derived from the pharyngeal arches. Parts of the platysma and sternocleidomastoid muscles have been removed to show the deeper muscles. Note that myoblasts from the second arch migrate from the neck to the head, where they give rise to the muscles of facial expression. These muscles are supplied by the facial nerve (cranial nerve VII), the nerve of the second pharyngeal arch.

pharyngeal arches have little cutaneous distribution (see Fig. 9-7*C*); however, they innervate the mucous membranes of the tongue, pharynx, and larynx.

PHARYNGEAL POUCHES

The primordial pharynx, derived from the foregut, widens cranially where it joins the stomodeum (see Figs. 9-3*A* and *B* and 9-4*B*), and narrows caudally where it joins the esophagus. The endoderm of the pharynx lines the internal aspects of the pharyngeal arches and passes into diverticula—the **pharyngeal pouches** (see Figs. 9-1*H* to *J* and 9-3*B* and *C*). The pouches develop in a craniocaudal sequence between the arches. The first pair of pouches, for example, lies between the first and second pharyngeal arches. There are four well-defined pairs of pharyngeal pouches; the fifth pair is rudimentary or absent. The endoderm of the pouches contacts the ectoderm of the pharyngeal grooves and together they form the double-layered **pharyngeal membranes** that separate the pharyngeal pouches from the pharyngeal grooves (see Figs. 9-1*H* and 9-3*C*).

Derivatives of the Pharyngeal Pouches

The endodermal epithelial lining of the pharyngeal pouches gives rise to important organs in the head and neck.

The First Pharyngeal Pouch

The first pharyngeal pouch expands into an elongate **tubotympanic recess** (Fig. 9-8*B*). The expanded distal part of this recess contacts the first pharyngeal groove, where it later contributes to the formation of the **tympanic membrane** (eardrum). The cavity of the tubotympanic recess becomes the **tympanic cavity** and **mastoid antrum**. The connection of the tubotympanic recess with the pharynx gradually elongates to form the **pharyngotympanic tube** (auditory tube).

The Second Pharyngeal Pouch

Although the second pharyngeal pouch is largely obliterated as the palatine tonsil develops, part of the cavity of this pouch remains as the **tonsillar sinus** or fossa (Figs. 9-8*C* and 9-9). The endoderm of the second pouch proliferates and grows into the underlying mesenchyme. The central parts of these buds break down, forming **tonsillar crypts** (pitlike depressions). The pouch endoderm forms the surface epithelium and the lining of the tonsillar crypts. At approximately 20 weeks, the mesenchyme around the crypts differentiates into lymphoid tissue, which soon organizes into the **lymphatic nodules** of the palatine tonsil.

The Third Pharyngeal Pouch

The third pharyngeal pouch expands and develops a solid, dorsal bulbar part and a hollow, elongate ventral part (see Fig. 9-8*B*). Its connection with the pharynx is reduced to a

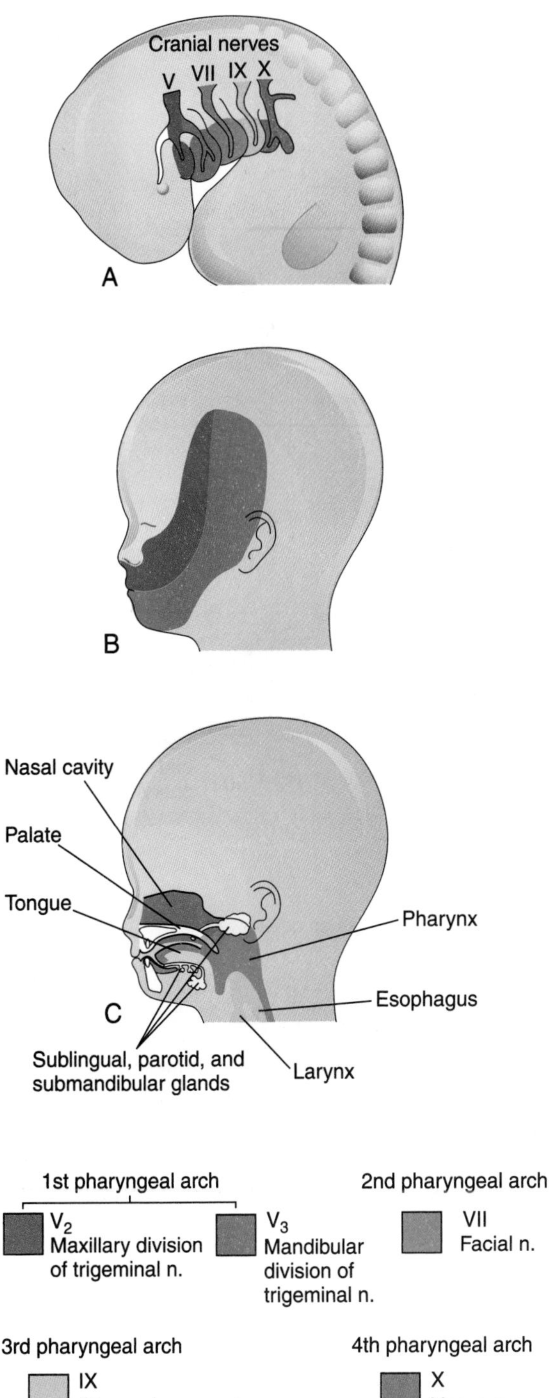

FIGURE 9-7. **A,** Lateral view of the head, neck, and thoracic regions of a 4-week embryo showing the cranial nerves supplying the pharyngeal arches. **B,** Sketch of the head and neck regions of a 20-week fetus showing the superficial distribution of the two caudal branches of the first arch nerve (cranial nerve V). **C,** Sagittal section of the fetal head and neck showing the deep distribution of sensory fibers of the nerves to the teeth and mucosa of the tongue, pharynx, nasal cavity, palate, and larynx.

narrow duct that soon degenerates. By the sixth week, the epithelium of each *dorsal bulbar part of the pouch* begins to differentiate into an inferior parathyroid gland. The epithelium of the elongate *ventral parts of the pouch* proliferates, obliterating their cavities. These come together in the median plane to form the **thymus**. The bilobed form of this lymphatic organ remains throughout life, discretely encapsulated; each lobe has its own blood supply, lymphatic drainage, and nerve supply. The developing thymus and **parathyroid glands** lose their connections with the pharynx. The brain and associated structures expand rostrally while the pharynx and cardiac structures generally expand caudally. This causes the derivatives of pharyngeal pouches two to four to become displaced caudally. Later, the parathyroid glands separate from the thymus and lie on the dorsal surface of the thyroid gland (see Figs. 9-8*C* and 9-9).

Histogenesis of the Thymus

This primary lymphoid organ develops from epithelial cells derived from endoderm of the third pair of pharyngeal pouches and from mesenchyme into which epithelial tubes grow. The tubes soon become solid cords that proliferate and give rise to side branches. Each side branch becomes the core of a lobule of the thymus. Some cells of the epithelial cords become arranged around a central point, forming small groups of cells—the **thymic corpuscles** (Hassall corpuscles). Other cells of the epithelial cords spread apart but retain connections with each other to form an epithelial reticulum. The mesenchyme between the epithelial cords forms thin incomplete septa between the lobules. **Lymphocytes** soon appear and fill the interstices between the epithelial cells. The lymphocytes are derived from **hematopoietic stem cells.**

The thymic primordium is surrounded by a thin layer of mesenchyme that is essential for its development. It also appears that **neural crest cells** play an important role in thymic organogenesis. Growth and development of the thymus are not complete at birth. It is a relatively large organ during the perinatal period and may extend through the superior thoracic aperture at the root of the neck. As puberty is reached, the thymus begins to diminish in relative size (i.e., undergoes involution). By adulthood, it is often scarcely recognizable because of fat infiltrating the cortex of the gland; however, it is still functional and important for the maintenance of health. In addition to secreting thymic hormones, the adult thymus primes thymocytes (T-cell precursors) before releasing them to the periphery.

The Fourth Pharyngeal Pouch

The fourth pharyngeal pouch also expands into dorsal bulbar and elongate ventral parts (see Figs. 9-8 and 9-9). Its connection with the pharynx is reduced to a narrow duct that soon degenerates. By the sixth week, each dorsal part develops into a **superior parathyroid gland**, which lies on the dorsal surface of the thyroid gland. Because the parathyroid glands derived from the third pouches accompany the thymus, they are in a more inferior position than the parathyroid glands derived from the fourth pouches (see Fig. 9-9).

Histogenesis of the Parathyroid Glands

The epithelium of the dorsal parts of the third and fourth pouches proliferates during the fifth week and forms small nodules on the dorsal aspect of each pouch. Vascular

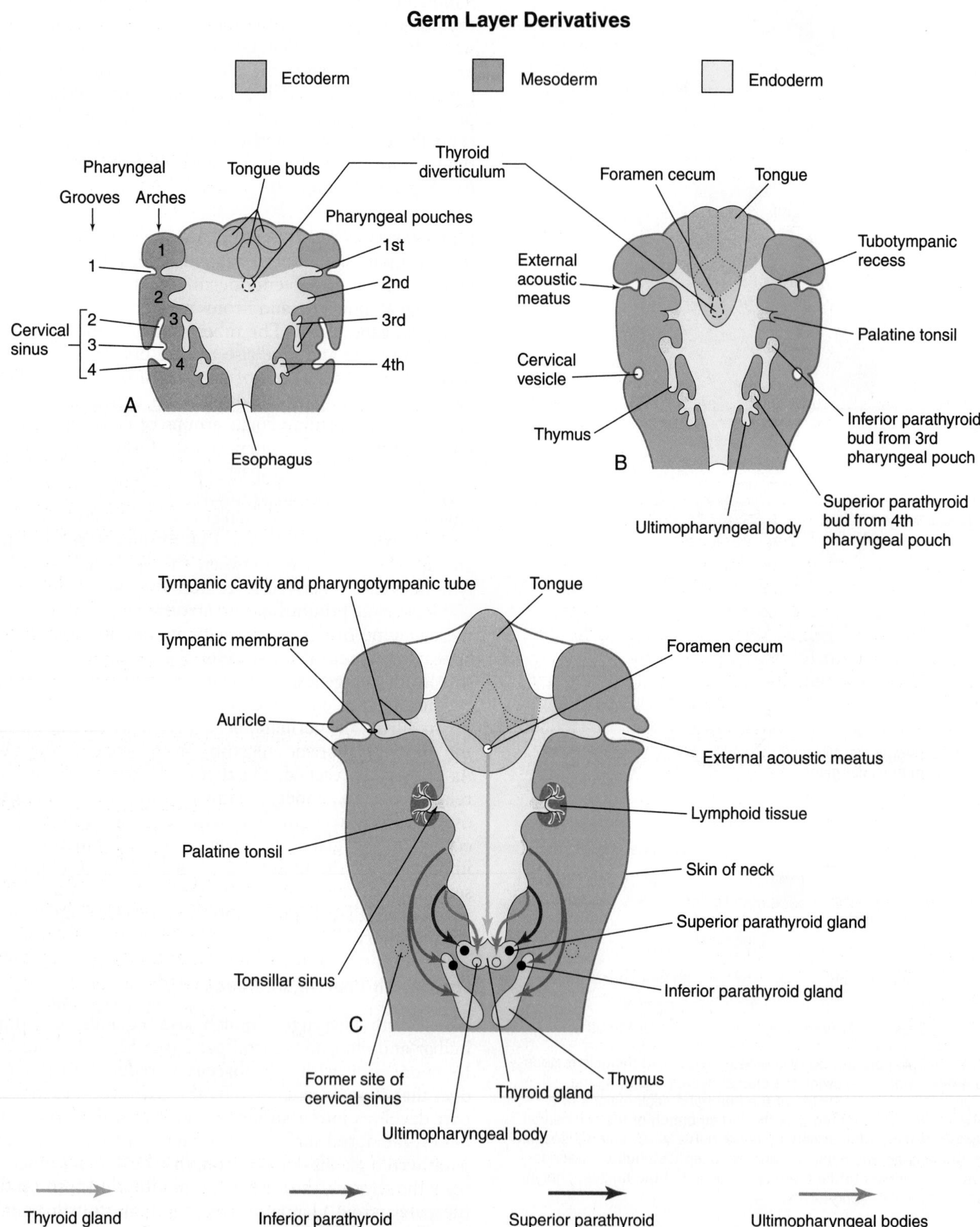

FIGURE 9-8. Schematic horizontal sections at the level shown in Figure 9-4*A* illustrating the adult derivatives of the pharyngeal pouches. **A,** At 5 weeks. Note that the second pharyngeal arch grows over the third and fourth arches, burying the second to fourth pharyngeal grooves in the cervical sinus. **B,** At 6 weeks. **C,** At 7 weeks. Note the migration of the developing thymus, parathyroid, and thyroid glands into the neck.

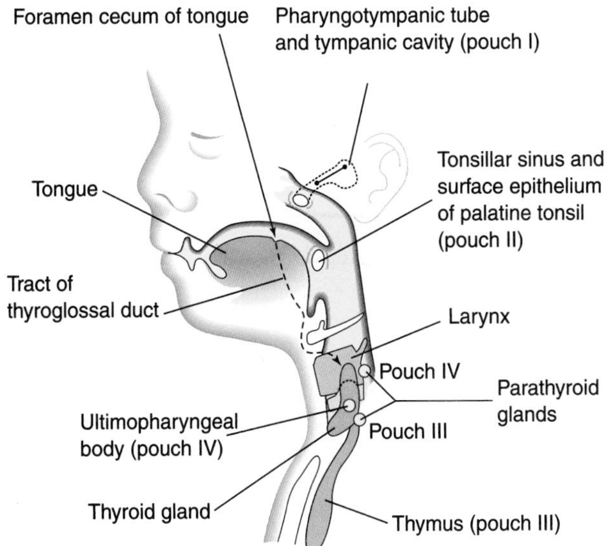

FIGURE 9-9. Schematic sagittal section of the head, neck, and upper thoracic regions of a 20-week fetus showing the adult derivatives of the pharyngeal pouches and the descent of the thyroid gland into the neck.

mesenchyme soon grows into these nodules, forming a capillary network. The *chief* or *principal cells* differentiate during the embryonic period and are believed to become functionally active in regulating fetal calcium metabolism. The **oxyphil cells** differentiate 5 to 7 years after birth.

The elongated ventral part of each fourth pouch develops into an **ultimopharyngeal body**, which fuses with the thyroid gland. Its cells disseminate within the thyroid, giving rise to the **parafollicular cells**. These cells are also called C cells to indicate that they produce calcitonin, a hormone involved in the regulation of calcium levels. **C cells** differentiate from **neural crest cells** that migrate from the pharyngeal arches into the fourth pair of pharyngeal pouches.

PHARYNGEAL GROOVES

The head and neck regions of the human embryo exhibit four pharyngeal grooves (clefts) on each side during the fourth and fifth weeks (see Figs. 9-1*B* to *D* and 9-2). These grooves separate the pharyngeal arches externally. Only one pair of grooves contributes to postnatal structures; the first pair persists as the **external acoustic meatus** or ear canals (see Fig. 9-8*C*). The other grooves lie in a slitlike depression—the **cervical sinus**—and are normally obliterated along with the sinus as the neck develops (see Fig. 9-4*B*, *D*, and *F*).

PHARYNGEAL MEMBRANES

The pharyngeal membranes appear in the floors of the pharyngeal grooves (see Figs. 9-1*H* and 9-3*C*). These membranes form where the epithelia of the grooves and pouches approach each other. The endoderm of the pouches and the ectoderm of the grooves are soon separated by mesenchyme. Only one pair of membranes contributes to the formation of adult structures; the first **pharyngeal membrane**, along with the intervening layer of mesenchyme, becomes the **tympanic membrane** (see Fig. 9-8C).

ATRESIA OF NASOLACRIMAL DUCT

Part of the nasolacrimal duct occasionally fails to canalize, resulting in a congenital anomaly—atresia of the nasolacrimal duct. Obstruction of this nasolacrimal duct with clinical symptoms occurs in approximately 6% of newborn infants.

CONGENITAL AURICULAR SINUSES AND CYSTS

Small auricular sinuses and cysts are usually located in a triangular area of skin anterior to the auricle of the external ear (Fig. 9-10*F*); however, they may occur in other sites around the auricle or in its lobule (earlobe). Although some sinuses and cysts are remnants of the first pharyngeal groove, others represent ectodermal folds sequestered during formation of the auricle from the auricular hillocks (swellings that contribute to the auricle). These sinuses and cysts are classified as minor anomalies that are of no serious medical consequence.

BRANCHIAL (CERVICAL) SINUSES

External branchial (cervical) sinuses are uncommon and almost all result from failure of the second pharyngeal groove and the cervical sinus to obliterate (Figs. 9-10*D* and 9-11*A* and *B*). The sinus typically opens along the anterior border of the sternocleidomastoid muscle in the inferior third of the neck. Anomalies of the other pharyngeal grooves occur in approximately 5% of cases. External branchial sinuses are commonly detected during infancy because of the discharge of mucous material from them (see Fig. 9-11*A*). These **lateral cervical sinuses** are bilateral in approximately 10% of cases and are commonly associated with auricular sinuses.

Internal branchial (cervical) sinuses open into the tonsillar sinus or near the palatopharyngeal arch (see Fig. 9-10*D* and *F*). These sinuses are very rare. Almost all these sinuses result from persistence of the proximal part of the second pharyngeal pouch. Normally this pouch disappears as the palatine tonsil develops; its normal remnant is the tonsillar sinus.

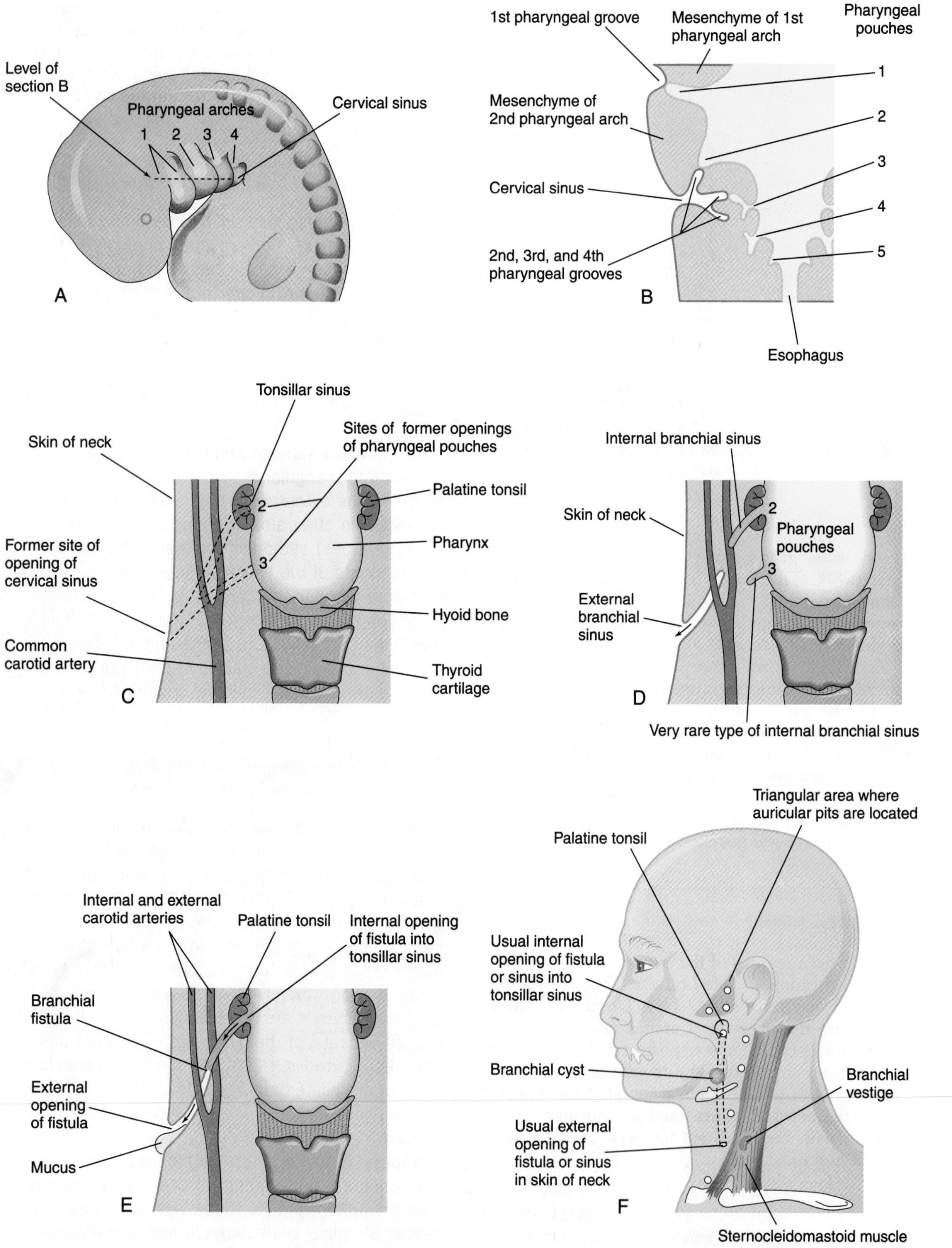

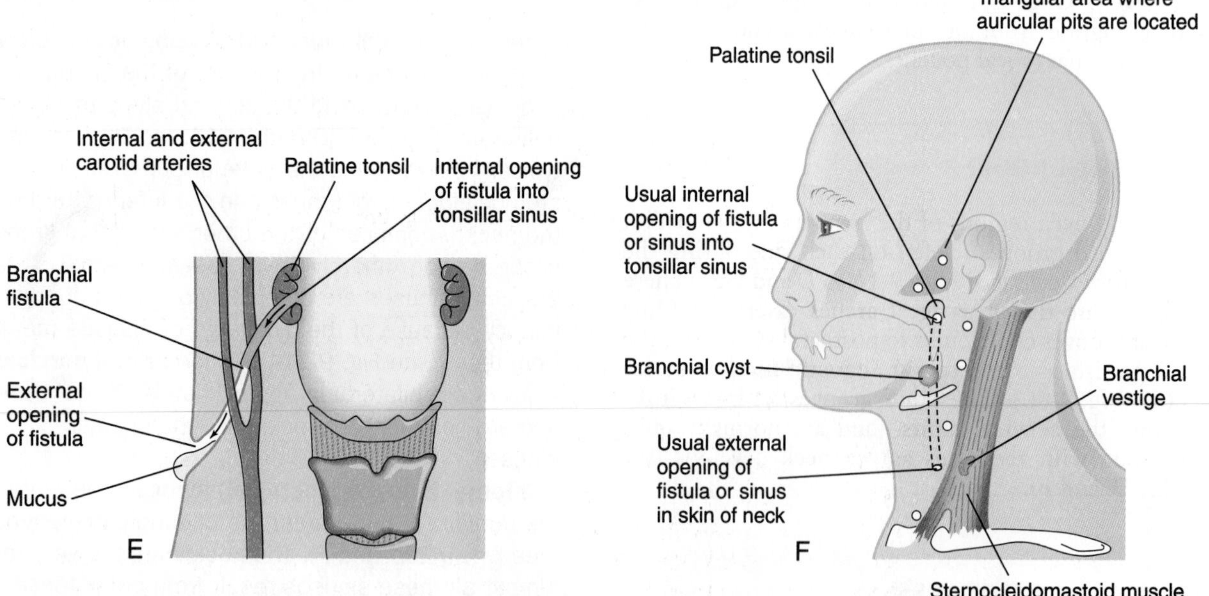

FIGURE 9-10. **A,** Lateral view of the head, neck, and thoracic regions of a 5-week embryo showing the cervical sinus that is normally present at this stage. **B,** Horizontal section of the embryo, at the level shown in **A,** illustrating the relationship of the cervical sinus to the pharyngeal arches and pouches. **C,** Diagrammatic sketch of the adult pharyngeal and neck regions indicating the former sites of openings of the cervical sinus and pharyngeal pouches. The *broken lines* indicate possible courses of branchial fistulas. **D,** Similar sketch showing the embryologic basis of various types of branchial sinus. **E,** Drawing of a branchial fistula resulting from persistence of parts of the second pharyngeal groove and second pharyngeal pouch. **F,** Sketch showing possible sites of branchial cysts and openings of branchial sinuses and fistulas. A branchial vestige is also illustrated (see also Fig. 9-14).

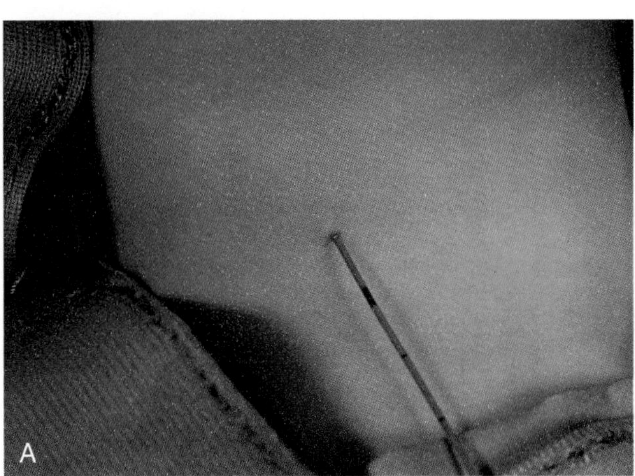

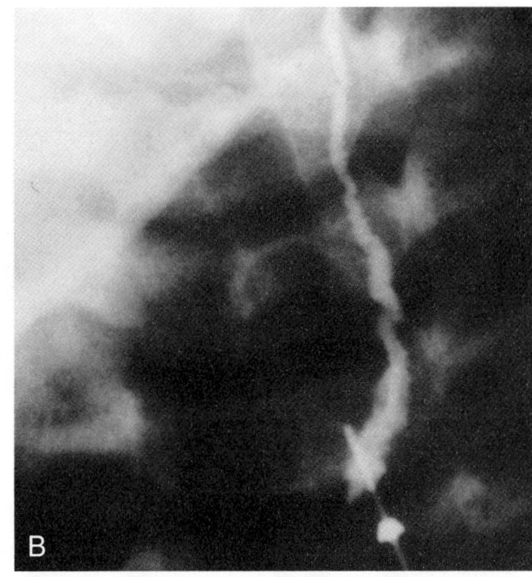

FIGURE 9-11. **A,** A child's neck showing a catheter inserted into the external opening of a branchial sinus. The catheter allows definition of the length of the tract, which facilitates surgical excision. **B,** A fistulogram of a complete branchial fistula. The radiograph was taken after injection of a contrast medium showing the course of the fistula through the neck. (Courtesy of Dr. Pierre Soucy, Division of Paediatric Surgery, Children's Hospital of Eastern Ontario, Ottawa, Ontario, Canada.)

BRANCHIAL FISTULA

An abnormal canal that opens internally into the tonsillar sinus and externally in the side of the neck is a branchial fistula. This canal results from persistence of parts of the second pharyngeal groove and second pharyngeal pouch (see Figs. 9-10*E* and *F* and 9-11*B*). The fistula ascends from its opening in the neck through the subcutaneous tissue and platysma muscle to reach the carotid sheath. The fistula then passes between the internal and external carotid arteries and opens into the tonsillar sinus.

PIRIFORM SINUS FISTULA

A piriform sinus fistula is thought to result from the persistence of remnants of the ultimopharyngeal body; the fistula traces the path of this embryonic body to the thyroid gland (see Fig. 9-8*C*).

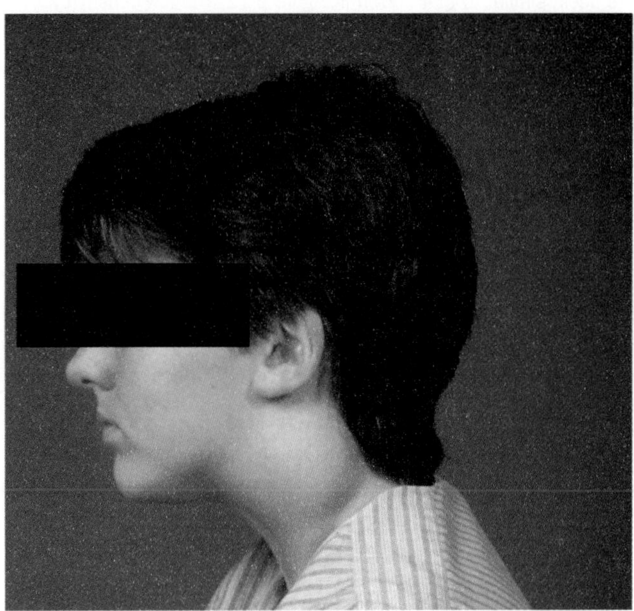

FIGURE 9-12. A boy showing the swelling in the neck produced by a branchial cyst. Branchial cysts often lie free in the neck just inferior to the angle of the mandible, or they may develop anywhere along the anterior border of the sternocleidomastoid muscle as in this case. (Courtesy of Dr. Pierre Soucy, Division of Paediatric Surgery, Children's Hospital of Eastern Ontario, Ottawa, Ontario, Canada.)

BRANCHIAL CYSTS

Remnants of parts of the cervical sinus and/or the second pharyngeal groove may persist and form a spherical or elongate cyst (see Fig. 9-10*F*). Although they may be associated with branchial sinuses and drain through them, branchial cysts often lie free in the neck just inferior to the angle of the mandible. However, they develop anywhere along the anterior border of the sternocleidomastoid muscle. Branchial cysts do not usually become apparent until late childhood or early adulthood, when they produce a slowly enlarging, painless swelling in the neck (Fig. 9-12). The cysts enlarge because of the accumulation of fluid and cellular debris derived from desquamation of their epithelial linings (Fig. 9-13). Branchial cysts have also been observed in the parathyroid glands.

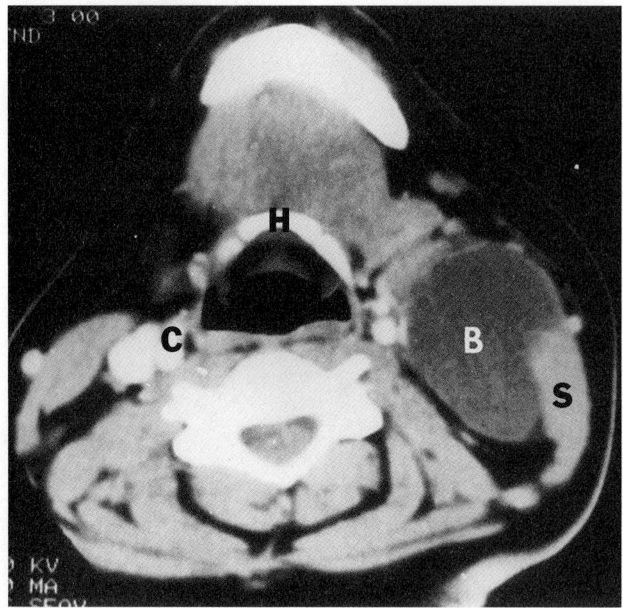

FIGURE 9-13. Branchial cyst (B). This is a computed tomography (CT) image of the neck region of a woman who presented with a "lump" in the neck, similar to that shown in Figure 9-12. The low-density cyst is anterior to the right sternocleidomastoid muscle (S) at the level of the hyoid bone (h). The normal appearance of the carotid sheath (c) is shown for comparison with the compressed sheath on the right side. (From McNab T, McLennan MK, Margolis M: Radiology rounds. Can Fam Physician 41:1673, 1995.)

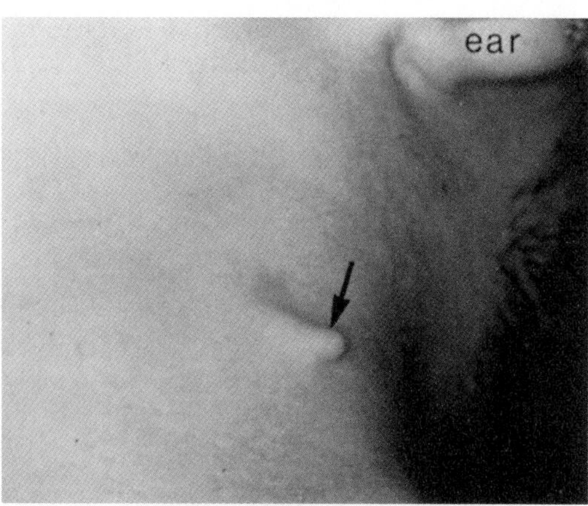

FIGURE 9-14. A cartilaginous branchial vestige under the skin of a child's neck. (From Raffensperger JG: Swenson's Pediatric Surgery, 5th ed. 1990. Courtesy of Appleton-Century-Crofts.)

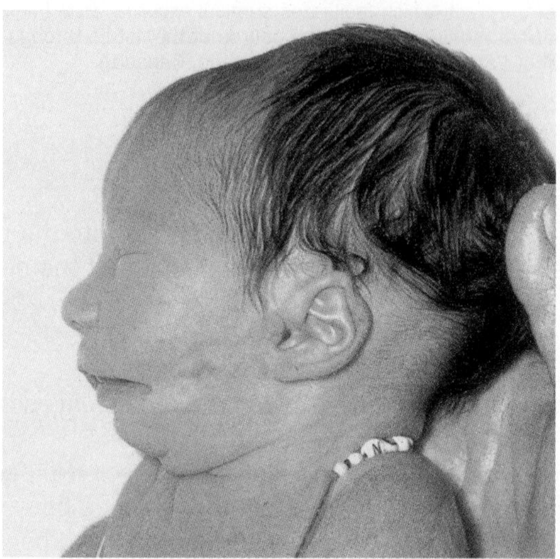

FIGURE 9-15. An infant with the first arch syndrome, a pattern of anomalies resulting from insufficient migration of neural crest cells into the first pharyngeal arch. Note the deformed auricle, the preauricular appendage, the defect in the cheek between the auricle and the mouth, hypoplasia of the mandible, and macrostomia (large mouth).

Branchial Vestiges

Normally the pharyngeal cartilages disappear, except for parts that form ligaments or bones; however, in unusual cases, cartilaginous or bony remnants of pharyngeal arch cartilages appear under the skin in the side of the neck (Fig. 9-14). These are usually found anterior to the inferior third of the sternocleidomastoid muscle (see Fig. 9-10*F*).

First Arch Syndrome

Abnormal development of the components of the first pharyngeal arch results in various congenital anomalies of the eyes, ears, mandible, and palate that together constitute the first arch syndrome (Fig. 9-15). This syndrome is believed to result from insufficient migration of neural crest cells into the first arch during the fourth week. There are two main manifestations of the first arch syndrome:

- In **Treacher Collins syndrome** (mandibulofacial dysostosis), caused by an autosomal dominant gene, there is malar hypoplasia (underdevelopment of the zygomatic bones of the face) with down-slanting palpebral fissures, defects of the lower eyelids, deformed external ears, and sometimes abnormalities of the middle and internal ears.
- In **Pierre Robin syndrome**, an autosomal recessive disorder, is associated with hypoplasia of the mandible, cleft palate, and defects of the eye and ear are present. Many cases of this syndrome are sporadic. In the Robin morphogenetic complex, the initiating defect is a small mandible (micrognathia), which results in posterior displacement of the tongue and obstruction to full closure of the palatal processes, resulting in a bilateral cleft palate (see Figs. 9-37 and 9-40).

DiGeorge Syndrome

Infants with **DiGeorge syndrome** are born without a thymus and parathyroid glands and have defects in their cardiac outflow tracts. In some cases, ectopic glandular tissue has been found. Clinically, the disease is characterized by *congenital hypoparathyroidism*, increased susceptibility to infections (from immune deficiency, specifically defective T-cell function), anomalies of the mouth (shortened philtrum of lip [fish-mouth deformity]), low-set notched ears, nasal clefts, *thyroid hypoplasia*, and cardiac abnormalities (defects of the arch of the aorta and heart). DiGeorge syndrome occurs because the third and fourth pharyngeal pouches fail to differentiate into the thymus and parathyroid glands. This is the result of a breakdown in signaling between pharyngeal endoderm and adjacent neural crest cells. The facial abnormalities result primarily from abnormal development of the first arch components because neural crest cells are disrupted, and the cardiac anomalies arise in those sites normally occupied by neural crest cells. In most cases of DiGeorge syndrome, there is a microdeletion in the q11.2 region of chromosome 22, HIRA and UFDIL gene mutation, and neural crest cell defects.

Accessory Thymic Tissue

An isolated mass of thymic tissue may persist in the neck, often close to an inferior parathyroid gland (Fig. 9-16). This tissue breaks free from the developing thymus as it shifts caudally in the neck.

Ectopic Parathyroid Glands

The location of the parathyroid glands is highly variable. They may be found anywhere near or within the thyroid gland or thymus. The superior glands are more constant in position than the inferior ones. Occasionally, an inferior parathyroid gland remains near the bifurcation of the common carotid artery. In other cases, it may be in the thorax.

Abnormal Number of Parathyroid Glands

Uncommonly there are more than four parathyroid glands. Supernumerary parathyroid glands probably result from division of the primordia of the original glands. Absence of a parathyroid gland results from failure of one of the primordia to differentiate or from atrophy of a gland early in development.

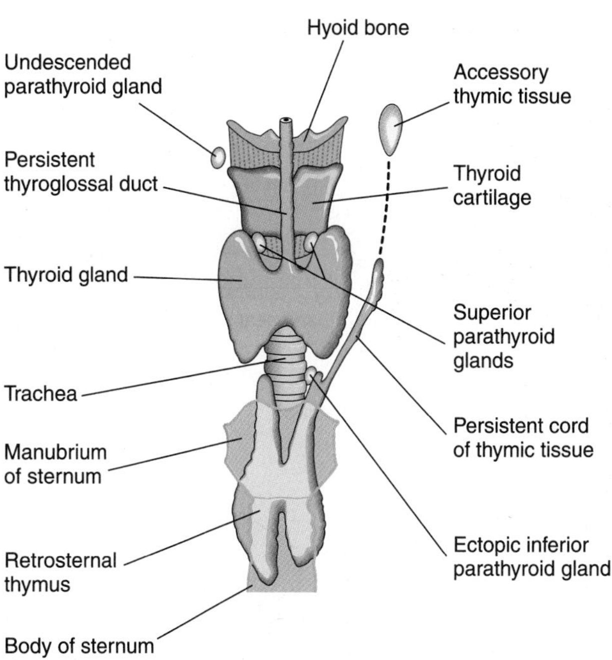

FIGURE 9-16. Anterior view of the thyroid gland, thymus, and parathyroid glands, illustrating various congenital anomalies that may occur.

DEVELOPMENT OF THE THYROID GLAND

The thyroid gland is the first endocrine gland to develop in the embryo. It begins to form approximately 24 days after fertilization from a median endodermal thickening in the floor of the primordial pharynx (Fig. 9-17). This thickening soon forms a small outpouching—the **thyroid primordium**. As the embryo and tongue grow, the developing thyroid gland descends in the neck, passing ventral to the developing hyoid bone and laryngeal cartilages. For a short time, the thyroid gland is connected to the tongue by a narrow tube, the **thyroglossal duct** (see Fig. 9-17*B* and *C*). At first the thyroid primordium is hollow, but soon becomes a solid mass of cells and divides into right and left lobes that are connected by the **isthmus of the thyroid gland** (Fig. 9-18), which lies anterior to the developing second and third tracheal rings.

By 7 weeks, the thyroid gland has assumed its definitive shape and is usually located in its final site in the neck (see Fig. 9-17*D*). By this time, the *thyroglossal duct* has normally degenerated and disappeared. The proximal opening of the thyroglossal duct persists as a small pit in the dorsum (posterosuperior surface) of the tongue—the **foramen cecum**. A pyramidal lobe of the thyroid gland extends superiorly from the isthmus in approximately 50% of people. A **pyramidal lobe** differentiates from the distal end of the thyroglossal duct and attaches to the hyoid bone by fibrous tissue and/or smooth muscle—the **levator muscle of thyroid gland** (see Fig. 9-18).

Histogenesis of the Thyroid Gland

The thyroid primordium consists of a solid mass of endodermal cells. This cellular aggregation later breaks up into

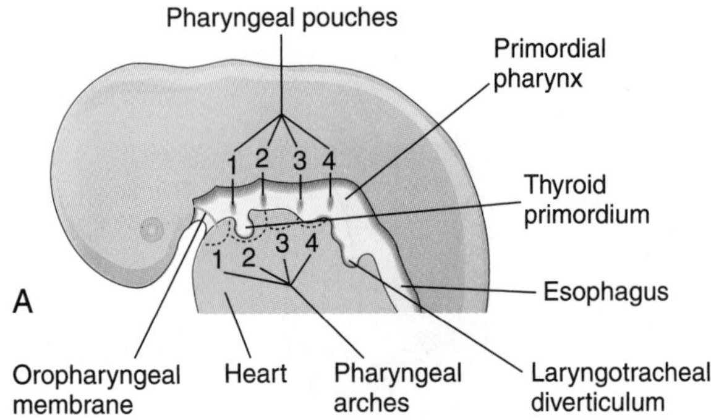

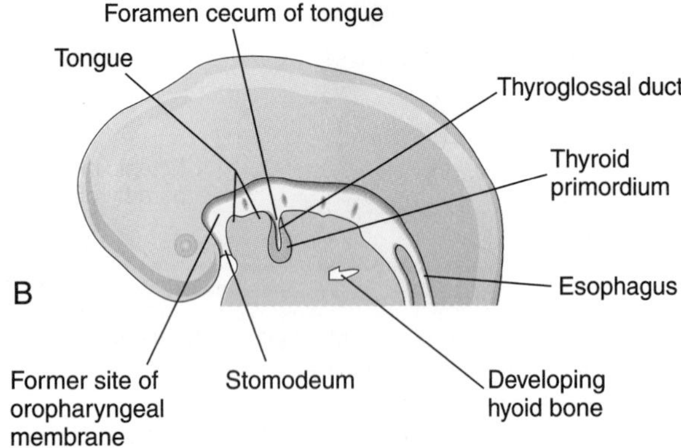

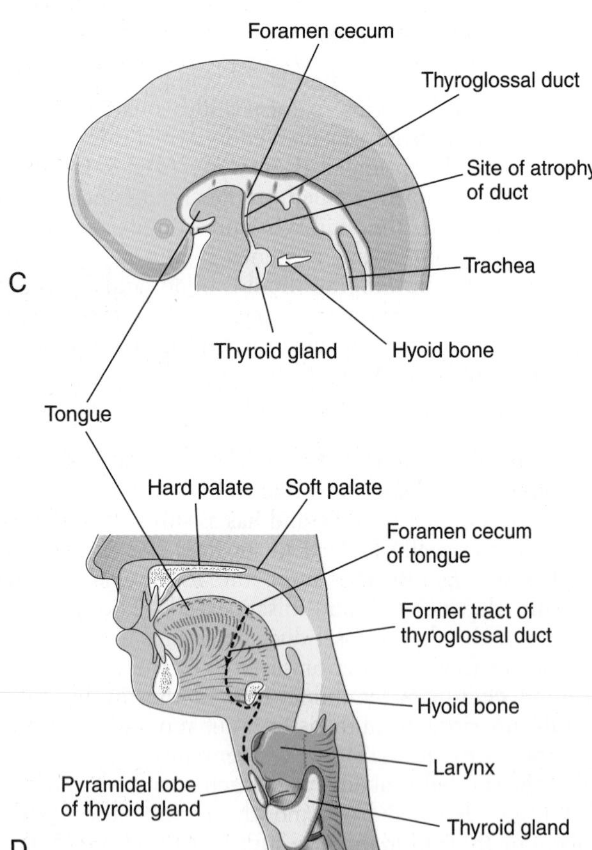

FIGURE 9-17. Development of the thyroid gland. **A, B,** and **C,** Schematic sagittal sections of the head and neck regions of embryos at 4, 5, and 6 weeks illustrating successive stages in the development of the thyroid gland. **D,** Similar section of an adult head and neck showing the path taken by the thyroid gland during its embryonic descent (indicated by the former tract of the thyroglossal duct).

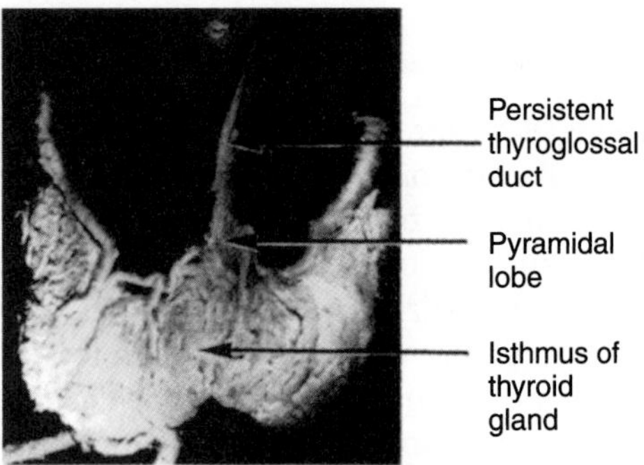

FIGURE 9-18. The anterior surface of a dissected adult thyroid gland showing persistence of the thyroglossal duct. Observe the pyramidal lobe ascending from the superior border of the isthmus. It represents a persistent portion of the inferior end of the thyroglossal duct that has formed thyroid tissue.

a network of epithelial cords as it is invaded by the surrounding vascular mesenchyme. By the 10th week, the cords have divided into small cellular groups. A lumen soon forms in each cell cluster and the cells become arranged in a single layer around a lumen. During the 11th week, colloid begins to appear in these structures—**thyroid follicles**; thereafter, iodine concentration and the synthesis of thyroid hormones can be demonstrated. By 20 weeks, the levels of fetal thyroid-stimulating hormone and thyroxine begin to increase, reaching adult levels by 35 weeks.

CONGENITAL HYPOTHYROIDISM

The primary cause of congenital hypothyroidism is a derangement in the development of the thyroid gland rather than central causes related to the hypothalamic-pituitary axis.

THYROGLOSSAL DUCT CYSTS AND SINUSES

Cysts may form anywhere along the course of the thyroglossal duct (Fig. 9-19). Normally, the thyroglossal duct atrophies and disappears, but a remnant of it may persist and form a cyst in the tongue or in the anterior part of the neck, usually just inferior to the hyoid bone (Fig. 9-20). Most thyroglossal duct cysts are observed by the age of 5 years. Unless the lesions become infected, most of them are asymptomatic. The swelling produced by a thyroglossal duct cyst usually develops as a painless, progressively enlarging, movable mass (Fig. 9-21). The cyst may contain some thyroid tissue. After infection of a cyst, a perforation of the skin occurs, forming a thyroglossal duct sinus that usually opens in the median plane of the neck, anterior to the laryngeal cartilages (see Fig. 9-19*A*).

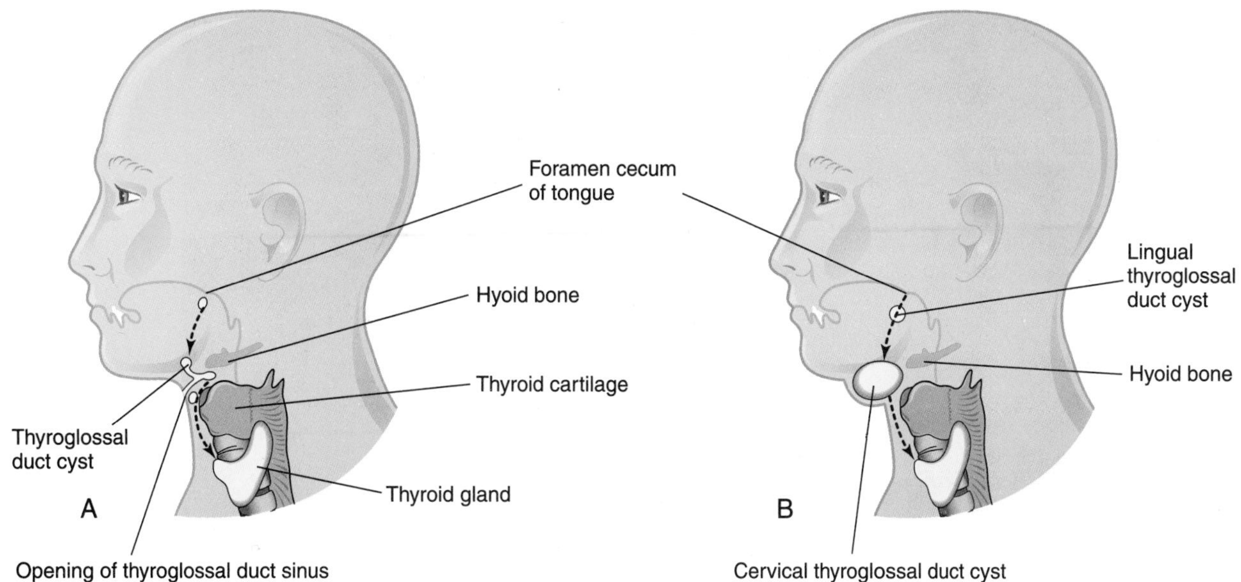

FIGURE 9-19. **A,** Sketch of the head and neck showing the possible locations of thyroglossal duct cysts. A thyroglossal duct sinus is also illustrated. The *broken line* indicates the course taken by the thyroglossal duct during descent of the developing thyroid gland from the foramen cecum to its final position in the anterior part of the neck. **B,** Similar sketch illustrating lingual and cervical thyroglossal duct cysts. Most thyroglossal duct cysts are located just inferior to the hyoid bone.

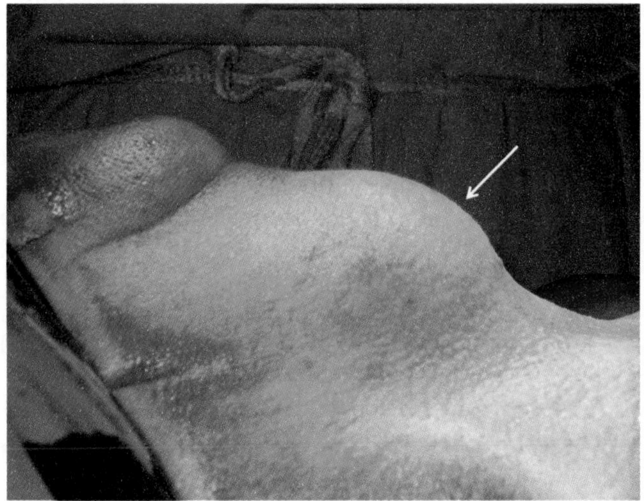

FIGURE 9-20. Large thyroglossal duct cyst (*arrow*) in a male patient. (Courtesy of Dr. Srinivasa Ramachandra, St. Georges University School of Medicine, Grenada.)

ECTOPIC THYROID GLAND

An ectopic thyroid gland is an infrequent congenital anomaly and is usually located along the course of the thyroglossal duct (see Fig. 9-17*C*). **Lingual thyroid tissue** is the most common of ectopic thyroid tissues; intralingual thyroid masses are found in as many as 10% of autopsies, although they are clinically relevant in only one in 4000 persons with thyroid disease. Incomplete movement of the thyroid gland results in the **sublingual thyroid gland** appearing high in the neck, at or just inferior to the hyoid bone (Figs. 9-22 and 9-23). As a rule, an ectopic sublingual thyroid gland in the neck is the only thyroid tissue present. It is clinically important to differentiate an ectopic thyroid gland from a thyroglossal duct cyst or accessory thyroid tissue to *prevent inadvertent surgical removal of the thyroid gland*. This may be the only thyroid tissue present. Failure to do so may leave the person permanently dependent on thyroid medication.

ACCESSORY THYROID TISSUE

Accessory thyroid tissue may also appear in the thymus inferior to the thyroid gland. Although this tissue may be functional, it is often of insufficient size to maintain normal function if the thyroid gland is removed. Accessory thyroid tissue may also develop in the neck lateral to the thyroid cartilage. It usually lies on the thyrohyoid muscle. Accessory thyroid tissue originates from remnants of the thyroglossal duct.

AGENESIS OF THYROID GLAND

Congenital hypothyroidism, resulting from defective development of the thyroid gland, occurs frequently. Absence of the thyroid gland, or one of its lobes, is a rare anomaly. In thyroid hemiagenesis (unilateral failure of formation), the left lobe is more commonly absent. Mutations in the receptor for thyroid-stimulating hormone is probably involved in some cases.

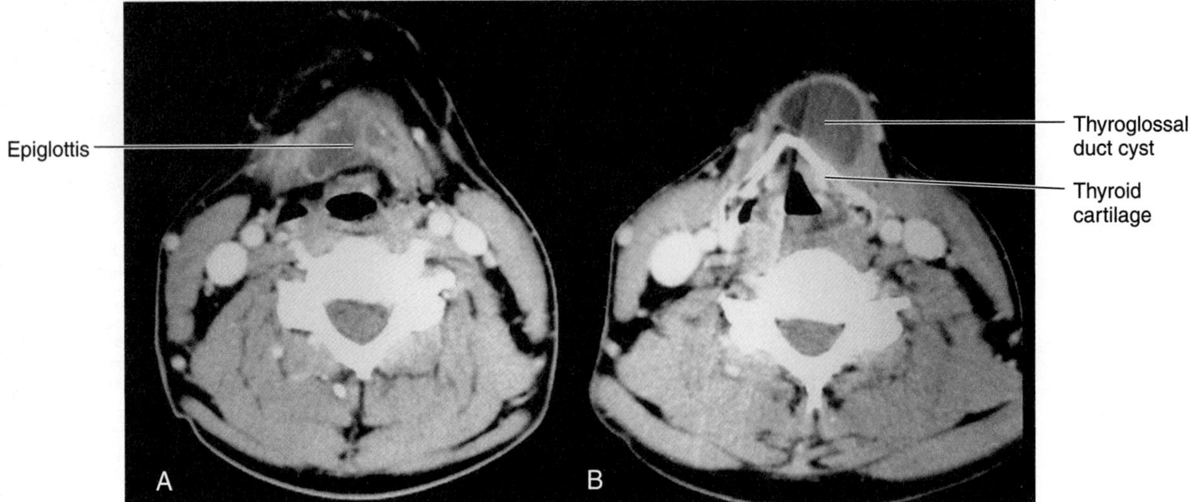

FIGURE 9-21. Computed tomography images. **A,** Level of the thyrohyoid membrane and base of the epiglottis. **B,** Level of thyroid cartilage, which is calcified. The thyroglossal duct cyst extends cranially to the margin of the hyoid bone. (Courtesy of Dr. Gerald S. Smyser, Altru Health System, Grand Forks, ND.)

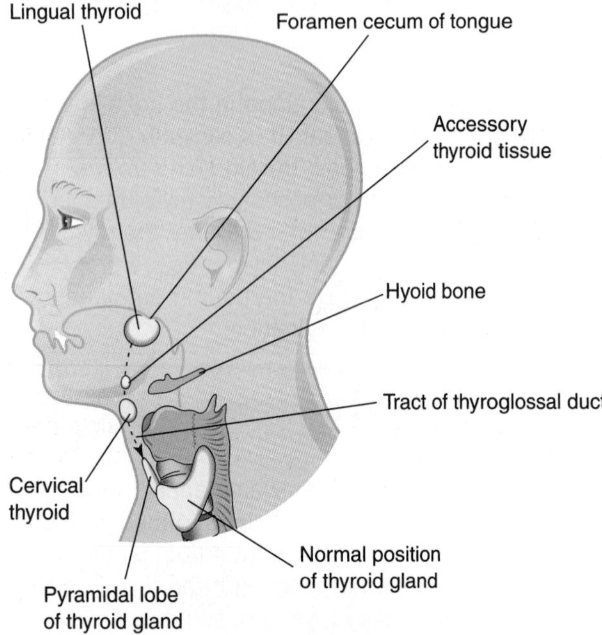

FIGURE 9-22. Sketch of the head and neck showing the usual sites of ectopic thyroid tissue. The *broken line* indicates the path followed by the thyroid gland during its descent and the former tract of the thyroglossal duct.

DEVELOPMENT OF THE TONGUE

Near the end of the fourth week, a median triangular elevation appears in the floor of the primordial pharynx, just rostral to the foramen cecum (Fig. 9-24*A*). This swelling—the **median lingual swelling** (tongue bud) (Latin, *tuberculum impar*)—is the first indication of tongue development. Soon, two oval **lateral lingual swellings** (distal tongue buds) develop on each side of the median tongue bud. The three lingual swellings result from the proliferation of mesenchyme in ventromedial parts of the first pair of pharyngeal arches. The lateral lingual swellings rapidly increase in size, merge with each other, and overgrow the median lingual swelling. The merged lateral lingual swellings form the anterior two thirds (oral part) of the tongue (see Fig. 9-24*C*). The fusion site of the lateral lingual swellings is indicated by the midline groove of the tongue and internally by the fibrous **lingual septum**. The median lingual swellings do not form a recognizable part of the adult tongue.

Formation of the posterior third (pharyngeal part) of the tongue is indicated in the fetus by two elevations that develop caudal to the foramen cecum (see Fig. 9-24*A*):

- The **copula** (Latin, bond, tie) forms by fusion of the ventromedial parts of the second pair of pharyngeal arches.
- The **hypopharyngeal eminence** develops caudal to the copula from mesenchyme in the ventromedial parts of the third and fourth pairs of arches.

As the tongue develops, the copula is gradually overgrown by the hypopharyngeal eminence and disappears (see Fig. 9-24*B* and *C*). As a result, the posterior third of the tongue develops from the rostral part of the hypopharyngeal eminence.

The line of fusion of the anterior and posterior parts of the tongue is roughly indicated by a V-shaped groove—the **terminal sulcus** (see Fig. 9-24*C*). Pharyngeal arch mesenchyme forms the connective tissue and vasculature of the tongue. Most of the tongue muscles are derived from myoblasts that migrate from the occipital myotomes (see Fig. 9-6*A*). The hypoglossal nerve (CN XII) accompanies the myoblasts during their migration and innervates the tongue muscles as they develop. Both the anterior and posterior portions of the tongue are located within the oral cavity at birth; the posterior third descends into the oropharynx by 4 years of age.

Lingual Papillae and Taste Buds

Lingual papillae appear toward the end of the eighth week. The *vallate* and *foliate papillae* appear first, close to

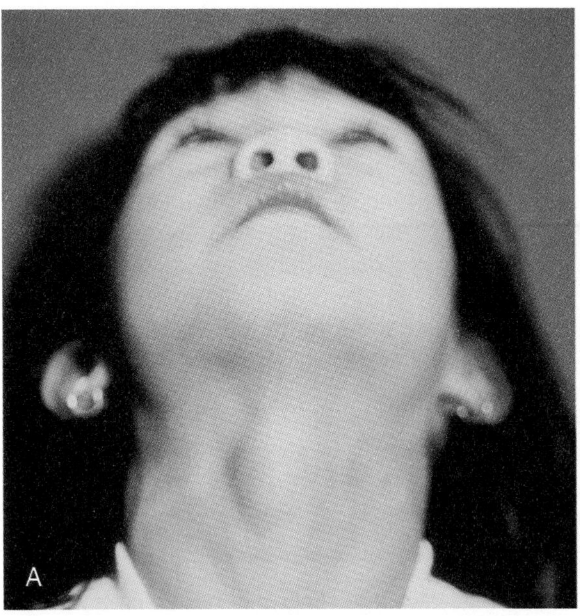

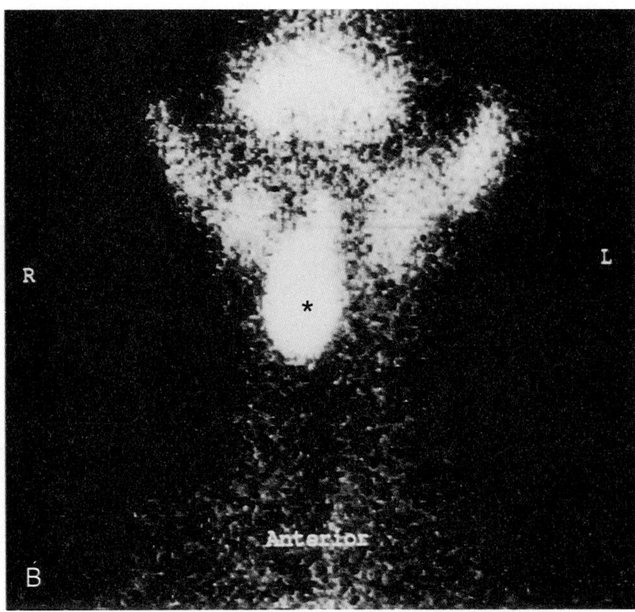

FIGURE 9-23. **A,** A sublingual thyroid mass in a 5-year-old girl. **B,** Technetium-99m pertechnetate scan showing a sublingual thyroid gland (*) without evidence of functioning thyroid tissue in the anterior part of the neck. (From Leung AKC, Wong AL, Robson WLLM: Ectopic thyroid gland simulating a thyroglossal duct cyst. Can J Surg 38:87, 1995.)

terminal branches of the glossopharyngeal nerve (CN IX). The *fungiform papillae* appear later near terminations of the chorda tympani branch of the facial nerve (CN VII). The most common lingual papillae, known as **filiform papillae** because of their threadlike shape, develop during the early fetal period (10–11 weeks). They contain afferent nerve endings that are sensitive to touch. **Taste buds** develop during weeks 11 to 13 by inductive interaction between the epithelial cells of the tongue and invading gustatory nerve cells from the chorda tympani, glossopharyngeal, and vagus nerves. Most taste buds form on the dorsal surface of the tongue, and some develop on the palatoglossal arches, palate, posterior surface of the epiglottis, and the posterior wall of the oropharynx. Fetal facial responses can be induced by bitter-tasting substances at 26 to 28 weeks, indicating that reflex pathways between taste buds and facial muscles are established by this stage.

Nerve Supply of the Tongue

The development of the tongue explains its nerve supply. The sensory supply to the mucosa of almost the entire anterior two thirds of the tongue is from the lingual branch of the mandibular division of the **trigeminal nerve** (CN V), the nerve of the first pharyngeal arch. This arch forms the median and lateral lingual swellings (see Fig. 9-24). Although the facial nerve is the nerve of the second pharyngeal arch, its chorda tympani branch supplies the taste buds in the anterior two thirds of the tongue, except for the vallate papillae. Because the second arch component, the copula, is overgrown by the third arch, the facial nerve (CN VII) does not supply any of the tongue mucosa, except for the taste buds in the anterior part of the tongue. The vallate papillae in the anterior part of the tongue are innervated by the **glossopharyngeal nerve** (CN IX) of the third pharyngeal arch (see Fig. 9-24*C*). The reason usually given for this is that the mucosa of the posterior third of the tongue is pulled slightly anteriorly as the tongue develops. The posterior third of the tongue is innervated mainly by the glossopharyngeal nerve of the third pharyngeal arch. The superior laryngeal branch of the vagus nerve (CN X) of the fourth arch supplies a small area of the tongue anterior to the epiglottis (see Fig. 9-24*C*). All muscles of the tongue are supplied by the **hypoglossal nerve** (CN XII), except for the palatoglossus, which is supplied from the pharyngeal plexus by fibers arising from the vagus nerve (CN X).

CONGENITAL ANOMALIES OF TONGUE

Abnormalities of the tongue are uncommon, except for fissuring of the tongue and hypertrophy of the lingual papillae, which are characteristics of infants with Down syndrome (see Chapter 20).

CONGENITAL LINGUAL CYSTS AND FISTULAS

Cysts in the tongue may be derived from remnants of the thyroglossal duct (see Fig. 9-19). They may enlarge and produce symptoms of pharyngeal discomfort and/or dysphagia (difficulty in swallowing). Fistulas are also derived from persistence of lingual parts of the thyroglossal duct; they open through the foramen cecum into the oral cavity.

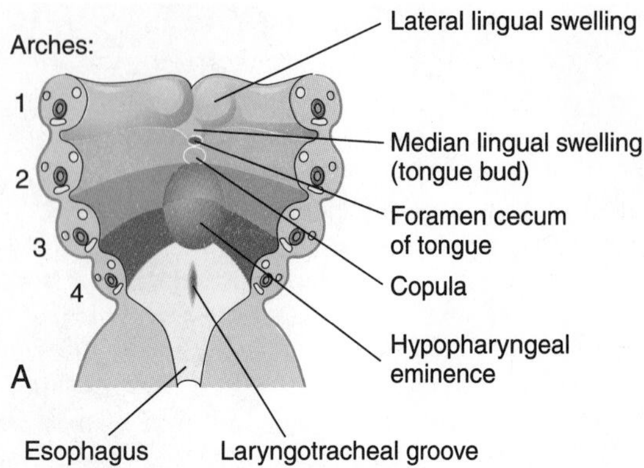

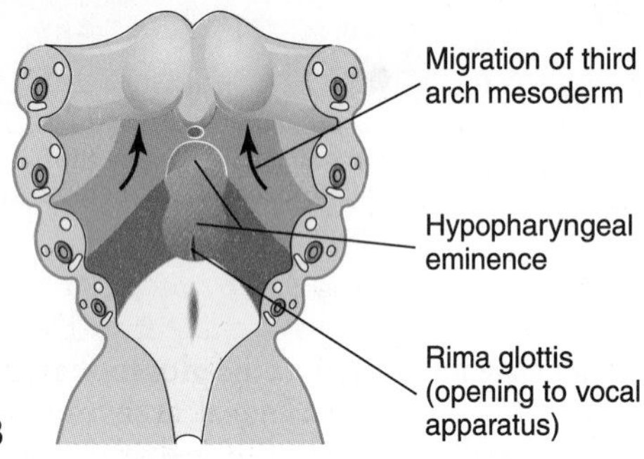

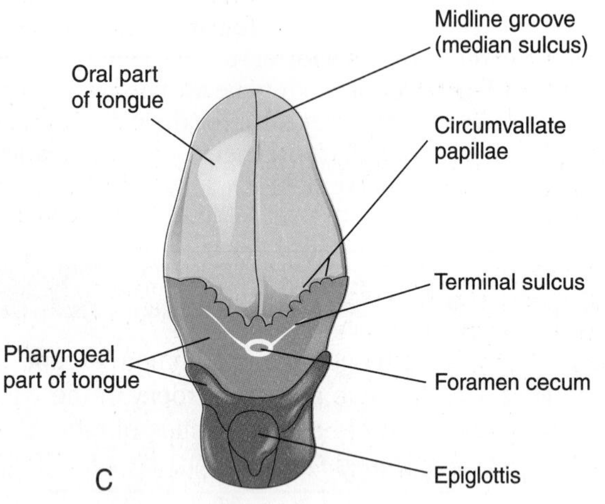

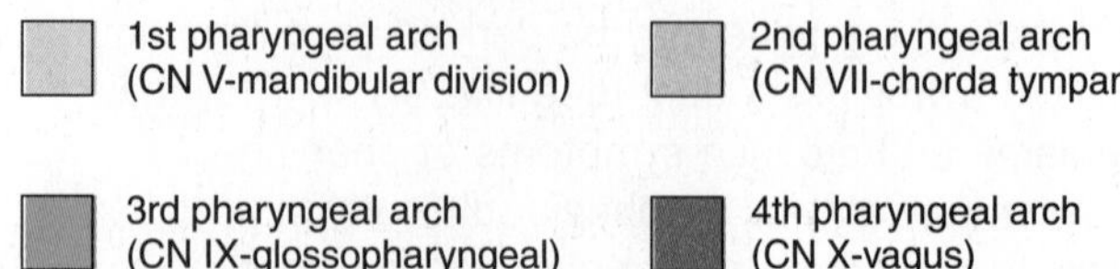

FIGURE 9-24. **A** and **B,** Schematic horizontal sections through the pharynx at the level shown in Figure 9-4*A* showing successive stages in the development of the tongue during the fourth and fifth weeks. **C,** Drawing of the adult tongue showing the pharyngeal arch derivation of the nerve supply of its mucosa.

ANKYLOGLOSSIA

The lingual frenulum normally connects the inferior surface of the tongue to the floor of the mouth. Sometimes the frenulum is short and extends to the tip of the tongue (Fig. 9-25). This interferes with its free protrusion and may make breast-feeding difficult. Ankyloglossia (tongue-tie) occurs in approximately one in 300 North American infants but is usually of no functional significance. A short frenulum usually stretches with time, making surgical correction of the anomaly unnecessary.

MACROGLOSSIA

An excessively large tongue is not common. It results from generalized hypertrophy of the developing tongue, usually resulting from lymphangioma (a lymph tumor) or muscular hypertrophy.

MICROGLOSSIA

An abnormally small tongue is extremely rare and is usually associated with micrognathia (underdeveloped mandible and recession of the chin) and limb defects (Hanhart's syndrome).

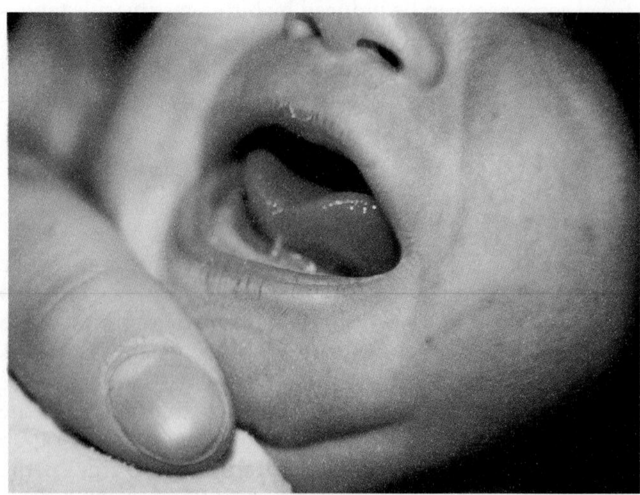

FIGURE 9-25. An infant with ankyloglossia or tongue-tie. Note the short frenulum, which extends to the tip of the tongue. Tongue-tie interferes with protrusion of the tongue and may make breast-feeding difficult. (Courtesy of Dr. Evelyn Jain, Lakeview Breastfeeding Clinic, Calgary, Alberta, Canada.)

Bifid or Cleft Tongue (Glossoschisis)

Incomplete fusion of the lateral lingual swellings results in a deep midline groove in the tongue; usually this cleft does not extend to the tip of the tongue. This is a very uncommon anomaly.

DEVELOPMENT OF THE SALIVARY GLANDS

During the sixth and seventh weeks of the embryonic period, the salivary glands begin as solid epithelial buds from the primordial oral cavity (see Fig. 9-7*C*). The club-shaped ends of these epithelial buds grow into the underlying mesenchyme. The connective tissue in the glands is derived from neural crest cells. All parenchymal (secretory) tissue arises by proliferation of the oral epithelium.

The **parotid glands** are the first to appear (early in the sixth week). They develop from buds that arise from the oral ectodermal lining near the angles of the stomodeum. Elongation of the jaws causes lengthening of the parotid duct, with the gland remaining close to its site of origin. Later the cords canalize—develop lumina—and become ducts by approximately 10 weeks. The rounded ends of the cords differentiate into **acini**. Secretions commence at 18 weeks. The capsule and connective tissue develop from the surrounding mesenchyme.

The **submandibular glands** appear late in the sixth week. They develop from endodermal buds in the floor of the stomodeum. Solid cellular processes grow posteriorly, lateral to the developing tongue. Later they branch and differentiate. Acini begin to form at 12 weeks and secretory activity begins at 16 weeks. Growth of the submandibular glands continues after birth with the formation of mucous acini. Lateral to the tongue, a linear groove forms that soon closes over to form the **submandibular duct**.

The **sublingual glands** appear in the eighth week, approximately 2 weeks later than the other salivary glands (see Fig. 9-7*C*). They develop from multiple endodermal epithelial buds in the **paralingual sulcus**. These buds branch and canalize to form 10 to 12 ducts that open independently into the floor of the mouth.

DEVELOPMENT OF THE FACE

The **facial primordia** appear early in the fourth week around the large primordial stomodeum (Fig. 9-26*A* and *B*). Facial development depends on the inductive influence of the prosencephalic and rhombencephalic organizing centers. The **prosencephalic organizing center** includes prechordal mesoderm located in the midline rostral to the notochord and overlying the presumptive prosencephalic neural plate (see Chapter 17). The midbrain-hindbrain boundary is a signaling center that directs the spatial organization of the caudal midbrain and the rostral hindbrain structures.

The **five facial primordia** that appear as prominences around the stomodeum (see Fig. 9-26*A*) are

- The single frontonasal prominence
- The paired maxillary prominences
- The paired mandibular prominences

The paired maxillary and mandibular prominences are derivatives of the first pair of pharyngeal arches. The prominences are produced mainly by the expansion of **neural crest populations** that originate from the mesencephalic and rostral rhombencephalic neural folds during the fourth week. These cells are the major source of connective tissue components, including cartilage, bone, and ligaments in the facial and oral regions. The results of experimental studies in chick and mouse embryos indicate that myoblasts, originating from paraxial and prechordal mesoderm, contribute to the craniofacial voluntary muscles.

The **frontonasal prominence** (FNP) surrounds the ventrolateral part of the forebrain, which gives rise to the **optic vesicles** that form the eyes (see Fig. 9-26*C*). The frontal part of the FNP forms the forehead; the nasal part of the FNP forms the rostral boundary of the stomodeum and nose. The paired maxillary prominences form the lateral boundaries of the **stomodeum**, and the paired mandibular prominences constitute the caudal boundary of the stomodeum (Fig. 9-27).

The five facial prominences are **active centers of growth** in the underlying mesenchyme. This embryonic connective tissue is continuous from one prominence to the other. Facial development occurs mainly between the fourth and eighth weeks (see Fig. 9-26*A* to *G*). By the end of the embryonic period, the face has an unquestionably human appearance. Facial proportions develop during the fetal period (see Fig. 9-26*H* and *I*). The lower jaw and lower lip are the first parts of the face to form. They result from merging of the medial ends of the mandibular prominences in the median plane.

By the end of the fourth week, bilateral oval thickenings of the surface ectoderm—**nasal placodes**—the primordia of the nasal epithelium, have developed on the inferolateral parts of the FNP (Figs. 9-28 and 9-29*A* and *B*). Initially these placodes are convex, but later they are stretched to produce a flat depression in each placode. Mesenchyme in the margins of the placodes proliferates, producing horseshoe-shaped elevations—the medial and lateral **nasal prominences**. As a result, the nasal placodes lie in depressions—the **nasal pits** (see Fig. 9-29*C* and *D*). These pits are the primordia of the anterior nares (nostrils) and nasal cavities (see Fig. 9-29*E*).

Proliferation of mesenchyme in the maxillary prominences causes them to enlarge and grow medially toward each other and the nasal prominences (see Figs. 9-26*D* to *G*, 9-27, and 9-28). This proliferation-driven expansion results in movement of the medial nasal prominences toward the median plane and each other. Each lateral nasal prominence is separated from the maxillary prominence by a cleft called the **nasolacrimal groove** (see Figs. 9-26*C* and *D*).

By the end of the fifth week, the primordia of the auricles (external part of the ears) have begun to develop (Figs. 9-26*E* and 9-30). **Six auricular hillocks** (three mesenchymal swellings on each side) form around the first pharyngeal groove (three on each side), the primordia of the auricle, and the external acoustic meatus, respectively.

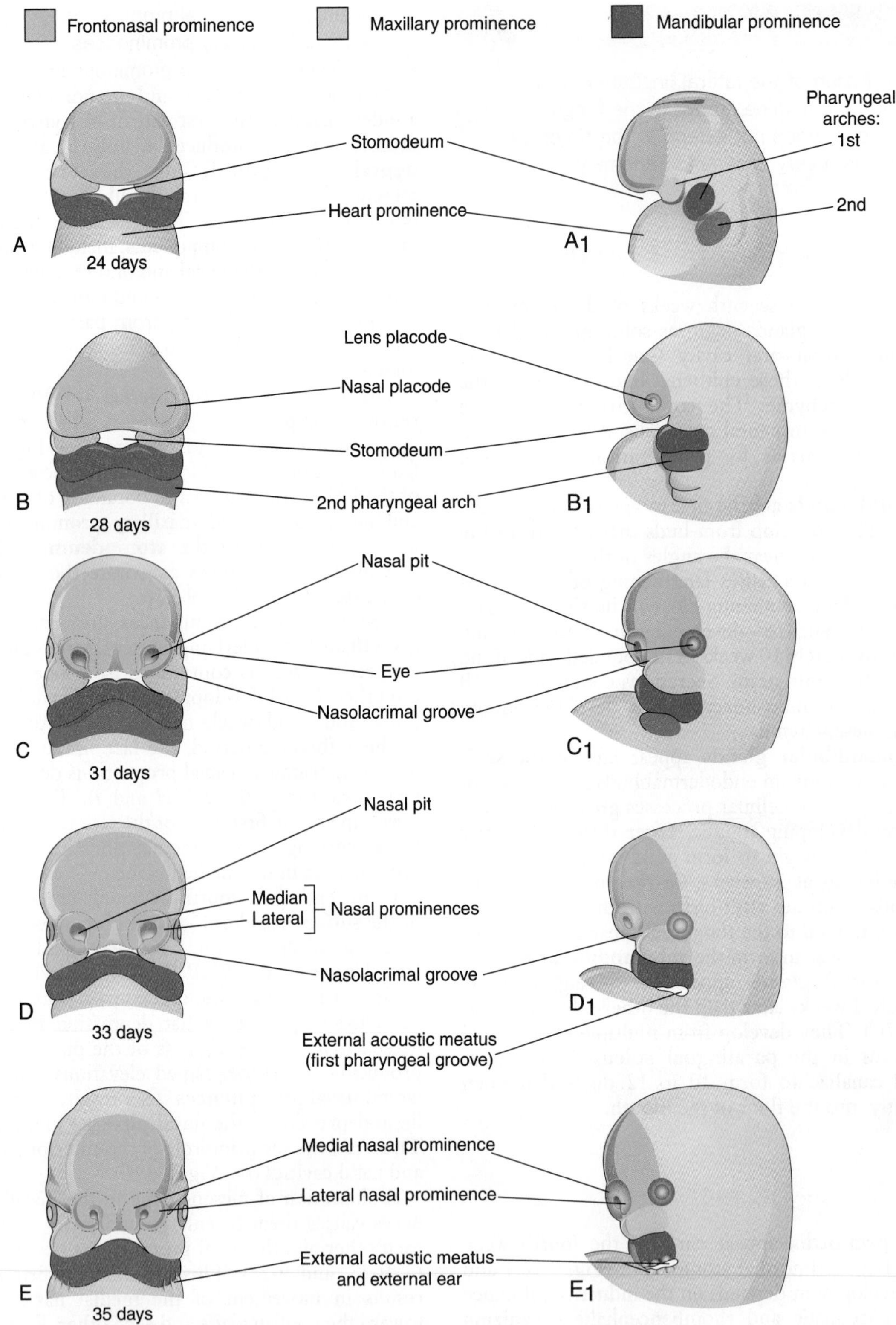

FIGURE 9-26. Diagrams illustrating progressive stages in the development of the human face.

Initially the external ears are located in the neck region (Fig. 9-31); however, as the mandible develops, they are located on the side of the head at the level of the eyes (see Fig. 9-26*H*).

By the end of the sixth week, each maxillary prominence has begun to merge with the lateral nasal prominence along the line of the nasolacrimal groove (Figs. 9-32 and 9-33). This establishes continuity between the side of the nose, formed by the lateral nasal prominence, and the cheek region formed by the maxillary prominence.

The **nasolacrimal duct** develops from a rodlike thickening of ectoderm in the floor of the nasolacrimal

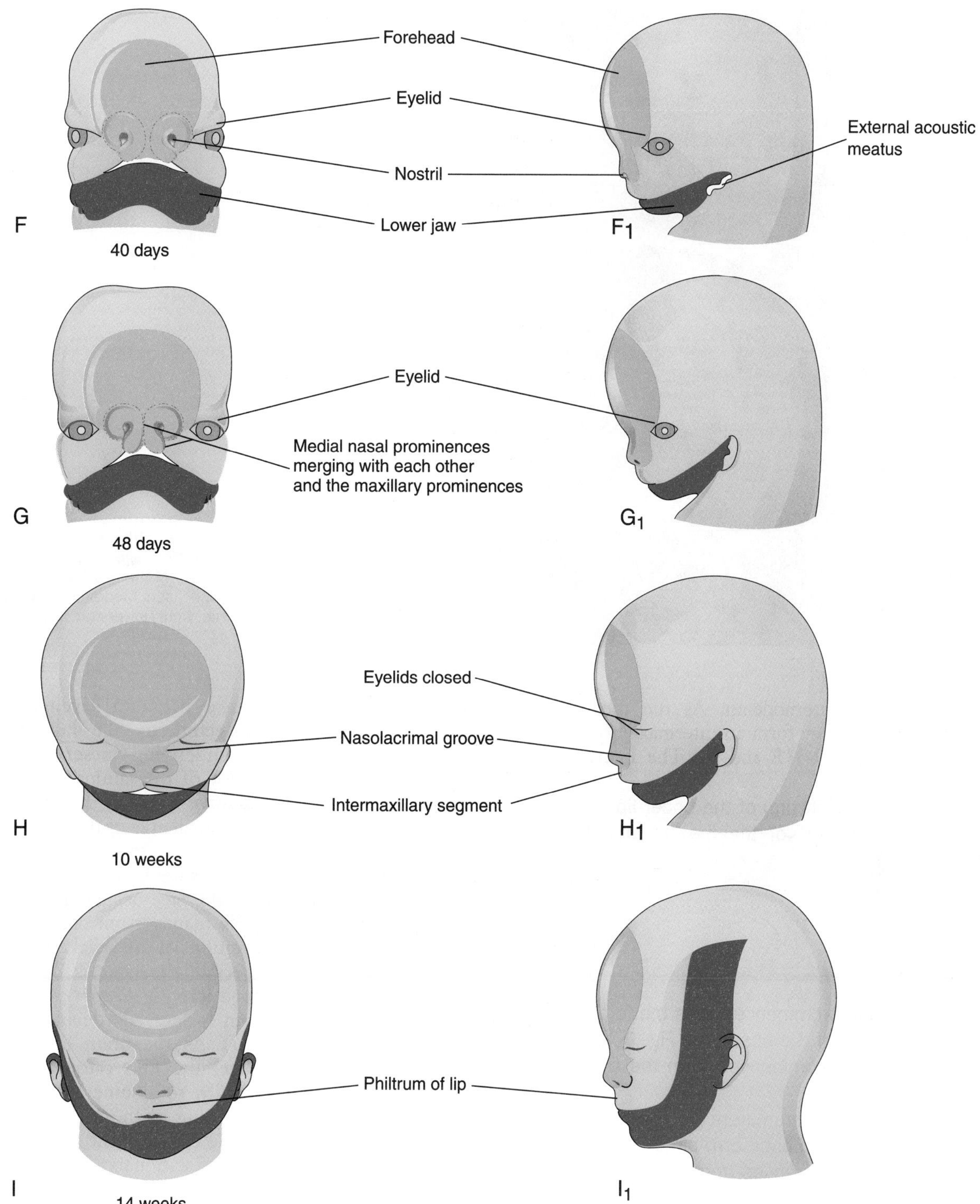

FIGURE 9-26, *CONT'D.*

groove. This thickening gives rise to a solid epithelial cord that separates from the ectoderm and sinks into the mesenchyme. Later, as a result of apoptosis, this epithelial cord canalizes to form a duct. The superior end of this duct expands to form the lacrimal sac. By the late fetal period, the nasolacrimal duct drains into the inferior meatus in the lateral wall of the nasal cavity. The duct usually becomes completely patent only after birth.

Between the 7th and 10th weeks, the medial nasal prominences merge with each other and with the maxillary and lateral nasal prominences (see Fig. 9-26*G* and *H*). Merging of these prominences requires disintegration of their contacting surface epithelia. This results in intermingling of the underlying mesenchymal cells. Merging of the medial nasal and maxillary prominences results in continuity of the upper jaw and lip and separation of the

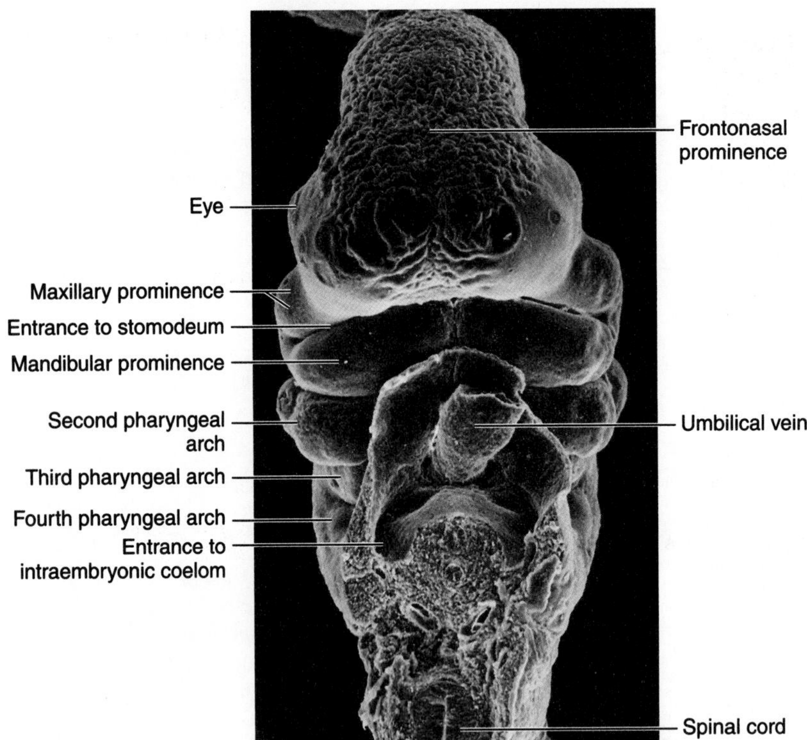

FIGURE 9-27. Scanning electron micrograph of a ventral view of a Carnegie stage 14 embryo (30–32 days). (Courtesy of the late Professor Emeritus Dr. K.V. Hinrichsen, Medizinische Fakultät, Institut für Anatomie, Ruhr-Universität Bochum, Bochum, Germany.)

nasal pits from the stomodeum. As the medial nasal prominences merge, they form an intermaxillary segment (see Figs. 9-26*H* and 9-33*E* and *F*). The intermaxillary segment gives rise to:

- The middle part (philtrum) of the upper lip
- The premaxillary part of the maxilla and its associated gingiva (gum)
- The primary palate

SUMMARY OF FACIAL DEVELOPMENT

- The frontal nasal prominence forms the forehead and dorsum and apex of the nose (see Fig. 9-26).
- The lateral nasal prominences form the alae (sides) of the nose.
- The medial nasal prominences form the nasal septum, ethmoid, and cribriform plate.
- The maxillary prominences form the upper cheek regions and the upper lip.
- The mandibular prominences give rise to the chin, lower lip, and lower cheek regions.

Recent clinical and embryologic studies indicate that the upper lip is formed entirely from the maxillary prominences. The lower parts of the medial nasal prominences appear to have become deeply positioned and covered by medial extensions of the maxillary prominences to form the philtrum.

In addition to connective tissue and muscular derivatives, various bones are derived from mesenchyme in the facial prominences. Until the end of the sixth week, the primordial jaws are composed of masses of mesenchymal tissue. The lips and gingivae begin to develop when a linear thickening of the ectoderm, the **labiogingival lamina**, grows into the underlying mesenchyme (see Fig. 9-37*B*). Gradually, most of the lamina degenerates, leaving a **labiogingival groove** between the lips and the gingivae (see Fig. 9-37*H*). A small area of the labiogingival lamina persists in the median plane to form the frenulum of the upper lip, which attaches the lip to the gingiva.

Further development of the face occurs slowly during the fetal period and results mainly from changes in the proportion and relative positions of the facial components. During the early fetal period, the nose is flat and the mandible is underdeveloped (see Fig. 9-26*H*); they obtain their characteristic form as facial development is completed (see Fig. 9-26*I*). As the brain enlarges, the cranial vault expands bilaterally. This causes the orbits, which were oriented laterally, to assume their forward-facing orientation. The opening of the external acoustic meatus (auditory canal) to the auricle of the ears appears to elevate, but in reality remains stationary. Rather, it is the elongation of the lower jaw that creates this impression. The smallness of the face prenatally results from:

- The rudimentary upper and lower jaws
- The unerupted primary (deciduous) teeth
- The small size of the nasal cavities and maxillary sinuses

DEVELOPMENT OF THE NASAL CAVITIES

As the face develops, the nasal placodes become depressed, forming **nasal pits** (see Figs. 9-28, 9-29, and 9-32). Proliferation of the surrounding mesenchyme forms the

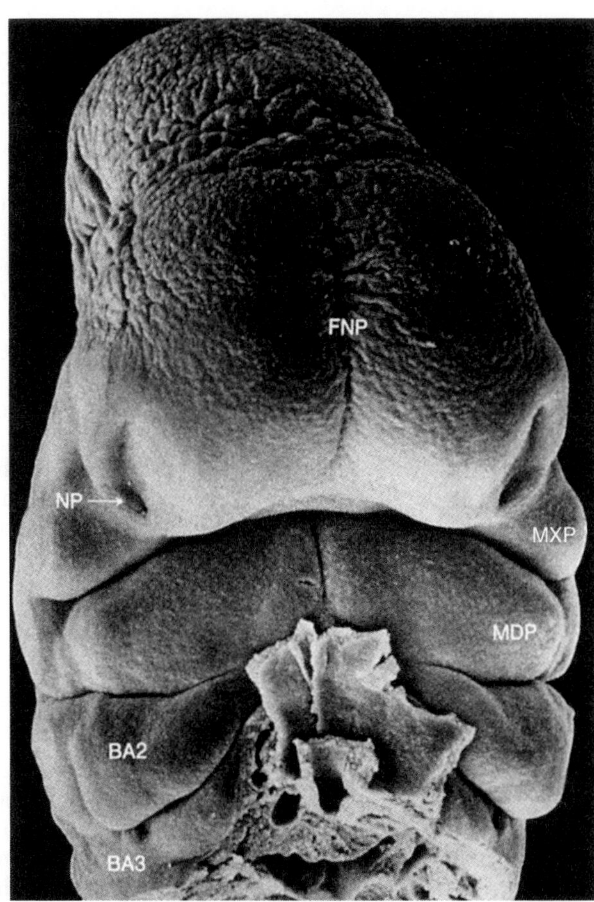

FIGURE 9-28. Scanning electron micrograph of a ventral view of a human embryo of approximately 33 days (Carnegie stage 15, crown-rump length 8 mm). Observe the prominent frontonasal process (FNP) surrounding the telencephalon (forebrain). Also observe the nasal pits (NP) located in the ventrolateral regions of the frontonasal prominence. Medial and lateral nasal prominences surround these pits. The maxillary prominences (MXP) form the lateral boundaries of the stomodeum. The fusing mandibular prominences (MDP) are located just caudal to the stomodeum. The second pharyngeal arch (BA2) is clearly visible and shows overhanging margins (opercula). The third pharyngeal arch (BA3) is also clearly visible. (From Hinrichsen K: The early development of morphology and patterns of the face in the human embryo. Adv Anat Embryol Cell Biol 98:1–79, 1985.)

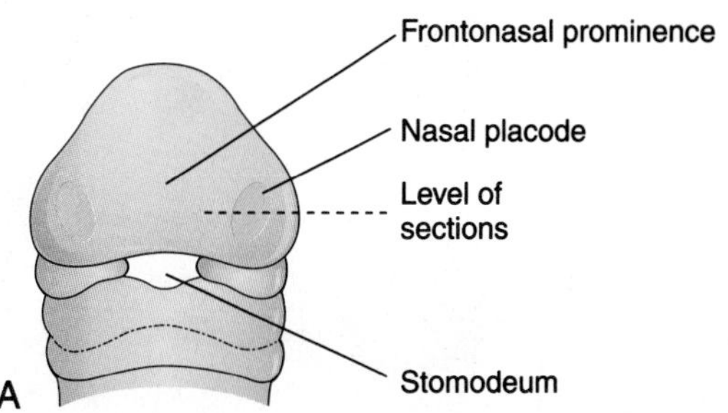

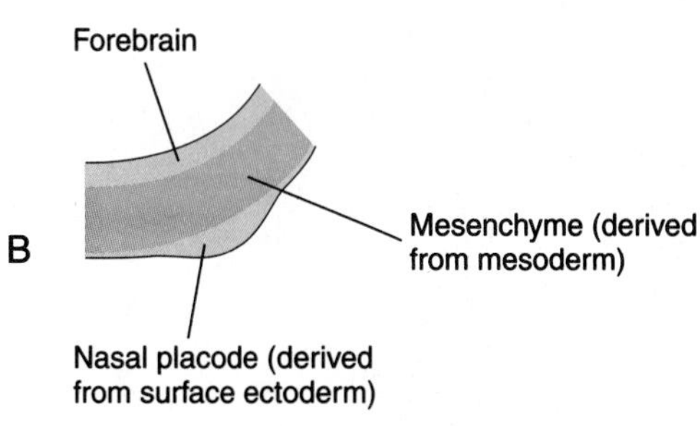

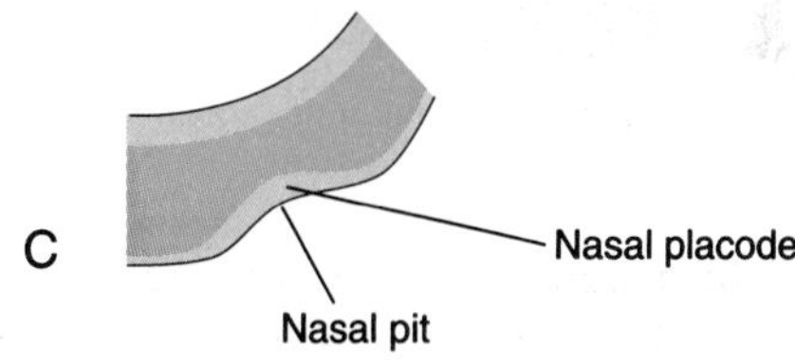

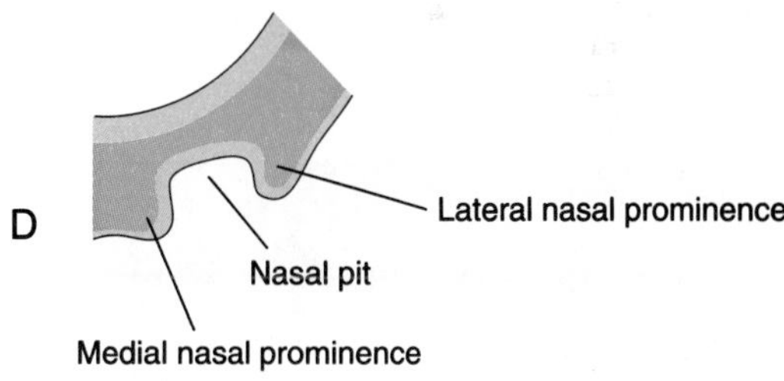

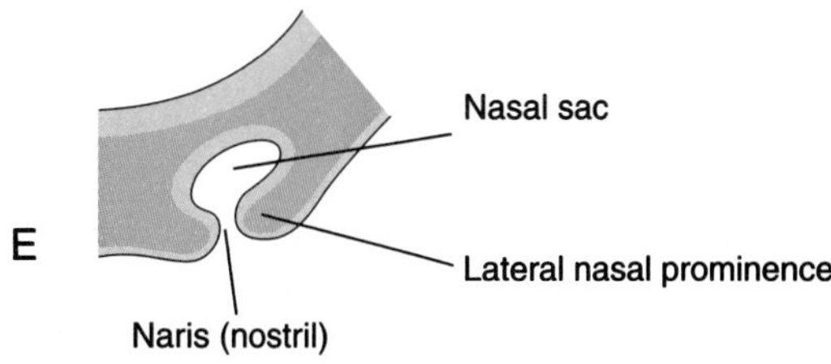

FIGURE 9-29. Progressive stages in the development of a human nasal sac (primordial nasal cavity). **A,** Ventral view of embryo of approximately 28 days. **B** to **E,** Transverse sections through the left side of the developing nasal sac.

medial and lateral nasal prominences, which results in deepening of the nasal pits and formation of primordial **nasal sacs**. Each nasal sac grows dorsally, ventral to the developing forebrain (Fig. 9-34*A*). At first, the nasal sacs are separated from the oral cavity by the **oronasal membrane**. This membrane ruptures by the end of the sixth week, bringing the nasal and oral cavities into communication (see Fig. 9-34*C*). Temporary epithelial plugs are formed in the nasal cavities from proliferation of the cells lining them. Between 13 to 15 weeks, the nasal plugs disappear.

The regions of continuity between the nasal and oral cavities are the **primordial choanae**, which lie posterior to the primary palate. After the secondary palate develops, the choanae are located at the junction of the nasal cavity and pharynx (see Figs. 9-34*D* and 9-37). While these changes are occurring, the superior, middle, and inferior

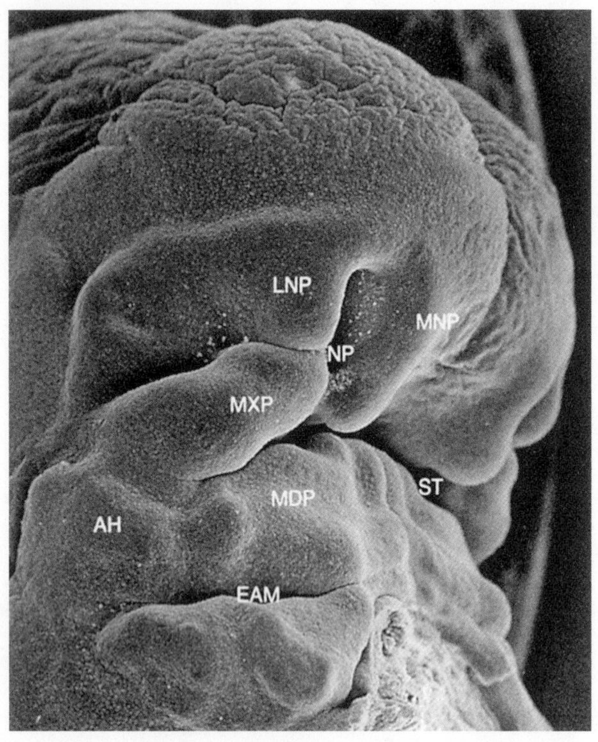

FIGURE 9-30. Scanning electron micrograph of the craniofacial region of a human embryo of approximately 41 days (Carnegie stage 16, crown-rump length 10.8 mm) viewed obliquely. The maxillary prominence (MXP) appears puffed up laterally and wedged between the lateral (LNP) and medial (MNP) nasal prominences surrounding the nasal pit (NP). The auricular hillocks (AH) can be seen on both sides of the pharyngeal groove between the first and second arches, which will form the external acoustic meatus (EAM). MDP, mandibular prominence; ST, stomodeum. (From Hinrichsen K: The early development of morphology and patterns of the face in the human embryo. Adv Anat Embryol Cell Biol 98:1–79, 1985.)

nasal conchae develop as elevations of the lateral walls of the nasal cavities (see Fig. 9-34*D*). Concurrently, the ectodermal epithelium in the roof of each nasal cavity becomes specialized to form the **olfactory epithelium**. Some epithelial cells differentiate into olfactory receptor cells (neurons). The axons of these cells constitute the **olfactory nerves**, which grow into the **olfactory bulbs** of the brain (see Fig. 9-34*C* and *D*).

Most of the upper lip, maxilla, and secondary palate form from the maxillary prominences (see Fig. 9-26*H*). These prominences merge laterally with the mandibular prominences. The primordial lips and cheeks are invaded by mesenchyme from the second pair of pharyngeal arches, which differentiates into the facial muscles (see Fig. 9-6, Table 9-1). These muscles of facial expression are supplied by the facial nerve (CN VII), the nerve of the second pharyngeal arch. The mesenchyme in the first pair of arches differentiates into the muscles of mastication and a few others, all of which are innervated by the trigeminal nerves (CN V), which supply the first pair of pharyngeal arches.

Paranasal Sinuses

Some paranasal sinuses begin to develop during late fetal life, such as the **maxillary sinuses**; the remainder of them develop after birth. They form from outgrowths or diverticula of the walls of the nasal cavities and become pneumatic (air-filled) extensions of the nasal cavities in the adjacent bones, such as the maxillary sinuses in the maxillae and the **frontal sinuses** in the frontal bones. The original openings of the diverticula persist as the orifices of the adult sinuses.

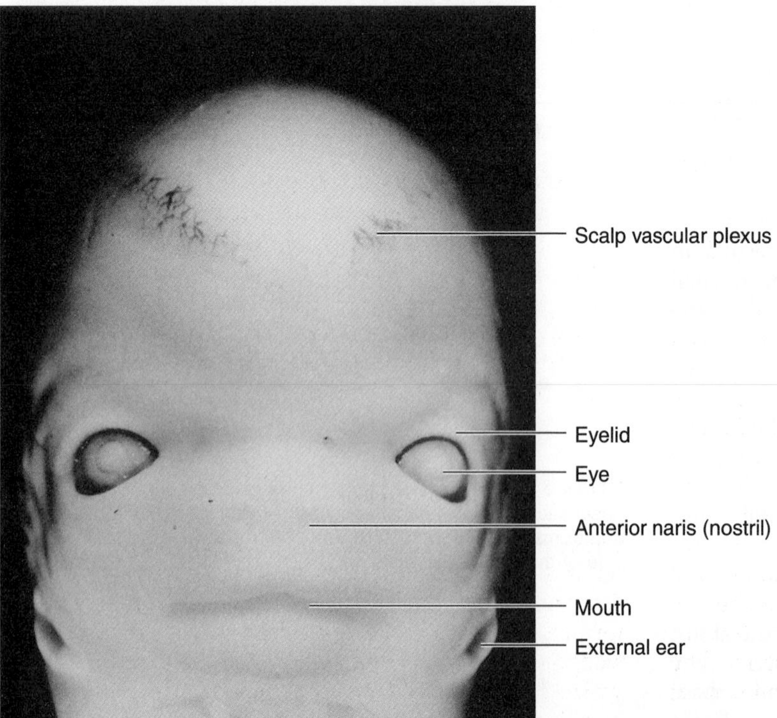

FIGURE 9-31. Ventral view of the face of an embryo at Carnegie stage 22, approximately 54 days. Observe that the eyes are widely separated and the ears are low-set at this stage. (From Nishimura H, Semba R, Tanimura T, Tanaka O: Prenatal Development of the Human with Special Reference to Craniofacial Structures: An Atlas. Bethesda, MD, U.S. Department of Health, Education, and Welfare, NIH, 1977.)

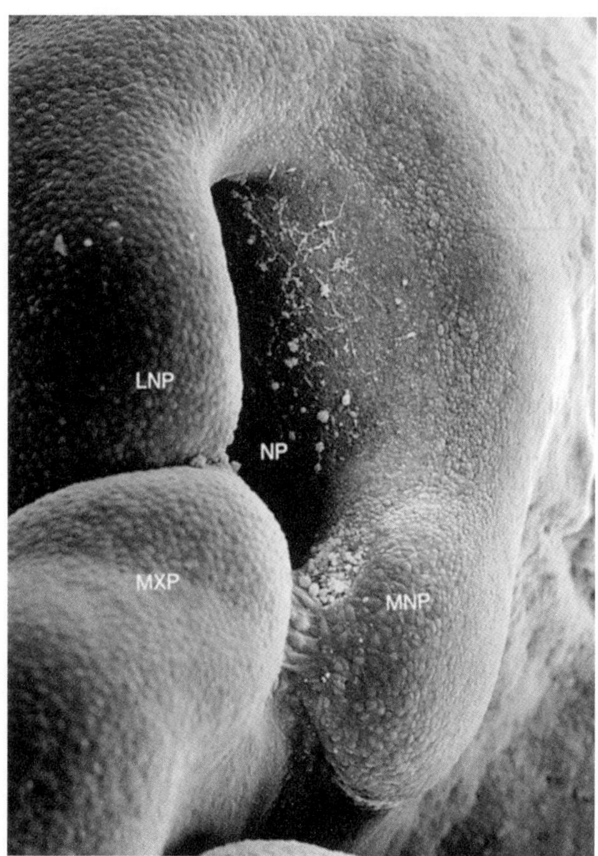

FIGURE 9-32. Scanning electron micrograph of the right nasal region of a human embryo of approximately 41 days (Carnegie stage 17, crown-rump length 10.8 mm) showing the maxillary prominence (MXP) fusing with the medial nasal prominence (MNP). Observe the large nasal pit (NP). Epithelial bridges can be seen between these prominences. Observe the furrow representing the nasolacrimal groove between the MXP and the lateral nasal prominence (LNP). (From Hinrichsen K: The early development of morphology and patterns of the face in the human embryo. Adv Anat Embryol Cell Biol 98:1–79, 1985.)

The first appearance of the **vomeronasal primordia** is in the form of bilateral epithelial thickenings on the nasal septum. Further invagination of the primordia and their breaking away from the nasal septal epithelium gives rise to a tubular **vomeronasal organ** ([VNO] of Jacobson) between days 37 and 43. This chemosensory structure, which ends blindly posteriorly, reaches its greatest development between 12 and 14 weeks. Later, a gradual replacement of the receptor population with patchy ciliated cells occurs. The VNO is consistently present in the form of a bilateral ductlike structure on the nasal septum, superior to the paraseptal cartilage (Fig. 9-35), at all ages. A paraseptal cartilage develops inferior to the VNO. The tubular human VNO with its minute anterior opening and the paraseptal cartilage are true homologs of the VNO in other animals. In other mammals, reptiles (snakes in particular), and amphibians, VNOs are lined by chemosensory epithelium similar to the olfactory epithelium, except that the VNO chemoreceptors lack cilia. A distinct VNO projects to the accessory olfactory bulb with connections to amygdala and other limbic centers. The vomeronasal nerves, accessory olfactory bulb, and central connections are lacking in humans.

Postnatal Development of Paranasal Sinuses

Most of the paranasal sinuses are rudimentary or absent in newborn infants. The maxillary sinuses are small at birth (3–4 mm in diameter). These sinuses grow slowly until puberty and are not fully developed until all the permanent teeth have erupted in early adulthood. No frontal or sphenoidal sinuses are present at birth. The ethmoidal cells are small before the age of 2 years and do not begin to grow rapidly until 6 to 8 years of age. At approximately 2 years of age, the two most anterior ethmoidal cells grow into the frontal bone, forming a frontal sinus on each side. Usually the frontal sinuses are visible in radiographs by the seventh year. The two most posterior ethmoidal cells grow into the sphenoid bone at approximately 2 years of age, forming two sphenoidal sinuses. Growth of the paranasal sinuses is important in altering the size and shape of the face during infancy and childhood and in adding resonance to the voice during adolescence.

Remnants of the Vomeronasal Organ

Well-developed VNOs are chemoreceptive sensory structures that are present on the nasal septum of amphibians, reptiles, and mammals. Recent studies have conclusively shown that VNOs appear in the human embryo and are present throughout life as intermittently ciliated, mucus-carrying ducts with a microscopic opening in the nasal septum. VNOs are well developed in animals serving as accessory chemoreceptor organs of importance in reproduction and feeding behavior.

DEVELOPMENT OF THE PALATE

The palate develops in two stages:

- The development of a primary palate
- The development of a secondary palate

Palatogenesis begins in the sixth week; however, development of the palate is not completed until the 12th week. The critical period of palate development is from the end of the sixth week until the beginning of the ninth week.

Primary Palate

Early in the sixth week, the primary palate—**median palatal process** (intermaxillary segment)—begins to develop (see Figs. 9-33*F* and 9-34). Initially, this segment, formed by merging of the medial nasal prominences, is a wedge-shaped mass of mesenchyme between the internal surfaces of the maxillary prominences of the developing maxillae. The primary palate forms the anterior/midline

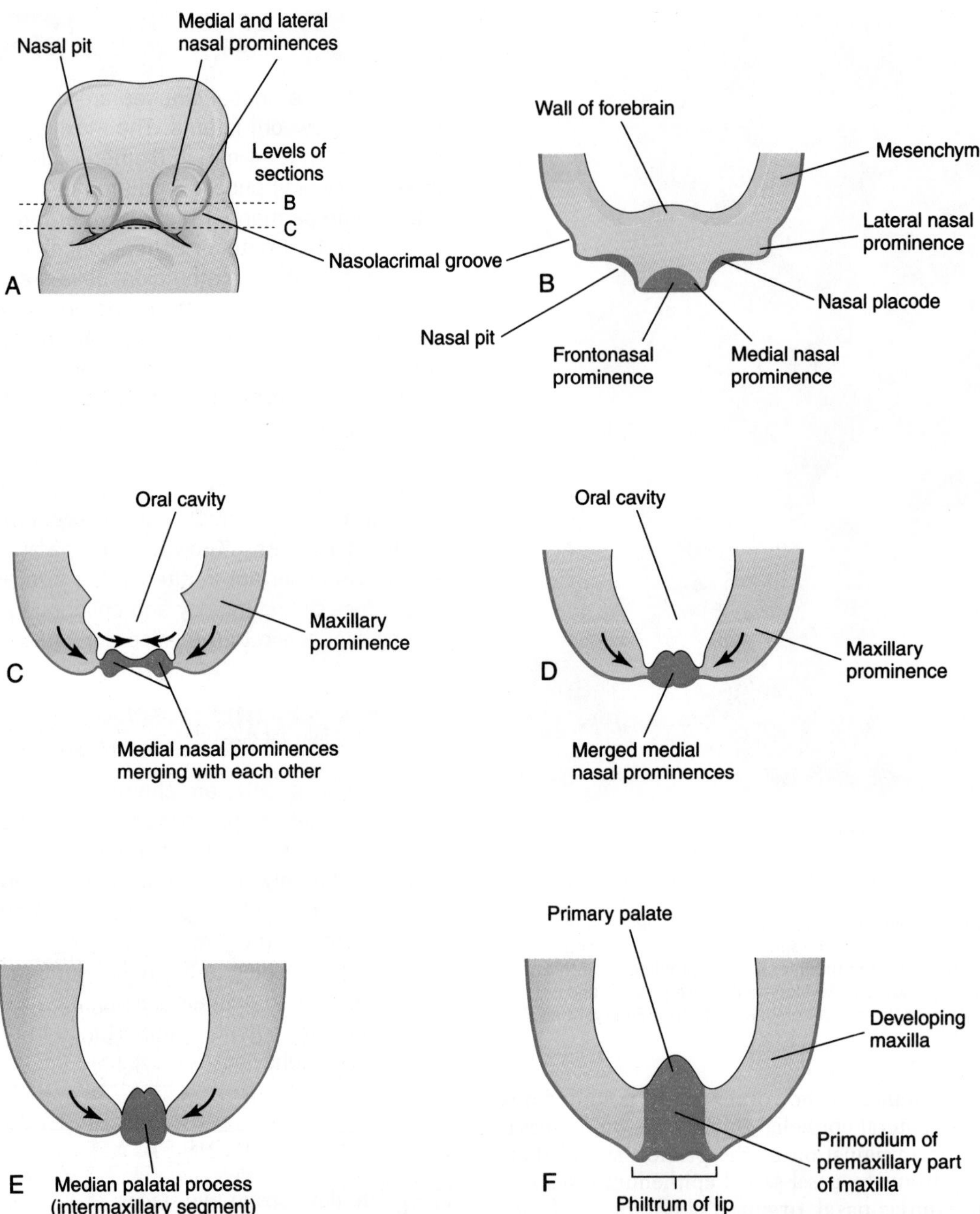

FIGURE 9-33. Early development of the maxilla, palate, and upper lip. **A,** Facial view of a 5-week embryo. **B** and **C,** Sketches of horizontal sections at the levels shown in **A**. The *arrows* in **C** indicate subsequent growth of the maxillary and medial nasal prominences toward the median plane and merging of the prominences with each other. **D** to **F,** Similar sections of older embryos illustrating merging of the medial nasal prominences with each other and the maxillary prominences to form the upper lip. Recent studies suggest that the upper lip is formed entirely from the maxillary prominences.

aspect of the maxilla, the premaxillary part of the maxilla. (Fig. 9-36). It represents only a small part of the adult hard palate (i.e., anterior to the incisive fossa).

Secondary Palate

The secondary palate is the primordium of the hard and soft parts of the palate (see Fig. 9-36). The secondary palate begins to develop early in the sixth week from two mesenchymal projections that extend from the internal aspects of the maxillary prominences. Initially these structures—the lateral palatal processes (shelves)—project inferomedially on each side of the tongue (Figs. 9-37*B* and 9-38*A* and *B*). As the jaws elongate, they pull the tongue away from its root, and, as a result, it is brought lower in the mouth. During the seventh and eighth weeks, the **lateral palatal processes** assume a horizontal position above the tongue (see Figs. 9-37*E* to *H* and 9-38*C*). This change in orientation occurs by a flowing process facilitated in part by the release of hyaluronic acid by the mesenchyme of the palatal processes.

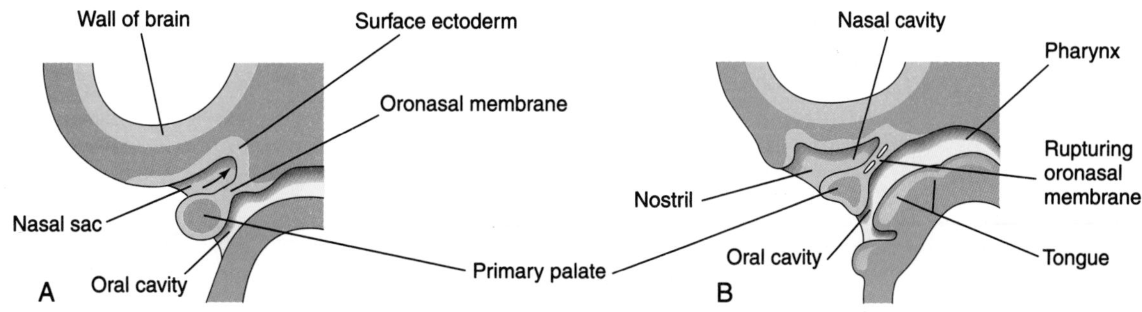

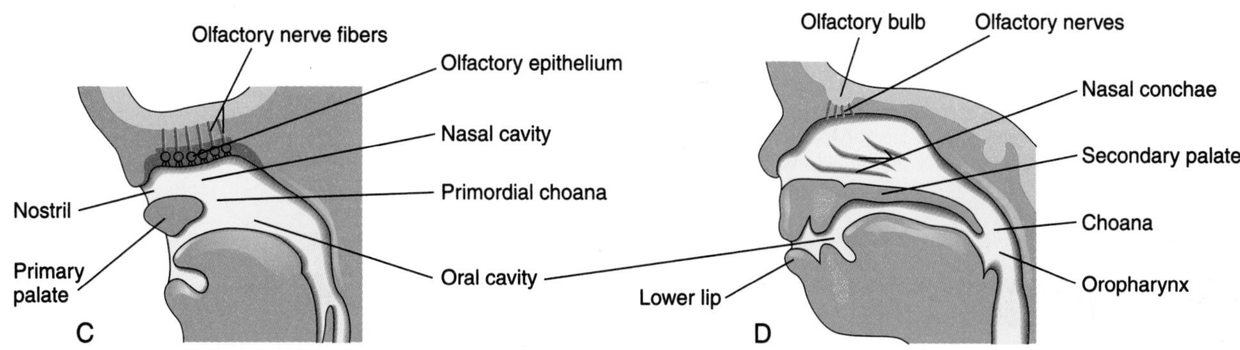

FIGURE 9-34. Sagittal sections of the head showing development of the nasal cavities. The nasal septum has been removed. **A,** 5 weeks. **B,** 6 weeks, showing breakdown of the oronasal membrane. **C,** 7 weeks, showing the nasal cavity communicating with the oral cavity and development of the olfactory epithelium. **D,** 12 weeks, showing the palate and the lateral wall of the nasal cavity.

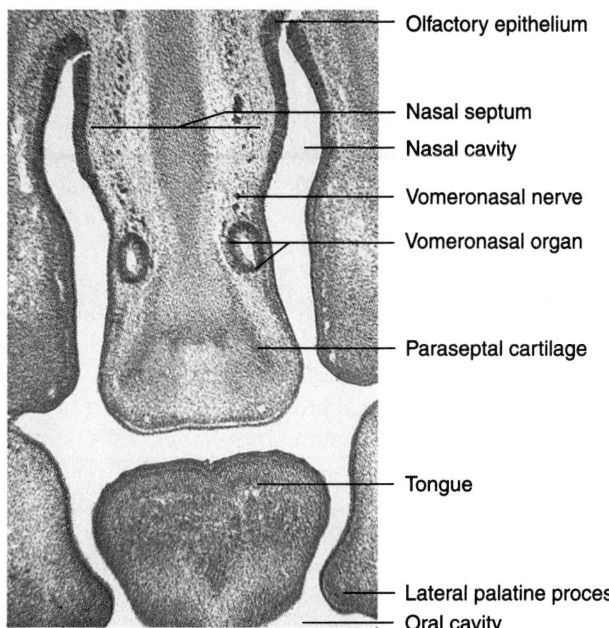

FIGURE 9-35. Photomicrograph of a frontal section through the developing oral cavity and nasal regions of a 22-mm human embryo of approximately 54 days. Observe the bilateral, tubular vomeronasal organ. (Courtesy of Dr. Kunwar Bhatnagar, Department of Anatomical Sciences and Neurobiology, School of Medicine, University of Louisville, Louisville, KY.)

Bone gradually develops in the primary palate, forming the premaxillary part of the maxilla, which lodges the incisor teeth (see Fig. 9-36*B*). Concurrently, bone extends from the maxillae and palatine bones into palatal processes to form the **hard palate** (see Fig. 9-37*E* and *G*). The posterior parts of these processes do not become ossified. They extend posteriorly beyond the nasal septum and fuse to form the **soft palate**, including its soft conical projection—the **uvula** (see Fig. 9-37*D*, *F*, and *H*). The median palatine raphe indicates the line of fusion of the palatal processes.

A small **nasopalatine canal** persists in the median plane of the palate between the anterior part of the maxilla and the palatal processes of the maxillae. This canal is represented in the adult hard palate by the **incisive fossa** (see Fig. 9-36*B*), which is the common opening for the small right and left incisive canals. An irregular suture runs on each side from the incisive fossa to the alveolar process of the maxilla, between the lateral incisor and canine teeth on each side (Fig. 9-36*B*). It is visible in the anterior region of the palates of young persons. This suture indicates where the embryonic primary and secondary palates fused.

The **nasal septum** develops as a downgrowth from internal parts of the merged medial nasal prominences (see Figs. 9-37 and 9-38). The fusion between the nasal septum and the palatal processes begins anteriorly during the ninth week and is completed posteriorly by the 12th week, superior to the primordium of the hard palate.

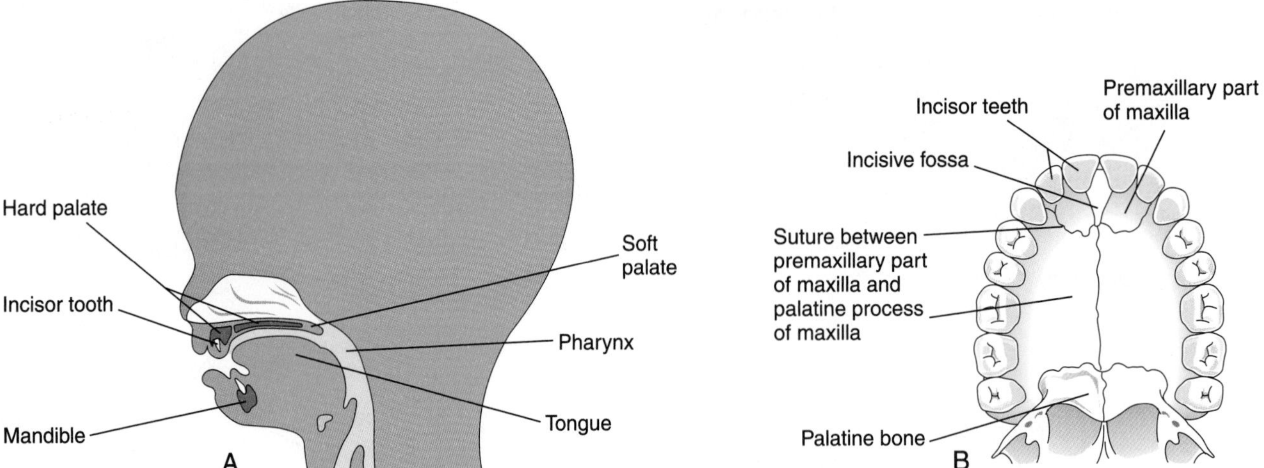

FIGURE 9-36. **A,** Sagittal section of the head of 20-week fetus illustrating the location of the palate. **B,** The bony palate and alveolar arch of a young adult. The suture between the premaxillary part of the maxilla and the fused palatal processes of the maxillae is usually visible in crania (skulls) of young persons. It is not visible in the hard palates of most dried crania because they are usually from old adults.

CLEFT LIP AND CLEFT PALATE

Clefts of the lip and palate are the most common craniofacial anomalies. The defects are usually classified according to developmental criteria, with the incisive fossa as a reference landmark. These clefts are especially conspicuous because they result in an abnormal facial appearance and defective speech. There are two major groups of cleft lip and cleft palate (Figs. 9-39 to 9-41):

Anterior cleft anomalies include cleft lip, with or without cleft of the alveolar part of the maxilla. A complete anterior cleft anomaly is one in which the cleft extends through the lip and alveolar part of the maxilla to the incisive fossa, separating the anterior and posterior parts of the palate (see Fig. 9-40*E* and *F*). Anterior cleft anomalies result from a deficiency of mesenchyme in the maxillary prominence(s) and the median palatal process (see Fig. 9-33*E*).

Posterior cleft anomalies include clefts of the secondary palate that extend through the soft and hard regions of the palate to the incisive fossa, separating the anterior and posterior parts of the palate (see Fig. 9-40*G* and *H*). Posterior cleft anomalies result from defective development of the secondary palate and growth distortions of the lateral palatal processes, which prevent their fusion. In addition, other factors such as width of the stomodeum, mobility of the shelves, and altered focal degeneration sites of the palatal epithelium may also contribute to these anomalies.

A cleft lip, with or without a cleft palate, occurs approximately once in 1000 births; however, the frequency varies widely among ethnic groups; 60% to 80% of affected infants are males. The clefts vary from small notches of the vermilion border of the lip to larger ones that extend into the floor of the nostril and through the alveolar part of the maxilla (see Figs. 9-39 and 9-41*A* and *B*). Cleft lip can be unilateral or bilateral.

A **unilateral cleft of the upper lip** (Figs. 9-39, 9-41*A*, and 9-42) results from failure of the maxillary prominence on the affected side to unite with the merged medial nasal prominences. This is the consequence of failure of the mesenchymal masses to merge and the mesenchyme to proliferate and smooth out the overlying epithelium. This results in a *persistent labial groove* (Fig. 9-43*D*). In addition, the epithelium in the labial groove becomes stretched and the tissues in the floor of the groove break down. As a result, the lip is divided into medial and lateral parts (see Fig. 9-43*G* and *H*). Sometimes a bridge of tissue, *Simonart band*, joins the parts of the incomplete cleft lip.

A **bilateral cleft lip** (Figs. 9-41*B* and 9-44*C* and *D*) results from failure of the mesenchymal masses in both maxillary prominences to meet and unite with the merged medial nasal prominences. The epithelium in both labial grooves becomes stretched and breaks down. In bilateral cases, the defects may be dissimilar, with varying degrees of defect on each side. When there is a complete bilateral cleft of the lip and alveolar part of the maxilla, the medial palatal process hangs free and projects anteriorly. These defects are especially deforming because of the loss of continuity of the orbicularis oris muscle, which closes the mouth and purses the lips.

A median cleft of the upper lip is an extremely rare defect that results from a mesenchymal deficiency. This defect causes partial or complete

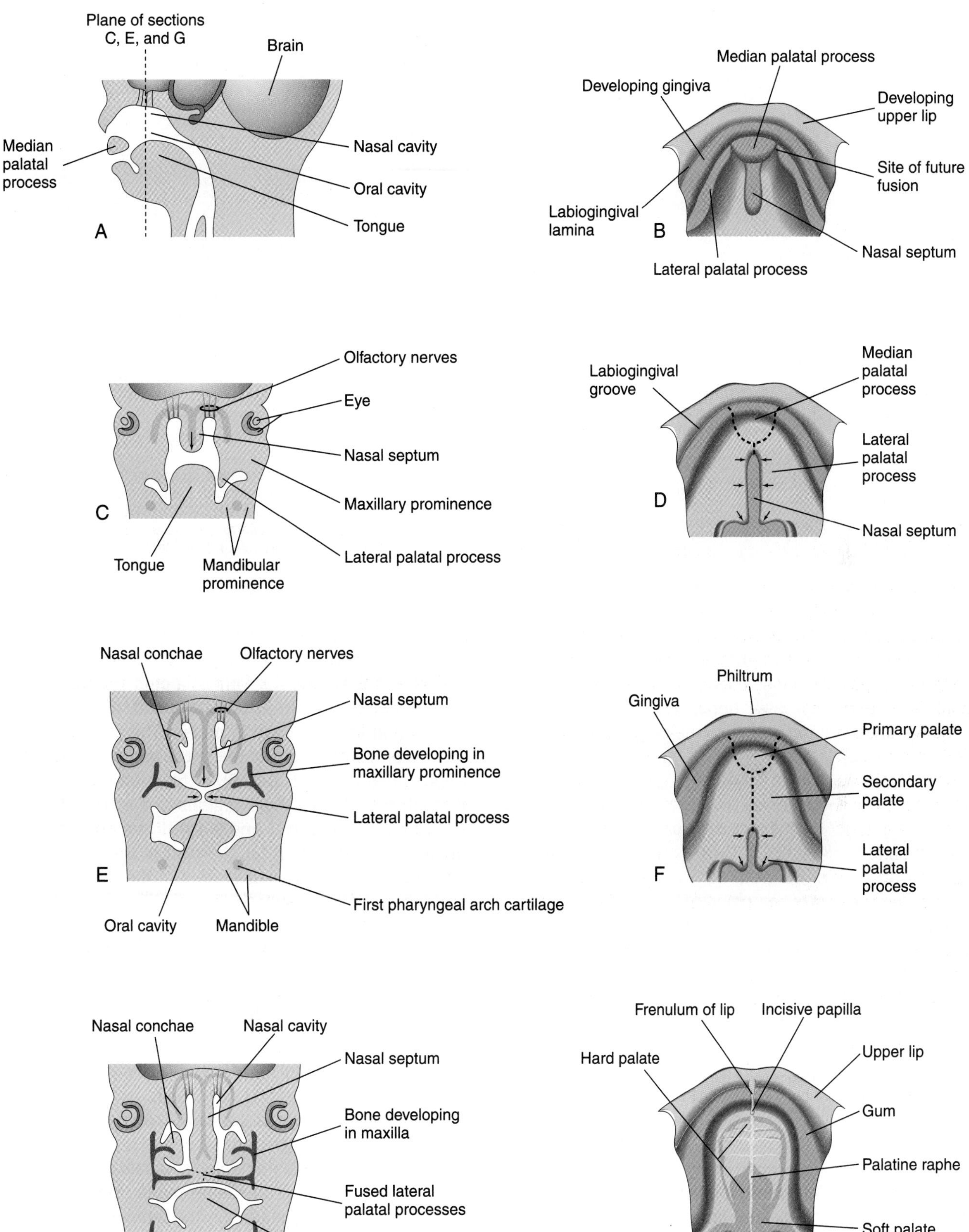

FIGURE 9-37. **A,** Sagittal section of the embryonic head at the end of the sixth week showing the median palatal process. **B, D, F,** and **H,** Roof of the mouth from the 6th to 12th weeks illustrating the development of the palate. The *broken lines* in **D** and **F** indicate sites of fusion of the palatal processes. The *arrows* indicate medial and posterior growth of the lateral palatal processes. **C, E,** and **G,** Frontal sections of the head illustrating fusion of the lateral palatal processes with each other and the nasal septum and separation of the nasal and oral cavities.

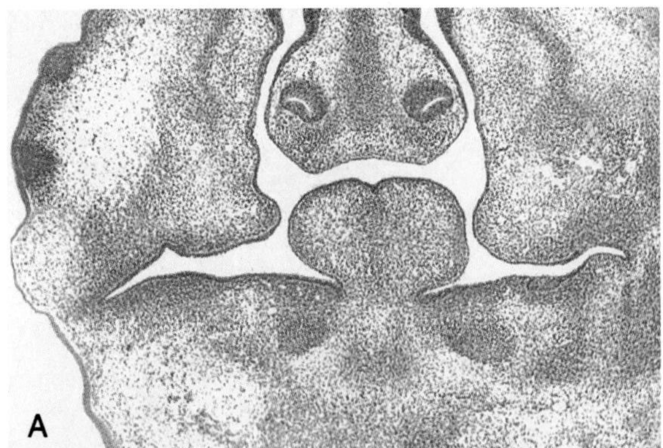

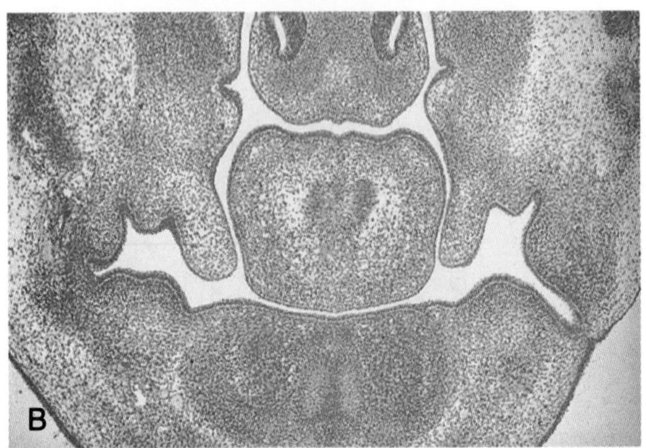

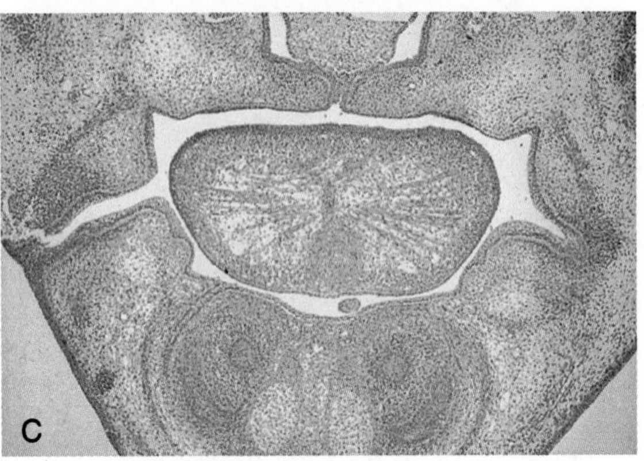

FIGURE 9-38. Frontal sections of human embryonic heads showing palatal process development during the eighth week. **A,** Embryo with a crown-rump length (CRL) of 24 mm. This section shows early development of the palatal processes. **B,** Embryo with a CRL of 27 mm. This section shows the palate just before palatal process elevation. **C,** Embryo with a CRL of 29 mm (near the end of the eighth week). The palatal processes are elevated and fused. (From Sandham A: Embryonic facial vertical dimension and its relationship to palatal shelf elevation. Early Hum Dev 12:241, 1985.)

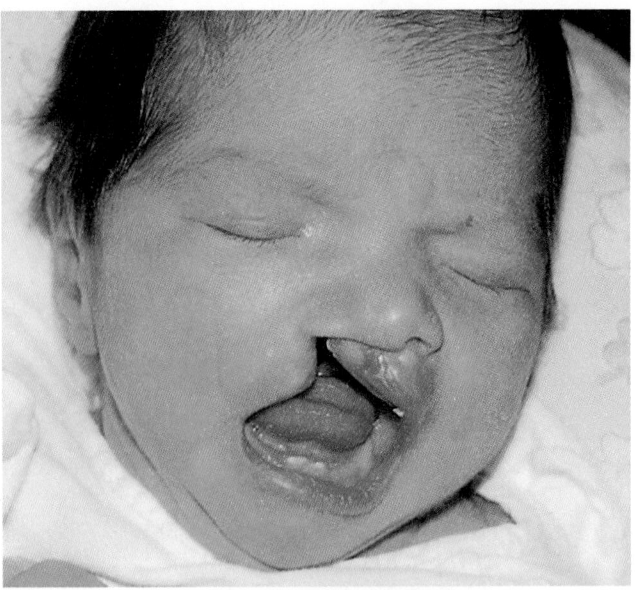

FIGURE 9-39. Infant with unilateral cleft lip and cleft palate. Clefts of the lip, with or without cleft palate, occur approximately once in 1000 births; most affected infants are males. (Courtesy of A.E. Chudley, Section of Genetics and Metabolism; Department of Pediatrics and Child Health, Children's Hospital, Winnipeg, Manitoba, Canada.)

failure of the medial nasal prominences to merge and form the median palatal process. A median cleft of the upper lip is a characteristic feature of the Mohr syndrome, which is transmitted as an autosomal recessive trait.

A median cleft of the lower lip is also very rare and results from failure of the mesenchymal masses in the mandibular prominences to merge completely and smooth out the embryonic cleft between them (see Fig. 9-26*A*)

A **cleft palate**, with or without a cleft lip, occurs approximately once in 2500 births and is more common in females than in males. The cleft may involve only the uvula; a cleft uvula has a fishtail appearance (see Fig. 9-40*B*), or the cleft may extend through the soft and hard regions of the palate (see Figs. 9-40*C* and *D* and 9-44). In severe cases associated with a cleft lip, the cleft in the palate extends through the alveolar part of the maxilla and the lips on both sides (see Figs. 9-40*G* and *H* and 9-41*B*).

A **complete cleft palate** indicates the maximum degree of clefting of any particular type; for example, a complete cleft of the posterior palate is an anomaly in which the cleft extends through the soft palate and anteriorly to the incisive fossa. The landmark for distinguishing anterior from posterior cleft anomalies is the incisive fossa.

Unilateral and bilateral clefts of the palate are classified into three groups:

- *Clefts of the primary or anterior palate* (i.e., clefts anterior to the incisive fossa) result from failure of mesenchymal masses in the lateral palatal processes to meet and fuse with the mesenchyme in the primary palate (see Fig. 9-40*E* and *F*).
- *Clefts of the secondary or posterior palate* (i.e., clefts posterior to the incisive fossa) result from failure of mesenchymal masses in the lateral palatal processes to meet and fuse with each

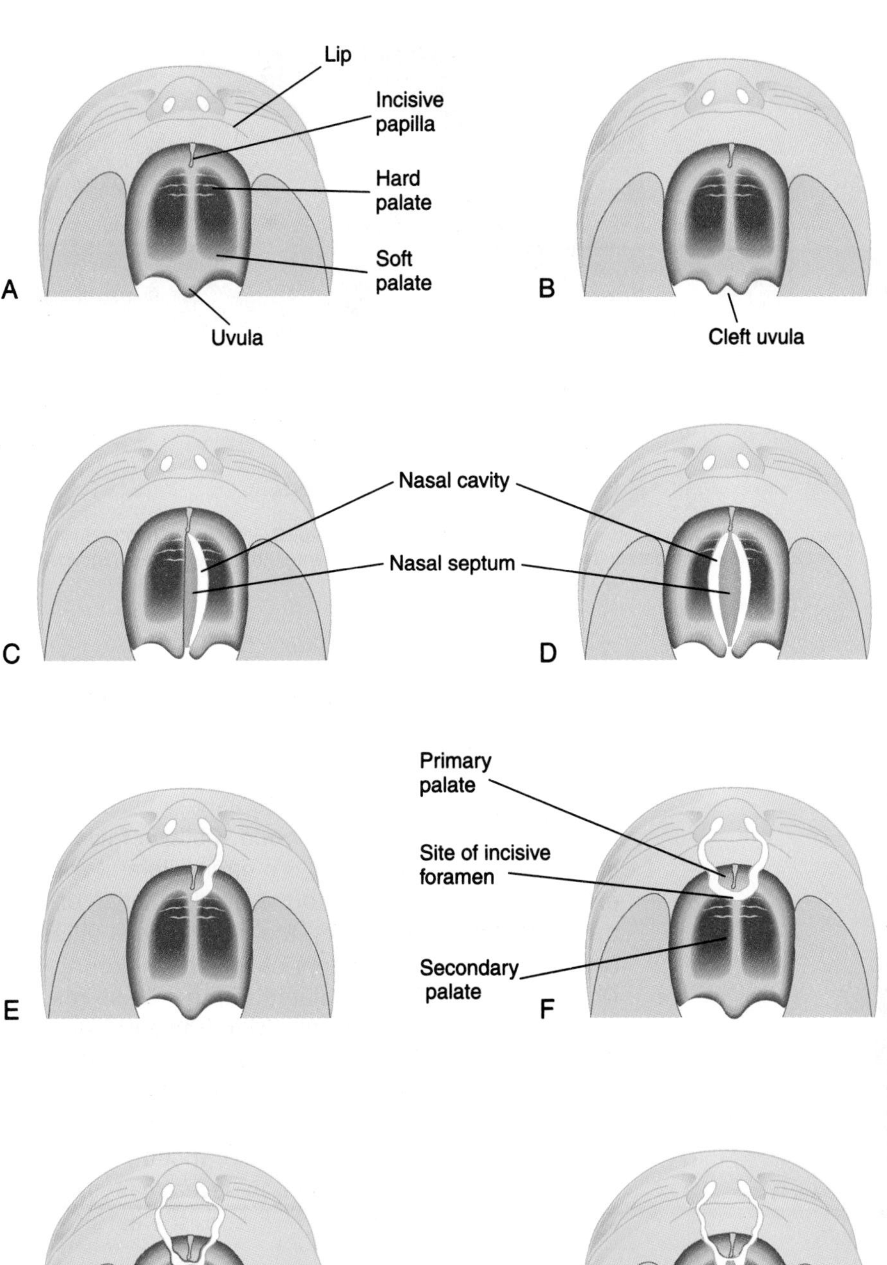

FIGURE 9-40. Various types of cleft lip and palate. **A,** Normal lip and palate. **B,** Cleft uvula. **C,** Unilateral cleft of the secondary (posterior) palate. **D,** Bilateral cleft of the posterior part of the palate. **E,** Complete unilateral cleft of the lip and alveolar process of the maxilla with a unilateral cleft of the primary (anterior) palate. **F,** Complete bilateral cleft of the lip and alveolar processes of the maxillae with bilateral cleft of the anterior part of the palate. **G,** Complete bilateral cleft of the lip and alveolar processes of the maxillae with bilateral cleft of the anterior part of the palate and unilateral cleft of the posterior part of the palate. **H,** Complete bilateral cleft of the lip and alveolar processes of the maxillae with complete bilateral cleft of the anterior and posterior palate.

other and the nasal septum (see Fig. 9-40*B*, *C*, and *D*).

- *Clefts of the primary and secondary parts of the palate* (i.e., clefts of the anterior and posterior palates) result from failure of the mesenchymal masses in the lateral palatal processes to meet and fuse with mesenchyme in the primary palate, with each other, and the nasal septum (see Figs. 9-4 and 9-40*G* and *H*).

Most clefts of the lip and palate result from multiple factors (*multifactorial inheritance*; see Chapter 20): genetic and nongenetic, each causing a minor developmental disturbance. How teratogenic factors induce cleft lip and palate is still unclear.

Some clefts of the lip and/or palate appear as part of syndromes determined by single mutant genes. Other clefts are parts of chromosomal syndromes, especially **trisomy 13** (see Chapter 20). A few cases of cleft lip and/or palate appear to have been caused by teratogenic agents (e.g., anticonvulsant drugs). Studies of twins indicate that genetic factors are of more importance in a cleft lip,

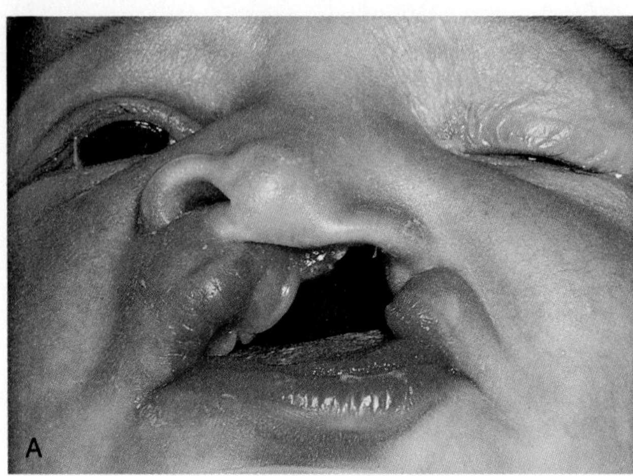

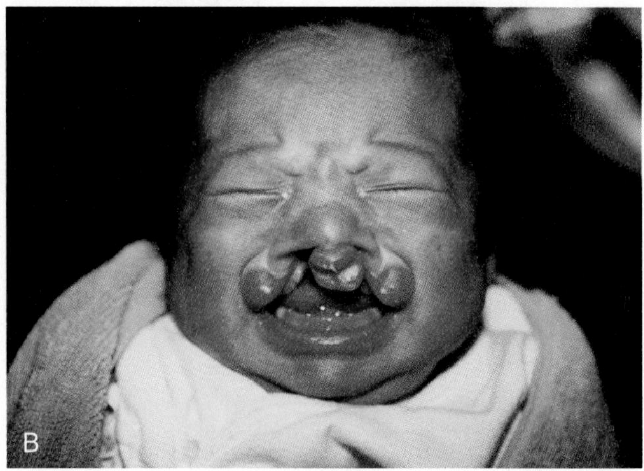

FIGURE 9-41. Congenital anomalies of the lip and palate. **A,** Infant with a left unilateral cleft lip and cleft palate. **B,** Infant with bilateral cleft lip and cleft palate. (Courtesy of Dr. Barry H. Grayson and Dr. Bruno L. Vendittelli, New York University Medical Center, Institute of Reconstructive Plastic Surgery, New York, NY.)

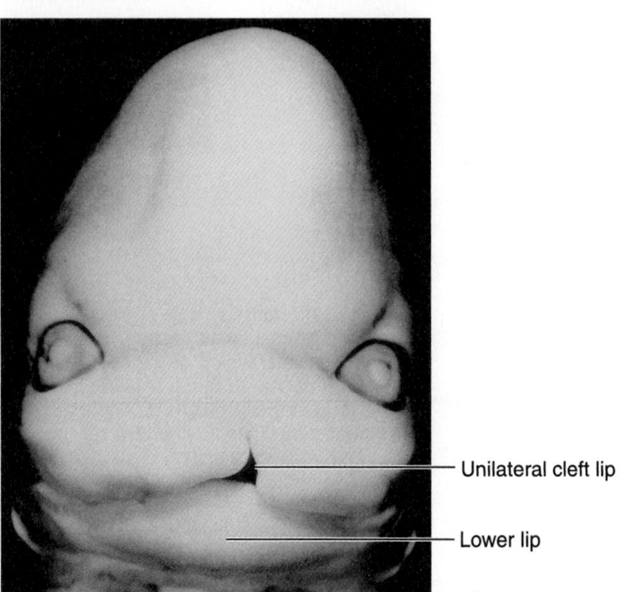

FIGURE 9-42. Ventral view of the face of an embryo at Carnegie stage 20 (approximately 51 days) with a unilateral cleft lip. (From Nishimura H, Semba R, Tanimura T, Tanaka O: Prenatal Development of the Human with Special Reference to Craniofacial Structures: An Atlas. Bethesda, MD, U.S. Department of Health, Education, and Welfare, NIH, 1977.)

with or without a cleft palate, than in a cleft palate alone. A sibling of a child with a cleft palate has an elevated risk of having a cleft palate, but no increased risk of having a cleft lip. A cleft of the lip and alveolar process of the maxilla that continues through the palate is usually transmitted through a male sex-linked gene. When neither parent is affected, the recurrence risk in subsequent siblings (brother or sister) is approximately 4%. The fact that the palatal processes fuse approximately a week later in females may explain why isolated cleft palate is more common in females than in males.

FACIAL CLEFTS

Various types of facial clefts occur, but they are all extremely rare. Severe clefts are usually associated with gross anomalies of the head. **Oblique facial clefts** (orbitofacial fissures) are often bilateral and extend from the upper lip to the medial margin of the orbit. When this occurs, the nasolacrimal ducts are open grooves (persistent nasolacrimal grooves). Oblique facial clefts associated with a cleft lip result from failure of the mesenchymal masses in the maxillary prominences to merge with the lateral and medial nasal prominences. Lateral or transverse facial clefts run from the mouth toward the ear. Bilateral clefts result in a very large mouth, a condition called **macrostomia**. In severe cases, the clefts in the cheeks extend almost to the ears.

OTHER FACIAL ANOMALIES

Congenital microstomia (small mouth) results from excessive merging of the mesenchymal masses in the maxillary and mandibular prominences of the first pharyngeal arch. In severe cases, the abnormality may be associated with underdevelopment (hypoplasia) of the mandible. Absence of the nose occurs when no nasal placodes form. A **single nostril** results when only one nasal placode forms. A **bifid nose** results when the medial nasal prominences do not merge completely; the nostrils are widely separated, and the nasal bridge is bifid. In mild forms of bifid nose, there is a groove in the tip of the nose.

By the beginning of the second trimester (see Fig. 9-26), features of the fetal face can be identified

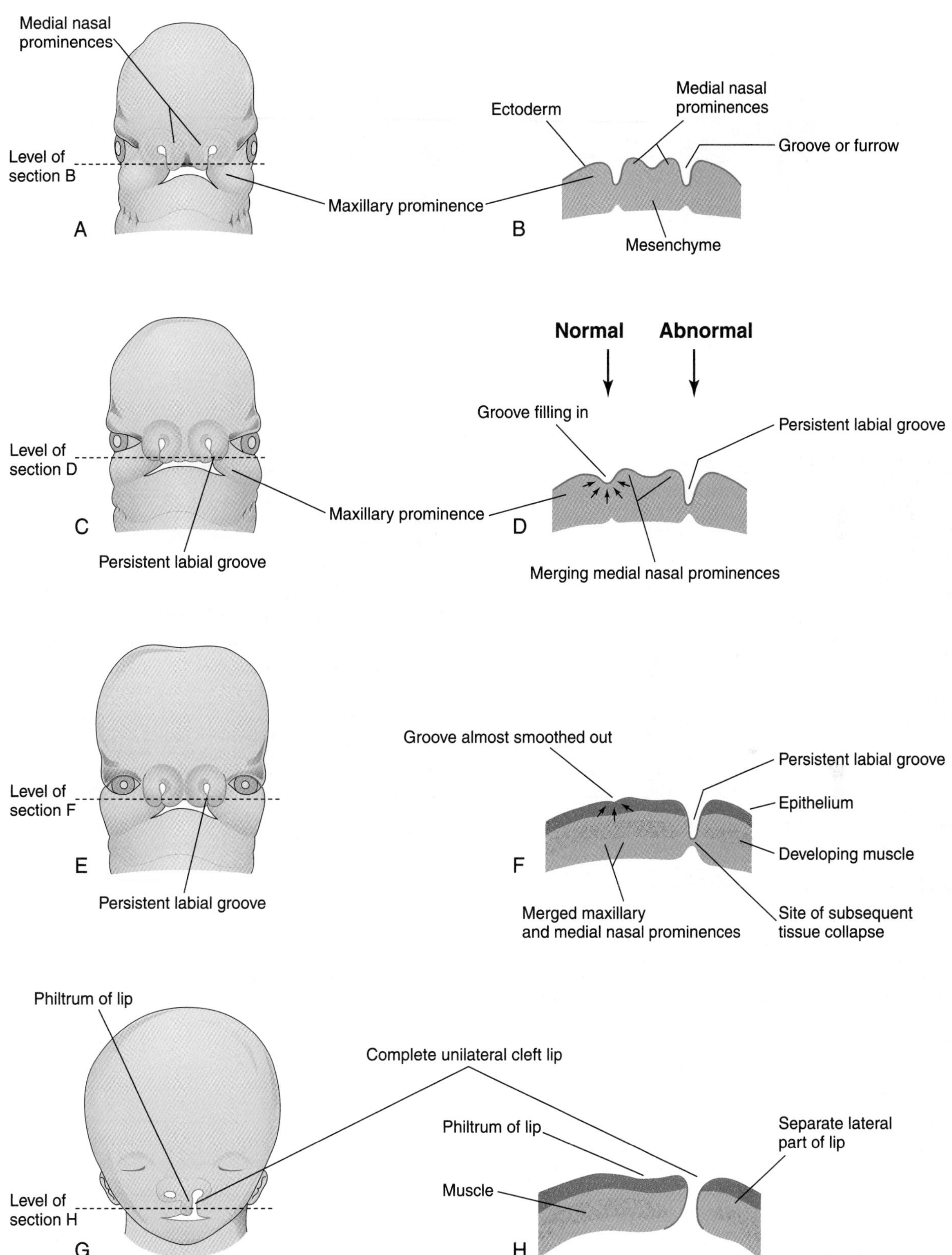

FIGURE 9-43. Drawings illustrating the embryologic basis of complete unilateral cleft lip. **A,** A 5-week embryo. **B,** Horizontal section through the head illustrating the grooves between the maxillary prominences and the merging medial nasal prominences. **C,** A 6-week embryo showing a persistent labial groove on the left side. **D,** Horizontal section through the head showing the groove gradually filling in on the right side after proliferation of mesenchyme (*arrows*). **E,** A 7-week embryo. **F,** Horizontal section through the head showing that the epithelium on the right has almost been pushed out of the groove between the maxillary and medial nasal prominences. **G,** A 10-week fetus with a complete unilateral cleft lip. **H,** Horizontal section through the head after stretching of the epithelium and breakdown of the tissues in the floor of the persistent labial groove on the left side, forming a complete unilateral cleft lip.

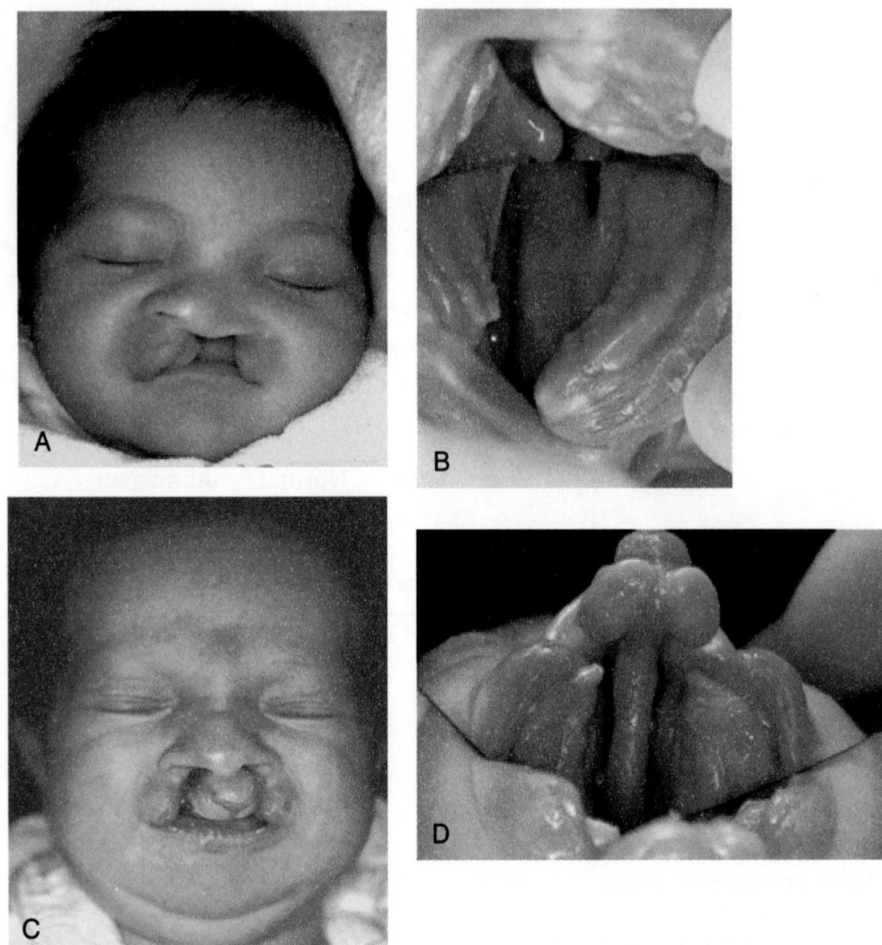

FIGURE 9-44. Congenital anomalies of the lip and palate. **A,** Newborn male infant with unilateral complete cleft lip and cleft palate. **B,** Intraoral photograph (taken with mirror) showing left unilateral complete cleft of the primary and secondary parts of palate. **C,** Newborn female infant with bilateral complete cleft lip and cleft palate. **D,** Intraoral photograph showing bilateral complete cleft palate. Note maxillary protrusion and natal tooth at gingival apex in each lesser segment. (Courtesy of Dr. John B. Mulliken, Children's Hospital Boston, Harvard Medical School, Boston, MA.)

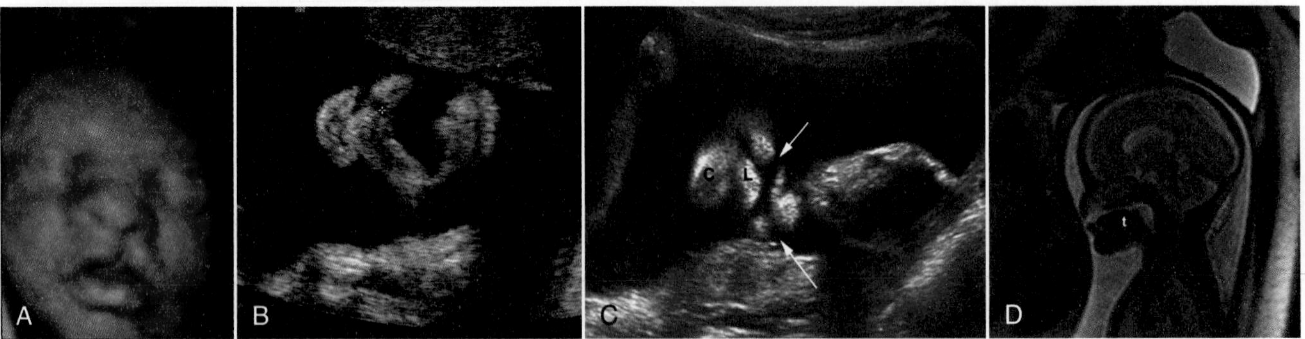

FIGURE 9-45. **A,** Three-dimensional ultrasound surface rendering of a fetus with unilateral cleft lip. **B,** Coronal sonogram of a fetal mouth with a cleft lip extending into the left nostril (+). Coronal plane. **C,** Coronal sonogram of a fetus showing a bilateral cleft lip (*arrows*), lower lip (L), and chin (C). **D,** Sagittal magnetic resonance image showing absence of the fetal midline palate. Note the fluid above the tongue (t) without the intervening palate. (**A** and **B**, Courtesy of Dr. G. J. Reid, Department of Obstetrics, Gynecology and Reproductive Sciences, University of Manitoba, Women's Hospital, Winnipeg, Manitoba, Canada; **C** and **D**, Courtesy of Deborah Levine, MD, Director of Obstetric and Gynecologic Ultrasound, Beth Israel Deaconess Medical Center, Boston, MA.)

sonographically. Using this imaging technique (Fig. 9-45), fetal facial anomalies such as a cleft lip are readily recognizable.

SUMMARY OF THE PHARYNGEAL APPARATUS

- The primordial pharynx is bounded laterally by **pharyngeal arches.** Each arch consists of a core of mesenchyme covered externally by ectoderm and internally by endoderm. The original mesenchyme of each arch is derived from mesoderm; later, **neural crest cells** migrate into the arches and are the major source of their connective tissue components, including cartilage, bone, and ligaments in the oral and facial regions. Each pharyngeal arch contains an artery, a cartilage rod, a nerve, and a muscular component.
- Externally the pharyngeal arches are separated by pharyngeal grooves. Internally the arches are separated by evaginations of the pharynx—**pharyngeal pouches.** Where the ectoderm of a groove contacts the endoderm of a pouch, **pharyngeal membranes** are formed. The adult derivatives of the various pharyngeal arch components are summarized in Table 9-1 and the derivatives of the pouches are illustrated in Figure 9-8.
- The **pharyngeal grooves** disappear except for the first pair, which persists as the external acoustic meatus. The pharyngeal membranes also disappear, except for the first pair, which becomes the tympanic membranes. The **first pharyngeal pouch** gives rise to the tympanic cavity, mastoid antrum, and pharyngotympanic tube. The **second pharyngeal pouch** is associated with the development of the palatine tonsil. The **thymus** is derived from the **third pair of pharyngeal pouches,** and the **parathyroid glands** are formed from the **third and fourth pairs of pharyngeal pouches.**
- The **thyroid gland** develops from a downgrowth from the floor of the primordial pharynx in the region where the tongue develops. The parafollicular cells (C cells) in the thyroid gland are derived from the **ultimopharyngeal bodies,** which are derived mainly from the fourth pair of pharyngeal pouches.
- Branchial cysts, sinuses, and fistulas may develop from parts of the second pharyngeal groove, the **cervical sinus,** or the second pharyngeal pouch that fail to obliterate.
- An **ectopic thyroid gland** results when the thyroid gland fails to descend completely from its site of origin in the tongue. The thyroglossal duct may persist or remnants of it may give rise to thyroglossal duct cysts and ectopic thyroid tissue masses. Infected cysts may perforate the skin and form thyroglossal duct sinuses that open anteriorly in the median plane of the neck.
- **Cleft lip** is a common congenital anomaly. Although frequently associated with cleft palate, cleft lip and cleft palate are etiologically distinct anomalies that involve different developmental processes occurring at different times. Cleft lip results from failure of mesenchymal masses in the medial nasal and maxillary prominences to merge, whereas cleft palate results from failure of mesenchymal masses in the palatal processes to meet and fuse. Most cases of cleft lip, with or without cleft palate, are caused by a combination of genetic and environmental factors (multifactorial inheritance).

CLINICALLY ORIENTED PROBLEMS

CASE 9-1

The mother of a 2-year-old boy consulted her pediatrician about an intermittent discharge of mucoid material from a small opening in the side of his neck. There was also extensive redness and swelling in the inferior third of the neck, just anterior to the sternocleidomastoid muscle.

- What is the most likely diagnosis?
- What is the probable embryologic basis of this intermittent mucoid discharge?
- Discuss the etiology of this congenital anomaly.

CASE 9-2

During a subtotal thyroidectomy, a surgeon could locate only one inferior parathyroid gland.

- Where might the other one be located?
- What is the embryologic basis for the ectopic location of this gland?

CASE 9-3

A young woman consulted her physician about a swelling in the anterior part of her neck, just inferior to the hyoid bone.

- What kind of a cyst might be present?
- Are they always in the median plane?
- Discuss the embryologic basis of these cysts.
- With what might such a swelling be confused?

CASE 9-4

A male infant was born with a unilateral cleft lip extending into the floor of his nose and through the alveolar process of his maxilla.

- What is the embryologic basis of these anomalies?
- Neither parent had a cleft lip or cleft palate. Are genetic factors likely involved?
- Are these anomalies more common in males?
- What is the chance that the next child will have a cleft lip?

CASE 9-5

An epileptic mother who was treated with an anticonvulsant drug during pregnancy gave birth to a child with cleft lip and cleft palate.

- Is there any evidence indicating that these drugs increase the incidence of these anomalies?
- Discuss the respective etiologies of these two birth defects.

Case 9-6

A mother consulted a pediatrician because her son was born with the tip of his tongue attached to the floor of his mouth.

- What is this condition called?
- Is this a common anomaly?
- Discuss the embryologic basis of this minor anomaly.
- What are the potential complications of this condition?

Discussion of these problems appears at the back of the book.

References and Suggested Reading

Aburezq H, Daskalogiannakis J, Forrest C: Management of the prominent bilateral cleft lip and palate. Cleft Palate Craniofac J 43:92, 2006.

Arnold JS, Werling U, Braunstein EM, et al: Inactivation of Tbx1 in the pharyngeal endoderm results in 22q11DS malformations. Development 133:977, 2006.

Avery JK, Chiego DJ Jr: Essentials of Oral Histology and Embryology. A Clinical Approach, 3rd ed. Philadelphia, Mosby, 2006.

Benacerraf BR: Ultrasound evaluation of the fetal face. In Callen PW (ed): Ultrasonography in Obstetrics and Gynecology, 4th ed. Philadelphia, WB Saunders, 2000.

Berkovitz BKB, Holland GR, Moxham B: Oral Anatomy, Histology, and Embryology, 3rd ed. Mosby, 2005.

Bhatnagar KP, Smith TD: The human vomeronasal organ. Part III: Postnatal development from infancy through the ninth decade. J Anat 199:289, 2001.

Breitsprecher L, Fanghanel J, Waite P, et al: Are there any new findings concerning the embryology and functional anatomy of the human muscles of facial expression? A contribution to the point selection, skin incision, and the muscle reconstruction for primary cheilo-rhinoplasties in patients with uni- and bilateral CLP. Mund Kiefer Gesichtschir 6:102, 2002.

Fisher DA, Polk DH: Development of the thyroid. Baillieres Clin Endocrinol Metab 3:627, 1989.

Francis-West PH, Robson L, Evans DJR. Craniofacial development: The tissue and molecular interactions that control development of the head. Adv Anat Embryol Cell Biol 169:1–138, 2003.

Garg V, Yamagishi C, Hu T, et al: Tbx1, a DiGeorge syndrome candidate gene, is regulated by Sonic hedgehog during pharyngeal arch development. Dev Biol 235:62, 2001.

Gartner LP, Hiatt JL: Color Textbook of Histology, 2nd ed. Philadelphia, WB Saunders, 2001.

Goldmuntz E: DiGeorge syndrome: New insights. Clin Perinatol 32:963, 2005.

Gorlin RJ, Cohen MM Jr, Levin LS: Syndromes of the Head and Neck, 3rd ed. New York, Oxford University Press, 1990.

Gross E, Sichel J-Y: Congenital neck lesions. Surg Clin North Am 86:383, 2006.

Hall BK: The Neural Crest in Development and Evolution. New York, Springer-Verlag, 1999.

Hall BK, Miyake T: Divide, accumulate, differentiate: Cell condensation in skeletal development revisited. Int J Dev Biol 39:881, 1995.

Helms JA, Cordero D, Tapadia MD: New insights into craniofacial morphogenesis. Development 132:851, 2005.

Hinrichsen K: The early development of morphology and patterns of the face in the human embryo. Adv Anat Embryol Cell Biol 98:1–79, 1985.

Jirásel JE: An Atlas of Human Prenatal Developmental Mechanics. Anatomy and Staging. London and New York, Taylor & Francis, 2004.

Jones KL: Smith's Recognizable Patterns of Human Malformation, 6th ed. Philadelphia, Elsevier/WB Saunders, 2005.

Jugessur A, Murray JC: Orofacial clefting: Recent insights into a complex trait. Curr Opin Genet Dev 15:270, 2005.

Lale SM, Lele MS, Anderson VM: The thymus in infancy and childhood. Chest Surg Clin N Am 11:233, 2001.

Leung AKC, Wong AL, Robson WLLM: Ectopic thyroid gland simulating a thyroglossal duct cyst: A case report. Can J Surg 38:87, 1995.

Mansilla MA, Cooper ME, Goldstein T, et al: Contributions of PTCH gene variants to isolated cleft lip and palate. Cleft Palate Craniofac J 43:21, 2006.

Marazita ML, Mooney MP: Current concepts in the embryology and genetics of cleft lip and cleft palate. Clin Plast Surg 31:125, 2004.

Mark M, Ghyselinck NB, Chambon P: Retinoic acid signaling in the development of branchial arches. Curr Opin Genet Dev 14: 591, 2004.

Moore KL, Dalley AD: Clinically Oriented Anatomy, 5th ed. Baltimore, Williams & Wilkins, 2006.

Moxham BJ: The development of the palate—a brief review. Eur J Anat 7(Suppl 1):53–74, 2003.

Neale D, Burrow G: Thyroid disease in pregnancy. Obstet Gynecol Clin North Am 31:893, 2004.

Nishimura Y: Embryological study of nasal cavity development in human embryos with reference to congenital nostril atresia. Acta Anat 147:140, 1993.

Noden DM: Cell movements and control of patterned tissue assembly during craniofacial development. J Craniofac Genet Dev Biol 11:192, 1991.

Noden DM: Vertebrate craniofacial development: novel approaches and new dilemmas. Curr Opin Genet Dev 2:576, 1992.

Noden DM, Francis-West P. The differentiation and morphogenesis of craniofacial muscles. Dev Dyn 235:1194–1218, 2006.

Ogawa GSH, Gonnering RS: Congenital nasolacrimal duct obstruction. J Pediatr 119:12, 1991.

Rodriguez-Vázquez JF: Development of the stapes and associated structures in human embryos. J Anat 207:165, 2005.

Santagati F, Minoux M, Ren S-Y, et al: Temporal requirement of Hoxa2 in cranial neural crest skeletal morphogenesis. Development 132:4927, 2005.

Sata I, Ishikawa H, Shimada K, et al: Morphology and analysis of the development of the human temporomandibular joint and masticatory muscle. Acta Anat 149:55, 1994.

Severtson M, Petruzzelli GJ: Macroglossia. Otolaryngol Head Neck Surg 114:501, 1996.

Smith TD, Bhatnagar KP: The human vomeronasal organ. Part II: Prenatal development. J Anat 197:421, 2000.

Smith TD, Siegel MI, Bonar CJ, Bhatnagar KP, et al: The existence of the vomeronasal organ in postnatal chimpanzees and evidence for its homology to that of humans. J Anat 198:77, 2001.

Sperber GH: Craniofacial Development. Hamilton, BC Decker, 2001.

Sulik KK: Craniofacial development. In Turvey TA, Vig KWL, Fonseca RJ (eds): Facial Clefts and Craniosynostosis. Principles and Management. Philadelphia, WB Saunders, 1996.

Vermeij-Keers C: Craniofacial embryology and morphogenesis: Normal and abnormal. In Stricker M, Van der Meulen JC, Raphael B, Mazzola R (eds): Craniofacial Malformations. Edinburgh, Churchill Livingstone, 1990.

Weinberg SM, Neiswanger K, Martin RA, et al: The Pittsburgh oral-facial cleft study: expanding the cleft phenotype. Background and justification. Cleft Palate Craniofac J 43:7, 2006.

Wyszynski DF, Sarkozi A, Czeizel AE: Oral clefts with associated anomalies: Methodological issues. Cleft Palate Craniofac J 43:1, 2006.

Zalel Y, Gamzu R, Mashiach S, et al: The development of the fetal thymus: An in utero sonographic evaluation. Prenat Diagn 22:114, 2002.

10

The Respiratory System

Respiratory Primordium 198

Development of the Larynx 198

Development of the Trachea 198

Development of the Bronchi and Lungs 202

Maturation of the Lungs 203

Summary of the Respiratory System 208

Clinically Oriented Problems 209

Development of the upper respiratory organs, the nasal cavities, for example, is described in Chapter 9. The lower respiratory organs (larynx, trachea, bronchi, and lungs) begin to form during the fourth week of development.

RESPIRATORY PRIMORDIUM

The **respiratory primordium** is indicated at approximately 28 days by a median outgrowth—the **laryngotracheal groove**—from the caudal end of the ventral wall of the primordial pharynx (Fig. 10-1*C*). This primordium of the tracheobronchial tree develops caudal to the fourth pair of pharyngeal pouches. The endoderm lining the laryngotracheal groove gives rise to the pulmonary epithelium and glands of the larynx, trachea, and bronchi. The connective tissue, cartilage, and smooth muscle in these structures develop from the splanchnic mesoderm surrounding the foregut (see Fig. 10-4*A*). By the end of the fourth week, the laryngotracheal groove has evaginated to form a pouchlike **laryngotracheal diverticulum**, which is located ventral to the caudal part of the foregut (Figs. 10-1*B* and 10-2*A*). As this diverticulum elongates, it is invested with splanchnic mesenchyme and its distal end enlarges to form a globular **respiratory bud** (see Fig. 10-2*B*). The laryngotracheal diverticulum soon separates from the primordial pharynx; however, it maintains communication with it through the **primordial laryngeal inlet** (see Fig. 10-2*C*). Longitudinal **tracheoesophageal folds** develop in the laryngotracheal diverticulum, approach each other, and fuse to form a partition—the **tracheoesophageal septum** (see Fig. 10-2*D* and *E*). This septum divides the cranial portion of the foregut into a ventral part, the **laryngotracheal tube** (primordium of larynx, trachea, bronchi, and lungs), and a dorsal part (primordium of oropharynx and esophagus (see Fig. 10-2*F*). The opening of the laryngotracheal tube into the pharynx becomes the **primordial laryngeal inlet** (Figs. 10-2*C* and 10-3*C*).

DEVELOPMENT OF THE LARYNX

The epithelial lining of the larynx develops from the endoderm of the cranial end of the laryngotracheal tube. The cartilages of the larynx develop from those in the fourth and sixth pairs of pharyngeal arches (see Chapter 9). The **laryngeal cartilages** develop from mesenchyme that is derived from *neural crest cells*. The mesenchyme at the cranial end of the laryngotracheal tube proliferates rapidly, producing paired **arytenoid swellings** (see Fig. 10-3*B*). These swellings grow toward the tongue, converting the slitlike aperture—the **primordial glottis**—into a T-shaped **laryngeal inlet** and reducing the developing laryngeal lumen to a narrow slit. The laryngeal epithelium proliferates rapidly, resulting in temporary *occlusion of the laryngeal lumen*. Recanalization of the larynx normally occurs by the 10th week. The laryngeal ventricles form during this recanalization process. These recesses are bounded by folds of mucous membrane that become the *vocal folds* (cords) and *vestibular folds*.

The **epiglottis** develops from the caudal part of the *hypopharyngeal eminence*, a prominence produced by proliferation of mesenchyme in the ventral ends of the third and fourth pharyngeal arches (see Fig. 10-3*B* to *D*). The rostral part of this eminence forms the posterior third or pharyngeal part of the tongue (see Chapter 9). Because the **laryngeal muscles** develop from myoblasts in the fourth and sixth pairs of pharyngeal arches, they are innervated by the laryngeal branches of the vagus nerves (cranial nerve X) that supply these arches (see Table 9-1). Growth of the larynx and epiglottis is rapid during the first 3 years after birth. By this time, the epiglottis has reached its adult form.

LARYNGEAL ATRESIA

This rare anomaly results from failure of recanalization of the larynx, which causes obstruction of the upper fetal airway—**congenital high airway obstruction syndrome**. Distal to the region of atresia (blockage) or stenosis (narrowing), the airways become dilated, the lungs are enlarged and echogenic (capable of producing echoes during ultrasound imaging studies because they are filled with fluid), the diaphragm is either flattened or inverted, and there is fetal ascites and/or hydrops (accumulation of serous fluid in the intracellular spaces causing severe edema).

Incomplete atresia (laryngeal web) results from incomplete recanalization of the larynx during the 10th week. A membranous web forms at the level of the vocal folds, partially obstructing the airway.

DEVELOPMENT OF THE TRACHEA

The endodermal lining of the laryngotracheal tube distal to the larynx differentiates into the epithelium and glands of the trachea and the pulmonary epithelium. The cartilage, connective tissue, and muscles of the trachea are derived from the splanchnic mesenchyme surrounding the laryngotracheal tube (Fig. 10-4).

TRACHEOESOPHAGEAL FISTULA

A fistula (abnormal passage) between the trachea and esophagus occurs once in 3000 to 4500 live births (Figs. 10-5 and 10-6); most affected infants are males. In more than 85% of cases, the tracheoesophageal fistula (TEF) is associated with esophageal atresia. A TEF results from incomplete division of the cranial part of the foregut into respiratory and esophageal parts during the fourth week. Incomplete fusion of the tracheoesophageal folds results in a defective tracheoesophageal septum and a TEF between the trachea and esophagus.

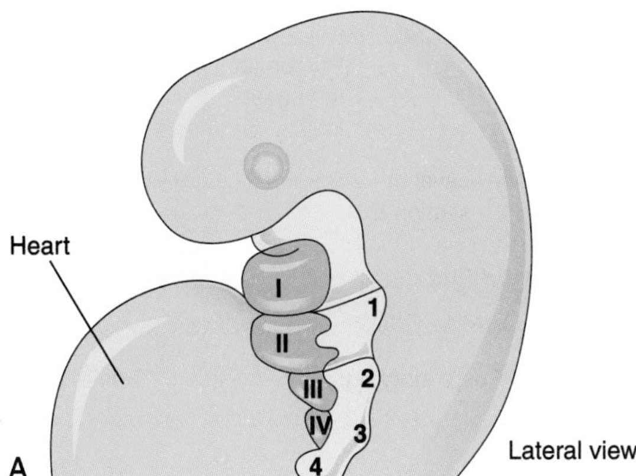

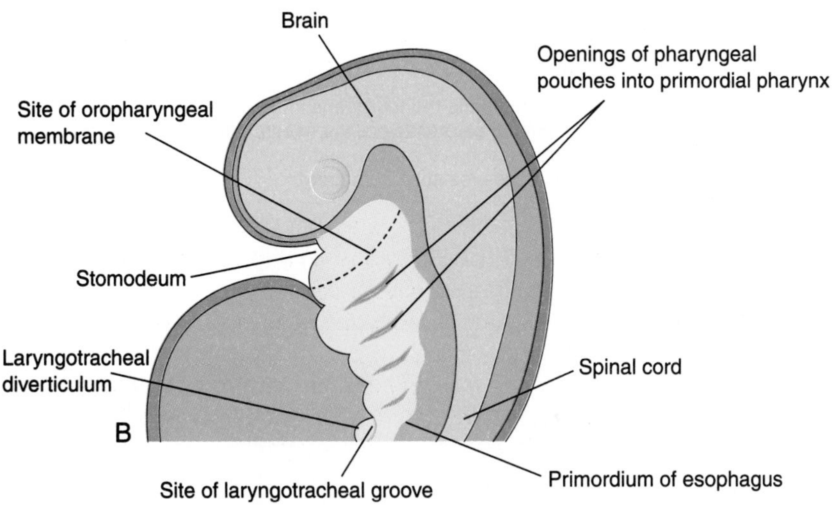

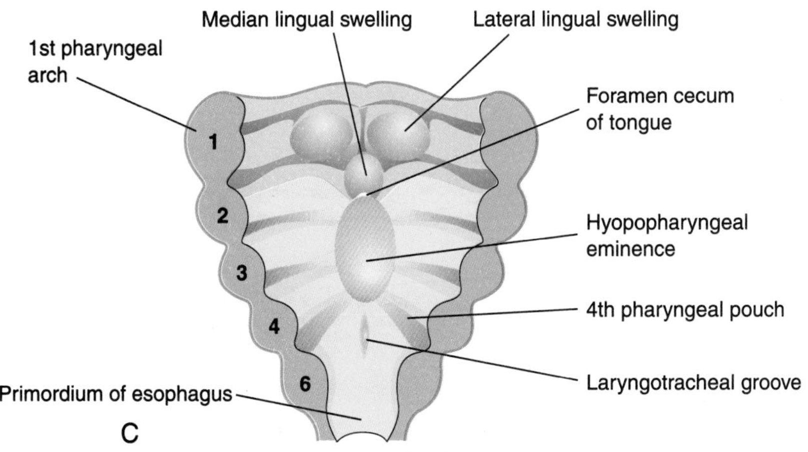

FIGURE 10-1. **A,** Lateral view of a 4-week embryo illustrating the relationship of the pharyngeal apparatus to the developing respiratory system. **B,** Sagittal section of the cranial half of the embryo. **C,** Horizontal section of the embryo illustrating the floor of the primordial pharynx and the location of the laryngotracheal groove.

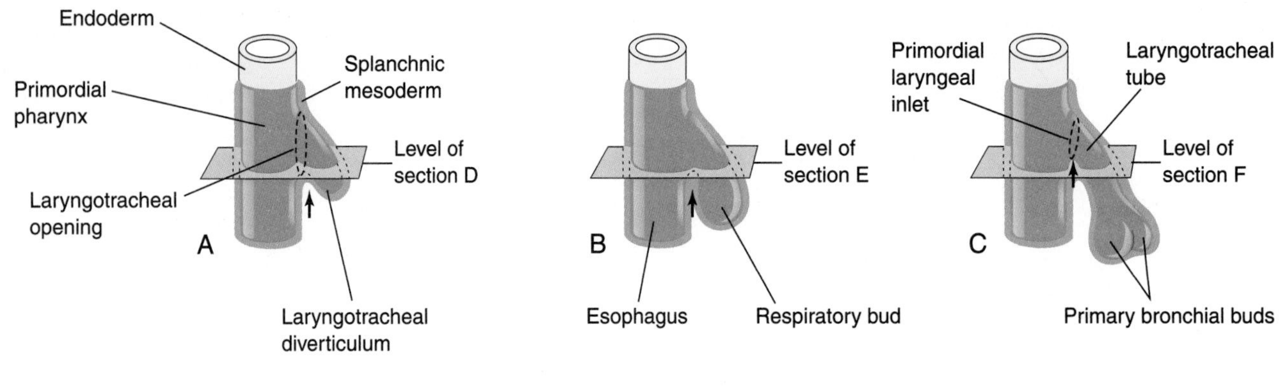

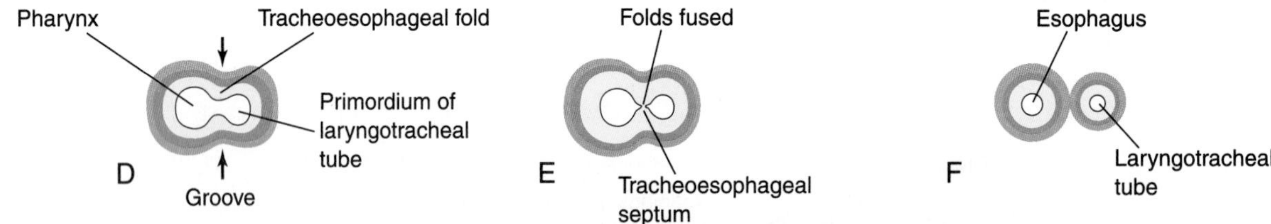

FIGURE 10-2. Successive stages in the development of the tracheoesophageal septum during the fourth and fifth weeks. **A** to **C,** Lateral views of the caudal part of the primordial pharynx showing the laryngotracheal diverticulum and partitioning of the foregut into the esophagus and laryngotracheal tube. **D** to **F,** Transverse sections illustrating formation of the tracheoesophageal septum and showing how it separates the foregut into the laryngotracheal tube and esophagus. The *arrows* indicate cellular changes resulting from growth.

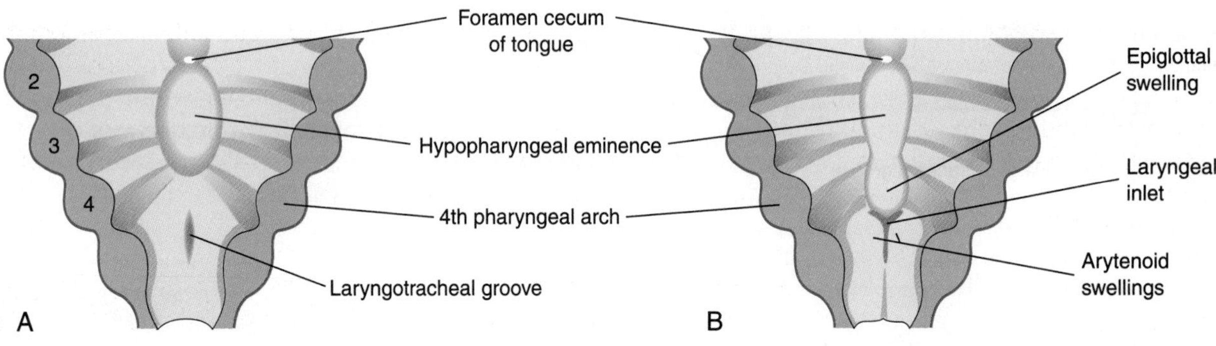

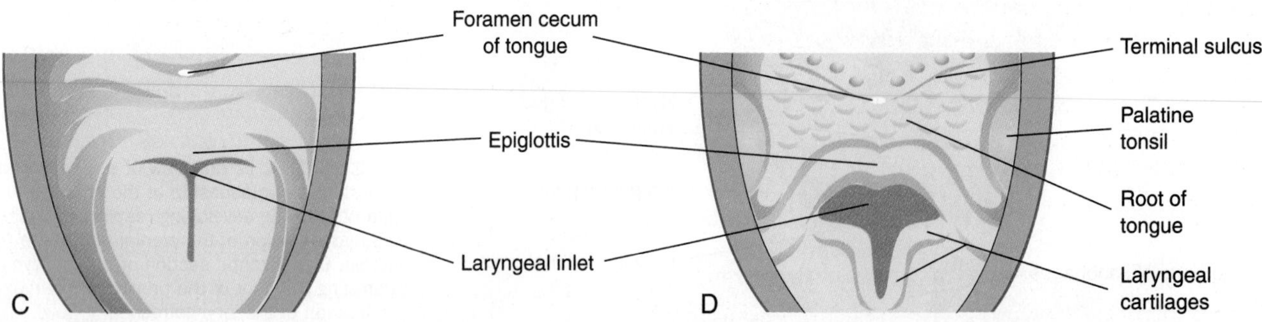

FIGURE 10-3. Successive stages in the development of the larynx. **A,** At 4 weeks. **B,** At 5 weeks. **C,** At 6 weeks. **D,** At 10 weeks. The epithelium lining the larynx is of endodermal origin. The cartilages and muscles of the larynx arise from mesenchyme in the fourth and sixth pairs of pharyngeal arches. Note that the laryngeal inlet changes in shape from a slitlike opening to a T-shaped inlet as the mesenchyme surrounding the developing larynx proliferates.

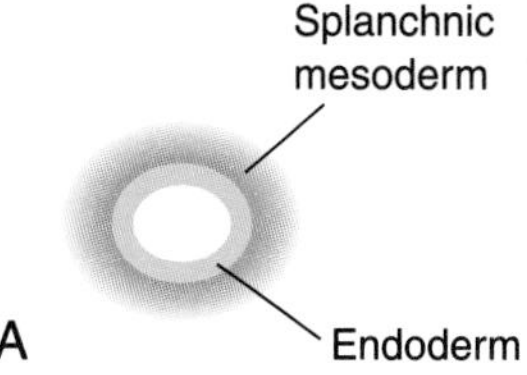

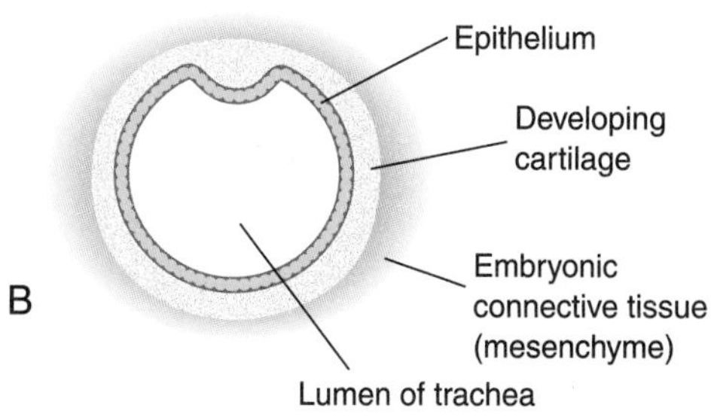

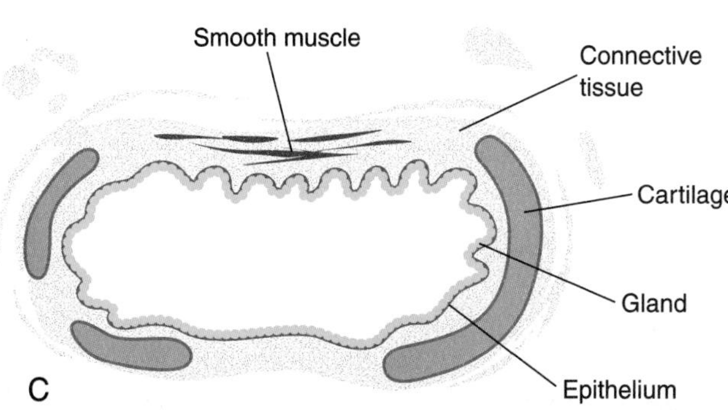

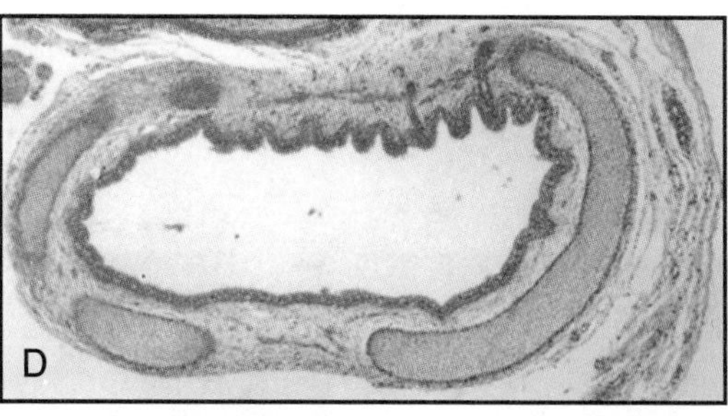

FIGURE 10-4. Transverse sections through the laryngotracheal tube illustrating progressive stages in the development of the trachea. **A,** At 4 weeks. **B,** At 10 weeks. **C,** At 11 weeks (drawing of micrograph in **D**). Note that endoderm of the tube gives rise to the epithelium and glands of the trachea and that mesenchyme surrounding the tube forms the connective tissue, muscle, and cartilage. **D,** Photomicrograph of a transverse section of the developing trachea at 12 weeks. (**D,** From Moore KL, Persaud TVN, Shiota K: Color Atlas of Clinical Embryology, 2nd ed. Philadelphia, WB Saunders, 2000.)

TEF is the most common anomaly of the lower respiratory tract. Four main varieties of TEF may develop (see Fig. 10-5). The usual anomaly is for the superior part of the esophagus to end blindly (**esophageal atresia**) and for the inferior part to join the trachea near its bifurcation (see Figs. 10-5*A* and 10-6). Other varieties of this anomaly are illustrated in Figure 10-5*B* to *D*. Infants with the common type of TEF and esophageal atresia cannot swallow so they frequently drool saliva at rest and immediately regurgitate milk when fed. Gastric and intestinal contents may also reflux from the stomach through the fistula into the trachea and lungs. This refluxed acid, and in some cases bile, can cause **pneumonitis** (inflammation of the lungs) leading to respiratory compromise. **Polyhydramnios** (see Chapter 7) is often associated with esophageal atresia. The excess amniotic fluid develops because fluid cannot pass to the stomach and intestines for absorption and subsequent transfer through the placenta to the mother's blood for disposal.

LARYNGOTRACHEOESOPHAGEAL CLEFT

Uncommonly, the larynx and upper trachea may fail to separate completely from the esophagus. This results in a persistent connection of variable lengths between these normally separated structures. Symptoms of this congenital anomaly are similar to those of tracheoesophageal fistula because of aspiration into the lungs, but aphonia (absence of voice) is a distinguishing feature.

TRACHEAL STENOSIS AND ATRESIA

Narrowing (stenosis) and obstruction (atresia) of the trachea are uncommon anomalies that are usually associated with one of the varieties of TEF. Stenoses and atresias probably result from unequal partitioning of the foregut into the esophagus and trachea. Sometimes there is a web of tissue obstructing airflow (incomplete tracheal atresia).

TRACHEAL DIVERTICULUM

This extremely rare anomaly consists of a blind, bronchus-like projection from the trachea. The outgrowth may terminate in normal-appearing lung tissue, forming a tracheal lobe of the lung.

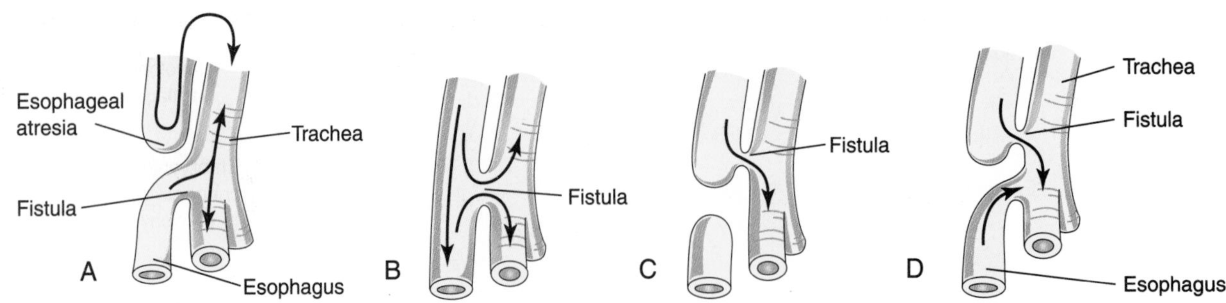

Figure 10-5. The four main varieties of tracheoesophageal fistula (TEF). Possible directions of the flow of the contents are indicated by *arrows*. Esophageal atresia, as illustrated in **A,** is associated with TEF in more than 85% of cases. **B,** Fistula between the trachea and esophagus. **C,** Air cannot enter the distal esophagus and stomach. **D,** Air can enter the distal esophagus and stomach, and the esophageal and gastric contents may enter the trachea and lungs.

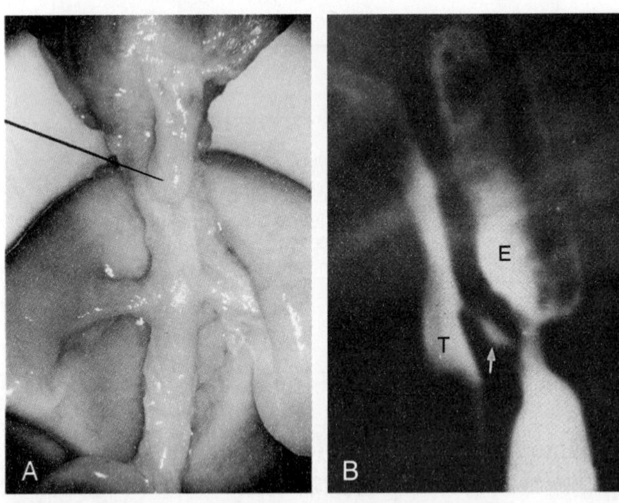

Figure 10-6. A, Tracheoesophageal fistula (TEF) in a 17-week male fetus. The upper esophageal segment ends blindly (*pointer*). **B,** Contrast radiograph of a newborn infant with TEF. Note the communication (*arrow*) between the esophagus (E) and trachea (T). (**A,** From Kalousek DK, Fitch N, Paradice B: Pathology of the Human Embryo and Previable Fetus. New York, Springer-Verlag, 1990; **B,** Courtesy of Dr. Prem S. Sahni, formerly of the Department of Radiology, Children's Hospital, Winnipeg, Manitoba, Canada.)

DEVELOPMENT OF THE BRONCHI AND LUNGS

The **respiratory bud** (lung bud) that developed at the caudal end of the laryngotracheal diverticulum during the fourth week (see Fig. 10-2*B*) soon divides into two outpouchings—the **primary bronchial buds** (Figs. 10-2*C* and 10-7*A*). These buds grow laterally into the pericardioperitoneal canals, the primordia of the pleural cavities (see Fig. 10-7*B*). **Secondary** and **tertiary bronchial buds** soon develop. Together with the surrounding splanchnic mesenchyme, the bronchial buds differentiate into the bronchi and their ramifications in the lungs. Early in the fifth week, the connection of each bronchial bud with the trachea enlarges to form the primordia of **main bronchi** (Fig. 10-8).

The embryonic right main bronchus is slightly larger than the left one and is oriented more vertically. This embryonic relationship persists in the adult; consequently, a foreign body is more liable to enter the right main bronchus than the left one. The main bronchi subdivide

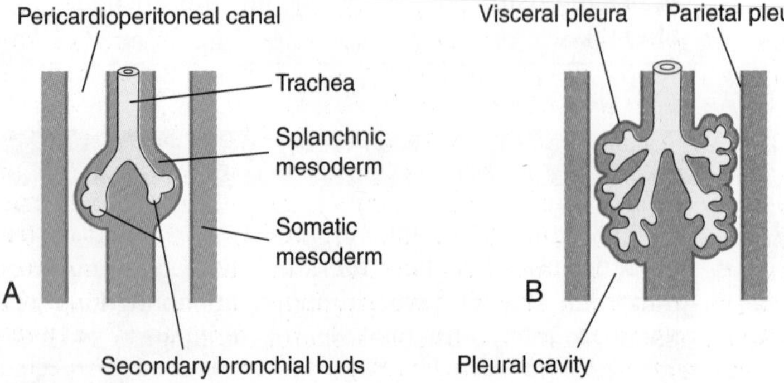

Figure 10-7. Illustrations of the growth of the developing lungs into the splanchnic mesenchyme adjacent to the medial walls of the pericardioperitoneal canals (primordial pleural cavities). Development of the layers of the pleura is also shown. **A,** At 5 weeks. **B,** At 6 weeks.

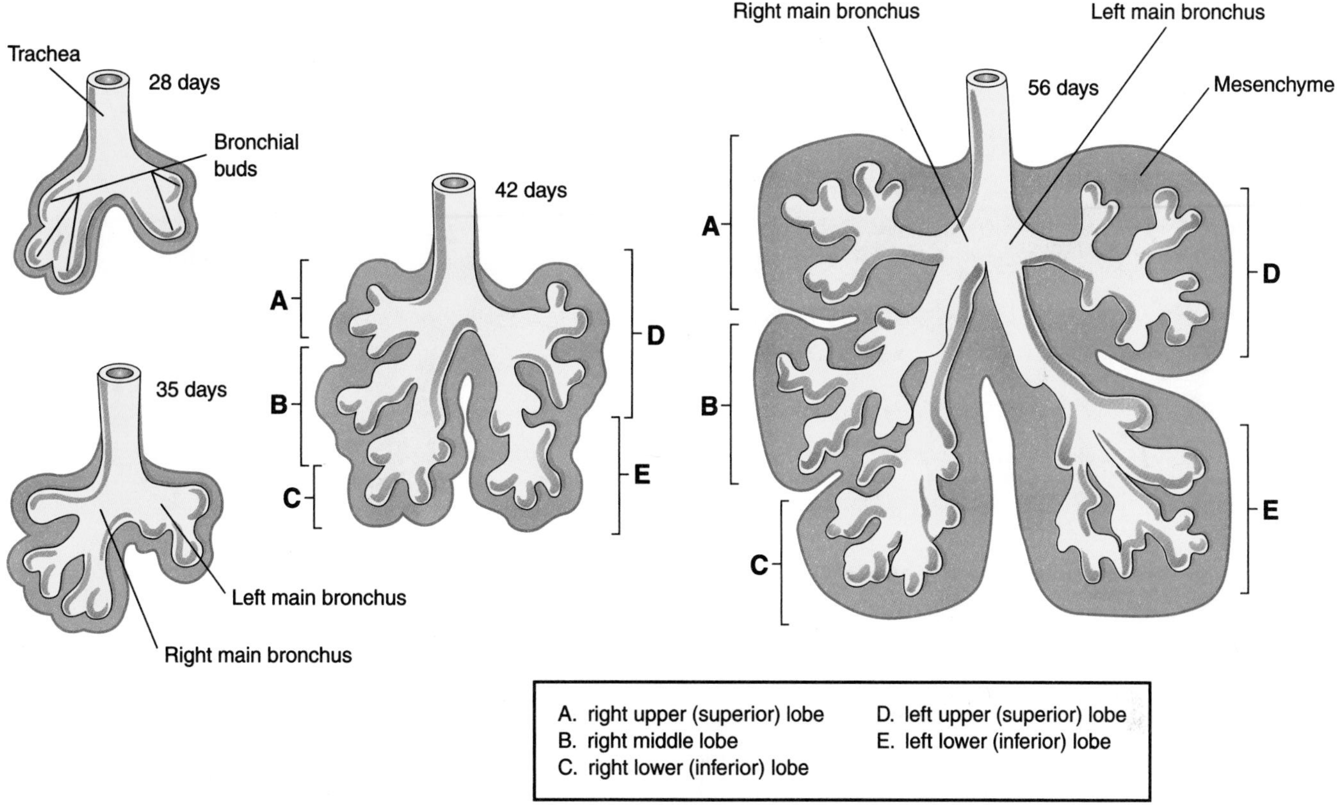

FIGURE 10-8. Successive stages in the development of the bronchial buds, bronchi, and lungs.

into **secondary bronchi** that form lobar, segmental, and intrasegmental branches (see Fig. 10-8). On the right, the superior lobar bronchus will supply the upper (superior) lobe of the lung, whereas the inferior bronchus subdivides into two bronchi, one to the middle lobe of the right lung and the other to the lower (inferior) lobe. On the left, the two secondary bronchi supply the upper and lower lobes of the lung. Each lobar bronchus undergoes progressive branching.

The **segmental bronchi**, 10 in the right lung and 8 or 9 in the left lung, begin to form by the seventh week. As this occurs, the surrounding mesenchyme also divides. Each segmental bronchus with its surrounding mass of mesenchyme is the primordium of a **bronchopulmonary segment**. By 24 weeks, approximately 17 orders of branches have formed and **respiratory bronchioles** have developed (Fig. 10-9*B*). An additional seven orders of airways develop after birth.

As the bronchi develop, cartilaginous plates develop from the surrounding splanchnic mesenchyme. The bronchial smooth muscle and connective tissue and the pulmonary connective tissue and capillaries are also derived from this mesenchyme. As the lungs develop, they acquire a layer of **visceral pleura** from the splanchnic mesenchyme (see Fig. 10-7). With expansion, the lungs and pleural cavities grow caudally into the mesenchyme of the body wall and soon lie close to the heart. The thoracic body wall becomes lined by a layer of **parietal pleura**, derived from the somatic mesoderm (see Fig. 10-7*B*).

Maturation of the Lungs

Maturation of the lungs is divided into four stages: pseudoglandular, canalicular, terminal sac, and alveolar.

Pseudoglandular Stage (6 to 16 Weeks)

The developing lungs somewhat histologically resemble exocrine glands during this stage (Figs. 10-9*A* and 10-10*A*). By 16 weeks, all major elements of the lung have formed, except those involved with gas exchange. Respiration is not possible; hence, *fetuses born during this period are unable to survive*.

Canalicular Stage (16 to 26 Weeks)

This period overlaps the pseudoglandular stage because cranial segments of the lungs mature faster than caudal ones. During the canalicular stage, the lumina of the bronchi and terminal bronchioles become larger, and the lung tissue becomes highly vascular (see Figs. 10-9*B* and 10-10*B*). By 24 weeks, each terminal bronchiole has given rise to two or more **respiratory bronchioles**, each of which then divides into three to six passages—primordial alveolar ducts. Respiration is possible at the end of the canalicular stage because some thin-walled **terminal sacs** (primordial alveoli) have developed at the ends of the respiratory bronchioles, and *the lung tissue is well vascularized.* Although a fetus born toward the end of this period

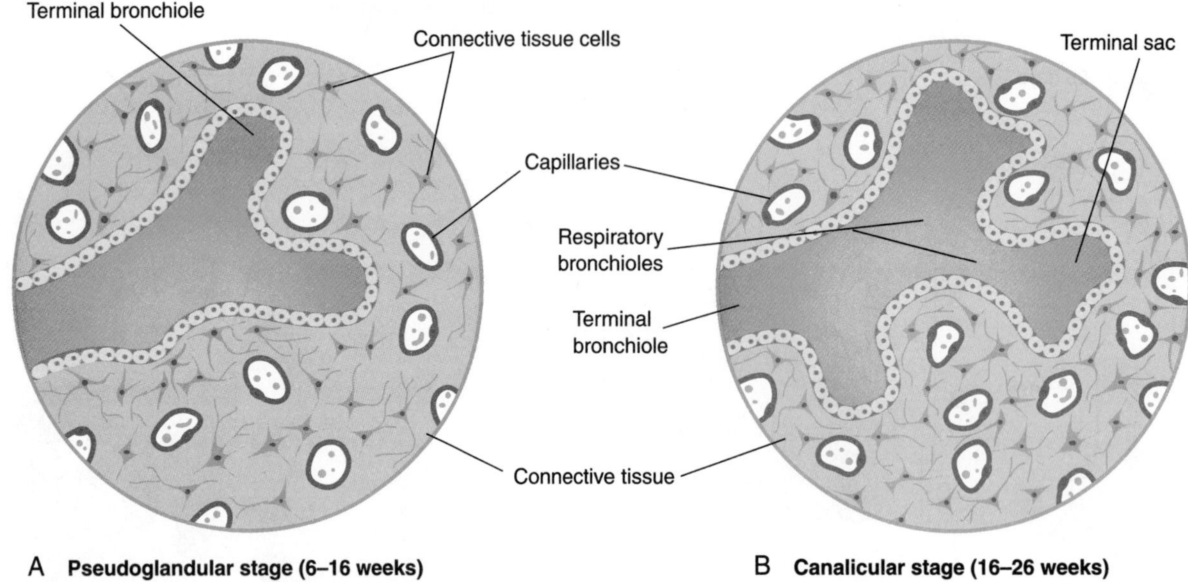

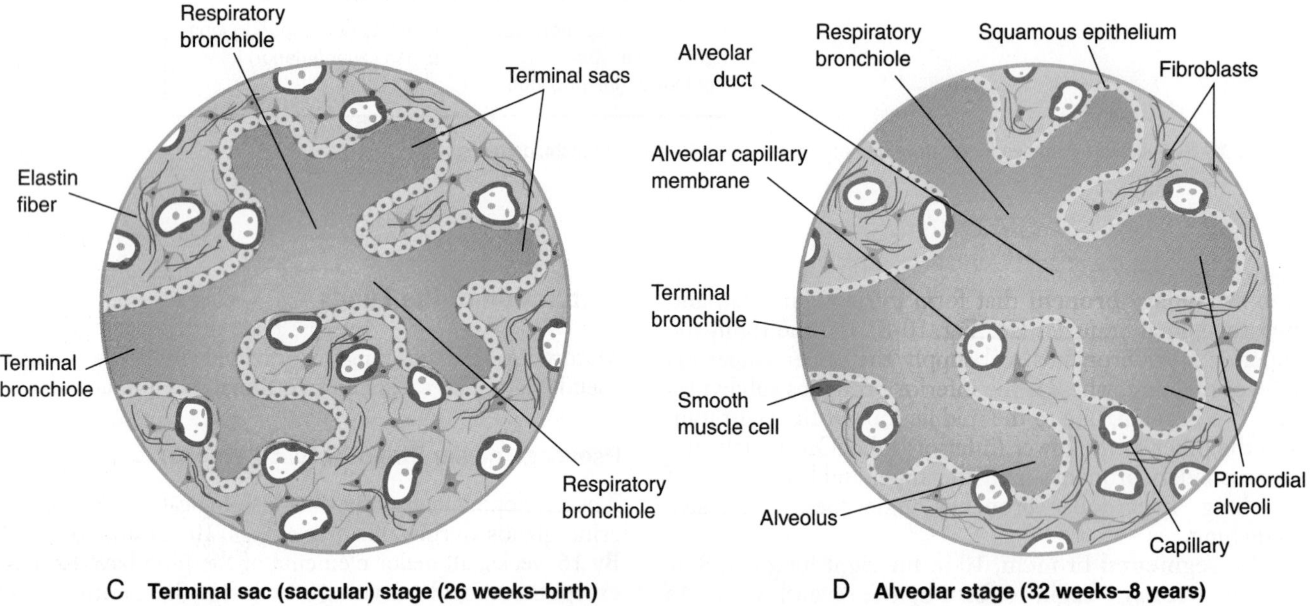

FIGURE 10-9. Diagrammatic sketches of histologic sections illustrating the stages of lung development. **A** and **B,** Early stages of lung development. **C** and **D,** Note that the alveolocapillary membrane is thin and that some capillaries bulge into the terminal sacs and alveoli.

may survive if given intensive care, it often dies because its respiratory and other systems are still relatively immature.

Terminal Sac Stage (26 Weeks to Birth)

During this period, many more terminal sacs or saccules develop (see Figs. 10-9*C* and 10-10*D*), and their *epithelium becomes very thin.* Capillaries begin to bulge into these sacs (developing alveoli). The intimate contact between epithelial and endothelial cells establishes the **blood-air barrier**, which permits adequate gas exchange for survival of the fetus if it is born prematurely. By 26 weeks, the terminal sacs are lined mainly by squamous epithelial cells of endodermal origin—**type I pneumocytes**—across which gas exchange occurs. The capillary network proliferates rapidly in the mesenchyme around the developing alveoli, and there is concurrent active development of lymphatic capillaries. Scattered among the squamous epithelial cells are rounded secretory epithelial cells—**type II pneumocytes**, *which secrete pulmonary surfactant*, a complex mixture of phospholipids and proteins. **Surfactant** forms as a monomolecular film over the internal walls of the **alveolar sacs** and counteracts surface tension forces at the air-alveolar interface. This facilitates expansion of the saccules (primordial alveoli) by preventing atelectasis (collapse of saccules during exhalation).

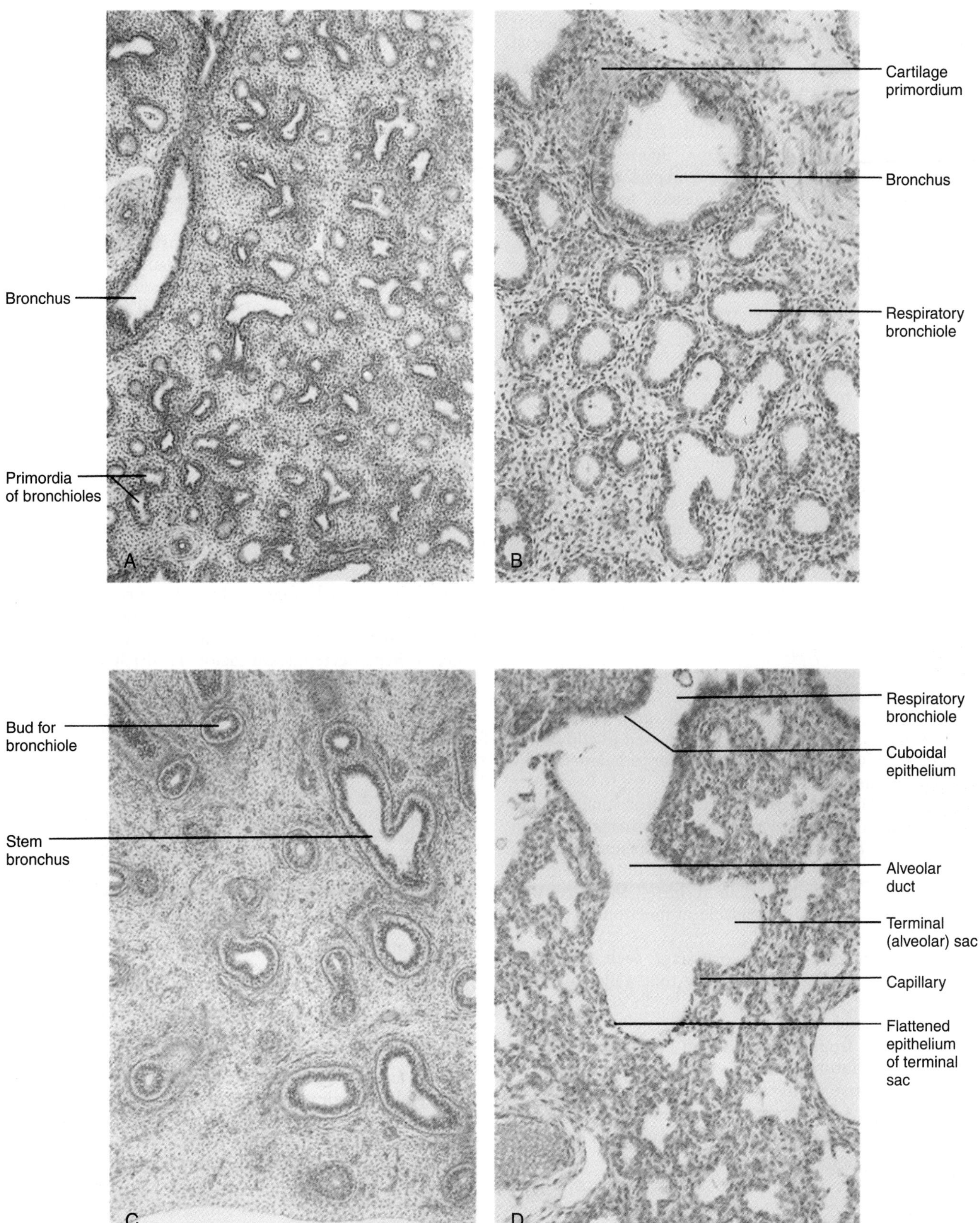

FIGURE 10-10. Photomicrographs of sections of developing human lungs. **A,** Pseudoglandular stage, 8 weeks. Note the "glandular" appearance of the lung. **B,** Canalicular stage, 16 weeks. The lumina of the bronchi and terminal bronchioles are enlarging. **C,** Canalicular stage, 18 weeks. **D,** Terminal sac stage, 24 weeks. Observe the thin-walled terminal sacs (primordial alveoli) that have developed at the ends of the respiratory bronchioles. Also observe that the number of capillaries have increased and that some of them are closely associated with the developing alveoli. (From Moore KL, Persaud TVN, Shiota K: Color Atlas of Clinical Embryology, 2nd ed. Philadelphia, WB Saunders, 2000.)

The maturation of type II pneumocytes and surfactant production varies widely in fetuses of different gestational ages. The production of surfactant increases during the terminal stages of pregnancy, particularly during the last 2 weeks.

Surfactant production begins by 20 weeks, but it is present in only small amounts in premature infants. It does not reach adequate levels until the late fetal period. By 26 to 28 weeks after fertilization, the fetus usually weighs approximately 1000 g and sufficient alveolar sacs and surfactant are present to permit survival of a prematurely born infant. Before this, the lungs are usually incapable of providing adequate gas exchange, partly because the alveolar surface area is insufficient and the vascularity underdeveloped. It is not the presence of thin terminal sacs or a primordial alveolar epithelium so much as the development of an adequate pulmonary vasculature and sufficient surfactant that is critical to the survival and neurodevelopmental outcome of premature infants. Consequently, fetuses born prematurely at 24 to 26 weeks after fertilization may survive if given intensive care; however, they may suffer from respiratory distress because of surfactant deficiency. Survival of these infants has improved with the use of antenatal corticosteroids, which induces surfactant production, and also with postnatal surfactant replacement therapy.

Alveolar Stage (32 Weeks to 8 Years)

Exactly when the terminal sac stage ends and the alveolar stage begins depends on the definition of the term **alveolus**. Sacs analogous to alveoli are present at 32 weeks. The epithelial lining of the terminal sacs attenuates to a thin squamous epithelial layer. The type I pneumocytes become so thin that the adjacent capillaries bulge into the alveolar saccules (see Figs. 10-9*D* and 10-10*D*). By the late fetal period, the lungs are capable of respiration because the **alveolocapillary membrane** (pulmonary diffusion barrier or respiratory membrane) is sufficiently thin to allow gas exchange. Although the lungs do not begin to perform this vital function until birth, they are well developed so that they are capable of functioning as soon as the baby is born.

At the beginning of the alveolar stage, each respiratory bronchiole terminates in a cluster of thin-walled **alveolar sacs**, separated from one another by loose connective tissue. These saccules represent future **alveolar ducts**. The transition from dependence on the placenta for gas exchange to autonomous gas exchange requires the following adaptive changes in the lungs:

- Production of surfactant in the alveolar sacs
- Transformation of the lungs from secretory into gas exchanging organs
- Establishment of parallel pulmonary and systemic circulations

Characteristic **mature alveoli** do not form until after birth; approximately 95% of mature alveoli develop postnatally. Before birth, the primordial alveoli appear as small bulges on the walls of respiratory bronchioles and alveolar sacs. After birth, the primordial alveoli enlarge as the lungs expand, but the greatest increase in the size of the lungs results from an increase in the number of respiratory bronchioles and primordial alveoli rather than from an increase in the size of the alveoli. Alveolar development is largely completed by 3 years of age, but new alveoli may be added until approximately 8 years of age. Unlike mature alveoli, immature alveoli have the potential for forming additional primordial alveoli. As these alveoli increase in size, they become mature alveoli. The major mechanism for increasing the number of alveoli is the formation of secondary connective tissue septa that subdivide existing primordial alveoli. Initially, the septa are relatively thick, but they are soon transformed into mature thin septa that are capable of gas exchange.

Lung development during the first few months after birth is characterized by an exponential increase in the surface area of the air-blood barrier through the multiplication of alveoli and capillaries. Approximately 150 million primordial alveoli, one half of the adult number, are present in the lungs of a full-term newborn infant. On chest radiographs, therefore, the lungs of newborn infants are denser than adult lungs. Between the third and the eighth years, the adult complement of 300 million alveoli is achieved.

Molecular studies indicate that lung development is controlled by a cascade of signaling pathways that are regulated by the temporal and sequential expression of highly conserved genes. The commitment and differentiation of endodermal foregut cells to form respiratory-type epithelial cells are associated with expression of several transcription factors, including thyroid transcription factor 1, hepatocyte nuclear factor (HNF) 3β, and GATA-6, as well as other Zinc-finger family members, retinoic acid receptors, and homeobox (Hox) domain-containing genes. Hox genes specify the anteroposterior axis in the embryo. Fibroblast growth factor 10 and other signals from splanchnic mesenchyme probably induce the outgrowth of the respiratory bud. Branching of this bud (branching morphogenesis) and its proliferation depend on epithelial (endodermal foregut)-mesenchymal (mesoderm) interactions. The Wnt signaling pathway plays an essential role in the inductive interactions between epithelium and mesenchyme. Recent studies suggest that Wnt7b signaling from the epithelium regulates mesenchymal proliferation and blood vessel formation in the lung. The patterning morphogen sonic hedgehog (Shh-Gli) modulates the expression of fibroblast growth factor 10, which controls the branching of the bronchial buds. Also, the morphogen retinoic acid regulates Hox a5, b5, and c4, which are expressed in the developing lung.

Fetal breathing movements (FBMs), which can be detected by real-time ultrasonography, occur before birth, exerting sufficient force to cause aspiration of some amniotic fluid into the lungs. FBMs occur intermittently (approximately 30% of them during rapid eye movement sleep) and are essential for normal lung development (Fig. 10-11). The pattern of FBMs is widely used in the diagnosis of labor and as a predictor of fetal outcome in a preterm delivery. By birth, the fetus has had the advantage of several months of breathing exercise. FBMs, which increase as the time of delivery approaches, probably condition the respiratory muscles. In addition, these movements stimulate lung development, possibly by creating a pressure gradient between the lungs and the amniotic fluid.

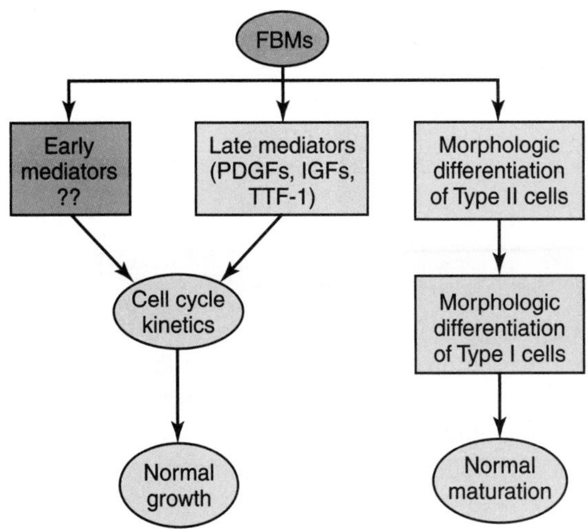

FIGURE 10-11. Fetal breathing movements (FBMs) seem to play a role in lung growth through their effects on lung cell cycle kinetics by regulating the expression of growth factors, such as platelet-derived growth factors (PDGFs) and insulin-like growth factors (IGFs), and establishing the gradient of thyroid transcription factor 1 (TTF-1) expression at the last stage of lung organogenesis (i.e., late mediators). It is also suggested that FBMs influence the expression of other unknown growth factors (i.e., early mediators) that are responsible for changes in cell cycle kinetics at earlier stages of lung development. FBMs appear to also be required for the accomplishment of the morphologic differentiation of type I and II pneumocytes. (From Inanlou MR, Baguma-Nibasheka M, Kablar B: The role of fetal breathing-like movements in lung organogenesis. Histol Histopathol 20:1261, 2005.)

At birth, the lungs are approximately half-filled with fluid derived from the amniotic cavity, lungs, and tracheal glands. Aeration of the lungs at birth is not so much the inflation of empty collapsed organs but rather the rapid replacement of intra-alveolar fluid by air. *The fluid in the lungs is cleared at birth by three routes:*

- Through the mouth and nose by pressure on the fetal thorax during vaginal delivery
- Into the pulmonary arteries, veins, and capillaries
- Into the lymphatics

In the near term fetus, the pulmonary lymphatic vessels are relatively larger and more numerous than in the adult. Lymph flow is rapid during the first few hours after birth and then diminishes. Three factors are important for normal lung development: adequate thoracic space for lung growth, FBMs, and an adequate amniotic fluid volume.

Oligohydramnios and Lung Development

When oligohydramnios (insufficient amount of amniotic fluid) is severe and chronic because of amniotic fluid leakage or decreased production, lung development is retarded and severe pulmonary hypoplasia results from restriction of the fetal thorax.

Lungs of Newborn Infants

Fresh healthy lungs always contain some air; consequently, pulmonary tissue removed from them will float in water. A diseased lung, partly filled with fluid, may not float. Of medicolegal significance is the fact that the lungs of a stillborn infant are firm and sink when placed in water because they contain fluid, not air.

Respiratory Distress Syndrome

This disease (RDS) affects *approximately* 2% of live newborn infants; those born prematurely are most susceptible. These infants develop rapid, labored breathing shortly after birth. RDS is also known as *hyaline membrane disease* (HMD). An estimated 30% of all neonatal disease results from HMD or its complications. *Surfactant deficiency is a major cause of RDS or HMD.* The lungs are underinflated, and the alveoli contain a fluid with a high protein content that resembles a glassy or hyaline membrane. This membrane is believed to be derived from a combination of substances in the circulation and from the injured pulmonary epithelium. It has been suggested that prolonged intrauterine asphyxia may produce irreversible changes in the type II alveolar cells, making them incapable of producing surfactant. There appear to be other causes for an absence or deficiency of surfactant in premature and full-term infants. All the growth factors and hormones controlling surfactant production have not been identified, but corticosteroids and thyroxine, which are involved in fetal lung maturation, are potent stimulators of surfactant production. *Maternal glucocorticoid treatment during pregnancy accelerates fetal lung development and surfactant production.* This finding has led to the routine clinical use of corticosteroids (betamethasone) for the prevention of RDS in preterm labor. In addition, administration of exogenous surfactant (*surfactant replacement therapy*) reduces the severity of RDS and neonatal mortality.

Lobe of Azygos Vein

This lobe appears in the right lung in *approximately* 1% of people. It develops when the apical bronchus grows superiorly, medial to the arch of the azygos vein, instead of lateral to it. As a result, the vein lies at the bottom of a fissure in the superior (upper) lobe, which produces a linear marking on a radiograph of the lungs.

Congenital Lung Cysts

Cysts (filled with fluid or air) are thought to be formed by the dilation of terminal bronchi. They probably result from a disturbance in bronchial development during late fetal life. If several cysts are present, the lungs have a honeycomb appearance on radiographs. Congenital lung cysts (Fig. 10-12) are usually located at the periphery of the lung.

Agenesis of Lungs

Absence of the lungs results from failure of the respiratory bud to develop. Agenesis of one lung is more common than bilateral agenesis, but both conditions are rare. Unilateral pulmonary agenesis is compatible with life. The heart and other mediastinal structures are shifted to the affected side, and the existing lung is hyperexpanded.

Lung Hypoplasia

In infants with congenital diaphragmatic hernia (see Chapter 8), the lung is unable to develop normally because it is compressed by the abnormally positioned abdominal viscera. Lung hypoplasia is characterized by a markedly reduced lung volume and hypertrophy of the smooth muscle in the pulmonary arteries. The pulmonary hypertension leads to decreased blood flow through the pulmonary vascular system as the blood continues to shunt through the ductus arteriosus. Many infants with congenital diaphragmatic hernia die of pulmonary insufficiency, despite optimal postnatal care, because their lungs are too hypoplastic for air exchange and there is too much resistance for pulmonary blood flow to support extrauterine life.

Accessory Lung

A small accessory lung (*pulmonary sequestration*) is very uncommon. It is almost always located at the base of the left lung. It does not communicate with the tracheobronchial tree, and its blood supply is usually systemic rather than pulmonary in origin.

SUMMARY OF THE RESPIRATORY SYSTEM

- By the fourth week, a laryngotracheal diverticulum develops from the floor of the primordial pharynx.
- The laryngotracheal diverticulum becomes separated from the foregut by tracheoesophageal folds that fuse to form a tracheoesophageal septum. This septum results in the formation of the esophagus and the laryngotracheal tube.
- The endoderm of the laryngotracheal tube gives rise to the epithelium of the lower respiratory organs and the tracheobronchial glands. The splanchnic mesenchyme surrounding the laryngotracheal tube forms the connective tissue, cartilage, muscle, and blood and lymphatic vessels of these organs.
- Pharyngeal arch mesenchyme contributes to formation of the epiglottis and connective tissue of the larynx. The laryngeal muscles are derived from mesenchyme in the caudal pharyngeal arches. The laryngeal cartilages are derived from neural crest cells.

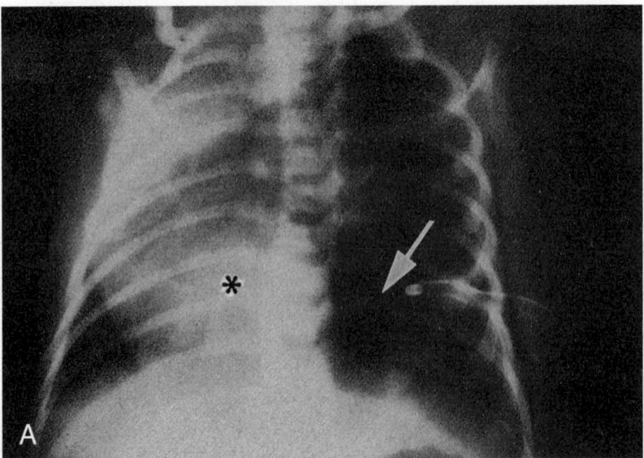

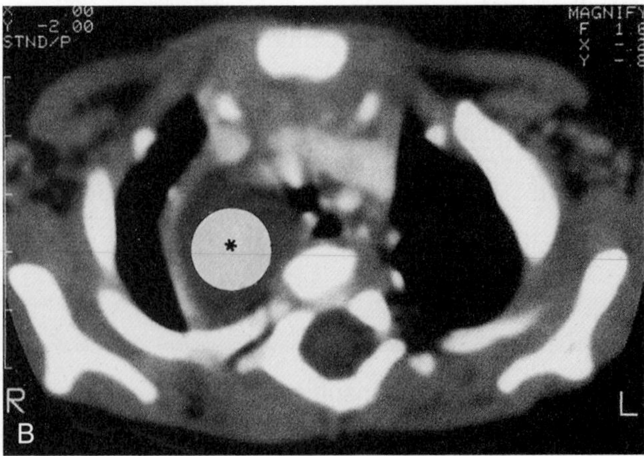

Figure 10-12. Congenital lung cysts. **A,** Chest radiograph (posteroanterior) of an infant showing a large left-sided congenital cystic adenomatoid malformation (*arrow*). The heart (*asterisk*) has shifted to the right. Note the chest tube on the left side, which was placed on the initial diagnosis of a pneumothorax (air in pleural cavity). **B,** Axial computed tomography image of the thorax in an infant with a large right-sided congenital bronchogenic cyst (*asterisk*). (Courtesy of Dr. Prem S. Sahni, formerly of the Department of Radiology, Children's Hospital, Winnipeg, Manitoba, Canada.)

- The distal end of the laryngotracheal diverticulum gives rise to a respiratory bud that divides into two bronchial buds. Each bronchial bud soon enlarges to form a main bronchus, and then the main bronchus subdivides to form lobar, segmental, and subsegmental branches.
- Each tertiary bronchial bud (segmental bronchial bud), with its surrounding mesenchyme, is the primordium of a bronchopulmonary segment. Branching continues until *approximately* 17 orders of branches have formed. Additional airways are formed after birth, until *approximately* 24 orders of branches are present.
- Lung development is divided into four stages: pseudoglandular (6–16 weeks), canalicular (16–26 weeks), terminal sac (26 weeks to birth), and alveolar (32 weeks to *approximately* 8 years of age).
- By 20 weeks, type II pneumocytes begin to secrete pulmonary surfactant. Deficiency of surfactant results in respiratory distress syndrome (RDS) or hyaline membrane disease (HMD).
- A tracheoesophageal fistula (TEF), which results from faulty partitioning of the foregut into the esophagus and trachea, is usually associated with esophageal atresia.

CLINICALLY ORIENTED PROBLEMS

Case 10-1

Choking and continuous coughing were observed in a newborn infant. There was an excessive amount of mucous secretion and saliva in the infant's mouth, and the infant experienced considerable difficulty in breathing. The pediatrician was unable to pass a catheter through the esophagus into the stomach.

- What congenital anomalies would be suspected?
- Discuss the embryologic basis of these defects.
- What kind of an examination do you think would be used to confirm the tentative diagnosis?

Case 10-2

A premature infant developed rapid, shallow respiration shortly after birth. A diagnosis of RDS was made.

- How do you think the infant might attempt to overcome his or her inadequate exchange of oxygen and carbon dioxide?
- What usually causes RDS?
- What treatment is currently used clinically to prevent RDS?
- A deficiency of what substance is associated with RDS?

Case 10-3

The parents of a newborn infant were told that their son had a fistula between his trachea and esophagus.

- What is the most common type of TEF?
- What is its embryologic basis?
- What anomaly of the digestive tract is frequently associated with this abnormality?

Case 10-4

A newborn infant with esophageal atresia experienced respiratory distress with cyanosis shortly after birth. Radiographs demonstrated air in the infant's stomach.

- How did the air enter the stomach?
- What other problem might result in an infant with this fairly common type of congenital anomaly?

Discussion of these problems is given at the back of the book.

References and Suggested Reading

Abel R, Bush A, Chitty RS, et al: Congenital lung disease. In Chernick V, Boat T, Wilmott R, Bush A (eds): Kendig's Disorders of the Respiratory Tract in Children, 7th ed. Philadelphia, WB Saunders, 2006.

Bizzarro MJ, Gross I: Effects of hormones on lung development. Obstet Gynecol Clin North Am 31:949, 2004.

Bratu I, Flageole H, Chen M-F, et al: The multiple facets of pulmonary sequestration. J Pediatr Surg 36:784, 2001.

Brunner HG, van Bokhoven H: Genetic players in esophageal atresia and tracheoesophageal fistula. Curr Opin Genet Dev 15:341, 2005.

Crelin ES: Development of the upper respiratory system. Clin Symp 28:3, 1976.

Goldstein RB: Ultrasound evaluation of the fetal thorax. In Callen PW (ed): Ultrasonography in Obstetrics and Gynecology, 4th ed. Philadelphia, WB Saunders, 2000.

Haddad GG, Fontán JJP: Development of the respiratory system. In Behrman RE, Kliegman Jenson HB (eds): Nelson Textbook of Pediatrics, 17th ed. Philadelphia, Elsevier/Saunders, 2004.

Holinger LD: Congenital anomalies of the larynx; congenital anomalies of the trachea and bronchi. In Behrman RE, Kliegman Jenson HB (eds): Nelson Textbook of Pediatrics, 17th ed. Philadelphia, WB Saunders, 2004.

Inanlou MR, Baguma-Nibasheka M, Kablar B: The role of fetal breathing-like movements in lung organogenesis. Histol Histopathol 20:1261, 2005.

Jobe AH: Lung development and maturation. In Martin RJ, Fanaroff AA, Walsh MC (eds): Fanaroff and Martin's Neonatal-Perinatal Medicine. Diseases of the Fetus and Infant, 8th ed. Philadelphia, Mosby, 2006.

Kays DW: Congenital diaphragmatic hernia and neonatal lung lesions. Surg Clin North Am 86:329, 2006.

Langston C: New concepts in the pathology of congenital lung malformations. Semin Pediatr Surg 12:17, 2003.

Moore KL, Dalley AF: Clinically Oriented Anatomy, 5th ed. Baltimore, Williams & Wilkins, 2005.

Moya FR, Lally KP: Evidence-based management of infants with congenital diaphragmatic hernia. Sem Perinatol 29:112, 2005.

O'Rahilly R, Boyden E: The timing and sequence of events in the development of the human respiratory system during the embryonic period proper. Z Anat Entwicklungsgesch 141:237, 1973.

Rottier R, Tibboel D: Fetal lung and diaphragm development in congenital diaphragmatic hernia. Semin Perinatol 29:86, 2005.

Sañudo JR, Domenech-Mateu JM: The laryngeal primordium and epithelial lamina. A new interpretation. J Anat 171:207, 1990.

Smith EI: The early development of the trachea and oesophagus in relation to atresia of the oesophagus and tracheo-oesophageal fistula. Contr Embryol Carnegie Inst 245:36, 1957.

Spencer C, Neales K: Antenatal corticosteroids to prevent neonatal respiratory distress syndrome. BMJ 320:325, 2000.

Turner BS, Bradshaw W, Brandon D: Neonatal lung remodeling. J Perinat Neonat Nurs 19:362, 2006.

Warburton D, Schwarz M, Tefft D, et al: The molecular basis of lung morphogenesis. Mech Dev 92:55, 2000.

Wells LJ, Boyden EA: The development of the bronchopulmonary segments in human embryos of horizons XVII and XIX. Am J Anat 95:163, 1954.

Whitsett JA, Wert SE: Molecular determinants of lung morphogenesis. In Chernick V (ed): Kendig's Disorders of the Respiratory Tract in Children, 7th ed. Philadelphia, WB Saunders, 2006.

11

The Digestive System

Foregut 212
- Development of the Esophagus 212
- Development of the Stomach 213
- Omental Bursa 216
- Development of the Duodenum 216
- Development of the Liver and Biliary Apparatus 218
- Development of the Pancreas 221
- Development of the Spleen 223

Midgut 224
- Rotation of the Midgut Loop 224
- Cecum and Appendix 227

Hindgut 235
- Cloaca 235
- The Anal Canal 236

Summary of the Digestive System 241

Clinically Oriented Problems 241

The **primordial gut** at the beginning of the fourth week is closed at its cranial end by the **oropharyngeal membrane** (see Fig. 9-1*E*) and at its caudal end by the **cloacal membrane** (Fig. 11-1*B*). The primordial gut forms during the fourth week as the head, tail, and lateral folds incorporate the dorsal part of the umbilical vesicle into the embryo (see Chapter 5). The endoderm of the primordial gut gives rise to most of its epithelium and glands. The epithelium at the cranial and caudal ends of the alimentary tract is derived from ectoderm of the **stomodeum** and **proctodeum**, respectively (see Fig. 11-1*A* and *B*).

Fibroblast growth factors (FGFs) are involved in early *anterior-posterior axial patterning*, and it appears that FGF-4 signals from the adjacent ectoderm and mesoderm induce the endoderm. Other secreted factors, such as activins, members of the transforming growth factor β superfamily, contribute to the formation of the endoderm. The endoderm specifies temporal and positional information, which is essential for the development of the gut. The muscular, connective tissue, and other layers of the wall of the digestive tract are derived from the splanchnic mesenchyme surrounding the primordial gut. Mesenchymal factors, FoxF proteins, control proliferation of the endodermal epithelium that secretes sonic hedgehog (Shh). For descriptive purposes, the primordial gut is divided into three parts: foregut, midgut, and hindgut. *Molecular studies* suggest that *Hox* and *ParaHox* genes, as well as Shh signals, regulate the regional differentiation of the primordial gut to form the different parts.

FOREGUT

The derivatives of the foregut are

- The primordial pharynx and its derivatives
- The lower respiratory system
- The esophagus and stomach
- The duodenum, distal to the opening of the bile duct
- The liver, biliary apparatus (hepatic ducts, gallbladder, and bile duct), and pancreas

These foregut derivatives, other than the pharynx, lower respiratory tract, and most of the esophagus, are supplied by the celiac trunk, the artery of the foregut (see Fig. 11-1*B*).

Development of the Esophagus

The esophagus develops from the foregut immediately caudal to the pharynx (see Fig. 11-1*B*). The partitioning of the trachea from the esophagus by the **tracheoesophageal septum** is described in Chapter 10. Initially, the esophagus is short, but it elongates rapidly, mainly because of the growth and relocation of the heart and lungs. The esophagus reaches its final relative length by the seventh week. Its epithelium and glands are derived from endoderm. The epithelium proliferates and partly or completely obliterates the lumen; however, recanalization of the esophagus normally occurs by the end of the eighth week. The striated muscle forming the muscularis externa of the superior third of the esophagus is derived from mesenchyme in the caudal pharyngeal arches. The smooth muscle, mainly in the inferior third of the esophagus, develops from the surrounding splanchnic mesenchyme. Recent studies indicate transdifferentiation of smooth muscle cells in the superior part of the esophagus to striated muscle, which is dependent on myogenic regulatory factors. Both types of muscle are innervated by branches of the vagus nerves (cranial nerve X), which supply the caudal pharyngeal arches (see Table 9-1).

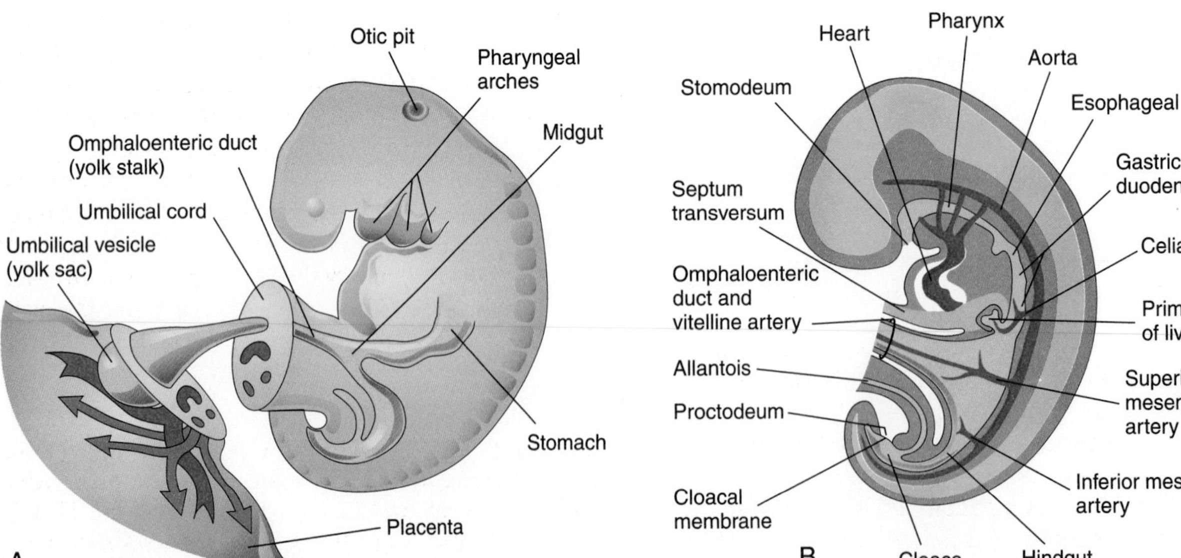

FIGURE 11-1. **A,** Lateral view of a 4-week embryo showing the relationship of primordial gut to omphaloenteric duct (yolk sac). **B,** Drawing of median section of the embryo showing early digestive system and its blood supply. The primordial gut is a long tube extending the length of the embryo. Its blood vessels are derived from the vessels that supplied the omphaloenteric duct.

Esophageal Atresia

Blockage of the esophagus occurs with an incidence of 1 in 3000 to 4500 live births. Approximately one third of affected infants are born prematurely. Esophageal atresia is associated with **tracheoesophageal fistula** in more than 85% of cases (see Fig. 10-5). Atresia may occur as a separate anomaly, but this is less common. **Esophageal atresia** results from deviation of the tracheoesophageal septum in a posterior direction (see Fig. 10-2); as a result, there is incomplete separation of the esophagus from the laryngotracheal tube. Isolated esophageal atresia may be associated with other congenital anomalies, e.g., anorectal atresia and anomalies of the urogenital system. In these cases, the atresia results from failure of recanalization of the esophagus during the eighth week of development. The cause of this arrest of development is thought to result from defective growth of endodermal cells.

A fetus with esophageal atresia is unable to swallow amniotic fluid; consequently, this fluid cannot pass to the intestine for absorption and transfer through the placenta to the maternal blood for disposal. This results in *polyhydramnios*, the accumulation of an excessive amount of amniotic fluid. Newborn infants with esophageal atresia usually appear healthy initially. Excessive drooling may be noted early on after birth, and the diagnosis of esophageal atresia should be considered if the infant fails oral feeding with immediate regurgitation and coughing. Inability to pass a catheter through the esophagus into the stomach strongly suggests esophageal atresia. A radiographic examination demonstrates the anomaly by imaging the nasogastric tube arrested in the proximal esophageal pouch. Surgical repair of esophageal atresia now results in survival rates of more than 85%.

Esophageal Stenosis

Narrowing of the lumen of the esophagus (stenosis) can be anywhere along the esophagus, but it usually occurs in its distal third, either as a web or as a long segment of esophagus with a threadlike lumen. Stenosis usually results from incomplete recanalization of the esophagus during the eighth week, or it may result from a failure of esophageal blood vessels to develop in the affected area. As a result, atrophy of a segment of the esophageal wall occurs.

Short Esophagus (Congenital Hiatal Hernia)

Initially the esophagus is very short. Its failure to elongate sufficiently as the neck and thorax develop results in displacement of part of the stomach superiorly through the esophageal hiatus into the thorax—**congenital hiatal hernia**. Most hiatal hernias occur long after birth, usually in middle-aged people, and result from weakening and widening of the esophageal hiatus in the diaphragm.

Development of the Stomach

The distal part of the foregut is initially a simple tubular structure (see Fig. 11-1*B*). Around the middle of the fourth week, a slight dilation indicates the site of the primordium of the stomach. It first appears as a fusiform enlargement of the caudal or distal part of the foregut and is initially oriented in the median plane (Figs. 11-1 and 11-2*B*). The primordial stomach soon enlarges and broadens ventrodorsally. During the next 2 weeks, the dorsal border of the stomach grows faster than its ventral border; this demarcates the greater curvature of the stomach (see Fig. 11-2*D*).

Rotation of the Stomach

As the stomach enlarges and acquires its final shape, it slowly rotates 90 degrees in a clockwise direction (viewed from the cranial end) around its longitudinal axis. The effects of rotation on the stomach are (Figs. 11-2 and 11-3):

- The ventral border (lesser curvature) moves to the right and the dorsal border (greater curvature) moves to the left.
- The original left side becomes the ventral surface and the original right side becomes the dorsal surface.
- Before rotation, the cranial and caudal ends of the stomach are in the median plane (see Fig. 11-2*B*). During rotation and growth of the stomach, its cranial region moves to the left and slightly inferiorly, and its caudal region moves to the right and superiorly.
- After rotation, the stomach assumes its final position with its long axis almost transverse to the long axis of the body (see Fig. 11-2*E*). The rotation and growth of the stomach explain why the left vagus nerve supplies the anterior wall of the adult stomach and the right vagus nerve innervates its posterior wall.

Mesenteries of the Stomach

The stomach is suspended from the dorsal wall of the abdominal cavity by a dorsal mesentery—the **primordial dorsal mesogastrium** (see Figs. 11-2*B* and *C* and 11-3*A*). This mesentery is originally in the median plane, but it is carried to the left during rotation of the stomach and formation of the **omental bursa** or lesser sac of peritoneum (see Fig. 11-3*A* to *E*). The **primordial ventral mesogastrium** attaches to the stomach. The ventral

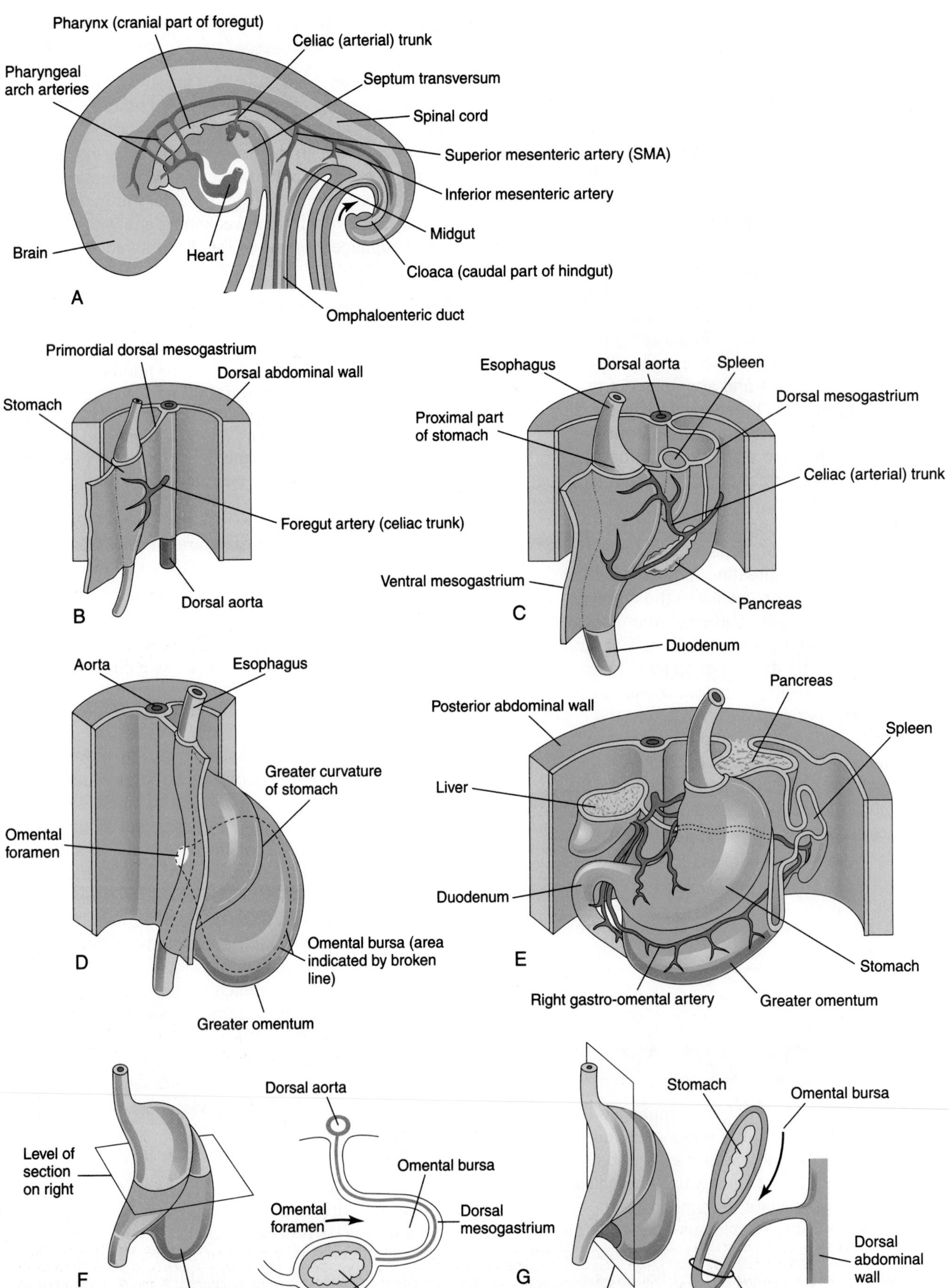

FIGURE 11-2. Development and rotation of stomach and formation of the omental bursa (lesser sac) and greater omentum. **A,** Median section of a 28-day embryo. **B,** Anterolateral view of a 28-day embryo. **C,** Embryo approximately 35 days. **D,** Embryo approximately 40 days. **E,** Embryo approximately 48 days. **F,** Lateral view of the stomach and greater omentum of an embryo at approximately 52 days. The transverse section shows the omental foramen and omental bursa. **G,** Sagittal section showing the omental bursa and greater omentum. The *arrow* in **F** and **G** indicates the site of the omental foramen.

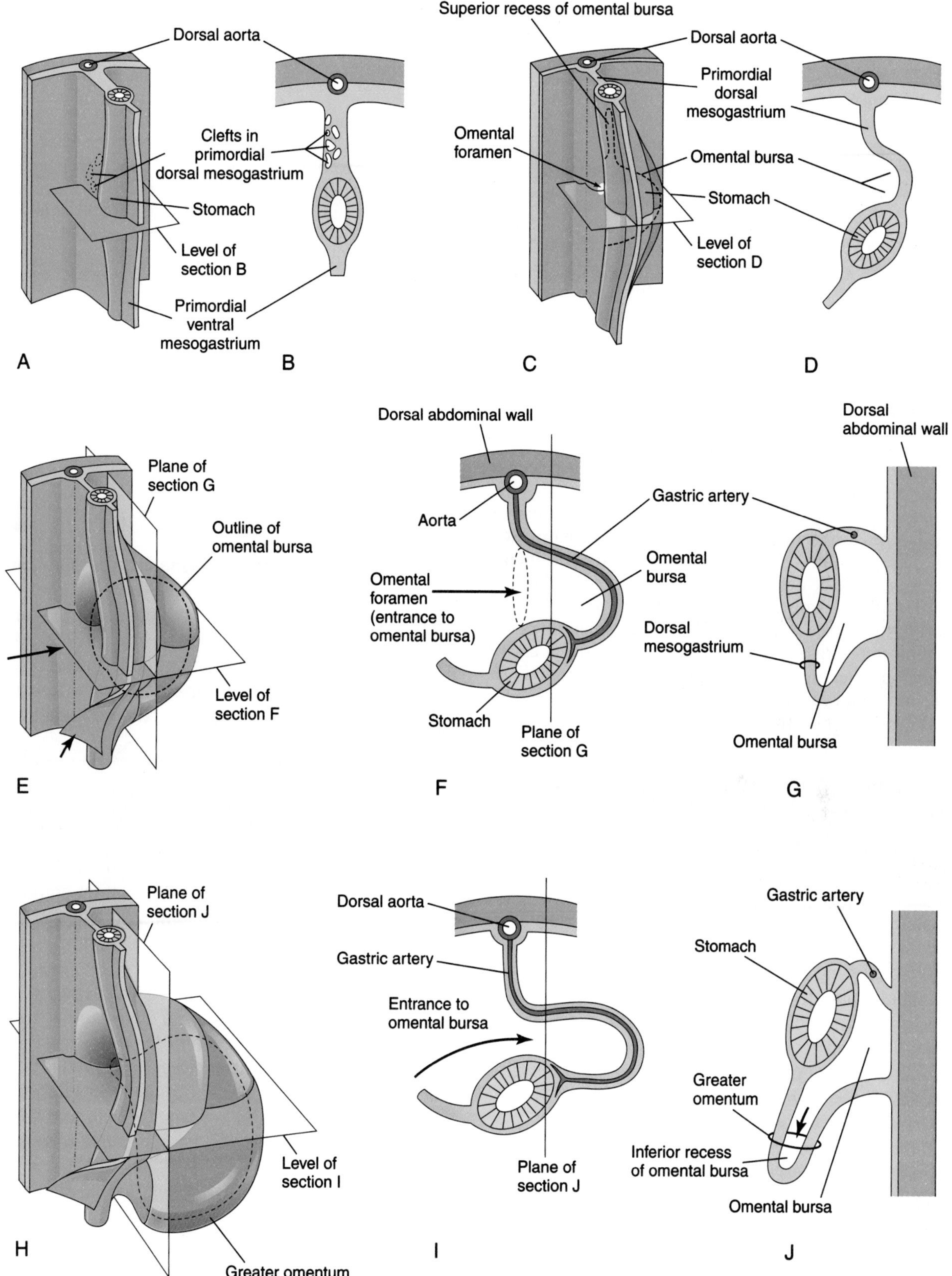

FIGURE 11-3. Development of stomach and its mesenteries and formation of omental bursa. **A,** At 5 weeks. **B,** Transverse section showing clefts in the dorsal mesogastrium. **C,** Later stage after coalescence of the clefts to form the omental bursa. **D,** Transverse section showing the initial appearance of the omental bursa. **E,** The dorsal mesentery has elongated and the omental bursa has enlarged. **F** and **G,** Transverse and sagittal sections, respectively, showing elongation of the dorsal mesogastrium and expansion of the omental bursa. **H,** At 6 weeks, showing the greater omentum and expansion of the omental bursa. **I** and **J,** Transverse and sagittal sections, respectively, showing the inferior recess of the omental bursa and the omental foramen. The *arrows* in **E**, **F**, and **I** indicate the site of the omental foramen. In **J**, the *arrow* indicates the inferior recess of the omental bursa.

mesogastrium also attaches the duodenum to the liver and the ventral abdominal wall (see Fig. 11-2*C*).

Omental Bursa

Isolated clefts develop in the mesenchyme forming the thick dorsal mesogastrium (see Fig. 11-3*A* and *B*). The clefts soon coalesce to form a single cavity, the **omental bursa** or lesser peritoneal sac (see Fig. 11-3*C* and *D*). Rotation of the stomach pulls the dorsal mesogastrium to the left, thereby enlarging the bursa, a large recess of the peritoneal cavity. The omental bursa expands transversely and cranially and soon lies between the stomach and the posterior abdominal wall. This pouchlike bursa facilitates movements of the stomach.

The superior part of the omental bursa is cut off as the diaphragm develops, forming a closed space—the **infracardiac bursa**. If it persists, it usually lies medial to the base of the right lung. The inferior part of the superior part of the omental bursa persists as the **superior recess of the omental bursa**. As the stomach enlarges, the omental bursa expands and acquires an **inferior recess of the omental bursa** between the layers of the elongated dorsal mesogastrium—the **greater omentum**. This membrane overhangs the developing intestines (see Fig. 11-3*J*). The inferior recess disappears as the layers of the greater omentum fuse (see Fig. 11-15*F*). The omental bursa communicates with the main part of the peritoneal cavity through an opening—the **omental foramen** (see Figs. 11-2*D* and *F* and 11-3*C* and *F*). In the adult, this foramen is located posterior to the free edge of the lesser omentum.

Congenital Hypertrophic Pyloric Stenosis

Anomalies of the stomach are uncommon except for hypertrophic pyloric stenosis. This anomaly affects one in every 150 males and one in every 750 females. In infants with this anomaly, there is a **marked muscular thickening of the pylorus**, the distal sphincteric region of the stomach (Fig. 11-4). The circular and, to a lesser degree, the longitudinal muscles in the pyloric region are hypertrophied. This results in severe stenosis of the pyloric canal and obstruction of the passage of food. As a result, the stomach becomes markedly distended (see Fig. 11-4*C*), and the infant expels the stomach's contents with considerable force (projectile vomiting). Surgical relief of the pyloric obstruction (*pyloromyotomy*) is the usual treatment. The cause of congenital pyloric stenosis is unknown, but the high rate of concordance in monozygotic twins suggests that genetic factors may be involved.

Development of the Duodenum

Early in the fourth week, the duodenum begins to develop from the caudal or distal part of the foregut, the cranial or proximal part of the midgut, and the splanchnic mesenchyme associated with these endodermal parts of the primordial gut (Fig. 11-5*A*). The junction of the two parts of the duodenum is just distal to the origin of the bile duct (see Fig. 11-5*D*). The developing duodenum grows rapidly, forming a C-shaped loop that projects ventrally (see Fig. 11-5*B* to *D*). As the stomach rotates, the duodenal loop rotates to the right and comes to lie retroperitoneally (external to peritoneum). Because of its derivation from the foregut and midgut, the duodenum is supplied by branches of the celiac and superior mesenteric arteries that supply these parts of the primordial gut (see Fig. 11-1). During the fifth and sixth weeks, the lumen of the duodenum becomes progressively smaller and is temporarily obliterated because of the proliferation of its epithelial cells. Normally vacuolation occurs as the epithelial cells degenerate; as a result, the duodenum normally becomes recanalized by the end of the embryonic period (Fig. 11-6*C* and *D*). By this time, most of the ventral mesentery of the duodenum has disappeared.

Duodenal Stenosis

Partial occlusion of the duodenal lumen—**duodenal stenosis** (see Fig. 11-6*A*)—usually results from incomplete recanalization of the duodenum resulting from defective vacuolization (see Fig. 11-6*E3*). Most stenoses involve the horizontal (third) and/or ascending (fourth) parts of the duodenum. Because of the stenosis, the stomach's contents (usually containing bile) are often vomited.

Duodenal Atresia

Complete occlusion of the lumen of the duodenum—**duodenal atresia** (see Fig. 11-6*B*)—is not common. During early duodenal development, the lumen is completely occluded by epithelial cells. If recanalization of the lumen fails to occur (see Fig. 11-6*D3*), a short segment of the duodenum is occluded (see Fig. 11-6*F3*). The blockage occurs nearly always at the junction of the bile and pancreatic ducts (**hepatopancreatic ampulla**) but occasionally involves the horizontal (third) part of the duodenum. Investigation of families with **familial duodenal atresia** suggests an autosomal recessive inheritance.

In infants with duodenal atresia, vomiting begins a few hours after birth. The vomitus almost always contains bile; often there is distention of the epigastrium—the upper central area of the abdomen—resulting from an overfilled stomach and superior part of the duodenum. Duodenal atresia may occur as an isolated anomaly, but other congenital anomalies are often associated with it, e.g., anular pancreas (see Fig. 11-11*C*),

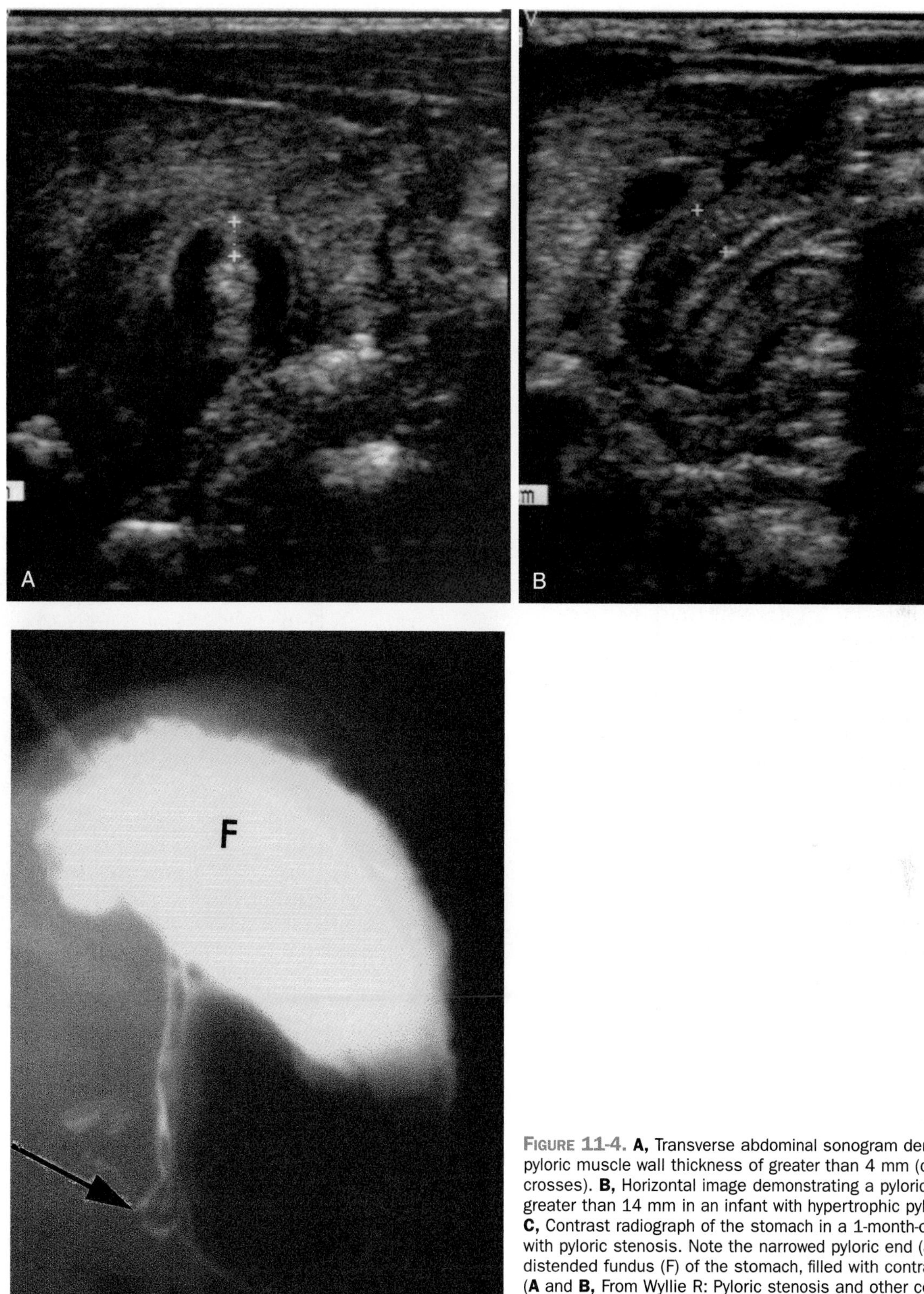

FIGURE 11-4. **A,** Transverse abdominal sonogram demonstrating a pyloric muscle wall thickness of greater than 4 mm (distance between crosses). **B,** Horizontal image demonstrating a pyloric channel length greater than 14 mm in an infant with hypertrophic pyloric stenosis. **C,** Contrast radiograph of the stomach in a 1-month-old male infant with pyloric stenosis. Note the narrowed pyloric end (*arrow*) and the distended fundus (F) of the stomach, filled with contrast material. (**A** and **B,** From Wyllie R: Pyloric stenosis and other congenital anomalies of the stomach. In Behrman RE, Kliegman RM, Arvin AM [eds]: Nelson Textbook of Pediatrics, 15th ed. Philadelphia, WB Saunders, 1996; **C,** Courtesy of Dr. Prem S. Sahni, formerly of the Department of Radiology, Children's Hospital, Winnipeg, Manitoba, Canada.)

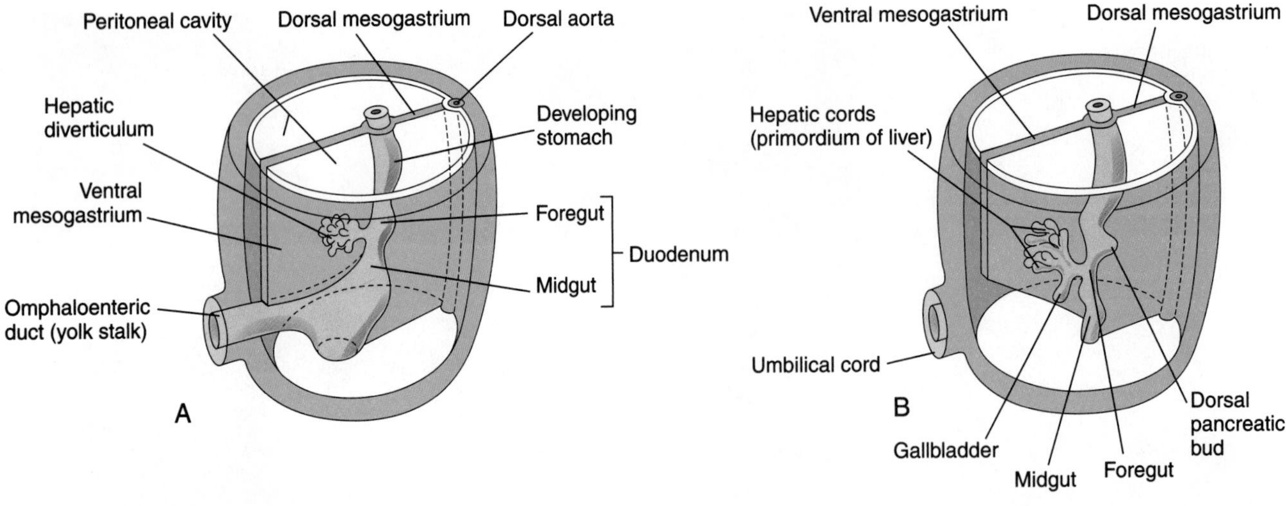

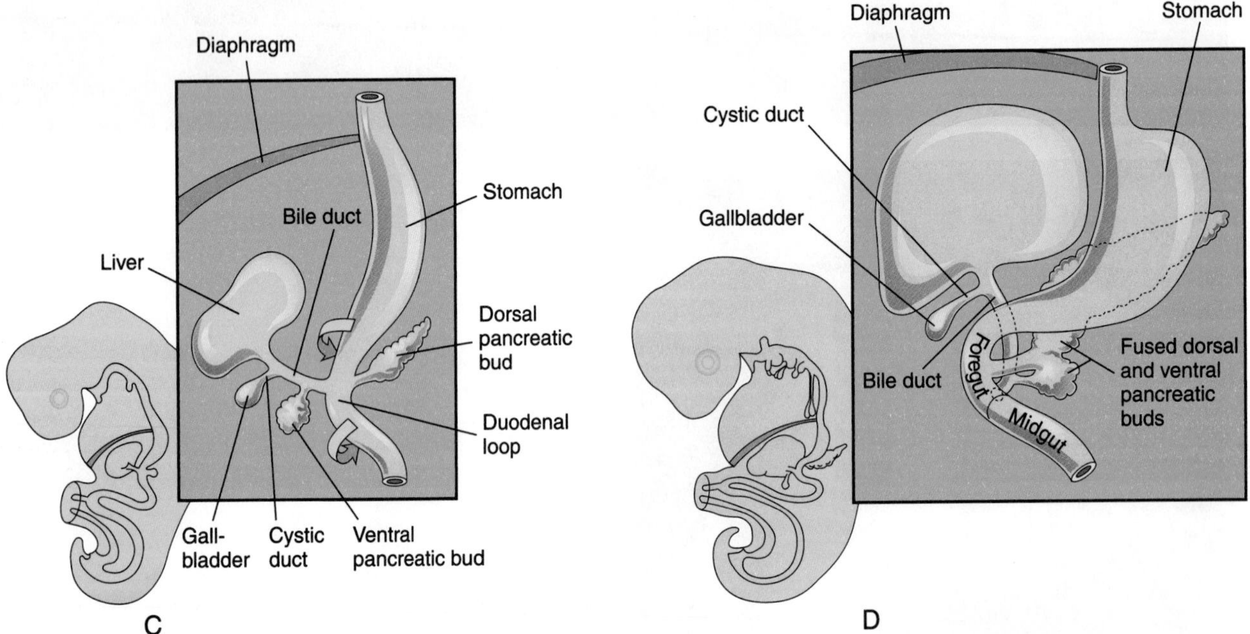

FIGURE 11-5. Progressive stages in the development of the duodenum, liver, pancreas, and extrahepatic biliary apparatus. **A,** At 4 weeks. **B** and **C,** At 5 weeks. **D,** At 6 weeks. The pancreas develops from dorsal and ventral pancreatic buds that fuse to form the pancreas. Note that the entrance of the bile duct into the duodenum gradually shifts from its initial position to a posterior one. This explains why the bile duct in the adult passes posterior to the duodenum and the head of the pancreas.

cardiovascular abnormalities, anorectal anomalies, and malrotation. Importantly, approximately one third of affected infants have Down syndrome and an additional 20% are premature. Duodenal atresia is associated with **bilious emesis** (vomiting of bile) because the blockage occurs distal to the opening of the bile duct.

Polyhydramnios also occurs because duodenal atresia prevents normal intestinal absorption of swallowed amniotic fluid. The diagnosis of duodenal atresia is suggested by the presence of a "double bubble" sign on plain radiographs or ultrasound scans (Fig. 11-7). This appearance is caused by a distended, gas-filled stomach and proximal duodenum.

Development of the Liver and Biliary Apparatus

The liver, gallbladder, and biliary duct system arise as a ventral outgrowth—**hepatic diverticulum**—from the caudal or distal part of the foregut early in the fourth week (Figs. 11-5*A* and 11-8*A*). Based on recent research findings, it has been suggested that both the hepatic diverticulum and the ventral bud of the pancreas develop

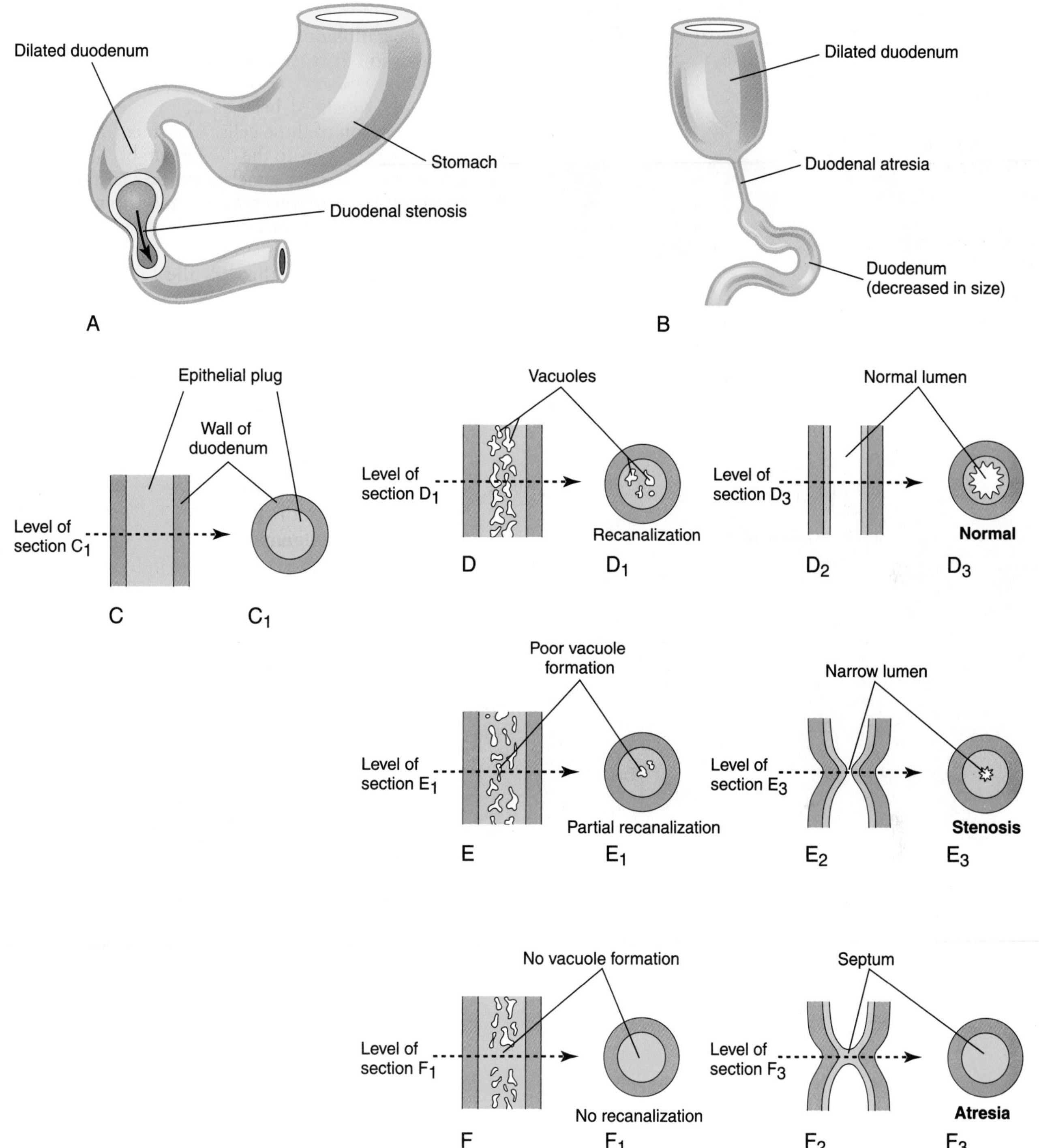

FIGURE 11-6. The embryologic basis of common types of congenital intestinal obstruction. **A,** Duodenal stenosis. **B,** Duodenal atresia. **C** to **F,** Diagrammatic longitudinal and transverse sections of the duodenum showing (1) normal recanalization (**D** to **D$_3$**), (2) stenosis (**E** to **E$_3$**), and atresia (**F** to **F$_3$**). Most duodenal atresias occur in the descending (second) and horizontal (third) parts of the duodenum.

from two cell populations in the embryonic endoderm. At sufficient levels, FGFs, secreted by the developing heart, interact with the bipotential cells and induce formation of the hepatic diverticulum. The diverticulum extends into the **septum transversum**, a mass of splanchnic mesoderm between the developing heart and midgut. The septum transversum forms the ventral mesentery in this region.

The hepatic diverticulum enlarges rapidly and divides into two parts as it grows between the layers of the **ventral mesogastrium** (see Fig. 11-5*A*). The larger cranial part of the hepatic diverticulum is the **primordium of the liver**. The proliferating endodermal cells give rise to interlacing cords of hepatocytes and to the epithelial lining of the intrahepatic part of the biliary apparatus. The **hepatic**

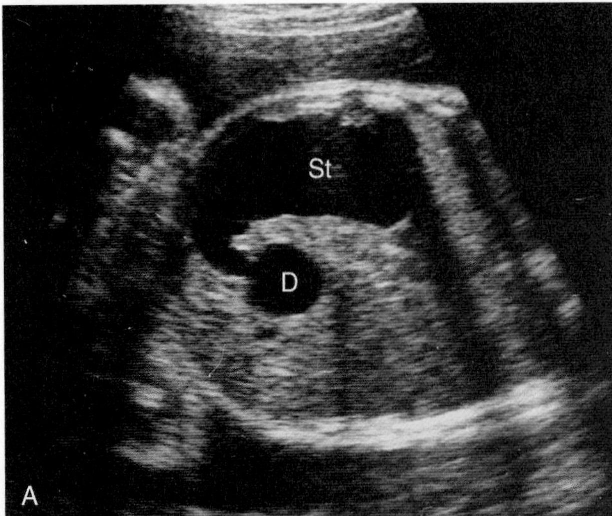

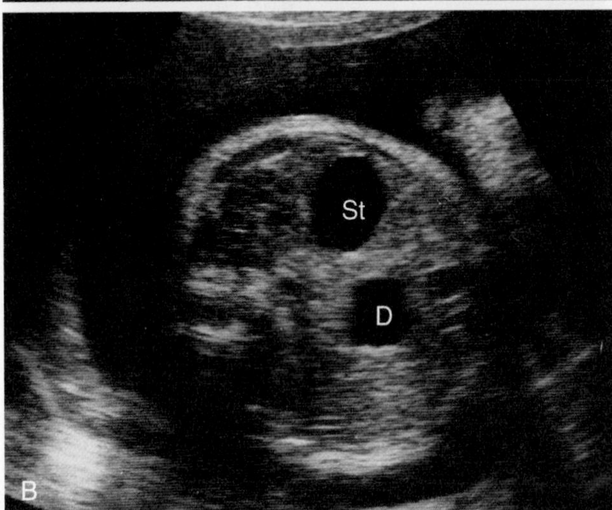

FIGURE 11-7. Ultrasound scans of a fetus at 33 weeks' gestation (31 weeks after fertilization) showing duodenal atresia. **A,** An oblique scan showing the dilated, fluid-filled stomach (St) entering the proximal duodenum (D), which is also enlarged because of the atresia (blockage) distal to it. **B,** Transverse scan illustrating the characteristic "double bubble" appearance of the stomach and duodenum when there is duodenal atresia. (Courtesy of Dr. Lyndon M. Hill, Magee-Women's Hospital, Pittsburgh, PA.)

cords anastomose around endothelium-lined spaces, the primordia of the **hepatic sinusoids**. The fibrous and hematopoietic tissue and Kupffer cells of the liver are derived from mesenchyme in the septum transversum.

The liver grows rapidly and, from the 5th to 10th weeks, fills a large part of the upper abdominal cavity (see Fig. 11-8*C* and *D*). The quantity of oxygenated blood flowing from the umbilical vein into the liver determines the development and functional segmentation of the liver. Initially, the right and left lobes are approximately the same size, but the right lobe soon becomes larger. **Hematopoiesis** begins during the sixth week, giving the liver a bright reddish appearance. By the ninth week, the liver accounts for approximately 10% of the total weight of the fetus. **Bile formation** by hepatic cells begins during the 12th week.

The small caudal part of the hepatic diverticulum becomes the **gallbladder**, and the stalk of the diverticulum forms the **cystic duct** (see Fig. 11-5*C*). Initially, the *extrahepatic biliary apparatus* is occluded with epithelial cells, but it is later canalized because of vacuolation resulting from degeneration of these cells. The stalk connecting the hepatic and cystic ducts to the duodenum becomes the **bile duct**. Initially, this duct attaches to the ventral aspect of the duodenal loop; however, as the duodenum grows and rotates, the entrance of the bile duct is carried to the dorsal aspect of the duodenum (see Fig. 11-5*C* and *D*). The bile entering the duodenum through the bile duct after the 13th week gives the *meconium* (intestinal contents) a dark green color.

Ventral Mesentery

This thin, double-layered membrane (see Fig. 11-8) gives rise to:

- The **lesser omentum**, passing from the liver to the lesser curvature of the stomach (**hepatogastric ligament**) and from the liver to the duodenum (**hepatoduodenal ligament**)
- The **falciform ligament**, extending from the liver to the ventral abdominal wall

The **umbilical vein** passes in the free border of the falciform ligament on its way from the umbilical cord to the liver. The ventral mesentery, derived from the mesogastrum, also forms the **visceral peritoneum of the liver**. The liver is covered by peritoneum except for the bare area that is in direct contact with the diaphragm (Fig. 11-9).

ANOMALIES OF THE LIVER

Minor variations of liver lobulation are common, but congenital anomalies of the liver are rare. Variations of the hepatic ducts, bile duct, and cystic duct are common and clinically significant. **Accessory hepatic ducts** may be present, and awareness of their possible presence is of surgical importance (Moore and Dalley, 2006). These accessory ducts are narrow channels running from the right lobe of the liver into the anterior surface of the body of the gallbladder. In some cases, the cystic duct opens into an accessory hepatic duct rather than into the common hepatic duct.

EXTRAHEPATIC BILIARY ATRESIA

This is the most serious anomaly of the extrahepatic biliary system and occurs in one in 10,000 to 15,000 live births. The most common form of extrahepatic biliary atresia (present in 85% of cases) is **obliteration of the bile ducts** at or superior to the *porta hepatis*—a deep transverse fissure on the visceral surface of the liver. Previous speculations

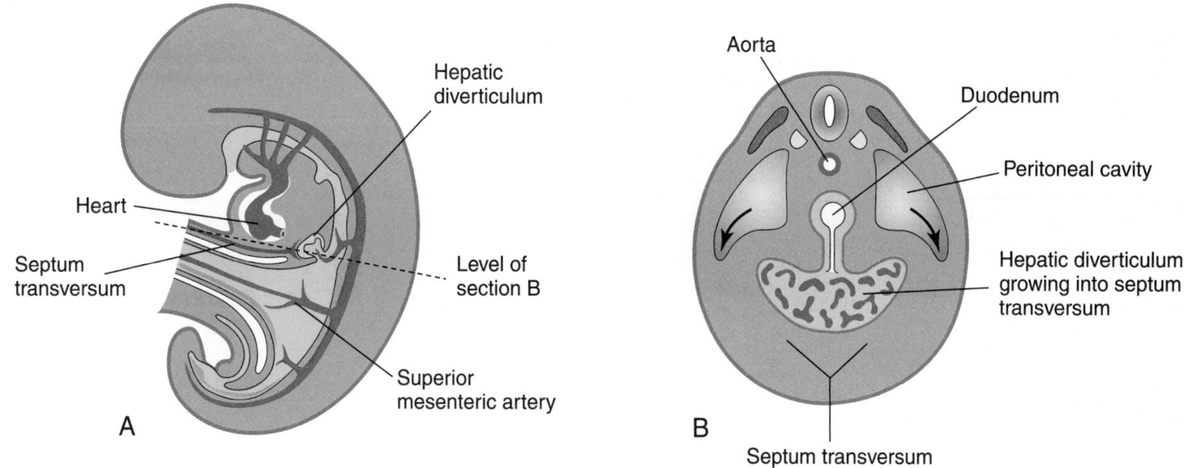

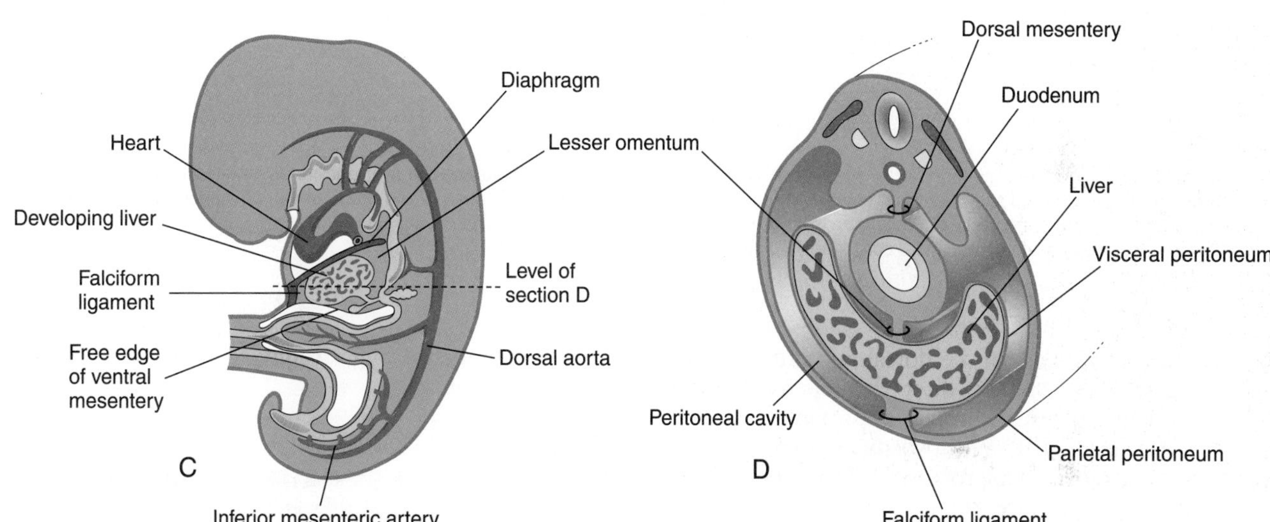

FIGURE 11-8. Illustrations showing how the caudal part of the septum transversum becomes stretched and membranous as it forms the ventral mesentery. **A,** Median section of a 4-week embryo. **B,** Transverse section of the embryo showing expansion of the peritoneal cavity (*arrows*). **C,** Sagittal section of a 5-week embryo. **D,** Transverse section of the embryo after formation of the dorsal and ventral mesenteries. Note that the liver is joined to the ventral abdominal wall and to the stomach and the duodenum by the falciform ligament and lesser omentum, respectively.

that there is a failure of the bile ducts to canalize may not be true. Biliary atresia could result from a failure of the remodeling process at the hepatic hilum or from infections or immunologic reactions during late fetal development. **Jaundice** occurs soon after birth and stools are acholic (clay colored). When biliary atresia cannot be corrected surgically (**Kasai hepatoportoenterostomy**), the child may die if a liver transplantation is not performed.

Development of the Pancreas

The pancreas develops between the layers of the mesentery from dorsal and ventral **pancreatic buds** of endodermal cells, which arise from the caudal or dorsal part of the foregut (Figs. 11-9 and 11-10*A* and *B*). Most of the pancreas is derived from the **dorsal pancreatic bud**. The larger dorsal pancreatic bud appears first and develops a slight distance cranial to the ventral bud. It grows rapidly between the layers of the dorsal mesentery. The **ventral pancreatic bud** develops near the entry of the bile duct into the duodenum and grows between the layers of the ventral mesentery. As the duodenum rotates to the right and becomes C shaped, the ventral pancreatic bud is carried dorsally with the bile duct (see Fig. 11-10*C* to *G*). It soon lies posterior to the dorsal pancreatic bud and later fuses with it.

The ventral pancreatic bud forms the **uncinate process** and part of the **head of the pancreas**. As the stomach, duodenum, and ventral mesentery rotate, the pancreas comes to lie along the dorsal abdominal wall. As the pancreatic buds fuse, their ducts anastomose. The **pancreatic duct** forms from the duct of the ventral bud and the distal part of the duct of the dorsal bud (see Fig. 11-10*G*). The

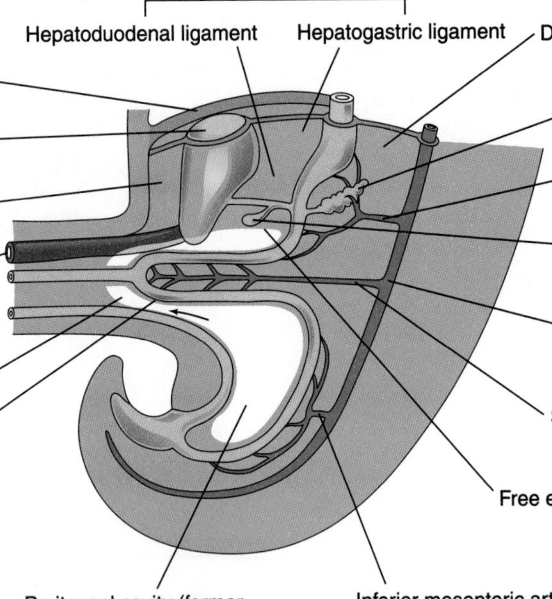

FIGURE 11-9. Median section of caudal half of an embryo at the end of the fifth week showing the liver and its associated ligaments. The *arrow* indicates the communication of the peritoneal cavity with the extraembryonic coelom. Because of the rapid growth of the liver and the midgut loop, the abdominal cavity temporarily becomes too small to contain the developing intestines; consequently, they enter the extraembryonic coelom in the proximal part of the umbilical cord (see Fig. 11-13).

proximal part of the duct of the dorsal bud often persists as an **accessory pancreatic duct** that opens into the minor duodenal papilla, located approximately 2 cm cranial to the main duct. The two ducts often communicate with each other. In approximately 9% of people, the pancreatic ducts fail to fuse, resulting in two ducts.

Molecular studies show that the ventral pancreas develops from a bipotential cell population in the ventral part of the endoderm. A default mechanism involving FGF-2, which is secreted by the developing heart, appears to play a role. Formation of the dorsal pancreatic bud depends on the notochord secreting activin and FGF-2, which block the expression of Shh in the endoderm.

Histogenesis of the Pancreas

The parenchyma of the pancreas is derived from the endoderm of the pancreatic buds, which forms a network of tubules. Early in the fetal period, **pancreatic acini** begin to develop from cell clusters around the ends of these tubules (primordial pancreatic ducts). The **pancreatic islets** develop from groups of cells that separate from the tubules and come to lie between the acini. **Insulin secretion** begins during the early fetal period (10 weeks). The glucagon- and somatostatin-containing cells develop before differentiation of the insulin-secreting cells. Glucagon has been detected in fetal plasma at 15 weeks. The connective tissue sheath and interlobular septa of the pancreas develop from the surrounding splanchnic mesenchyme. When there is *maternal diabetes mellitus*, the insulin-secreting beta cells in the fetal pancreas are chronically exposed to high levels of glucose. As a result, these cells undergo hypertrophy to increase the rate of insulin secretion.

ACCESSORY PANCREATIC TISSUE

Accessory pancreatic tissue is most often located in the wall of the stomach or duodenum or in an ileal diverticulum (e.g., a Meckel diverticulum; see Fig. 11-21).

ANULAR PANCREAS

Although an anular pancreas is uncommon, the anomaly warrants description because it may cause duodenal obstruction (Fig. 11-11C). The ringlike or anular part of the pancreas consists of a thin, flat band of pancreatic tissue surrounding the descending or second part of the duodenum. An anular pancreas may cause obstruction of the duodenum either shortly after birth or later. Infants present with symptoms of complete or partial bowel obstruction. Blockage of the duodenum develops if inflammation (pancreatitis) develops in the anular pancreas. An anular pancreas may be associated with Down syndrome, intestinal atresia, imperforate anus, pancreatitis, and malrotation. Males are

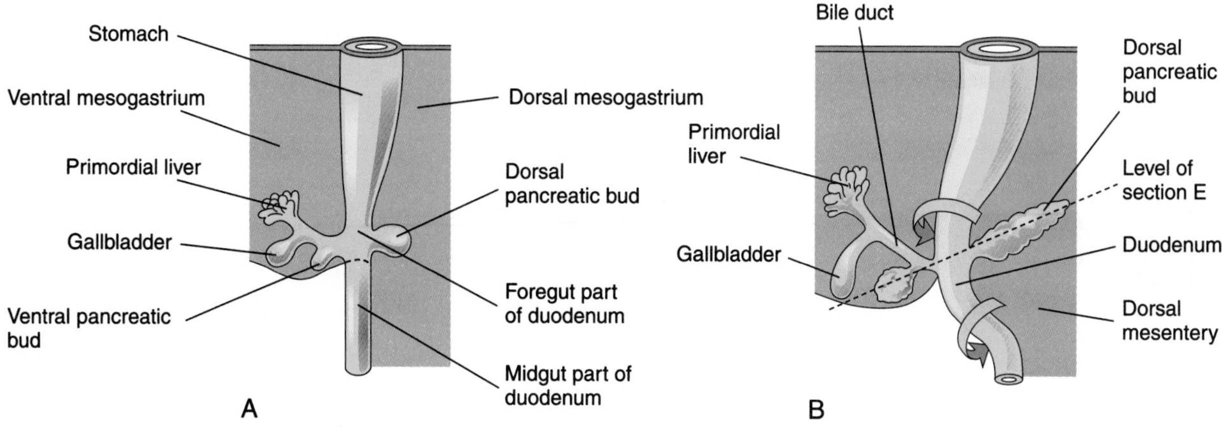

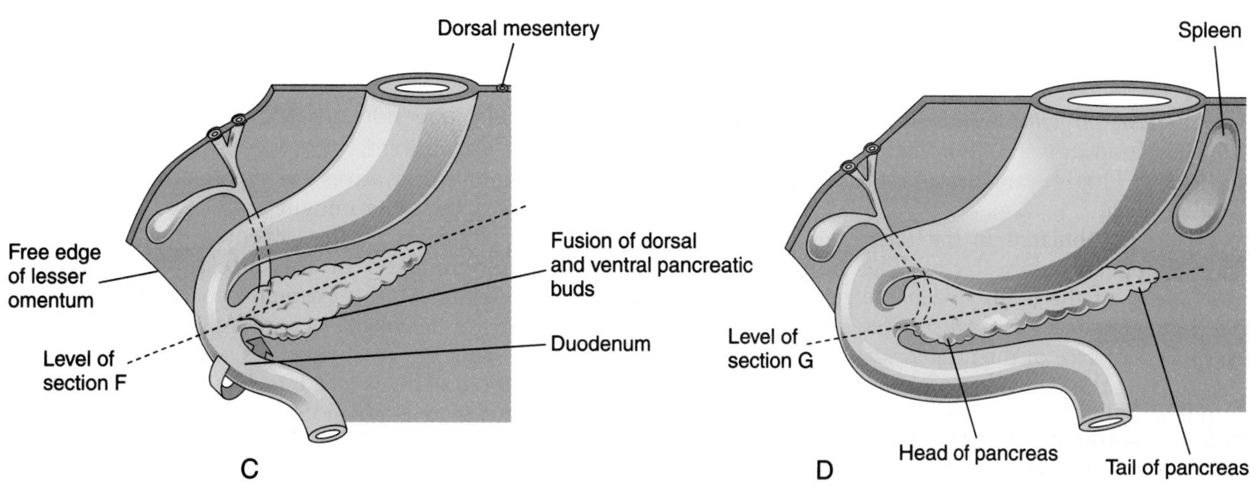

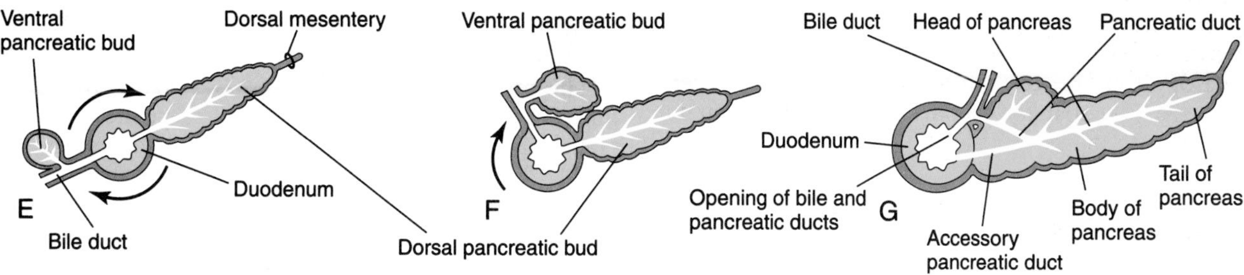

FIGURE 11-10. **A** to **D,** Successive stages in the development of the pancreas from the fifth to the eighth weeks. **E** to **G,** Diagrammatic transverse sections through the duodenum and developing pancreas. Growth and rotation (*arrows*) of the duodenum bring the ventral pancreatic bud toward the dorsal bud; they subsequently fuse. Note that the bile duct initially attaches to the ventral aspect of the duodenum and is carried around to the dorsal aspect as the duodenum rotates. The pancreatic duct is formed by the union of the distal part of the dorsal pancreatic duct and the ventral pancreatic duct. The proximal part of the dorsal pancreatic duct usually obliterates, but it may persist as an accessory pancreatic duct.

affected much more frequently than females. An anular pancreas probably results from the growth of a bifid ventral pancreatic bud around the duodenum (see Fig. 11-11*A* to *C*). The parts of the bifid ventral bud then fuse with the dorsal bud, forming a pancreatic ring (Latin, *anulus*).

Development of the Spleen

Development of the spleen is described with the digestive system because this organ is derived from a mass of mesenchymal cells located between the layers of the dorsal mesogastrium (Fig. 11-12). The spleen, a vascular lymphatic organ, begins to develop during the fifth week but does not acquire its characteristic shape until early in the

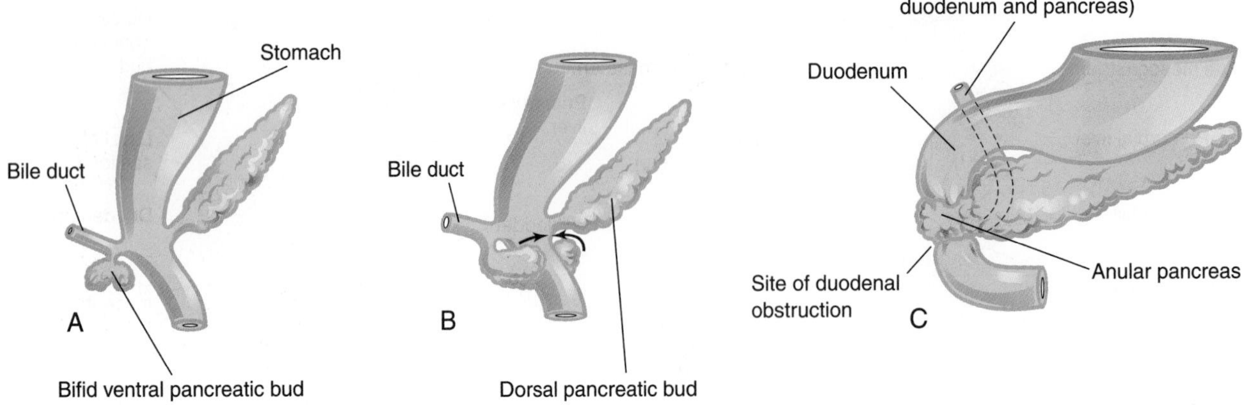

FIGURE 11-11. **A** and **B,** Probable basis of an anular pancreas. **C,** An anular pancreas encircling the duodenum. This anomaly produces complete obstruction (atresia) or partial obstruction (stenosis) of the duodenum. In most cases, the anular pancreas encircles the second part of the duodenum, distal to the hepatopancreatic ampulla.

fetal period. *Gene-targeting experiments* show that capsulin, a basic helix-loop transcription factor, and homeobox genes NKx2-5, Hox11, and Bapx1 regulate the development of the spleen.

The spleen is lobulated in the fetus, but the lobules normally disappear before birth. The notches in the superior border of the adult spleen are remnants of the grooves that separated the fetal lobules. As the stomach rotates, the left surface of the mesogastrium fuses with the peritoneum over the left kidney. This fusion explains the dorsal attachment of the **splenorenal ligament** and why the adult splenic artery, the largest branch of the celiac trunk, follows a tortuous course posterior to the omental bursa and anterior to the left kidney (see Fig. 11-12*C*).

Histogenesis of the Spleen

The mesenchymal cells in the splenic primordium differentiate to form the capsule, connective tissue framework, and parenchyma of the spleen. The spleen functions as a **hematopoietic center** until late fetal life; however, it retains its potential for blood cell formation even in adult life.

ACCESSORY SPLEENS (POLYSPLENIA)

One or more small splenic masses of fully functional splenic tissue may exist in one of the peritoneal folds, commonly near the hilum of the spleen, in the tail of the pancreas, or within the gastrosplenic ligament. These accessory spleens are usually isolated but may be attached to the spleen by thin bands. An accessory spleen occurs in approximately 10% of people and is usually approximately 1 cm in diameter.

MIDGUT

The derivatives of the midgut are

- The small intestine, including the duodenum distal to the opening of the bile duct
- The cecum, appendix, ascending colon, and the right one half to two thirds of the transverse colon

These midgut derivatives are supplied by the **superior mesenteric artery**, the midgut artery (see Fig. 11-1). As the midgut elongates, it forms a ventral, U-shaped loop of gut—the **midgut loop of the intestine**—that projects into the remains of the extraembryonic coelom in the proximal part of the umbilical cord. At this stage, the intraembryonic coelom communicates with extraembryonic coelom at the umbilicus (see Fig. 11-9). This midgut loop of the intestine is a **physiologic umbilical herniation**, which occurs at the beginning of the sixth week (Figs. 11-13 and 11-14). The loop communicates with the umbilical vesicle through the narrow **omphaloenteric duct** (yolk stalk) until the 10th week. The physiologic umbilical herniation occurs because there is not enough room in the abdominal cavity for the rapidly growing midgut. The shortage of space is caused mainly by the relatively massive liver and the kidneys that exist during this period of development.

The midgut loop of intestine has a cranial (proximal) limb and a caudal (distal) limb and is suspended from the dorsal abdominal wall by an elongated mesentery (see Fig. 11-13*A*). The omphaloenteric duct is attached to the apex of the midgut loop where the two limbs join (see Fig. 11-13*A*). The cranial limb grows rapidly and forms small intestinal loops, but the caudal limb undergoes very little change except for development of the **cecal swelling** (diverticulum), the primordium of the cecum, and appendix (see Fig. 11-13*C*).

Rotation of the Midgut Loop

While it is in the umbilical cord, the midgut loop rotates 90 degrees counterclockwise (looking from the ventral side) around the axis of the **superior mesenteric artery** (see Fig. 11-13*B*). This brings the cranial limb (small intestine) of the midgut loop to the right and the caudal limb (large intestine) to the left. During rotation, the cranial limb elongates and forms intestinal loops (e.g., primordia of jejunum and ileum).

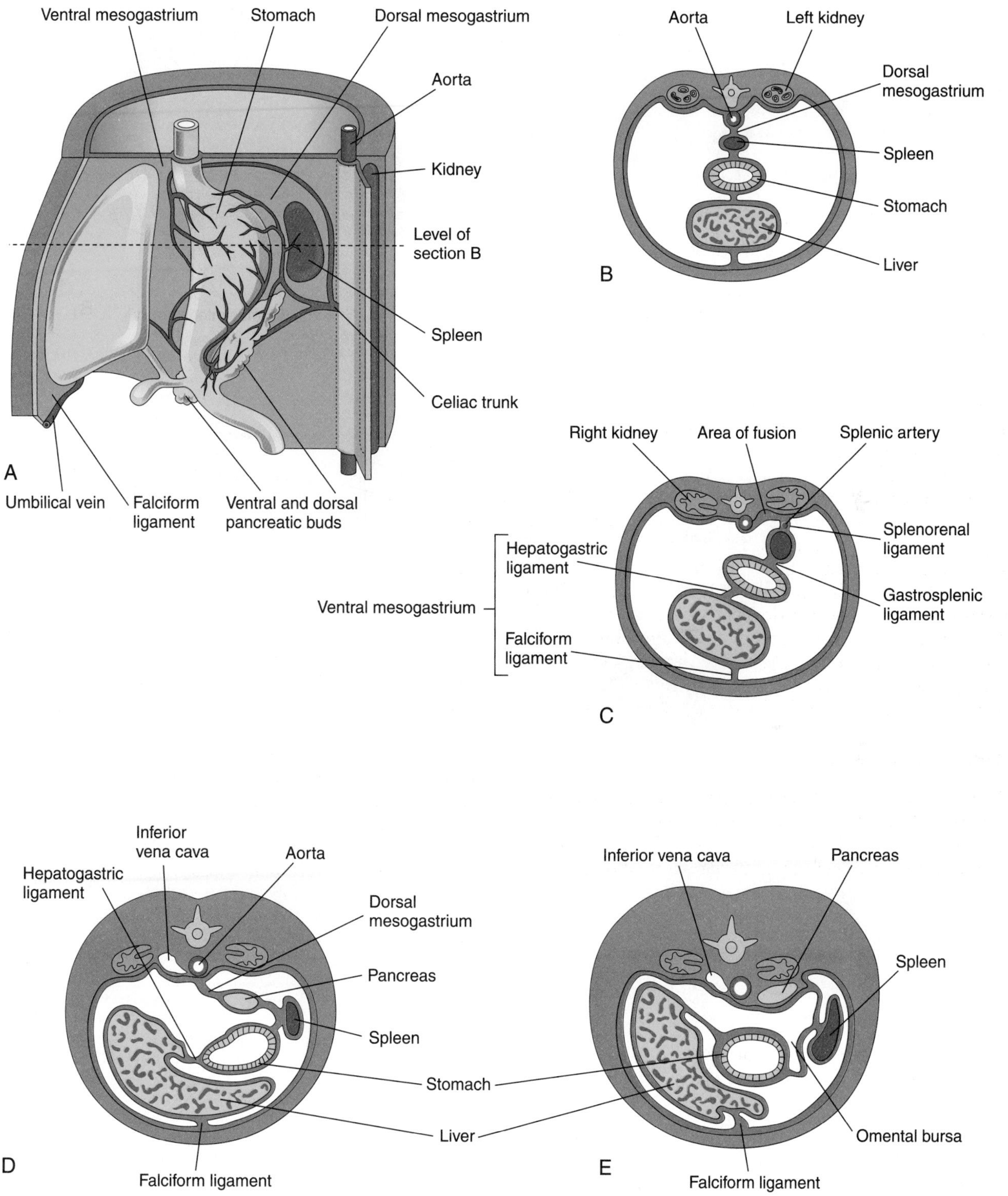

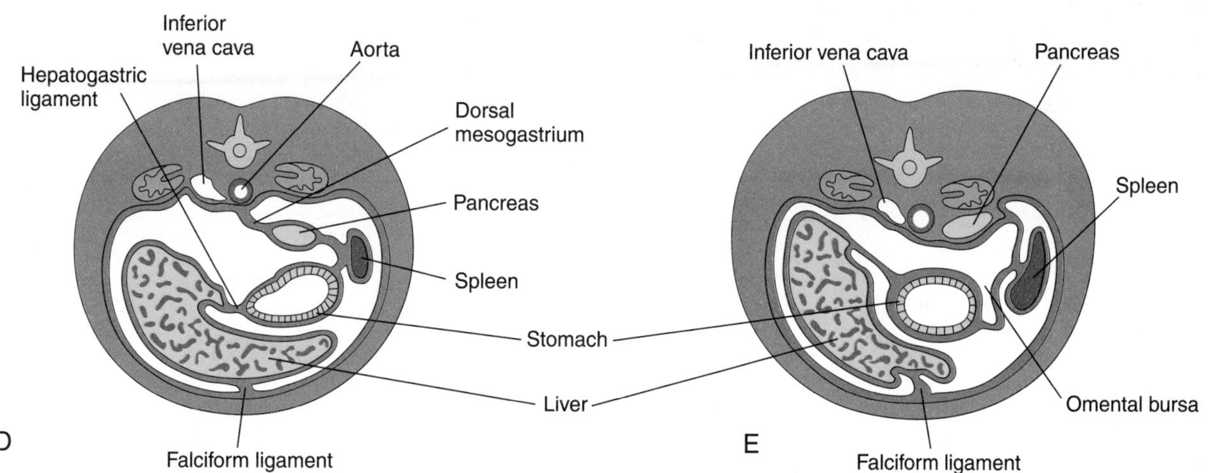

FIGURE 11-12. **A,** Left side of the stomach and associated structures at the end of the fifth week. Note that the pancreas, spleen, and celiac trunk are between the layers of the dorsal mesogastrium. **B,** Transverse section of the liver, stomach, and spleen at the level shown in **A**, illustrating their relationship to the dorsal and ventral mesenteries. **C,** Transverse section of a fetus showing fusion of the dorsal mesogastrium with the peritoneum on the posterior abdominal wall. **D** and **E,** Similar sections showing movement of the liver to the right and rotation of the stomach. Observe the fusion of the dorsal mesogastrium to the dorsal abdominal wall. As a result, the pancreas becomes retroperitoneal.

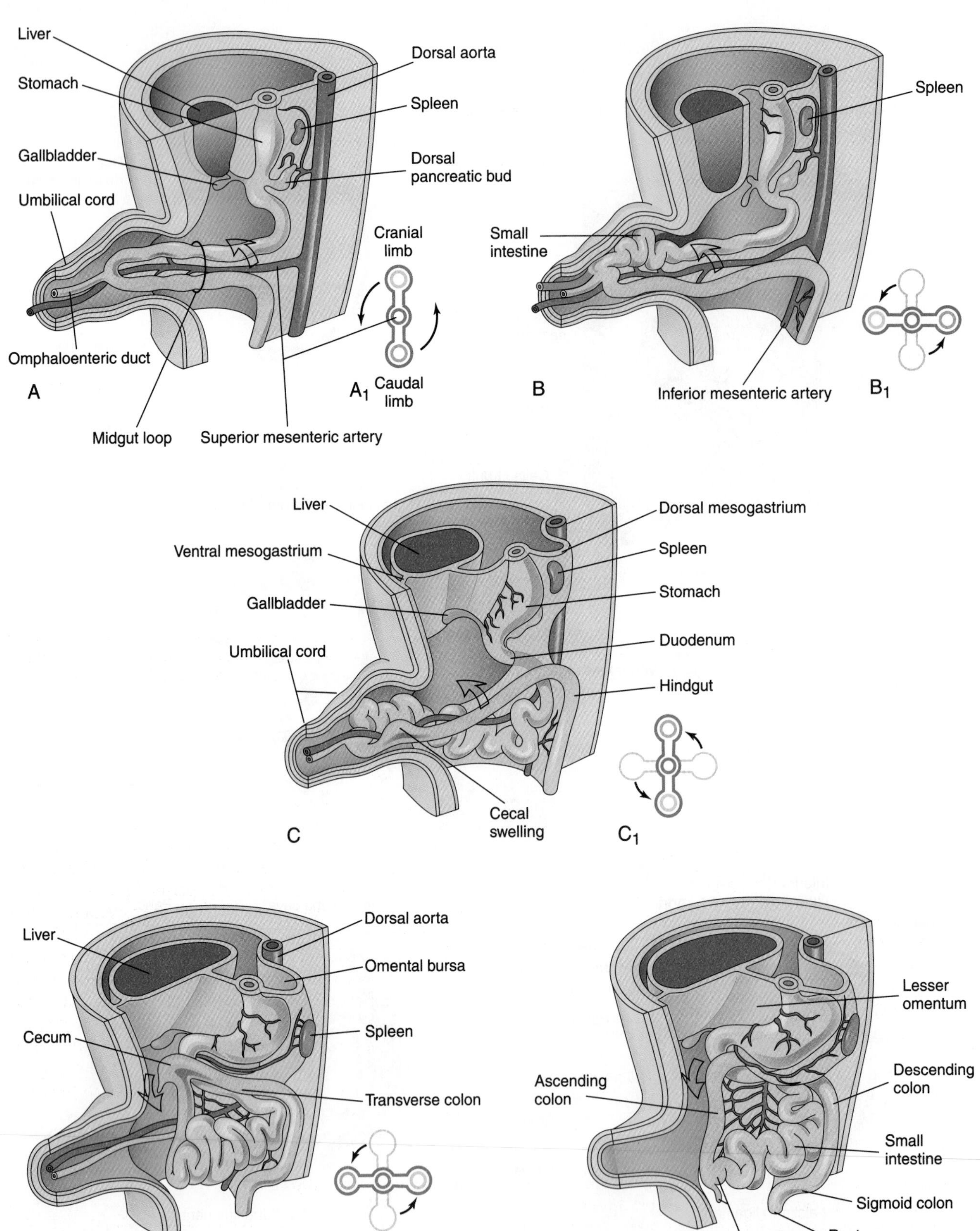

FIGURE 11-13. Drawings illustrating rotation of the midgut, as seen from the left, from the beginning of the 6th week to the 12th week. The midgut loop is in the proximal part of the umbilical cord. **A,** Transverse section through the midgut loop, illustrating the initial relationship of the limbs of the loop to the artery. **B,** Later stage showing the beginning of midgut rotation. **B_1,** Illustration of the 90-degree counterclockwise rotation that carries the cranial limb of the midgut to the right. **C,** At approximately 10 weeks, showing the intestines returning to the abdomen. **C_1,** Illustration of a further rotation of 90 degrees. **D,** At approximately 11 weeks, after return of intestines to the abdomen. **D_1,** Illustration of a further 90-degree rotation of the gut, for a total of 270 degrees. **E,** Later fetal period, showing the cecum rotating to its normal position in the lower right quadrant of the abdomen.

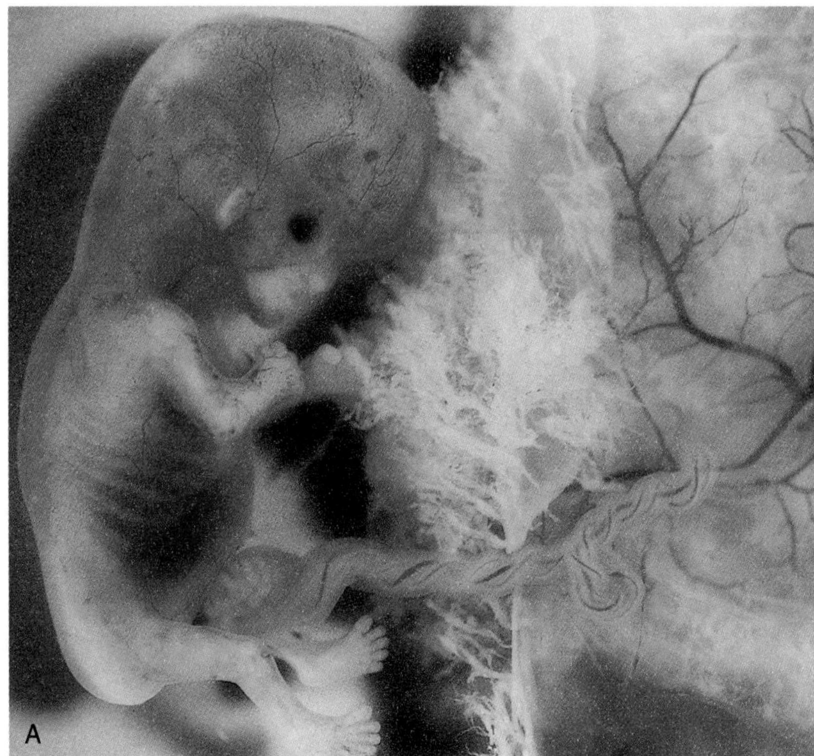

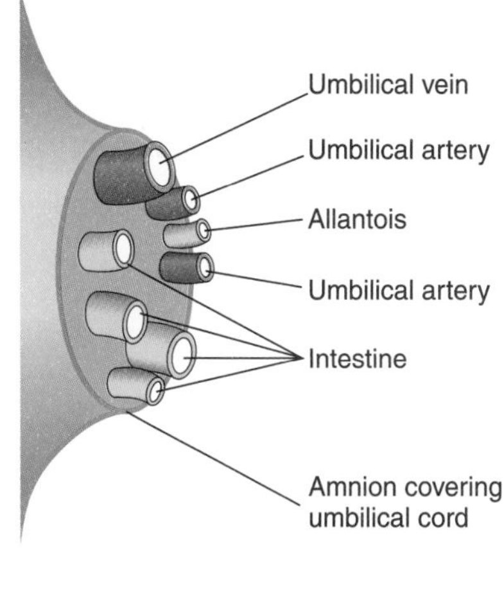

FIGURE 11-14. **A,** Physiologic hernia in a fetus (approximately 58 days) attached to its chorionic sac. Note the herniated intestine derived from the midgut loop in the proximal part of the umbilical cord. Also note the umbilical blood vessels. **B,** Schematic drawing showing the structures in the proximal part of the umbilical cord. (**A,** Courtesy of Dr. D.K. Kalousek, Department of Pathology, University of British Columbia, Children's Hospital, Vancouver, British Columbia, Canada.)

Return of the Midgut to the Abdomen

During the 10th week, the intestines return to the abdomen (reduction of the midgut hernia) (see Fig. 11-13*C* and *D*). It is not known what causes the intestine to return; however, the enlargement of the abdominal cavity, and the relative decrease in the size of the liver and kidneys are important factors. The small intestine (formed from the cranial limb) returns first, passing posterior to the superior mesenteric artery and occupies the central part of the abdomen. As the large intestine returns, it undergoes a further 180-degree counterclockwise rotation (see Fig. 11-13*C1* and *D1*). Later it comes to occupy the right side of the abdomen. The ascending colon becomes recognizable as the posterior abdominal wall progressively elongates (see Fig. 11-13*E*).

Fixation of the Intestines

Rotation of the stomach and duodenum causes the duodenum and pancreas to fall to the right. The enlarged colon presses the duodenum and pancreas against the posterior abdominal wall; as a result, most of the duodenal mesentery is absorbed (Fig. 11-15*C*, *D*, and *F*). Consequently, the duodenum, except for approximately the first 2.5 cm (derived from foregut), has no mesentery and lies retroperitoneally. Similarly, the head of the pancreas becomes retroperitoneal (posterior to peritoneum). The attachment of the dorsal mesentery to the posterior abdominal wall is greatly modified after the intestines return to the abdominal cavity. At first, the dorsal mesentery is in the median plane. As the intestines enlarge, lengthen, and assume their final positions, their mesenteries are pressed against the posterior abdominal wall. The mesentery of the ascending colon fuses with the parietal peritoneum on this wall and disappears; consequently, the ascending colon also becomes retroperitoneal (see Fig. 11-15*B* and *E*).

Other derivatives of the midgut loop (e.g., the jejunum and ileum) retain their mesenteries. The mesentery is at first attached to the median plane of the posterior abdominal wall (see Fig. 11-13*B* and *C*). After the mesentery of the ascending colon disappears, the fan-shaped mesentery of the small intestines acquires a new line of attachment that passes from the duodenojejunal junction inferolaterally to the ileocecal junction.

The Cecum and Appendix

The primordium of the cecum and wormlike (Latin, *vermiform*) appendix—the **cecal swelling** (diverticulum)—appears in the sixth week as an elevation on the antimesenteric border of the caudal limb of the midgut loop (Fig. 11-13*C* and 11-16*A*). The apex of the cecal swelling does not grow as rapidly as the rest of it; thus, the appendix is initially a small diverticulum of the cecum (see Fig. 11-16*B*). The appendix increases rapidly in length so

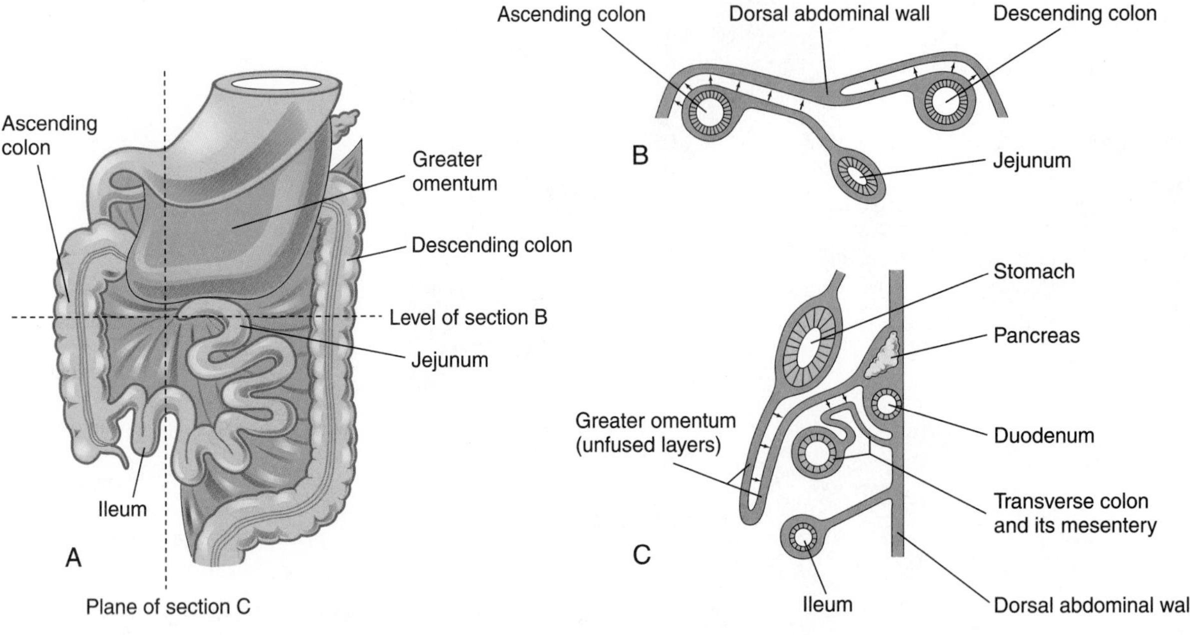

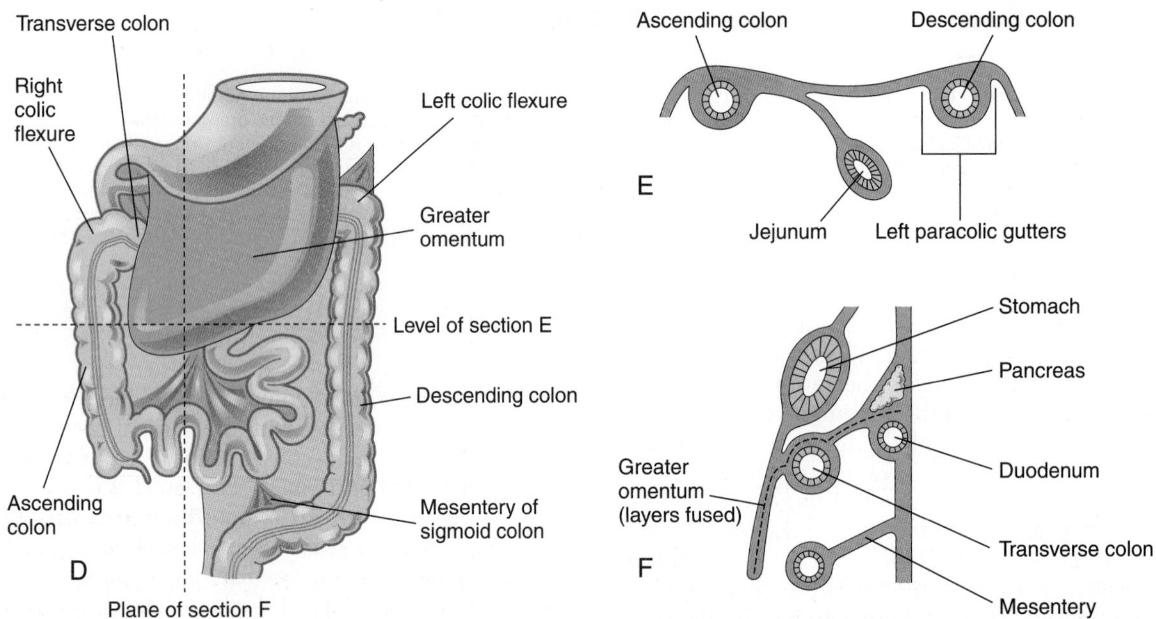

FIGURE 11-15. Fixation of the intestines. **A,** Ventral view of the intestines before their fixation. **B,** Transverse section at the level shown in **A.** The *arrows* indicate areas of subsequent fusion. **C,** Sagittal section at the plane shown in **A,** illustrating the greater omentum overhanging the transverse colon. The *arrows* indicate areas of subsequent fusion. **D,** Ventral view of the intestines after their fixation. **E,** Transverse section at the level shown in **D** after disappearance of the mesentery of the ascending and descending colon. **F,** Sagittal section at the plane shown in **D,** illustrating fusion of the greater omentum with the mesentery of the transverse colon and fusion of the layers of the greater omentum.

that at birth it is a relatively long tube arising from the distal end of the cecum (see Fig. 11-16*D*). After birth, the wall of the cecum grows unequally, with the result that the appendix comes to enter its medial side. The appendix is subject to considerable variation in position. As the ascending colon elongates, the appendix may pass posterior to the cecum (retrocecal appendix) or colon (retrocolic appendix). It may also descend over the brim of the pelvis (pelvic appendix). In approximately 64% of people, the appendix is located retrocecally (Fig. 11-16*E*).

CONGENITAL OMPHALOCELE

This anomaly is a persistence of the herniation of abdominal contents into the proximal part of the umbilical cord (Figs. 11-17 and 11-18). Herniation of intestines into the cord occurs in approximately 1 in 5000 births and herniation of liver and intestines in 1 in approximately 10,000 births. The abdominal

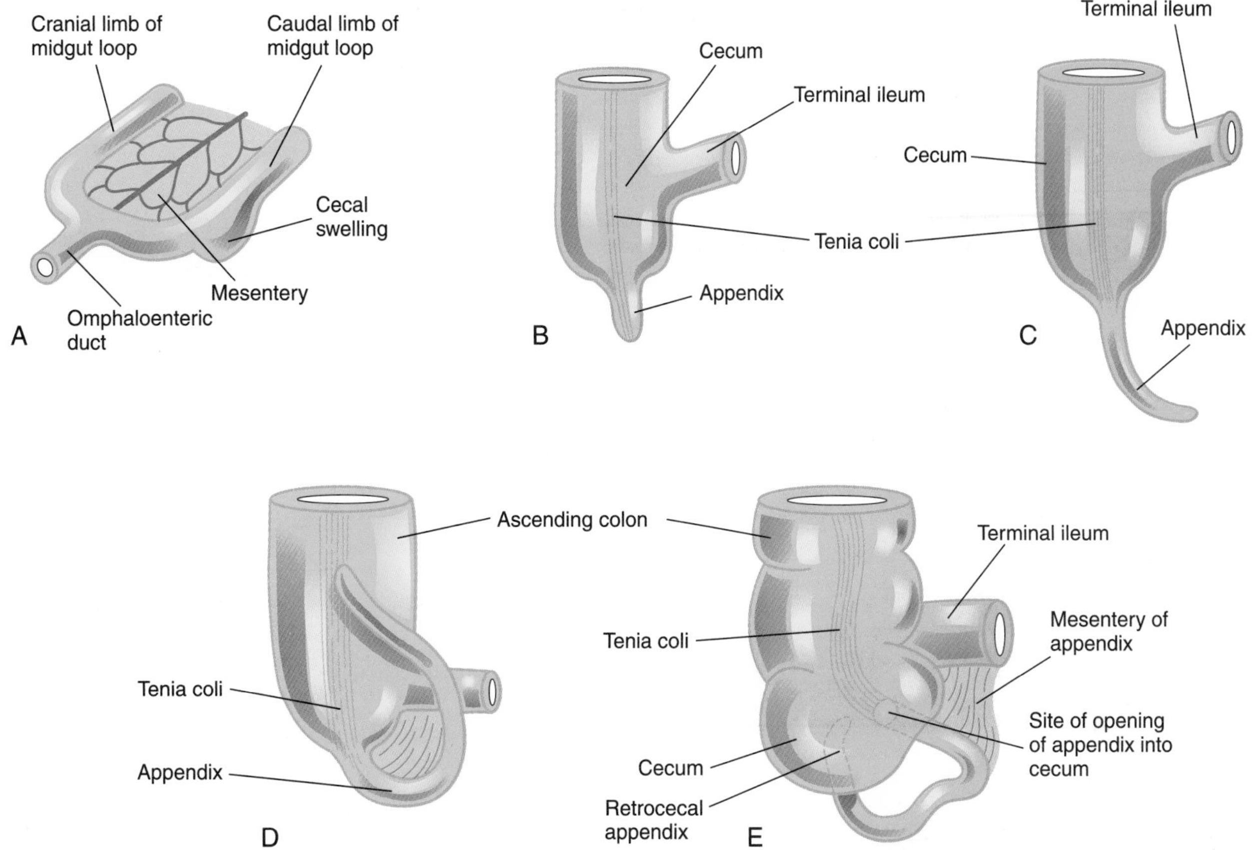

FIGURE 11-16. Successive stages in the development of the cecum and appendix. **A,** At 6 weeks. **B,** At 8 weeks. **C,** At 12 weeks. **D,** At birth. Note that the appendix is relatively long and is continuous with the apex of the cecum. **E,** Adult. Note the appendix is now shorter and lies on the medial side of the cecum. In approximately 64% of people, the appendix is located posterior to the cecum (retrocecal) or posterior to the ascending colon (retrocolic). The tenia coli is a thickened band of longitudinal muscle in the wall of the colon; it ends at the base of the appendix.

cavity is proportionately small when there is an omphalocele because the impetus for it to grow is absent. Surgical repair is required and is often delayed if the defect is very large. Infants with these large omphaloceles often suffer from pulmonary and thoracic hypoplasia and a delayed closure is a better clinical decision. Omphalocele results from impaired growth of the four components of the abdominal wall. Because the formation of the abdominal compartment occurs during gastrulation, a critical failure of growth at this time is often associated with other congenital anomalies involving the cardiac and urogenital systems. The covering of the hernial sac is the epithelium of the umbilical cord, a derivative of the amnion.

UMBILICAL HERNIA

When the intestines return to the abdominal cavity during the 10th week and then herniate through an imperfectly closed umbilicus, an umbilical hernia forms. This common type of hernia is different from an omphalocele. In an umbilical hernia, the protruding mass (usually the greater omentum and part of the small intestine) is covered by subcutaneous tissue and skin. The hernia usually does not reach its maximum size until the end of the first month after birth. It usually ranges in diameter from 1 to 5 cm. The defect through which the hernia occurs is in the linea alba (fibrous band in the median line of the anterior abdominal wall between the rectus muscles). The hernia protrudes during crying, straining, or coughing and can be easily reduced through the fibrous ring at the umbilicus. Surgery is not usually performed unless the hernia persists to the age of 3 to 5 years.

GASTROSCHISIS

This anomaly is a relatively uncommon congenital abdominal wall defect (Fig. 11-19). Gastroschisis results from a defect lateral to the median plane of

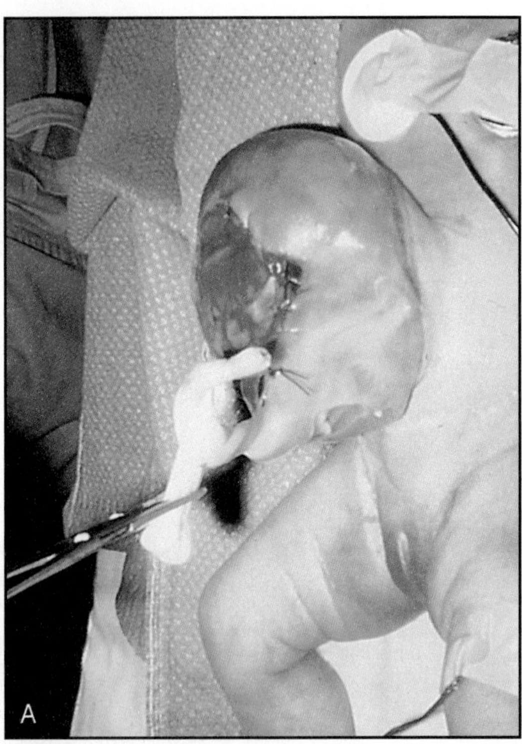

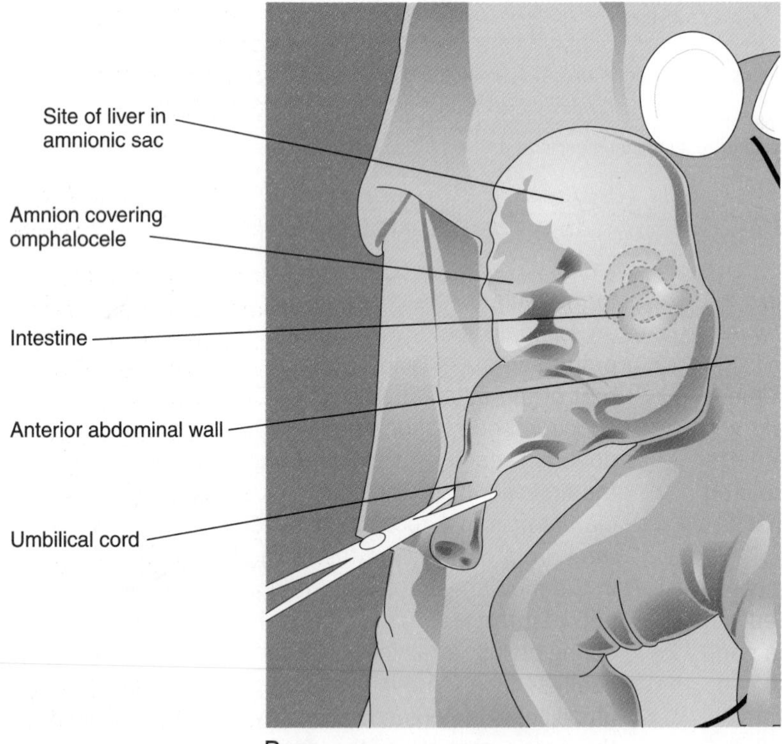

FIGURE 11-17. **A,** An infant with a large omphalocele. **B,** Drawing of the infant with an omphalocele resulting from a median defect of the abdominal muscles, fascia, and skin near the umbilicus. This defect resulted in the herniation of intra-abdominal structures (liver and intestine) into the proximal end of the umbilical cord. It is covered by a membrane composed of peritoneum and amnion. (**A,** Courtesy of Dr. N.E. Wiseman, Pediatric Surgeon, Children's Hospital, Winnipeg, Manitoba, Canada.)

the anterior abdominal wall. The linear defect permits extrusion of the abdominal viscera without involving the umbilical cord. The viscera protrude into the amniotic cavity and are bathed by amniotic fluid. The term *gastroschisis*, which literally means a "split or open stomach," is a misnomer because it is the anterior abdominal wall that is split, not the stomach. The defect usually occurs on the right side lateral to the umbilicus and is more common in males than females. The exact cause of gastroschisis is uncertain, but various causes have been proposed including ischemic injury to the

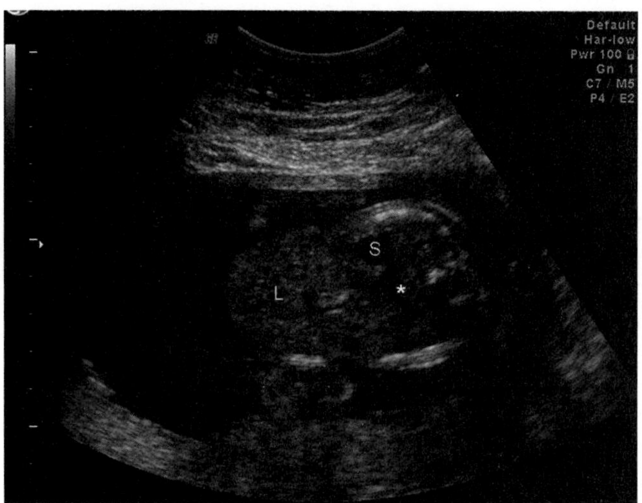

FIGURE 11-18. Sonogram of the abdomen of a fetus showing a large omphalocele, with the liver (L) protruding (herniating) from the abdomen (*). Also observe the stomach (S). (Courtesy of Dr. G.J. Reid, Department of Obstetrics, Gynecology and Reproductive Sciences, University of Manitoba, Women's Hospital, Winnipeg, Manitoba, Canada.)

anterior abdominal wall (absence of the right omphalomesenteric artery), rupture of the anterior abdominal wall, weakness of the wall caused by abnormal involution of the right umbilical vein, and perhaps rupture of an omphalocele before the anterior abdominal wall has folded.

ANOMALIES OF THE MIDGUT

Congenital abnormalities of the intestine are common; most of them are anomalies of gut rotation—**nonrotation or malrotation of the gut**—that result from incomplete rotation and/or fixation of the intestines. **Nonrotation** occurs when the intestine does not rotate as it reenters the abdomen. As a result, the caudal limb of the midgut loop returns to the abdomen first and the small intestines lie on the right side of the abdomen and the entire large intestine is on the left. The usual 270-degree counterclockwise rotation is not completed, and the cecum lies just inferior to the pylorus of the stomach. The cecum is fixed to the posterolateral abdominal wall by peritoneal bands that pass over the duodenum (Fig. 11-20*B*). These bands and the volvulus (twisting) of the intestines cause **duodenal obstruction**. This type of malrotation results from failure of the midgut loop to complete the final 90 degrees of rotation (see Fig. 11-13*D*). Only two parts of the intestine are attached to the posterior abdominal wall: the duodenum and proximal colon. This improperly positioned and incompletely fixed intestine may lead to a catastrophic twisting of the midgut—**midgut volvulus** (see Fig. 11-20*F*). The small intestine hangs by a narrow stalk that contains the superior mesenteric artery and vein.

When midgut volvulus occurs, the superior mesenteric artery may be obstructed, resulting in infarction and **gangrene of the intestine** supplied by it (Fig. 11-20*A* and *B*). Infants with intestinal malrotation are prone to volvulus and present with **bilious emesis** (vomiting bile). A simple contrast study can determine the presence of rotational abnormalities.

REVERSED ROTATION

In very unusual cases, the midgut loop rotates in a clockwise rather than a counterclockwise direction (see Fig. 11-20*C*). As a result, the duodenum lies anterior to the superior mesenteric artery rather than posterior to it, and the transverse colon lies posterior instead of anterior to it. In these infants, the transverse colon may be obstructed by pressure from the superior mesenteric artery. In more unusual cases, the small intestine lies on the left side of the abdomen and the large intestine lies on the right side, with the cecum in the center. This unusual situation results from malrotation of the midgut followed by failure of fixation of the intestines.

SUBHEPATIC CECUM AND APPENDIX

If the cecum adheres to the inferior surface of the liver when it returns to the abdomen, it will be drawn superiorly as the liver diminishes in size; as a result, the cecum remains in its fetal position (see Fig. 11-20*D*). A subhepatic cecum and appendix are more common in males and occur in approximately 6% of fetuses. A subhepatic cecum and "high-riding" appendix may be seen in adults; however, when it occurs, it may create a problem in the diagnosis of appendicitis and during the surgical removal of the appendix (*appendectomy*).

MOBILE CECUM

In approximately 10% of people, the cecum has an abnormal amount of freedom. In very unusual cases, it may herniate into the right inguinal canal. A mobile cecum results from incomplete fixation of the ascending colon. This condition is clinically significant because of the possible variations in position of the appendix and because twisting (volvulus) of the cecum may occur.

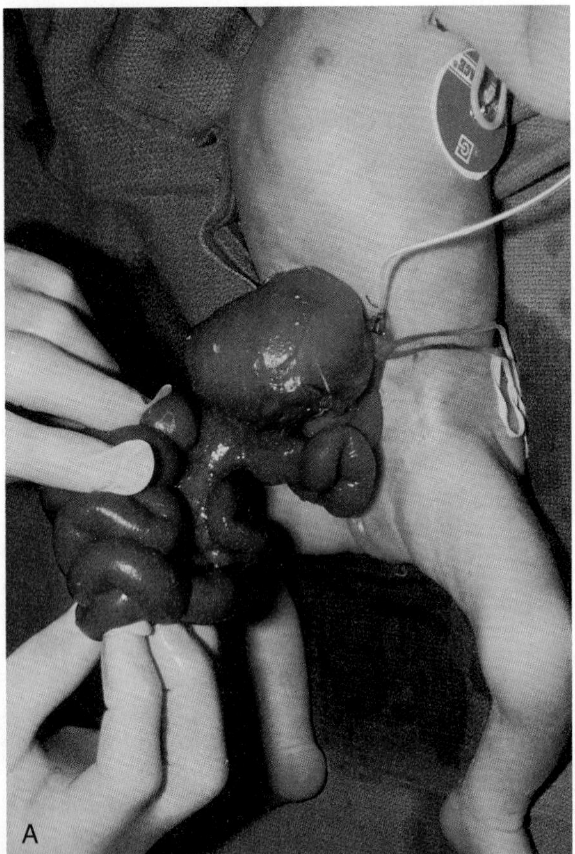

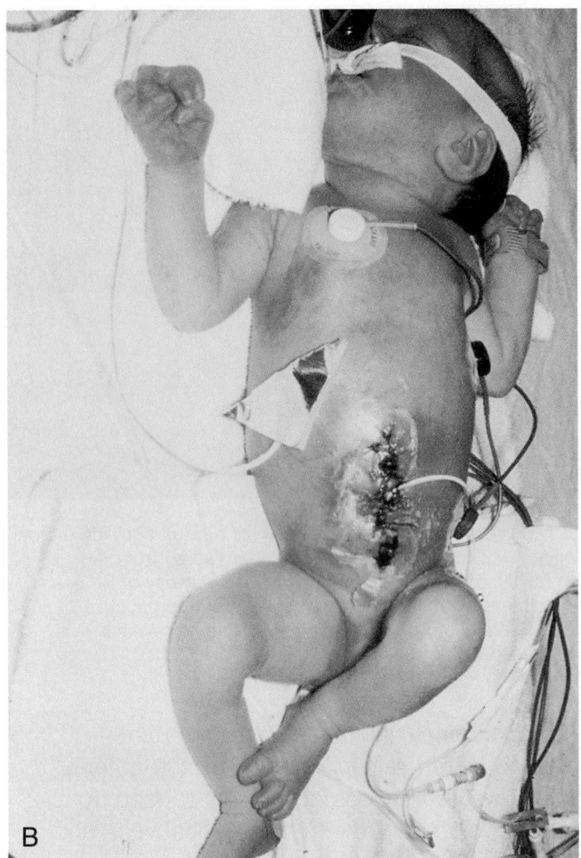

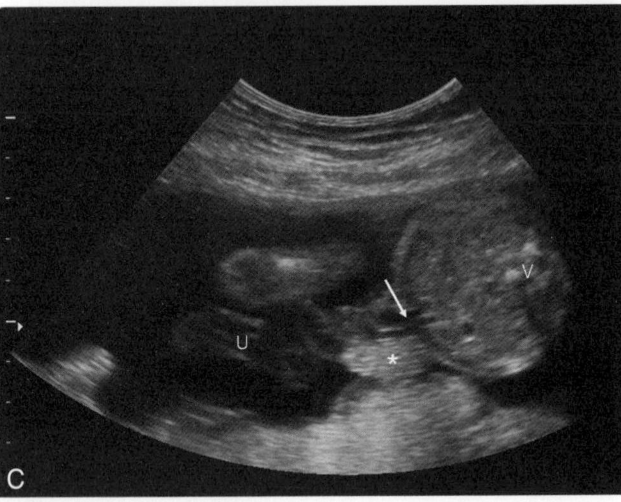

FIGURE 11-19. **A,** Newborn infant with an anterior abdominal wall defect—gastroschisis—showing the protruding viscera. The defect was 2 to 4 cm long and involved all layers of the abdominal wall. It was located to the right of the umbilicus. **B,** Photograph of the infant after the viscera were returned to the abdomen and the defect was surgically closed. **C,** Sonogram of a fetus at (21 weeks' gestation) with gastroschisis. Note that the intestines (*) are herniated on the right side of the attachment (*arrow*) of the umbilical cord (U). Also note the fetal vertebrae (V). (**A** and **B,** Courtesy of A.E. Chudley, MD, Section of Genetics and Metabolism, Department of Pediatrics and Child Health, Children's Hospital, Winnipeg, Manitoba, Canada. **C,** Courtesy of Dr. G.J. Reid, Department of Obstetrics, Gynecology and Reproductive Sciences, University of Manitoba, Women's Hospital, Winnipeg, Manitoba, Canada.)

INTERNAL HERNIA

In this very uncommon anomaly, the small intestine passes into the mesentery of the midgut loop during the return of the intestines to the abdomen (see Fig. 11-20*E*). As a result, a hernia-like sac forms. This condition usually does not produce symptoms and is often detected at autopsy or during an anatomic dissection.

STENOSIS AND ATRESIA OF THE INTESTINE

Partial occlusion (stenosis) and complete occlusion (atresia) of the intestinal lumen (see Fig. 11-6) account for approximately one third of cases of intestinal obstruction. The obstructive lesion occurs most often in the duodenum (25%) and ileum (50%). The length of the area affected varies. These anomalies result from failure of an adequate number

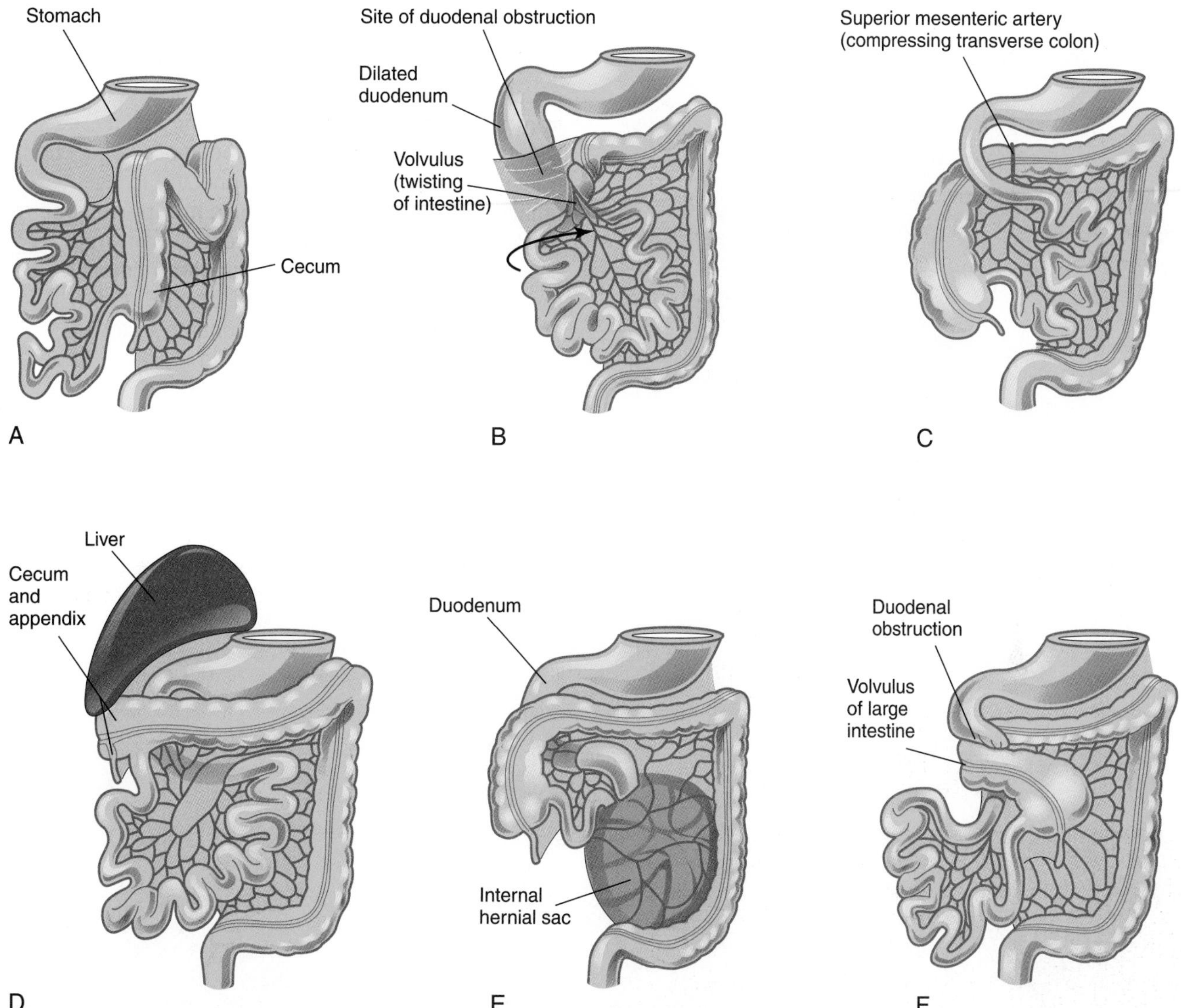

FIGURE 11-20. Anomalies of midgut rotation. **A,** Nonrotation. **B,** Mixed rotation and volvulus. **C,** Reversed rotation. **D,** Subhepatic cecum and appendix. **E,** Internal hernia. **F,** Midgut volvulus.

of vacuoles to form during recanalization of the intestine. In some cases, a transverse septum or web forms, producing the blockage or atresia (see Fig. 11-6*F2*). Another possible cause of stenoses and atresias is interruption of the blood supply to a loop of fetal intestine resulting from a *fetal vascular accident* caused by impaired microcirculation that is associated with fetal distress, drug exposure, or a volvulus. The loss of blood supply leads to necrosis of the bowel and the development of a fibrous cord connecting the proximal and distal ends of normal intestine. Malfixation of the gut predisposes it to volvulus, strangulation, and impairment of its blood supply. This disability most likely occurs during the 10th week as the intestines return to the abdomen.

ILEAL DIVERTICULUM AND OTHER OMPHALOENTERIC REMNANTS

This outpouching of the ileum is one of the most common anomalies of the digestive tract (Fig. 11-21). A congenital ileal diverticulum (Meckel diverticulum) occurs in 2% to 4% of people and is three to five times more prevalent in males than females. An ileal diverticulum is of clinical significance because it may become inflamed and cause symptoms that mimic appendicitis.

The wall of the diverticulum contains all layers of the ileum and may contain small patches of gastric and pancreatic tissues. This ectopic gastric mucosa often secretes acid, producing ulceration and bleeding (Fig. 11-22*A*). An ileal diverticulum is the

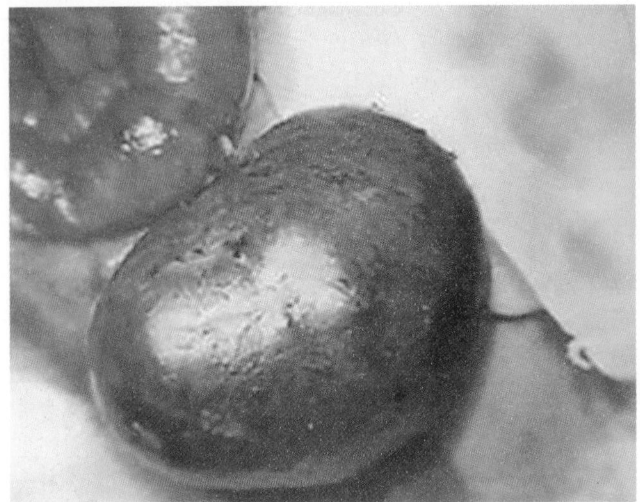

Figure 11-21. A large ileal diverticulum, commonly referred to clinically as a Meckel diverticulum. Only a small percentage of these diverticula produce symptoms. Ileal diverticula are one of the most common anomalies of the digestive tract. (Courtesy of Dr. M.N. Golarz De Bourne, St. Georges University Medical School, Grenada.)

remnant of the proximal part of the omphaloenteric duct (yolk stalk). It typically appears as a fingerlike pouch approximately 3 to 6 cm long that arises from the antimesenteric border of the ileum (see Fig. 11-21), 40 to 50 cm from the ileocecal junction. An ileal diverticulum may be connected to the umbilicus by a fibrous cord (which may predispose to intestinal obstruction as the intestine can wrap around this cord) or an **omphaloenteric fistula** (omphalomesenteric duct) (Figs. 11-22*B* and *C*, and 11-23*B*); other possible remnants of the omphaloenteric duct are illustrated in Figure 11-22*D* to *F*.

Duplication of the Intestine

Most intestinal duplications are cystic or tubular duplications. *Cystic duplications* are more common (Fig. 11-24*A* and *B*). *Tubular duplications* usually

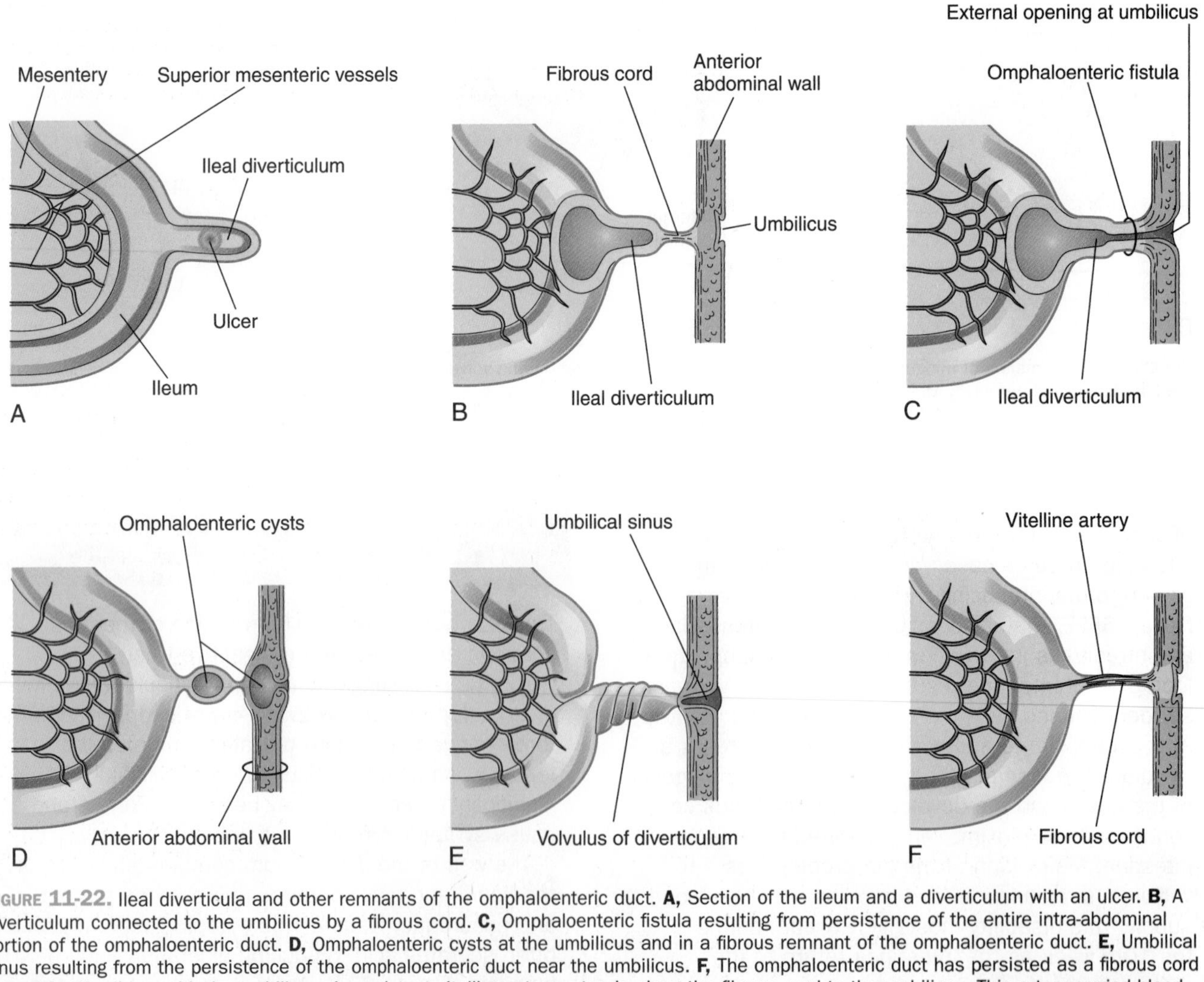

Figure 11-22. Ileal diverticula and other remnants of the omphaloenteric duct. **A,** Section of the ileum and a diverticulum with an ulcer. **B,** A diverticulum connected to the umbilicus by a fibrous cord. **C,** Omphaloenteric fistula resulting from persistence of the entire intra-abdominal portion of the omphaloenteric duct. **D,** Omphaloenteric cysts at the umbilicus and in a fibrous remnant of the omphaloenteric duct. **E,** Umbilical sinus resulting from the persistence of the omphaloenteric duct near the umbilicus. **F,** The omphaloenteric duct has persisted as a fibrous cord connecting the ileum with the umbilicus. A persistent vitelline artery extends along the fibrous cord to the umbilicus. This artery carried blood from the embryo to the omphaloenteric duct (yolk stalk).

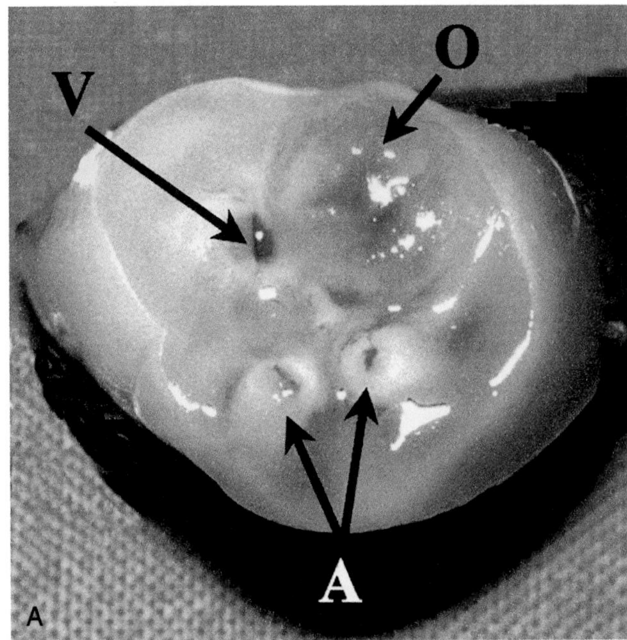

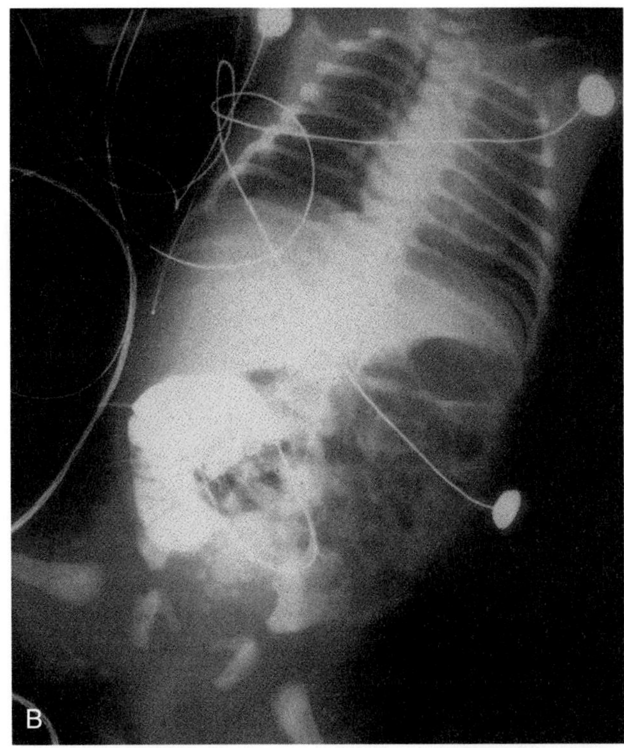

FIGURE 11-23. Newborn male infant with a patent omphaloenteric duct (omphalomesenteric duct). **A,** The transected umbilical cord shows two umbilical arteries (A), an umbilical vein (V), and a larger lumen (O) of the omphaloenteric duct. **B,** An abdominal radiograph identifies contrast material injected through the omphaloenteric duct into the ileum. (From Hinson RM, Biswas A, Mizelelle KM, Tunnessen WW Jr: Picture of the month (persistent omphalomesenteric duct). Arch Pediatr Adolesc Med 151:1161, 1997. Copyright 1997, American Medical Association.)

communicate with the intestinal lumen (see Fig. 11-24*C*). Almost all duplications are caused by failure of normal recanalization of the intestines; as a result, two lumina form (see Fig. 11-24*H* and *I*). The duplicated segment of the intestine lies on the mesenteric side of the intestine. The duplication of the intestine often contains ectopic gastric mucosa, which may result in local peptic ulceration and lower gastrointestinal bleeding.

HINDGUT

The derivatives of the hindgut are

- The left one third to one half of the transverse colon, the descending colon and sigmoid colon, the rectum, and the superior part of the anal canal
- The epithelium of the urinary bladder and most of the urethra (see Chapter 12)

All hindgut derivatives are supplied by the **inferior mesenteric artery**, the artery of the hindgut. The junction between the segment of transverse colon derived from the midgut and that originating from the hindgut is indicated by the change in blood supply from a branch of the superior mesenteric artery (midgut artery) to a branch of the inferior mesenteric artery (hindgut artery). The descending colon becomes retroperitoneal as its mesentery fuses with the peritoneum on the left posterior abdominal wall and then disappears (see Fig. 11-15*B* and *E*). The mesentery of the sigmoid colon is retained, but it is shorter than in the embryo.

Cloaca

The expanded terminal part of the hindgut, the **cloaca**, is an endoderm-lined chamber that is in contact with the surface ectoderm at the **cloacal membrane** (Fig. 11-25*A* and *B*). This membrane is composed of endoderm of the cloaca and ectoderm of the **proctodeum** or anal pit (see Fig. 11-25*D*). The cloaca receives the **allantois** ventrally (Fig. 11-25*A*), which is a fingerlike diverticulum.

Partitioning of the Cloaca

The cloaca is divided into dorsal and ventral parts by a wedge of mesenchyme—the **urorectal septum**—that develops in the angle between the allantois and hindgut. As the septum grows toward the cloacal membrane, it develops forklike extensions that produce infoldings of the lateral walls of the cloaca (see Fig. 11-25*B1*). These folds grow toward each other and fuse, forming a partition that divides the cloaca into two parts (see Fig. 11-25*D1* and *F1*):

- The *rectum* and cranial part of the *anal canal* dorsally
- The *urogenital sinus* ventrally

By the seventh week, the urorectal septum has fused with the cloacal membrane, dividing it into a dorsal **anal**

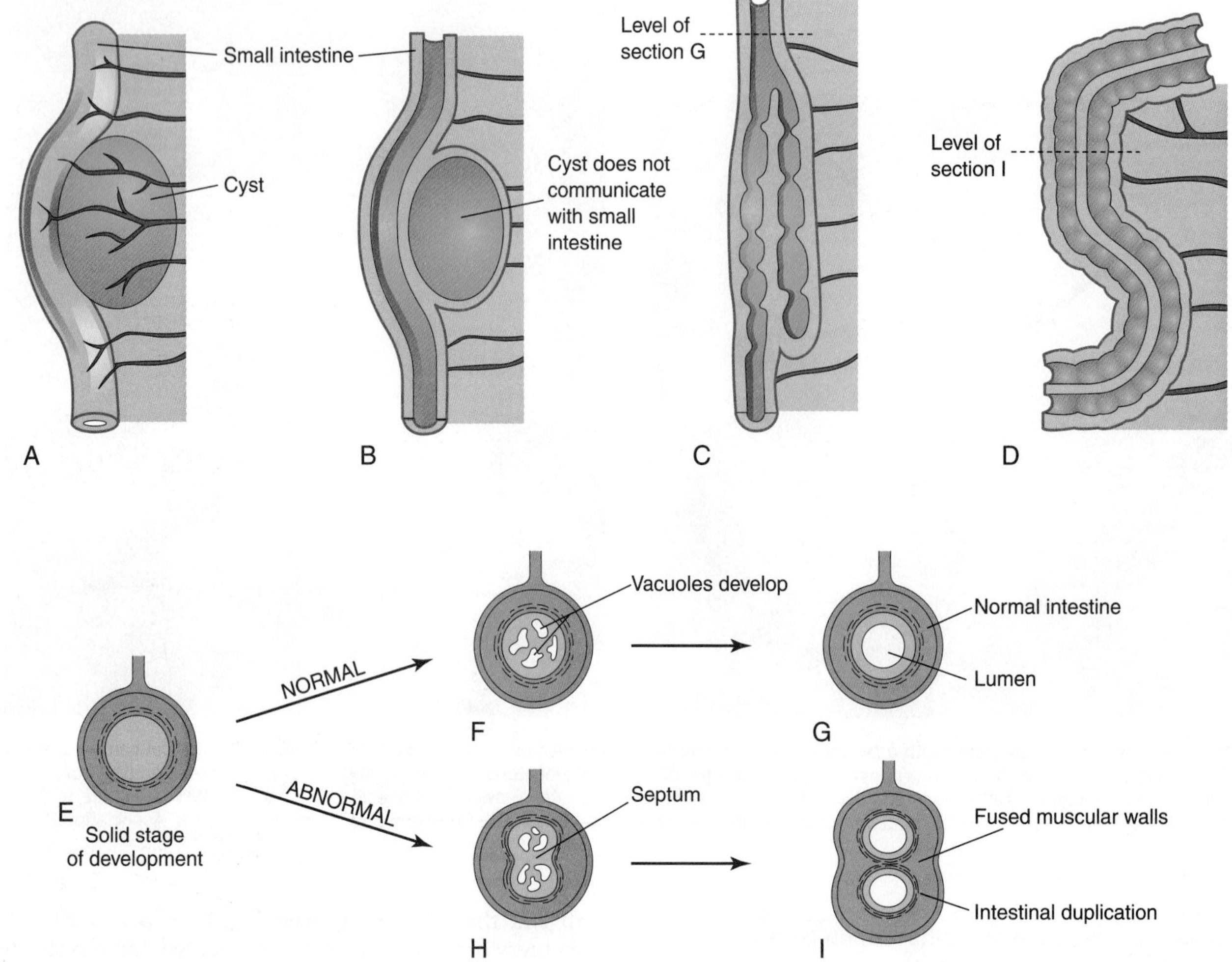

FIGURE 11-24. **A,** Cystic duplication of the small intestine. Note that it is on the mesenteric side of the intestine and receives branches from the arteries supplying the intestine. **B,** Longitudinal section of the duplication shown in **A**; its musculature is continuous with the gut wall. **C,** A short tubular duplication. **D,** A long duplication showing a partition consisting of the fused muscular walls. **E,** Transverse section of the intestine during the solid stage. **F,** Normal vacuole formation. **G,** Coalescence of the vacuoles and reformation of the lumen. **H,** Two groups of vacuoles have formed. **I,** Coalescence of the vacuoles illustrated in **H** results in intestinal duplication.

membrane and a larger ventral **urogenital membrane** (see Fig. 11-25*E* and *F*). The area of fusion of the urorectal septum with the cloacal membrane is represented in the adult by the **perineal body**, the tendinous center of the perineum. This fibromuscular node is the landmark of the perineum where several muscles converge and attach. The urorectal septum also divides the cloacal sphincter into anterior and posterior parts. The posterior part becomes the external anal sphincter, and the anterior part develops into the superficial transverse perineal, bulbospongiosus, and ischiocavernosus muscles. This developmental fact explains why one nerve, the *pudendal nerve*, supplies all these muscles. Mesenchymal proliferations produce elevations of the surface ectoderm around the **anal membrane**. As a result, this membrane is soon located at the bottom of an ectodermal depression—the **proctodeum** or anal pit (see Fig. 11-25*E* and *F*). The anal membrane usually ruptures at the end of the eighth week, bringing the distal part of the digestive tract (anal canal) into communication with the amniotic cavity.

The Anal Canal

The superior two thirds (approximately 25 mm) of the adult anal canal are derived from the **hindgut**; the inferior one third (approximately 13 mm) develops from the **proctodeum** (Fig. 11-26). The junction of the epithelium derived from the ectoderm of the proctodeum and the endoderm of the hindgut is roughly indicated by the irregular **pectinate line**, located at the inferior limit of the anal valves. This line indicates the approximate former site of the anal membrane. Approximately 2 cm superior to the anus is an **anocutaneous line** ("white line"). This is approximately where the composition of the anal epithelium changes from columnar to stratified squamous cells. At the anus, the epithelium is keratinized and continuous with the skin around the anus. The other layers of the wall of the anal canal are derived from splanchnic mesenchyme. Similar to the pyloric sphincter and the ileocecal valve (sphincter), the formation of the anal sphincter appears to be under Hox D genetic control.

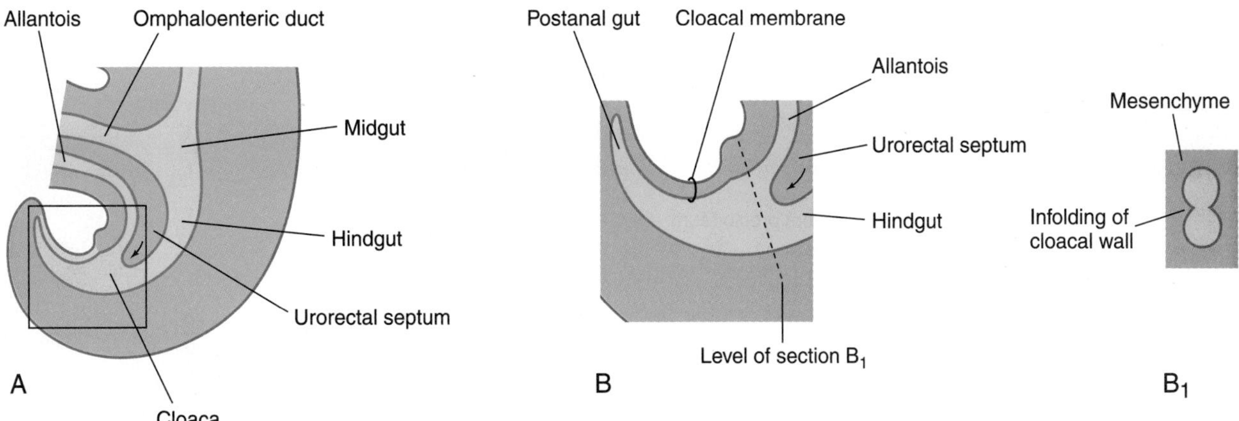

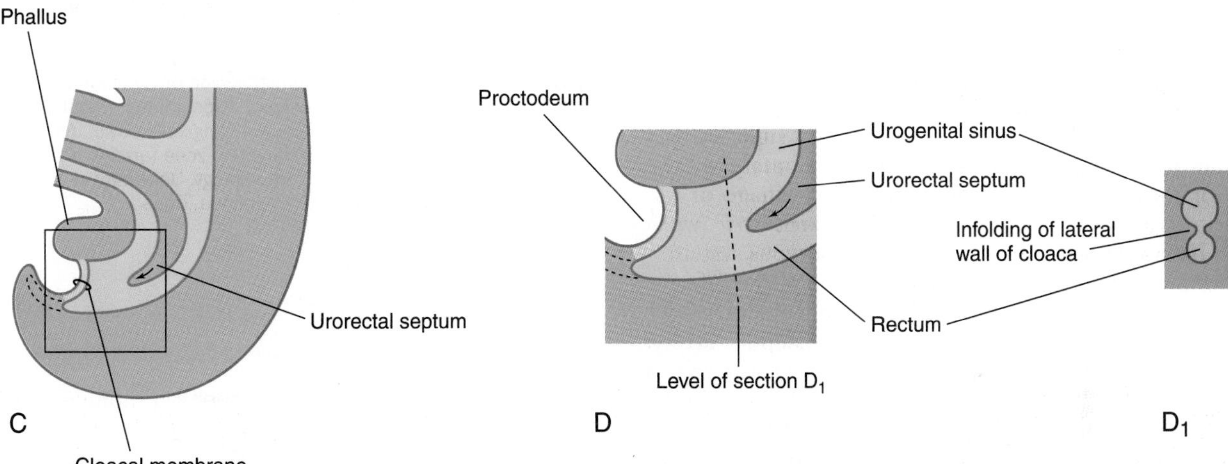

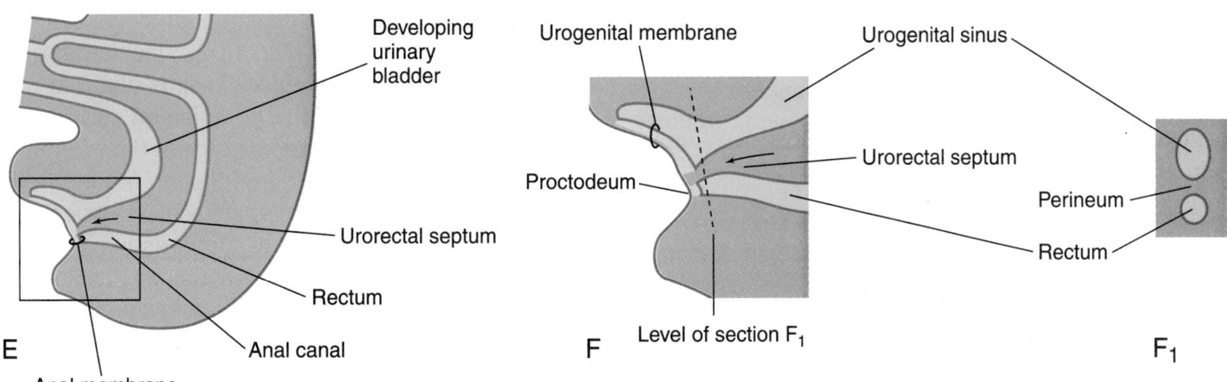

FIGURE 11-25. Successive stages in the partitioning of the cloaca into the rectum and urogenital sinus by the urorectal septum. **A, C,** and **E,** Views from the left side at 4, 6, and 7 weeks, respectively. **B, D,** and **F,** Enlargements of the cloacal region. **B_1, D_1,** and **F_1,** Transverse sections of the cloaca at the levels shown in **B, D,** and **F,** respectively. Note that the postanal portion (shown in **B**) degenerates and disappears as the rectum forms from the dorsal part of the cloaca (shown in **C** and **D**).

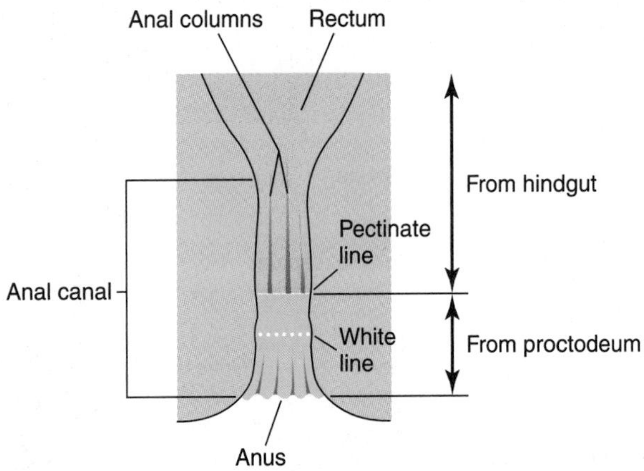

FIGURE 11-26. Sketch of the rectum and anal canal showing their developmental origins. Note that the superior two thirds of the anal canal are derived from the hindgut, whereas the inferior one third of the canal is derived from the proctodeum. Because of their different embryologic origins, the superior and inferior parts of the anal canal are supplied by different arteries and nerves and have different venous and lymphatic drainages.

Because of its hindgut origin, the superior two thirds of the anal canal are mainly supplied by the *superior rectal artery*, the continuation of the inferior mesenteric artery (hindgut artery). The venous drainage of this superior part is mainly via the *superior rectal vein*, a tributary of the inferior mesenteric vein. The lymphatic drainage of the superior part is eventually to the *inferior mesenteric lymph nodes*. Its nerves are from the autonomic nervous system.

Because of its origin from the proctodeum, the inferior one third of the anal canal is supplied mainly by the *inferior rectal arteries*, branches of the internal pudendal artery. The venous drainage is through the *inferior rectal vein*, a tributary of the internal pudendal vein that drains into the internal iliac vein. The *lymphatic drainage* of the inferior part of the anal canal is to the *superficial inguinal lymph nodes*. Its nerve supply is from the *inferior rectal nerve*; hence, it is sensitive to pain, temperature, touch, and pressure.

The differences in blood supply, nerve supply, and venous and lymphatic drainage of the anal canal are important clinically, e.g., when considering the metastasis (spread) of cancer cells. The characteristics of carcinomas in the two parts also differ. Tumors in the superior part are painless and arise from columnar epithelium, whereas those in the inferior part are painful and arise from stratified squamous epithelium.

ANOMALIES OF THE HINDGUT

Most anomalies of the hindgut are located in the anorectal region and result from **abnormal development of the urorectal septum**. Clinically, they are divided into high and low anomalies depending on whether the rectum terminates superior or inferior to the puborectal sling formed by the puborectalis, a part of the levator ani muscle (see Moore and Dalley, 2006).

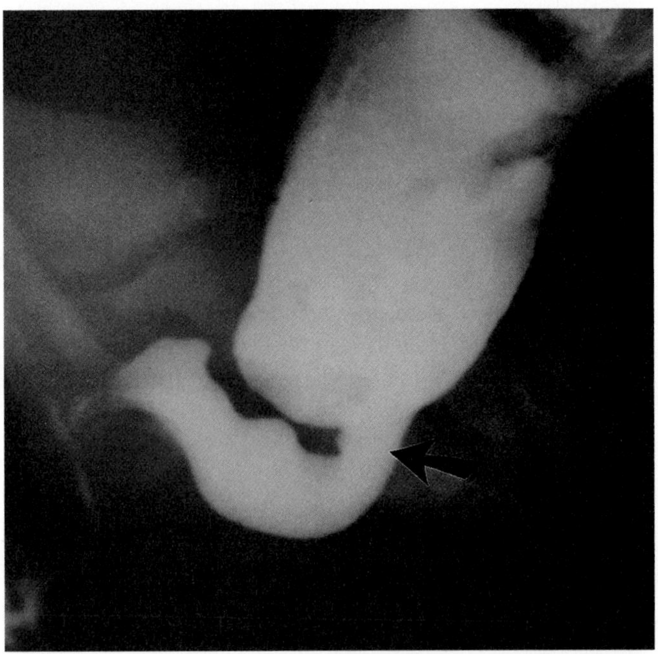

FIGURE 11-27. Radiograph of the colon after a barium enema in a 1-month-old infant with congenital megacolon or Hirschsprung's disease. The aganglionic distal segment (rectum and distal sigmoid colon) is narrow, with distended normal ganglionic bowel, full of fecal material, proximal to it. Note the transition zone (*arrow*). (Courtesy of Dr. Martin H. Reed, Department of Radiology, University of Manitoba and Children's Hospital, Winnipeg, Manitoba, Canada.)

CONGENITAL MEGACOLON OR HIRSCHSPRUNG DISEASE

This disease is a dominantly inherited multigenic disorder with incomplete penetrance and variable expressivity. Of the genes so far identified, the RET proto-oncogene is the major susceptibility gene and accounts for most cases. This disease affects one in 5000 newborns and is defined as an absence of ganglion cells (**aganglionosis**) in a variable length of distal bowel. Infants with congenital megacolon or Hirschsprung's disease (Fig. 11-27) lack autonomic ganglion cells in the myenteric plexus distal to the dilated segment of colon. The enlarged colon—**megacolon** (Greek, *megas*, big)—has the normal number of ganglion cells. The dilation results from failure of relaxation of the aganglionic segment, which prevents movement of the intestinal contents, resulting in dilation. In most cases, only the rectum and sigmoid colon are involved; occasionally, ganglia are also absent from more proximal parts of the colon.

Congenital megacolon is the most common cause of neonatal obstruction of the colon and accounts for 33% of all neonatal obstructions; males are affected more often than females (4:1). Megacolon results from failure of neural crest cells to migrate into the wall of the colon during the fifth to seventh

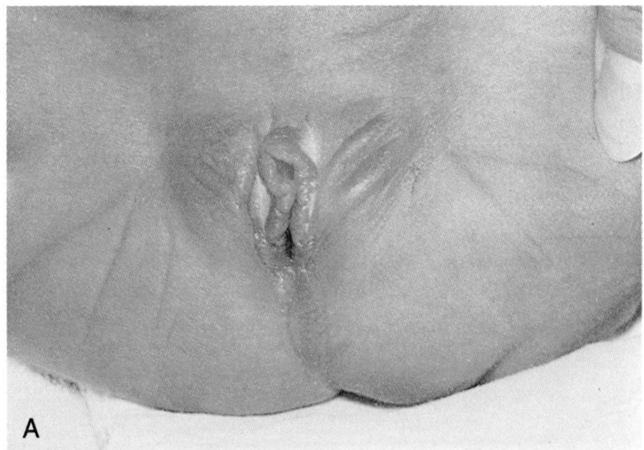

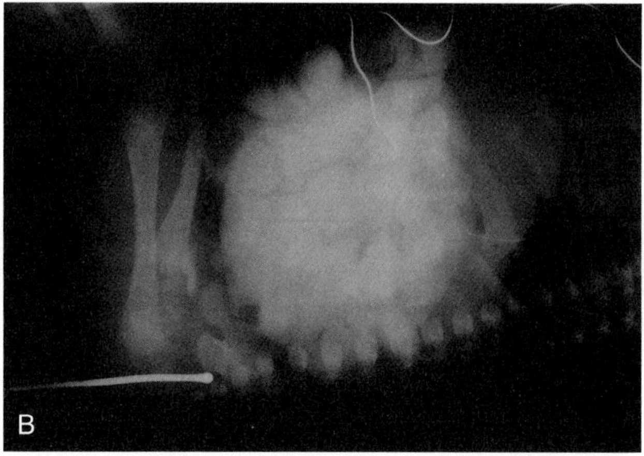

FIGURE 11-28. Imperforate anus. **A,** Female neonate with membranous anal atresia (imperforate anus). In most cases of anal atresia, a thin layer of tissue separates the anal canal from the exterior. Some form of imperforate anus occurs approximately once in every 5000 neonates; it is more common in males. **B,** Radiograph of an infant with an imperforate anus. The dilated end of the radiopaque probe is at the bottom of the blindly ending anal membrane. The large intestine is distended with feces and contrast material. (**A,** Courtesy of A.E. Chudley, MD, Section of Genetics and Metabolism, Department of Pediatrics and Child Health, Children's Hospital, Winnipeg, Manitoba, Canada. **B,** Courtesy of Dr. Prem S. Sahni, formerly of the Department of Radiology, Children's Hospital, Winnipeg, Manitoba, Canada.)

weeks. This results in failure of parasympathetic ganglion cells to develop in the *Auerbach* and *Meissner plexuses*. The cause of failure of some neural crest cells to complete their migration is unknown.

IMPERFORATE ANUS AND ANORECTAL ANOMALIES

Imperforate anus occurs approximately once in every 5000 newborn infants and is more common in males (Figs. 11-28 and 11-29*C*). *Most anorectal anomalies result from abnormal development of the urorectal septum*, resulting in incomplete separation of the cloaca into urogenital and anorectal portions (see Fig. 11-29*A*). There is normally a temporary communication between the rectum and anal canal dorsally from the bladder and urethra ventrally (see Fig. 11-25*C*), but it closes when the urorectal septum fuses with the cloacal membrane (see Fig. 11-25*E*). Lesions are classified as low or high depending on whether the rectum ends superior or inferior to the puborectalis muscle. The following are **low anomalies of the anorectal region**.

ANAL AGENESIS, WITH OR WITHOUT A FISTULA

The anal canal may end blindly or there may be an **ectopic anus** or an **anoperineal fistula** that opens into the perineum (see Fig. 11-29*D* and *E*). The abnormal canal may, however, open into the vagina in females or the urethra in males (see Figs. 11-29*F* and G). More than 90% of low anorectal anomalies are associated with an external fistula. Anal agenesis with a fistula results from incomplete separation of the cloaca by the urorectal septum. Constipation often occurs with low lesions.

ANAL STENOSIS

The anus is in the normal position, but the anus and anal canal are narrow (see Fig. 11-29*B*). This anomaly is probably caused by a slight dorsal deviation of the urorectal septum as it grows caudally to fuse with the cloacal membrane. As a result, the anal canal and anal membrane are small. Sometimes only a small probe can be inserted into the anal canal.

MEMBRANOUS ATRESIA OF ANUS

The anus is in the normal position, but a thin layer of tissue separates the anal canal from the exterior (see Figs. 11-28 and 11-29*C*). The anal membrane is thin enough to bulge on straining and appears blue from the presence of *meconium* (feces of newborn) superior to it. This anomaly results from failure of the anal membrane to perforate at the end of the eighth week.

ANORECTAL AGENESIS, WITH OR WITHOUT A FISTULA

This anomaly and those that follow are classified as **high anomalies of the anorectal region**. The rectum ends superior to the puborectalis muscle when there is anorectal agenesis. This is the most common

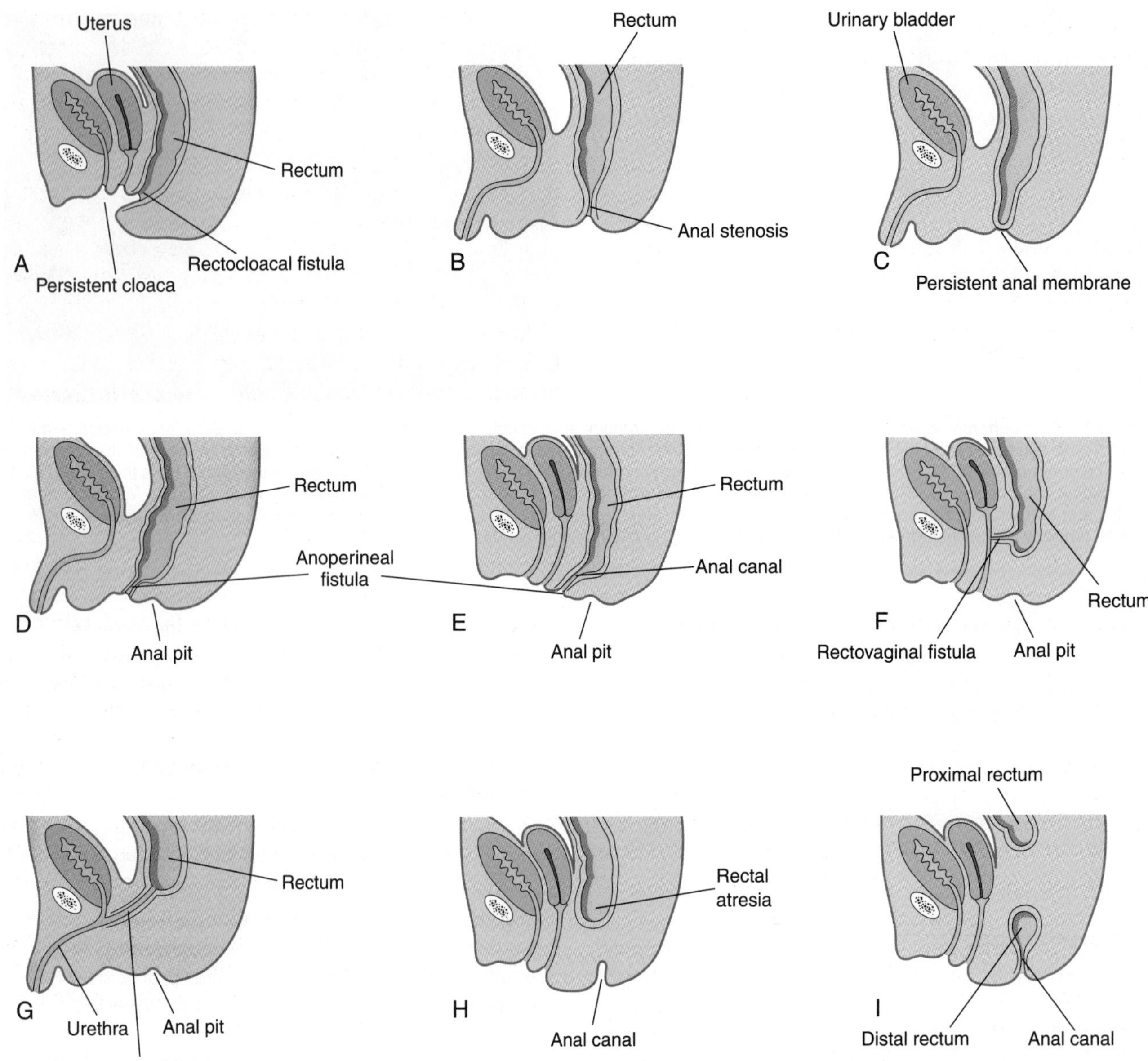

FIGURE 11-29. Various types of anorectal anomalies. **A,** Persistent cloaca. Note the common outlet for the intestinal, urinary, and reproductive tracts. **B,** Anal stenosis. **C,** Membranous anal atresia (imperforate anus). **D** and **E,** Anal agenesis with a perineal fistula. **F,** Anorectal agenesis with a rectovaginal fistula. **G,** Anorectal agenesis with a rectourethral fistula. **H** and **I,** Rectal atresia.

type of anorectal anomaly, which accounts for approximately two thirds of anorectal defects. Although the rectum ends blindly, there is usually a fistula to the bladder (*rectovesical fistula*) or urethra (*rectourethral fistula*) in males or to the vagina (*rectovaginal fistula*) or the vestibule of the vagina (*rectovestibular fistula*) in females (see Fig. 11-29*F* and G). Passage of **meconium** (a dark green material in the fetal intestines) or flatus (gas) in the urine is diagnostic of a rectourinary fistula. *Anorectal agenesis with a fistula* is the result of incomplete separation of the cloaca by the urorectal septum. In newborn males with this condition, meconium (feces) may be observed in the urine, whereas fistulas in females result in the presence of meconium in the vestibule of the vagina. Children with high malformations tend to have a poorer outcome, with higher rates of fecal incontinence (inability to control defecation).

RECTAL ATRESIA

The anal canal and rectum are present but are separated (see Fig. 11-29*H* and *I*). Sometimes the two segments of bowel are connected by a fibrous cord, the remnant of an atretic portion of the rectum. The cause of rectal atresia may be abnormal recanalization of the colon or more likely defective blood supply.

SUMMARY OF THE DIGESTIVE SYSTEM

- The **primordial gut** forms from the dorsal part of the umbilical vesicle (yolk sac) that becomes incorporated into the embryo. The endoderm of the primordial gut gives rise to the epithelial lining of the digestive tract, except for the cranial and caudal extremities, which are derived from the ectoderm of the stomodeum and proctodeum, respectively. The muscular and connective tissue components of the digestive tract are derived from the splanchnic mesenchyme surrounding the primordial gut.
- The **foregut** gives rise to the pharynx, lower respiratory system, esophagus, stomach, proximal part of the duodenum, liver, pancreas, and biliary apparatus. Because the trachea and esophagus have a common origin from the foregut, incomplete partitioning by the tracheoesophageal septum results in stenoses or atresias, with or without fistulas between them.
- The **hepatic diverticulum**, the primordium of the liver, gallbladder, and biliary duct system, is an outgrowth of the endodermal epithelial lining of the foregut. Epithelial liver cords develop from the hepatic diverticulum and grow into the septum transversum. Between the layers of the ventral mesentery derived from the septum transversum, primordial cells differentiate into the hepatic tissues and the lining of the ducts of the biliary system.
- **Congenital duodenal atresia** results from failure of the vacuolization and recanalization process to occur after the normal solid developmental stage of the duodenum. Usually the epithelial cells degenerate and the lumen of the duodenum is restored. Obstruction of the duodenum can also be caused by an anular pancreas.
- The **pancreas** develops from pancreatic buds that form from the endodermal lining of the foregut. When the duodenum rotates to the right, the **ventral pancreatic bud** moves dorsally and fuses with the dorsal pancreatic bud. The ventral pancreatic bud forms most of the head of the pancreas, including the uncinate process. The **dorsal pancreatic bud** forms the remainder of the pancreas. In some fetuses, the duct systems of the two buds fail to fuse, and an accessory pancreatic duct forms.
- The **midgut** gives rise to the duodenum (the part distal to the entrance of the bile duct), jejunum, ileum, cecum, appendix, ascending colon, and the right one half to two thirds of the transverse colon. The midgut forms a U-shaped **umbilical loop of the intestine** that herniates into the umbilical cord during the sixth week because there is no room for it in the abdomen. While in the umbilical cord, the midgut loop rotates counterclockwise 90 degrees. During the 10th week, the intestines return to the abdomen, rotating a further 180 degrees during this process.
- **Omphaloceles, malrotations, and abnormal fixation of the gut** result from failure of return or abnormal rotation of the intestine in the abdomen. Because the gut is normally occluded during the fifth and sixth weeks, stenosis (partial obstruction), atresia (complete obstruction), and duplications result if recanalization fails to occur or occurs abnormally. Remnants of the omphaloenteric duct may persist. **Ileal diverticula** are common; however, only a few of them become inflamed and produce pain.
- The **hindgut** gives rise to the left one third to one half of the transverse colon, the descending and sigmoid colon, the rectum, and the superior part of the anal canal. The inferior part of the anal canal develops from the proctodeum. The caudal part of the hindgut, the **cloaca**, is divided by the urorectal septum into the urogenital sinus and rectum. The urogenital sinus gives rise to the urinary bladder and urethra. The rectum and superior part of the anal canal are separated from the exterior by the anal membrane. This membrane normally breaks down by the end of the eighth week.
- Most anorectal anomalies result from abnormal partitioning of the cloaca by the **urorectal septum** into the rectum and anal canal posteriorly and the urinary bladder and urethra anteriorly. Arrested growth and/or deviation of the urorectal septum in a dorsal direction causes most **anorectal abnormalities**, such as rectal atresia and fistulas between the rectum and the urethra, urinary bladder, or vagina.

CLINICALLY ORIENTED PROBLEMS

Case 11-1

A female infant was born prematurely at 32 weeks' gestation to a 39-year-old woman whose pregnancy was complicated by polyhydramnios. Amniocentesis at 16 weeks showed that the infant had trisomy 21. The baby began to vomit within a few hours after birth. Marked dilation of the epigastrium was noted. Radiographs of the abdomen showed gas in the stomach and the superior part of the duodenum, but no other intestinal gas was observed. A diagnosis of duodenal atresia was made.

- Where does obstruction of the duodenum usually occur?
- What is the embryologic basis of this congenital anomaly?
- What caused distention of the infant's epigastrium?

- Is duodenal atresia commonly associated with malformations such as the Down syndrome?
- What is the embryologic basis of the polyhydramnios in this case?

CASE 11-2

The umbilicus of a newborn infant failed to heal normally. It was swollen, and there was a persistent discharge from the umbilical stump. A sinus tract was outlined with radiopaque oil during fluoroscopy. The tract was resected on the ninth day after birth and its distal end was found to terminate in a diverticulum of the ileum.

- What is the embryologic basis of the sinus tract?
- What is the usual clinical name given to this type of ileal diverticulum?
- Is this anomaly common?

CASE 11-3

A female infant was born with a small dimple where the anus should have been. Examination of the infant's vagina revealed meconium and an opening of a sinus tract in the posterior wall of the vagina. Radiographic examination using a contrast medium injected through a tiny catheter inserted into the opening revealed a fistulous connection with the lower bowel.

- With which part of the lower bowel would the fistula probably be connected?
- Name this anomaly.
- What is the embryologic basis of this condition?

CASE 11-4

A newborn infant was born with a light gray, shiny mass measuring the size of an orange that protruded from the umbilical region. The mass was covered by a thin transparent membrane.

- What is this congenital anomaly called?
- What is the origin of the membrane covering the mass?
- What would be the composition of the mass?
- What is the embryologic basis of this protrusion?

CASE 11-5

A newborn infant appeared normal at birth; however, excessive vomiting and abdominal distention developed after a few hours. The vomitus contained bile, and only a little meconium was passed. Radiographic examination showed a gas-filled stomach and dilated, gas-filled loops of small bowel, but no air was present in the large intestine. This indicated a congenital obstruction of the small bowel.

- What part of the small bowel was probably obstructed?
- What would the condition be called?
- Why was only a little meconium passed?
- What would likely be observed at operation?
- What was the probable embryologic basis of the condition?

Discussion of these problems appears at the back of the book.

References and Suggested Reading

Bates MD, Balistreri WF: Development and function of the liver and biliary system. In Behrman RE, Kliegman RM, Jenson HB (eds): Nelson Textbook of Pediatrics, 17th ed. Philadelphia, WB Saunders, 2004.

Beck F, Tata F, Chawengsaksophak K: Homeobox genes and gut development. Bioessays 22:431, 2000.

Brunner HG, van Bokhoven H: Genetic players in esophageal atresia and tracheoesophageal fistula. Curr Opin Genet Dev 15:341, 2005.

Gosche JR, Vick L, Boulanger SC, Islam S: Midgut abnormalities. Surg Clin North Am 86:285, 2006.

Hill LM: Ultrasound of fetal gastrointestinal tract. In Callen PW (ed): Ultrasonography in Obstetrics and Gynecology, 4th ed. Philadelphia, WB Saunders, 2000.

Jirásek JE: An Atlas of Human Prenatal Developmental Mechanics. Anatomy and Staging, London and New York, Taylor & Francis, 2004.

Kablar B, Tajbakhsh S, Rudnick MA: Transdifferentiation of esophageal smooth muscle is myogenic bHLH factor-dependent. Development 127:1627, 2000.

Kumar M, Melton D: Pancreas specification: A budding question. Curr Opin Genet Dev 13:401, 2003.

Lau ST, Caty MG: Hindgut abnormalities. Surg Clin North Am 86:285, 2006.

Ledbetter DJ: Gastroschisis and omphalocele. Surg Clin North Am 86:249, 2006.

Magnuson DK, Parry RL, Chwals WJ: Selected abdominal gastrointestinal anomalies. In Martin RJ, Fanaroff AA, Walsh MC (eds): Fanaroff and Martin's Neonatal-Perinatal Medicine. Diseases of the Fetus and Infant, 8th ed. Philadelphia, Mosby, 2006.

Martucciello G, Ceccherinil, Lerone M, et al: Pathogenesis of Hirschsprung's disease. J Pediatr Surg 35:1017, 2000.

Meizner I, Levy A, Barnhard Y: Cloacal exstrophy sequence: an exceptional ultrasound diagnosis. Obstet Gynecol 86:446, 1995.

Moore KL, Dalley AF: Clinically Oriented Anatomy, 5th ed. Baltimore, Williams & Wilkins, 2006.

Naik-Mathuria B, Olutoye OO: Foregut abnormalities. Surg Clin North Am 86:261, 2006.

Orenstein S, Peters J, Khan S, et al: Congenital anomalies: Esophageal atresia and tracheoesophageal fistula and function of the esophagus. In Behrman RE, Kliegman RM, Jenson HB (eds): Nelson Textbook of Pediatrics, 17th ed. Philadelphia, Elsevier/Saunders, 2004.

Patterson KD, Drysdale TA, Krieg PA: Embryonic origins of spleen asymmetry. Development 127:167, 2000.

Wyllie R: Pyloric stenosis and other congenital anomalies of the stomach; intestinal atresia, stenosis, and malformations; intestinal duplications, Meckel diverticulum, and other remnants of the omphalomesenteric duct. In Behrman RE, Kliegman RM, Jenson HB (eds): Nelson Textbook of Pediatrics, 17th ed. Philadelphia, WB Saunders, 2004.

Young HM, Newgreen D: Enteric neural crest-derived cells: Origin, identification, migration, and differentiation. Anat Rec 262:1, 2001.

Zona JZ: Umbilical anomalies. In Raffensperger JG (ed): Swenson's Pediatric Surgery, 5th ed. Norwalk, CT, Appleton & Lange, 1990.

12

The Urogenital System

Development of the Urinary System 244
Development of the Kidneys and Ureters 244
Development of the Urinary Bladder 256
Development of the Urethra 260
Development of the Suprarenal Glands 260
Development of the Genital System 262
Development of the Gonads 263
Development of the Genital Ducts 265
Development of the Male Genital Ducts and Glands 265
Development of the Female Genital Ducts and Glands 269
Development of the Uterus and Vagina 269
Development of External Genitalia 271
Development of Male External Genitalia 271
Development of Female External Genitalia 273
Development of the Inguinal Canals 277
Relocation of the Testes and Ovaries 279
Descent of the Testes 279
Descent of the Ovaries 281
Summary of the Urogenital System 282
Clinically Oriented Problems 283

The urogenital system can be divided functionally into the urinary system and the genital system. Embryologically, these systems are closely associated with one another, especially during their early stages of development. They are also associated anatomically, especially in adult males (e.g., the urethra conveys both urine and semen). Although these systems are separate in normal adult females, the urethra and vagina open into a small common space—the vestibule of the vagina—between the labia minora.

The **urogenital system** develops from the intermediate mesenchyme derived from the dorsal body wall of the embryo (Fig. 12-1*A* and *B*). During folding of the embryo in the horizontal plane (see Chapter 5), this mesoderm is carried ventrally and loses its connection with the somites (see Fig. 12-1*C* and *D*). A longitudinal elevation of mesoderm—the **urogenital ridge**—forms on each side of the dorsal aorta (see Fig. 12-1*F*). The part of the urogenital ridge giving rise to the urinary system is the **nephrogenic cord** (see Fig. 12-1*C* to *F*); the part giving rise to the genital system is the **gonadal ridge** (see Fig. 12-29*C*). The following genes are important for the formation of the urogenital ridge: Wilms' tumor suppressor 1 (WT1), steroidogenic factor 1, and DAX1 gene, mutations of which result in X-linked adrenal hypoplasia congenita.

DEVELOPMENT OF THE URINARY SYSTEM

The urinary system begins to develop before the genital system and consists of:

- The kidneys, which excrete urine
- The ureters, which convey urine from the kidneys to the urinary bladder
- The urinary bladder, which stores urine temporarily
- The urethra, which carries urine from the bladder to the exterior of the body

Development of the Kidneys and Ureters

Three sets of kidneys develop in human embryos. The first set—the pronephroi—is rudimentary, and the structures are never functional. The second set—the mesonephroi—is well developed and functions briefly. The third set—the metanephroi—becomes the permanent kidneys.

Pronephroi

These bilateral transitory, nonfunctional structures appear in human embryos early in the fourth week. They are represented by a few cell clusters and tubular structures in the neck region (Fig. 12-2*A*). The pronephric ducts run caudally and open into the *cloaca* (see Fig. 12-2*B*). The pronephroi soon degenerate; however, most of the length of the pronephric ducts persists and is used by the next set of kidneys.

Mesonephroi

These large, elongated excretory organs appear late in the fourth week, caudal to the rudimentary pronephroi (see Fig. 12-2). The mesonephroi are well developed and function as interim kidneys for approximately four weeks, until the permanent kidneys develop (Fig. 12-3). The mesonephric kidneys consist of glomeruli and tubules (Figs. 12-3 to 12-5). The **mesonephric tubules** open into bilateral mesonephric ducts, which were originally the pronephric ducts. The **mesonephric ducts** open into the cloaca. The mesonephroi degenerate toward the end of the first trimester; however, their tubules become the efferent ductules of the testes. The mesonephric ducts have several adult derivatives in males (Table 12-1).

Metanephroi

Metanephroi—**the primordia of permanent kidneys**—begin to develop early in the fifth week and start to function approximately 4 weeks later. Urine formation continues throughout fetal life. Urine is excreted into the amniotic cavity and mixes with the amniotic fluid. A mature fetus swallows several hundred milliliters of amniotic fluid every day, which is absorbed by its intestines. The fetal waste products are transferred through the *placental membrane* into the maternal blood for elimination by the maternal kidneys. The permanent kidneys develop from two sources (Fig. 12-6):

- The metanephric diverticulum (ureteric bud)
- The metanephrogenic blastema or metanephric mass of mesenchyme

The **metanephric diverticulum** is an outgrowth from the mesonephric duct near its entrance into the cloaca, and the **metanephrogenic blastema** is derived from the caudal part of the **nephrogenic cord** (see Fig. 12-6). As it elongates, the metanephric diverticulum penetrates the metanephrogenic blastema—a mass of mesenchyme (see Fig. 12-6*B*). The *stalk of the metanephric diverticulum* becomes the **ureter**, and the cranial portion of the diverticulum undergoes repetitive branching events, forming the branches which differentiate into the **collecting tubules** of the metanephros (see Fig. 12-6*C* to *E*).

The first four generations of tubules enlarge and become confluent to form the **major calices** (see Fig. 12-6*C* to *E*), and the second four generations coalesce to form the **minor calices**. The end of each arched collecting tubule induces clusters of mesenchymal cells in the metanephrogenic blastema to form small metanephric vesicles (Fig. 12-7*A*). These vesicles elongate and become **metanephric tubules** (see Fig. 12-7*B* and *C*). The proximal ends of these tubules are invaginated by **glomeruli**. The tubules differentiate into proximal and distal convoluted tubules, and the **nephron loop** (Henle loop), together with the glomerulus and its capsule, constitute a **nephron** (see Fig. 12-7*D*). Each distal convoluted tubule contacts an arched collecting tubule, and the tubules become confluent.

Between the 10th and 18th weeks of gestation, the number of glomeruli increases gradually and then increases rapidly until the 32nd week, when an upper limit is reached. The **fetal kidneys** are subdivided into lobes (Fig. 12-8). The lobulation usually disappears during infancy as the nephrons increase and grow. At term, nephron formation is complete, with each kidney containing 400,000 to 2,000,000 nephrons. The increase in kidney size after birth results mainly from the elongation of the

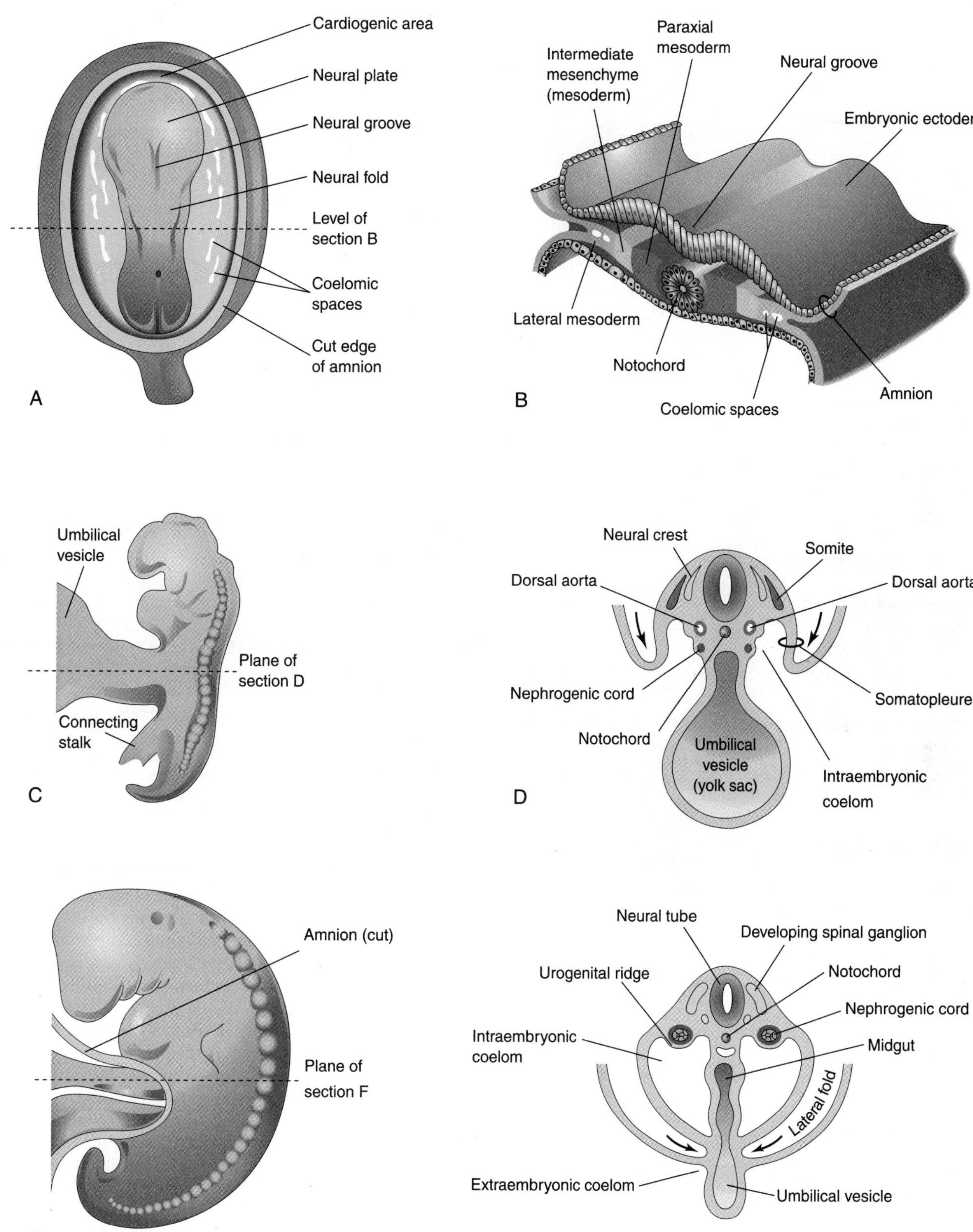

FIGURE 12-1. **A,** Dorsal view of an embryo during the third week (approximately 18 days). **B,** Transverse section of the embryo showing the position of the intermediate mesenchyme before lateral folding of the embryo. **C,** Lateral view of an embryo during the fourth week (approximately 24 days). **D,** Transverse section of the embryo after the commencement of folding, showing the nephrogenic cords. **E,** Lateral view of an embryo later in the fourth week (approximately 26 days). **F,** Transverse section of the embryo showing the lateral folds meeting each other ventrally. Observe the position of the urogenital ridges and nephrogenic cords.

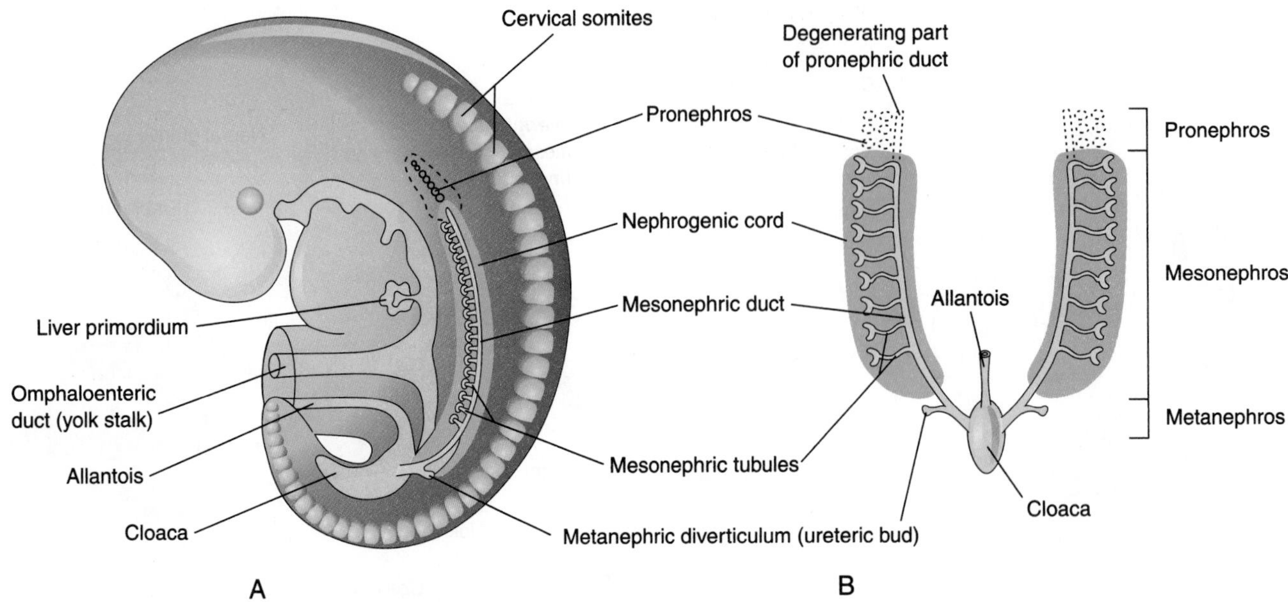

FIGURE 12-2. Illustrations of the three sets of excretory systems in an embryo during the fifth week. **A,** Lateral view. **B,** Ventral view. The mesonephric tubules have been pulled laterally; their normal position is shown in **A**.

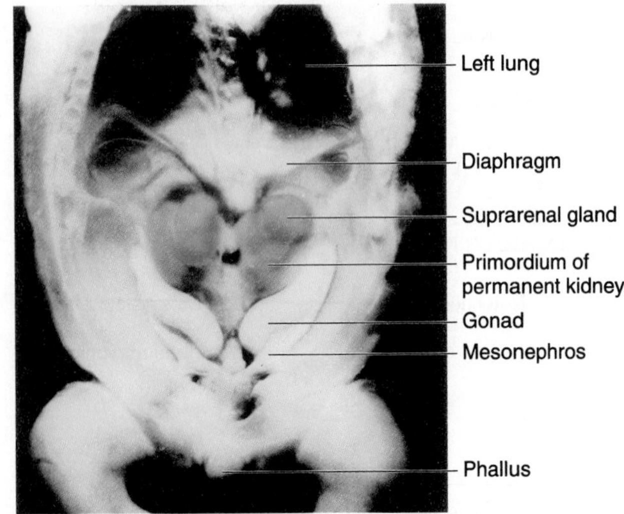

FIGURE 12-3. Dissection of the thorax, abdomen, and pelvis of an embryo at Carnegie stage 22, approximately 54 days. Observe the large suprarenal (adrenal) glands and the elongated mesonephroi (mesonephric kidneys). Also observe the gonads (testes or ovaries). The phallus will develop into a penis or a clitoris depending on the genetic sex of the embryo. (From Nishimura H [ed]: Atlas of Human Prenatal Histology. Tokyo, Igaku-Shoin, 1983.)

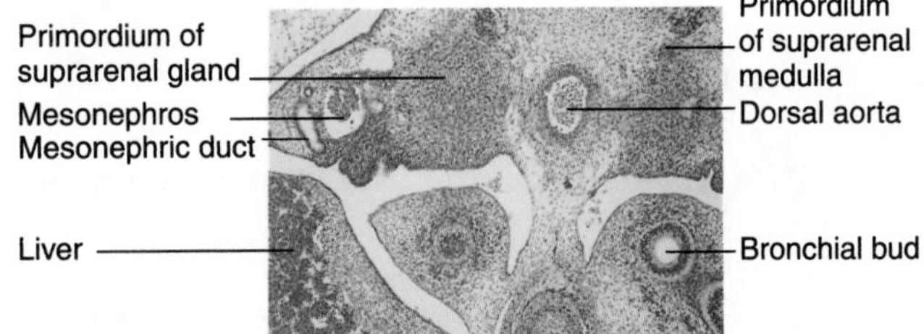

FIGURE 12-4. Photomicrograph of a transverse section of an embryo at Carnegie stage 17, approximately 42 days, primarily to show the mesonephros and developing suprarenal (adrenal) glands. Observe that the mesonephros extends into the thorax at this stage (see also Fig. 12-5*A*). (From Moore KL, Persaud TVN, Shiota K: Color Atlas of Clinical Embryology, 2nd ed. Philadelphia, WB Saunders, 2000.)

proximal convoluted tubules as well as an increase of interstitial tissue. Nephron formation is complete at birth except in premature infants. Although glomerular filtration begins at approximately the ninth fetal week, functional maturation of the kidneys and increasing rates of filtration occur after birth.

A **uriniferous tubule** consists of two embryologically different parts (see Figs. 12-6 and 12-7):

- A nephron derived from the metanephrogenic blastema
- A collecting tubule derived from the metanephric diverticulum (ureteric bud)

Branching of the metanephric diverticulum is dependent on induction by the metanephric mesenchyme. Differentiation of the nephrons depends on induction by the collecting tubules. The metanephric diverticulum and the metanephrogenic blastema interact and induce each other, a process known as **reciprocal induction**, to form the permanent kidneys. Molecular studies, especially knockout and transgenic analyses in the mouse, show that this process involves two principal signaling systems that use conserved molecular pathways. Recent research has provided insight into the complex interrelated molecular events regulating the development of the kidneys (Fig. 12-9). Before induction, a transcription factor WT1 is expressed in the metanephrogenic blastema supporting the survival of the as yet uninduced mesenchyme. Expression of Pax2, Eya1, and Sall1 is required for the expression of glial-derived neurotropic factor (GDNF) in the metanephric mesenchyme. GDNF plays an essential role in the induction and branching of the metanephric diverticulum (**branching morphogenesis**). The receptor for GDNF, c-ret, is first expressed in the mesonephric duct, but later becomes localized on the tip of the meta-

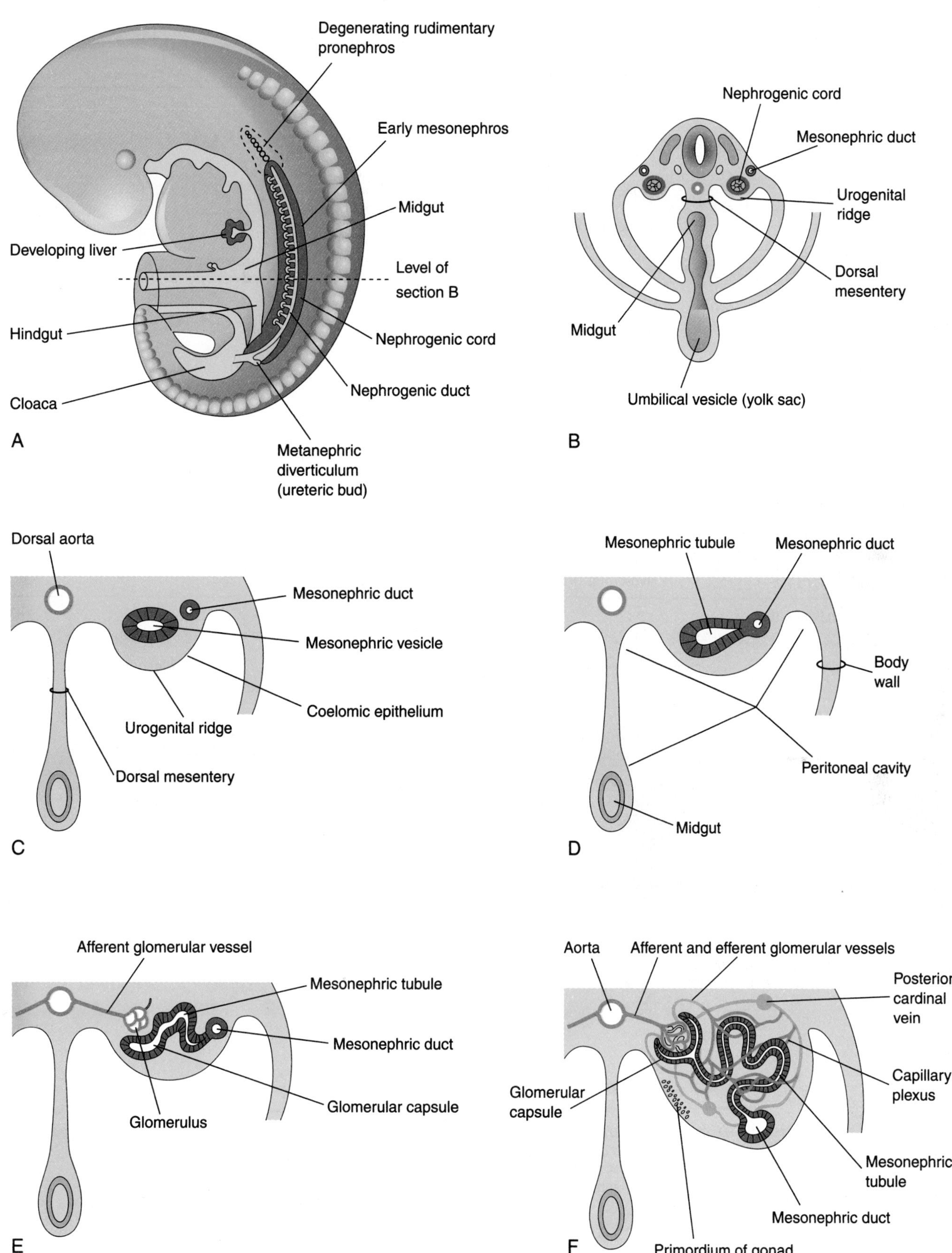

FIGURE 12-5. **A,** Lateral view of a 5-week embryo showing the extent of the early mesonephros and the primordium of the metanephros (primordium of permanent kidney.) **B,** Transverse section of the embryo showing the nephrogenic cords from which the mesonephric tubules develop. **C** to **F,** Successive stages in the development of a mesonephric tubule between the 5th and 11th weeks. Note that the mesenchymal cell cluster in the nephrogenic cord develops a lumen, thereby forming a mesonephric vesicle. The vesicle soon becomes an S-shaped mesonephric tubule and extends laterally to join the mesonephric duct. The expanded medial end of the mesonephric tubule is invaginated by blood vessels to form a glomerular capsule.

TABLE 12–1. Adult Derivatives and Vestigial Remains of Embryonic Urogenital Structures*

MALE	EMBRYONIC STRUCTURE	FEMALE
Testis	Indifferent gonad	Ovary
Seminiferous tubules	Cortex	*Ovarian follicles*
Rete testis	Medulla	*Rete ovarii*
Gubernaculum testis	Gubernaculum	*Ovarian ligament*
		Round ligament of uterus
Efferent ductules of testis	Mesonephric tubules	Epoophoron
Paradidymis		Paroophoron
Appendix of epididymis	Mesonephric duct	Appendix vesiculosa
Duct of epididymis		Duct of epoophoron
Ductus deferens		Longitudinal duct; Gartner duct
Ureter, pelvis, calices, and collecting tubules		*Ureter, pelvis, calices, and collecting tubules*
Ejaculatory duct and seminal gland		
Appendix of testis	Paramesonephric duct	Hydatid (of Morgagni)
		Uterine tube
		Uterus
Urinary bladder	Urogenital sinus	*Urinary bladder*
Urethra (except navicular fossa)		*Urethra*
Prostatic utricle		*Vagina*
Prostate gland		*Urethral and paraurethral glands*
Bulbourethral glands		*Greater vestibular glands*
Seminal colliculus	Sinus tubercle	Hymen
Penis	Phallus	*Clitoris*
Glans penis		*Glans of clitoris*
Corpora cavernosa of penis		*Corpora cavernosa of clitoris*
Corpus spongiosum of penis		*Bulb of vestibule*
Ventral aspect of penis	Urogenital folds	*Labia minora*
Scrotum	Labioscrotal swellings	*Labia majora*

*Functional derivatives are in italics.

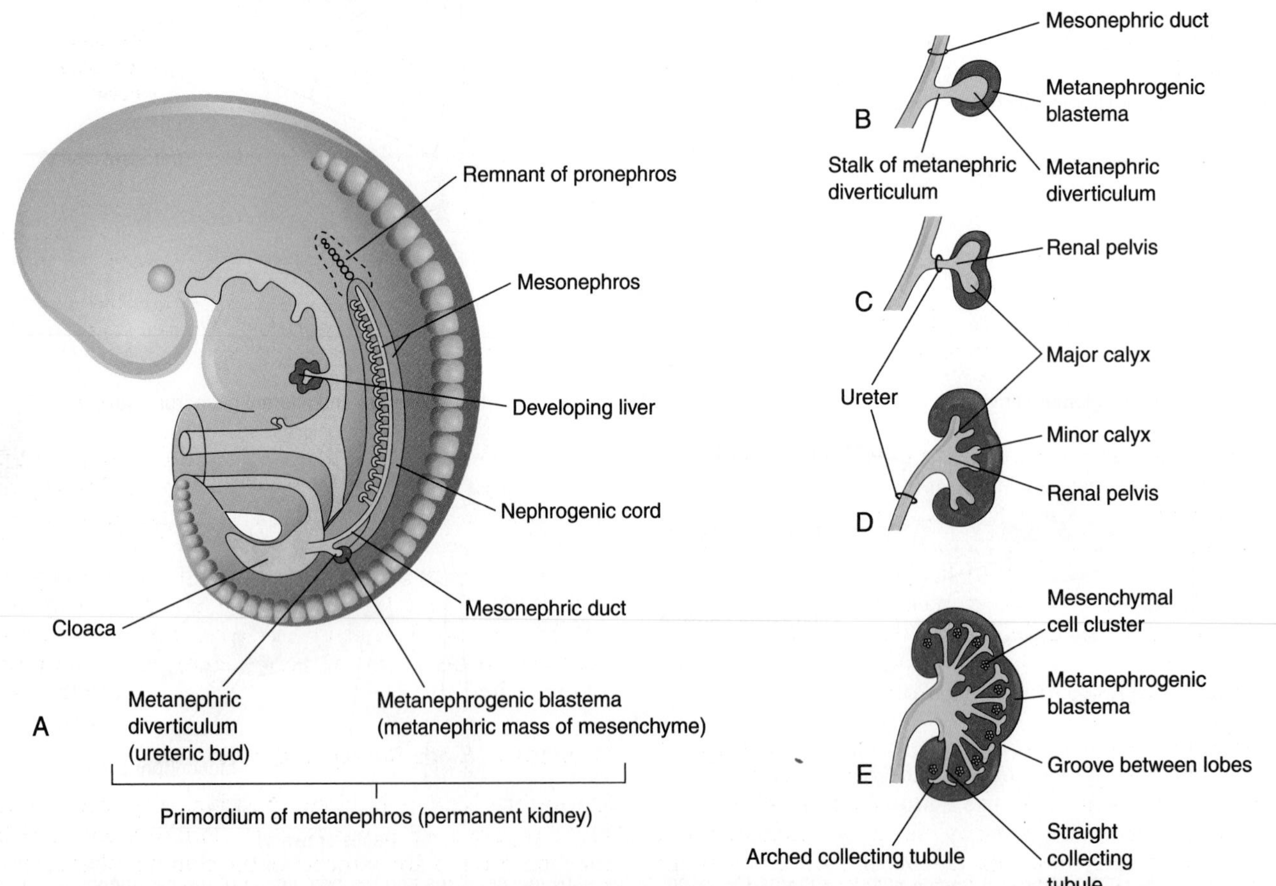

FIGURE 12-6. Development of the permanent kidney. **A,** Lateral view of a 5-week embryo showing the primordium of the metanephros. **B** to **E,** Successive stages in the development of the metanephric diverticulum (fifth to eighth weeks). Observe the development of the ureter, renal pelvis, calices, and collecting tubules.

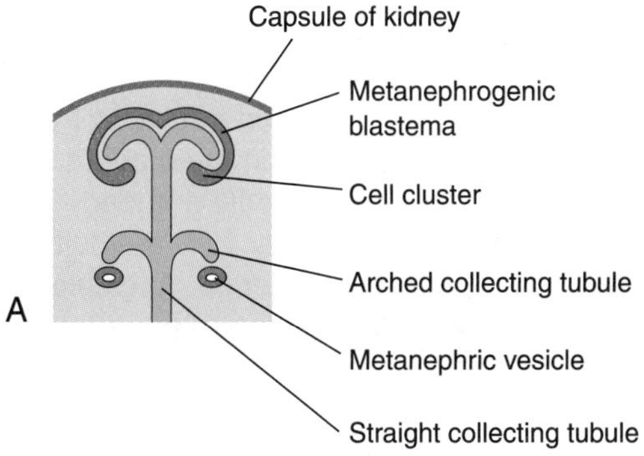

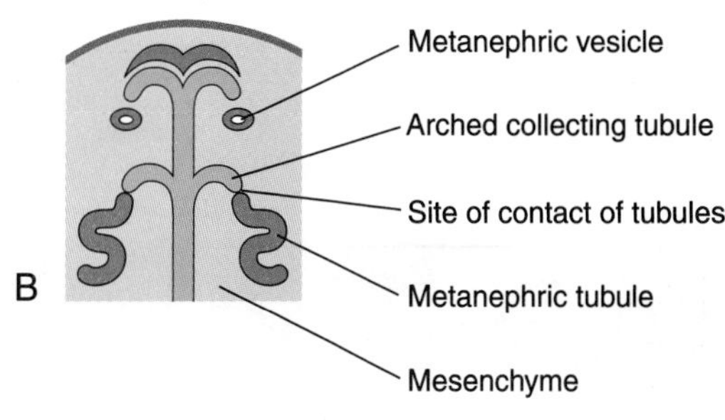

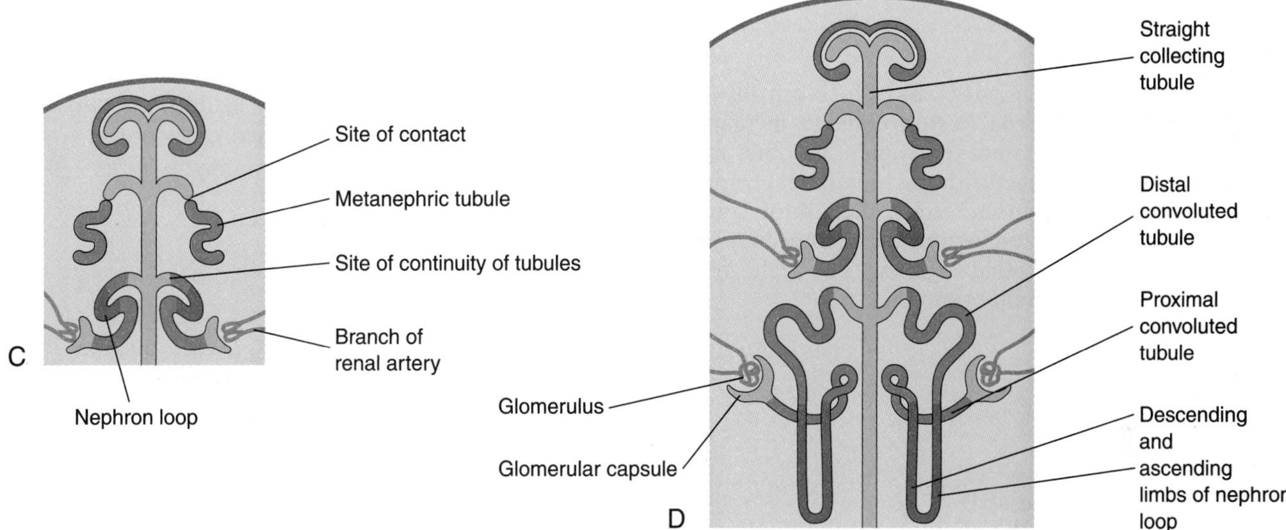

FIGURE 12-7. Development of nephrons. **A,** Nephrogenesis commences around the beginning of the eighth week. **B** and **C,** Note that the metanephric tubules, the primordia of the nephrons, become continuous with the collecting tubules to form uriniferous tubules. **D,** Observe that nephrons are derived from the metanephrogenic blastema and that the collecting tubules are derived from the metanephric diverticulum.

nephric diverticulum. Subsequent branching is controlled by transcription factors including Emx2 and Pax2 and growth factor signals including members of the Wnt, FGF, and BMP families. Transformation of the metanephric mesenchyme to the epithelial cells of the nephron—**mesenchymal-epithelial transition**—is regulated by mesenchyme factors including Wnt4.

Positional Changes of the Kidneys

Initially the metanephric kidneys (primordial permanent kidneys) lie close to each other in the pelvis, ventral to the sacrum (Fig. 12-10*A*). As the abdomen and pelvis grow, the kidneys gradually come to lie in the abdomen and move farther apart (see Fig. 12-10*B* and *C*). They attain their adult position by the ninth week (see Fig. 12-10*D*). This relative ascent results mainly from the growth of the embryo's body caudal to the kidneys. In effect, the caudal part of the embryo grows away from the kidneys so that they progressively occupy more cranial levels. Initially the **hilum of the kidney**, where vessels and nerves enter and leave, faces ventrally; however, as the kidney relocates (ascends), it rotates medially almost 90 degrees. By the ninth week, the hilum is directed anteromedially (see Fig. 12-10*C* and *D*). Eventually the kidneys become retroperitoneal (external to the peritoneum) on the posterior abdominal wall.

Changes in Blood Supply of the Kidneys

During the changes in kidney position, they receive their blood supply from vessels that are close to them. Initially the renal arteries are branches of the common iliac arteries (see Fig. 12-10*A* and *B*). Later, the kidneys receive their blood supply from the distal end of the aorta. When they are located at a higher level, they receive new branches

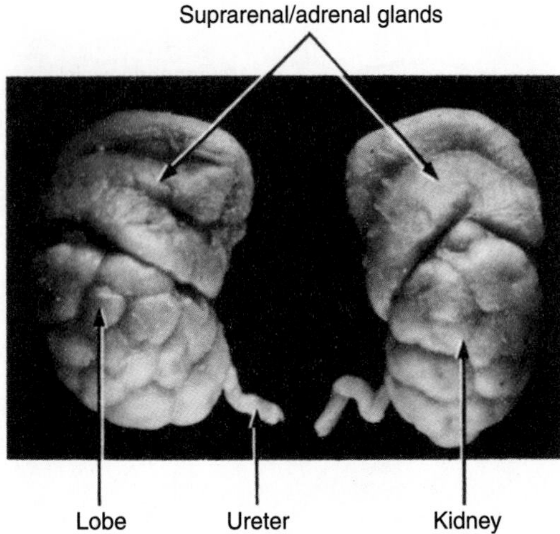

FIGURE 12-8. The kidneys and suprarenal glands of a 28-week fetus (×2). The external evidence of the lobes usually disappears by the end of the first postnatal year. Note the large size of the suprarenal glands at this age.

from the aorta (see Fig. 12-10*C* and *D*). Normally the caudal branches of the renal vessels undergo involution and disappear. The position of the kidneys becomes fixed once they come into contact with the suprarenal glands in the ninth week. The kidneys receive their most cranial arterial branches from the abdominal aorta; these branches become the permanent renal arteries. The right renal artery is longer and often more superior.

ACCESSORY RENAL ARTERIES

The common variations in the blood supply to the kidneys reflect the manner in which the blood supply continually changed during embryonic and early fetal life (see Fig. 12-10). Approximately 25% of adult kidneys have two to four renal arteries. **Accessory (supernumerary) renal arteries** usually arise from the aorta superior or inferior to the main renal artery and follow the main renal artery to the hilum of the kidney (Fig. 12-11*A*, *C*, and *D*). Accessory renal arteries may also enter the kidneys directly, usually into the superior or inferior poles. An accessory artery to the inferior pole (polar renal artery) may cross anterior to the ureter and obstruct it, causing **hydronephrosis**—distention of the renal pelvis and calices with urine (see Fig. 12-11*B*). If the artery enters the inferior pole of the right kidney, it usually crosses anterior to the inferior vena cava and ureter.

It is important to be aware that accessory renal arteries are end arteries; consequently, if an accessory artery is damaged or ligated, the part of the kidney supplied by it will become ischemic. Accessory arteries are approximately twice as common as accessory veins.

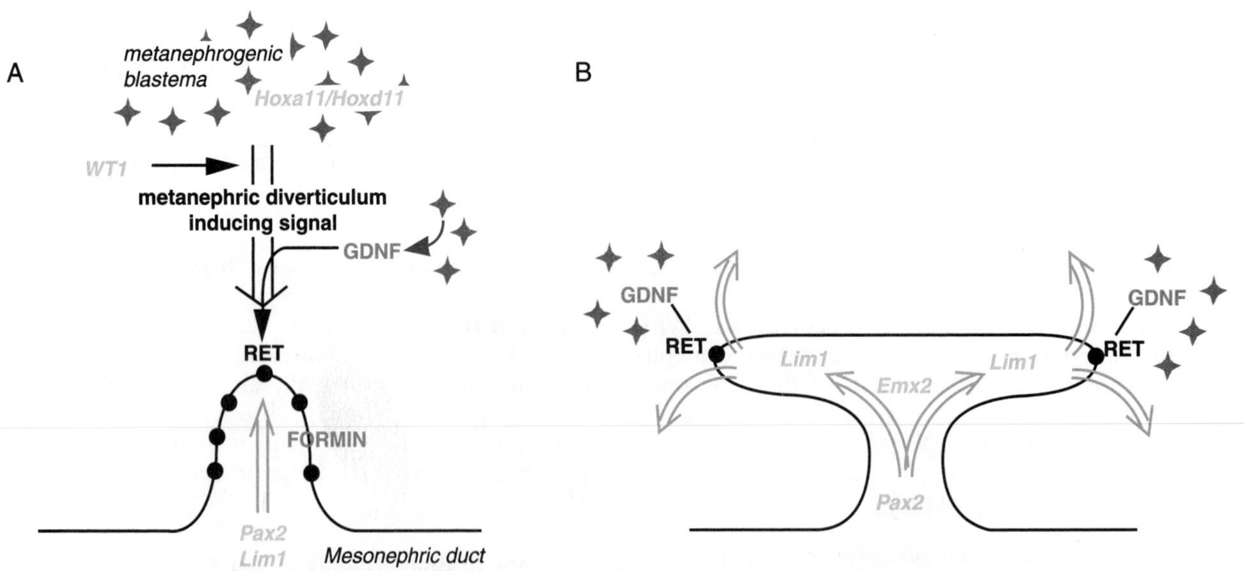

FIGURE 12-9. Molecular control of kidney development. **A,** The metanephric diverticulum requires inductive signals derived from metanephrogenic blastema (mesenchyme) under control of transcription factors (orange text) such as WT1 and signaling molecules (red text) including glial-derived neurotropic factor (GDNF) and its epithelial receptor, RET. The normal metanephric diverticulum (ureteric bud) response to these inductive signals is under the control of transcription factors such as Pax2, Lim1, and the FORMIN gene. **B,** Branching of the metanephric diverticulum is initiated and maintained by interaction with the mesenchyme under the regulation of genes such as *Emx2* and specified expression of GDNF and RET at the tips of the invading metanephric diverticulum. (From Piscione TD, Rosenblum ND: The malformed kidney: Disruption of glomerular and tubular development. Clin Genet 56:341–356, 1999.)

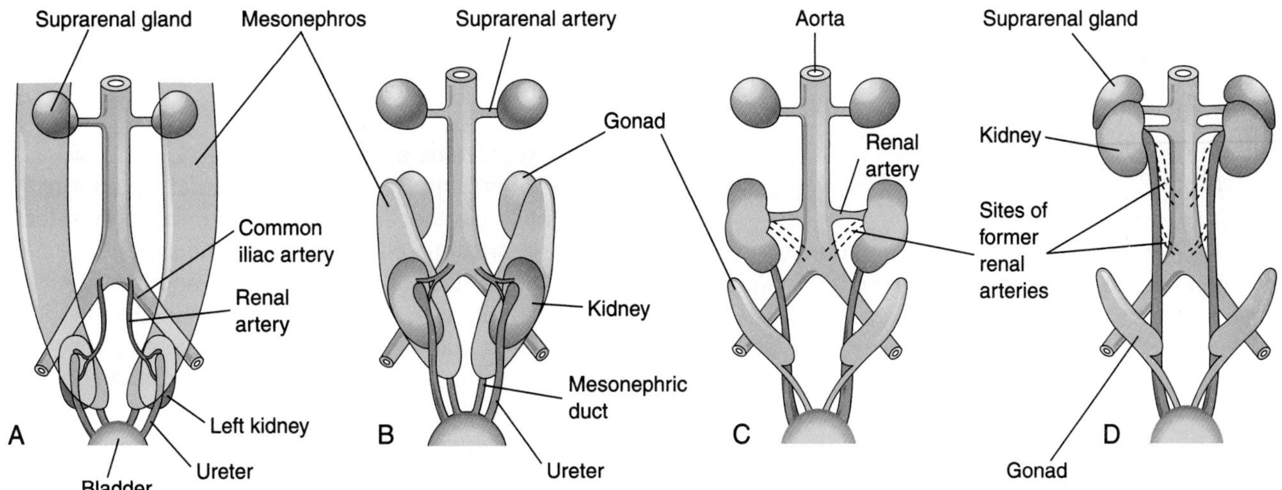

FIGURE 12-10. **A** to **D,** Diagrammatic ventral views of the abdominopelvic region of embryos and fetuses (sixth to ninth weeks) showing medial rotation and relocation of the kidneys from the pelvis to the abdomen. **A** and **B,** Observe also the size regression of the mesonephroi. **C** and **D,** Note that as the kidneys relocate, they are supplied by arteries at successively higher levels and that the hilum of the kidney is eventually directed anteromedially.

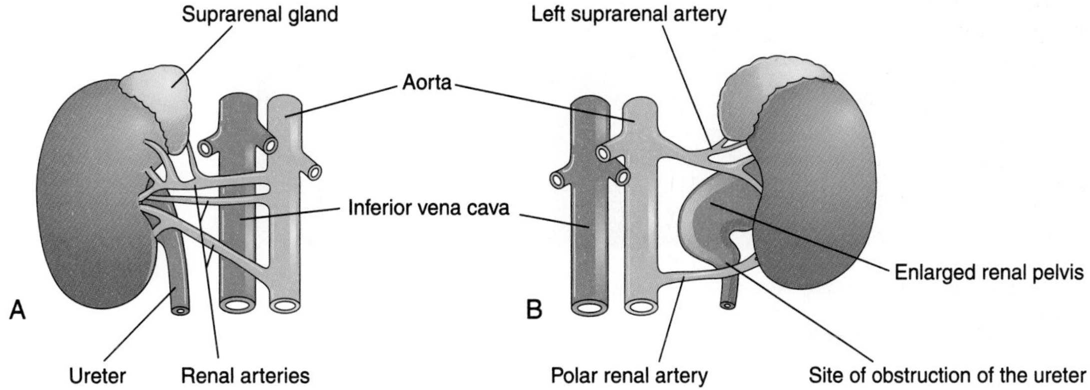

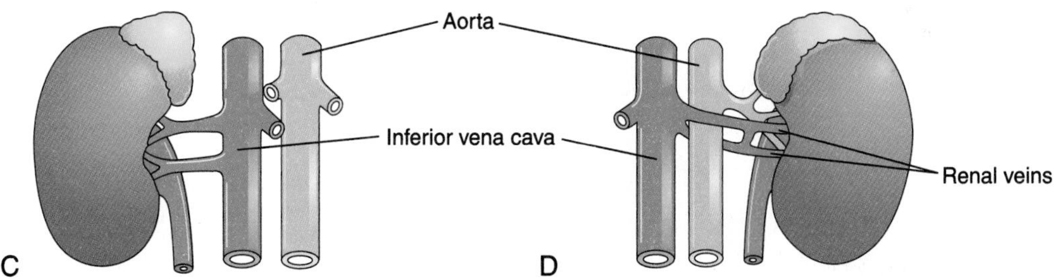

FIGURE 12-11. Common variations of renal vessels. **A** and **B,** Multiple renal arteries. Note the accessory vessels entering the poles of the kidney. The polar renal artery, illustrated in **B**, has obstructed the ureter and produced an enlarged renal pelvis. **C** and **D,** Multiple renal veins are less common than accessory arteries.

Congenital Anomalies of Kidneys and Ureters

Some type of abnormality of the kidneys and ureters occurs in 3% to 4% of newborn infants. Anomalies in shape and position are most common. Many fetal urinary tract abnormalities can be detected before birth by ultrasonography.

Renal Agenesis

Unilateral renal agenesis occurs approximately once in every 1000 newborn infants. Males are affected more often than females, and the left kidney is usually the one that is absent (Figs. 12-12*A* and *B* and 12-13*A*). Unilateral renal agenesis often causes no symptoms and is usually not discovered during infancy because the other kidney usually undergoes compensatory hypertrophy and performs the function of the missing kidney. Unilateral renal agenesis should be suspected in infants with a *single umbilical artery* (see Chapter 7).

Bilateral renal agenesis (see Fig. 12-12*C*) is associated with *oligohydramnios* (small amount of amniotic fluid) because little or no urine is excreted into the amniotic cavity. This condition occurs approximately once in 3000 births, and is incompatible with postnatal life because of the associated pulmonary hypoplasia. These infants have a characteristic facial appearance: the eyes are

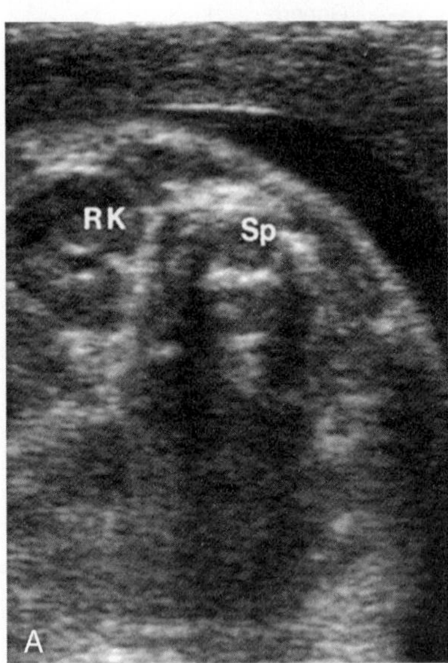

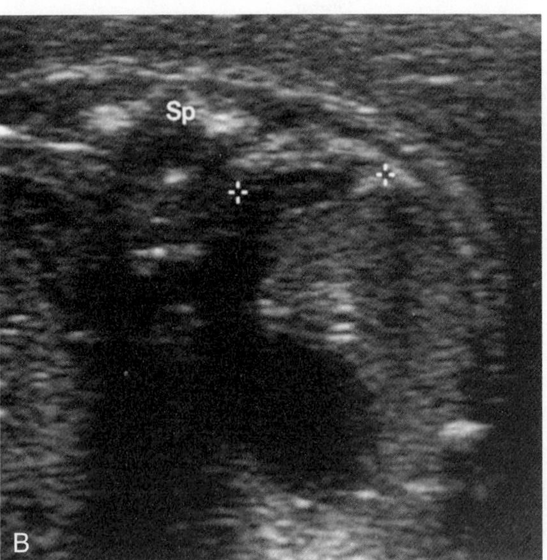

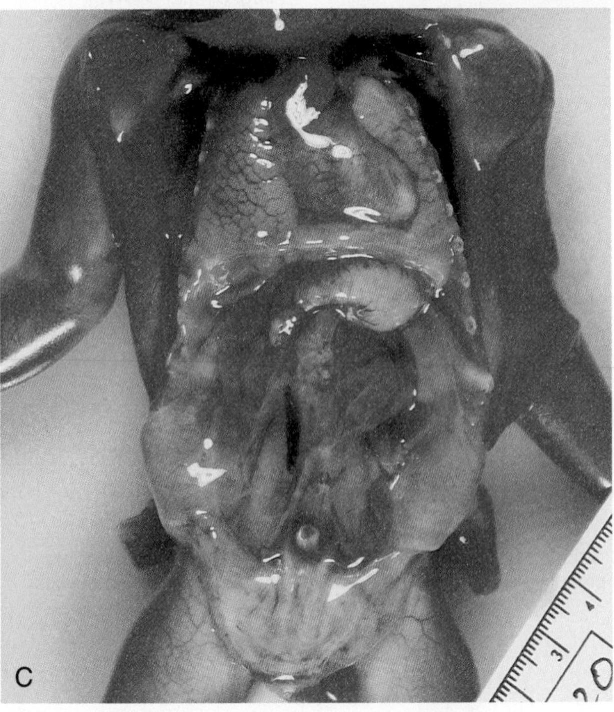

FIGURE 12-12. Sonograms of a fetus with unilateral renal agenesis. **A,** Transverse scan at the level of the lumbar region of the vertebral column or spine (Sp) showing the right kidney (RK) but not the left kidney. **B,** Transverse scan at a slightly higher level showing the left suprarenal gland (between cursors) within the left renal fossa. **C,** Bilateral renal agenesis. Note prominent suprarenal glands. Male fetus of 19.5 developmental weeks. (**A** and **B,** From Mahony BS: Ultrasound evaluation of the fetal genitourinary system. In Callen PW [ed]: Ultrasonography in Obstetrics and Gynecology, 3rd ed. Philadelphia, WB Saunders, 1994. **C,** Courtesy of Dr. D.K. Kalousek, Department of Pathology, University of British Columbia, Children's Hospital, Vancouver, British Columbia, Canada.)

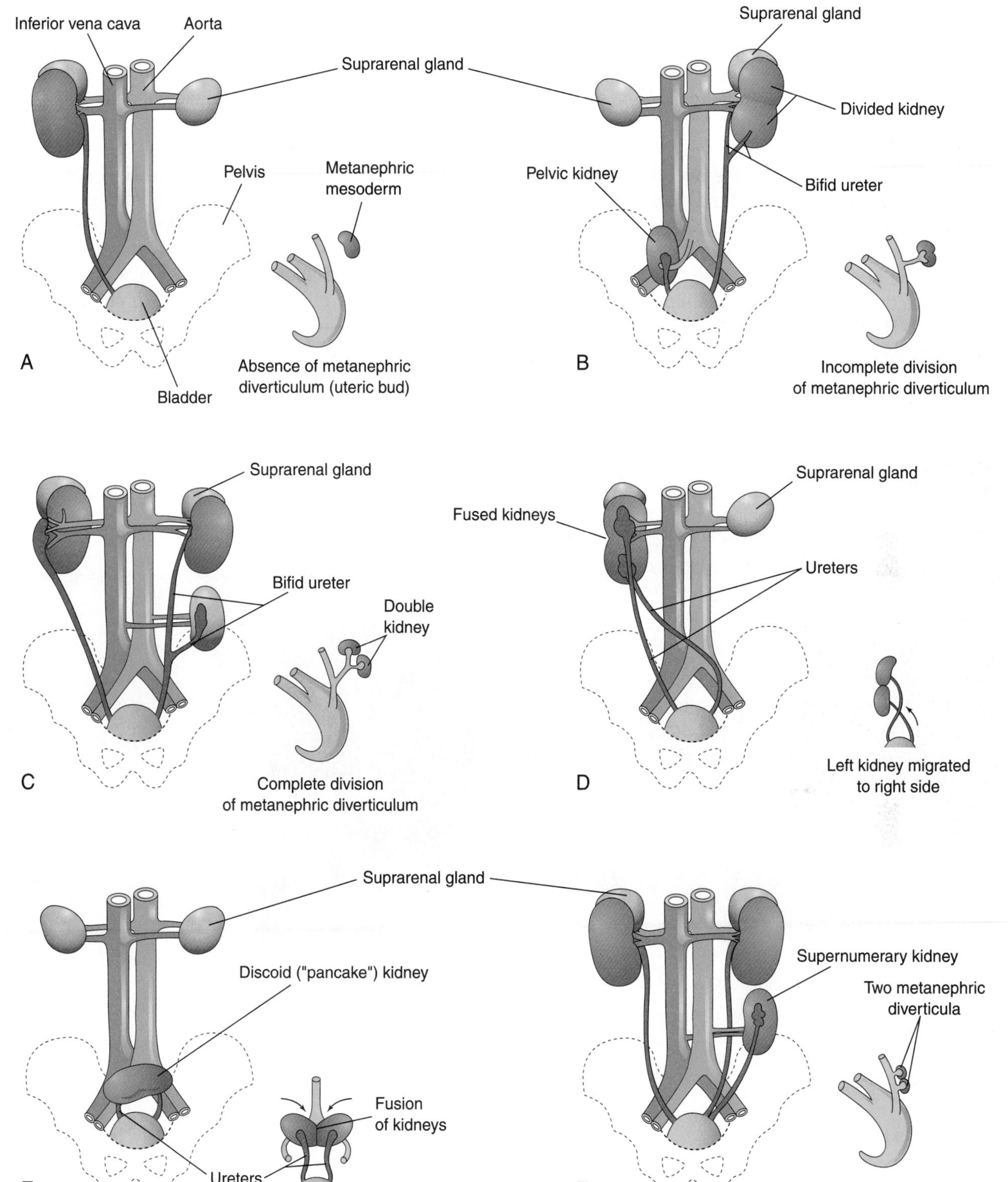

FIGURE 12-13. Illustrations of various anomalies of the urinary system. The small sketch to the lower right of each drawing illustrates the probable embryologic basis of the anomaly. **A,** Unilateral renal agenesis. **B,** Right side, pelvic kidney; left side, divided kidney with a bifid ureter. **C,** Right side, malrotation of the kidney; left side, bifid ureter and supernumerary kidney. **D,** Crossed renal ectopia. The left kidney crossed to the right side and fused with the right kidney. **E,** Discoid kidney resulting from fusion of the kidneys while they were in the pelvis. **F,** Supernumerary left kidney resulting from the development of two metanephric diverticula.

widely separated and have epicanthic folds, the ears are low-set, the nose is broad and flat, the chin is receding, and there are limb defects. Most infants with bilateral renal agenesis die shortly after birth or during the first months of life.

Renal agenesis results when the metanephric diverticula fail to develop or the primordia of the ureters degenerate. Failure of the metanephric diverticula to penetrate the metanephrogenic blastema results in failure of kidney development because no nephrons are induced by the collecting tubules to develop from the metanephrogenic blastema. Renal agenesis probably has a multifactorial etiology. There is clinical evidence that complete in utero involution of polycystic kidneys could lead to renal agenesis with a blind ending ureter on the same side.

Malrotated Kidney

If a kidney fails to rotate, the hilum faces anteriorly, that is, the fetal kidney retains its embryonic position (see Figs. 12-10*A* and 12-13*C*). If the hilum faces posteriorly, rotation of the kidney proceeded too far; if it faces laterally, lateral instead of medial rotation occurred. Abnormal rotation of the kidneys is often associated with ectopic kidneys.

Ectopic Kidneys

One or both kidneys may be in an abnormal position (see Fig. 12-13*B*, *E*, and *F*). Most ectopic kidneys are located in the pelvis (Fig. 12-14), but some lie in the inferior part of the abdomen. Pelvic kidneys and other forms of ectopia result from failure of the kidneys to alter position during embryo growth.

Pelvic kidneys are close to each other and may fuse to form a discoid ("pancake") kidney (see Fig. 12-13*E*). Ectopic kidneys receive their blood supply from blood vessels near them (internal or external iliac arteries and/or aorta). They are often supplied by multiple vessels. Sometimes a kidney crosses to the other side resulting in crossed renal ectopia (Fig. 12-15, showing both kidneys on the right side of the abdomen). Sometimes a kidney crosses to the other side, resulting in **crossed renal ectopia** with or without fusion. An unusual type of abnormal kidney is unilateral fused kidney. In such cases, the developing kidneys fuse while they are in the pelvis, and one kidney attains its normal position, carrying the other kidney with it (see Fig. 12-13*D*).

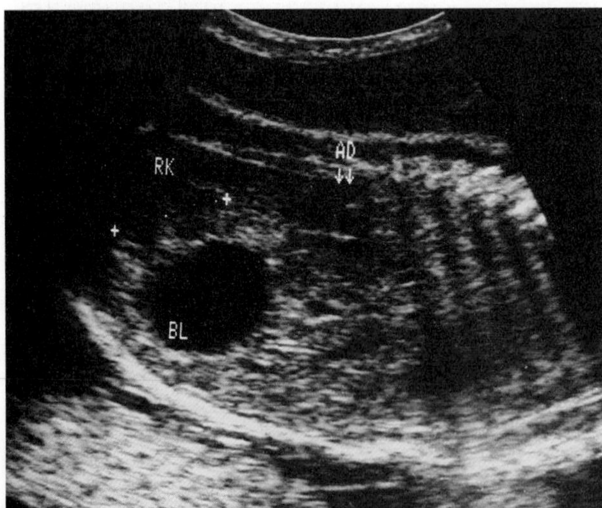

FIGURE 12-14. Sonogram of the pelvis of a fetus at 31 weeks' gestation (29 weeks after fertilization). Observe the abnormally low position of the right kidney (RK) near the urinary bladder (BL). This pelvic kidney resulted from its failure to ascend during the sixth to ninth weeks. Also observe the normal location of the suprarenal or adrenal gland (AD), which develops separately from the kidney. (Courtesy of Dr. Lyndon M. Hill, Director of Ultrasound, Magee-Women's Hospital, Pittsburgh, PA.)

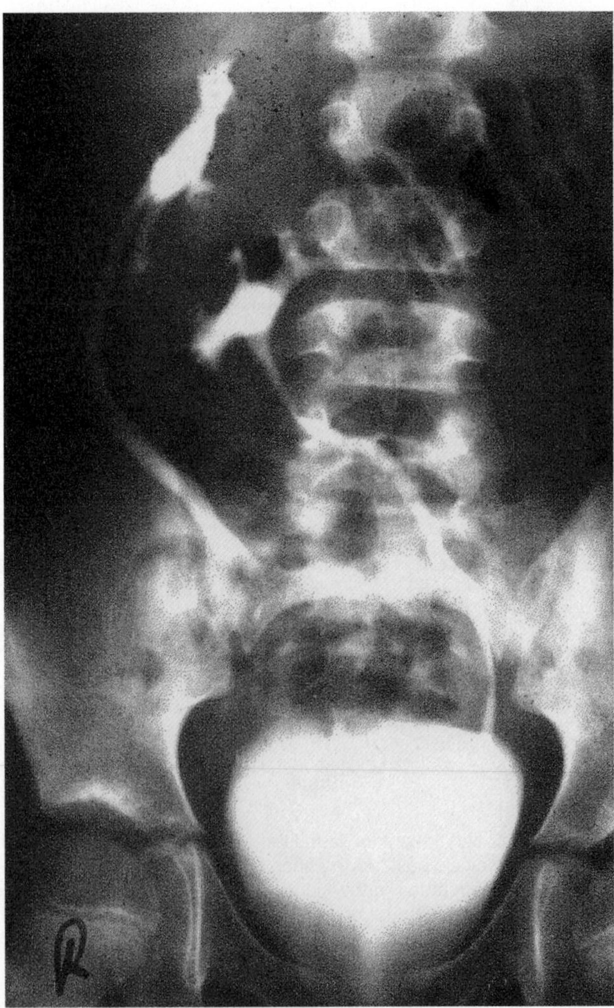

FIGURE 12-15. Intravenous pyelogram showing crossed renal ectopia. (Courtesy of Dr. Prem S. Sahni, formerly of the Department of Radiology, Children's Hospital, Winnipeg, Manitoba, Canada.)

Horseshoe Kidney

In 0.2% of the population, the poles of the kidneys are fused; usually the inferior poles fuse. The large U-shaped kidney usually lies in the hypogastrium, anterior to the inferior lumbar vertebrae (Fig. 12-16). Normal ascent of these fused kidneys is prevented because they are caught by the root of the inferior mesenteric artery. *A horseshoe kidney usually produces no symptoms* because its collecting system develops normally and the ureters enter the bladder. If urinary flow is impeded, signs and symptoms of obstruction and/or infection may appear. Approximately 7% of persons with Turner's syndrome have horseshoe kidneys.

Duplications of the Urinary Tract

Duplications of the abdominal part of the ureter and the renal pelvis are common (see Fig. 12-13*F*). These anomalies result from division of the metanephric diverticulum. The extent of the duplication depends on how complete the division of the diverticulum was. Incomplete division of the metanephric diverticulum results in a divided kidney with a bifid ureter (see Fig. 12-13*B*). Complete division results in a double kidney with a bifid ureter (see Fig. 12-13*B*) or separate ureters (Fig. 12-17). A **supernumerary kidney** (see Fig. 12-13*F*) with its own ureter, which is rare, probably results from the formation of two metanephric diverticula.

Ectopic Ureter

An ectopic ureter does not enter the urinary bladder. In males, ectopic ureters usually open into the neck of the bladder or into the prostatic part of the urethra, but they may enter the ductus deferens, prostatic utricle, or seminal gland. In females, ectopic ureters may open into the bladder neck, urethra, vagina, or vestibule of the vagina (Fig. 12-18). Incontinence is the common complaint resulting from an ectopic ureter because the urine flowing from the orifice does not enter the bladder; instead it continually dribbles from the urethra in males and the urethra and/or vagina in females.

An ectopic ureter results when the ureter is not incorporated into the trigone in the posterior part of the urinary bladder. Instead it is carried caudally with the mesonephric duct and is incorporated into the middle pelvic portion of the vesical part of the urogenital sinus. Because this part of the sinus becomes the prostatic urethra in males and the urethra in females, the location of ectopic ureteric orifices is understandable. When two ureters form on one side (see Fig. 12-17), they usually open into the urinary bladder (see Fig. 12-13*F*).

Cystic Kidney Diseases

In **autosomal recessive polycystic kidney disease**, diagnosed at birth or in utero by ultrasonography, both kidneys contain many hundreds of small cysts

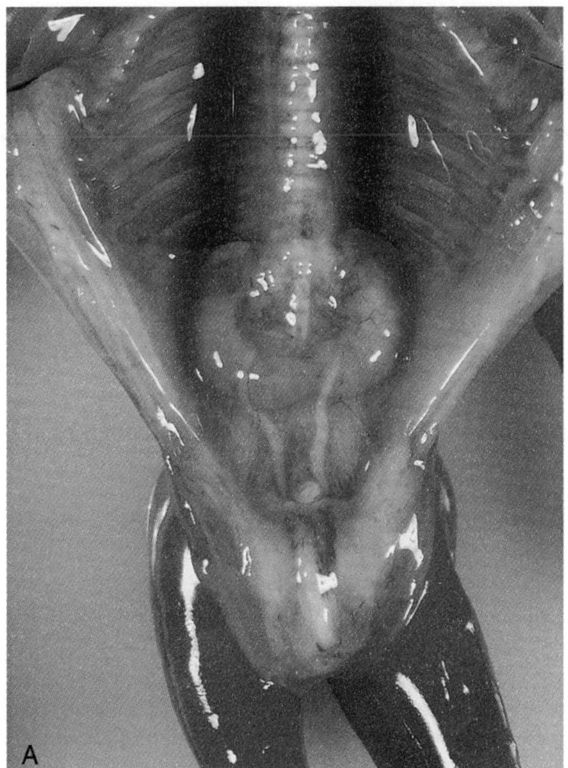

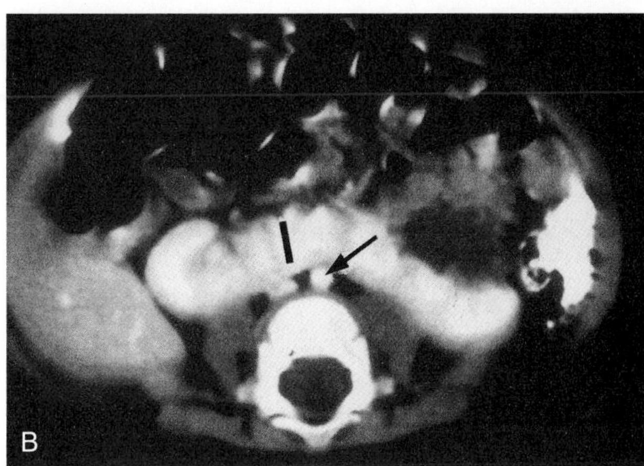

FIGURE 12-16. **A,** Horseshoe kidney in a 13-week female fetus. **B,** Contrast-enhanced computed tomography scan of the abdomen of an infant with a horseshoe kidney. Note the isthmus (vascular) of renal tissue (I) connecting the right and left kidneys just anterior to the aorta (*arrow*) and inferior vena cava. (**A,** Courtesy of Dr. D.K. Kalousek, Department of Pathology, University of British Columbia, Children's Hospital, Vancouver, British Columbia, Canada; **B,** Courtesy of Dr. Prem S. Sahni, formerly of the Department of Radiology, Children's Hospital, Winnipeg, Manitoba, Canada.)

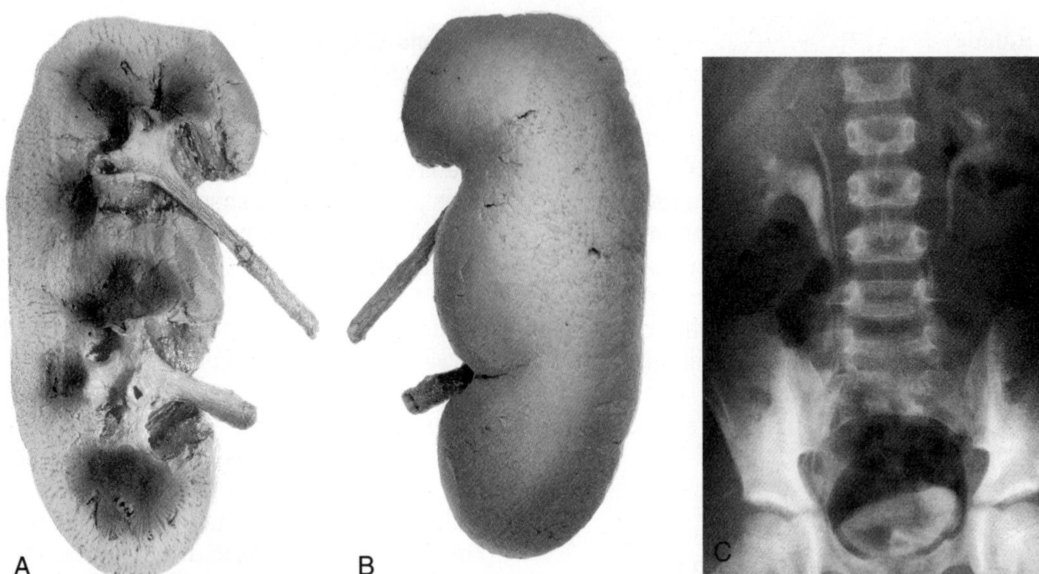

FIGURE 12-17. A duplex kidney with two ureters and renal pelves. **A,** Longitudinal section through the kidney showing two renal pelves and calices. **B,** Anterior surface of the kidney. **C,** Intravenous urography showing duplication of the right kidney and ureter in a 10-year-old male. The distal ends of the right ureter are fused at the level of the first sacral vertebra. The left kidney is normal. (Courtesy of Dr. Prem S. Sahni, Department of Radiology, Children's Hospital, Winnipeg, Manitoba, Canada.)

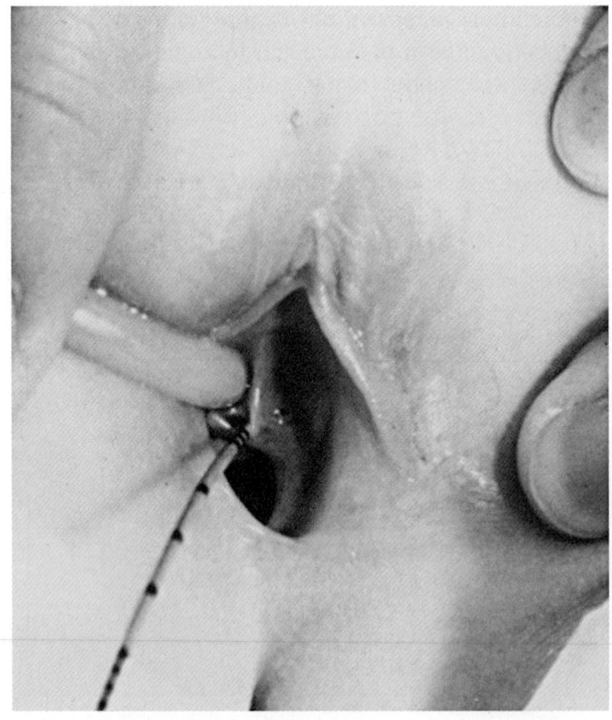

FIGURE 12-18. Ectopic ureter. This girl has an ectopic ureter entering the vestibule of the vagina near the external urethral orifice. The thin ureteral catheter with transverse marks has been introduced through the ureteric orifice into the ectopic ureter. This girl had a normal voiding pattern and constant urinary dribbling. (From Behrman RE, Kliegman RM, Arvin AM [eds]: Nelson Textbook of Pediatrics, 15th ed. Philadelphia, WB Saunders, 1996.)

(Fig. 12-19*A*), which result in renal insufficiency. Death of the infant usually occurs shortly after birth; however, an increasing number of these infants are surviving because of postnatal dialysis and **kidney transplantation**.

Multicystic dysplastic kidney disease results from dysmorphology during development of the renal system (see Fig. 12-19*B*). The outcome for children with multicystic dysplastic kidney disease is generally good because the disease is unilateral in 75% of the cases. In multicystic dysplastic kidney disease, fewer cysts are seen than in autosomal recessive polycystic kidney disease and they range in size from a few millimeters to many centimeters in the same kidney. For many years it was thought that the cysts were the result of failure of the metanephric diverticulum derivatives to join the tubules derived from the metanephrogenic blastema. It is now believed that the cystic structures are wide dilations of parts of the otherwise continuous nephrons, particularly the nephron loops (loops of Henle).

Development of the Urinary Bladder

Division of the cloaca by the urorectal septum (Fig. 12-20*A*) into a dorsal rectum and a ventral urogenital sinus was explained in Chapter 11. For descriptive purposes, the **urogenital sinus** is divided into three parts (see Fig. 12-20*C*):

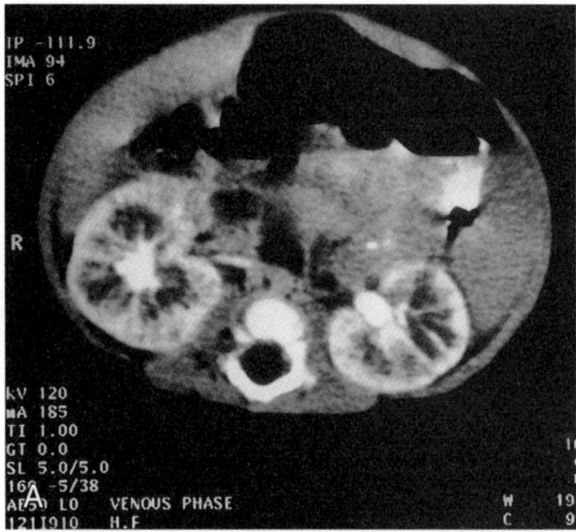

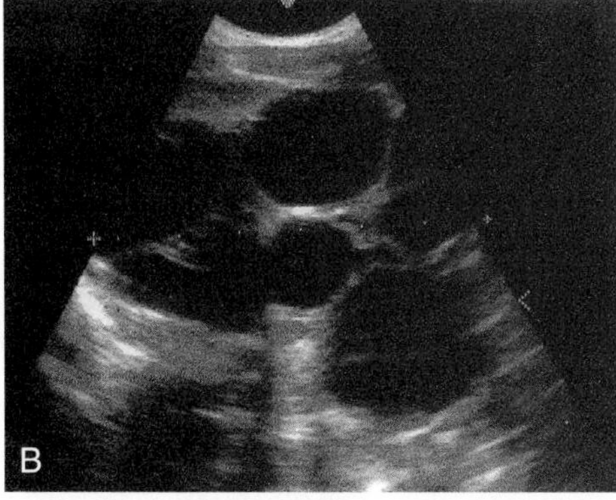

FIGURE 12-19. Cystic kidney disease. **A,** Computed tomography scan (contrast enhanced) of the abdomen of a 5-month-old male infant with infantile polycystic kidney disease. Note the linear ectasia (cysts) of collecting tubules. **B,** Ultrasound scan of the left kidney of a 15-day-old male infant showing multiple noncommunicating cysts with no renal tissue (unilateral multicystic dysplastic kidney). (Courtesy of Dr. Prem S. Sahni, formerly of the Department of Radiology, Children's Hospital, Winnipeg, Manitoba, Canada.)

- A cranial vesical part that forms most of the bladder and is continuous with the allantois
- A middle pelvic part that becomes the urethra in the bladder neck, the prostatic part of the urethra in males, and the entire urethra in females
- A caudal phallic part that grows toward the genital tubercle (primordium of the penis or clitoris)

The bladder develops mainly from the **vesical part of the urogenital sinus**, but its trigone region is derived from the caudal ends of the mesonephric ducts (see Fig. 12-20*A*). The entire epithelium of the bladder is derived from the endoderm of the vesical part. The other layers of its wall develop from adjacent splanchnic mesenchyme.

Initially the bladder is continuous with the **allantois**, a vestigial structure (see Fig. 12-20*C*). The allantois soon constricts and becomes a thick fibrous cord, the **urachus.** It extends from the apex of the bladder to the umbilicus (Figs. 12-20*G* and 12-21). In the adult, the urachus is represented by the **median umbilical ligament**. As the bladder enlarges, distal parts of the mesonephric ducts are incorporated into its dorsal wall (see Fig. 12-20*B* to *H*). These ducts contribute to the formation of the connective tissue in the **trigone of the bladder**. As the mesonephric ducts are absorbed, the ureters come to open separately into the urinary bladder (see Fig. 12-20*C* to *H*). Partly because of traction exerted by the kidneys during their positional change, the orifices of the ureters move superolaterally and the ureters enter obliquely through the base of the bladder. The orifices of the mesonephric ducts move close together and enter the prostatic part of the urethra as the caudal ends of these ducts develop into the ejaculatory ducts. In females, the distal ends of the mesonephric ducts degenerate.

In infants and children, the urinary bladder, even when empty, is in the abdomen. It begins to enter the greater pelvis at approximately 6 years of age, but it does not enter the lesser pelvis and become a pelvic organ until after puberty.

The apex of the urinary bladder in adults is continuous with the median umbilical ligament, which extends posteriorly along the posterior surface of the anterior abdominal wall. The median umbilical ligament lies between the medial umbilical ligaments, which are the fibrous remnants of the umbilical arteries (see Chapter 13).

URACHAL ANOMALIES

In infants, a remnant of the lumen may persist in the inferior part of the urachus. In approximately 50% of cases, the lumen is continuous with the cavity of the bladder. Remnants of the epithelial lining of the urachus may give rise to **urachal cysts** (Fig. 12-22*A*), which are not usually detected except during a postmortem unless they become infected and enlarge. The patent inferior end of the urachus may dilate to form a **urachal sinus** that opens into the bladder. The lumen in the superior part of the urachus may also remain patent and form a urachal sinus that opens at the umbilicus (see Fig. 12-22*B*). Very rarely the entire urachus remains patent and forms a **urachal fistula** that allows urine to escape from its umbilical orifice (see Fig. 12-22*C*).

CONGENITAL MEGACYSTIS

A pathologically large urinary bladder—**megacystis** or megalocystis—may result from a congenital disorder of the metanephric diverticulum, which may be associated with dilation of the renal pelvis. The large bladder may result from posterior urethral valves (Fig. 12-23). Absolute renal failure and pulmonary hypoplasia of lethal degree are the consequences of this anomaly, unless intrauterine treatment is effected.

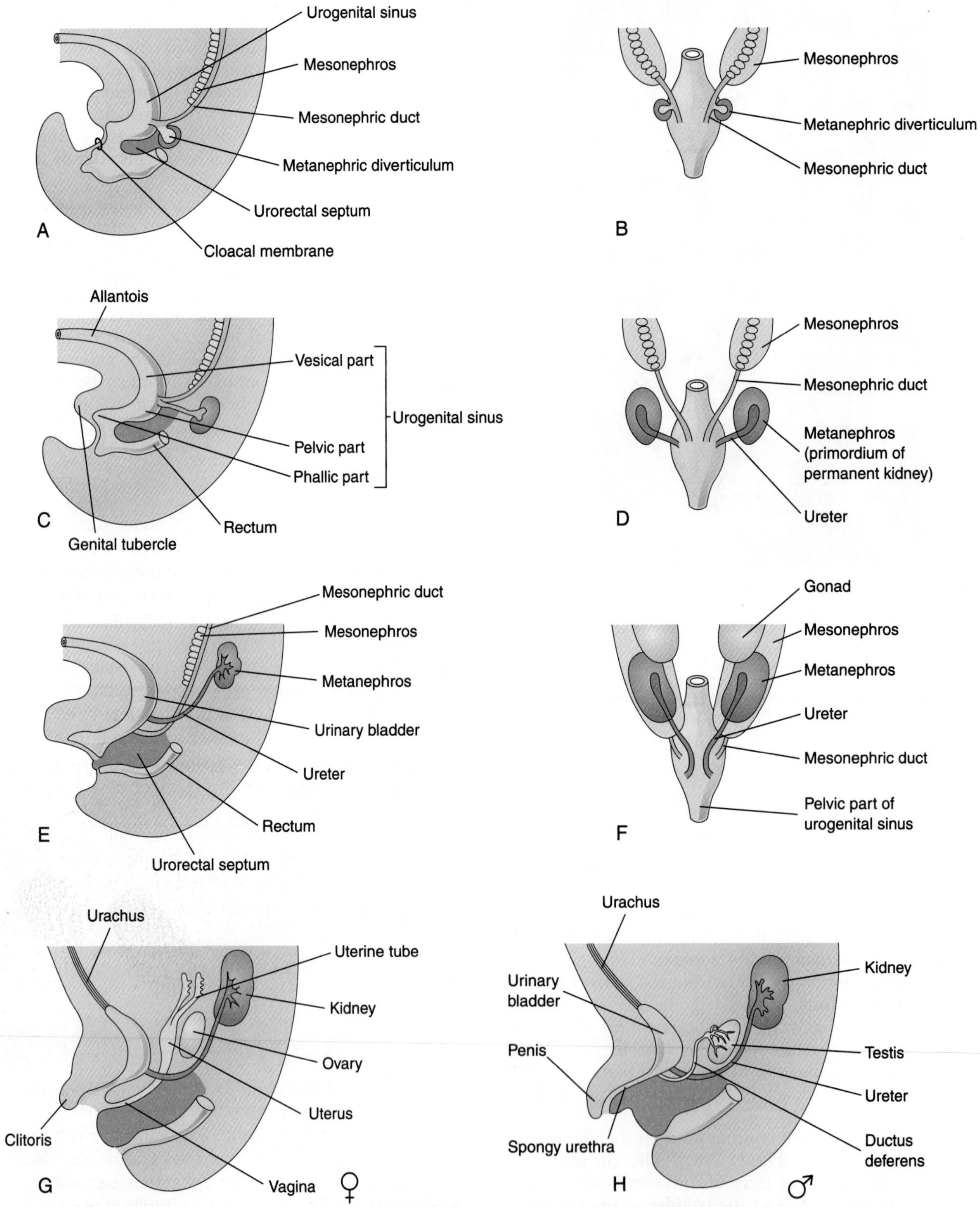

FIGURE 12-20. Diagrams showing division of the cloaca into the urogenital sinus and rectum; absorption of the mesonephric ducts; development of the urinary bladder, urethra, and urachus, and changes in the location of the ureters. **A,** Lateral view of the caudal half of a 5-week embryo. **B, D,** and **F,** Dorsal views. **C, E, G,** and **H,** Lateral views. The stages shown in **G** and **H** are reached by the 12th week.

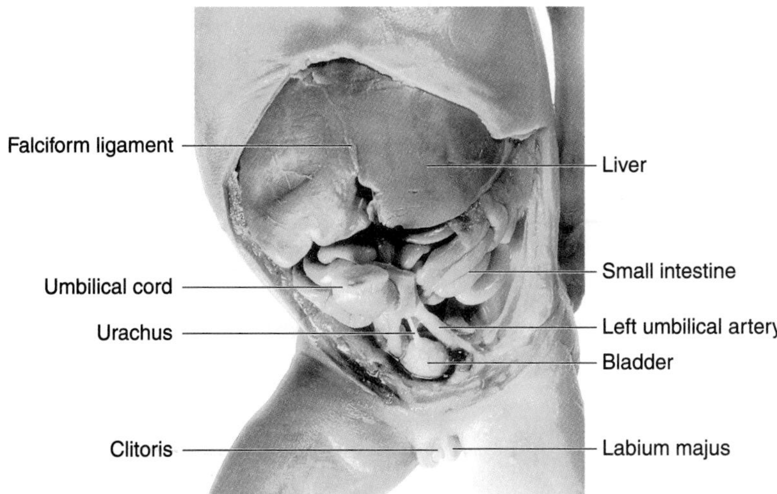

FIGURE 12-21. Dissection of the abdomen and pelvis of an 18-week female fetus showing the relation of the urachus to the urinary bladder and umbilical arteries. Note that the clitoris is relatively large at this stage.

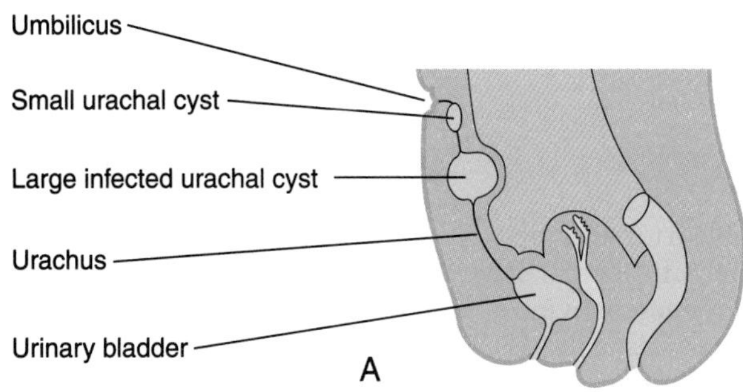

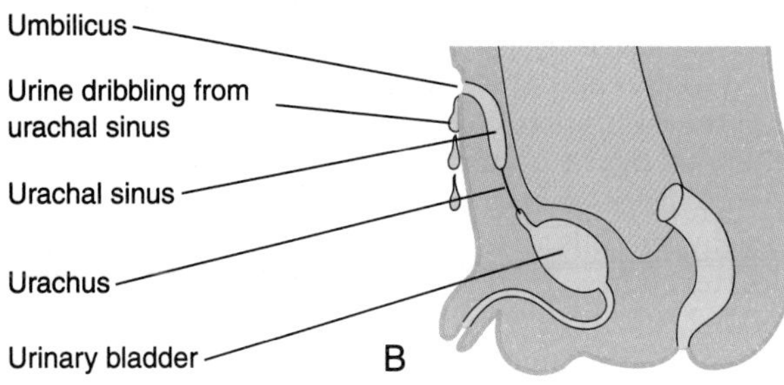

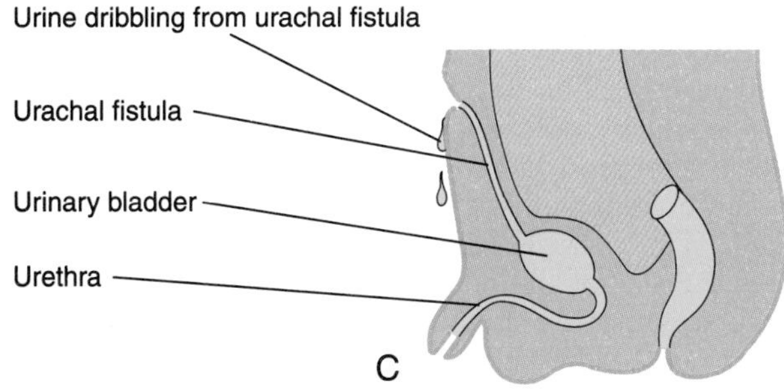

FIGURE 12-22. Illustrations of urachal anomalies. **A,** Urachal cysts. The most common site is in the superior end of the urachus just inferior to the umbilicus. **B,** Two types of urachal sinus are shown: One opens into the bladder and the other opens at the umbilicus. **C,** Patent urachus or urachal fistula connecting the bladder and the umbilicus.

EXSTROPHY OF BLADDER

This severe anomaly occurs approximately once in every 10,000 to 40,000 births. Exstrophy of the bladder (Fig. 12-24) usually occurs in males. Exposure and protrusion of the mucosal surface of the posterior wall of the bladder characterize this congenital anomaly. The trigone of the bladder and the ureteric orifices are exposed, and urine dribbles intermittently from the everted bladder. **Epispadias** and wide separation of the pubic bones are associated with complete exstrophy of the bladder. In some cases, the penis is divided into two parts

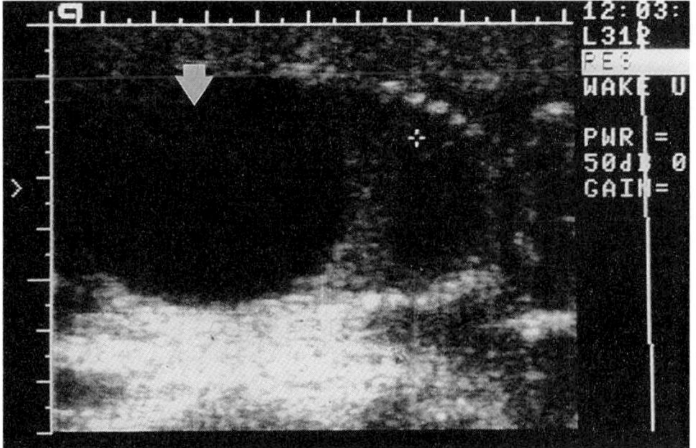

FIGURE 12-23. Sonogram of an 18-week male fetus with megacystis (enlarged bladder) caused by posterior urethral valves. The *cross* is placed on the fourth intercostal space, the level to which the diaphragm has been elevated by this very large fetal bladder (*arrow*, black = urine). Absolute renal failure and pulmonary hypoplasia of a lethal degree are consequences of this presentation, unless intrauterine treatment is effected. In this case, the fetus survived because of the placement of a pigtail catheter within the fetal bladder, allowing drainage of urine into the amniotic cavity. (Courtesy of Dr. C.R. Harman, Department of Obstetrics, Gynecology and Reproductive Sciences, Women's Hospital and University of Manitoba, Winnipeg, Manitoba, Canada.)

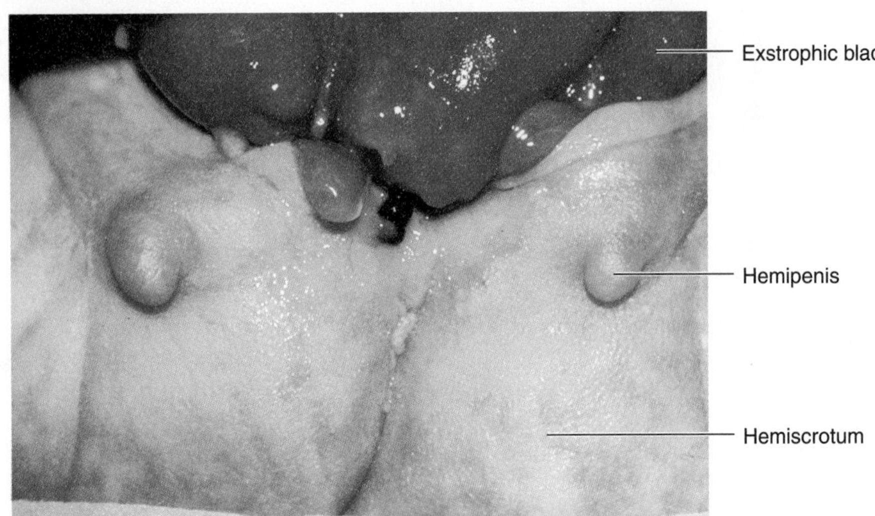

FIGURE 12-24. Exstrophy of the bladder and bifid penis in a male infant. The bladder mucosa is visible, and the halves of the penis and scrotum are widely separated. (Courtesy of A.E. Chudley, MD, Section of Genetics and Metabolism, Department of Pediatrics and Child Health, Children's Hospital and University of Manitoba, Winnipeg, Manitoba, Canada.)

and the halves of the scrotum are widely separated (Figs. 12-24 and 12-25).

Exstrophy of the bladder is caused by incomplete median closure of the inferior part of the anterior abdominal wall (see Fig. 12-25). The defect involves both the anterior abdominal wall and the anterior wall of the urinary bladder and results from failure of mesenchymal cells to migrate between the ectoderm and endoderm of the abdominal wall (cloacal membrane) (see Fig. 12-25*B* and *C*). As a result, the inferior parts of the rectus muscles are absent, and the external and internal oblique and the transverse abdominal muscles are deficient. No muscle and connective tissue form in the anterior abdominal wall over the urinary bladder. Rupture of the fragile cloacal membrane results in wide communication between the exterior and the mucous membrane of the bladder. Rupture of the membrane before division of the cloaca by the urorectal septum results in exstrophy of the cloaca, resulting in exposure of both the bladder and the hindgut.

Development of the Urethra

The epithelium of most of the male urethra and the entire female urethra is derived from endoderm of the urogenital sinus (Figs. 12-20*E* and *H* and 12-26). In males, the distal part of the urethra in the glans of the penis is derived from a solid cord of ectodermal cells that grows inward from the tip of the glans and joins the rest of the spongy urethra (see Fig. 12-26*A* to *C*); consequently, the epithelium of the terminal part of the urethra is derived from the surface ectoderm. The connective tissue and smooth muscle of the urethra in both sexes are derived from splanchnic mesenchyme.

DEVELOPMENT OF THE SUPRARENAL GLANDS

The cortex and medulla of the suprarenal (adrenal) glands have different origins (Fig. 12-27). The **cortex** develops from mesenchyme and the **medulla** differentiates from neural crest cells. During the sixth week, the cortex begins as an aggregation of mesenchymal cells on each side of the embryo between the root of the dorsal mesentery and the developing gonad (see Fig. 12-29*C*). The cells that form the medulla are derived from an adjacent sympathetic ganglion, which is derived from **neural crest cells**. Initially the neural crest cells form a mass on the medial side of the embryonic cortex (see Fig. 12-27*B*). As they are surrounded by the cortex, these cells differentiate into the secretory cells of the suprarenal medulla. Later, more mesenchymal cells arise from the mesothelium and enclose the cortex. These cells give rise to the permanent cortex (Fig. 12-27*C*).

Recently, immunohistochemical studies revealed a "transitional zone" that is located between the permanent cortex and the fetal cortex. It has been suggested that the **zona fasciculata** is derived from this third layer. The **zona glomerulosa** and zona fasciculata are present at birth, but the zona reticularis is not recognizable until the end of the third year (see Fig. 12-27*H*).

Relative to body weight, the suprarenal glands of the human fetus are 10 to 20 times larger than in the adult and are large compared with the kidneys (see Figs. 12-3 and 12-8). These large suprarenal glands result from the extensive size of the fetal cortex, which produces steroid precursors that are used by the placenta for the synthesis of estrogen. The suprarenal medulla remains relatively small until after birth. The suprarenal glands rapidly become smaller as the fetal cortex regresses during the first year of infancy. The glands lose approximately one third of their weight during the first 2 or 3 weeks after birth and do not regain their original weight until the end of the second year.

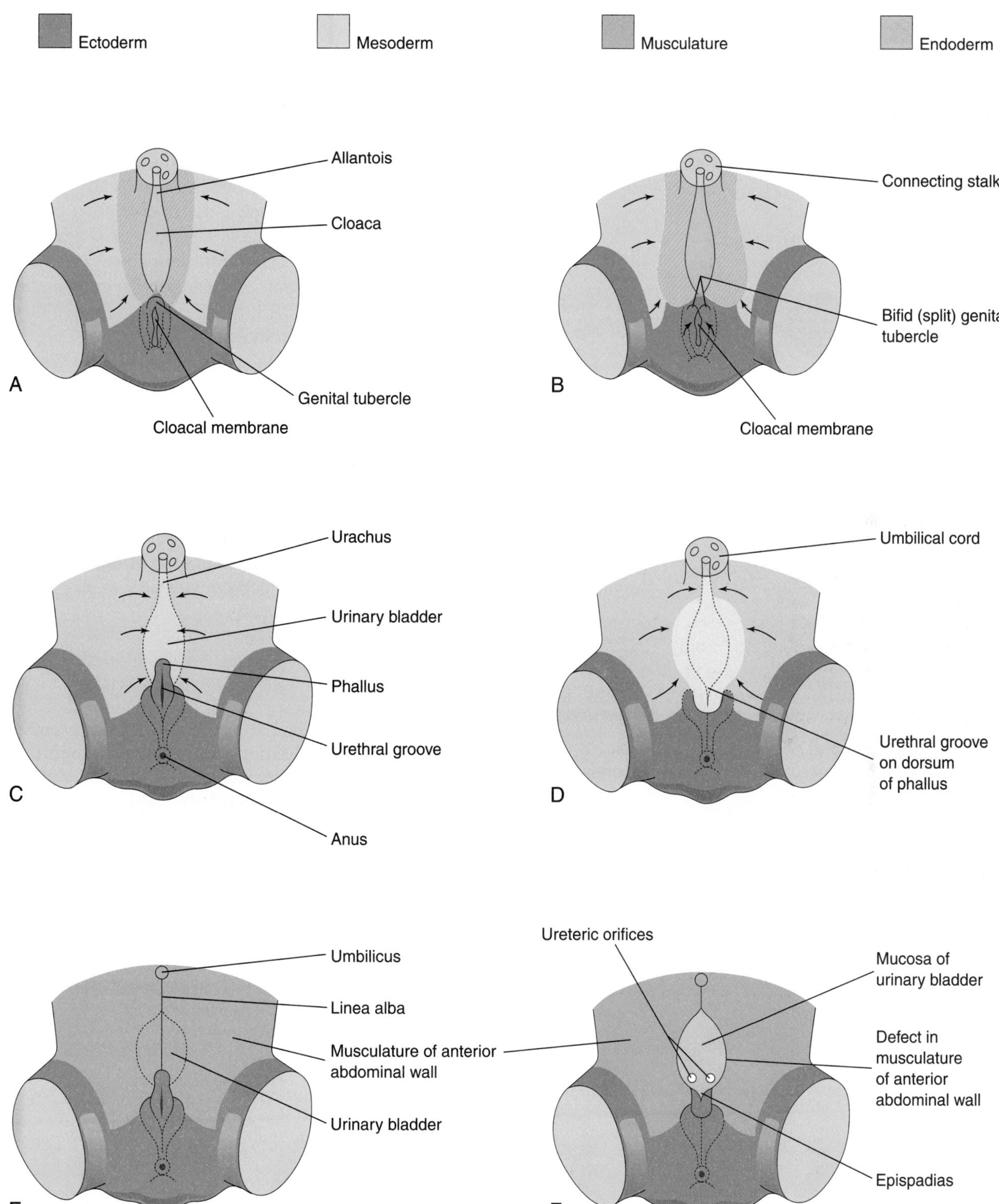

FIGURE 12-25. **A, C,** and **E,** Normal stages in the development of the infraumbilical abdominal wall and the penis during the fourth to eighth weeks. Note that mesoderm and later muscle reinforce the ectoderm of the developing anterior abdominal wall. **B, D,** and **F,** Probable stages in the development of exstrophy of the bladder and epispadias. **B** and **D,** Note that the mesenchyme fails to extend into the anterior abdominal wall anterior to the urinary bladder. Also note that the genital tubercle is located in a more caudal position than usual and that the urethral groove has formed on the dorsal surface of the penis. **F,** The surface ectoderm and anterior wall of the bladder have ruptured, resulting in exposure of the posterior wall of the bladder. Note that the musculature of the anterior abdominal wall is present on each side of the defect. (Based on Patten BM, Barry A: The genesis of exstrophy of the bladder and epispadias. Am J Anat 90:35, 1952.)

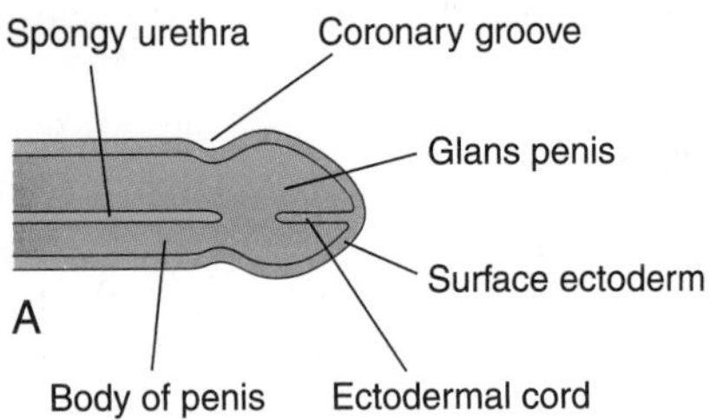

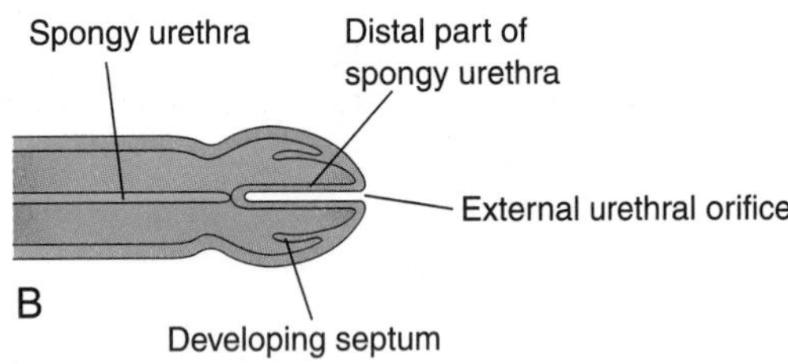

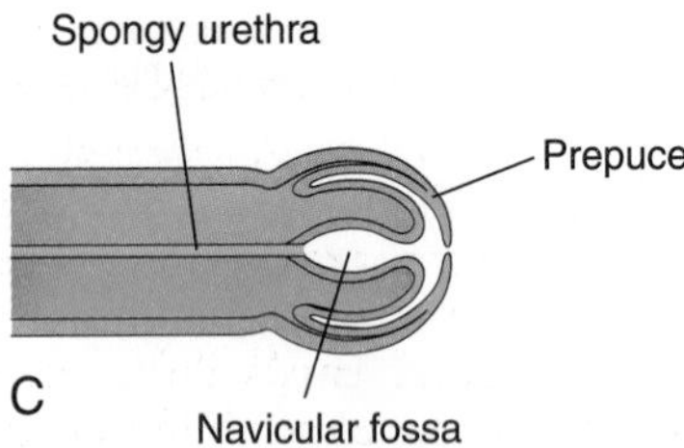

FIGURE 12-26. Schematic longitudinal sections of the developing penis illustrating development of the prepuce (foreskin) and the distal part of the spongy urethra. **A,** At 11 weeks. **B,** At 12 weeks. **C,** At 14 weeks. The epithelium of the spongy urethra has a dual origin; most of it is derived from endoderm of the phallic part of the urogenital sinus. The distal part of the urethra lining the navicular fossa is derived from surface ectoderm.

CONGENITAL ADRENAL HYPERPLASIA AND ADRENOGENITAL SYNDROME

An abnormal increase in the cells of the suprarenal cortex results in excessive androgen production during the fetal period. In females, this usually causes masculinization of the external genitalia (Fig. 12-28). Affected male infants have normal external genitalia, and the syndrome may go undetected in early infancy. Later in childhood in both sexes, androgen excess leads to rapid growth and accelerated skeletal maturation. The **adrenogenital syndrome** associated with congenital adrenal hyperplasia (CAH) manifests itself in various forms that can be correlated with enzymatic deficiencies of cortisol biosynthesis. CAH is a group of *autosomal recessive disorders* that result in virilization of female fetuses. CAH is caused by a genetically determined mutation in the cytochrome P450c21-steroid 21-hydroxylase gene, which causes a deficiency of suprarenal cortical enzymes that are necessary for the biosynthesis of various steroid hormones. The reduced hormone output results in an increased release of **adrenocorticotropin** from the anterior pituitary, which causes CAH and overproduction of androgens.

DEVELOPMENT OF THE GENITAL SYSTEM

Although the chromosomal or genetic sex of an embryo is determined at fertilization by the kind of sperm that fertilizes the secondary oocyte (see Chapter 2). Male and female morphologic characteristics do not begin to develop until the seventh week. The early genital systems in the two sexes are similar; therefore, the initial period of genital development is referred to as the *indifferent stage of sexual development*.

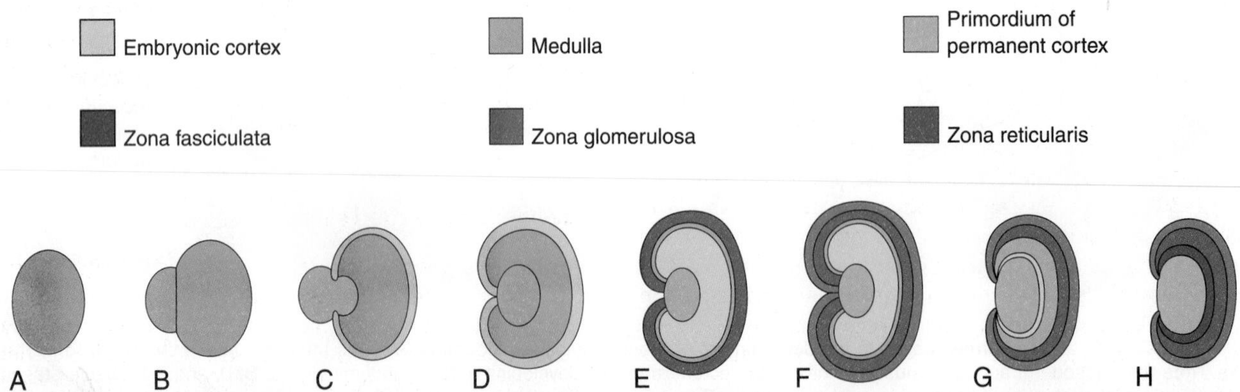

FIGURE 12-27. Schematic drawings illustrating development of the suprarenal glands. **A,** At 6 weeks, showing the mesodermal primordium of the fetal cortex. **B,** At 7 weeks, showing the addition of neural crest cells. **C,** At 8 weeks, showing the fetal cortex and the early permanent cortex beginning to encapsulate the medulla. **D** and **E,** Later stages of encapsulation of the medulla by the cortex. **F,** Newborn infant showing the fetal cortex and two zones of the permanent cortex. **G,** At 1 year, the fetal cortex has almost disappeared. **H,** At 4 years, showing the adult pattern of cortical zones. Note that the fetal cortex has disappeared and that the gland is much smaller than it was at birth (**F**).

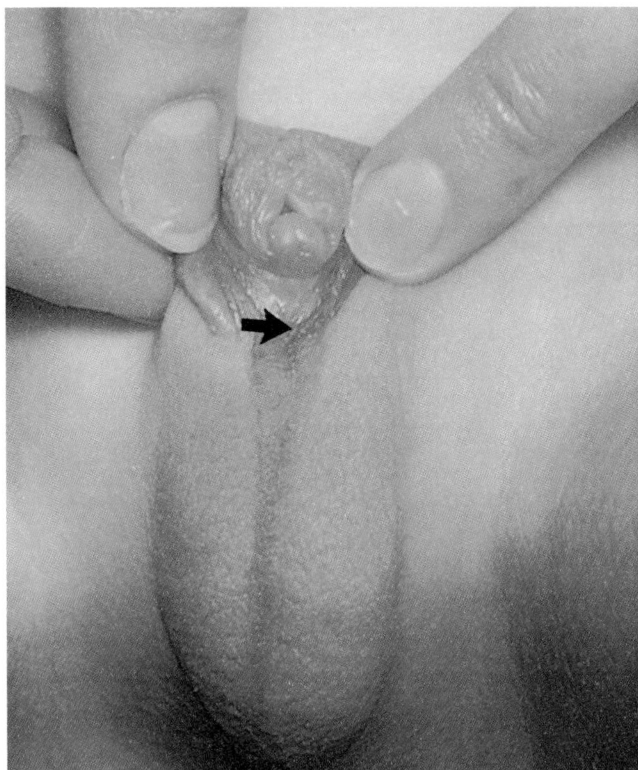

FIGURE 12-28. External genitalia of a 6-year-old girl showing an enlarged clitoris and fused labia majora that have formed a scrotum-like structure. The *arrow* indicates the opening into the urogenital sinus. This extreme masculinization is the result of congenital adrenal hyperplasia. (Courtesy of Dr. Heather Dean, Department of Pediatric and Child Health, University of Manitoba, Winnipeg, Manitoba, Canada.)

Development of the Gonads

The gonads (testes and ovaries) are derived from three sources (Fig. 12-29):

- Mesothelium (mesodermal epithelium) lining the posterior abdominal wall
- Underlying mesenchyme (embryonic connective tissue)
- Primordial germ cells

Indifferent Gonads

The initial stages of gonadal development occur during the fifth week when a thickened area of mesothelium develops on the medial side of the mesonephros (see Fig. 12-29). Proliferation of this epithelium and the underlying mesenchyme produces a bulge on the medial side of the mesonephros—the **gonadal ridge** (Fig. 12-30). Fingerlike epithelial cords—the **gonadal cords**—soon grow into the underlying mesenchyme (see Fig. 12-29*D*). The indifferent gonad now consists of an external cortex and an internal medulla.

In embryos with an XX sex chromosome complex, the cortex of the indifferent gonad differentiates into an ovary, and the medulla regresses. In embryos with an XY sex chromosome complex, the medulla differentiates into a testis, and the cortex regresses, except for vestigial remnants (see Table 12-1).

Primordial Germ Cells

These large, spherical sex cells are visible early in the fourth week among the endodermal cells of the umbilical vesicle (yolk sac) near the origin of the allantois (see Fig. 12-29A). During folding of the embryo (see Chapter 5), the dorsal part of the umbilical vesicle is incorporated into the embryo. As this occurs, the primordial germ cells migrate along the dorsal mesentery of the hindgut to the gonadal ridges (see Fig. 12-29*C*). During the sixth week, the primordial germ cells enter the underlying mesenchyme and are incorporated in the **gonadal cords** (see Fig. 12-29*D*). The migration of the primordial germ cells is regulated by the genes *stella*, *fragilis*, and *BMP-4*.

Sex Determination

Chromosomal and genetic sex depends on whether an X-bearing sperm or a Y-bearing sperm fertilizes the X-bearing oocyte. Before the seventh week, the gonads of the two sexes are identical in appearance and are called **indifferent gonads** (see Figs. 12-29*E* and 12-30).

Development of the male phenotype requires a Y chromosome. The **SRY gene for a testis-determining factor** (TDF) has been localized in the sex-determining, short arm region of the Y chromosome. It is the TDF regulated by the Y chromosome that determines testicular differentiation (Fig. 12-31). Under the influence of this organizing factor, the **gonadal cords** differentiate into **seminiferous cords** (primordia of seminiferous tubules). Expression of the *Sox9* and *Fgf9* genes is involved in the formation of the seminiferous cords. The absence of a Y chromosome results in the formation of an ovary.

Two X chromosomes are required for the development of the female phenotype. A number of genes and regions of the X chromosome have special roles in sex determination. Consequently, the type of sex chromosome complex established at fertilization determines the type of gonad that differentiates from the indifferent gonad. The type of gonads present then determines the type of sexual differentiation that occurs in the genital ducts and external genitalia. **Testosterone**, produced by the fetal testes, dihydrotestosterone, a metabolite of testosterone, and the antimüllerian hormone (AMH), determines normal male sexual differentiation. Primary female sexual differentiation in the fetus does not depend on hormones; it occurs even if the ovaries are absent and apparently is not under hormonal influence.

Development of the Testes

The **SRY gene for TDF** on the short arm of the Y chromosome acts as the switch that directs development of the indifferent gonad into a testis. Expression of the transcription factor SOX9 is also essential for testicular determination. TDF induces the gonadal cords to condense and extend into the medulla of the indifferent gonad, where they branch and anastomose to form the **rete testis** (see Fig. 12-31). The connection of the gonadal cords—*seminiferous cords*—with the surface epithelium is lost when a

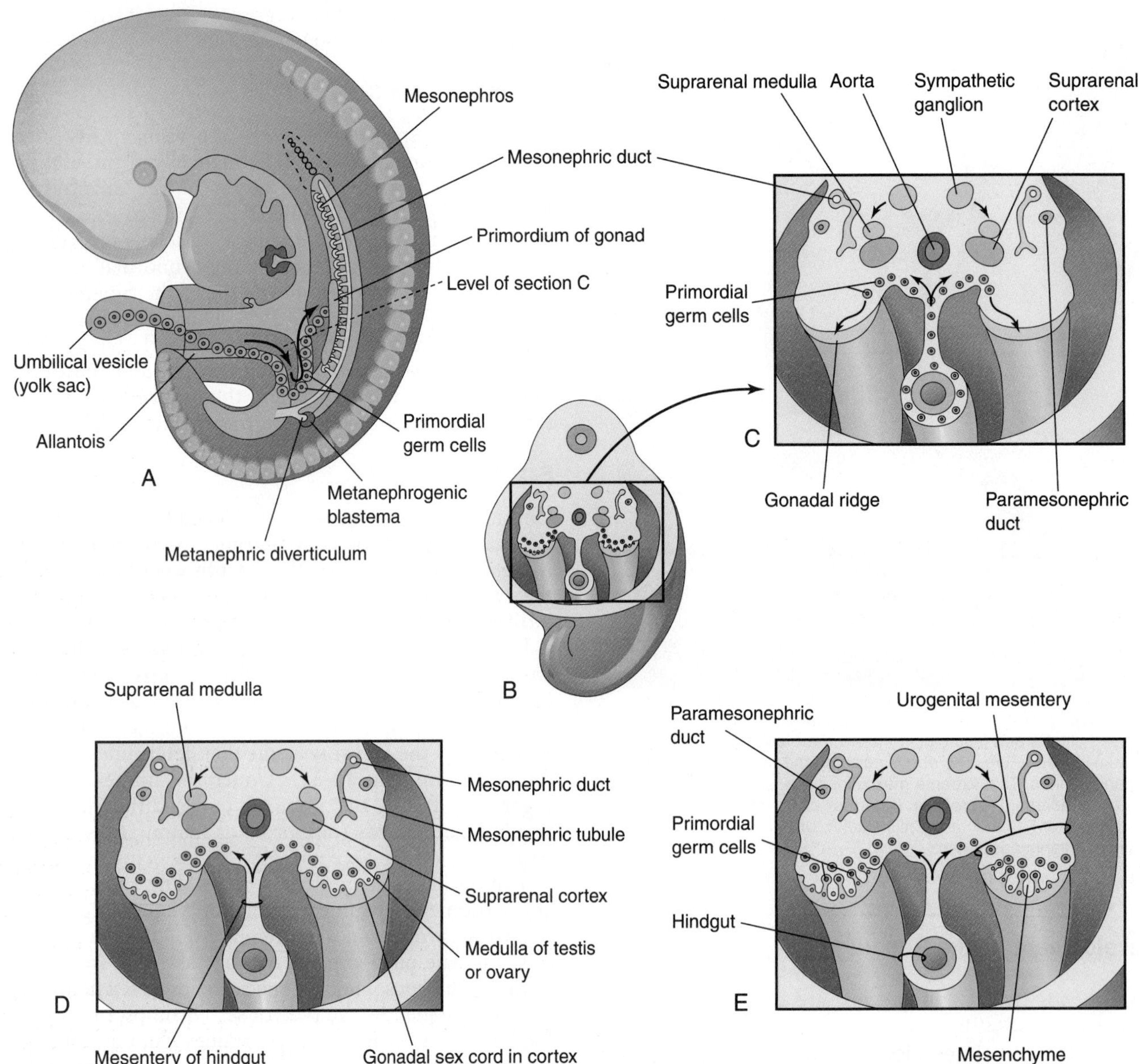

FIGURE 12-29. **A,** Sketch of a 5-week embryo illustrating the migration of primordial germ cells from the umbilical vesicle (yolk sac) into the embryo. **B,** Three-dimensional sketch of the caudal region of a 5-week embryo showing the location and extent of the gonadal ridges. **C,** Transverse section showing the primordium of the suprarenal glands, the gonadal ridges, and the migration of primordial germ cells into the developing gonads. **D,** Transverse section of a 6-week embryo showing the gonadal cords. **E,** Similar section at a later stage showing the indifferent gonads and paramesonephric ducts.

thick fibrous capsule, the tunica albuginea, develops. The development of the dense **tunica albuginea** is the characteristic feature of testicular development. Gradually the enlarging testis separates from the degenerating mesonephros and becomes suspended by its own mesentery, the **mesorchium**. The seminiferous cords develop into the seminiferous tubules, tubuli recti, and rete testis.

The **seminiferous tubules** are separated by mesenchyme that gives rise to the **interstitial cells** (Leydig cells). By the eighth week, these cells begin to secrete androgenic hormones—**testosterone** and **androstenedione**, which induce masculine differentiation of the mesonephric ducts and the external genitalia. Testosterone production is stimulated by human chorionic gonadotropin, which reaches peak amounts during the 8- to 12-week period. In addition to testosterone, the fetal testes produce a glycoprotein, AMH, or müllerian-inhibiting substance (MIS). AMH is produced by the **sustentacular cells** (Sertoli cells), which continues to puberty, after which the levels of AMH decrease. AMH suppresses development of the paramesonephric ducts, which form the uterus and uterine tubes.

The seminiferous tubules remain solid (i.e., no lumina) until puberty, at which time lumina begin to develop. The walls of the seminiferous tubules are composed of two kinds of cells (see Fig. 12-31):

- Sertoli cells, supporting cells derived from the surface epithelium of the testis
- Spermatogonia, primordial sperm cells derived from the primordial germ cells

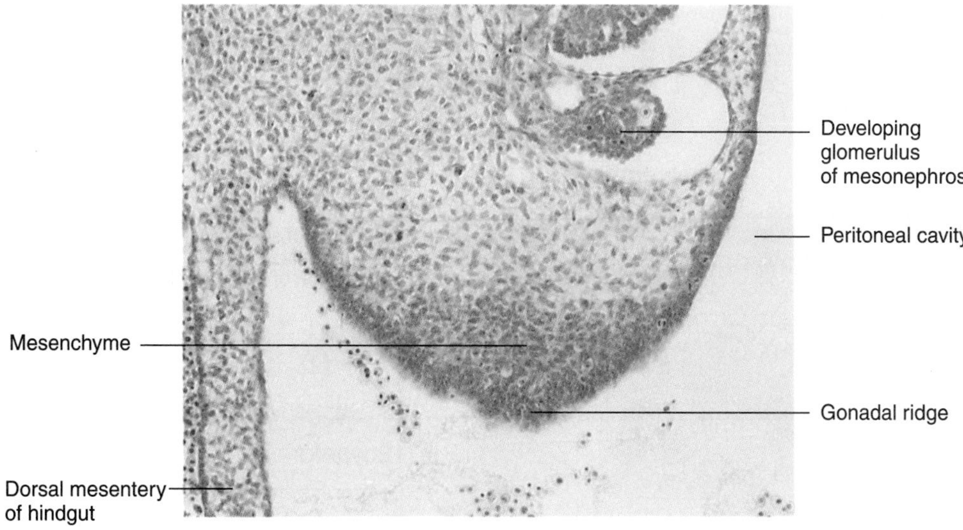

FIGURE 12-30. Photomicrograph of a transverse section of the abdomen of an embryo at Carnegie stage 16, approximately 40 days, showing the gonadal ridge, which will develop into a testis or an ovary depending on the genetic sex of the embryo. Most of the developing gonad is composed of mesenchyme derived from the coelomic epithelium of the gonadal ridge. The large round cells in the gonad are primordial germ cells. (From Moore KL, Persaud TVN, Shiota K: Color Atlas of Clinical Embryology, 2nd ed. Philadelphia, WB Saunders, 2000.)

Sertoli cells constitute most of the seminiferous epithelium in the fetal testis (Figs. 12-31 and 12-32*C*). During later fetal development, the surface epithelium of the testis flattens to form the mesothelium on the external surface of the adult testis. The *rete testis* becomes continuous with 15 to 20 mesonephric tubules that become **efferent ductules** (Latin, *ductuli efferentes*). These ductules are connected with the mesonephric duct, which becomes the **duct of the epididymis** (Figs. 12-31 and 12-33*A*).

Development of the Ovaries

Gonadal development occurs slowly in female embryos. The X chromosomes bear genes for ovarian development, and an autosomal gene also appears to play a role in ovarian organogenesis. The ovary is not identifiable histologically until approximately the 10th week. **Gonadal cords** do not become prominent, but they extend into the medulla and form a rudimentary **rete ovarii**. This structure and the gonadal cords normally degenerate and disappear (see Fig. 12-31). Cortical cords extend from the surface epithelium of the developing ovary into the underlying mesenchyme during the early fetal period. This epithelium is derived from the mesothelium. As the cortical cords increase in size, **primordial germ cells** are incorporated in them. At approximately 16 weeks, these cords begin to break up into isolated cell clusters—**primordial follicles—**each of which consists of an oogonium, derived from a primordial germ cell, surrounded by a single layer of flattened follicular cells derived from the surface epithelium (see Fig. 12-31). Active mitosis of oogonia occurs during fetal life producing primordial follicles (see Fig. 12-32*D*).

No oogonia form postnatally. Although many oogonia degenerate before birth, the two million or so that remain enlarge to become **primary oocytes** before birth. After birth, the surface epithelium of the ovary flattens to a single layer of cells continuous with the mesothelium of the peritoneum at the hilum of the ovary. The surface epithelium of the ovary was once called the germinal epithelium, which was inappropriate because it is now well established that the germ cells differentiate from the primordial germ cells (see Fig. 12-31). The surface epithelium becomes separated from the follicles in the cortex by a thin fibrous capsule, the tunica albuginea. As the ovary separates from the regressing mesonephros, it is suspended by a mesentery—the **mesovarium** (see Fig. 12-31).

Development of the Genital Ducts

During the fifth and sixth weeks, the genital system is in an indifferent state, and two pairs of genital ducts are present. The mesonephric ducts (Wolffian ducts) play an important part in the development of the male reproductive system (see Fig. 12-33*A*), and the paramesonephric ducts (müllerian ducts) have a leading role in the development of the female reproductive system.

The **paramesonephric ducts** develop lateral to the gonads and mesonephric ducts (see Fig. 12-31) on each side from longitudinal invaginations of the mesothelium on the lateral aspects of the mesonephroi. The edges of these paramesonephric grooves approach each other and fuse to form the **paramesonephric ducts** (see Fig. 12-29*C* and *E*). The funnel-shaped cranial ends of these ducts open into the peritoneal cavity (see Fig. 12-33*B* and *C*). Caudally, the paramesonephric ducts run parallel to the mesonephric ducts until they reach the future pelvic region of the embryo. Here they cross ventral to the mesonephric ducts, approach each other in the median plane, and fuse to form a Y-shaped **uterovaginal primordium** (Fig. 12-34*A*). This tubular structure projects into the dorsal wall of the urogenital sinus and produces an elevation—the **sinus tubercle** (see Fig. 12-34*B*).

Development of the Male Genital Ducts and Glands

The fetal testes produce **masculinizing hormones** (e.g., testosterone) and MIS. The Sertoli cells begin to produce MIS at 6 to 7 weeks. The interstitial cells begin producing

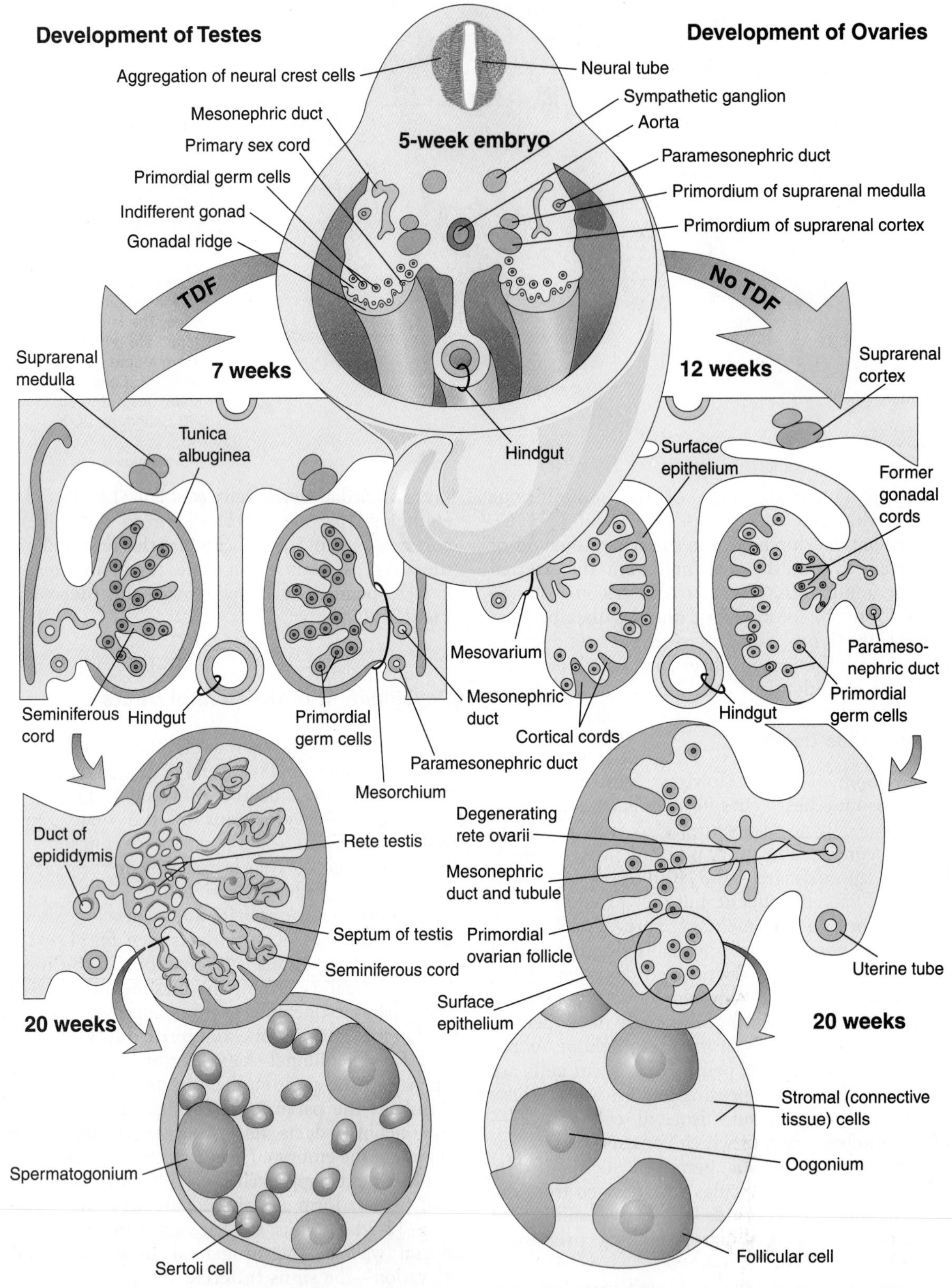

FIGURE 12-31. Schematic illustrations showing differentiation of the indifferent gonads of a 5-week embryo (*top*) into ovaries or testes. The left side of the drawing shows the development of testes resulting from the effects of the testis-determining factor (TDF) located on the Y chromosome. Note that the gonadal cords become seminiferous cords, the primordia of the seminiferous tubules. The parts of the gonadal cords that enter the medulla of the testis form the rete testis. In the section of the testis at the bottom left, observe that there are two kinds of cells, spermatogonia, derived from the primordial germ cells, and sustentacular or Sertoli cells, derived from mesenchyme. The right side shows the development of ovaries in the absence of TDF. Cortical cords have extended from the surface epithelium of the gonad and primordial germ cells have entered them. They are the primordia of the oogonia. Follicular cells are derived from the surface epithelium of the ovary.

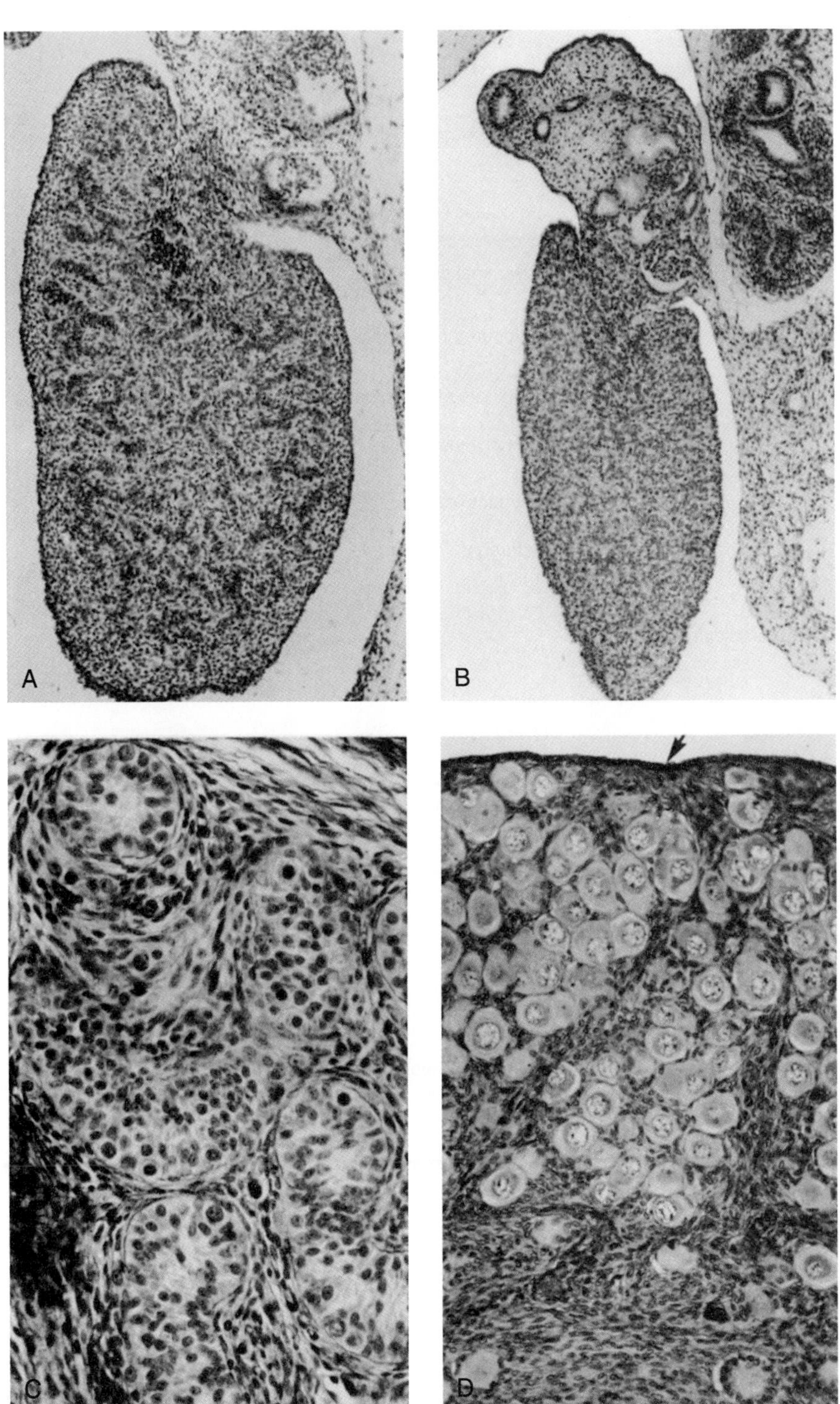

FIGURE 12-32. Transverse sections of gonads of human embryos and fetuses. **A,** Testis from an embryo of approximately 43 days showing prominent seminiferous cords (×175). **B,** From an embryo of approximately the same age, a gonad that may be assumed to be an ovary because of the absence of gonadal cords (×125). **C,** Section of a testis from a male fetus born prematurely at 21 weeks showing seminiferous tubules composed mostly of Sertoli cells. A few large spermatogonia are visible (×475). **D,** Section of an ovary from a 14-day-old female infant showing numerous primordial follicles in the cortex, each of which contains a primary oocyte. The *arrow* indicates the relatively thin surface epithelium of the ovary (×275). (From van Wagenen G, Simpson ME: Embryology of the Ovary and Testis. Homo sapiens and Macaca mulatta. New Haven, CT, Yale University Press, 1965. Courtesy of Yale University Press.)

testosterone in the eighth week. Testosterone, the production of which is stimulated by human chorionic gonadotropin, stimulates the mesonephric ducts to form male genital ducts, whereas MIS causes the paramesonephric ducts to disappear by epithelial-mesenchymal transformation. Under the influence of testosterone produced by the fetal testes in the eighth week, the proximal part of each mesonephric duct becomes highly convoluted to form the **epididymis**. As the mesonephros degenerates, some mesonephric tubules persist and are transformed into **efferent ductules** (see Fig. 12-33*A*). These ductules open into the **duct of the epididymis** (Latin, *ductus epididymis*) in this region. Distal to the epididymis, the mesonephric duct acquires a thick investment of smooth muscle and becomes the **ductus deferens**.

Seminal Glands

Lateral outgrowths from the caudal end of each mesonephric duct gives rise to the seminal glands (vesicles). These glands produce a secretion that makes up the majority of the fluid in ejaculate and nourishes the sperms.

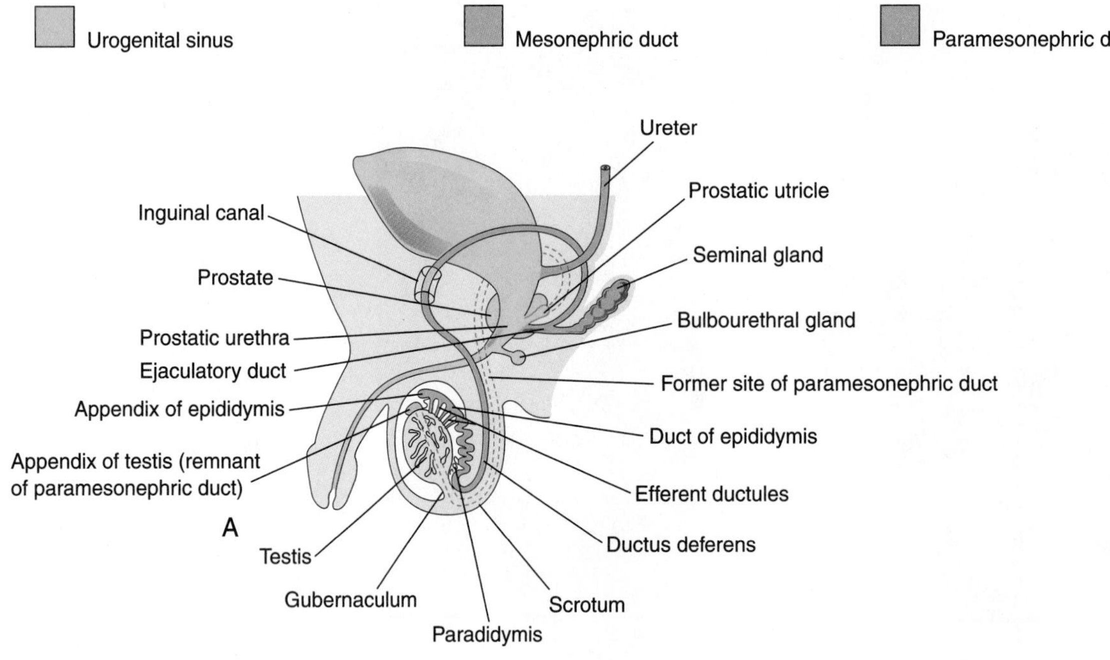

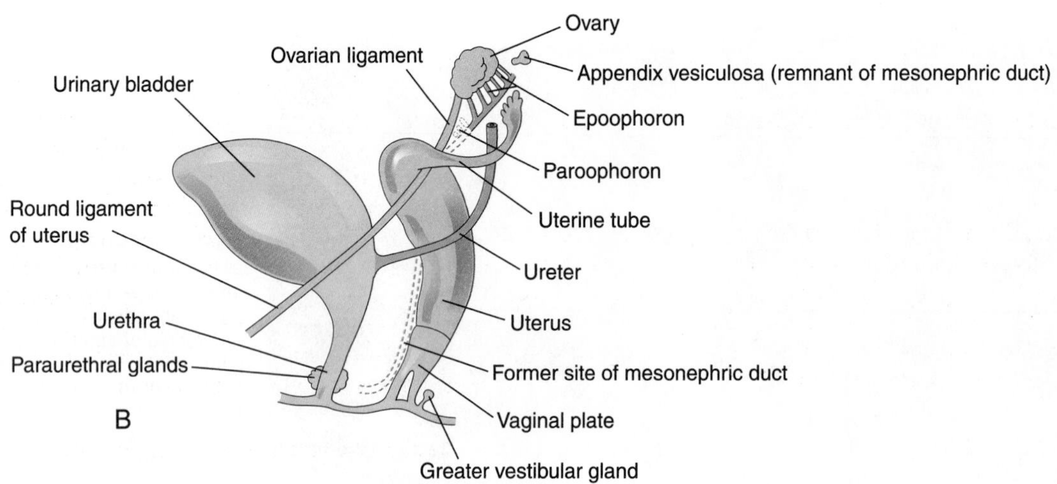

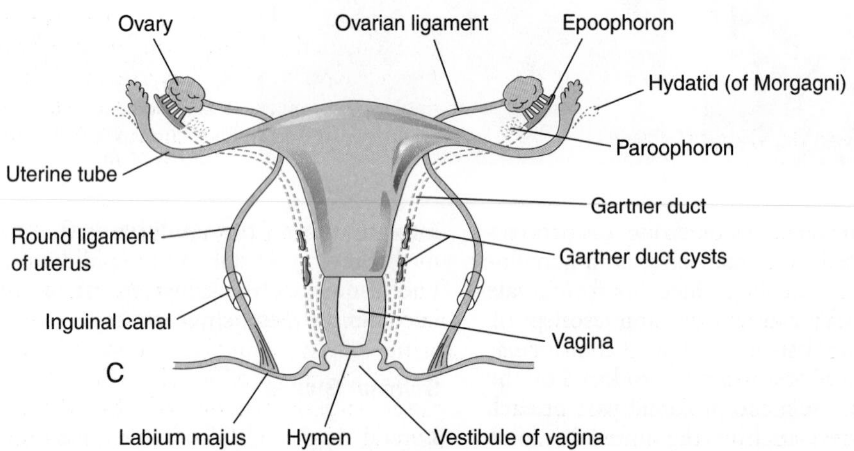

FIGURE 12-33. Schematic drawings illustrating development of the male and female reproductive systems from the genital ducts and urogenital sinus. Vestigial structures are also shown. **A,** Reproductive system in a newborn male. **B,** Female reproductive system in a 12-week fetus. **C,** Reproductive system in a newborn female.

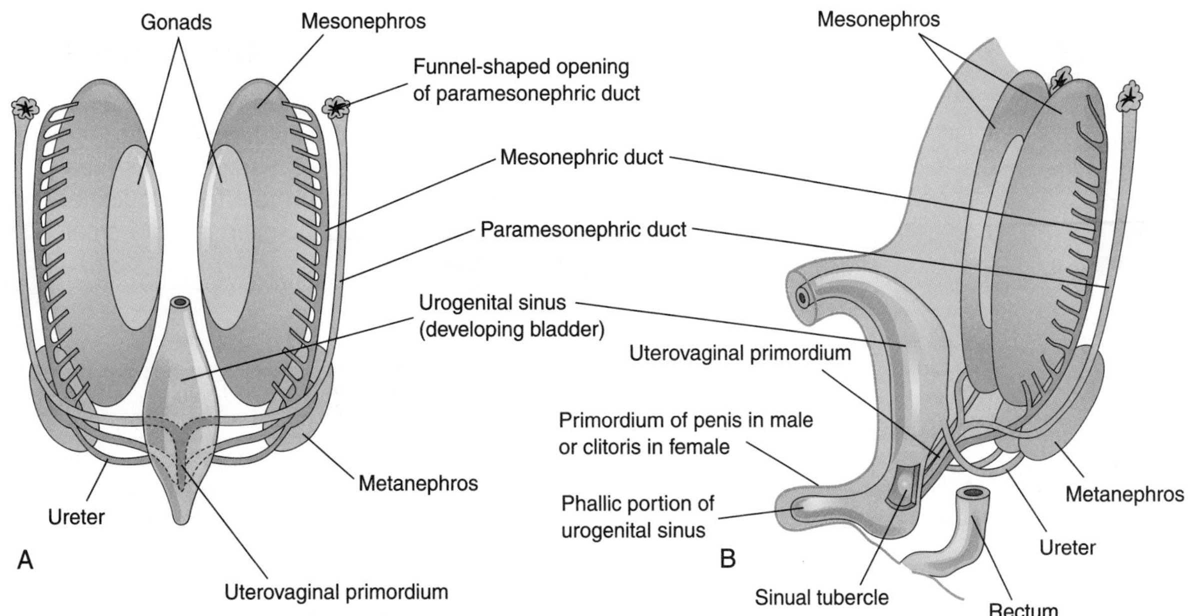

FIGURE 12-34. **A,** Sketch of a ventral view of the posterior abdominal wall of a 7-week embryo showing the two pairs of genital ducts present during the indifferent stage of sexual development. **B,** Lateral view of a 9-week fetus showing the sinus tubercle on the posterior wall of the urogenital sinus. It becomes the hymen in females and the seminal colliculus in males. The colliculus is an elevated part of the urethral crest on the posterior wall of the prostatic urethra.

The part of the mesonephric duct between the duct of this gland and the urethra becomes the **ejaculatory duct.**

Prostate

Multiple endodermal outgrowths arise from the prostatic part of the urethra and grow into the surrounding mesenchyme (Fig. 12-35*A* to *C*). The glandular epithelium of the prostate differentiates from these endodermal cells, and the associated mesenchyme differentiates into the dense stroma and smooth muscle of the prostate.

Bulbourethral Glands

These pea-sized structures develop from paired outgrowths from the spongy part of the urethra (see Fig. 12-33*A*). The smooth muscle fibers and the stroma differentiate from the adjacent mesenchyme. The secretions of these glands contribute to the semen.

Development of the Female Genital Ducts and Glands

In female embryos, the mesonephric ducts regress because of the absence of testosterone and only a few nonfunctional remnants persist (see Fig. 12-33*B* and *C*, Table 12-1). The **paramesonephric ducts** develop because of the absence of MIS. Female sexual development does not depend on the presence of ovaries or hormones. The paramesonephric ducts form most of the female genital tract. The uterine tubes develop from the unfused cranial parts of these ducts (see Figs. 12-33*B* and *C* and 12-34). The caudal fused portions of these ducts form the **uterovaginal primordium.** As the name of this structure indicates, it gives rise to the **uterus** and **vagina** (superior part). The endometrial stroma and myometrium are derived from splanchnic mesenchyme.

Fusion of the paramesonephric ducts also brings together a peritoneal fold that forms the **broad ligament,** and two peritoneal compartments—the **rectouterine pouch** and the **vesicouterine pouch** (Fig. 12-36*A* to *D*). Along the sides of the uterus, between the layers of the broad ligament, the mesenchyme proliferates and differentiates into cellular tissue—the **parametrium,**—which is composed of loose connective tissue and smooth muscle.

Auxiliary Genital Glands in Females

Buds grow from the urethra into the surrounding mesenchyme and form the bilateral mucus secreting **urethral glands** and **paraurethral glands.** These glands correspond to the prostate in the male. Outgrowths from the urogenital sinus form the **greater vestibular glands** in the lower third of the labia majora. These tubuloalveolar glands also secrete mucus and are homologous to the bulbourethral glands in the male (see Table 12-1).

Development of the Uterus and Vagina

The fibromuscular wall of the vagina develops from the surrounding mesenchyme. Contact of the **uterovaginal primordium** with the urogenital sinus, forming the **sinus tubercle** (see Fig. 12-34*B*), induces the formation of paired endodermal outgrowths—the **sinovaginal bulbs** (see Fig. 12-36*A*). They extend from the urogenital sinus to the caudal end of the uterovaginal primordium. The sinovaginal bulbs fuse to form a **vaginal plate** (see Fig. 12-33*B*). Later the central cells of this plate break

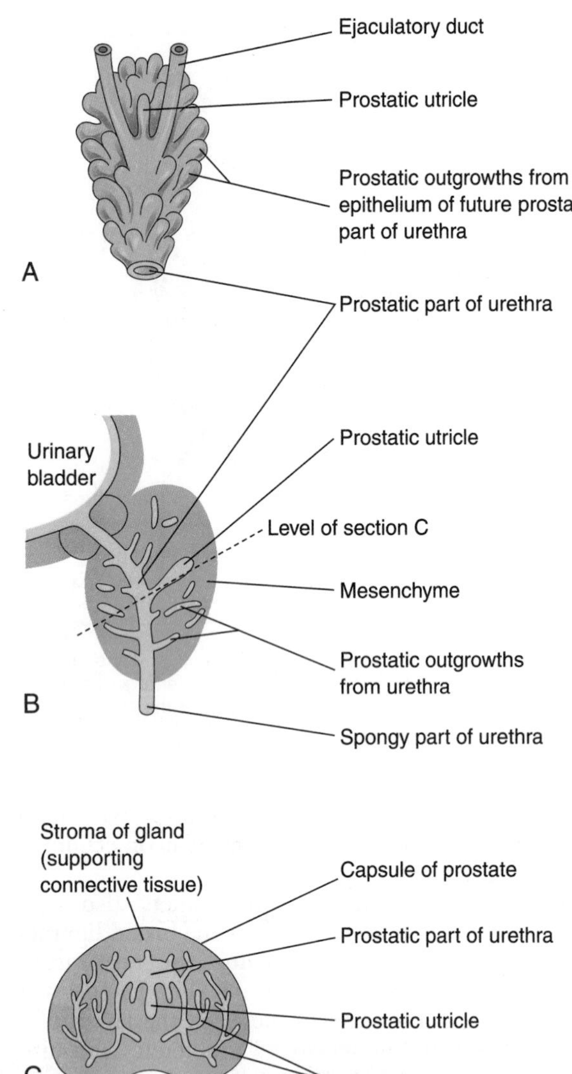

FIGURE 12-35. **A,** Dorsal view of the developing prostate in an 11-week fetus. **B,** Sketch of a median section of the developing urethra and prostate showing numerous endodermal outgrowths from the prostatic urethra. The vestigial prostatic utricle is also shown. **C,** Section of the prostate (16 weeks) at the level shown in **B**.

down, forming the lumen of the vagina. The epithelium of the vagina is derived from the peripheral cells of the vaginal plate (see Fig. 12-33*C*).

Until late fetal life, the lumen of the vagina is separated from the cavity of the urogenital sinus by a membrane—the **hymen** (Figs. 12-33*C* and 12-37*H*). The membrane is formed by invagination of the posterior wall of the urogenital sinus, resulting from expansion of the caudal end of the vagina. The hymen usually ruptures during the perinatal period and remains as a thin fold of mucous membrane just within the vaginal orifice.

Vestigial Structures Derived from Embryonic Genital Ducts

During conversion of the mesonephric and paramesonephric ducts into adult structures, parts of them remain as vestigial structures (see Fig. 12-1). These vestiges are rarely seen unless pathologic changes develop in them.

MESONEPHRIC DUCT REMNANTS IN MALES

The cranial end of the mesonephric duct may persist as an **appendix of the epididymis**, which is usually attached to the head of the epididymis (see Fig. 12-33*A*). Caudal to the efferent ductules, some mesonephric tubules may persist as a small body, the **paradidymis**.

MESONEPHRIC DUCT REMNANTS IN FEMALES

The cranial end of the mesonephric duct may persist as an **appendix vesiculosa** (see Fig. 12-33*B*). A few blind tubules and a duct, the **epoophoron**, correspond to the efferent ductules and duct of the epididymis in the male. The epoophoron may persist in the **mesovarium** between the ovary and uterine tube (see Fig. 12-33*B* and *C*). Closer to the uterus, some rudimentary tubules may persist as the **paroophoron**. Parts of the mesonephric duct, corresponding to the ductus deferens and ejaculatory duct, may persist as *Gartner's duct cysts* between the layers of the broad ligament along the lateral wall of the uterus and in the wall of the vagina (see Fig. 12-33*C*).

PARAMESONEPHRIC DUCT REMNANTS IN MALES

The cranial end of the paramesonephric duct may persist as a vesicular **appendix of the testis**, which is attached to the superior pole of the testis (see Fig. 12-33*A*). The **prostatic utricle**, a small saclike structure that opens into the prostatic urethra, is homologous to the vagina. The lining of the prostatic utricle is derived from the epithelium of the urogenital sinus. Within its epithelium, endocrine cells containing neuron-specific enolase and serotonin have been detected. The **seminal colliculus**, a small elevation in the posterior wall of the prostatic urethra, is the adult derivative of the sinus tubercle (see Fig. 12-34*B*). It is homologous to the hymen in the female (see Table 12-1 and Fig. 12-46*A*).

PARAMESONEPHRIC DUCT REMNANTS IN FEMALES

Part of the cranial end of the paramesonephric duct that does not contribute to the infundibulum of the uterine tube may persist as a **vesicular appendage** (see Fig. 12-33*C*), called a *hydatid (of Morgagni)*.

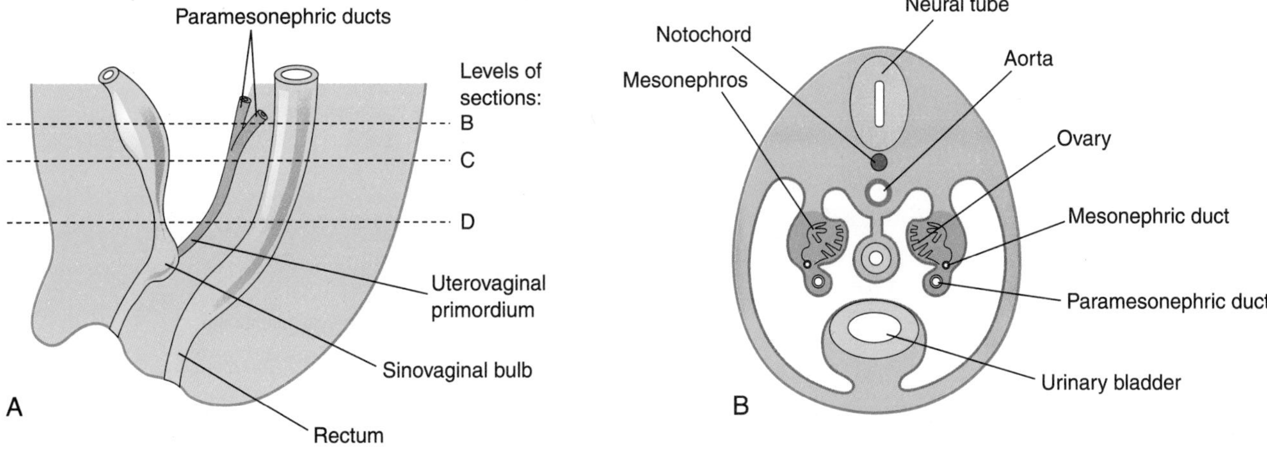

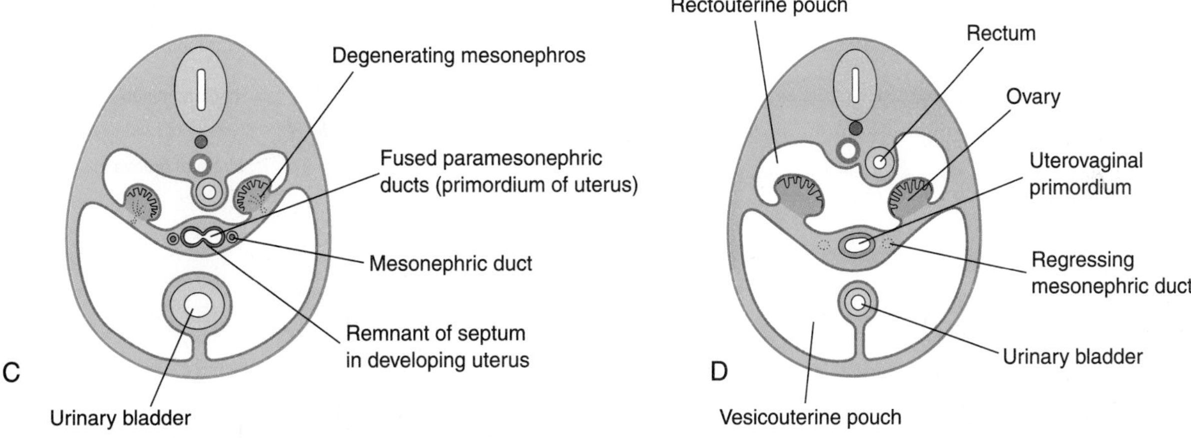

FIGURE 12-36. Early development of the ovaries and uterus. **A,** Schematic drawing of a sagittal section of the caudal region of an 8-week female embryo. **B,** Transverse section showing the paramesonephric ducts approaching each other. **C,** Similar section at a more caudal level illustrating fusion of the paramesonephric ducts. A remnant of the septum that initially separates them is shown. **D,** Similar section showing the uterovaginal primordium, broad ligament, and pouches in the pelvic cavity. Note that the mesonephric ducts have regressed.

DEVELOPMENT OF EXTERNAL GENITALIA

Up to the seventh week, the external genitalia are similar in both sexes (see Fig. 12-37*A* and *B*). Distinguishing sexual characteristics begin to appear during the 9th week, but the external genitalia are not fully differentiated until the 12th week.

Early in the fourth week, proliferating mesenchyme produces a **genital tubercle** in both sexes at the cranial end of the cloacal membrane. Labioscrotal swellings and urogenital folds soon develop on each side of the cloacal membrane. The genital tubercle soon elongates to form a **primordial phallus**. When the urorectal septum fuses with the cloacal membrane at the end of the sixth week, it divides the cloacal membrane into a dorsal anal membrane and a ventral **urethral membrane** (see Fig. 12-37*B*). The urogenital membrane lies in the floor of a median cleft, the **urethral groove**, which is bounded by the **urethral folds.** The anal and urogenital membranes rupture a week or so later, forming the anus and urogenital orifice, respectively. In the female fetus the urethra and vagina open into a common cavity, the **vestibule**.

Development of Male External Genitalia

Masculinization of the indifferent external genitalia is induced by **testosterone** produced by the interstitial cells of the fetal testes (see Fig. 12-37*C*, *E*, and *G*). As the phallus enlarges and elongates to become the penis, the urethral folds form the lateral walls of the urethral groove on the ventral surface of the penis (Fig. 12-38*A* and *B*). This groove is lined by a proliferation of endodermal cells, the **urethral plate**, which extends from the phallic portion of the urogenital sinus. The urethral folds fuse with each other along the ventral surface of the penis to form the **spongy urethra** (see Fig. 12-38*C1* and *C3*). The surface ectoderm fuses in the median plane of the penis, forming the **penile raphe** and enclosing the spongy urethra within the penis. At the tip of the **glans penis**, an ectodermal ingrowth forms a cellular ectodermal cord, which grows toward the root of the penis to meet the spongy urethra (see Fig. 12-26*A*). This cord canalizes and its lumen joins the previously formed spongy urethra. This completes the terminal part of the urethra and moves the external urethral orifice to the tip of the glans of the penis (see Fig. 12-26*C*).

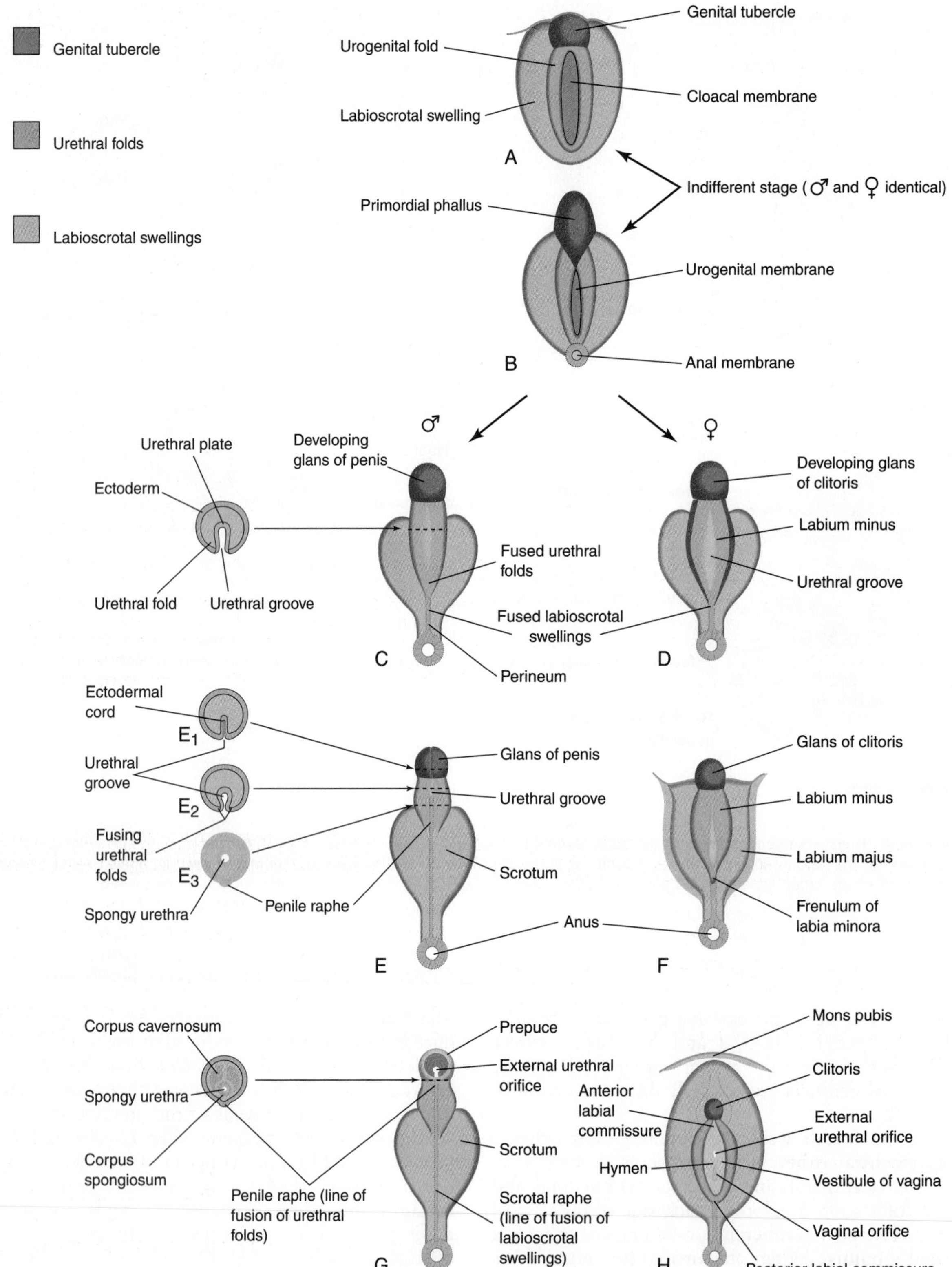

FIGURE 12-37. Development of the external genitalia. **A** and **B,** Diagrams illustrating the appearance of the genitalia during the indifferent stage (fourth to seventh weeks). **C, E,** and **G,** Stages in the development of male external genitalia at 9, 11, and 12 weeks, respectively. To the left are schematic transverse sections of the developing penis illustrating formation of the spongy urethra. **D, F,** and **H,** Stages in the development of female external genitalia at 9, 11, and 12 weeks, respectively.

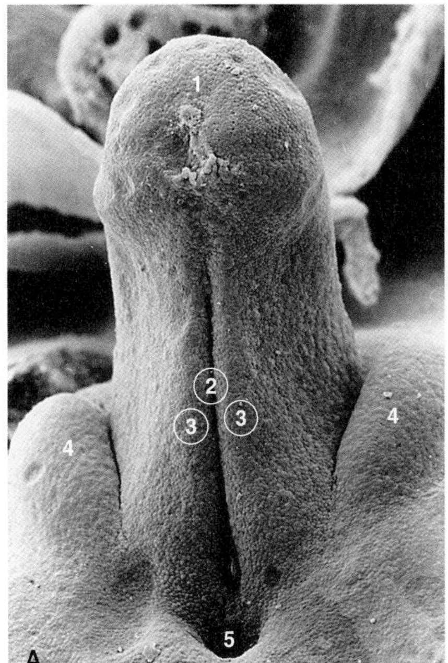

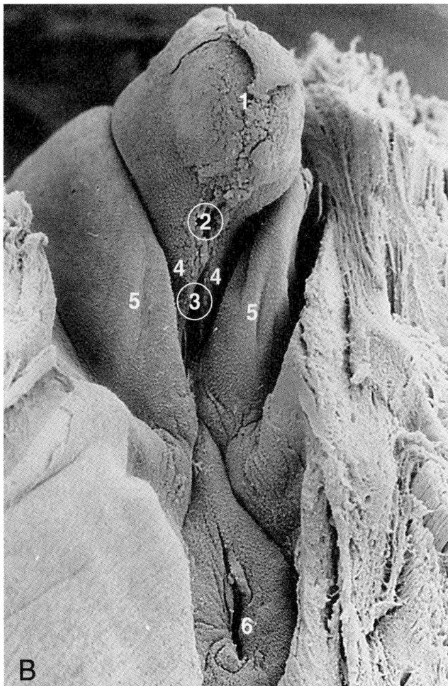

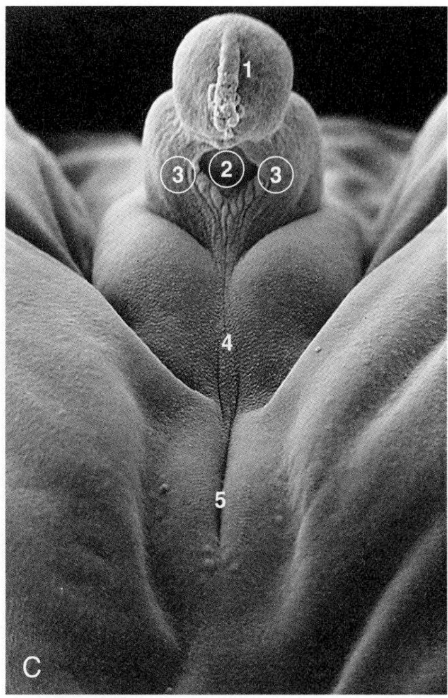

FIGURE 12-38. Scanning electron micrographs of the developing external genitalia. **A,** The perineum during the indifferent stage of a 17-mm, 7-week embryo (×100). 1, developing glans of penis with the ectodermal cord; 2, urethral groove continuous with the urogenital sinus; 3, urethral folds; 4, labioscrotal swellings; 5, anus. **B,** The external genitalia of a 7.2-cm, 10-week female fetus (×45). 1, glans of clitoris; 2, external urethral orifice; 3, opening into urogenital sinus; 4, urethral fold (primordium of labium minus); 5, labioscrotal swelling (labium majus); 6, anus. **C,** The external genitalia of a 5.5-cm, 10-week male fetus (×40). 1, glans of penis with ectodermal cord; 2, remains of urethral groove; 3, urethral folds in the process of closing; 4, labioscrotal swellings fusing to form the raphe of the scrotum; 5, anus. (From Hinrichsen KV: Embryologische Grundlagen. In Sohn C, Holzgreve W [eds]: Ultraschall in Gynäkologie und Geburtshilfe. New York, Georg Thieme Verlag, 1995.)

During the 12th week, a circular ingrowth of ectoderm occurs at the periphery of the glans penis (see Fig. 12-26*B*). When this ingrowth breaks down, it forms the **prepuce** (foreskin)—a covering fold of skin (see Fig. 12-26*C*). The corpora cavernosa and corpus spongiosum of the penis develop from mesenchyme in the phallus. The **labioscrotal swellings** grow toward each other and fuse to form the **scrotum** (see Fig. 12-37*E* and *G*). The line of fusion of these folds is clearly visible as the **scrotal raphe** (see Figs. 12-37*G* and 12-38*C*). Agenesis of the scrotum is an extremely rare anomaly.

Development of Female External Genitalia

The primordial phallus in the female fetus gradually becomes the clitoris (see Fig. 12-37*D*, *F*, and *H*). The clitoris is still relatively large at 18 weeks (see Fig. 12-21). The **urethral folds** do not fuse, except posteriorly, where they join to form the **frenulum of the labia minora**. The unfused parts of the urogenital folds form the **labia minora**. The labioscrotal folds fuse posteriorly to form the **posterior labial commissure** and anteriorly to form the **anterior labial commissure** and **mons pubis** (see Fig. 12-37*H*). Most parts of the labioscrotal folds remain unfused and form two large folds of skin, the **labia majora**.

DETERMINATION OF FETAL SEX

Visualization of the external genitalia during ultrasonography (Fig. 12-39) is clinically important for several reasons, including detection of fetuses at risk of severe X-linked disorders. Careful examination of the perineum may detect **ambiguous genitalia** (Fig. 12-40*B*). Documentation of testes in the scrotum provides the only 100% gender determination, which is not possible in utero until 22 to 36 weeks. Fetal position prevents good visualization of the perineum in 30% of fetuses.

When there is normal sexual differentiation, the appearance of the external and internal genitalia is consistent with the sex chromosome complement. Errors in sex determination and differentiation result in various degrees of intermediate sex—**intersexuality** or hermaphroditism. Intersex implies a discrepancy between the morphology of the gonads (testes/ovaries) and the appearance of the external genitalia. Intersexual conditions are classified according to the histologic appearance of the gonads:

- True hermaphrodites have ovarian and testicular tissue either in the same or in opposite gonads.

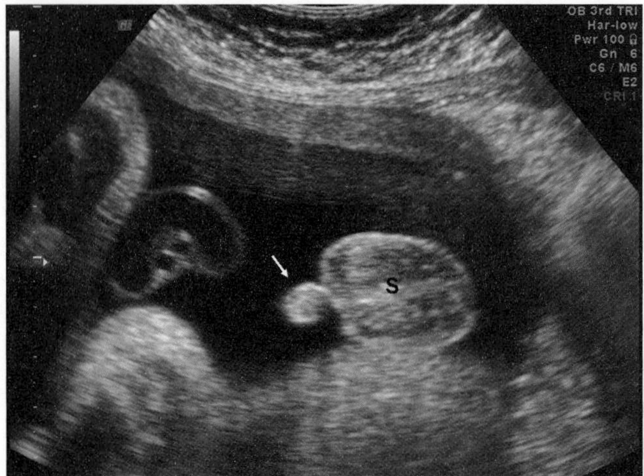

FIGURE 12-39. Sonogram of a 33-week male fetus showing normal external genitalia. Observe the penis (*arrow*) and scrotum (S). Also note the testis within the scrotum. (Courtesy of Dr. G.J. Reid, Department of Obstetrics, Gynecology and Reproductive Sciences, University of Manitoba, Women's Hospital, Winnipeg, Manitoba, Canada)

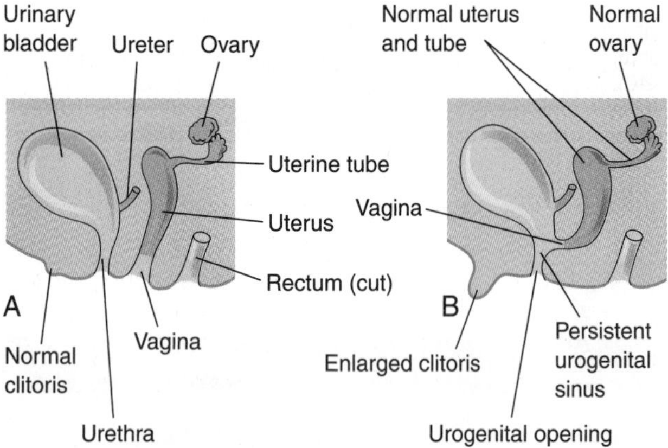

FIGURE 12-40. Schematic lateral views of the female urogenital system. **A,** Normal. **B,** Female pseudohermaphrodite caused by congenital adrenal hyperplasia (CAH). Note the enlarged clitoris and persistent urogenital sinus that were induced by androgens produced by the hyperplastic suprarenal glands.

- Female pseudohermaphrodites have ovaries.
- Male pseudohermaphrodites have testes.

True Hermaphroditism

Persons with this extremely rare intersexual condition usually have chromatin-positive nuclei (contain sex chromatin in cells observed in a buccal smear). Approximately 70% of them have a 46, XX chromosome constitution; approximately 20% have 46, XX/46, XY **mosaicism** (presence of two or more cell lines), and approximately 10% have a 46, XY chromosome constitution. The causes of true hermaphroditism are still poorly understood. Most true hermaphrodites have both testicular and ovarian tissue or an ovotestis. These tissues are not usually functional. An ovotestis (containing both testicular and ovarian tissue) forms if both the medulla and cortex of the indifferent gonads develop. True hermaphroditism results from an error in sex determination. The phenotype may be male or female but the external genitalia are always ambiguous.

Female Pseudohermaphroditism

Persons with this intersexual condition have chromatin-positive nuclei and a 46, XX chromosome constitution. This anomaly results from exposure of the female fetus to excessive androgens, causing virilization of the external genitalia (clitoral enlargement and labial fusion [see Figs. 12-28 and 12-40]). A common cause of female pseudohermaphroditism is CAH. There is no ovarian abnormality, but the excessive production of androgens by the fetal suprarenal glands causes varying degrees of masculinization of the external genitalia. Commonly there is clitoral hypertrophy, partial fusion of the labia majora, and a persistent urogenital sinus (see Fig. 12-40). In very unusual cases, the masculinization may be so intense that a complete clitoral urethra results. The administration of androgenic agents to women during early pregnancy may cause similar anomalies of the fetal external genitalia (see Chapter 20). Most cases have resulted from the use of certain progestational compounds for the treatment of threatened abortion. Masculinizing maternal tumors can also cause virilization of female fetuses.

Male Pseudohermaphroditism

Persons with this intersexual condition have chromatin-negative nuclei (do not contain sex chromatin) and a 46, XY chromosome constitution. The external genitalia are developmentally variable as is the development of the internal genitalia due to varying degrees of development of the paramesonephric ducts. These anomalies are caused by inadequate production of testosterone and MIS by the fetal testes. Testicular development in these males ranges from rudimentary to normal. Genetic defects in the enzymatic synthesis of testosterone by the fetal testes and in interstitial cells produce male pseudohermaphroditism through inadequate virilization of the male fetus.

ANDROGEN INSENSITIVITY SYNDROME

Persons with androgen insensitivity syndrome (AIS)—previously called testicular feminization syndrome—(1 in 20,000 live births) are normal-appearing females, despite the presence of testes and a 46, XY chromosome constitution (Fig. 12-41). The

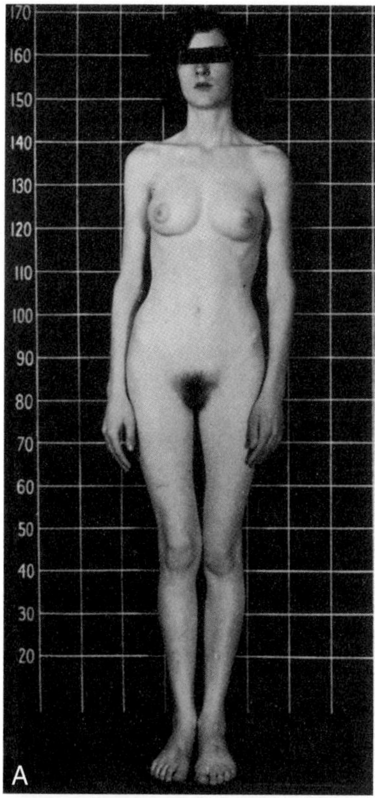

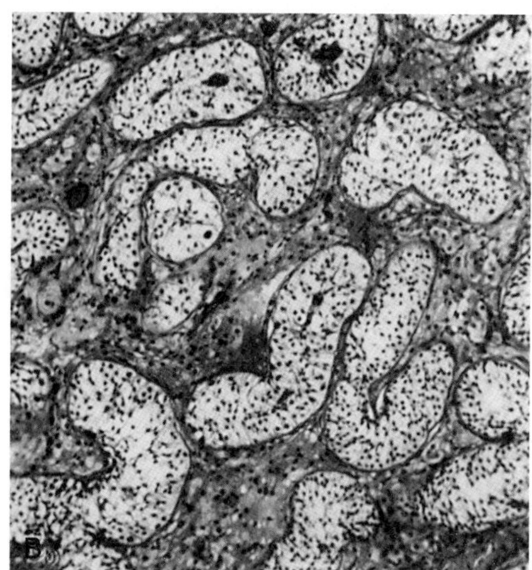

FIGURE 12-41. **A,** Photograph of a 17-year-old woman with androgen insensitivity syndrome (AIS). The external genitalia are female, but the patient has a 46, XY karyotype and testes. **B,** Photomicrograph of a section through a testis removed from the inguinal region of this woman showing seminiferous tubules lined by Sertoli cells. There are no germ cells, and the interstitial cells are hypoplastic. (From Jones HW, Scott WW: Hermaphroditism, Genital Anomalies and Related Endocrine Disorders. Baltimore, Williams & Wilkins, 1958. Courtesy of Williams & Wilkins.)

external genitalia are female, but the vagina usually ends in a blind pouch and the uterus and uterine tubes are absent or rudimentary. At puberty there is normal development of breasts and female characteristics, but menstruation does not occur. The testes are usually in the abdomen or the inguinal canals, but they may be within the labia majora. The failure of masculinization to occur in these individuals results from a resistance to the action of testosterone at the cellular level in the genital tubercle and labioscrotal and urethral folds.

Persons with **partial AIS** exhibit some masculinization at birth, such as ambiguous external genitalia, and may have an enlarged clitoris. The vagina ends blindly and the uterus is absent. Testes are in the inguinal canals or the labia majora. There are usually point mutations in the sequence that codes for the androgen receptor. Usually the testes are removed as soon as they are discovered because, in approximately one third of these individuals, malignant tumors develop by 50 years of age. AIS follows X-linked recessive inheritance, and the gene encoding the androgen receptor has been localized.

MIXED GONADAL DYSGENESIS

Persons with this very rare condition usually have chromatin-negative nuclei, a testis on one side, and an undifferentiated gonad on the other side. The internal genitalia are female, but male derivatives of the mesonephric ducts are sometimes present. The external genitalia range from normal female through intermediate states to normal male. At puberty, neither breast development nor menstruation occurs, but varying degrees of virilization are common.

HYPOSPADIAS

Hypospadias is the most common anomaly of the penis. There are four main types of hypospadias:

- Glanular hypospadias—the most common type
- Penile hypospadias
- Penoscrotal hypospadias
- Perineal hypospadias

In 1 of every 300 male infants, the external urethral orifice is on the ventral surface of the glans of the penis (**glanular hypospadias**) or on the ventral surface of the body of the penis (**penile hypospadias**). Usually the penis is underdeveloped and curved ventrally—**chordee**.

Glanular hypospadias and penile hypospadias constitute approximately 80% of cases (Fig. 12-42). In **penoscrotal hypospadias**, the urethral orifice is at the junction of the penis and scrotum. In **perineal hypospadias,** the labioscrotal folds fail to fuse and the external urethral orifice is located between the

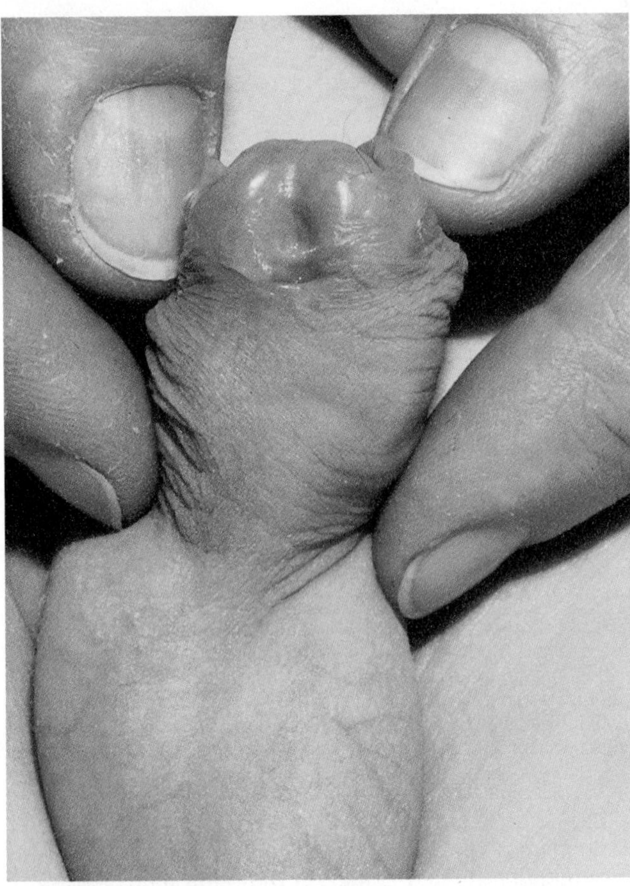

FIGURE 12-42. Glanular hypospadias in an infant. The external urethral orifice is on the ventral surface of the glans of the penis. (Courtesy of A.E. Chudley, MD, Section of Genetics and Metabolism, Department of Pediatrics and Child Health, University of Manitoba, Children's Hospital, Winnipeg, Manitoba, Canada.)

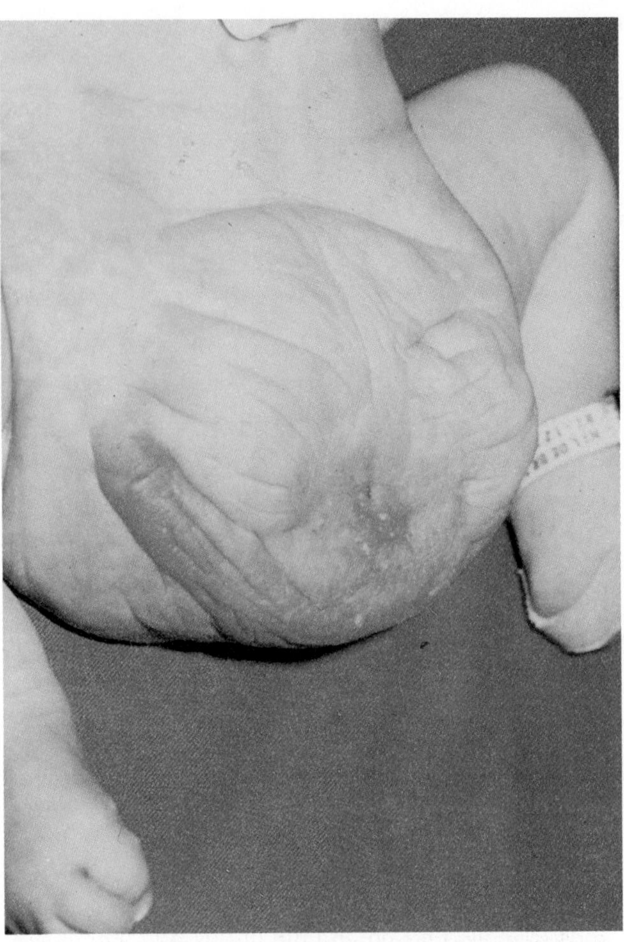

FIGURE 12-43. Perineum of an infant. No external genitalia are present. (Courtesy of Dr. A.E. Chudley, Section of Genetics and Metabolism, Department of Pediatrics and Child Health, Children's Hospital and University of Manitoba, Winnipeg, Manitoba, Canada.)

unfused halves of the scrotum. Because the external genitalia in this severe type of hypospadias are ambiguous, persons with perineal hypospadias and cryptorchidism (undescended testes) are sometimes misdiagnosed as male pseudohermaphrodites.

Hypospadias results from inadequate production of androgens by the fetal testes and/or inadequate receptor sites for the hormones. These defects result in failure of canalization of the ectodermal cord in the glans and/or failure of fusion of the urethral folds; as a consequence, there is incomplete formation of the spongy urethra. Differences in the timing and degree of hormonal failure and/or in the failure of the development of receptor sites account for the different types of hypospadias.

EPISPADIAS

In one of every 30,000 male infants, the urethra opens on the dorsal surface of the penis. Although epispadias may occur as a separate entity, it is often associated with exstrophy of the bladder (see Figs. 12-24 and 12-25). Epispadias may result from inadequate ectodermal-mesenchymal interactions during development of the genital tubercle. As a consequence, the genital tubercle develops more dorsally than in normal embryos. Consequently, when the urogenital membrane ruptures, the urogenital sinus opens on the dorsal surface of the penis. Urine is expelled at the root of the malformed penis.

AGENESIS OF EXTERNAL GENITALIA

Congenital absence of the penis or clitoris is an extremely rare condition (Fig. 12-43). Failure of the genital tubercle to develop may result from inadequate ectodermal-mesenchymal interactions during the seventh week. The urethra usually opens into the perineum near the anus.

Bifid Penis and Double Penis

These anomalies are very rare. Bifid penis is usually associated with exstrophy of the bladder (see Fig. 12-24). It may also be associated with urinary tract abnormalities and imperforate anus. Double penis results when two genital tubercles develop.

Micropenis

In this condition, the penis is so small that it is almost hidden by the suprapubic pad of fat. Micropenis results from fetal testicular failure and is commonly associated with hypopituitarism.

Anomalies of Uterine Tubes, Uterus, and Vagina

Anomalies of the uterine tubes occur infrequently, and only a few types have been reported. These include hydatid cysts, accessory ostia (openings), complete and segmental absence, duplication of a uterine tube, lack of the muscular layer, and failure of the tube to canalize.

Various types of uterine duplication and vaginal anomalies result from arrests of development of the uterovaginal primordium during the eighth week (Fig. 12-44) by:

- Incomplete development of a paramesonephric duct
- Failure of parts of one or both paramesonephric ducts to develop
- Incomplete fusion of the paramesonephric ducts
- Incomplete canalization of the vaginal plate to form the vagina

Abnormal Development of Uterus

Double uterus (Latin, *uterus didelphys*) results from failure of fusion of the inferior parts of the paramesonephric ducts. It may be associated with a double or a single vagina (see Fig. 12-44*B* to *D*). In some cases, the uterus appears normal externally but is divided internally by a thin septum (see Fig. 12-44*F*). If the duplication involves only the superior part of the body of the uterus, the condition is called **bicornuate uterus** (Figs. 12-44*D* and *E* and 12-45). If one paramesonephric duct is retarded in its growth and does not fuse with the other one, a **bicornuate uterus with a rudimentary horn** (cornu) develops (see Fig. 12-44*E*). The rudimentary horn may not communicate with the cavity of the uterus. A **unicornuate uterus** develops when one paramesonephric duct fails to develop; this results in a uterus with one uterine tube (see Fig. 12-44*G*). In many cases, the individuals are fertile but may have an increased incidence of premature delivery.

Absence of the Vagina and Uterus

Once in approximately every 5000 female births, absence of the vagina occurs. This results from failure of the sinovaginal bulbs to develop and form the vaginal plate (see Figs. 12-33*B* and 12-36*A*). When the vagina is absent, the uterus is usually absent also because the developing uterus (uterovaginal primordium) induces the formation of sinovaginal bulbs, which fuse to form the vaginal plate. Other anomalies involving the urogenital tract and the skeletal system may also be present (Mayer-Rokitansky-Küster-Hauser syndrome).

Vaginal Atresia

Failure of canalization of the vaginal plate results in atresia (blockage) of the vagina. A transverse vaginal septum occurs in approximately one in 80,000 women. Usually the septum is located at the junction of the middle and superior thirds of the vagina. Failure of the inferior end of the vaginal plate to perforate results in an **imperforate hymen.** Variations in the appearance of the hymen are common (Fig. 12-46). The vaginal orifice varies in diameter from very small to large, and there may be more than one orifice.

DEVELOPMENT OF THE INGUINAL CANALS

The inguinal canals form pathways for the testes to descend from the dorsal abdominal wall through the anterior abdominal wall into the scrotum. Inguinal canals develop in both sexes because of the morphologically indifferent stage of sexual development. As the mesonephros degenerates, a ligament—the **gubernaculum**—develops on each side of the abdomen from the caudal pole of the gonad (Fig. 12-47*A*). The gubernaculum passes obliquely through the developing anterior abdominal wall at the site of the future inguinal canal (see Fig. 12-47*B* to *D*) and attaches caudally to the internal surface of the *labioscrotal swellings* (future halves of the scrotum or labia majora).

The **processus vaginalis**, an evagination of peritoneum, develops ventral to the gubernaculum and herniates through the abdominal wall along the path formed by the gubernaculum (see Fig. 12-47*B*). The vaginal process carries along extensions of the layers of the abdominal wall before it, which form the walls of the inguinal canal. These layers also form the coverings of the spermatic cord and testis (see Fig. 12-47*D* to *F*). The opening in the transversalis fascia produced by the processus vaginalis becomes the **deep inguinal ring**, and the opening created in the external oblique aponeurosis forms the **superficial inguinal ring**.

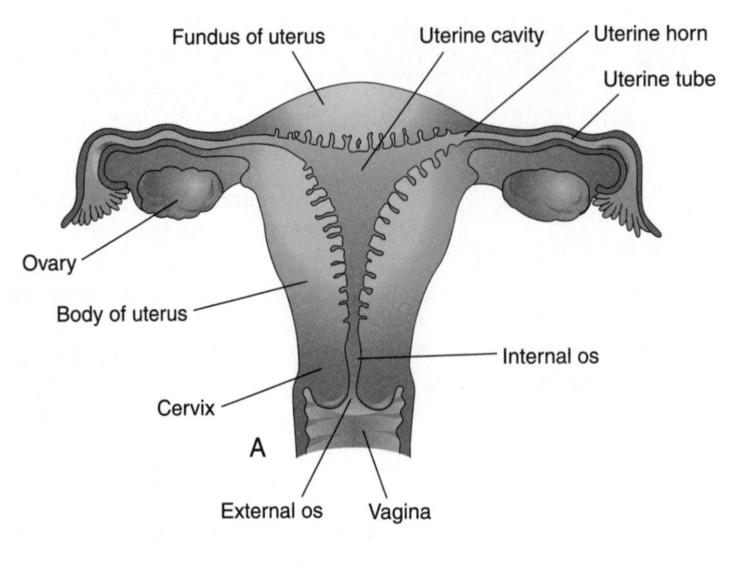

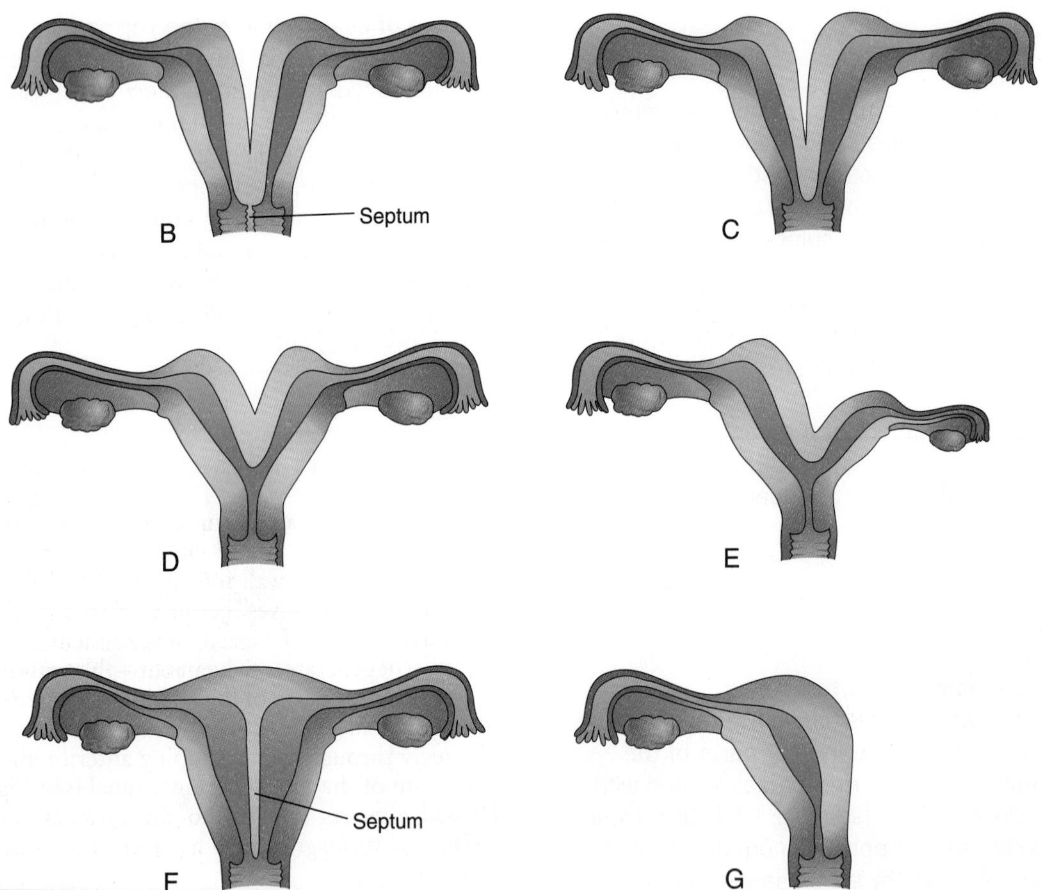

FIGURE 12-44. Various types of uterine anomaly. **A,** Normal uterus and vagina. **B,** Double uterus (Latin, *uterus didelphys*) and double vagina (Latin, *vagina duplex*). **C,** Double uterus with single vagina. **D,** Bicornuate uterus (two uterine horns). **E,** Bicornuate uterus with a rudimentary left horn. **F,** Septate uterus. **G,** Unicornuate uterus.

ABNORMAL SEX CHROMOSOME COMPLEXES

In embryos with abnormal sex chromosome complexes, such as XXX or XXY, the number of X chromosomes appears to be unimportant in sex determination. If a normal Y chromosome is present, the embryo develops as a male. If no Y chromosome is present or the testis-determining region of the Y chromosome is absent, female development occurs. The loss of an X chromosome does not appear to interfere with the migration of primordial germ cells to the gonadal ridges because some germ cells have

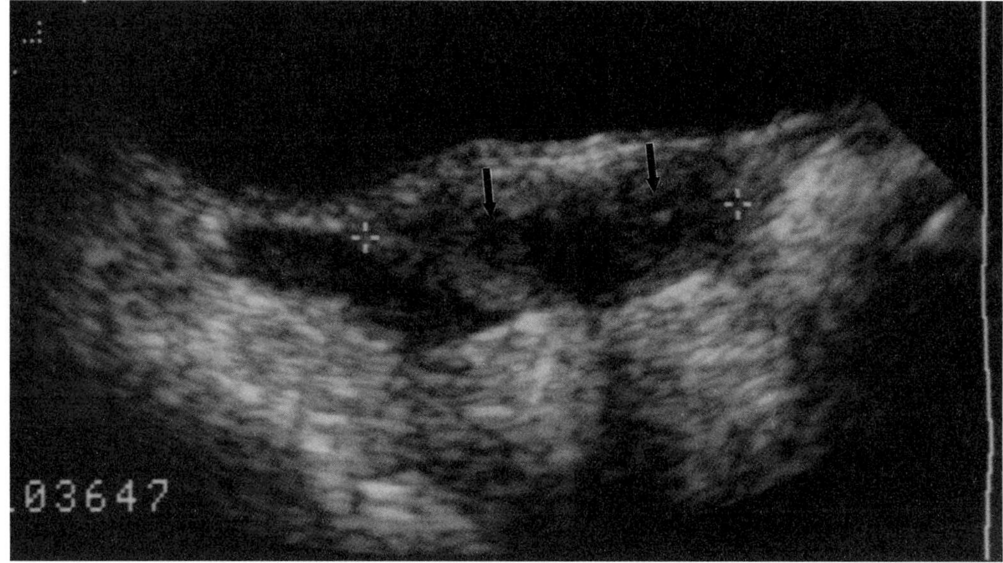

FIGURE 12-45. Sonogram of a bicornuate uterus. The transverse diameter of the uterine fundus (4 cm) is wider than normal (see electronic calipers ·:·) on left. Two separate uterine cavities are marked with *arrows*. (Courtesy of Dr. Anna Nussbaum Blask and Dr. Julianne Byrne, Children's National Medical Center, Washington, DC.)

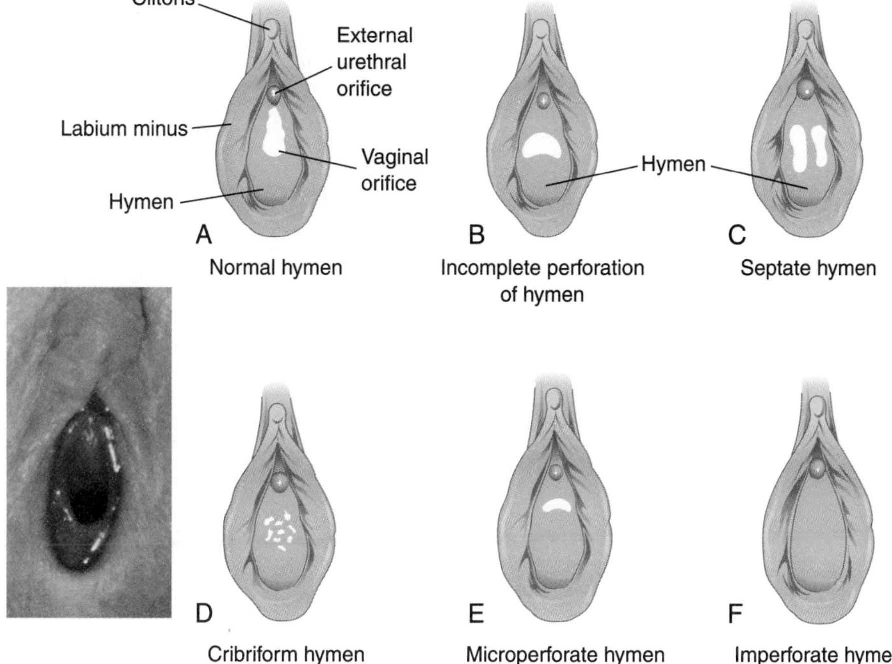

FIGURE 12-46. **A** to **F**, Congenital anomalies of the hymen. The normal appearance of the hymen is illustrated in **A** and in the inset photograph. *Inset*, Normal crescentic hymen in a prepubertal child. (Courtesy of Dr. Margaret Morris, Associate Professor of Obstetrics, Gynaecology and Reproductive Sciences, Women's Hospital and University of Manitoba, Winnipeg, Manitoba, Canada.)

been observed in the fetal gonads of 45, X females with Turner syndrome. Two X chromosomes are needed, however, to bring about normal ovarian development.

RELOCATION OF THE TESTES AND OVARIES

Descent of the Testes

Testicular descent is associated with:

- Enlargement of the testes and atrophy of the mesonephroi (mesonephric kidneys), allowing movement of the testes caudally along the posterior abdominal wall
- Atrophy of the paramesonephric ducts induced by the müllerian-inhibiting syndrome (MIS), enabling the testes to move transabdominally to the deep inguinal rings
- Enlargement of the processus vaginalis guiding the testis through the inguinal canal into the scrotum

By 26 weeks, the testes have descended retroperitoneally (external to the peritoneum) from the posterior abdominal wall to the deep inguinal rings (see Fig. 12-47*B* and *C*). This change in position occurs as the fetal pelvis enlarges and the trunk of the embryo elongates. Transabdominal movement of the testes is largely a relative movement that results from growth of the cranial part of the abdomen away from the future pelvic region. Little is known about the cause of testicular descent through the inguinal

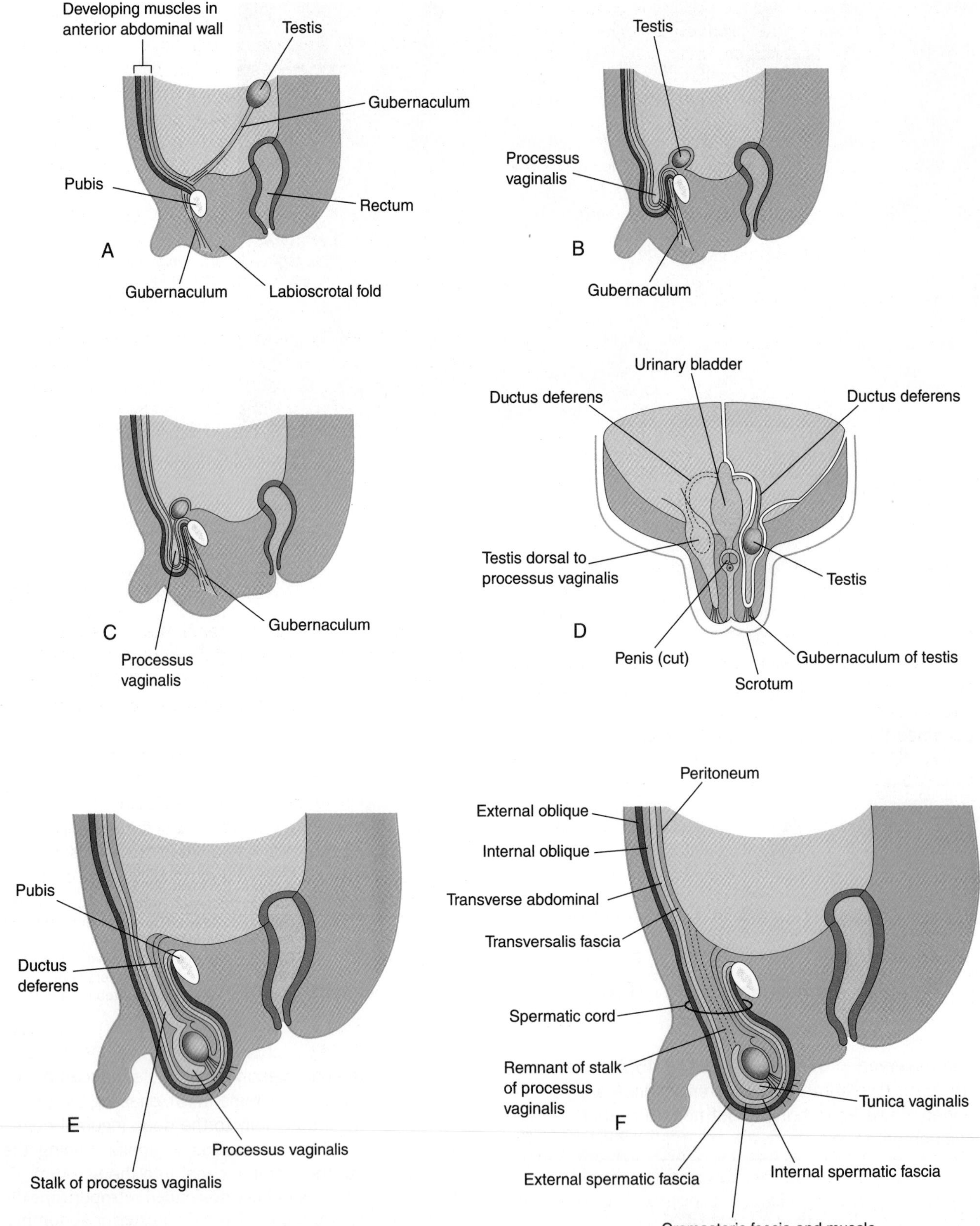

FIGURE 12-47. Formation of the inguinal canals and descent of the testes. **A,** Sagittal section of a 7-week embryo showing the testis before its descent from the dorsal abdominal wall. **B** and **C,** Similar sections at approximately 28 weeks showing the processus vaginalis and the testis beginning to pass through the inguinal canal. Note that the processus vaginalis carries fascial layers of the abdominal wall before it. **D,** Frontal section of a fetus approximately 3 days later illustrating descent of the testis posterior to the processus vaginalis. The processus vaginalis has been cut away on the left side to show the testis and ductus deferens. **E,** Sagittal section of a newborn male infant showing the processus vaginalis communicating with the peritoneal cavity by a narrow stalk. **F,** Similar section of a 1-month-old male infant after obliteration of the stalk of the processus vaginalis. Note that the extended fascial layers of the abdominal wall now form the coverings of the spermatic cord.

canals into the scrotum, but the process is controlled by androgens (e.g., testosterone) produced by the fetal testes. The role of the gubernaculum in testicular descent is uncertain. Initially it forms a path through the anterior abdominal wall for the processus vaginalis to follow during formation of the inguinal canal. The gubernaculum also anchors the testis to the scrotum and appears to guide its descent into the scrotum. Passage of the testis through the inguinal canal may also be aided by the increase in intra-abdominal pressure resulting from the growth of abdominal viscera.

Descent of the testes through the inguinal canals into the scrotum usually begins during the 26th week and takes 2 or 3 days. The testes pass external to the peritoneum and processus vaginalis. After the testes enter the scrotum, the inguinal canal contracts around the spermatic cord. More than 97% of full-term newborn males have both testes in the scrotum. During the first 3 months after birth, most undescended testes descend into the scrotum.

The mode of descent of the testis explains why the ductus deferens crosses anterior to the ureter (see Fig. 12-33*A*); it also explains the course of the testicular vessels. These vessels form when the testis is high on the posterior abdominal wall. When the testis descends, it carries its ductus deferens and vessels with it. As the testis and ductus deferens descend, they are ensheathed by the fascial extensions of the abdominal wall (see Fig. 12-47*F*).

- The extension of the transversalis fascia becomes the **internal spermatic fascia.**
- The extensions of the internal oblique muscle and fascia become the **cremasteric muscle** and **fascia.**
- The extension of the external oblique aponeurosis becomes the **external spermatic fascia.**

Within the scrotum, the testis projects into the distal end of the **processus vaginalis.** During the perinatal period, the connecting stalk of the processus normally obliterates, forming a serous membrane—**tunica vaginalis,**—which covers the front and sides of the testis (see Fig. 12-47*F*).

Descent of the Ovaries

The ovaries also descend from the posterior abdominal wall to the pelvis; however, they do not pass from the pelvis and enter the inguinal canals. The **gubernaculum** is also attached to the uterus near the attachment of the uterine tube. The cranial part of the gubernaculum becomes the **ovarian ligament,** and the caudal part forms the **round ligament of the uterus** (see Fig. 12-33*C*). The round ligaments pass through the inguinal canals and terminate in the labia majora. The relatively small processus vaginalis in the female usually obliterates and disappears long before birth. A processus vaginalis that persists after birth is called a **canal of Nuck.**

Cryptorchidism or Undescended Testes

Cryptorchidism (Greek, *kryptos*, hidden) occurs in up to 30% of premature males and in approximately 3% to 4% of full-term males. This reflects the fact that the testes begin to descend into the scrotum by the end of the second trimester. Cryptorchidism may be unilateral or bilateral. In most cases, undescended testes descend into the scrotum by the end of the first year. If both testes remain within or just outside the abdominal cavity, they fail to mature and sterility is common. If uncorrected, these men have a significantly higher risk of developing **germ cell tumors**, especially in cases of *abdominal cryptorchidism*. Undescended testes are often histologically normal at birth, but failure of development and atrophy are detectable by the end of the first year. Cryptorchid testes may be in the abdominal cavity or anywhere along the usual path of descent of the testis, but they are usually in the inguinal canal (Fig. 12-48*A*). The cause of most cases of cryptorchidism is unknown, but a deficiency of androgen production by the fetal testes is an important factor.

Ectopic Testes

After traversing the inguinal canal, the testis may deviate from its usual path of descent and lodge in various abnormal locations (see Fig. 12-48*B*):

- Interstitial (external to aponeurosis of external oblique muscle)
- In the proximal part of the medial thigh
- Dorsal to the penis
- On the opposite side (crossed ectopia)

All types of ectopic testis are rare, but **interstitial ectopia** occurs most frequently. An ectopic testis occurs when a part of the gubernaculum passes to an abnormal location and the testis follows it.

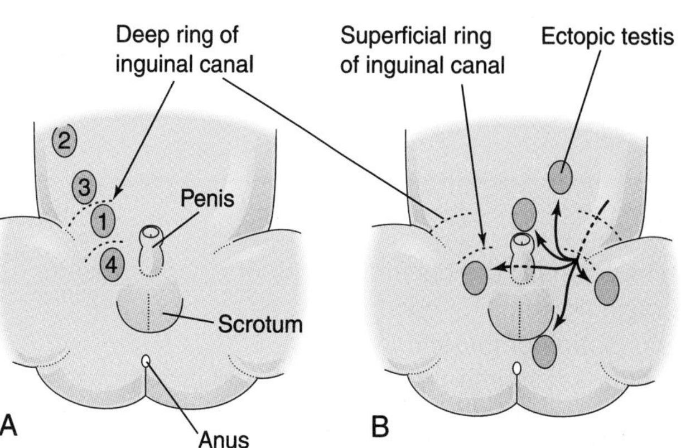

FIGURE 12-48. Possible sites of cryptorchid and ectopic testes. **A,** Positions of cryptorchid testes, numbered in order of frequency. **B,** Usual locations of ectopic testes.

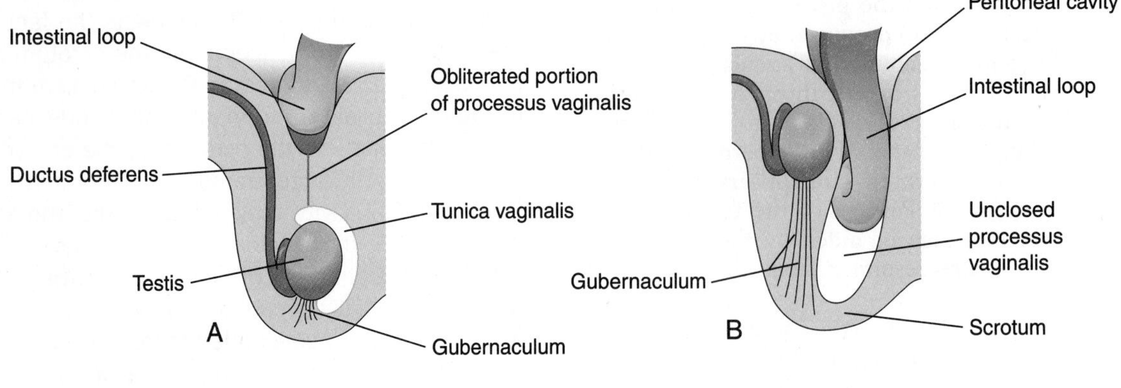

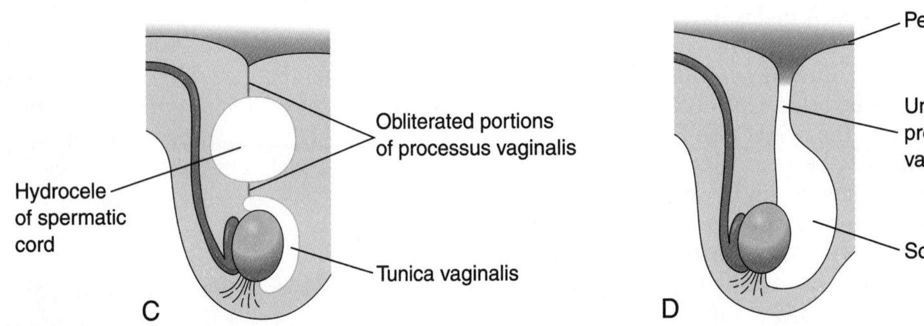

FIGURE 12-49. Diagrams of sagittal sections illustrating conditions resulting from failure of closure of the processus vaginalis. **A,** Incomplete congenital inguinal hernia resulting from persistence of the proximal part of the processus vaginalis. **B,** Complete congenital inguinal hernia into the scrotum resulting from persistence of the processus vaginalis. Cryptorchidism, a commonly associated anomaly, is also illustrated. **C,** Large hydrocele that resulted from an unobliterated portion of the processus vaginalis. **D,** Hydrocele of the testis and spermatic cord resulting from peritoneal fluid passing into an unclosed processus vaginalis.

CONGENITAL INGUINAL HERNIA

If the communication between the tunica vaginalis and the peritoneal cavity fails to close (Fig. 12-49*A* and *B*), a **persistent processus vaginalis** exists. A loop of intestine may herniate through it into the scrotum or labium majus (see Fig. 12-49*B*). Embryonic remnants resembling the ductus deferens or epididymis are often found in inguinal hernial sacs. Congenital inguinal hernia is much more common in males, especially when there are undescended testes. Congenital inguinal hernias are also common with ectopic testes and in females with AIS (Fig. 12-41).

HYDROCELE

Occasionally the abdominal end of the processus vaginalis remains open but is too small to permit herniation of intestine (see Fig. 12-49*D*). Peritoneal fluid passes into the patent processus vaginalis and forms a **scrotal hydrocele.** If the middle part of the processus vaginalis remains open, fluid may accumulate and give rise to a **hydrocele of the spermatic cord** (see Fig. 12-49*C*).

SUMMARY OF THE UROGENITAL SYSTEM

- Development of the urinary and genital systems is intimately associated.
- The urinary system develops before the genital system.
- Three successive kidney systems develop: pronephroi (nonfunctional), mesonephroi (temporary excretory organs), and metanephroi (permanent kidneys).
- The **metanephroi** develop from two sources: the metanephric diverticulum (ureteric bud), which gives rise to the ureter, renal pelvis, calices, and collecting tubules, and the metanephrogenic blastema (metanephric mass of mesenchyme), which gives rise to the nephrons.
- At first, the kidneys are located in the pelvis, but they gradually shift position to the abdomen. This apparent migration results from disproportionate growth of the fetal lumbar and sacral regions.
- Developmental abnormalities of the kidneys and ureters are common. Incomplete division of the metanephric diverticulum results in a double ureter and supernumerary kidney. An ectopic kidney that is abnormally rotated results if the developing kidney remains in its embryonic position in the pelvis.
- The **urinary bladder** develops from the urogenital sinus and the surrounding splanchnic mesenchyme.

The female urethra and most of the male urethra have a similar origin.

- **Exstrophy of the bladder** results from a rare ventral body wall defect through which the posterior wall of the urinary bladder protrudes onto the abdominal wall. **Epispadias** is a common associated anomaly in males; the urethra opens on the dorsum of the penis.
- The **genital system** develops in close association with the urinary system. Genetic sex is established at fertilization, but the gonads do not begin to attain sexual characteristics until the seventh week.
- **Primordial germ cells** form in the wall of the umbilical vesicle (yolk sac) during the fourth week and migrate into the developing gonads, where they differentiate into germ cells (oogonia/spermatogonia).
- The **external genitalia** do not acquire distinct masculine or feminine characteristics until the 12th week. The genitalia develop from primordia that are identical in both sexes.
- **Gonadal sex** is determined by the testes-determining factor (TDF), which is located on the Y chromosome. TDF directs testicular differentiation. The **interstitial cells** (Leydig cells) produce **testosterone**, which stimulates development of the **mesonephric ducts** into male genital ducts. Testosterone also stimulates development of the indifferent external genitalia into the penis and scrotum. MIS, produced by the **Sertoli cells**, inhibits development of the paramesonephric ducts (primordia of female genital ducts).
- In the absence of a Y chromosome and the presence of two X chromosomes, ovaries develop, the mesonephric ducts regress, the **paramesonephric ducts** develop into the uterus and uterine tubes, the vagina develops from the vaginal plate derived from the **urogenital sinus**, and the indifferent external genitalia develop into the clitoris and labia (majora and minora).
- Persons with true hermaphroditism have both ovarian and testicular tissue and variable internal and external genitalia. Errors in sexual differentiation cause **pseudohermaphroditism**. Male pseudohermaphroditism results from failure of the fetal testes to produce adequate amounts of masculinizing hormones or from the tissue insensitivity of the sexual structures. Female pseudohermaphroditism usually results from **congenital adrenal hyperplasia** (CAH), a disorder of the fetal suprarenal (adrenal) glands that causes excessive production of androgens and masculinization of the external genitalia.
- Most anomalies of the female genital tract, such as double uterus, result from incomplete fusion of the paramesonephric ducts. **Cryptorchidism** and **ectopic testes** result from abnormalities of testicular descent.
- **Congenital inguinal hernia** and **hydrocele** result from persistence of the processus vaginalis. Failure of the urethral folds to fuse in males results in various types of **hypospadias**.

CLINICALLY ORIENTED PROBLEMS

Case 12-1

A 4-year-old girl was still in diapers because she was continually wet. The pediatrician saw urine coming from the infant's vagina. An intravenous urogram showed two renal pelves and two ureters on the right side. One ureter was clearly observed to enter the bladder, but the termination of the other one was not clearly seen. A pediatric urologist examined the child under general anesthesia and observed a small opening in the posterior wall of the vagina. He passed a tiny catheter into it and injected a radiopaque solution. This procedure showed that the opening in the vagina was the orifice of the second ureter.

- What is the embryologic basis for the two renal pelves and ureters?
- Describe the embryologic basis of the ectopic ureteric orifice.
- What is the anatomic basis of the continual dribbling of urine into the vagina?

Case 12-2

A seriously injured young man suffered a cardiac arrest. After cardiopulmonary resuscitation, his heart began to beat again, but spontaneous respirations did not occur. Artificial respiration was instituted, but there was no electroencephalographic evidence of brain activity. After 2 days, the man's family agreed that there was no hope of his recovery and asked that his kidneys be donated for transplantation. The radiologist carried out femoral artery catheterization and aortography (radiographic visualization of the aorta and its branches). This technique showed a single large renal artery on the right, but two renal arteries on the left, one medium in size and the other small. Only the right kidney was used for transplantation because it is more difficult to implant small arteries than large ones. Grafting of the small accessory renal artery into the aorta would be difficult because of its size, and part of the kidney would die if one of the arteries was not successfully grafted.

- Are accessory renal arteries common?
- What is the embryologic basis of the two left renal arteries?
- In what other circumstance might an accessory renal artery be of clinical significance?

Case 12-3

A 32-year-old woman with a short history of cramping lower abdominal pain and tenderness underwent a laparotomy because of a suspected ectopic pregnancy. The operation revealed a pregnancy in a rudimentary right uterine horn. The gravid uterine horn was totally removed.

- Is this type of uterine anomaly common?
- What is the embryologic basis of the rudimentary uterine horn?

CASE 12-4

During the physical examination of a newborn male infant, it was observed that the urethra opened on the ventral surface of the penis at the junction of the glans and body. The penis was curved toward the undersurface of the penis.

- Give the medical terms for the anomalies described.
- What is the embryologic basis of the abnormal urethral orifice?
- Is this anomaly common? Discuss its etiology.

CASE 12-5

A 20-year-old woman was prevented from competing in the Olympics because her buccal smear test was chromatin negative, indicating that she had a male sex chromosome complement.

- Is she a male or a female?
- What is the probable basis for her failing to pass the sex chromatin test?
- Is there an anatomic basis for not allowing her to compete in the Olympics?

CASE 12-6

A 10-year-old boy suffered pain in his left groin while attempting to lift a heavy box. Later he noticed a lump in his groin. When he told his mother about the lump, she arranged an appointment with the family physician. After a physical examination, a diagnosis of indirect inguinal hernia was made.

- Explain the embryologic basis of this type of inguinal hernia.
- Based on your embryologic knowledge, list the layers of the spermatic cord that would cover the hernial sac.

Discussion of problems appears at the back of the book.

References and Suggested Reading

American Academy of Pediatrics: Evaluation of the newborn with developmental anomalies of the external genitalia. Pediatrics 106:138, 2000.

Bendon RW: Oligohydramnios. Front Fetal Health 2:10, 2000.

Billmire DF: Germ cell tumors. Surg Clin North Am 86:489, 2006.

de Santa-Barbara P, Moniot B, Poulat F, et al: Expression and subcellular localization of SF-1, SOX9, WTN1, and AMH proteins during early human testicular development. Dev Dyn 217:293, 2000.

Elder JS: Urologic disorders in infants and children. In Behrman RE, Kliegman RM, Jenson HB (eds): Nelson Textbook of Pediatrics, 17th ed. Philadelphia, WB Saunders, 2004.

Filly RA, Feldstein VA: Ultrasound evaluation of the genitourinary system. In Callen PW (ed): Ultrasonography in Obstetrics and Gynecology, 4th ed. Philadelphia, WB Saunders, 2000.

Gasser B, Mauss Y, Ghnassia JP, et al: A quantitative study of normal nephrogenesis in the human fetus: its implication in the natural history of kidney changes due to low obstructive uropathies. Fetal Diagn Ther 8:371, 1993.

Habert R, Lejeune H, Saez JM: Origin, differentiation and regulation of fetal and adult Leydig cells. Mol Cell Endocrinol 179:47, 2001.

Hay ED: Epithelial-mesenchymal transitions. Semin Dev Biol 1:347, 1990.

Hecht NB: Molecular mechanism of male germ cell differentiation. BioEssays 20:555, 1998.

Haynes JH: Inguinal and scrotal disorders. Surg Clin North Am 86:371, 2006.

Hyun SJ: Cloacal exstrophy. J Neonat Netwk 25:101, 2006.

Josso N, di Clemente N, Gouedard L: Anti-müllerian hormone and its receptors. Mol Cell Endocrinol 179:25, 2001.

Kuure S, Vuolteenaho R, Vainio S: Kidney morphogenesis: cellular and molecular regulation. Mech Dev 92:19, 2000.

Levine LS, White PC: Disorders of the adrenal glands. In Behrman RE, Kliegman RM, Jenson HB (eds): Nelson Textbook of Pediatrics, 17th ed. Philadelphia, WB Saunders, 2004.

McElreavey K, Fellous M: Sex determination and the Y chromosome. Am J Med Genet (Semin Med Genet) 89:176, 1999.

Moore KL: The development of clinical sex chromatin tests. In Moore KL (ed): The Sex Chromatin. Philadelphia, WB Saunders, 1966.

Moore KL, Dalley AF: Clinically Oriented Anatomy, 6th ed. Baltimore, Williams & Wilkins, 2006.

Nebot-Cegarra J, Fàbregas PJ, Sánchez-Pérez I: Cellular proliferation in the urorectal septation complex of the human embryo at Carnegie stages 13–18: A nuclear area-based morphometric analysis. J Anat 207:353, 2005.

Neri G, Opitz J: Syndromal (and nonsyndromal) forms of male pseudohermaphroditism. Am J Med Genet (Semin Med Genet) 89:201, 1999.

Palmert MR, Dahms WT: Abnormalities of sexual differentiation. In Martin RJ, Fanaroff AA, Walsh MC (eds): Fanaroff and Martin's Neonatal-Perinatal Medicine. Diseases of the Fetus and Infant, 8th ed. Philadelphia, Mosby, 2006.

Persaud TVN: Embryology of the female genital tract and gonads. In Copeland LJ, Jarrell J (eds): Textbook of Gynecology, 2nd ed. Philadelphia, WB Saunders, 2000.

Piscione TD, Rosenblum ND: The malformed kidney: How gene mutations perturb developmental pathways. Front Fetal Health 2:14, 2000.

Powell DM, Newman KD, Randolph J: A proposed classification of vaginal anomalies and their surgical correction. J Pediatr Surg 30:271, 1995.

Rainey WE, Rehman K, Carr BR: Fetal and maternal adrenals in human pregnancy. Obstet Gynecol Clin North Am 31:817, 2004.

Schedl A, Hastie ND: Cross-talk in kidney development. Curr Opin Genet Dev 10:543, 2000.

Sobel V, Zhu Y-S, Imperato-McGinley J: Fetal hormones and sexual differentiation. Obstet Gynecol Clin North Am 31:837, 2004.

Soffer SZ, Rosen NG, Hong AR, et al: Cloacal exstrophy: A unified management plan. J Pediatr Surg 35:932, 2000.

Trimble EL: Update on diethylstilbestrol. Obstet Gynecol 56:187, 2001.

Veitia RA, Salas-Cortes L, Ottolenghi C, et al: Testis determination in mammals: more questions than answers. Mol Cell Endocrinol 179:3, 2001.

Vogt BA, Dell KM, Davis ID: The kidney and urinary tract. In Martin RJ, Fanaroff AA, Walsh MC (eds): Fanaroff and Martin's Neonatal-Perinatal Medicine. Diseases of the Fetus and Infant, 8th ed. Philadelphia, Mosby, 2006.

Ward CJ, Hogan MC, Rossetti S, et al: The gene mutated in autosomal recessive polycystic kidney disease encodes a large, receptor-like protein. Nat Genet 30:259, 2002.

Wensing CJG: The embryology of testicular descent. Horm Res 30:144, 1988.

Witschi E: Migration of the germ cells of human embryos from the yolk sac to the primitive gonadal folds. Contr Embryol Carnegie Inst 32:67, 1948.

Woolf AS: A molecular and genetic view of human renal and urinary tract malformations. Kidney Int 58:500, 2000.

Woolf AS: The life of the human kidney before birth: Its secrets unfold. Pediatr Res 49:8, 2001.

13

The Cardiovascular System

Early Development of the Heart and Blood Vessels 286
- Development and Fate of Veins Associated with the Heart 286
- Fate of the Vitelline and Umbilical Arteries 292

Later Development of the Heart 292
- Circulation through the Primordial Heart 292
- Partitioning of the Primordial Heart 292
- Changes in the Sinus Venosus 297
- Conducting System of the Heart 308

Anomalies of the Heart and Great Vessels 309

Derivatives of the Pharyngeal Arch Arteries 317
- Derivatives of the First Pair of Pharyngeal Arch Arteries 318
- Derivatives of the Second Pair of Pharyngeal Arch Arteries 318
- Derivatives of the Third Pair of Pharyngeal Arch Arteries 318
- Derivatives of the Fourth Pair of Pharyngeal Arch Arteries 319
- Fate of the Fifth Pair of Pharyngeal Arch Arteries 319
- Derivatives of the Sixth Pair of Pharyngeal Arch Arteries 319
- Pharyngeal Arch Arterial Anomalies 319

Fetal and Neonatal Circulation 325
- Fetal Circulation 325
- Transitional Neonatal Circulation 327
- Derivatives of Fetal Vascular Structures 330

Development of the Lymphatic System 333
- Development of Lymph Sacs and Lymphatic Ducts 333
- Thoracic Duct 333
- Development of the Lymph Nodes 333
- Development of the Lymphocytes 333
- Development of the Spleen and Tonsils 334

Summary of the Cardiovascular System 335

Clinically Oriented Problems 336

The cardiovascular system is the first major system to function in the embryo. The primordial heart and vascular system appear in the middle of the third week. This precocious cardiac development is necessary because the rapidly growing embryo can no longer satisfy its nutritional and oxygen requirements by diffusion alone. Consequently, there is a need for an efficient method of acquiring oxygen and nutrients from the maternal blood and disposing of carbon dioxide and waste products. The cardiovascular system is derived mainly from:

- *Splanchnic mesoderm*, which forms the primordium of the heart (Fig. 13-1*A* and *B*)
- *Paraxial and lateral mesoderm* near the otic placodes from which the internal ears develop
- *Neural crest cells* from the region between the otic vesicles and the caudal limits of the third pair of somites

Blood vessel development—**angiogenesis**—is described in Chapter 4. Primordial blood vessels cannot be distinguished structurally as arteries or veins, but are named according to their future fates and relationship to the heart.

EARLY DEVELOPMENT OF THE HEART AND BLOOD VESSELS

The earliest sign of the heart is the appearance of paired endothelial strands—**angioblastic cords**—in the cardiogenic mesoderm during the third week (see Fig. 13-1*B* and *C*). An inductive influence from the anterior endoderm stimulates early formation of the heart. These cords canalize to form thin heart tubes. As lateral embryonic folding occurs, the endocardial tubes approach each other and fuse to form a *heart tube* (see Figs. 13-7*C* and 13-9*C*). Fusion of the heart tubes begins at the cranial end of the developing heart and extends caudally. *Molecular studies* in mouse and chick embryos have demonstrated the presence of two *bHLH* (basic helix-loop-helix) genes, *dHAND* and *eHAND*, in the paired primordial endocardial tubes and in later stages of cardiac morphogenesis. The murine *MEF2C* gene, which is expressed in cardiogenic precursor cells before formation of the heart tubes, appears to be an essential regulator in early cardiac development. *The heart begins to beat at 22 to 23 days* (Fig. 13-2). Blood flow begins during the fourth week and can be visualized by Doppler ultrasonography (Fig. 13-3).

Development and Fate of Veins Associated with the Heart

Three paired veins drain into the tubular heart of a 4-week embryo (see Fig. 13-2):

- *Vitelline veins* return poorly oxygenated blood from the umbilical vesicle.
- *Umbilical veins* carry well-oxygenated blood from the chorion.
- *Common cardinal veins* return poorly oxygenated blood from the body of the embryo.

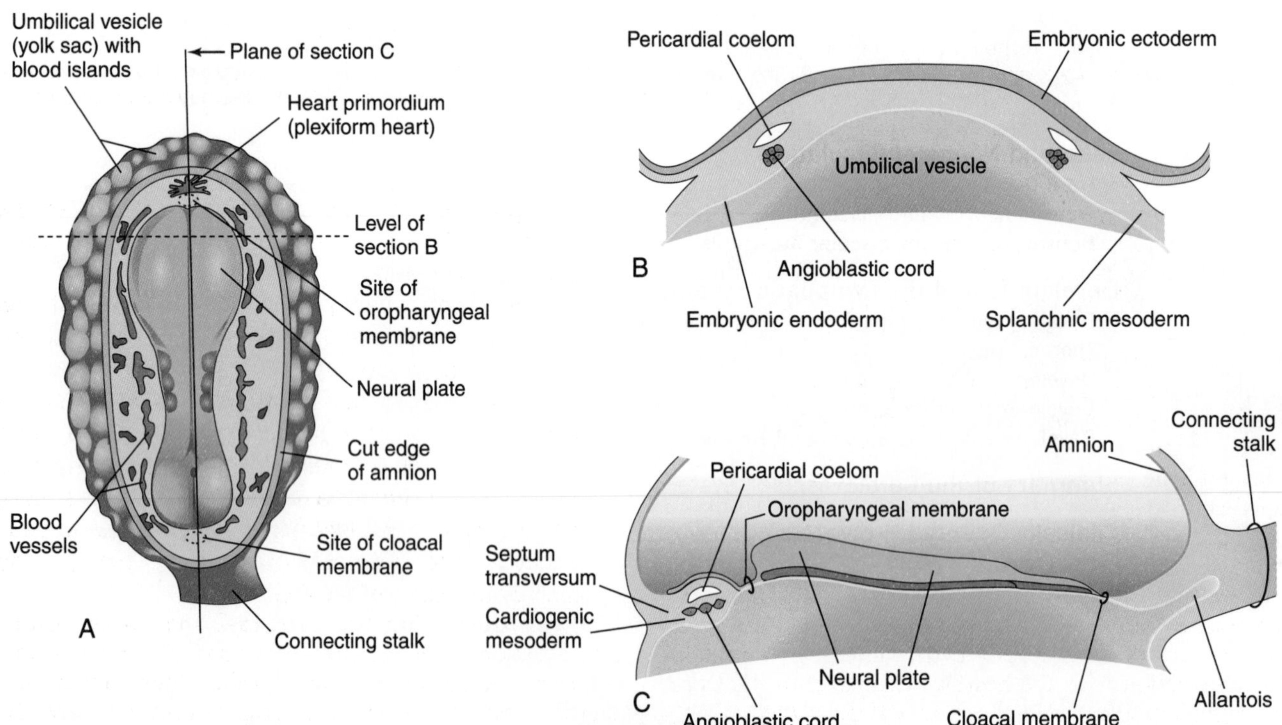

FIGURE 13-1. Early development of the heart. **A,** Drawing of a dorsal view of an embryo (approximately 18 days). **B,** Transverse section of the embryo demonstrating the angioblastic cords in the cardiogenic mesoderm and their relationship to the pericardial coelom. **C,** Longitudinal section through the embryo illustrating the relationship of the angioblastic cords to the oropharyngeal membrane, pericardial coelom, and septum transversum.

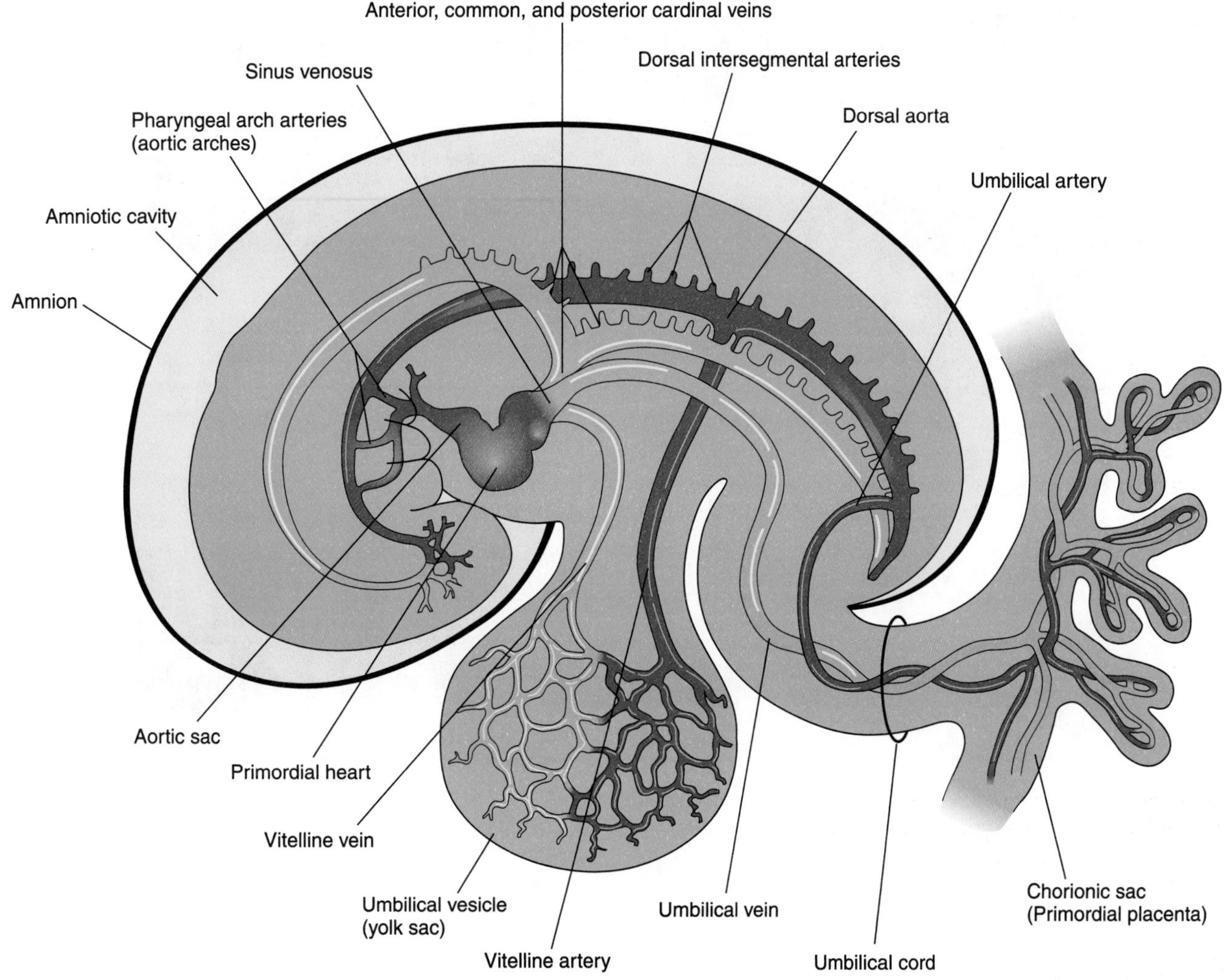

FIGURE 13-2. Drawing of the embryonic cardiovascular system (approximately 26 days) showing vessels on the left side only. The umbilical vein carries well-oxygenated blood and nutrients from the chorion sac to the embryo. The umbilical arteries carry poorly oxygenated blood and waste products from the embryo to the chorion.

The **vitelline veins** follow the omphaloenteric duct (yolk stalk) into the embryo. The duct is the narrow tube connecting the umbilical vesicle (yolk sac) with the midgut (see Fig. 11-1). After passing through the septum transversum, the vitelline veins enter the venous end of the heart—the **sinus venosus** (Figs. 13-2 and 13-4*A*). The left vitelline vein regresses while the right vitelline vein forms most of the **hepatic portal system** (Fig. 13-5*B*) as well as a portion of the inferior vena cava. As the liver primordium grows into the septum transversum (see Chapter 11), the **hepatic cords** anastomose around preexisting endothelium-lined spaces. These spaces, the primordia of the **hepatic sinusoids**, later become linked to the vitelline veins.

The **umbilical veins** run on each side of the liver and carry well-oxygenated blood from the placenta to the sinus venosus. As the liver develops, the umbilical veins lose their connection with the heart and empty into the liver. The right umbilical vein disappears during the seventh week, leaving the left umbilical vein as the only vessel carrying well-oxygenated blood from the placenta to the embryo. Transformation of the umbilical veins may be summarized as follows (see Fig. 13-5):

- The right umbilical vein and the cranial part of the left umbilical vein between the liver and the sinus venosus degenerate.
- The persistent caudal part of the left umbilical vein becomes the **umbilical vein**, which carries all the blood from the placenta to the embryo.
- A large venous shunt—the **ductus venosus (DV)**—develops within the liver (see Fig. 13-5*B*) and connects the umbilical vein with the inferior vena cava (IVC). The DV forms a bypass through the liver, enabling most of the blood from the placenta to pass directly to the heart without passing through the capillary networks of the liver.

The **cardinal veins** (see Figs. 13-2 and 13-4*A*) constitute the main venous drainage system of the embryo. The anterior and posterior cardinal veins drain cranial and caudal parts of the embryo, respectively, and are the earliest veins to develop. They join the **common cardinal veins**, which enter the sinus venosus (see Fig. 13-2). During the eighth week, the **anterior cardinal veins** become connected by an anastomosis (see Fig. 13-5*A* and

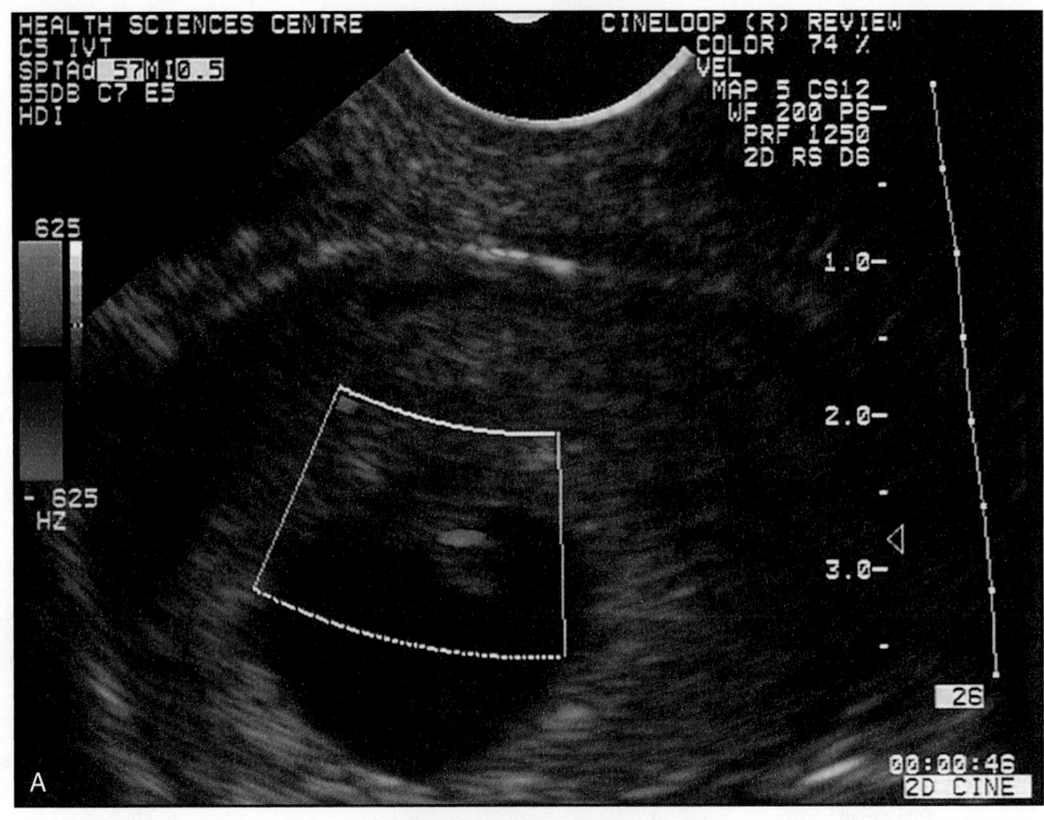

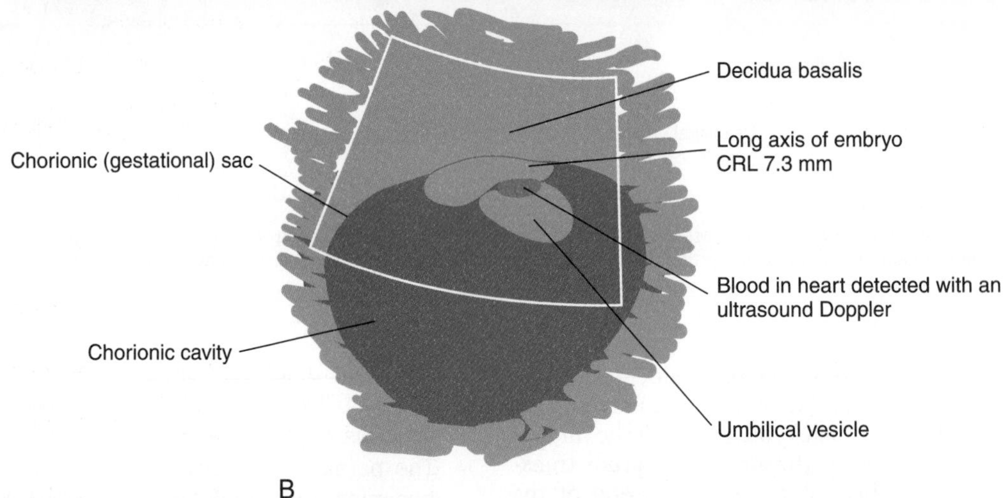

FIGURE 13-3. **A,** Sonogram of a 5-week embryo (crown-rump length: 7.3 mm) and its umbilical vesicle (yolk sac) within its chorionic sac. The pulsating heart of the embryo was visualized using Doppler ultrasonography. **B,** Sketch of the sonogram for orientation and identification of structures. (Courtesy of E.A. Lyons, MD, Professor of Radiology and Obstetrics and Gynecology, University of Manitoba, Winnipeg, Manitoba, Canada.)

B), which shunts blood from the left to the right anterior cardinal vein. This anastomotic shunt becomes the **left brachiocephalic vein** when the caudal part of the left anterior cardinal vein degenerates (see Figs. 13-4*D* and 13-5*C*). The **superior vena cava** (SVC) forms from the right anterior cardinal vein and the right common cardinal vein.

The **posterior cardinal veins** develop primarily as the vessels of the mesonephroi (interim kidneys) and largely disappear with these transitory kidneys (see Chapter 12). The only adult derivatives of the posterior cardinal veins are the root of the azygos vein and the common iliac veins (see Fig. 13-4*D*). The subcardinal and supracardinal veins gradually develop and replace and supplement the posterior cardinal veins.

The **subcardinal veins** appear first (see Fig. 13-4*A*). They are connected with each other through the subcardinal anastomosis and with the posterior cardinal veins through the mesonephric sinusoids. The subcardinal veins form the stem of the left renal vein, the suprarenal veins, the gonadal veins (testicular and ovarian), and a segment of the IVC (see Fig. 13-4*D*).

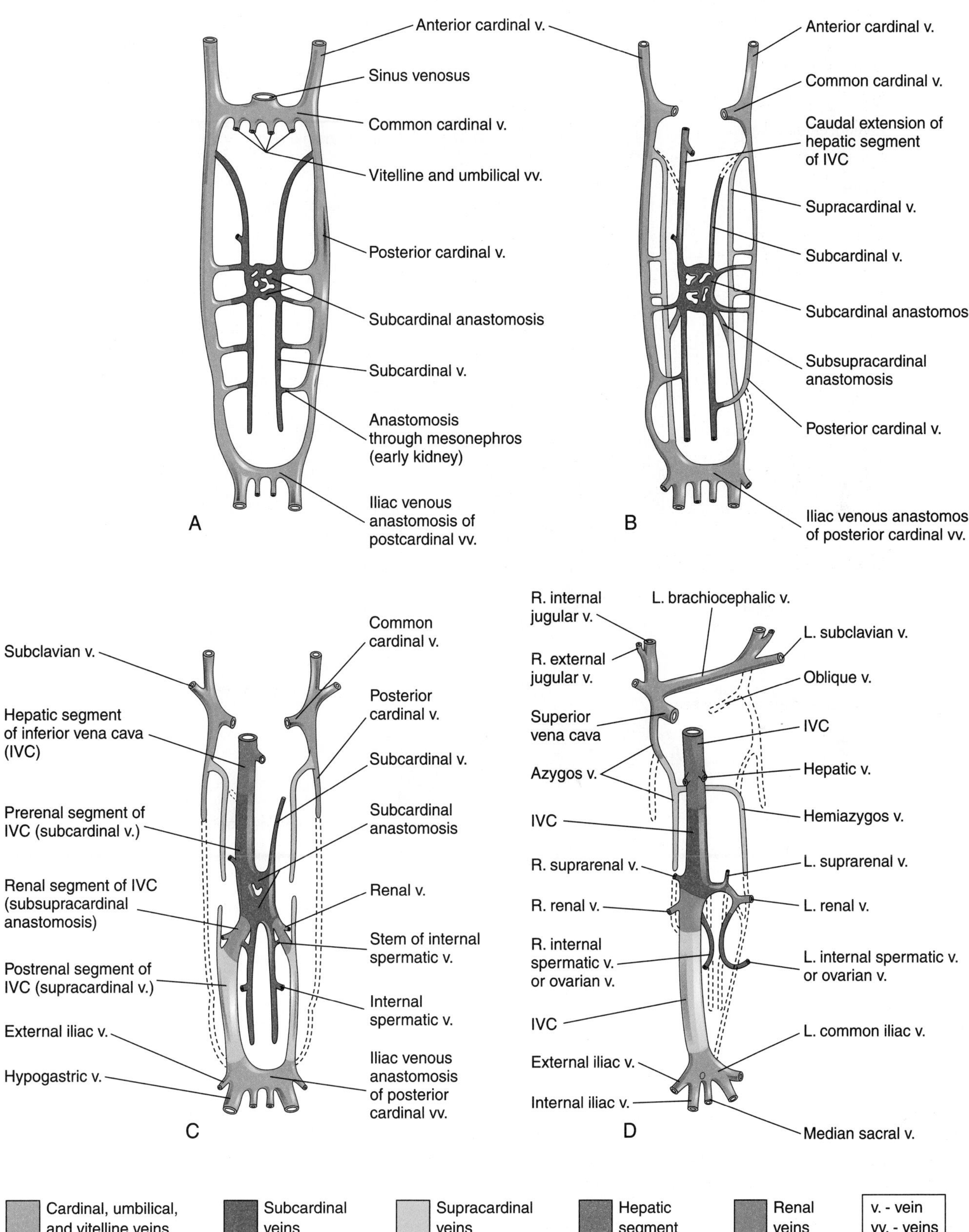

FIGURE 13-4. Illustrations of the primordial veins of the trunk in the human embryo (ventral views). Initially, three systems of veins are present: the umbilical veins from the chorion, the vitelline veins from the umbilical vesicle (yolk sac), and the cardinal veins from the body of the embryo. Next the subcardinal veins appear, and finally the supracardinal veins develop. **A,** At 6 weeks. **B,** At 7 weeks. **C,** At 8 weeks. **D,** Adult. This drawing illustrates the transformations that produce the adult venous pattern. (Modified from Arey LB: Developmental Anatomy, revised 7th ed. Philadelphia, WB Saunders, 1974.)

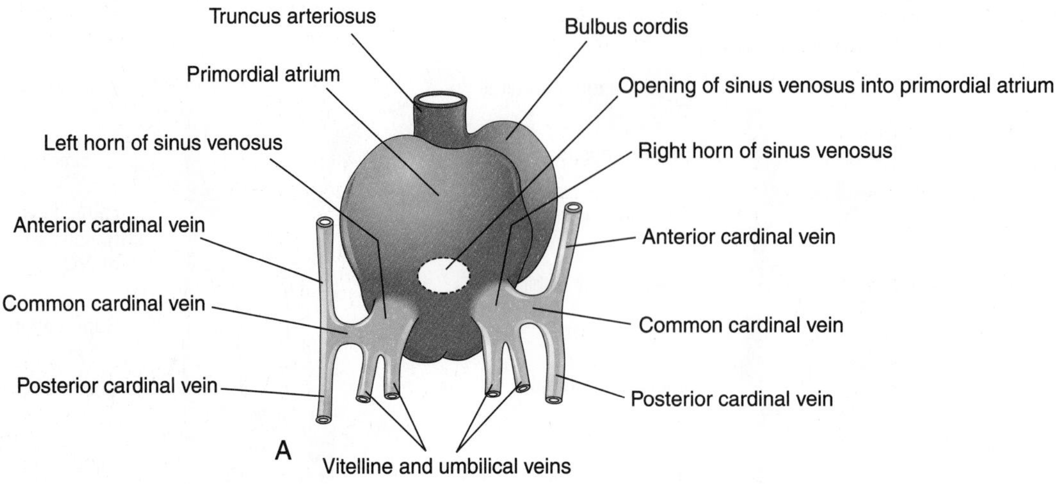

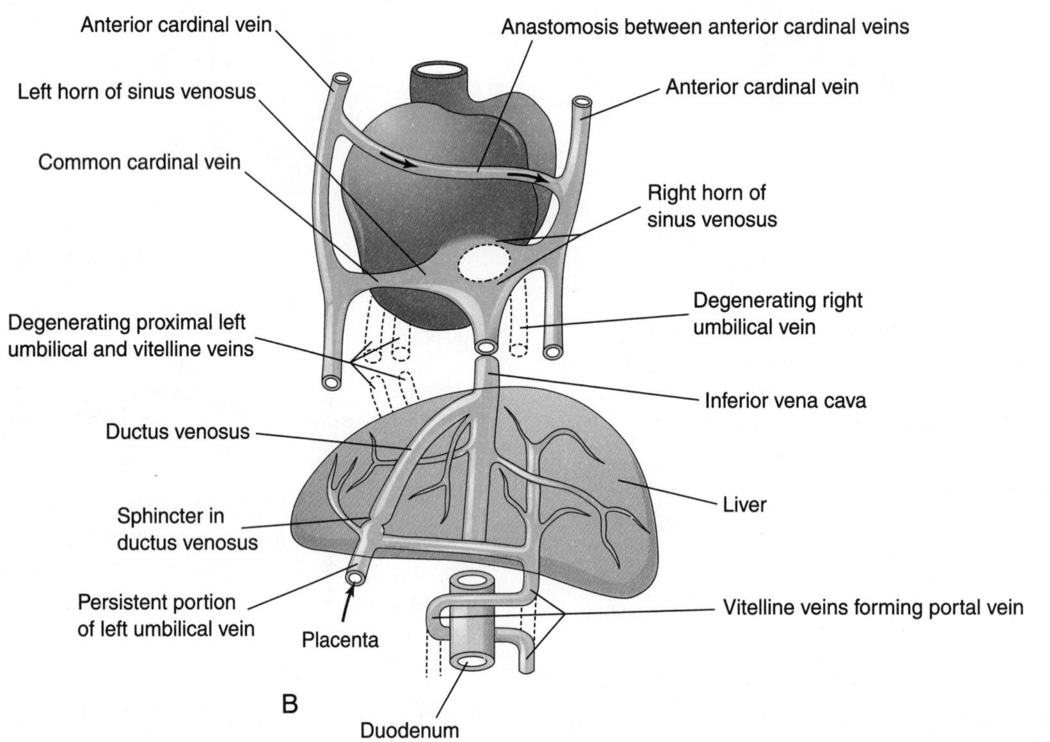

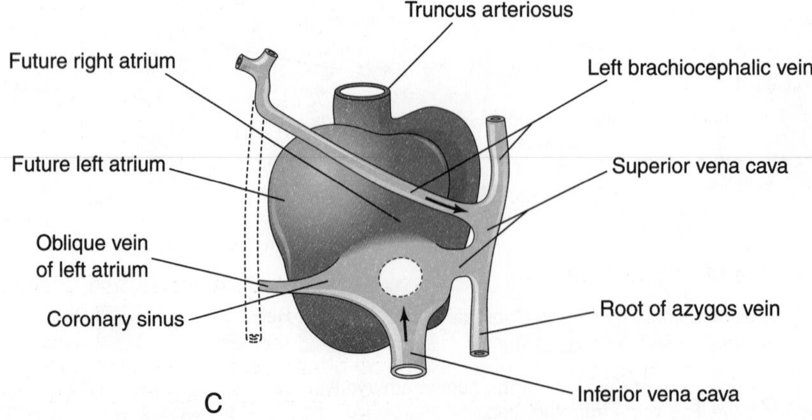

FIGURE 13-5. Dorsal views of the developing heart. **A,** During the fourth week (approximately 24 days), showing the primordial atrium and sinus venosus and veins draining into them. **B,** At 7 weeks, showing the enlarged right sinus horn and venous circulation through the liver. The organs are not drawn to scale. **C,** At 8 weeks, indicating the adult derivatives of the cardinal veins.

The **supracardinal veins** are the last pair of vessels to develop. They become disrupted in the region of the kidneys (see Fig. 13-4*C*). Cranial to this they become united by an anastomosis that is represented in the adult by the **azygos** and **hemiazygos veins** (see Figs. 13-4*D* and 13-5*C*). Caudal to the kidneys, the left supracardinal vein degenerates, but the right supracardinal vein becomes the inferior part of the IVC (see Fig. 13-4*D*).

Development of the Inferior Vena Cava

The IVC forms during a series of changes in the primordial veins of the trunk that occur as blood, returning from the caudal part of the embryo, is shifted from the left to the right side of the body. The IVC is composed of four main segments (see Fig. 13-4*C*):

- A *hepatic segment* derived from the hepatic vein (proximal part of right vitelline vein) and hepatic sinusoids
- A *prerenal segment* derived from the right subcardinal vein
- A *renal segment* derived from the subcardinal-supracardinal anastomosis
- A *postrenal segment* derived from the right supracardinal vein

ANOMALIES OF VENAE CAVAE

Because of the many transformations that occur during the formation of the SVC and IVC, variations in their adult form occur, but they are not common (Fig. 13-6). The most common anomaly of the IVC is for its abdominal course to be interrupted; as a result, blood drains from the lower limbs, abdomen, and pelvis to the heart through the azygos system of veins.

DOUBLE SUPERIOR VENAE CAVAE

Persistence of the left anterior cardinal vein results in a **persistent left SVC**; hence, there are two superior venae cavae (see Fig. 13-6). The anastomosis that usually forms the left brachiocephalic vein is small or absent. The abnormal left SVC, derived from the left anterior cardinal and common cardinal veins, opens into the right atrium through the coronary sinus.

LEFT SUPERIOR VENA CAVA

The left anterior cardinal vein and common cardinal vein may form a left SVC, and the right anterior cardinal vein and common cardinal vein, which usually form the SVC, degenerate. As a result, blood from the right side is carried by the brachiocephalic vein to the unusual left SVC, which empties into the coronary sinus.

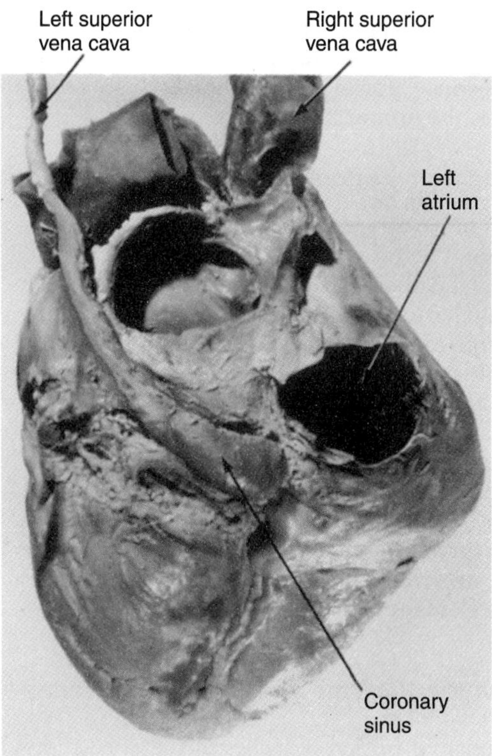

FIGURE 13-6. The posterior aspect of a dissected adult heart with double superior venae cavae. The small anomalous left superior vena cava opens into the coronary sinus.

ABSENCE OF THE HEPATIC SEGMENT OF THE INFERIOR VENA CAVA

Occasionally the hepatic segment of the IVC fails to form. As a result, blood from inferior parts of the body drains into the right atrium through the azygos and hemiazygos veins. The hepatic veins open separately into the right atrium.

DOUBLE INFERIOR VENAE CAVAE

In unusual cases, the IVC inferior to the renal veins is represented by two vessels. Usually the left one is much smaller. This condition probably results from failure of an anastomosis to develop between the veins of the trunk (see Fig. 13-4*B*). As a result, the inferior part of the left supracardinal vein persists as a second IVC.

Pharyngeal Arch Arteries and Other Branches of the Dorsal Aorta

As the pharyngeal arches form during the fourth and fifth weeks, they are supplied by arteries—the **pharyngeal arch arteries**—that arise from the **aortic sac** and terminate in the **dorsal aortas** (see Fig. 13-2). Initially, the paired dorsal aortas run through the entire length of the embryo.

Later, the caudal portions of the dorsal aortas fuse to form a single lower thoracic/abdominal aorta. Of the remaining paired dorsal aortas, the right regresses and the left becomes the primordial aorta.

Intersegmental Arteries

Thirty or so branches of the dorsal aorta, the **intersegmental arteries**, pass between and carry blood to the somites and their derivatives (see Fig. 13-2). The intersegmental arteries in the neck join to form a longitudinal artery on each side, the **vertebral artery**. Most of the original connections of the intersegmental arteries to the dorsal aorta disappear. In the thorax, the intersegmental arteries persist as **intercostal arteries**. Most of the intersegmental arteries in the abdomen become **lumbar arteries**, but the fifth pair of lumbar intersegmental arteries remains as the **common iliac arteries**. In the sacral region, the intersegmental arteries form the **lateral sacral arteries**. The caudal end of the dorsal aorta becomes the **median sacral artery**.

Fate of the Vitelline and Umbilical Arteries

The unpaired ventral branches of the dorsal aorta supply the umbilical vesicle (yolk sac), allantois, and chorion (see Fig. 13-2). The **vitelline arteries** pass to the vesicle and later the primordial gut, which forms from the incorporated part of the umbilical vesicle. Only three vitelline arteries remain: celiac arterial trunk to foregut, superior mesenteric artery to midgut, and inferior mesenteric artery to hindgut.

The paired **umbilical arteries** pass through the connecting stalk (primordial umbilical cord) and become continuous with vessels in the chorion, the embryonic part of the placenta (see Chapter 7). The umbilical arteries carry poorly oxygenated blood to the placenta (see Fig. 13-2). Proximal parts of the umbilical arteries become the **internal iliac arteries** and **superior vesical arteries**, whereas distal parts obliterate after birth and become the **medial umbilical ligaments**. The major changes leading to the definitive arterial system, especially the transformation of the pharyngeal arch arteries, are described later.

LATER DEVELOPMENT OF THE HEART

As the heart tubes fuse, the external layer of the embryonic heart—the **primordial myocardium**—is formed from splanchnic mesoderm surrounding the pericardial coelom (Fig. 13-7*B*). At this stage, the developing heart is composed of a thin endothelial tube, separated from a thick primordial myocardium by gelatinous connective tissue—**cardiac jelly** (see Fig. 13-7*C* and *D*). The endothelial tube becomes the internal endothelial lining of the heart—**endocardium**—and the primordial **myocardium** becomes the muscular wall of the heart or myocardium. The visceral pericardium or **epicardium** is derived from mesothelial cells that arise from the external surface of the sinus venosus and spread over the myocardium (see Fig. 13-7*D* and *F*).

As folding of the head region occurs, the heart and pericardial cavity come to lie ventral to the foregut and caudal to the oropharyngeal membrane (Fig. 13-8). Concurrently, the tubular heart elongates and develops alternate dilations and constrictions (Fig. 13-9*C* to *E*): the **bulbus cordis** (composed of the **truncus arteriosus** [TA], the conus arteriosus, and the conus cordis), ventricle, atrium, and sinus venosus.

The **TA** is continuous cranially with the **aortic sac** (Fig. 13-10*A*), from which the pharyngeal arch arteries arise. The **sinus venosus** receives the umbilical, vitelline, and common cardinal veins from the chorion, umbilical vesicle, and embryo, respectively (see Fig. 13-10*B*). The arterial and venous ends of the heart are fixed by the pharyngeal arches and septum transversum, respectively. Because the bulbus cordis and ventricle grow faster than other regions, the heart bends upon itself, forming a U-shaped **bulboventricular loop** (see Fig. 13-7*E*). The signaling molecule(s) and cellular mechanisms responsible for cardiac looping are largely unknown. As the primordial heart bends, the atrium and sinus venosus come to lie dorsal to the TA, bulbus cordis, and ventricle (see Fig. 13-10*A* and *B*). By this stage the sinus venosus has developed lateral expansions, the right and left **sinus horns**.

As the heart elongates and bends, it gradually invaginates into the **pericardial cavity** (see Figs. 13-7*C* and *D* and 13-8*C*). The heart is initially suspended from the dorsal wall by a mesentery, the **dorsal mesocardium**, but the central part of this mesentery soon degenerates, forming a communication, the **transverse pericardial sinus**, between the right and left sides of the pericardial cavity (see Fig. 13-7*E* and *F*). The heart is now attached only at its cranial and caudal ends.

Circulation through the Primordial Heart

The initial contractions of the heart are of myogenic origin. The muscle layers of the atrium and ventricle are continuous, and contractions occur in peristalsis-like waves that begin in the sinus venosus. At first, circulation through the primordial heart is an ebb-and-flow type; however, by the end of the fourth week, coordinated contractions of the heart result in unidirectional flow. Blood enters the sinus venosus (see Fig. 13-10*A* and *B*) from the:

- Embryo through the common cardinal veins
- Developing placenta through the umbilical veins
- Umbilical vesicle through the vitelline veins

Blood from the sinus venosus enters the **primordial atrium**; flow from it is controlled by **sinuatrial (SA) valves** (Fig. 13-11*A* to *D*). The blood then passes through the **atrioventricular canal** into the **primordial ventricle**. When the ventricle contracts, blood is pumped through the bulbus cordis and TA into the **aortic sac**, from which it is distributed to the pharyngeal arch arteries in the pharyngeal arches (see Fig. 13-10*C*). The blood then passes into the dorsal **aortas** for distribution to the embryo, umbilical vesicle, and placenta (see Fig. 13-2).

Partitioning of the Primordial Heart

Partitioning of the atrioventricular canal, primordial atrium, and ventricle begins around the middle of the

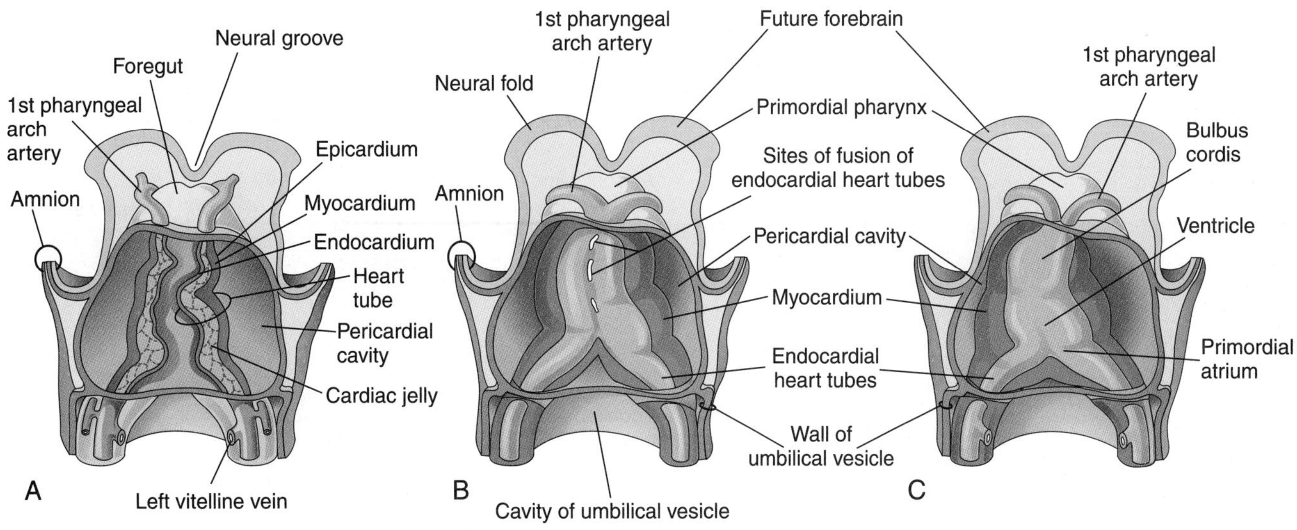

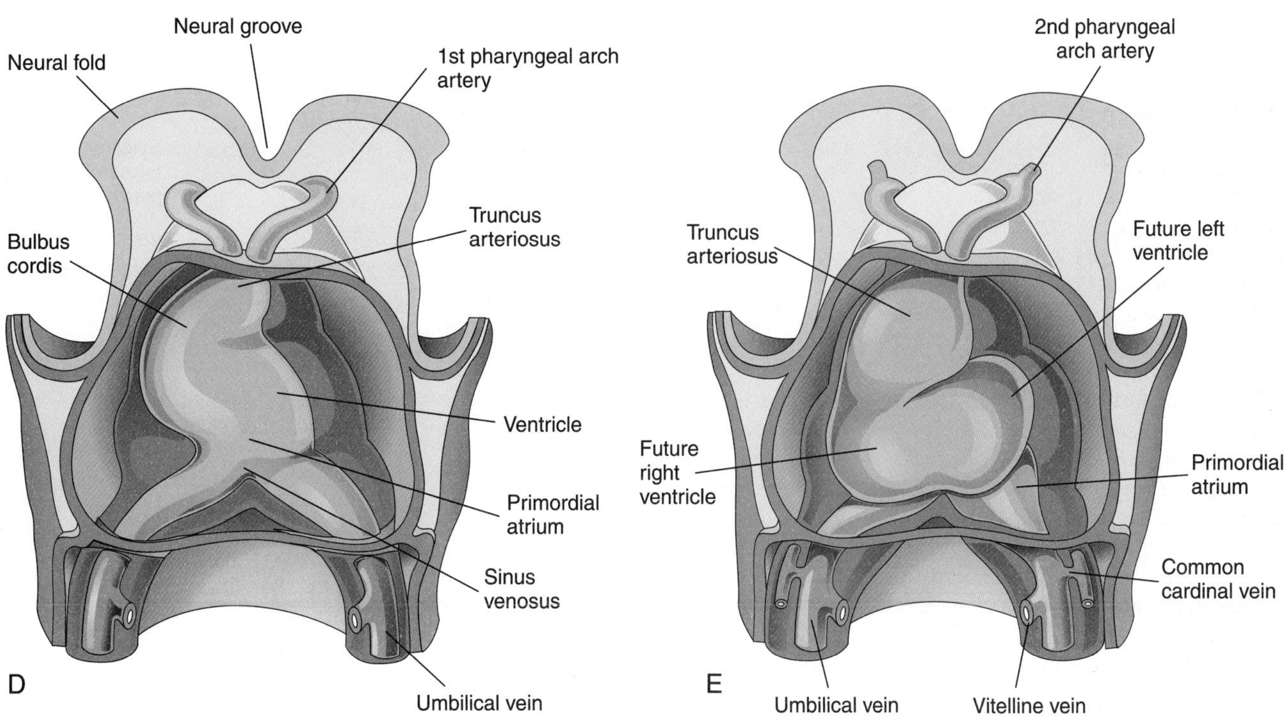

FIGURE 13-7. **A** to **C**, Ventral views of the developing heart and pericardial region (22–35 days). The ventral pericardial wall has been removed to show the developing myocardium and fusion of the two heart tubes to form a single tube. The fusion begins at the cranial ends of the heart tubes and extends caudally until a single tubular heart is formed. The endothelium of the heart tube forms the endocardium of the heart. As the heart elongates, it forms regional segments and bends upon itself, giving rise to an S-shaped heart (**D** and **E**).

fourth week and is essentially completed by the end of the eighth week. Although described separately, these processes occur concurrently.

Partitioning of the Atrioventricular Canal

Toward the end of the fourth week, **endocardial cushions** form on the dorsal and ventral walls of the **atrioventricular (AV) canal**. As these masses of tissue are invaded by mesenchymal cells during the fifth week (see Fig. 13-11*B*), the **AV endocardial cushions** approach each other and fuse, dividing the AV canal into right and left **AV canals** (see Fig. 13-11*C* and *D*). These canals partially separate the primordial atrium from the primordial ventricle, and the endocardial cushions function as AV valves.

The endocardial cushions develop from a specialized extracellular matrix or cardiac jelly. After **inductive signals** from the myocardium of the AV canal, a segment of the inner endocardial cells undergoes **epithelial-mesenchymal transformation**, which then invades the

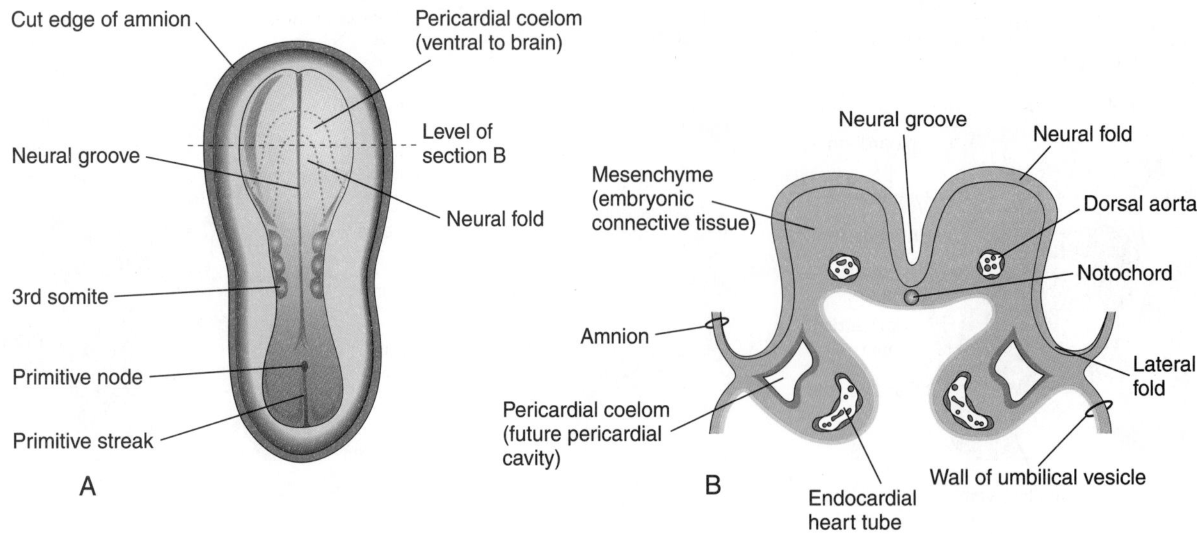

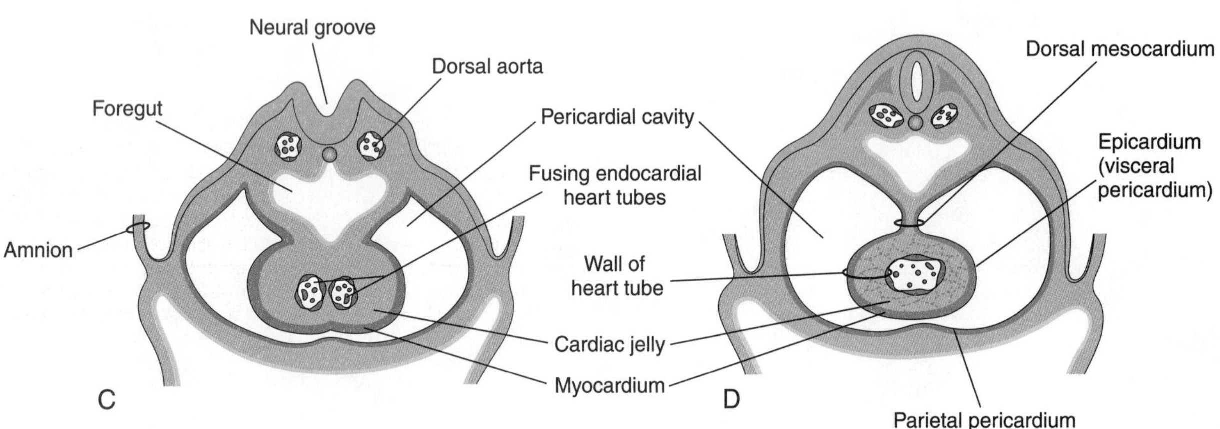

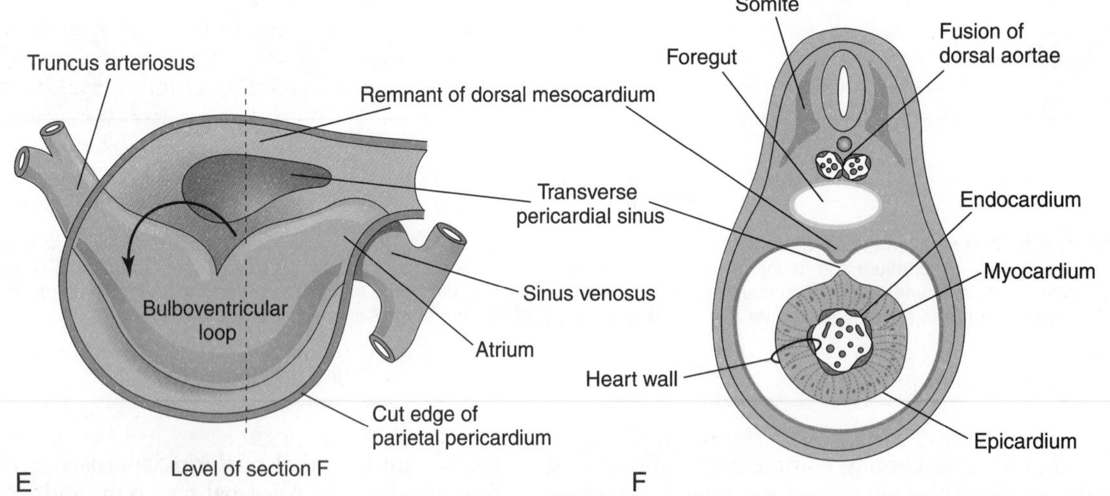

FIGURE 13-8. **A,** Dorsal view of an embryo (approximately 20 days). **B,** Schematic transverse section of the heart region of the embryo illustrated in **A** showing the two endocardial heart tubes and the lateral folds of the body. **C,** Transverse section of a slightly older embryo showing the formation of the pericardial cavity and the fusing heart tubes. **D,** Similar section (approximately 22 days) showing the single heart tube suspended by the dorsal mesocardium. **E,** Schematic drawing of the heart (approximately 28 days) showing degeneration of the central part of the dorsal mesocardium and formation of the transverse sinus of the pericardium. **F,** Transverse section of the embryo at the level shown in **E** showing the layers of the heart wall.

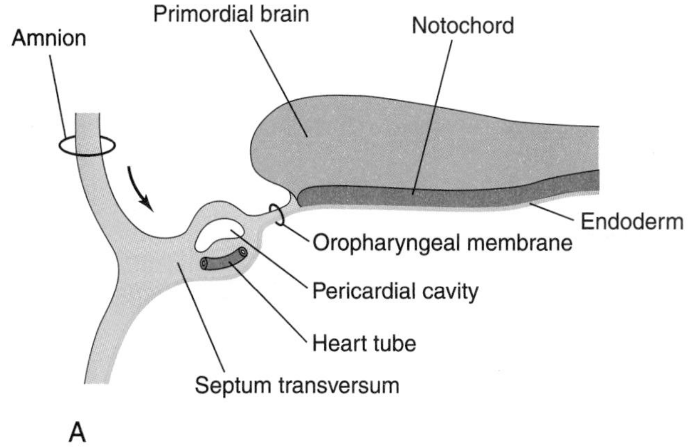

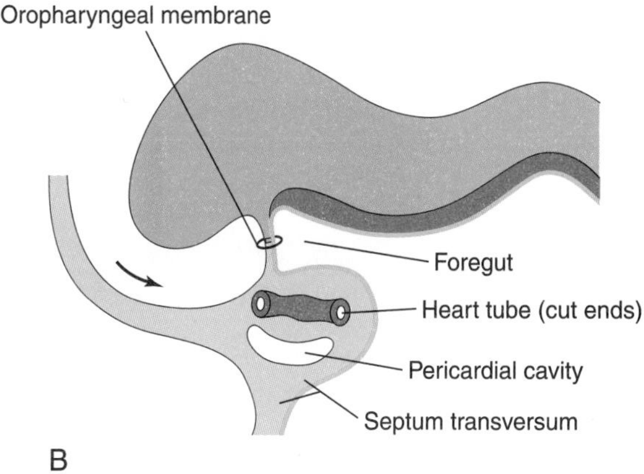

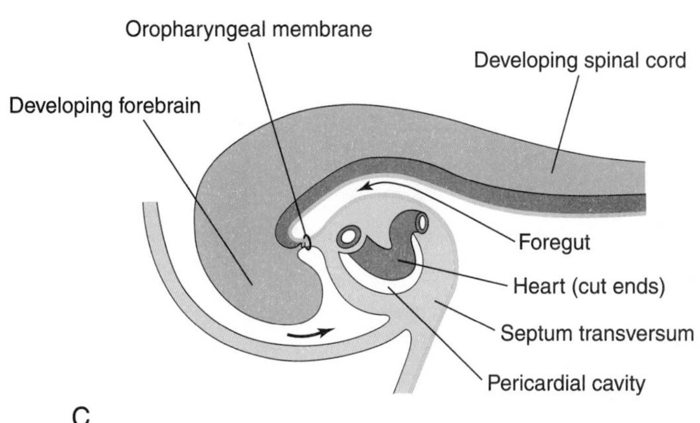

FIGURE 13-9. Longitudinal sections through the cranial half of human embryos during the fourth week showing the effect of the head fold (*arrow*) on the position of the heart and other structures. **A** and **B,** As the head fold develops, the heart tube and pericardial cavity come to lie ventral to the foregut and caudal to the oropharyngeal membrane. **C,** Note that the positions of the pericardial cavity and septum transversum have reversed with respect to each other. The septum transversum now lies posterior to the pericardial cavity, where it will form the central tendon of the diaphragm.

extracellular matrix. The transformed endocardial cushions contribute to the formation of the valves and the membranous septa of the heart. Transforming growth factor β (TGF-β_1 and TGF-β_2), bone morphogenetic proteins (BMP-2A and BMP-4), the zinc finger protein Slug, and an activin-receptor-like kinase (ChALK2) have been reported to be involved in the epithelial-mesenchymal transformation and formation of the endocardial cushions.

Partitioning of the Primordial Atrium

Beginning at the end of the fourth week, the primordial atrium is divided into right and left atria by the formation and subsequent modification and fusion of two septa: the septum primum and septum secundum (Figs. 13-12 and 13-13).

The **septum primum**, a thin crescent-shaped membrane, grows toward the fusing endocardial cushions from the roof of the primordial atrium, partially dividing the common atrium into right and left halves. As this curtain-like septum grows, a large opening, the **foramen primum**, is located between its crescentic free edge and the endocardial cushions (see Figs. 13-12*C* and 13-13*A* to *C*). The foramen primum serves as a shunt, enabling oxygenated blood to pass from the right to the left atrium. The foramen primum becomes progressively smaller and disappears as the septum primum fuses with the fused endocardial cushions to form a **primordial AV septum** (see Fig. 13-13*D* and D_1).

Before the foramen primum disappears, perforations, produced by **apoptosis,** appear in the central part of the septum primum. As the septum fuses with the fused endocardial cushions, these perforations coalesce to form another opening in the septum primum, the **foramen secundum**. Concurrently, the free edge of the septum primum fuses with the left side of the fused endocardial cushions, obliterating the foramen primum (see Figs. 13-12*D* and 13-13*D*). The foramen secundum ensures continued shunting of oxygenated blood from the right to the left atrium.

The **septum secundum**, a thick crescentic muscular fold, grows from the ventrocranial wall of the right atrium, immediately adjacent to the septum primum (see Fig. 13-13D_1). As this thick septum grows during the fifth and sixth weeks, it gradually overlaps the foramen secundum in the septum primum (see Fig. 13-13*E*). The septum secundum forms an incomplete partition between the atria; consequently, an **oval foramen** (Latin [L.], *foramen ovale*) forms. The cranial part of the septum primum, initially attached to the roof of the left atrium, gradually disappears (see Fig. 13-13G_1 and H_1). The remaining part of the septum primum, attached to the fused endocardial cushions, forms the flaplike **valve of the oval foramen**.

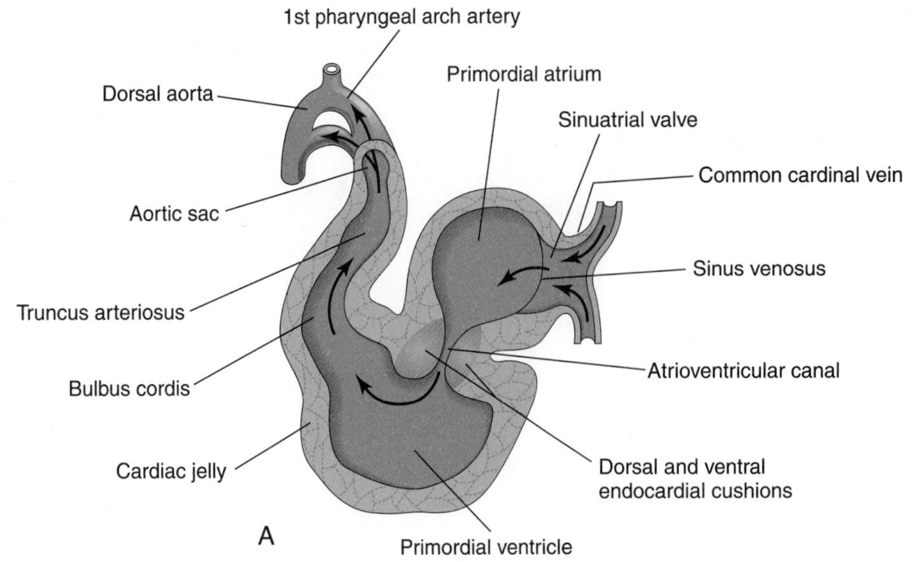

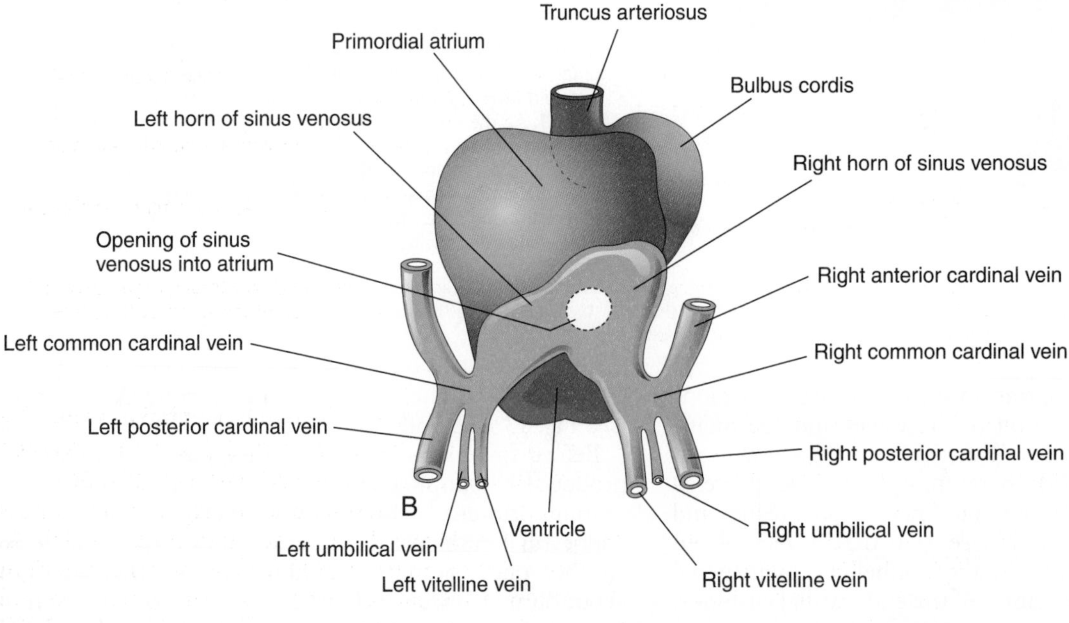

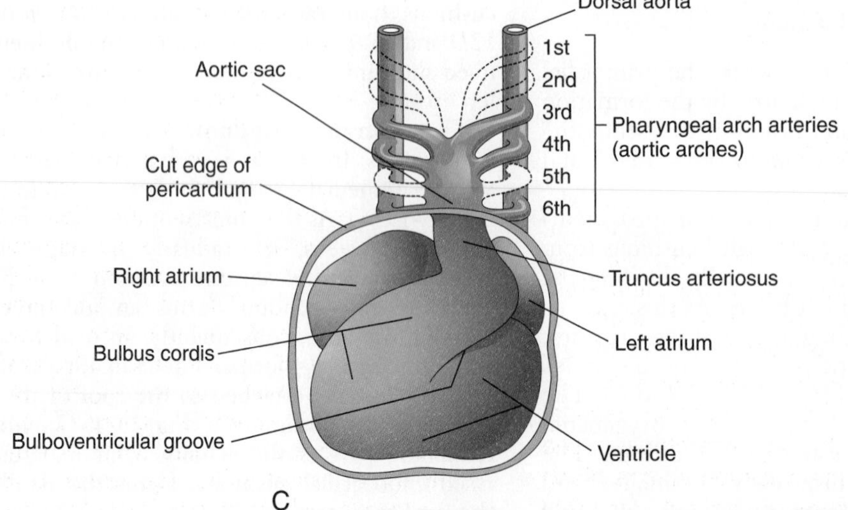

FIGURE 13-10. A, Sagittal section of the primordial heart (approximately 24 days) showing blood flow through it (*arrows*). **B,** Dorsal view of the heart (approximately 26 days) illustrating the horns of the sinus venosus and the dorsal location of the primordial atrium. **C,** Ventral view of the heart and pharyngeal arch arteries (approximately 35 days). The ventral wall of the pericardial sac has been removed to show the heart in the pericardial cavity.

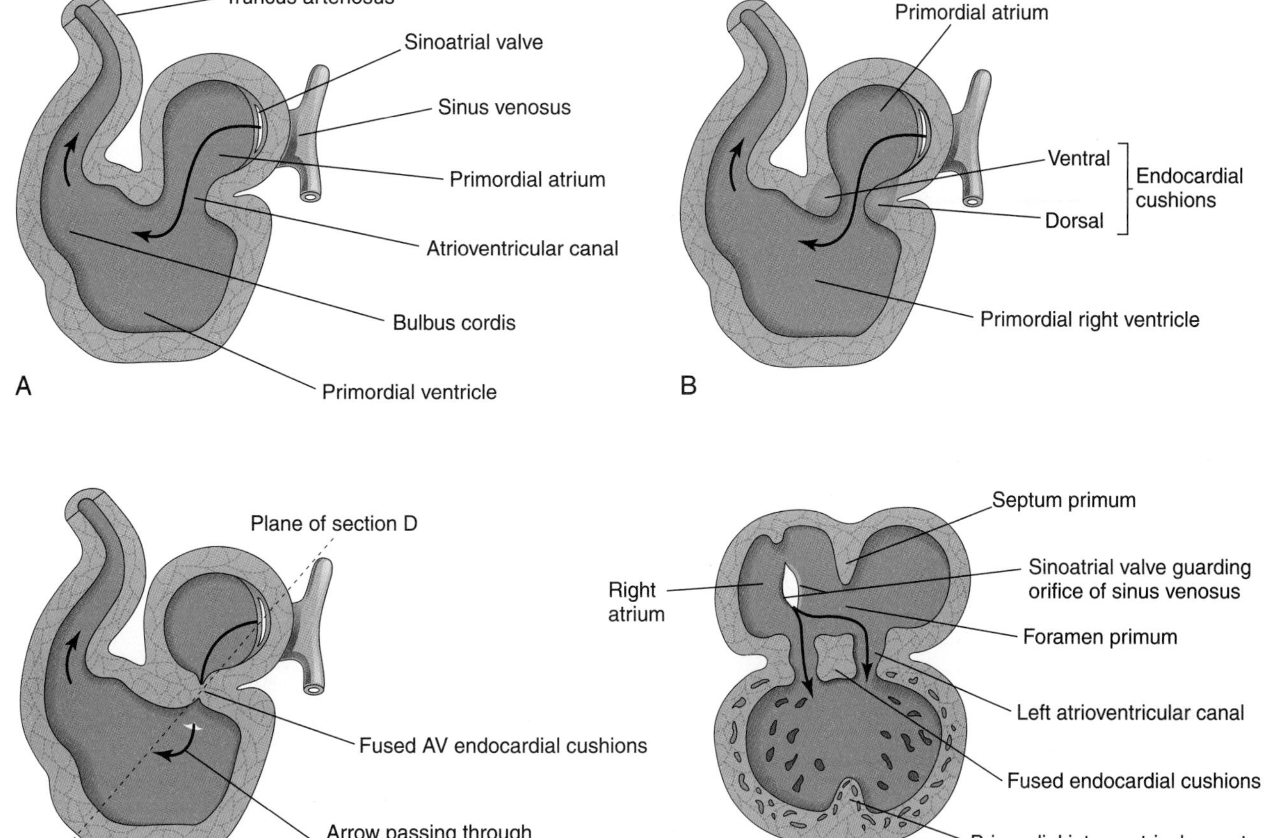

FIGURE 13-11. **A** to **C,** Sagittal sections of the primordial heart during the fourth and fifth weeks illustrating blood flow through the heart and division of the atrioventricular canal. The *arrows* are passing through the sinuatrial (SA) orifice. **D,** Coronal section of the heart at the plane shown in **C**. Note that the interatrial and interventricular septa have started to develop.

Before birth the oval foramen allows most of the oxygenated blood entering the right atrium from the IVC to pass into the left atrium (Fig. 13-14*A*) and prevents the passage of blood in the opposite direction because the septum primum closes against the relatively rigid septum secundum (see Fig. 13-14*B*). After birth, the oval foramen functionally closes due to higher pressure in the left atrium that the right. Approximately 3 months of age, the valve of the oval foramen fuses with the septum secundum, forming the **oval fossa** (see Fig. 13-52).

Changes in the Sinus Venosus

Initially, the sinus venosus opens into the center of the dorsal wall of the primordial atrium, and its right and left sinual horns are approximately the same size (see Fig. 13-5*A*). Progressive enlargement of the right sinus horn results from two **left-to-right shunts of blood**:

- The *first shunt* results from transformation of the vitelline and umbilical veins, discussed previously.
- The *second shunt* occurs when the anterior cardinal veins become connected by an anastomosis (see Fig. 13-5*B* and *C*). This communication shunts blood from the left to the right anterior cardinal vein. This shunt becomes the **left brachiocephalic vein**. The right anterior cardinal vein and the right common cardinal vein become the SVC (see Fig. 13-15*C*).

By the end of the fourth week, the right sinual horn is noticeably larger than the left sinus horn (Fig. 13-15*A*). As this occurs, the **sinuatrial (SA) orifice** moves to the right and opens in the part of the primordial atrium that will become the adult right atrium (see Figs. 13-11 and 13-15*C*). As the right sinual horn enlarges, it receives all the blood from the head and neck through the SVC and from the placenta and caudal regions of the body through the IVC. Initially, the **sinus venosus** is a separate chamber of the heart and opens into the dorsal wall of the right atrium (see Fig. 13-10*A* and *B*). The left horn becomes the **coronary sinus**, and the right sinus horn becomes incorporated into the wall of the right atrium (see Fig. 13-15*B* and *C*).

Because it is derived from the sinus venosus, the smooth part of the wall of the right atrium is called the **sinus venarum** (see Fig. 13-15*B* and *C*). The remainder of the anterior internal surface of the wall of the atrium and the conical muscular pouch, the **right auricle**, have a rough trabeculated appearance. These two parts are derived from the primordial atrium. The smooth part and the rough part are demarcated internally in the right atrium by a vertical ridge, the **crista terminalis**, and externally by a shallow groove, the **sulcus terminalis**.

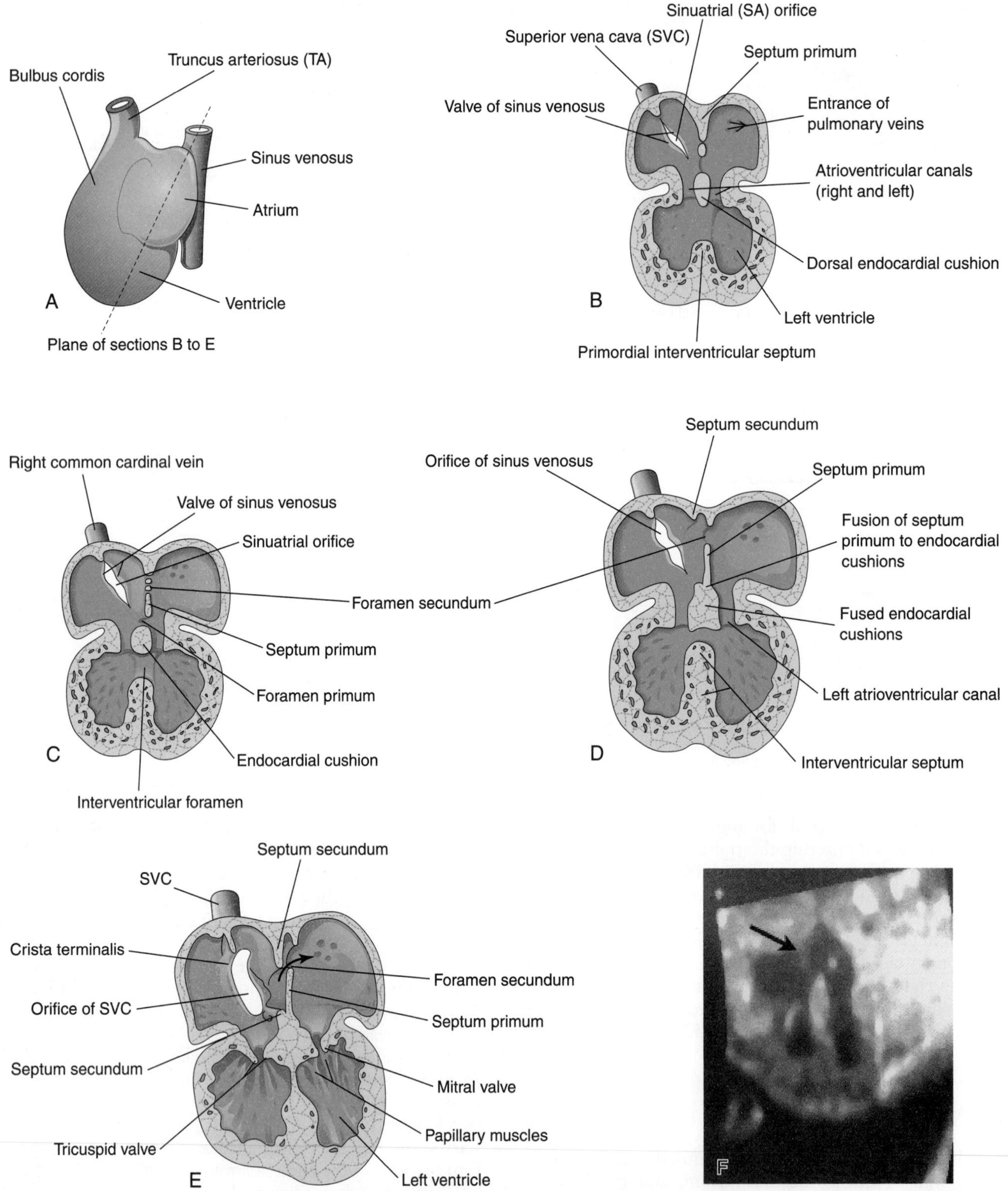

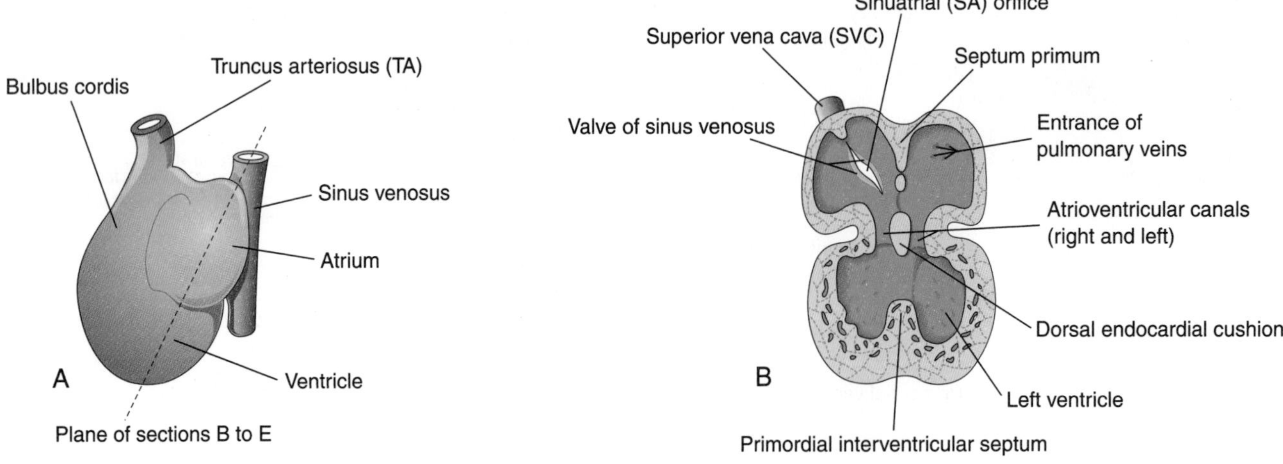

FIGURE 13-12. Drawings of the developing heart showing partitioning of the atrioventricular canal, primordial atrium and ventricle. **A,** Sketch showing the plane of the sections. **B,** Frontal section of the heart during the fourth week (approximately 28 days) showing the early appearance of the septum primum, interventricular septum, and dorsal endocardial cushion. **C,** Similar section of the heart (approximately 32 days) showing perforations in the dorsal part of the septum primum. **D,** Section of the heart (approximately 35 days) showing the foramen secundum. **E,** At approximately 8 weeks, showing the heart after it is partitioned into four chambers. The *arrow* indicates the flow of well-oxygenated blood from the right to the left atrium. **F,** Sonogram of a second trimester fetus showing the four chambers of the heart. Note the septum secundum (*arrow*) and the descending aorta. (Courtesy of Dr. G. J. Reid, Department of Obstetrics, Gynecology and Reproductive Sciences, University of Manitoba, Women's Hospital, Winnipeg, Manitoba, Canada.)

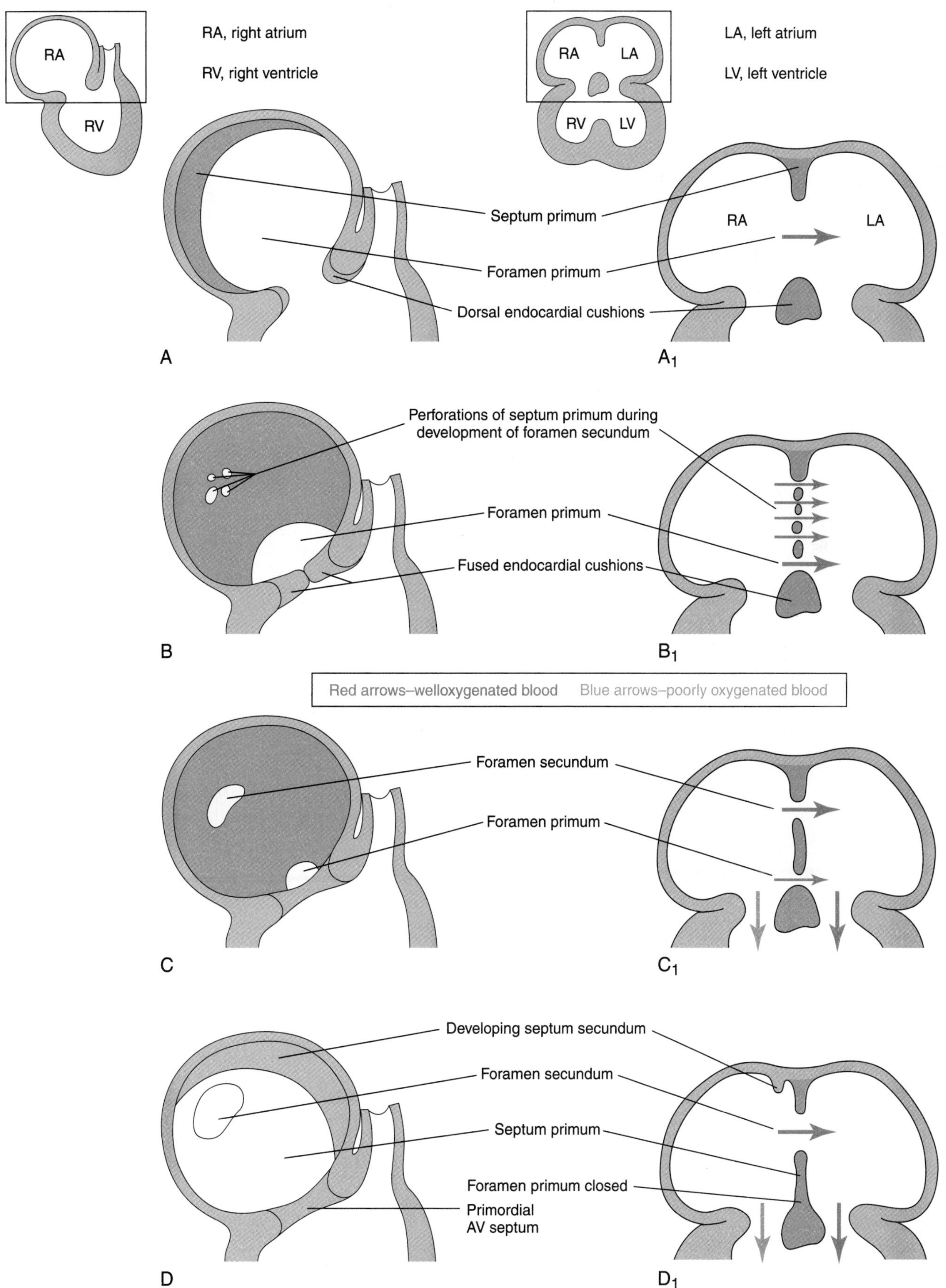

FIGURE 13-13. Diagrammatic sketches illustrating progressive stages in partitioning of the primordial atrium. **A** to **H,** Views of the developing interatrial septum as viewed from the right side. $\mathbf{A_1}$ to $\mathbf{H_1}$ are coronal sections of the developing interatrial septum. As the septum secundum grows, note that it overlaps the opening in the septum primum (foramen secundum). Observe the valve of the oval foramen in $\mathbf{G_1}$ and $\mathbf{H_1}$. When pressure in the right atrium exceeds that in the left atrium, blood passes from the right to the left side of the heart. When the pressures are equal or higher in the left atrium, the valve closes the oval foramen ($\mathbf{G_1}$). *Continued*

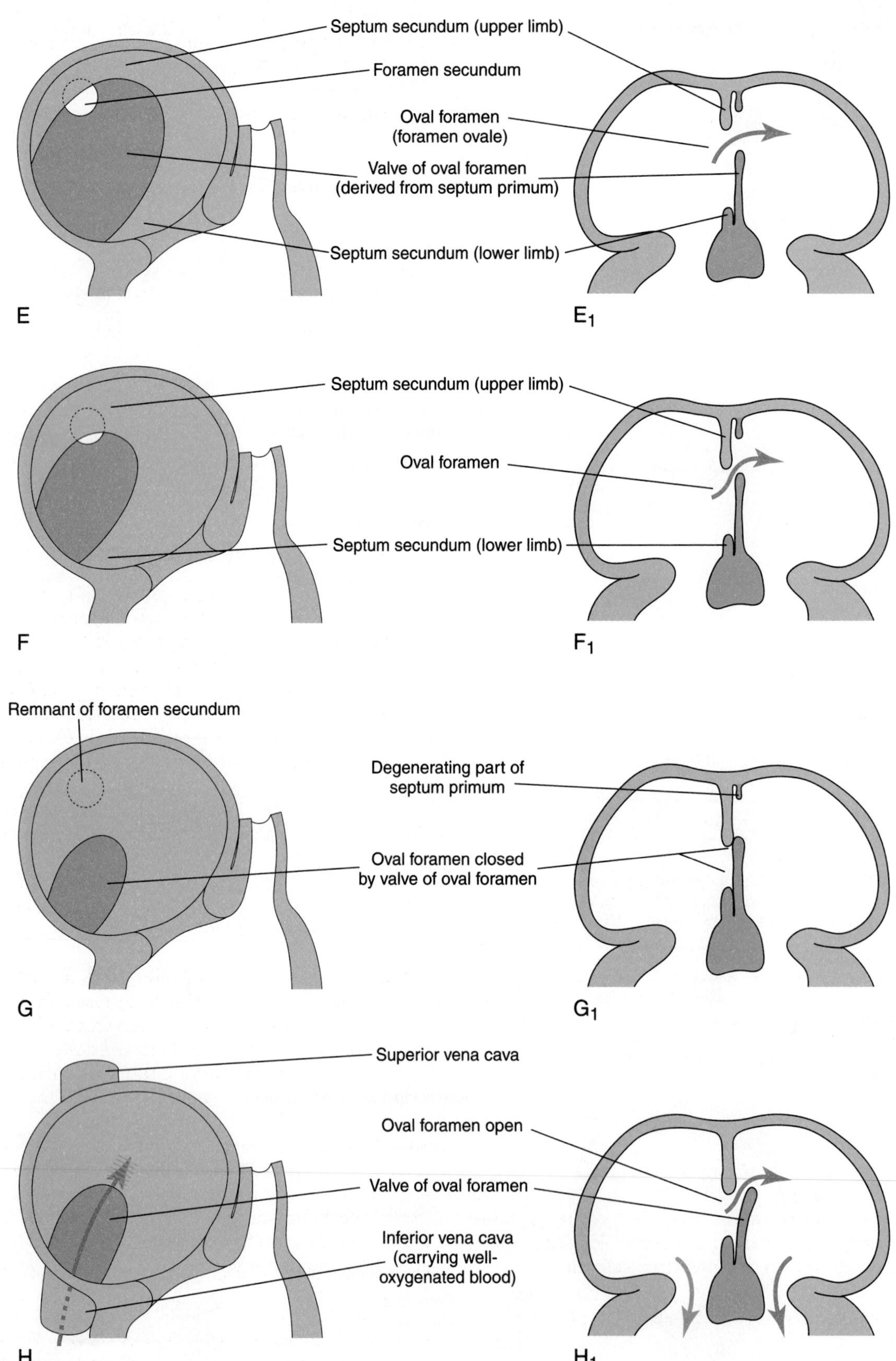

Figure 13-13, *cont'd*.

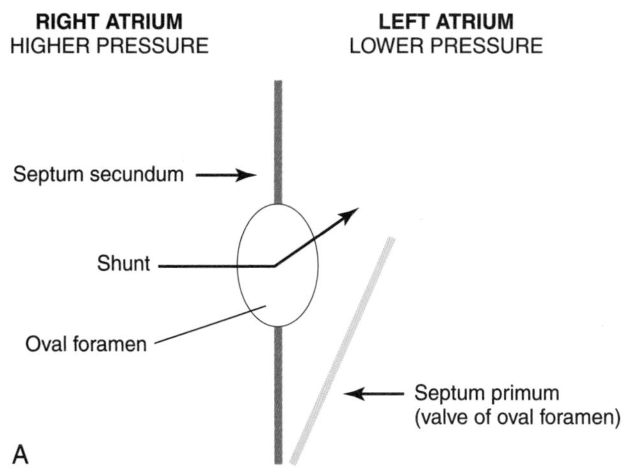

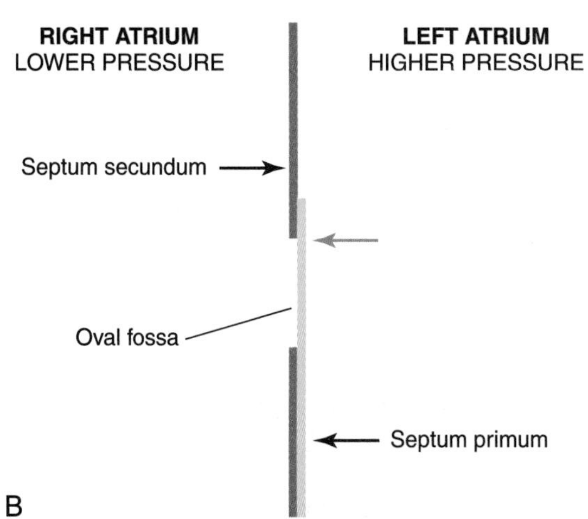

FIGURE 13-14. Diagrams illustrating the relationship of the septum primum to the oval foramen and septum secundum. **A,** Before birth, well-oxygenated blood is shunted from the right atrium through the oval foramen into the left atrium when the pressure increases. When the pressure decreases in the right atrium, the flaplike valve of the oval foramen is pressed against the relatively rigid septum secundum. This closes the oval foramen. **B,** After birth, the pressure in the left atrium increases as the blood returns from the lungs. Eventually the septum primum is pressed against the septum secundum and adheres to it, permanently closing the oval foramen and forming the oval fossa.

The *crista terminalis* represents the cranial part of the right SA valve (see Fig. 13-15*C*); the caudal part of this valve forms the valves of the IVC and coronary sinus. The left SA valve fuses with the septum secundum and is incorporated with it into the interatrial septum.

Primordial Pulmonary Vein and Formation of the Left Atrium

Most of the wall of the left atrium is smooth because it is formed by incorporation of the **primordial pulmonary vein** (Fig. 13-16). This vein develops as an outgrowth of the dorsal atrial wall, just to the left of the septum primum. As the atrium expands, the primordial pulmonary vein and its main branches are incorporated into the wall of the left atrium. As a result, four pulmonary veins are formed (see Fig. 13-16*C* and *D*).

Molecular studies have confirmed that atrial myoblasts migrate into the walls of the pulmonary veins. The functional significance of this pulmonary cardiac muscle (pulmonary myocardium) is uncertain. The small left auricle is derived from the primordial atrium; its internal surface has a rough trabeculated appearance.

ANOMALOUS PULMONARY VENOUS CONNECTIONS

In total anomalous pulmonary venous connections, none of the pulmonary veins connects with the left atrium. They open into the right atrium or into one of the systemic veins or into both. In partial anomalous pulmonary venous connections, one or more pulmonary veins have similar anomalous connections; the others have normal connections.

Partitioning of the Primordial Ventricle

Division of the primordial ventricle is first indicated by a median ridge—the muscular **interventricular (IV) septum**—in the floor of the ventricle near its apex (see Fig. 13-12*B*). The IV septum has a concave free edge (Fig. 13-17*A*). Initially, the IV septum attains most of its height from dilation of the ventricles on each side of the muscular IV septum (see Fig. 13-17*B*). Later, there is active proliferation of myoblasts in the septum, which increase its size. Until the seventh week, there is a crescent-shaped **IV foramen** between the free edge of the IV septum and the fused endocardial cushions. The IV foramen permits communication between the right and left ventricles (Figs. 13-17 and 13-18*B*). The IV foramen usually closes by the end of the seventh week as the bulbar ridges fuse with the endocardial cushion (Fig. 13-18*C* to *E*).

Closure of the IV foramen and formation of the membranous part of the IV septum result from the fusion of tissues from three sources: the right bulbar ridge, the left bulbar ridge, and the endocardial cushion.

The **membranous part of the IV septum** is derived from an extension of tissue from the right side of the endocardial cushion to the muscular part of the IV septum. This tissue merges with the **aorticopulmonary septum** and the thick muscular part of the IV septum (Figs. 13-18*E* and 13-19*C*). After closure of the IV foramen and formation of the membranous part of the IV septum, the pulmonary trunk is in communication with the right ventricle and the aorta communicates with the left ventricle (see Fig. 13-18*E*).

Cavitation of the ventricular walls forms a spongework of muscular bundles—**trabeculae carneae**. Some of these bundles become the **papillary muscles** and **tendinous cords** (L. *chordae tendineae*). The tendinous cords run from the papillary muscles to the AV valves (see Fig. 13-19*C* and *D*).

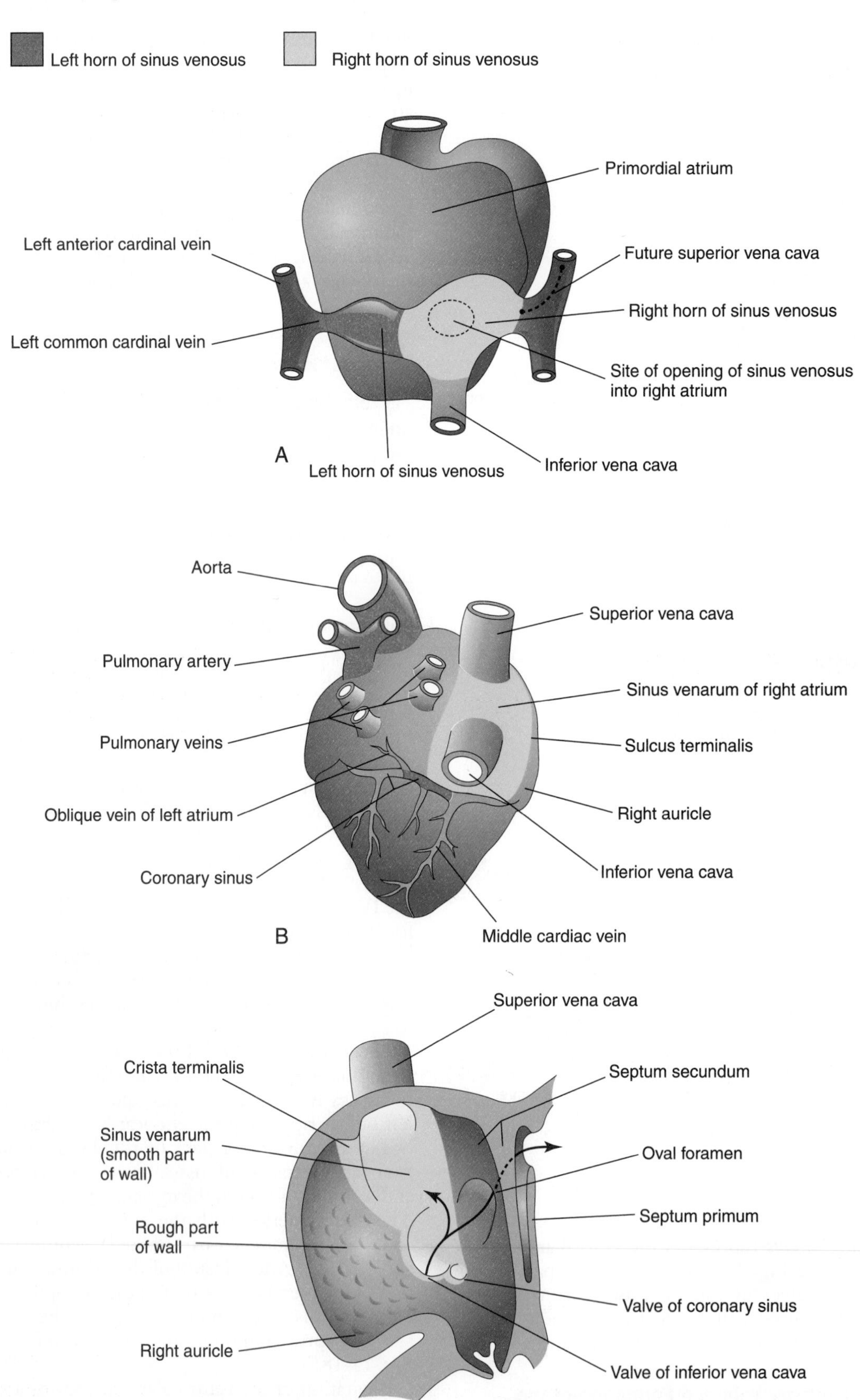

FIGURE 13-15. Diagrams illustrating the fate of the sinus venosus. **A,** Dorsal view of the heart (approximately 26 days) showing the primordial atrium and sinus venosus. **B,** Dorsal view at 8 weeks after incorporation of the right sinus horn into the right atrium. The left sinus horn has become the coronary sinus. **C,** Internal view of the fetal right atrium showing (1) the smooth part of the wall of the right atrium (sinus venarum) derived from the right sinus horn and (2) the crista terminalis and the valves of the inferior vena cava and coronary sinus derived from the right sinuatrial valve. The primordial right atrium becomes the right auricle, a conical muscular pouch.

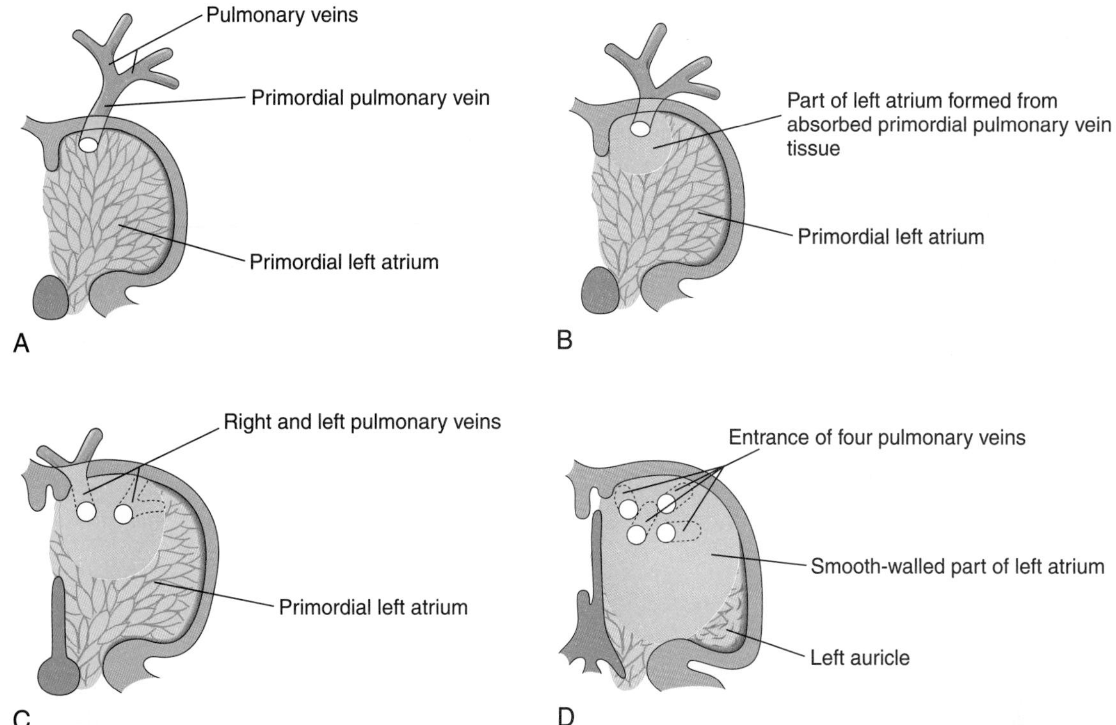

FIGURE 13-16. Diagrammatic sketches illustrating absorption of the pulmonary vein into the left atrium. **A,** At 5 weeks, showing the primordial pulmonary vein opening into the primordial left atrium. **B,** Later stage showing partial absorption of the primordial pulmonary vein. **C,** At 6 weeks, showing the openings of two pulmonary veins into the left atrium resulting from absorption of the primordial pulmonary vein. **D,** At 8 weeks, showing four pulmonary veins with separate atrial orifices. The primordial left atrium becomes the left auricle, a tubular appendage of the atrium. Most of the left atrium is formed by absorption of the primordial pulmonary vein and its branches.

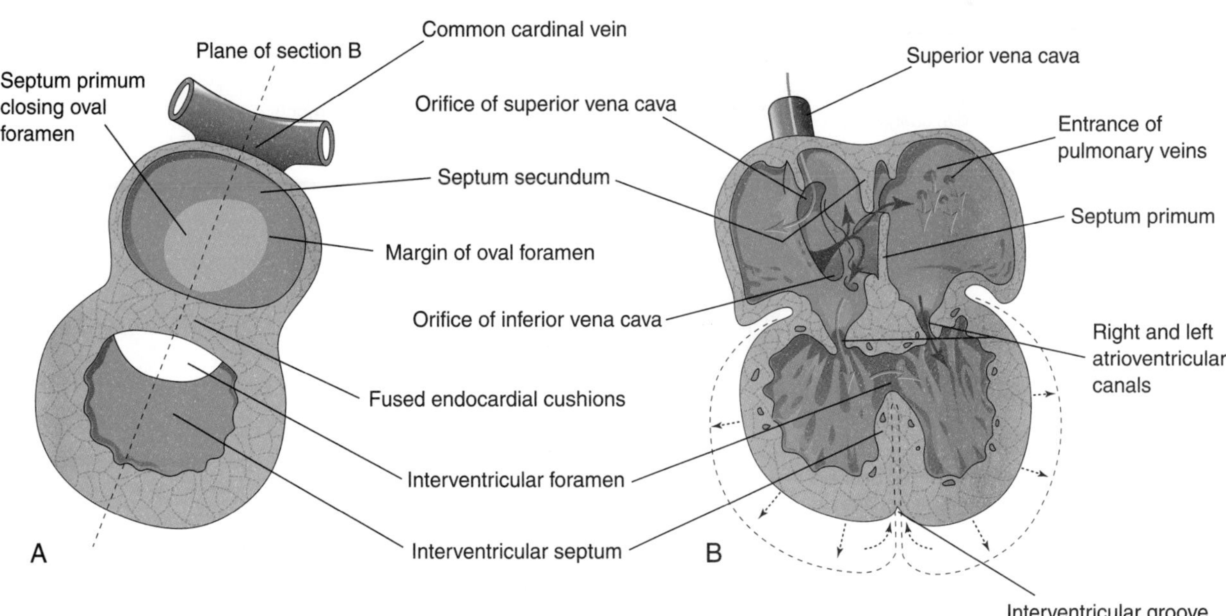

FIGURE 13-17. Schematic diagrams illustrating partitioning of the primordial heart. **A,** Sagittal section late in the fifth week showing the cardiac septa and foramina. **B,** Coronal section at a slightly later stage illustrating the directions of blood flow through the heart (*blue arrows*) and expansion of the ventricles (*black arrows*).

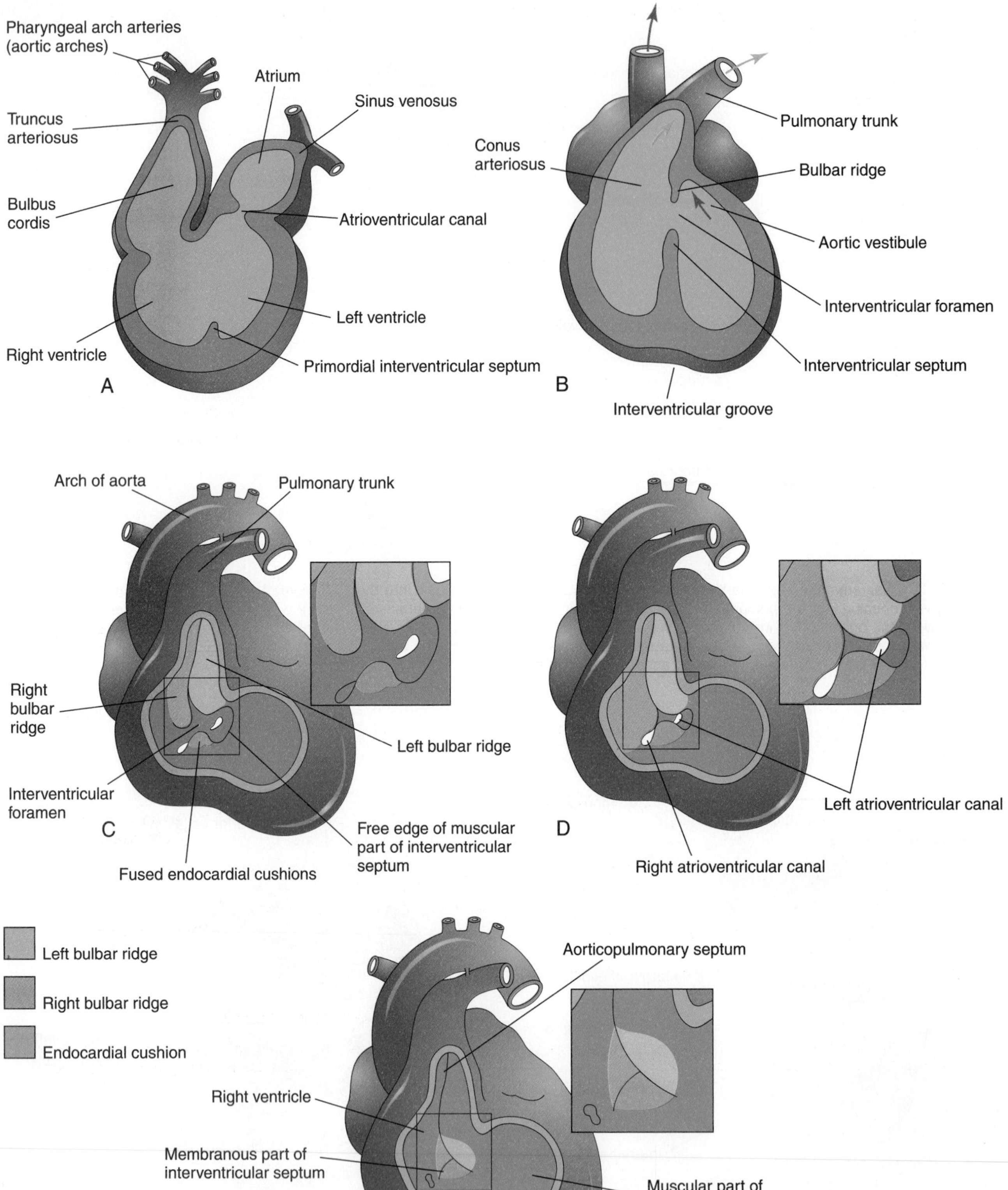

FIGURE 13-18. Sketches illustrating incorporation of the bulbus cordis into the ventricles and partitioning of the bulbus cordis and truncus arteriosus into the aorta and pulmonary trunk. **A,** Sagittal section at 5 weeks showing the bulbus cordis as one of the chambers of the primordial heart. **B,** Schematic coronal section at 6 weeks, after the bulbus cordis has been incorporated into the ventricles to become the conus arteriosus (infundibulum) of the right ventricle and the aortic vestibule of the left ventricle. The *arrow* indicates blood flow. **C** to **E,** Schematic drawings illustrating closure of the interventricular foramen and formation of the membranous part of the interventricular septum. The walls of the truncus arteriosus, bulbus cordis, and right ventricle have been removed. **C,** At 5 weeks, showing the bulbar ridges and fused endocardial cushions. **D,** At 6 weeks, showing how proliferation of subendocardial tissue diminishes the interventricular foramen. **E,** At 7 weeks, showing the fused bulbar ridges, the membranous part of the interventricular septum formed by extensions of tissue from the right side of the endocardial cushions, and closure of the interventricular foramen.

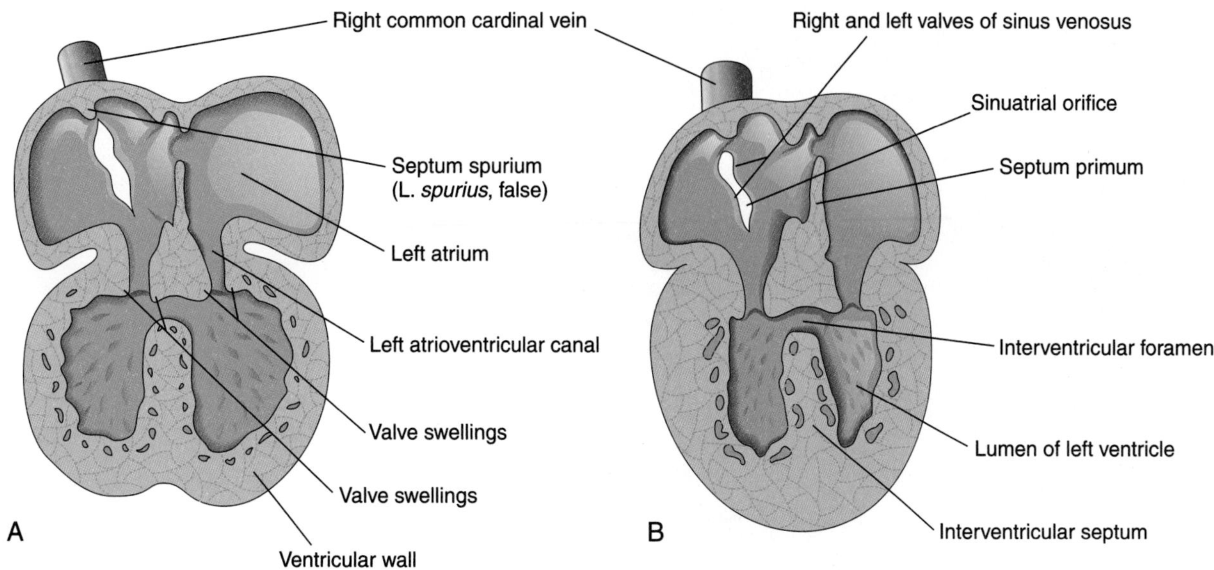

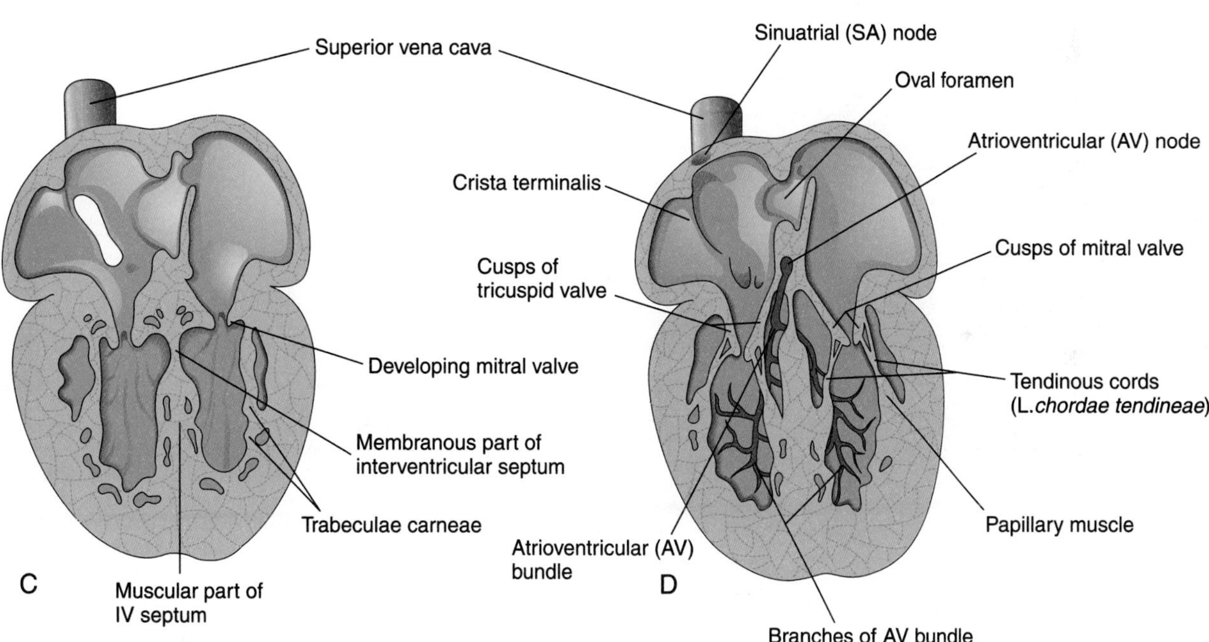

FIGURE 13-19. Schematic sections of the heart illustrating successive stages in the development of the atrioventricular valves, tendinous cords, and papillary muscles. **A,** At 5 weeks. **B,** At 6 weeks. **C,** At 7 weeks. **D,** At 20 weeks, showing the conducting system of the heart.

FETAL CARDIAC ULTRASONOGRAPHY

Cardiac screening using high-resolution real-time ultrasonography is usually performed between 18 and 22 weeks of gestation (Fig. 13-20) because the heart is large enough to examine easily; however, fetal cardiac anatomy can be studied as early as 16 weeks if necessary.

Partitioning of the Bulbus Cordis and Truncus Arteriosus

During the fifth week, active proliferation of mesenchymal cells in the walls of the bulbus cordis results in the formation of **bulbar ridges** (conotruncal ridges) (Figs. 13-18*C* and *D* and 13-21*B* and *C*). Similar ridges that are continuous with the bulbar ridges form in the TA. The bulbar and **truncal ridges** are derived largely from neural crest mesenchyme. **Neural crest cells** migrate through the

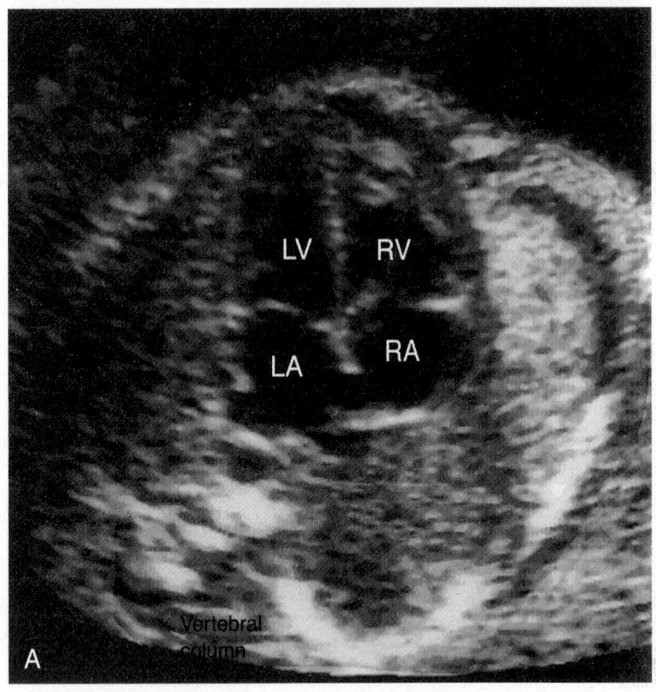

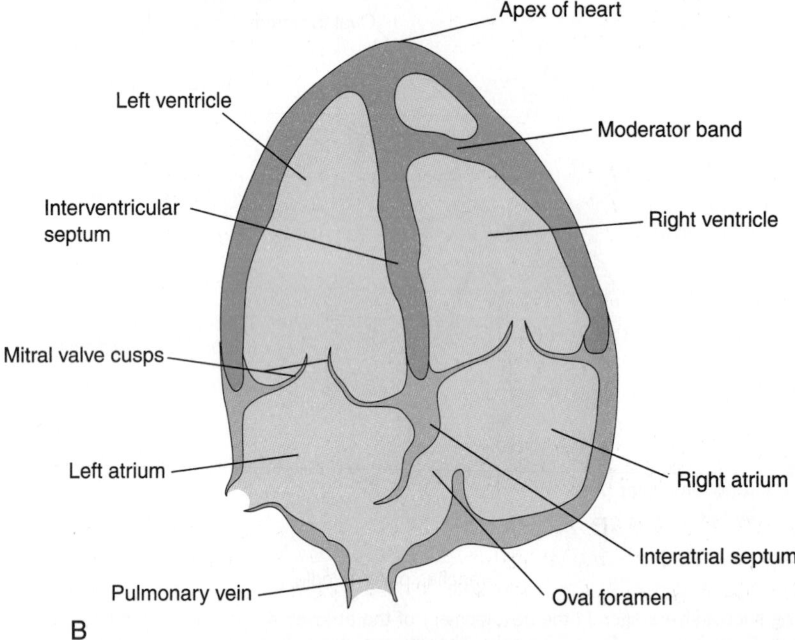

FIGURE 13-20. **A,** Ultrasound image showing the four-chamber view of the heart in a fetus of approximately 20 weeks' gestation. **B,** Orientation sketch (modified from the AIUM Technical Bulletin, Performance of the Basic Fetal Cardiac Ultrasound Examination). The scan was obtained across the fetal thorax. The ventricles and atria are well formed and two atrioventricular (AV) valves are present. The moderator band is one of the trabeculae carneae that carries part of the right branch of the AV bundle. LA, left atrium; LV, left ventricle; RA, right atrium; RV, right ventricle. (Courtesy of Wesley Lee, MD, Division of Fetal Imaging, William Beaumont Hospital, Royal Oak, MI.)

primordial pharynx and pharyngeal arches to reach the ridges. As this occurs, the bulbar and truncal ridges undergo a 180-degree spiraling. The spiral orientation of the bulbar and truncal ridges, possibly caused in part by the streaming of blood from the ventricles, results in the formation of a spiral **aorticopulmonary septum** when the ridges fuse (see Fig. 13-21*D* to *G*). This septum divides the bulbus cordis and TA into two arterial channels, the ascending aorta and pulmonary trunk. Because of the spiraling of the aorticopulmonary septum, the **pulmonary trunk** twists around the **ascending aorta** (see Fig. 13-21*H*). The bulbus cordis is incorporated into the walls of the definitive ventricles (see Fig. 13-18*A* and *B*):

- In the right ventricle, the bulbus cordis is represented by the **conus arteriosus** (infundibulum), which gives origin to the pulmonary trunk.
- In the left ventricle, the bulbus cordis forms the walls of the **aortic vestibule**, the part of the ventricular cavity just inferior to the aortic valve.

Development of the Cardiac Valves

When partitioning of the TA is nearly completed (see Fig. 13-21*A* to *C*), the **semilunar valves** begin to develop from three swellings of subendocardial tissue around the orifices of the aorta and pulmonary trunk. These swellings

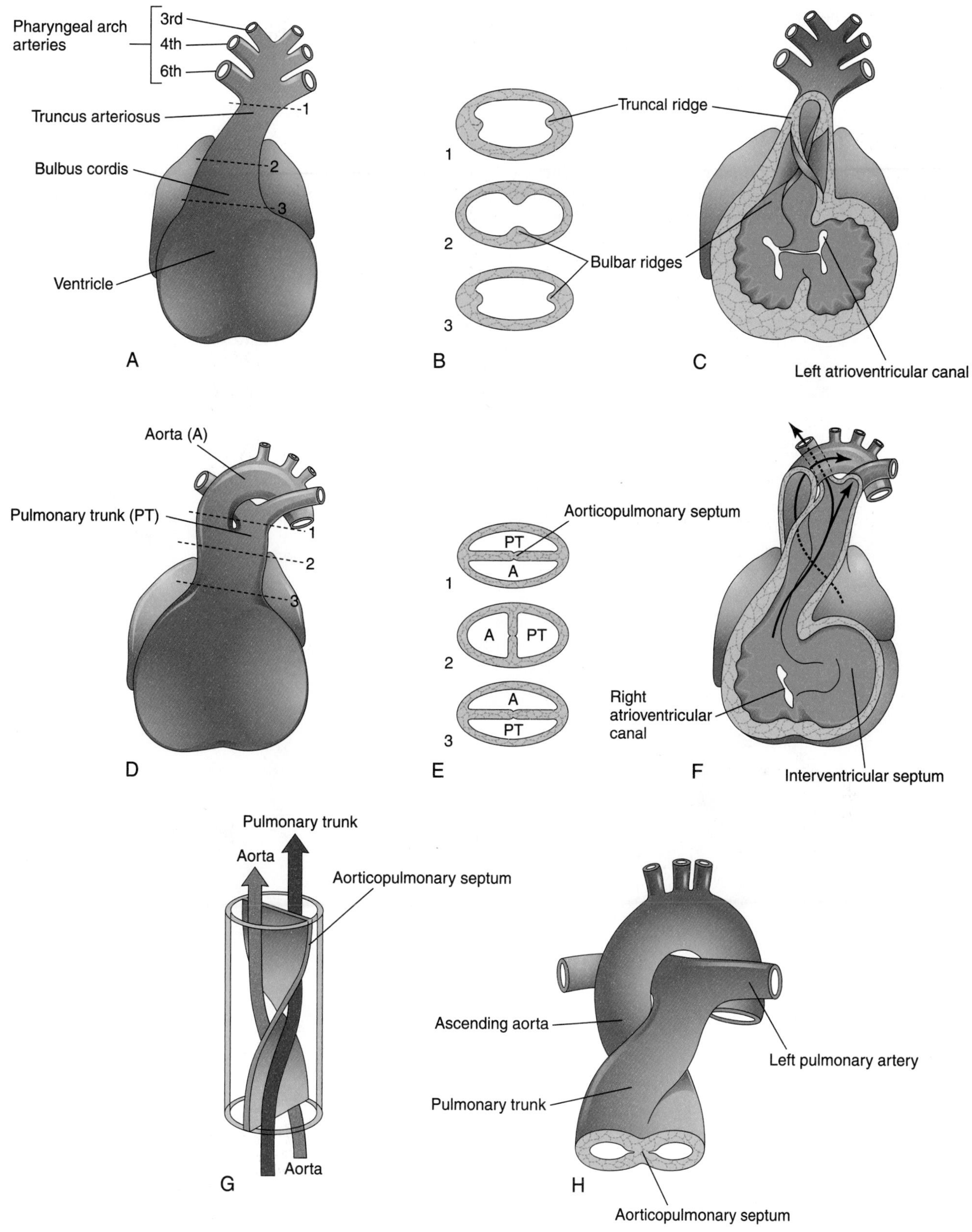

FIGURE 13-21. Partitioning of the bulbus cordis and truncus arteriosus. **A,** Ventral aspect of heart at 5 weeks. The *broken lines* and *arrows* indicate the levels of the sections shown in **B. B,** Transverse sections of the truncus arteriosus and bulbus cordis, illustrating the truncal and bulbar ridges. **C,** The ventral wall of the heart and truncus arteriosus has been removed to demonstrate these ridges. **D,** Ventral aspect of heart after partitioning of the truncus arteriosus. The *broken lines* and *arrows* indicate the levels of the sections shown in **E. E,** Sections through the newly formed aorta (A) and pulmonary trunk (PT), showing the aorticopulmonary septum. **F,** 6 weeks. The ventral wall of the heart and pulmonary trunk have been removed to show the aorticopulmonary septum. **G,** Diagram illustrating the spiral form of the aorticopulmonary septum. **H,** Drawing showing the great arteries (ascending aorta and pulmonary trunk) twisting around each other as they leave the heart.

are hollowed out and reshaped to form three thin-walled cusps (Figs. 13-19*C* and *D* and 13-22). The **AV valves** (tricuspid and mitral valves) develop similarly from localized proliferations of tissue around the AV canals.

Conducting System of the Heart

Initially, the muscle in the primordial atrium and ventricle is continuous. The atrium acts as the interim pacemaker of the heart, but the sinus venosus soon takes over this function. The **SA node** develops during the fifth week. It is originally in the right wall of the sinus venosus, but it is incorporated into the wall of the right atrium with the sinus venosus (see Fig. 13-19*D*). The SA node is located high in the right atrium, near the entrance of the SVC. After incorporation of the sinus venosus, cells from its left wall are found in the base of the interatrial septum just anterior to the opening of the coronary sinus. Together with cells from the AV region, they form the **AV node and bundle**, which are located just superior to the endocardial cushions. The fibers arising from the AV bundle pass from the atrium into the ventricle and split into right and left **bundle branches**. The bundle branches are distributed throughout the ventricular myocardium (see Fig. 13-19*D*).

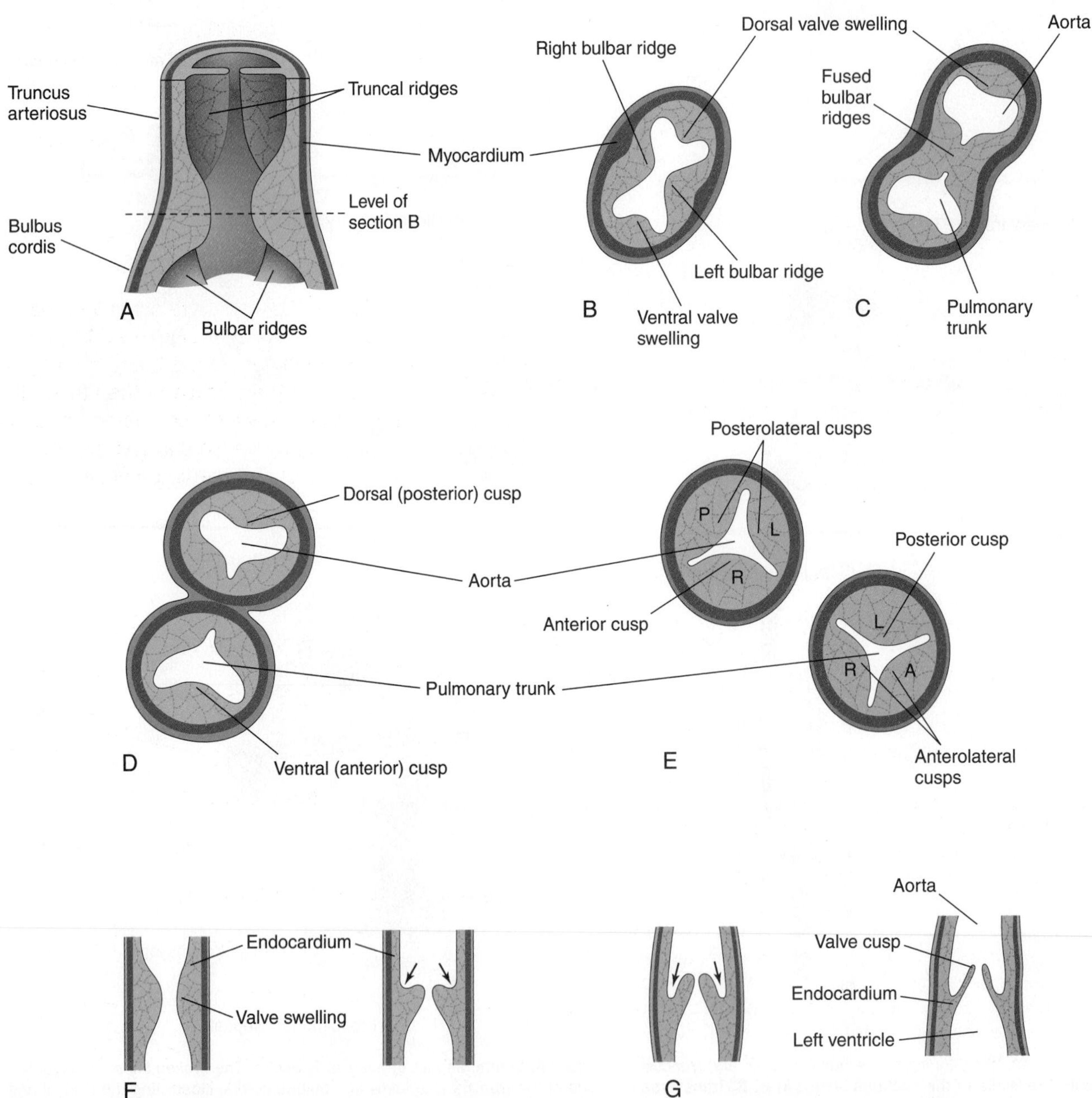

FIGURE 13-22. Development of the semilunar valves of the aorta and pulmonary trunk. **A,** Sketch of a section of the truncus arteriosus and bulbus cordis showing the valve swellings. **B,** Transverse section of the bulbus cordis. **C,** Similar section after fusion of the bulbar ridges. **D,** Formation of the walls and valves of the aorta and pulmonary trunk. **E,** Rotation of the vessels has established the adult relations of the valves. **F** and **G,** Longitudinal sections of the aorticoventricular junction illustrating successive stages in the hollowing (*arrows*) and thinning of the valve swellings to form the valve cusps.

The SA node, AV node, and AV bundle are richly supplied by nerves; however, the conducting system is well developed before these nerves enter the heart. This specialized tissue is normally the only signal pathway from the atria to the ventricles. As the four chambers of the heart develop, a band of connective tissue grows in from the epicardium, subsequently separating the muscle of the atria from that of the ventricles. This connective tissue forms part of the **cardiac skeleton** (fibrous skeleton of the heart).

ABNORMALITIES OF THE CONDUCTING SYSTEM

Abnormalities of the conducting tissue may cause unexpected death during infancy. Conducting tissue abnormalities have been observed in the hearts of several infants who died unexpectedly from a disorder known as **sudden infant death syndrome** (SIDS). These abnormalities are the most common cause of infant deaths in developed countries, generally accounting for 40% to 50% of infant deaths during the first year. Most likely, no single mechanism is responsible for the sudden and unexpected deaths of these apparently healthy infants. There is some suggestion that they have an abnormality in the autonomic nervous system. A **brain stem developmental abnormality** or maturational delay related to neuroregulation of cardiorespiratory control appears to be the most compelling hypothesis.

ANOMALIES OF THE HEART AND GREAT VESSELS

Congenital heart defects (CHDs) are common, with a frequency of six to eight cases per 1000 births. Some CHDs are caused by single-gene or chromosomal mechanisms. Other defects result from exposure to teratogens such as the rubella virus (see Chapter 20); however, in many cases, the cause is unknown. Most CHDs are thought to be caused by multiple factors, genetic and environmental (i.e., **multifactorial inheritance**), each of which has a minor effect. The molecular aspects of abnormal cardiac development are poorly understood, and gene therapy for infants with CHDs is at present a remote prospect. Imaging technology, such as real-time two-dimensional echocardiography, permits detection of fetal CHDs as early as the 17th or 18th week.

Most CHDs are well tolerated during fetal life; however, at birth, when the fetus loses contact with the maternal circulation, the impact of CHDs becomes apparent. Some types of CHD cause very little disability; others are incompatible with extrauterine life. Because of recent advances in cardiovascular surgery, many types of CHD can be corrected surgically, and fetal cardiac surgery may soon be possible for complex CHDs. Not all CHDs are described in this book. Emphasis is on those that are compatible with life or are currently amenable to surgery. The subsequent discussion of cardiac anomalies is understandably brief.

DEXTROCARDIA

If the heart tube bends to the left instead of to the right (Fig. 13-23), the heart is displaced to the right and there is transposition—the heart and its vessels are reversed left to right as in a mirror image. Dextrocardia is the most frequent positional abnormality of the heart. In dextrocardia with situs inversus (transposition of abdominal viscera), the incidence of accompanying cardiac defects is low. If there is no other associated vascular abnormalities, these hearts function normally. In isolated dextrocardia, the abnormal position of the heart is not accompanied by displacement of other viscera. This anomaly is usually complicated by severe cardiac anomalies (e.g., single ventricle and arterial transposition). The TGF-β factor Nodal is involved in looping of the heart tube, but its role in dextrocardia is unclear.

ECTOPIA CORDIS

In ectopia cordis, an extremely rare condition, the heart is in an abnormal location (Fig. 13-24). In the thoracic form of ectopia cordis, the heart is partly or completely exposed on the surface of the thorax. It is usually associated with widely separated halves of the sternum and an open pericardial sac. Death occurs in most cases during the first few days after

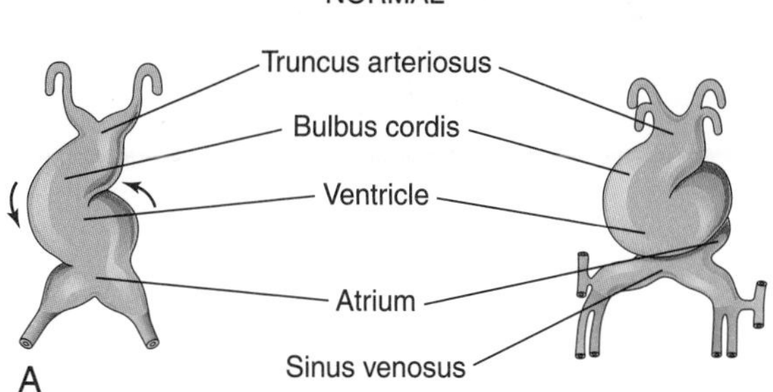

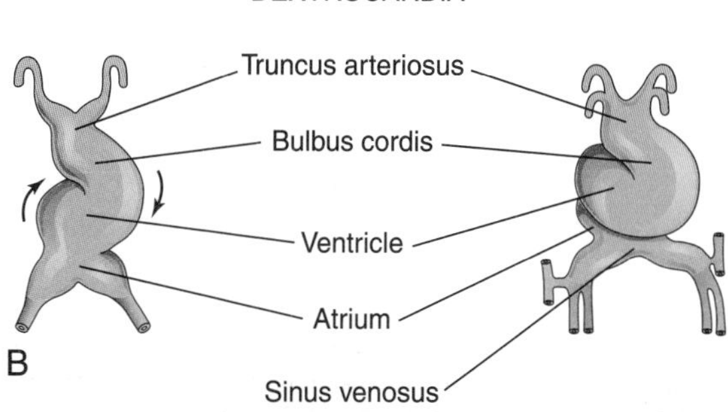

FIGURE 13-23. The primordial heart tube during the fourth week. **A,** Normal bending to the right. **B,** Abnormal bending to the left.

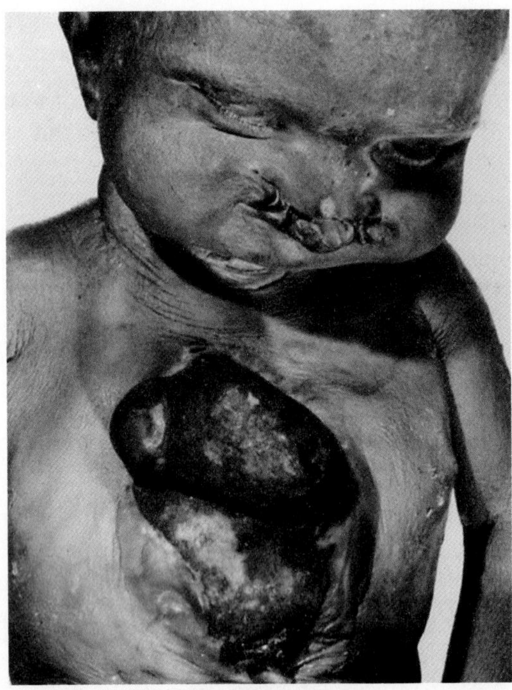

FIGURE 13-24. Newborn infant with ectopia cordis, cleft sternum, and bilateral cleft lip. Death occurred in the first days of life from infection, cardiac failure, and hypoxia.

birth, usually from infection, cardiac failure, or hypoxemia. If there are not severe cardiac defects, surgical therapy usually consists of covering the heart with skin. In some cases of ectopia cordis, the heart protrudes through the diaphragm into the abdomen.

The clinical outcome for patients with ectopia cordis has improved, and many have survived to adulthood. The most common thoracic form of ectopia cordis results from faulty development of the sternum and pericardium because of failure of complete fusion of the lateral folds in the formation of the thoracic wall during the fourth week.

ATRIAL SEPTAL DEFECTS

An atrial septal defect (ASD) is a common congenital heart anomaly and occurs more frequently in females than in males. The most common form of ASD is **patent oval foramen** (Fig. 13-25*B*). A small isolated patent oval foramen is of no hemodynamic significance; however, if there are other defects (e.g., pulmonary stenosis or atresia), blood is shunted through the oval foramen into the left atrium and produces **cyanosis** (deficient oxygenation of blood).

A **probe patent oval foramen** is present in up to 25% of people (see Fig. 13-25*B*). In this circumstance, a probe can be passed from one atrium to the other through the superior part of the floor of the oval fossa. This defect is not clinically significant, but a probe patent oval foramen may be forced open because of other cardiac defects and contribute to the functional pathology of the heart. Probe patent oval foramen results from incomplete adhesion between the flaplike valve of the oval foramen and the septum secundum after birth.

There are four clinically significant types of ASD (Figs. 13-26 and 13-27): ostium secundum defect, endocardial cushion defect with ostium primum defect, sinus venosus defect, and common atrium. The first two types of ASD are relatively common.

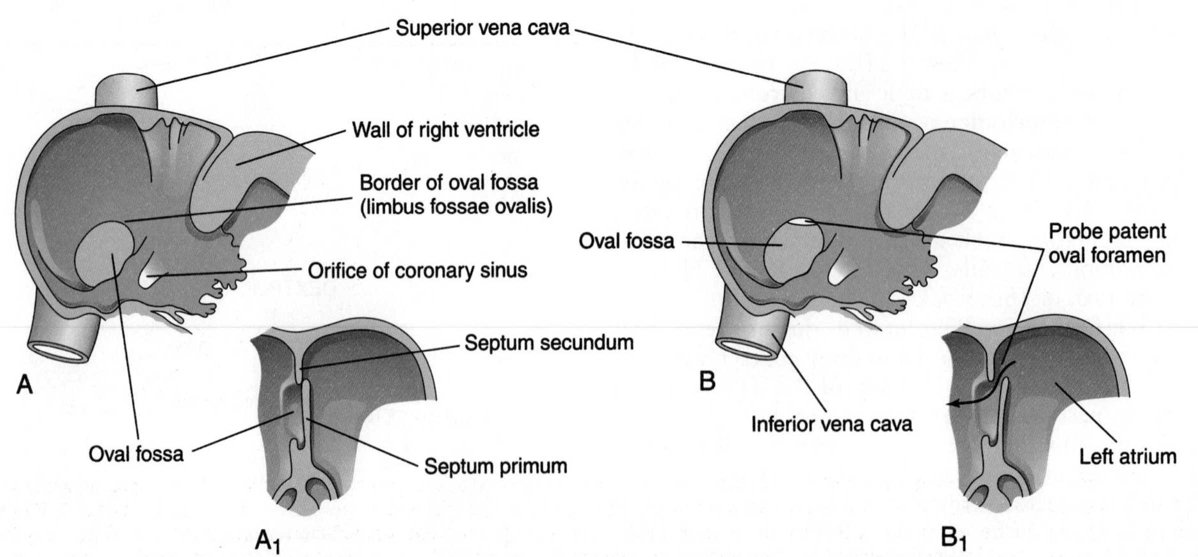

FIGURE 13-25. **A,** Normal postnatal appearance of the right side of the interatrial septum after adhesion of the septum primum to the septum secundum. **A_1,** Sketch of a section of the interatrial septum illustrating formation of the oval fossa in the right atrium. Note that the floor of this fossa is formed by the septum primum. **B** and **B_1,** Similar views of a probe patent oval foramen resulting from incomplete adhesion of the septum primum to the septum secundum.

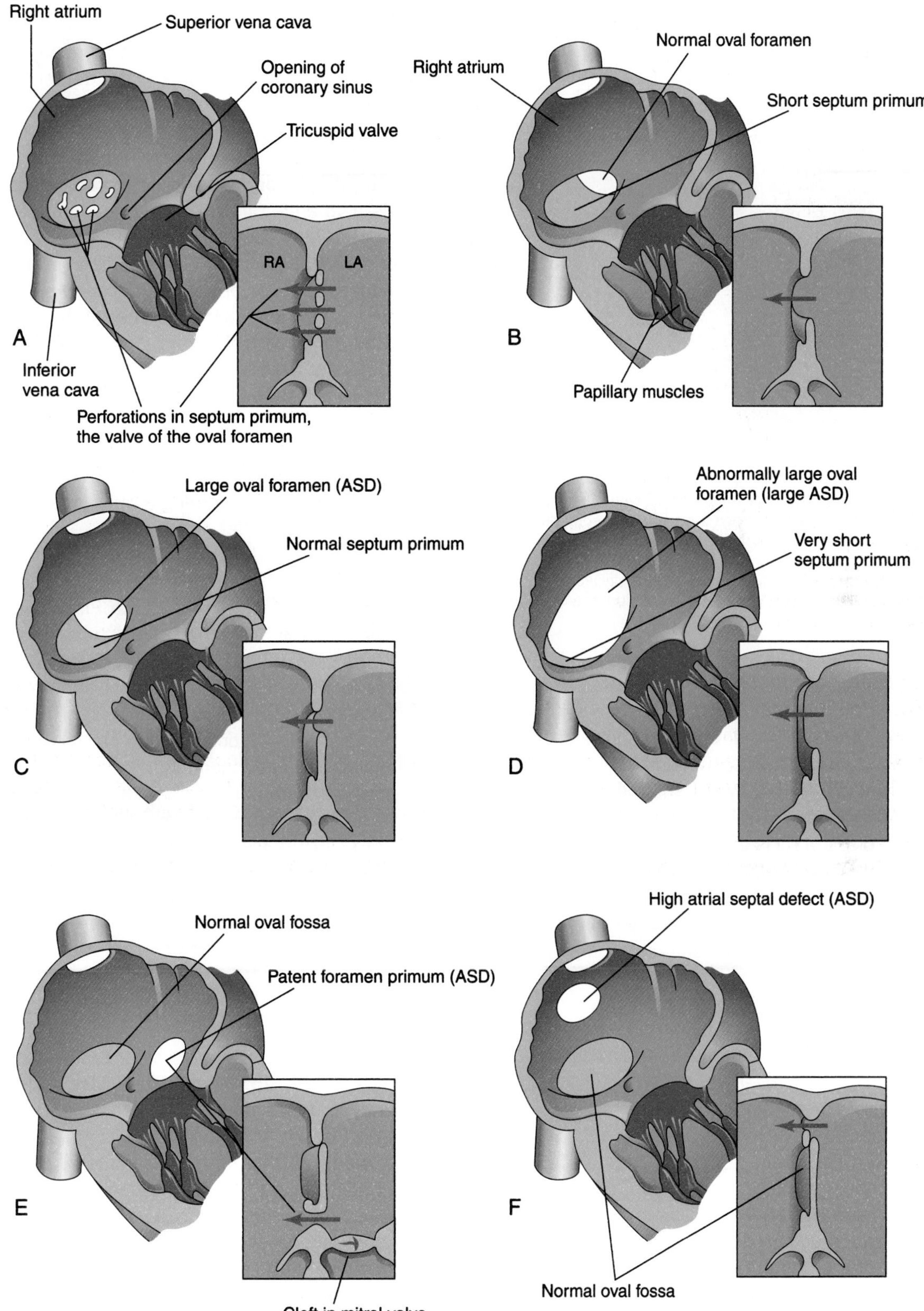

FIGURE 13-26. Drawings of the right aspect of the interatrial septum (**A** to **F**). The adjacent sketches of sections of the septa illustrate various types of atrial septal defect (ASD). **A,** Patent oval foramen resulting from resorption of the septum primum in abnormal locations. **B,** Patent oval foramen caused by excessive resorption of the septum primum (short flap defect). **C,** Patent oval foramen resulting from an abnormally large oval foramen. **D,** Patent oval foramen resulting from an abnormally large oval foramen and excessive resorption of the septum primum. **E,** Endocardial cushion defect with primum-type ASD. The adjacent section shows the cleft in the anterior cusp of the mitral valve. **F,** Sinus venosus ASD. The high septal defect resulted from abnormal absorption of the sinus venosus into the right atrium. In **E** and **F,** note that the oval fossa has formed normally.

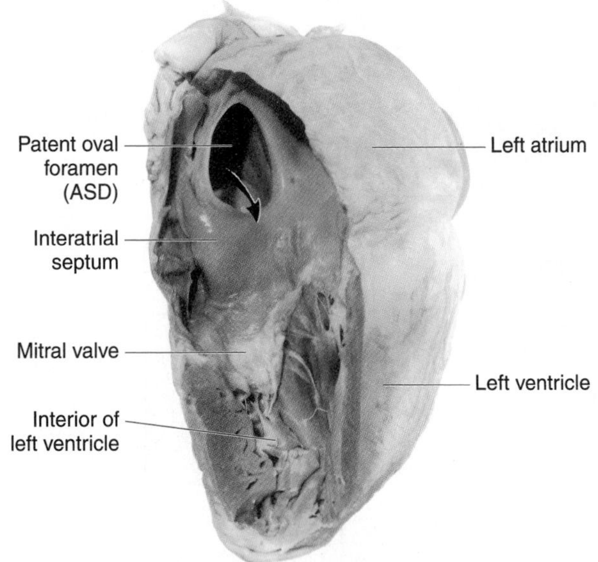

FIGURE 13-27. Dissection of an adult male heart with a large patent oval foramen. The arrow passes through a large atrial septal defect (ASD), which resulted from an abnormally large oval foramen and excessive resorption of the septum primum. This is referred to as a secundum type ASD and is one of the most common types of congenital heart disease. The right ventricle and atrium are enlarged.

Ostium secundum ASDs (see Figs. 13-26*A* to *D* and 13-27) are in the area of the oval fossa and include both defects of the septum primum and septum secundum. Ostium secundum ASDs are well tolerated during childhood; symptoms such as pulmonary hypertension usually appear in the 30s or later. Closure of the ASD is carried out at open heart surgery, and the mortality rate is less than 1%. The defects may be multiple and, in symptomatic older children, defects of 2 cm or more in diameter are not unusual. Females with ASD outnumber males 3:1. Ostium secundum ASDs are one of the most common types of CHD, yet the least severe.

The patent oval foramen usually results from abnormal resorption of the septum primum during the formation of the foramen secundum. If resorption occurs in abnormal locations, the septum primum is fenestrated or netlike (see Fig. 13-26*A*). If excessive resorption of the septum primum occurs, the resulting short septum primum will not close the oval foramen (see Fig. 13-26*B*). If an abnormally large oval foramen occurs because of defective development of the septum secundum, a normal septum primum will not close the abnormal oval foramen at birth (see Fig. 13-26*C*). Large ostium secundum ASDs may also occur because of a combination of excessive resorption of the septum primum and a large oval foramen (see Figs. 13-26*D* and 13-27).

Endocardial cushion defects with ostium primum ASDs are less common forms of ASD (see Fig. 13-26*E*). Several cardiac abnormalities are grouped together under this heading because they result from the same developmental defect, a deficiency of the endocardial cushions and the AV septum. The septum primum does not fuse with the endocardial cushions; as a result, there is a **patent foramen primum–ostium primum defect**. Usually there is also a cleft in the anterior cusp of the mitral valve. In the less common complete type of endocardial cushion and AV septal defects, fusion of the endocardial cushions fails to occur. As a result, there is a large defect in the center of the heart known as an **AV septal defect** (Fig. 13-28). This type of ASD occurs in approximately 20% of persons with Down syndrome; otherwise, it is a relatively uncommon cardiac defect. It consists of a continuous interatrial and interventricular defect with markedly abnormal AV valves. This severe cardiac defect can be detected during an ultrasound examination of the fetal heart.

All **sinus venosus ASDs** (high ASDs) are located in the superior part of the interatrial septum close to the entry of the SVC (see Fig. 13-26*F*). A sinus venosus defect is one of the rarest types of ASD. It results from incomplete absorption of the sinus venosus into the right atrium and/or abnormal development of the septum secundum. This type of ASD is commonly associated with partial anomalous pulmonary venous connections.

Common atrium is a rare cardiac defect in which the interatrial septum is absent. This situation is the result of failure of the septum primum and septum secundum to develop (combination of ostium secundum, ostium primum, and sinus venosus defects).

VENTRICULAR SEPTAL DEFECTS

VSDs are the most common type of CHD, accounting for approximately 25% of defects. VSDs occur more frequently in males than in females. VSDs may occur in any part of the IV septum (see Fig. 13-28*B*), but **membranous VSD** is the most common type (Figs. 13-28*B* and 13-29*A*). Frequently, during the first year, 30% to 50% of small VSDs close spontaneously. Most people with a large VSD have massive left-to-right shunting of blood.

Incomplete closure of the IV foramen results from failure of the membranous part of the IV septum to develop. It also results from failure of an extension of subendocardial tissue to grow from the right side of the endocardial cushion and fuse with the aorticopulmonary septum and the muscular part of the IV septum (see Fig. 13-18*C* to *E*). Large VSDs with excessive pulmonary blood flow (Fig. 13-30)

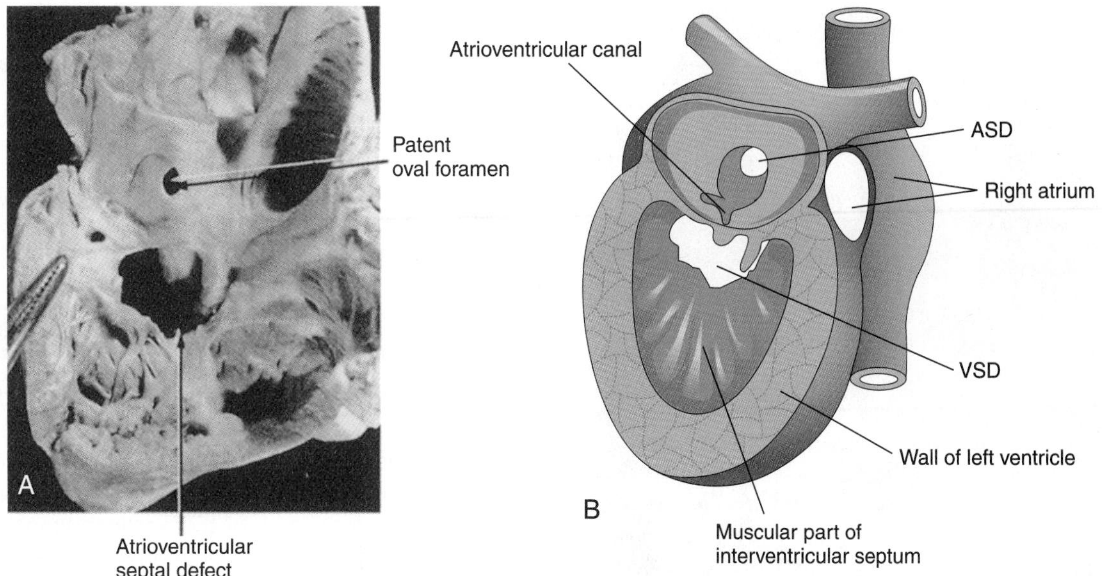

FIGURE 13-28. **A,** An infant's heart, sectioned and viewed from the right side, showing a patent oval foramen and an atrioventricular (canal) septal defect. **B,** Schematic drawing of a heart illustrating various septal defects. ASD, atrial septal defect; VSD, ventricular septal defect. (**A,** From Lev M: Autopsy Diagnosis of Congenitally Malformed Hearts. Springfield, IL: Charles C Thomas, 1953.)

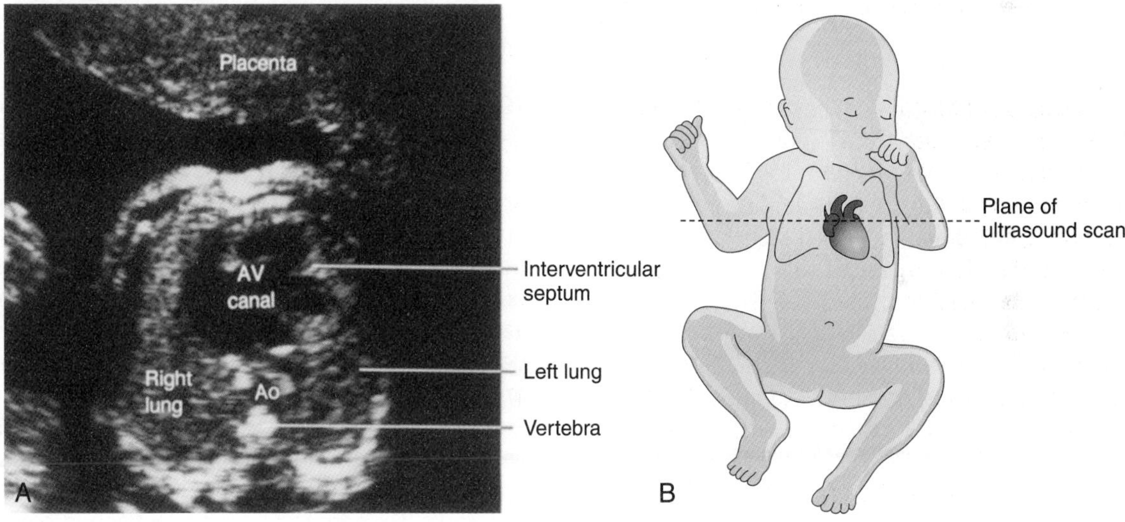

FIGURE 13-29. **A,** Ultrasound image of the heart of a second-trimester fetus with an atrioventricular (AV) canal (atrioventricular septal) defect. An atrial septal defect and ventricular septal defect are also present. Ao, aorta. **B,** Orientation drawing. (**A,** Courtesy of B. Benacerraf, MD, Diagnostic Ultrasound Associates, P.C., Boston, MA.)

and pulmonary hypertension result in dyspnea (difficult breathing) and cardiac failure early in infancy.

Muscular VSD is a less common type of defect and may appear anywhere in the muscular part of the interventricular septum. Sometimes there are multiple small defects, producing what is sometimes called the **"Swiss cheese" VSD**. Muscular VSDs probably occur because of excessive cavitation of myocardial tissue during formation of the ventricular walls and the muscular part of the interventricular septum.

Absence of the IV septum—**single ventricle** or common ventricle—resulting from failure of the IV septum to form, is extremely rare and results in a **three-chambered heart** (L. *cor triloculare biatriatum*). When there is a single ventricle, the atria empty through a single common valve or two separate AV valves into a single ventricular chamber. The aorta and pulmonary trunk arise from the ventricle. **TGA** (transposition of the great arteries) (see Fig. 13-32) and a rudimentary outlet chamber are present in most infants with a single ventricle. Some children die during infancy from congestive heart failure.

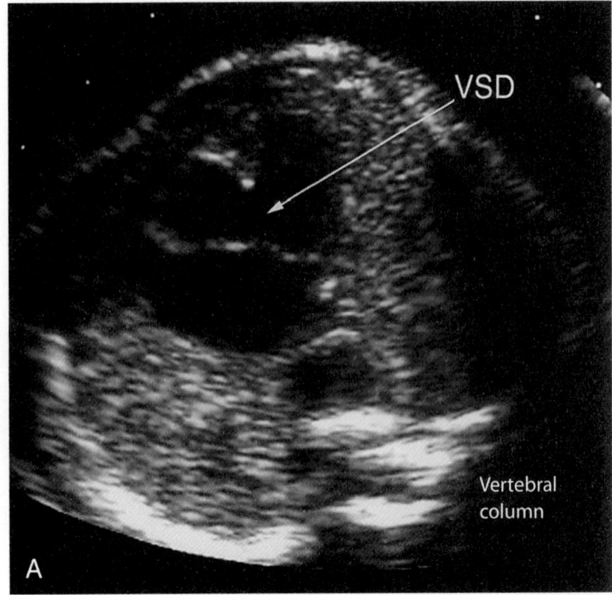

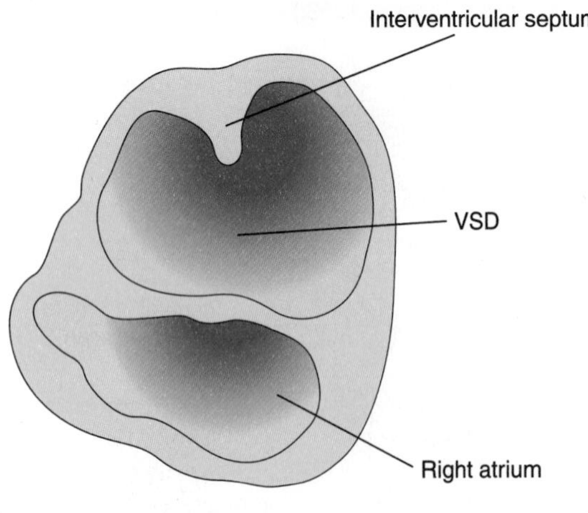

FIGURE 13-30. Ultrasound scan of a fetal heart at 23.4 weeks' gestation with an atrioventricular septal defect and a large ventricular septal defect (VSD). (**A,** Courtesy of Wesley Lee, MD, Division of Fetal Imaging, William Beaumont Hospital, Royal Oak, MI.)

PERSISTENT TRUNCUS ARTERIOSUS

Persistent TA results from failure of the truncal ridges and aorticopulmonary septum to develop normally and divide the TA into the aorta and pulmonary trunk (Fig. 13-31). In this defect, a **single arterial trunk**, the TA, arises from the heart and supplies the systemic, pulmonary, and coronary circulations. A VSD is always present with a TA anomaly and the TA straddles the VSD (see Fig. 13-31*B*). Recent studies indicate that developmental arrest of the outflow tract, semilunar valves, and aortic sac in the early embryo (days 31–32) is involved in the pathogenesis of TA anomalies. The most common type of TA is a single arterial vessel that branches to form the pulmonary trunk and ascending aorta (see Fig. 13-31*A* and *B*.) In the next most common type, the right and left pulmonary arteries arise close together from the dorsal wall of the TA (see Fig. 13-31*C*). Less common types are illustrated in Figure 13-31*D* and *E*.

AORTICOPULMONARY SEPTAL DEFECT

Aorticopulmonary septal defect is a rare condition in which there is an opening (**aortic window**) between the aorta and pulmonary trunk near the aortic valve. The aorticopulmonary defect results from localized defect in the formation of the aorticopulmonary septum. The presence of pulmonary and aortic valves and an intact IV septum distinguishes this anomaly from the persistent truncus arteriosus defect.

TRANSPOSITION OF THE GREAT ARTERIES

TGA is the most common cause of **cyanotic heart disease** in newborn infants (Fig. 13-32). TGA is often associated with other cardiac anomalies (e.g., ASD and VSD). In typical cases, the aorta lies anterior and to the right of the pulmonary trunk and arises from the morphologic right ventricle, whereas the pulmonary trunk arises from the morphologic left ventricle. The associated ASD and VSD defects permit some interchange between the pulmonary and systemic circulations. Because of these anatomic abnormalities, deoxygenated systemic venous blood returning to the right atrium enters the right ventricle and then passes to the body through the aorta. Oxygenated pulmonary venous blood passes through the left ventricle back into the pulmonary circulation. Because of the patent oval foramen, there is some mixing of the blood. Without surgical correction of the transposition of great vessels (TGA), these infants usually die within a few months.

Many attempts have been made to explain the basis of TGA, but the conal growth hypothesis is favored by most investigators. According to this explanation, the aorticopulmonary septum fails to pursue a spiral course during partitioning of the bulbus cordis and TA. This defect is thought to result from failure of the conus arteriosus to develop normally during incorporation of the bulbus cordis into the ventricles. Recent studies suggest that defective migration of neural crest cells may also be involved.

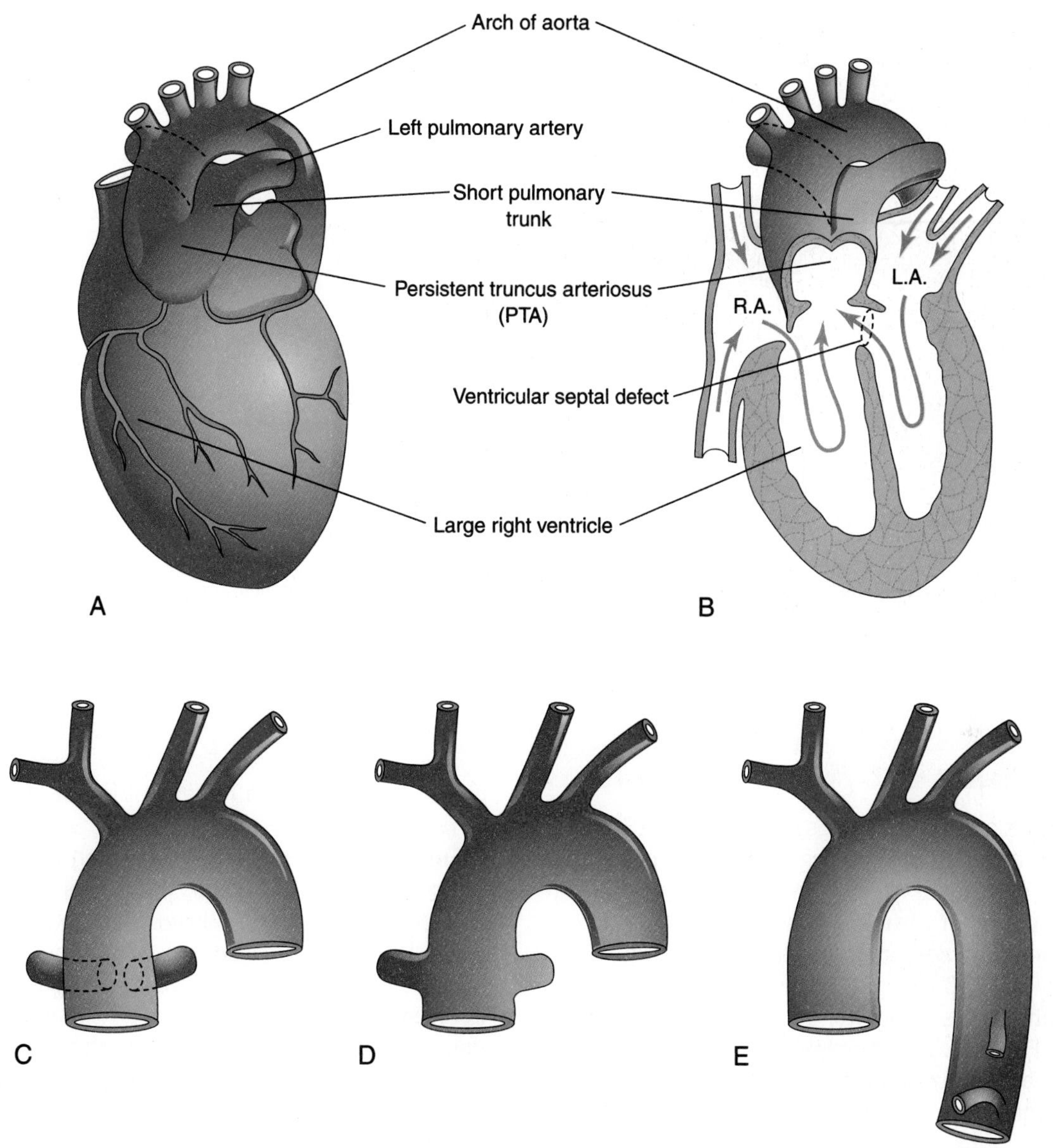

Arch of aorta
Left pulmonary artery
Short pulmonary trunk
Persistent truncus arteriosus (PTA)
Ventricular septal defect
Large right ventricle
R.A.
L.A.
A
B
C
D
E

FIGURE 13-31. Illustrations of the common types of persistent truncus arteriosus (PTA). **A,** The common trunk divides into the aorta and a short pulmonary trunk. **B,** Coronal section of the heart shown in **A**. Observe the circulation in this heart (*arrows*) and the ventral septal defect. **C,** The right and left pulmonary arteries arise close together from the truncus arteriosus. **D,** The pulmonary arteries arise independently from the sides of the truncus arteriosus. **E,** No pulmonary arteries are present; the lungs are supplied by the bronchial arteries. L.A., left atrium; R.A., right atrium.

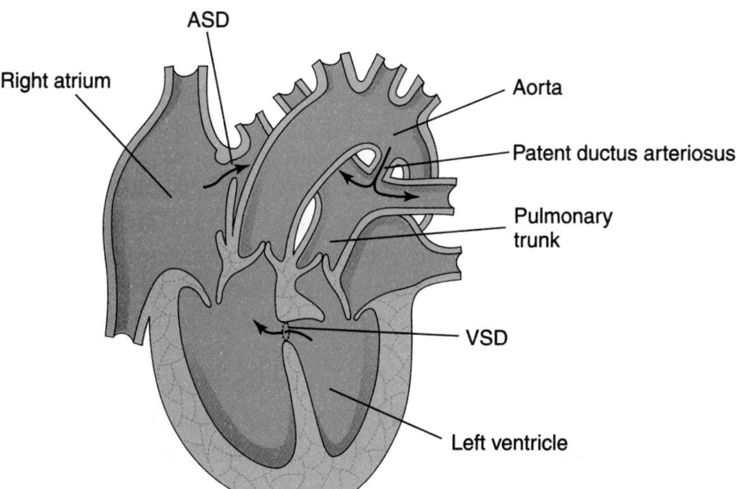

FIGURE 13-32. Diagram of a malformed heart illustrating transposition of the great arteries (TGA). The ventricular and atrial septal defects allow mixing of the arterial and venous blood. TGA is the most common single cause of cyanotic heart disease in newborn infants. As here, it is often associated with other cardiac anomalies (ventricular septal defect [VSD] and atrial septal defect [ASD]).

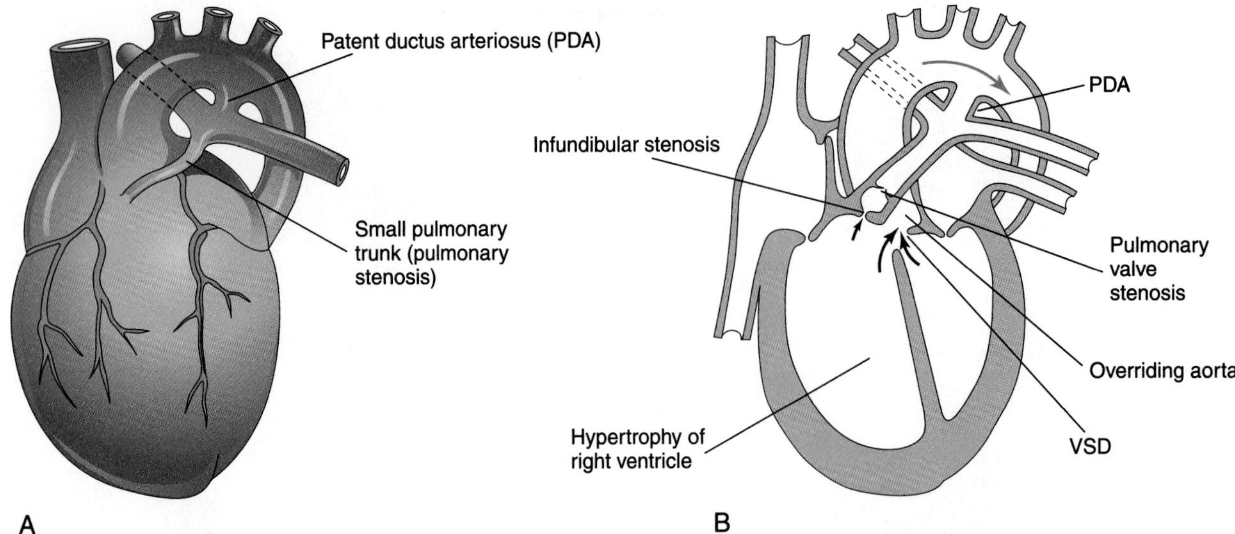

FIGURE 13-33. **A,** Drawing of an infant's heart showing a small pulmonary trunk (pulmonary stenosis) and a large aorta resulting from unequal partitioning of the truncus arteriosus. There is also hypertrophy of the right ventricle and a patent ductus arteriosus (PDA). **B,** Frontal section of a heart illustrating tetralogy of Fallot. Observe the four cardiac deformities of this tetralogy: pulmonary valve stenosis, ventricular septal defect (VSD), overriding aorta, and hypertrophy of the right ventricle. In this case, there is also infundibular stenosis.

UNEQUAL DIVISION OF THE TRUNCUS ARTERIOSUS

Unequal division of the TA (Figs. 13-33*A* and 13-34*B* and *C*) results when partitioning of the TA superior to the valves is unequal. One of the great arteries is large and the other is small. As a result, the aorticopulmonary septum is not aligned with the IV septum and a VSD results—of the two vessels, the one with the largest diameter usually straddles the VSD (see Fig. 13-33*B*). In **pulmonary valve stenosis**, the cusps of the pulmonary valve are fused to form a dome with a narrow central opening (see Fig. 13-34*D*). In **infundibular stenosis**, the conus arteriosus (infundibulum) of the right ventricle is underdeveloped. The two types of pulmonary stenosis may occur together. Depending on the degree of obstruction to blood flow, there is a variable degree of hypertrophy of the right ventricle (see Fig. 13-33*A* and *B*).

TETRALOGY OF FALLOT

This classic group of four cardiac defects (Figs. 13-33*B*, 13-35, and 13-36) consists of:

- Pulmonary stenosis (obstruction of right ventricular outflow)
- VSD
- Dextroposition of aorta (overriding or straddling aorta)
- Right ventricular hypertrophy

The pulmonary trunk is usually small (see Fig. 13-33*A*), and there may be various degrees of pulmonary artery stenosis as well. *Cyanosis* is an obvious sign of the tetralogy but is not often present at birth.

This anomaly results when division of the TA is so unequal that the pulmonary trunk has no lumen, or there is no orifice at the level of the pulmonary valve. Pulmonary atresia may or may not be associated with a VSD. Pulmonary atresia with VSD is an extreme form of tetralogy of Fallot. The entire right ventricular output is through the aorta. Pulmonary blood flow is dependent on a PDA (patent ductus arteriosus) or on bronchial collateral vessels. Initial treatment may require surgical placement of a temporary shunt, but in many cases, primary surgical repair is the treatment of choice in early infancy.

AORTIC STENOSIS AND AORTIC ATRESIA

In **aortic valve stenosis**, the edges of the valve are usually fused to form a dome with a narrow opening (see Fig. 13-34*D*). This anomaly may be congenital or may develop after birth. The valvular stenosis causes extra work for the heart and results in hypertrophy of the left ventricle and abnormal heart sounds (*heart murmurs*). In subaortic stenosis, there is often a band of fibrous tissue just inferior to the aortic valve. The narrowing of the aorta results from persistence of tissue that normally degenerates as the valve forms. **Aortic atresia** is present when obstruction of the aorta or its valve is complete.

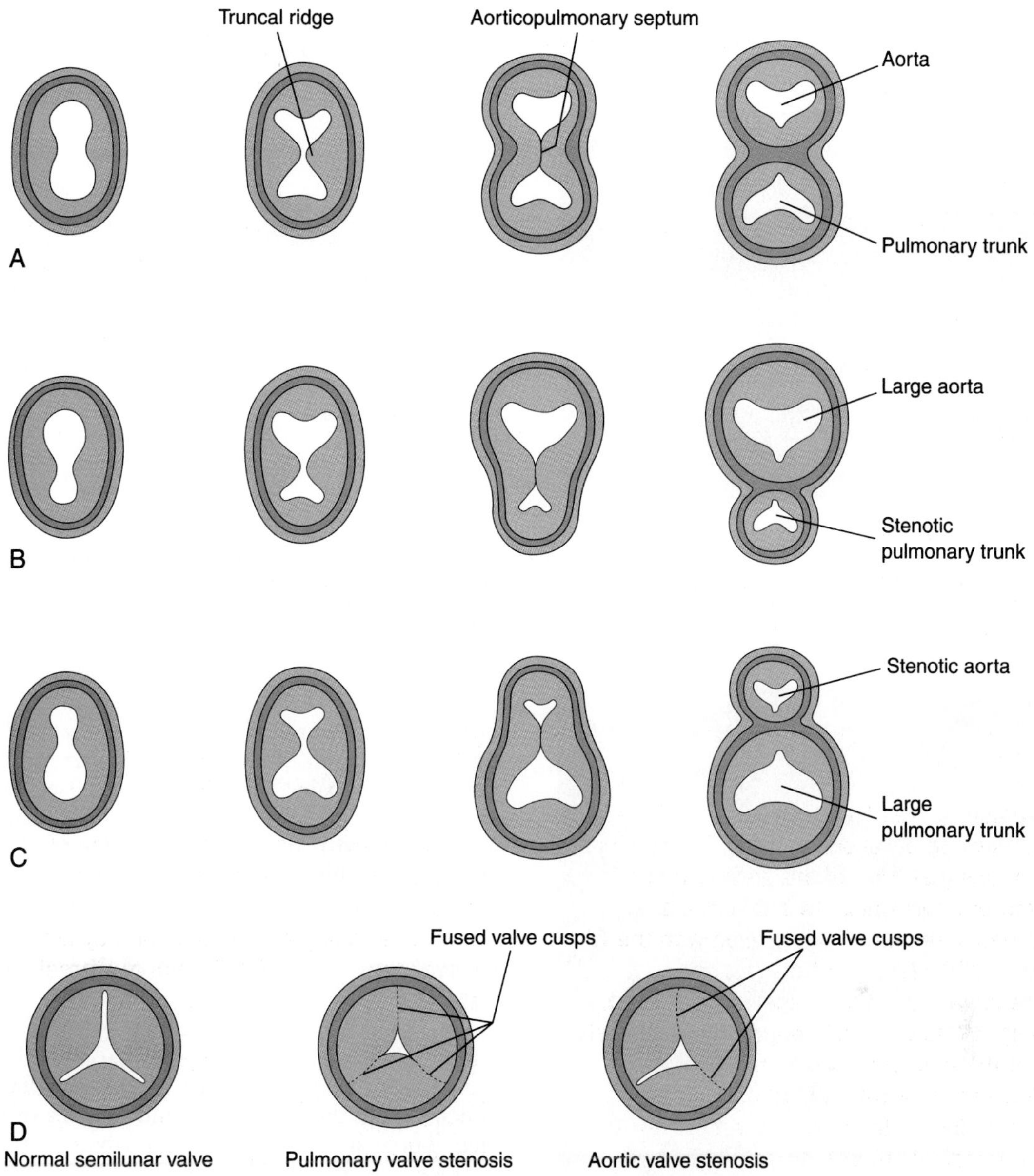

FIGURE 13-34. Abnormal division of the truncus arteriosus (TA). **A** to **C,** Sketches of transverse sections of the TA illustrating normal and abnormal partitioning of the TA. **A,** Normal. **B,** Unequal partitioning of the TA resulting in a small pulmonary trunk. **C,** Unequal partitioning resulting in a small aorta. **D,** Sketches illustrating a normal semilunar valve and stenotic pulmonary and aortic valves.

HYPOPLASTIC LEFT HEART SYNDROME

The left ventricle is small and nonfunctional (Fig. 13-37); the right ventricle maintains both pulmonary and systemic circulations. The blood passes through an atrial septal defect or a dilated oval foramen from the left to the right side of the heart, where it mixes with the systemic venous blood. In addition to the underdeveloped left ventricle, there are atresia of the aortic or mitral orifice and hypoplasia of the ascending aorta. Infants with this severe anomaly usually die during the first few weeks after birth. Disturbances in the migration of neural crest cells, in hemodynamic function, in apoptosis, and in the proliferation of the extracellular matrix are likely responsible for the pathogenesis of many CHDs such as this syndrome.

DERIVATIVES OF THE PHARYNGEAL ARCH ARTERIES

As the pharyngeal arches develop during the fourth week, they are supplied by arteries—the pharyngeal arch arteries—from the *aortic sac* (Fig. 13-38*B*). These arteries terminate in the dorsal aorta of the ipsilateral side. Although six pairs of pharyngeal arch arteries usually

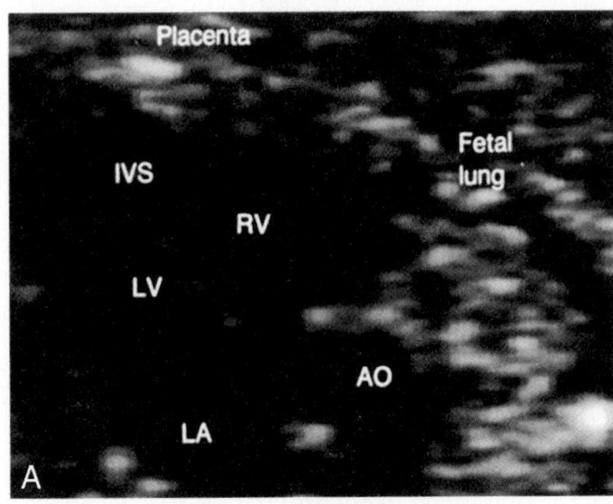

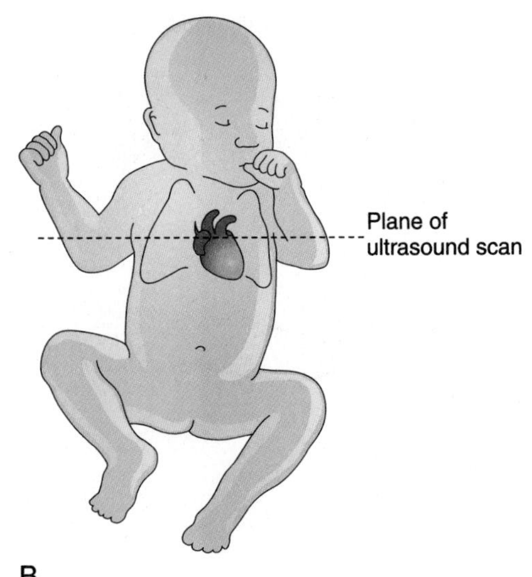

FIGURE 13-35. **A,** Ultrasound image of the heart of a 20-week fetus with tetralogy of Fallot. Note that the large overriding aorta (AO) straddles the interventricular septum. As a result, it receives blood from the left (LV) and right (RV) ventricles. IVS, interventricular septum; LA, left atrium) **B,** Orientation drawing. (**A,** Courtesy of B. Benacerraf, MD, Diagnostic Ultrasound Associates, P.C., Boston, MA.)

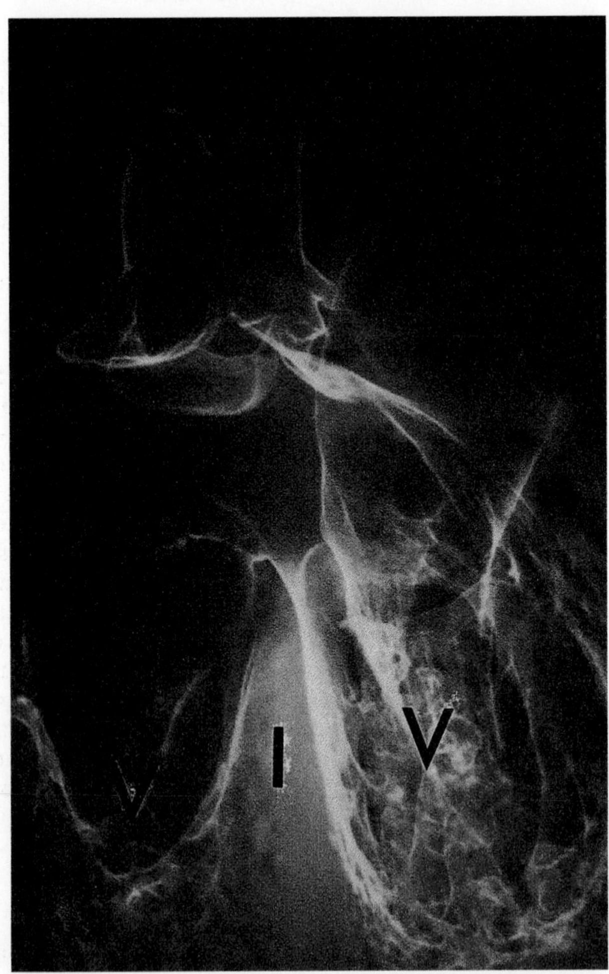

FIGURE 13-36. Tetralogy of Fallot. Fine barium powder was injected into the heart. Note the two ventricles (V), interventricular septum (I), interventricular septal defect at the superior margin, and origin of the aorta above the right ventricle (overriding aorta). The main pulmonary artery is not visualized. (Courtesy of Dr. Joseph R. Siebert, Children's Hospital & Regional Medical Center, Seattle, WA.)

develop, they are not all present at the same time. By the time the sixth pair of pharyngeal arch arteries has formed, the first two pairs have disappeared (see Fig. 13-38*C*). During the eighth week, the primordial pharyngeal arch arterial pattern is transformed into the final fetal arterial arrangement (Fig. 13-39*C*).

Derivatives of the First Pair of Pharyngeal Arch Arteries

These pharyngeal arch arteries largely disappear, but remnants of them form part of the **maxillary arteries**, which supply the ears, teeth, and muscles of the eye and face. These arteries may also contribute to the formation of the **external carotid arteries**.

Derivatives of the Second Pair of Pharyngeal Arch Arteries

Dorsal parts of these arteries persist and form the stems of the **stapedial arteries**, which are small vessels that run through the ring of the stapes, a small bone in the middle ear.

Derivatives of the Third Pair of Pharyngeal Arch Arteries

Proximal parts of these arteries form the **common carotid arteries**, which supply structures in the head (see Fig. 13-39*D*). Distal parts of the third pair of pharyngeal arch arteries join with the dorsal **aortas** to form the **internal carotid arteries**, which supply the middle ears, orbits, brain and its meninges, and pituitary gland.

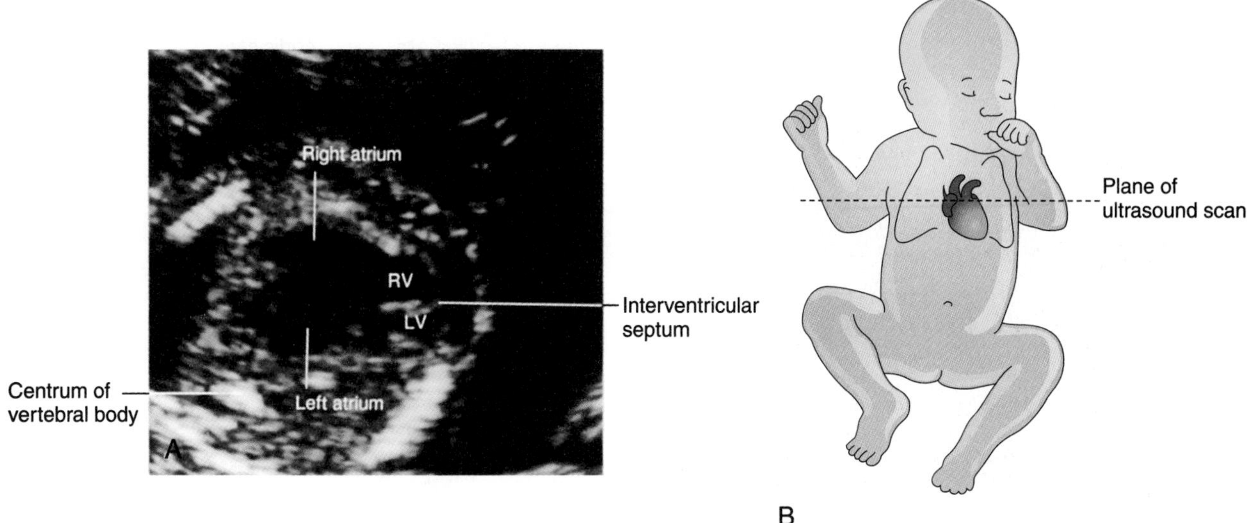

FIGURE 13-37. **A,** Ultrasound image of the heart of a second-trimester fetus with a hypoplastic left heart. Note that the left ventricle (LV) is much smaller than the right ventricle (RV). This is an oblique scan of the fetal thorax through the long axis of the ventricles. **B,** Orientation drawing. (**A,** Courtesy of B. Benacerraf, MD, Diagnostic Ultrasound Associates, P.C., Boston, MA.)

Derivatives of the Fourth Pair of Pharyngeal Arch Arteries

The left fourth pharyngeal arch artery forms **part of the arch of the aorta** (see Fig. 13-39*C*). The proximal part of the artery develops from the **aortic sac** and the distal part is derived from the **left dorsal aorta.**

The *right fourth pharyngeal arch artery* becomes the **proximal part of the right subclavian artery.** The distal part of the right subclavian artery forms from the **right dorsal aorta** and **right seventh intersegmental artery.** The left subclavian artery is not derived from a pharyngeal arch artery; it forms from the left seventh intersegmental artery (see Fig. 13-39*A*). As development proceeds, differential growth shifts the origin of the left subclavian artery cranially. Consequently, it comes to lie close to the origin of the left common carotid artery (see Fig. 13-39*D*).

Fate of the Fifth Pair of Pharyngeal Arch Arteries

Approximately 50% of the time, the fifth pair of pharyngeal arch arteries are rudimentary vessels that soon degenerate, leaving no vascular derivatives. In the other 50%, these arteries do not develop.

Derivatives of the Sixth Pair of Pharyngeal Arch Arteries

The **left sixth pharyngeal arch artery** develops as follows (see Fig. 13-39*B* and *C*):

- The proximal part of the artery persists as the proximal part of the left pulmonary artery.
- The distal part of the artery passes from the left pulmonary artery to the dorsal aorta and forms a prenatal shunt, the ductus arteriosus (DA).

The **right sixth pharyngeal arch artery** develops as follows:

- The proximal part of the artery persists as the proximal part of the right pulmonary artery.
- The distal part of the artery degenerates.

The transformation of the sixth pair of pharyngeal arch arteries explains why the course of the **recurrent laryngeal nerves** differs on the two sides. These nerves supply the sixth pair of pharyngeal arches and hook around the sixth pair of pharyngeal arch arteries on their way to the developing larynx (Fig. 13-40*A*). **On the right,** because the distal part of the right sixth artery degenerates, the right recurrent laryngeal nerve moves superiorly and hooks around the proximal part of the right subclavian artery, the derivative of the fourth pharyngeal arch artery (see Fig. 13-40*B*). **On the left,** the left recurrent laryngeal nerve hooks around the DA formed by the distal part of the sixth pharyngeal arch artery. When this arterial shunt involutes after birth, the nerve remains around the ligamentum arteriosum (remnant of DA), and the arch of the aorta (see Fig. 13-40*C*).

Pharyngeal Arch Arterial Anomalies

Because of the many changes involved in transformation of the embryonic pharyngeal arch arterial system into the adult arterial pattern, it is understandable that many anomalies may occur. Most abnormalities result from the persistence of parts of the pharyngeal arch arteries that usually disappear or from disappearance of parts that normally persist.

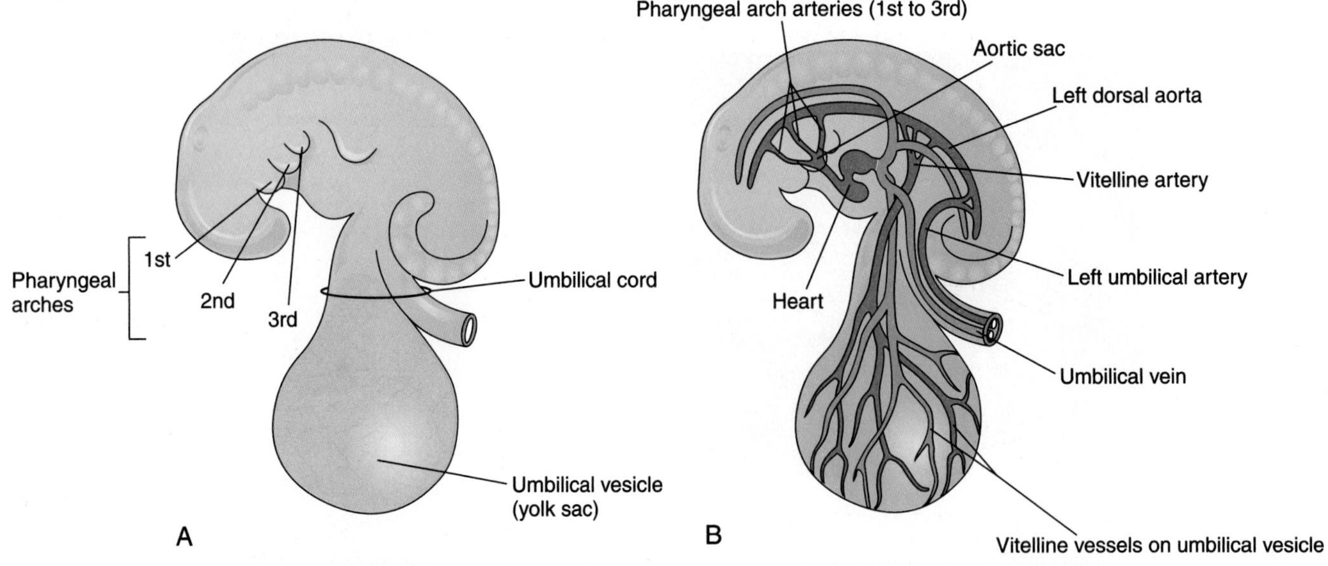

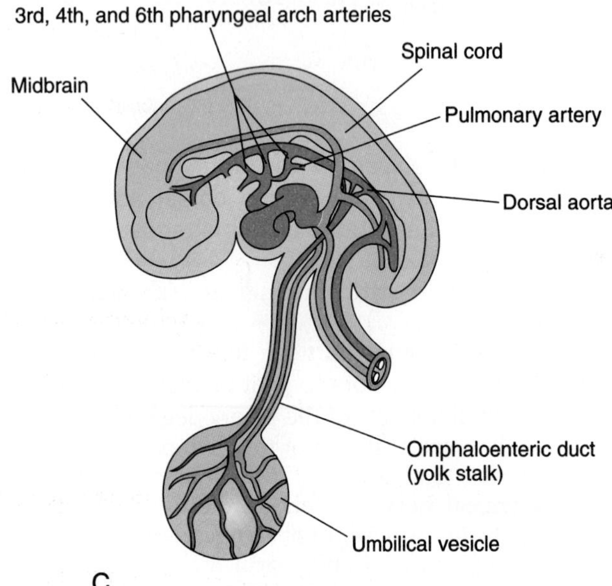

FIGURE 13-38. Pharyngeal and pharyngeal arch arteries. **A,** Left side of an embryo (approximately 26 days). **B,** Schematic drawing of this embryo showing the left pharyngeal arch arteries arising from the aortic sac, running through the pharyngeal arches, and terminating in the left dorsal aorta. **C,** An embryo (approximately 37 days) showing the single dorsal aorta and that most of the first two pairs of pharyngeal arch arteries have degenerated.

COARCTATION OF THE AORTA

Aortic coarctation (constriction) occurs in approximately 10% of children and adults with CHDs. Coarctation is characterized by an aortic constriction of varying length (Fig. 13-41). Most coarctations occur distal to the origin of the left subclavian artery at the entrance of the DA (juxtaductal coarctation). The classification into preductal and postductal coarctations is commonly used; however, in 90% of instances, the coarctation is directly opposite the DA. Coarctation of the aorta occurs twice as often in males as in females and is associated with a bicuspid aortic valve in 70% of cases.

In **postductal coarctation** (see Fig. 13-41*A* and *B*), the constriction is just distal to the DA. This permits development of a collateral circulation during the fetal period (see Fig. 13-41*B*), thereby assisting with passage of blood to inferior parts of the body.

In **preductal coarctation** (see Fig. 13-41*C*), the constriction is proximal to the DA. The narrowed segment may be extensive (see Fig. 13-41*D*); before birth, blood flows through the DA to the descending aorta for distribution to the lower body.

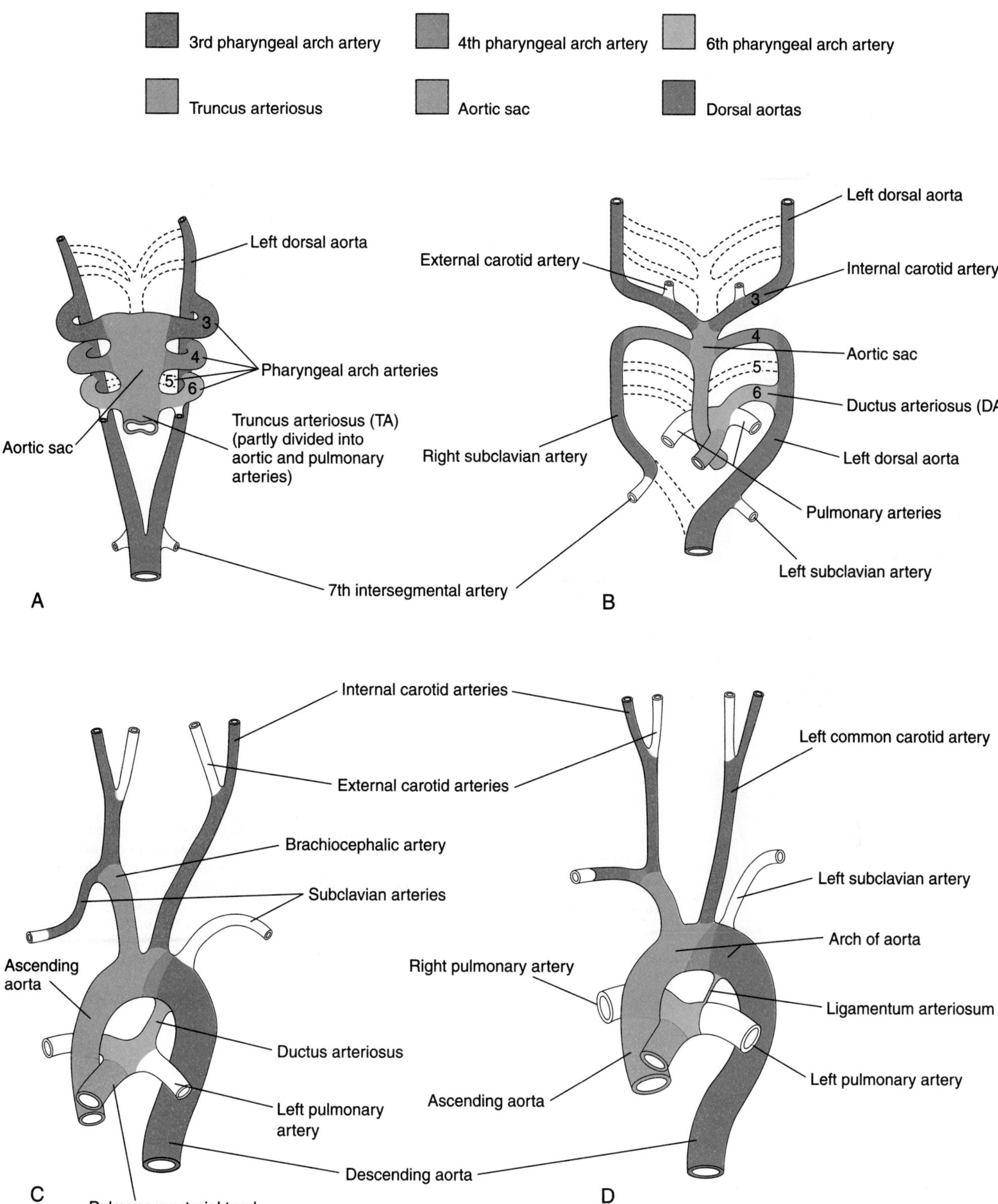

FIGURE 13-39. Schematic drawings illustrating the arterial changes that result during transformation of the truncus arteriosus, aortic sac, pharyngeal arch arteries, and dorsal aortas into the adult arterial pattern. The vessels that are not colored are not derived from these structures. **A,** Pharyngeal arch arteries at 6 weeks; by this stage, the first two pairs of arteries have largely disappeared. **B,** Pharyngeal arch arteries at 7 weeks; the parts of the dorsal aortas and pharyngeal arch arteries that normally disappear are indicated with *broken lines*. **C,** Arterial arrangement at 8 weeks. **D,** Sketch of the arterial vessels of a 6-month-old infant. Note that the ascending aorta and pulmonary arteries are considerably smaller in **C** than in **D**. This represents the relative flow through these vessels at the different stages of development. Observe the large size of the ductus arteriosus in **C** and that it is essentially a direct continuation of the pulmonary trunk. The DA normally becomes functionally closed within the first few days after birth. Eventually the ductus arteriosus becomes the ligamentum arteriosum, as shown in **D**.

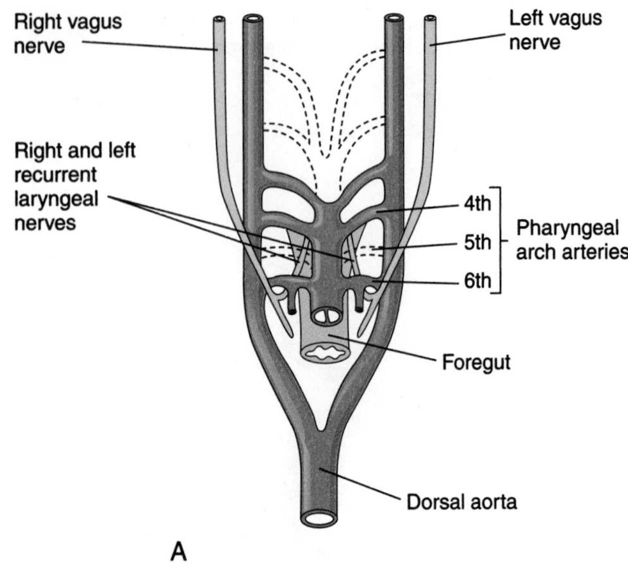

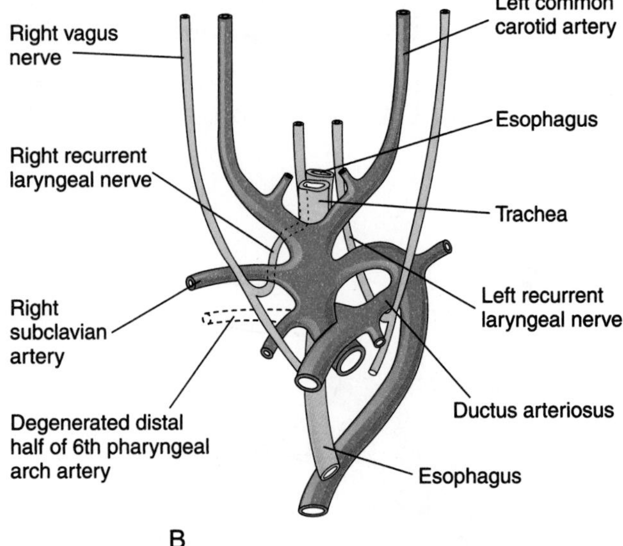

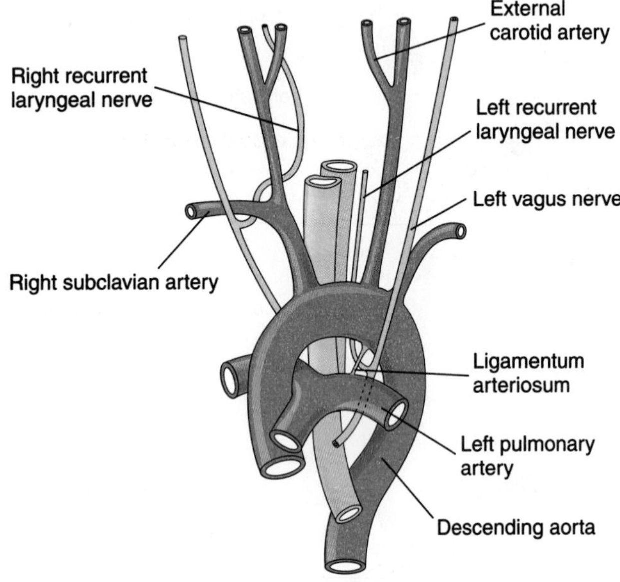

FIGURE 13-40. The relation of the recurrent laryngeal nerves to the pharyngeal arch arteries. **A,** At 6 weeks, showing the recurrent laryngeal nerves hooked around the sixth pair of pharyngeal arch arteries. **B,** At 8 weeks, showing the right recurrent laryngeal nerve hooked around the right subclavian artery and the left recurrent laryngeal nerve hooked around the ductus arteriosus and the arch of the aorta. **C,** After birth, showing the left recurrent nerve hooked around the ligamentum arteriosum and the arch of the aorta.

In an infant with severe aortic coarctation, closure of the DA results in hypoperfusion and rapid deterioration of the infant. These babies usually receive PGE_2, in an attempt to reopen the DA and establish an adequate blood flow to the lower limbs. Aortic coarctation may be a feature of Turner syndrome (see Chapter 20). This and other observations suggest that genetic and/or environmental factors cause coarctation. There are three main views about the embryologic basis of coarctation of the aorta:

- During formation of the arch of the aorta, muscle tissue of the DA may be incorporated into the wall of the aorta; then, when the DA constricts at birth, the ductal muscle in the aorta also constricts, forming a coarctation.
- There may be abnormal involution of a small segment of the left dorsal aorta (see Fig. 13-41*F*). Later, this stenotic segment (area of coarctation) moves cranially with the left subclavian artery (see Fig. 13-41G).
- During fetal life, the segment of the arch of the aorta between the left subclavian artery and the DA is normally narrow because it carries very little blood. After closure of the DA, this narrow area (isthmus) normally enlarges until it is the same diameter as the aorta. If the isthmus persists, a coarctation forms.

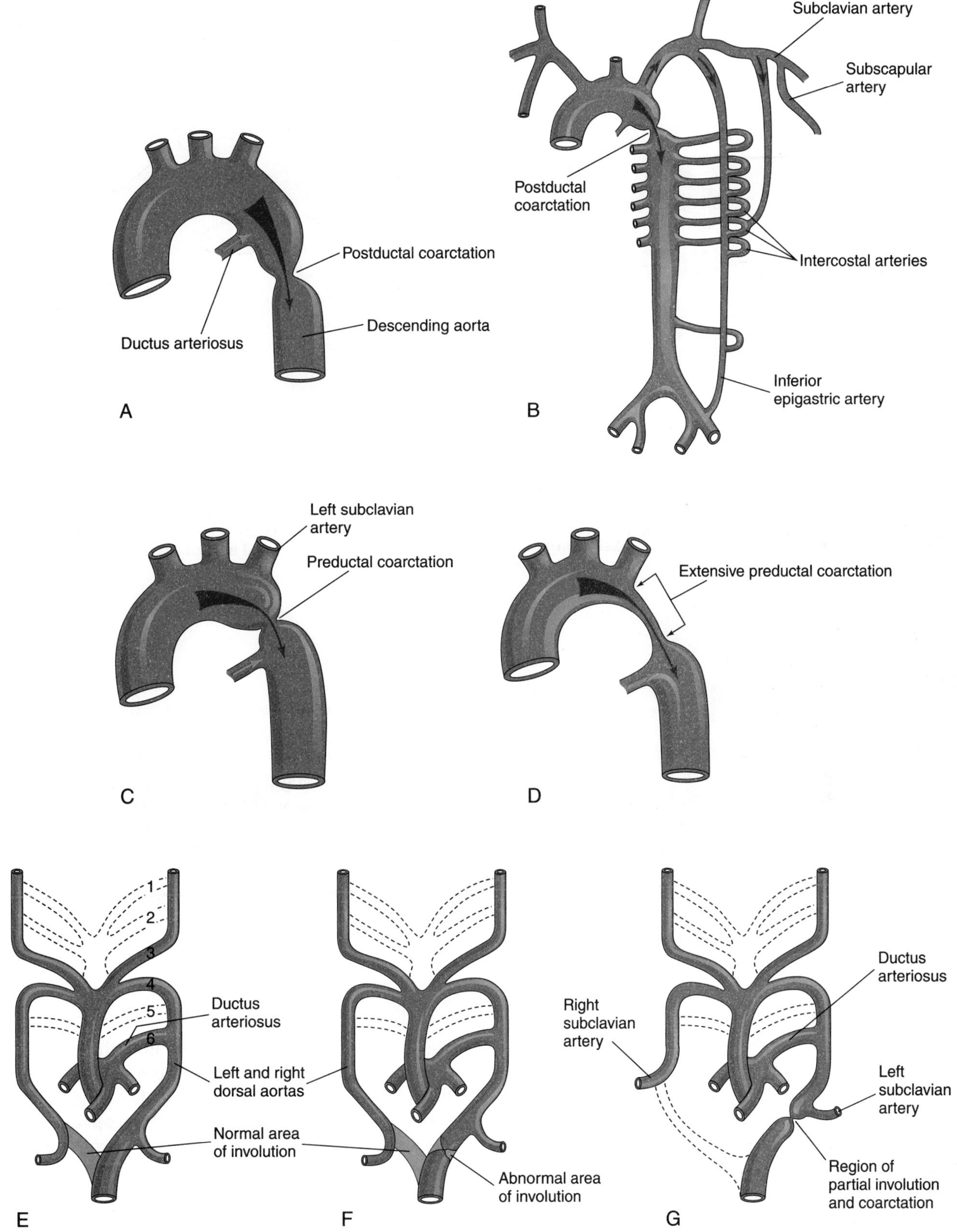

FIGURE 13-41. **A,** Postductal coarctation of the aorta. **B,** Diagrammatic representation of the common routes of collateral circulation that develop in association with postductal coarctation of the aorta. **C** and **D,** Preductal coarctation. **E,** Sketch of the pharyngeal arch arterial pattern in a 7-week embryo showing the areas that normally involute. Note that the distal segment of the right dorsal aorta normally involutes as the right subclavian artery develops. **F,** Abnormal involution of a small distal segment of the left dorsal aorta. **G,** Later stage showing the abnormally involuted segment appearing as a coarctation of the aorta. This moves to the region of the ductus arteriosus with the left subclavian artery. These drawings (**E** to **G**) illustrate one hypothesis about the embryologic basis of coarctation of the aorta.

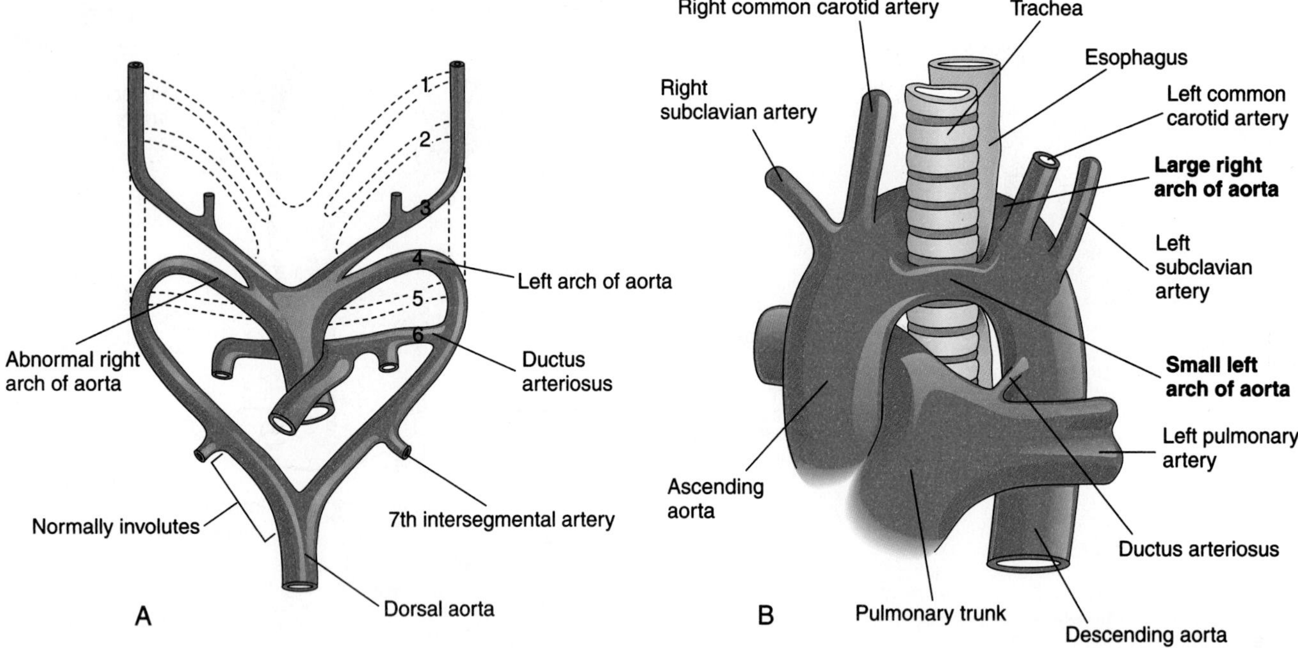

FIGURE 13-42. **A,** Drawing of the embryonic pharyngeal arch arteries illustrating the embryologic basis of the right and left arches of the aorta (double arch of the aorta). **B,** A large right arch of the aorta and a small left arch of the aorta arise from the ascending aorta and form a vascular ring around the trachea and esophagus. Observe that there is compression of the esophagus and trachea. The right common carotid and subclavian arteries arise separately from the large right arch of the aorta.

DOUBLE PHARYNGEAL ARCH ARTERY

This rare anomaly is characterized by a **vascular ring** around the trachea and esophagus (Fig. 13-42*B*). Varying degrees of compression of these structures may occur in infants. If the compression is significant, it causes wheezing respirations that are aggravated by crying, feeding, and flexion of the neck. The vascular ring results from failure of the distal part of the right dorsal aorta to disappear (see Fig. 13-42*A*); as a result, right and left arches form. Usually the right arch of the aorta is larger and passes posterior to the trachea and esophagus (see Fig. 13-42*B*).

RIGHT ARCH OF THE AORTA

When the entire right dorsal aorta persists (Fig. 13-43*A* and *B*) and the distal part of the left dorsal aorta involutes, a right arch of the aorta results. There are two main types:

- **Right arch of the aorta without a retroesophageal component** (see Fig. 13-43*B*). The DA (or ligamentum arteriosum) passes from the right pulmonary artery to the right arch of the aorta. Because no vascular ring is formed, this condition is usually asymptomatic.
- **Right arch of the aorta with a retroesophageal component** (see Fig. 13-43*C*). Originally, there was probably a small left arch of the aorta that involuted, leaving the right arch of the aorta posterior to the esophagus. The DA (or ligamentum arteriosum) attaches to the distal part of the arch of the aorta and forms a ring, which may constrict the esophagus and trachea.

ANOMALOUS RIGHT SUBCLAVIAN ARTERY

The right subclavian artery arises from the distal part of the arch of the aorta and passes posterior to the trachea and esophagus to supply the right upper limb (Figs. 13-44 and 13-45). A **retroesophageal right subclavian artery** occurs when the right fourth pharyngeal arch artery and the right dorsal aorta disappear cranial to the seventh intersegmental artery. As a result, the right subclavian artery forms from the right seventh intersegmental artery and the distal part of the right dorsal aorta. As development proceeds, differential growth shifts the origin of the right subclavian artery cranially until it comes to lie close to the origin of the left subclavian artery.

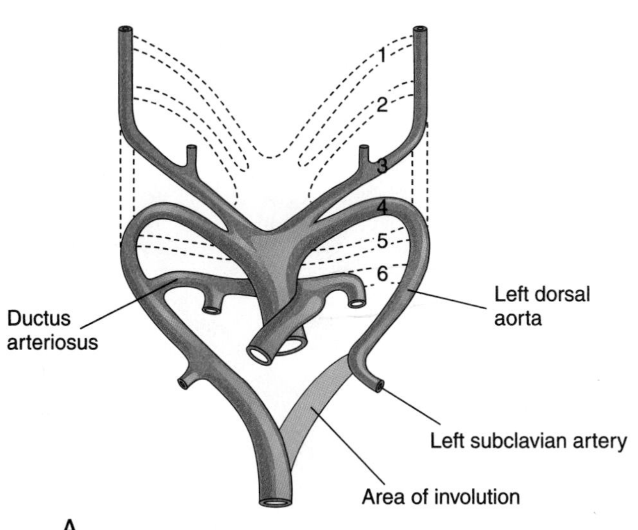

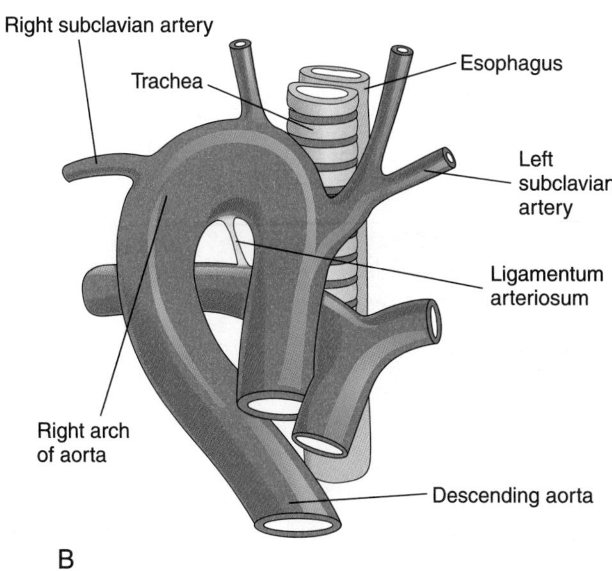

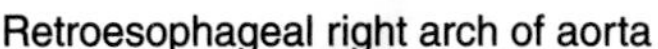

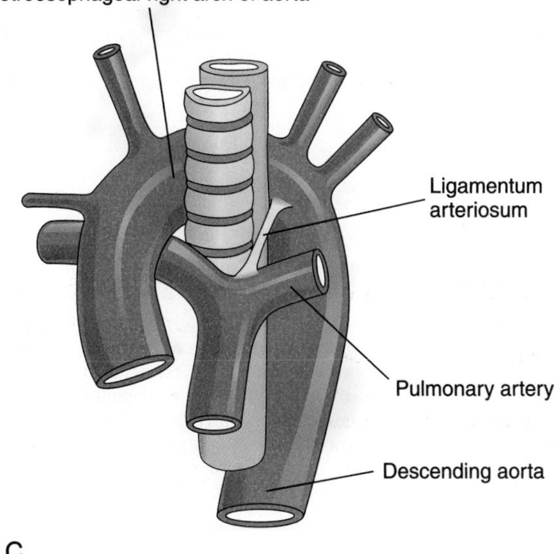

FIGURE 13-43. **A,** Sketch of the pharyngeal arch arteries showing the normal involution of the distal portion of the left dorsal aorta. There is also persistence of the entire right dorsal aorta and the distal part of the right sixth pharyngeal arch artery. **B,** Right pharyngeal arch artery without a retroesophageal component. **C,** Right arch of the aorta with a retroesophageal component. The abnormal right arch of the aorta and the ligamentum arteriosum (postnatal remnant of the ductus arteriosus) form a ring that compresses the esophagus and trachea.

Although an anomalous right subclavian artery is fairly common and always forms a vascular ring, it is rarely clinically significant because the ring is usually not tight enough to constrict the esophagus and trachea.

FETAL AND NEONATAL CIRCULATION

The fetal cardiovascular system (Fig. 13-46) is designed to serve prenatal needs and permit modifications at birth that establish the neonatal circulatory pattern (Fig. 13-47). Good respiration in the newborn infant is dependent on normal circulatory changes occurring at birth, which result in oxygenation of the blood occurring in the lungs when fetal blood flow through the placenta ceases. Prenatally, the lungs do not provide gas exchange and the pulmonary vessels are vasoconstricted. The three vascular structures most important in the transitional circulation are the DV, foramen ovale, and DA.

Fetal Circulation

Highly oxygenated, nutrient-rich blood returns under high pressure from the placenta in the **umbilical vein** (see Fig. 13-46). On approaching the liver, approximately half of the blood passes directly into the **DV**, a fetal vessel connecting the umbilical vein to the IVC (Figs. 13-48 and 13-49); consequently, this blood bypasses the liver. The other half of the blood in the umbilical vein flows into

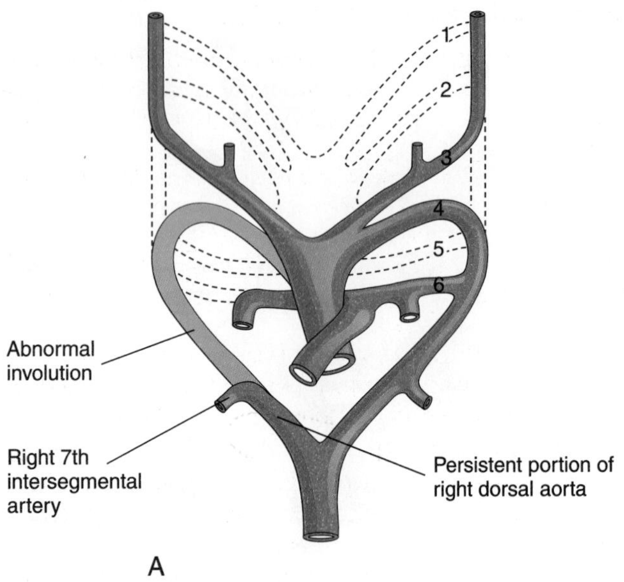

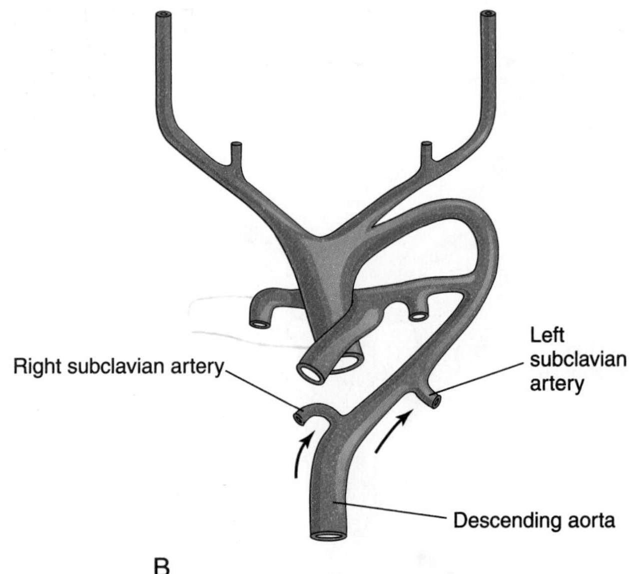

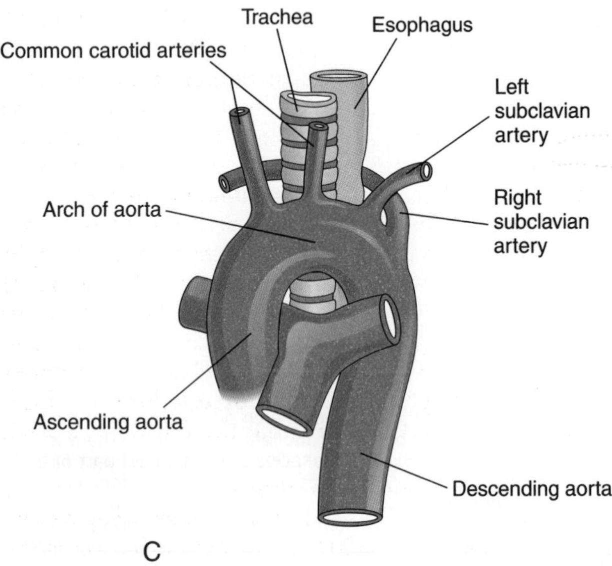

FIGURE 13-44. Sketches illustrating the possible embryologic basis of abnormal origin of the right subclavian artery. **A,** The right fourth pharyngeal arch artery and the cranial part of the right dorsal aorta have involuted. As a result, the right subclavian artery forms from the right seventh intersegmental artery and the distal segment of the right dorsal aorta. **B,** As the arch of the aorta forms, the right subclavian artery is carried cranially (*arrows*) with the left subclavian artery. **C,** The abnormal right subclavian artery arises from the aorta and passes posterior to the trachea and esophagus.

the sinusoids of the liver and enters the IVC through the **hepatic veins**.

Blood flow through the DV is regulated by a sphincter mechanism close to the umbilical vein. When the sphincter contracts, more blood is diverted to the portal vein and hepatic sinusoids and less to the DV (see Fig. 13-49). Although an anatomic sphincter in the DV has been described, its presence is not universally accepted. However, it is generally agreed that there is a physiologic sphincter that prevents overloading of the heart when venous flow in the umbilical vein is high (e.g., during uterine contractions).

After a short course in the IVC, the blood enters the right atrium of the heart. Because the IVC also contains poorly oxygenated blood from the lower limbs, abdomen, and pelvis, the blood entering the right atrium is not as well oxygenated as that in the umbilical vein, but it still has a high oxygen content (see Fig. 13-46). Most blood from the IVC is directed by the **crista dividens** (inferior border of the septum secundum), through the oval foramen into the left atrium (Fig. 13-50). Here it mixes with the relatively small amount of poorly oxygenated blood returning from the lungs through the pulmonary veins. The fetal lungs use oxygen from the blood instead of replenishing it. From the left atrium, the blood then passes to the left ventricle and leaves through the ascending aorta.

The arteries to the heart, neck, head, and upper limbs receive well-oxygenated blood from the ascending aorta. The liver also receives well-oxygenated blood from the umbilical vein (see Figs. 13-48 and 13-49). The small amount of well-oxygenated blood from the IVC in the right atrium that does not enter the foramen ovale mixes

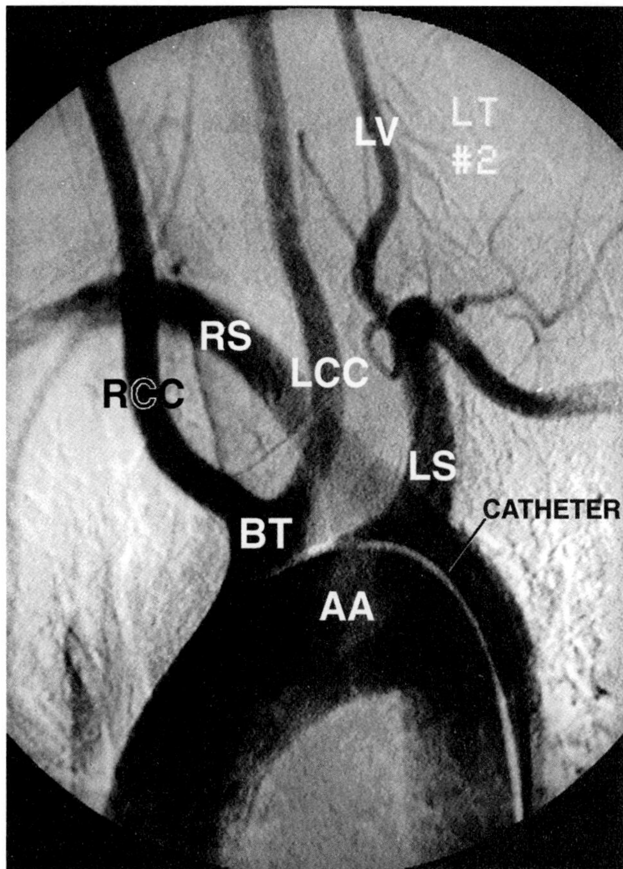

FIGURE 13-45. Abnormal origin of right subclavian artery. This left anterior oblique view of an aortic arch arteriogram shows both common carotid arteries arising from a common stem of the arch of the aorta (BT). The origin of the right subclavian artery (RS) is distal to the separate origin of the left subclavian artery (LS), but is superimposed in this view. The right subclavian artery then courses cranially and to the right, posterior to the esophagus and trachea. AA, arch of aorta; BT, brachiocephalic trunk; RCC, right common carotid artery; LCC, left common carotid artery; LV, left vertebral artery. (Courtesy of Gerald S. Smyser, MD, Altru Health System, Grand Forks, ND.)

with poorly oxygenated blood from the SVC and coronary sinus and passes into the right ventricle. This blood, with a medium oxygen content, leaves through the pulmonary trunk.

Approximately 10% of this blood flow goes to the lungs; most blood passes through the **DA** into the descending aorta to the fetal body and returns to the placenta through the umbilical arteries (see Fig. 13-46). The DA protects the lungs from circulatory overloading and allows the right ventricle to strengthen in preparation for functioning at full capacity at birth. Because of the high pulmonary vascular resistance in fetal life, pulmonary blood flow is low. Approximately 10% of blood from the ascending aorta enters the descending aorta; 65% of the blood in the descending aorta passes into the umbilical arteries and is returned to the placenta for reoxygenation. The remaining 35% of the blood in the descending aorta supplies the viscera and the inferior part of the body.

Transitional Neonatal Circulation

Important circulatory adjustments occur at birth when the circulation of fetal blood through the placenta ceases and the infant's lungs expand and begin to function (see Fig. 13-47).

As soon as the baby is born, the oval foramen, DA, DV, and umbilical vessels are no longer needed. The sphincter in the DV constricts, so that all blood entering the liver passes through the hepatic sinusoids. Occlusion of the placental circulation causes an immediate decrease in blood pressure in the IVC and right atrium.

Aeration of the lungs at birth is associated with a:

- Dramatic decrease in pulmonary vascular resistance
- Marked increase in pulmonary blood flow
- Progressive thinning of the walls of the pulmonary arteries; the thinning of the walls of these arteries results mainly from stretching as the lungs increase in size with the first few breaths

Because of increased pulmonary blood flow and loss of flow from the umbilical vein, the pressure in the left atrium is higher than in the right atrium. The increased left atrial pressure functionally closes the **oval foramen** by pressing the valve of the oval foramen against the septum secundum (see Fig. 13-47). The output from the right ventricle now flows into the pulmonary trunk. Because pulmonary vascular resistance is lower than the systemic vascular resistance, blood flow in the DA reverses, passing from the descending aorta to the pulmonary trunk.

The right ventricular wall is thicker than the left ventricular wall in fetuses and newborn infants because the right ventricle has been working harder in utero. By the end of the first month, the left ventricular wall thickness is greater than the right because the left ventricle is now working harder. The right ventricular wall becomes thinner because of the atrophy associated with its lighter workload.

The **DA constricts at birth** but there is often a small shunt of blood via the DA from the aorta to the pulmonary trunk for 24 to 48 hours in a normal full-term infant. At the end of 24 hours, 20% of ducts are functionally closed, 82% by 48 hours, and 100% at 96 hours. In premature infants and in those with persistent hypoxia, the DA may remain open much longer. In full-term infants, oxygen is the most important factor in controlling closure of the DA and appears to be mediated by **bradykinin**, a substance released from the lungs during their initial inflation. Bradykinin has potent contractile effects on smooth muscle. The action of this substance appears to be dependent on the high oxygen content of the blood in the aorta resulting from aeration of the lungs at birth. When the Po_2 of the blood passing through the DA reaches approximately 50 mm Hg, the wall of the ductus constricts. The mechanisms by which oxygen causes ductal constriction are not well understood. The effects of oxygen on the ductal smooth muscle may be direct or may be mediated by its effects on prostaglandin E_2 (PGE_2) secretion. Transforming growth factor β (TGF-β) is probably involved in the anatomic closure of the DA after birth. During fetal life, the patency of the DA before birth is controlled by the lower content of oxygen in the blood passing through it and by endogenously produced prostaglandins (**PGs**) that act on the smooth muscle in the wall of the DA. The

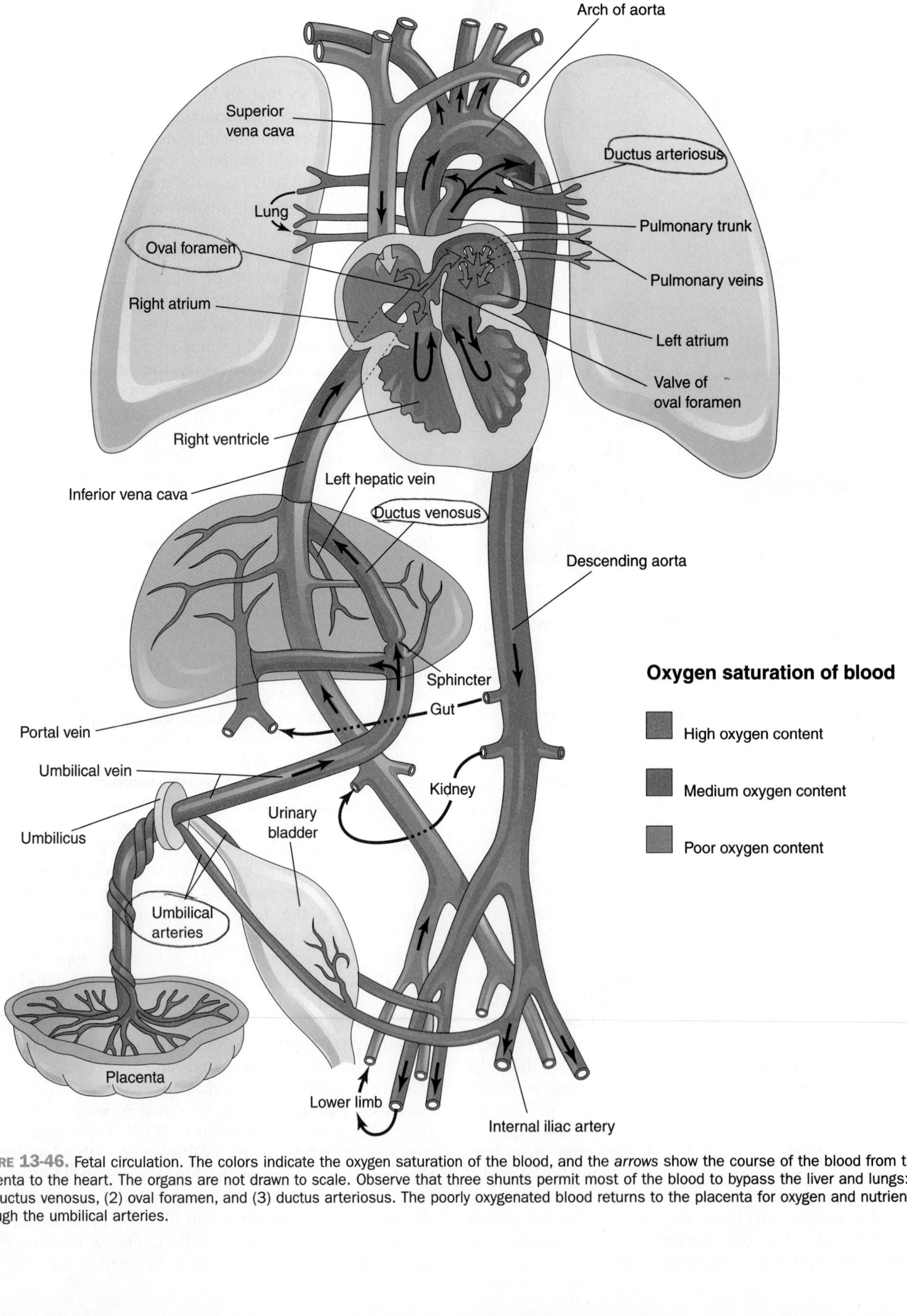

FIGURE 13-46. Fetal circulation. The colors indicate the oxygen saturation of the blood, and the *arrows* show the course of the blood from the placenta to the heart. The organs are not drawn to scale. Observe that three shunts permit most of the blood to bypass the liver and lungs: (1) ductus venosus, (2) oval foramen, and (3) ductus arteriosus. The poorly oxygenated blood returns to the placenta for oxygen and nutrients through the umbilical arteries.

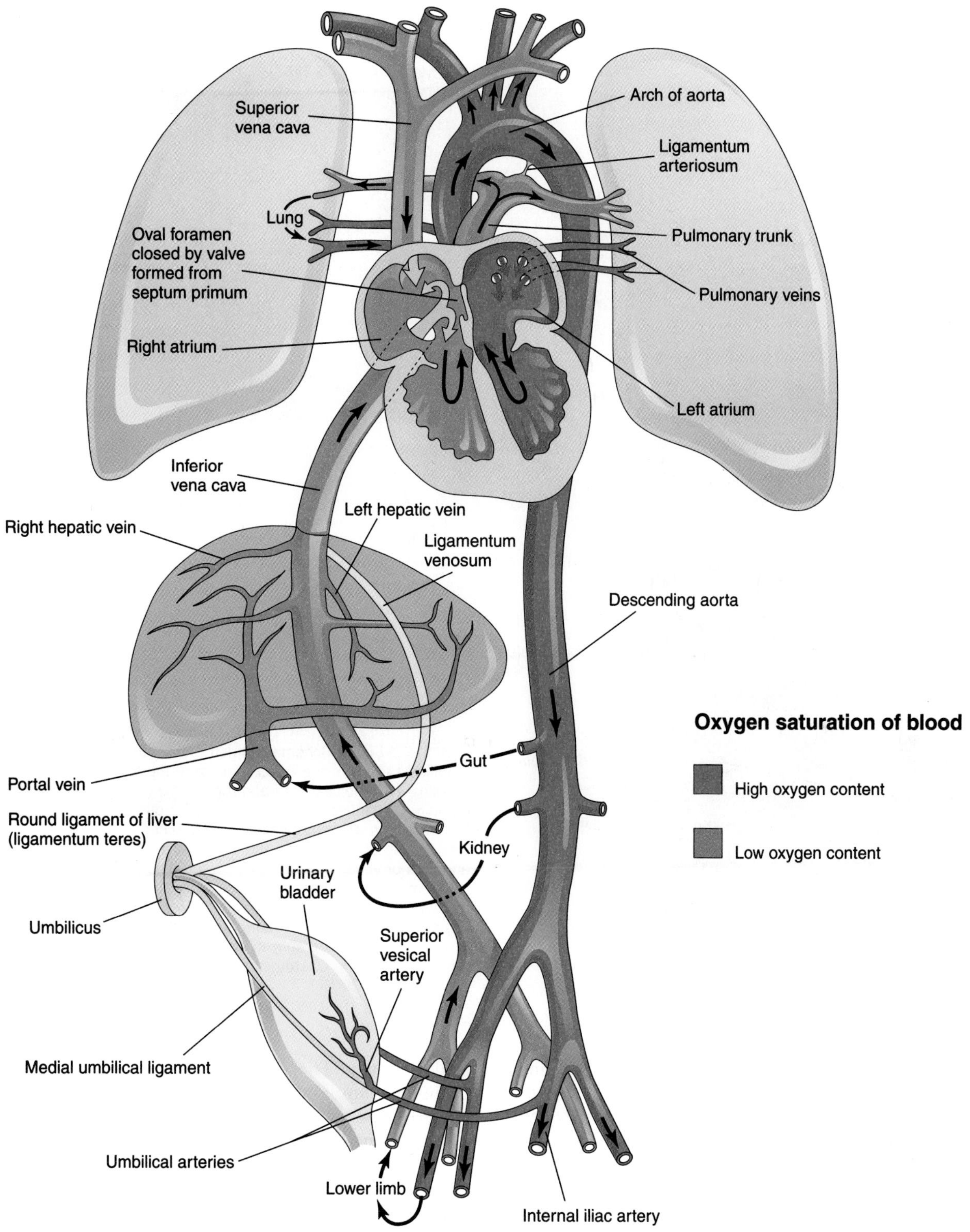

FIGURE 13-47. Neonatal circulation. The adult derivatives of the fetal vessels and structures that become nonfunctional at birth are shown. The *arrows* indicate the course of the blood in the infant. The organs are not drawn to scale. After birth, the three shunts that short-circuited the blood during fetal life cease to function, and the pulmonary and systemic circulations become separated.

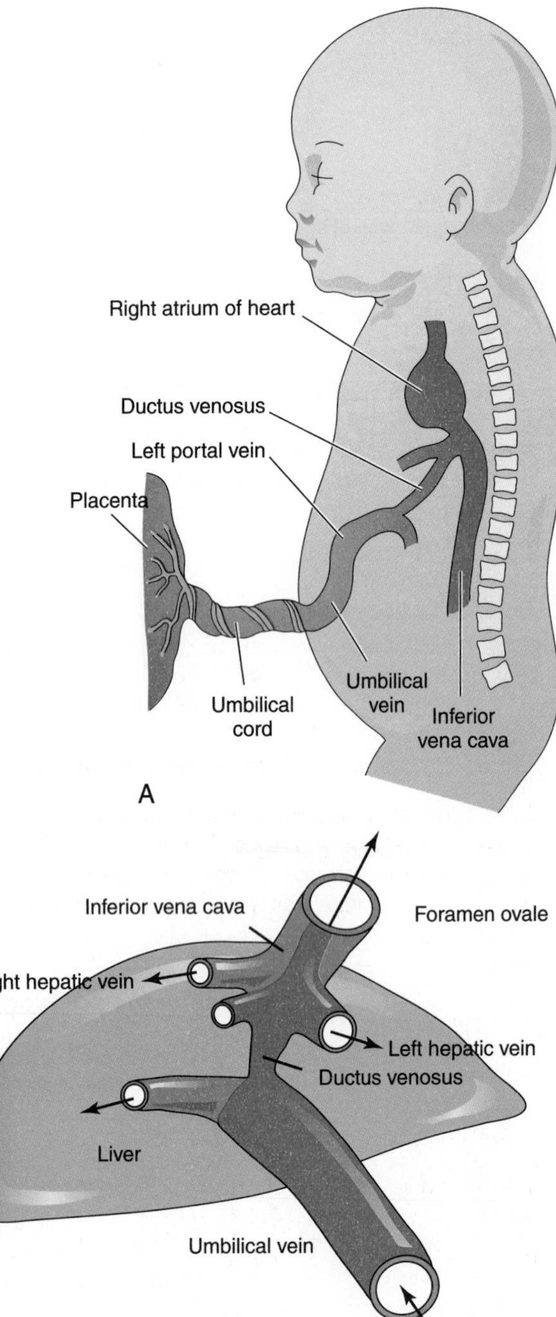

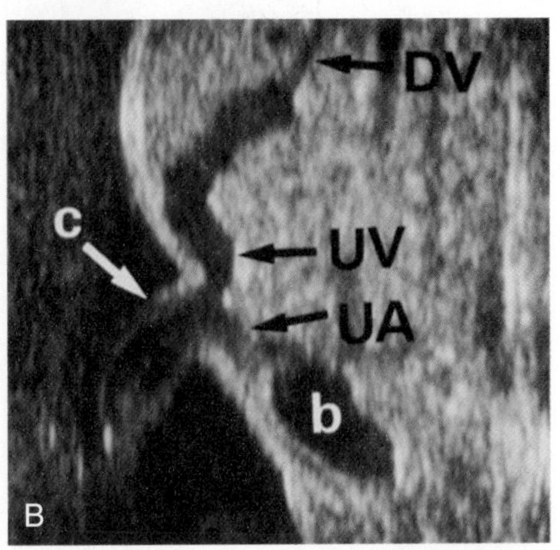

FIGURE 13-48. **A,** Schematic illustration of the course of the umbilical vein from the umbilical cord to the liver. **B,** Ultrasound scan showing the umbilical cord and the course of its vessels in the embryo. b, bladder; c, umbilical cord; DV, ductus venosus; UV, umbilical vein; UA, umbilical artery. **C,** Schematic presentation of the relationship among the ductus venosus, umbilical vein, hepatic veins, and inferior vena cava. The oxygenated blood is coded with red. (**B,** From Goldstein RB: Ultrasound evaluation of the fetal abdomen. In Callen PW [ed]: Ultrasonography in Obstetrics and Gynecology, 3rd ed. Philadelphia, WB Saunders, 1996. **C,** From Tekay A, Campbell S: Doppler ultrasonography in obstetrics. In Callen PW [ed]: Ultrasonography in Obstetrics and Gynecology, 4th ed. Philadelphia, WB Saunders, 2000.)

PGs cause the DA to relax. Hypoxia and other ill-defined influences cause the local production of PGE_2 and prostacyclin (PGI_2), which keep the DA open. Inhibitors of PG synthesis, such as **indomethacin**, can cause constriction of a patent DA (PDA) in premature infants.

The umbilical arteries constrict at birth, preventing loss of the infant's blood. Because the umbilical cord is not tied for a minute or so, blood flow through the umbilical vein continues, transferring well-oxygenated fetal blood from the placenta to the infant. The change from the fetal to the adult pattern of blood circulation is not a sudden occurrence. Some changes occur with the first breath; others take place over hours and days. During the transitional stage, there may be a right-to-left flow through the oval foramen. The closure of fetal vessels and the oval foramen is initially a functional change. Later, anatomic closure results from proliferation of endothelial and fibrous tissues.

Derivatives of Fetal Vascular Structures

Because of the changes in the cardiovascular system at birth, certain vessels and structures are no longer required. Over a period of months, these fetal vessels form nonfunctional ligaments. Fetal structures, such as the oval foramen, persist as anatomic vestiges (e.g., oval fossa; see Fig. 13-52).

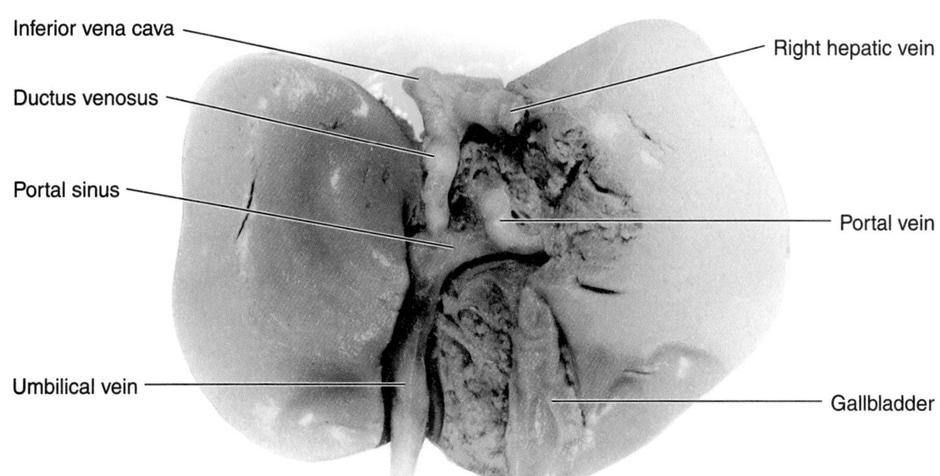

FIGURE 13-49. Dissection of the visceral surface of the fetal liver. Approximately 50% of umbilical venous blood bypasses the liver and joins the inferior vena cava through the ductus venosus.

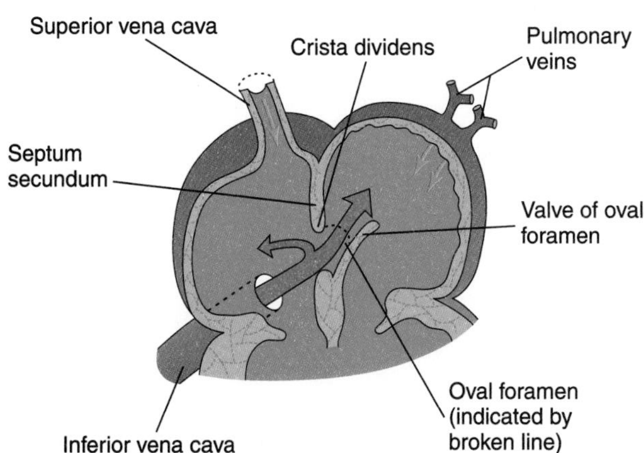

FIGURE 13-50. Schematic diagram of blood flow through the fetal atria illustrating how the crista dividens (lower edge of septum secundum) separates the blood coming from the inferior vena cava into two streams. The larger stream passes through the oval foramen into the left atrium, where it mixes with the small amount of poorly oxygenated blood coming from the lungs through the pulmonary veins. The smaller stream of blood from the inferior vena cava remains in the right atrium and mixes with poorly oxygenated blood from the superior vena cava and coronary sinus.

Umbilical Vein and the Round Ligament of the Liver

The umbilical vein remains patent for a considerable period and may be used for exchange transfusions of blood during early infancy. These transfusions are often done to prevent brain damage and death in infants with anemia from *erythroblastosis fetalis*. In exchange transfusions, most of the infant's blood is replaced with donor blood. The lumen of the umbilical vein usually does not disappear completely; in these people, the round ligament can be cannulated, if necessary, for the injection of contrast media or chemotherapeutic drugs.

The intra-abdominal part of the *umbilical vein* eventually becomes the **round ligament of liver** (L. *ligamentum teres*) (see Fig. 13-47), which passes from the umbilicus to the porta hepatis; here it is attached to the left branch of the portal vein (Fig. 13-51).

Ductus Venosus and Ligamentum Venosum

The DV becomes the ligamentum venosum. This ligament passes through the liver from the left branch of the portal vein and attaches to the IVC (see Fig. 13-51).

Umbilical Arteries and Abdominal Ligaments

Most of the intra-abdominal parts of the umbilical arteries become the **medial umbilical ligaments** (see Fig. 13-47); the proximal parts of these vessels persist as the **superior vesical arteries**, which supply the urinary bladder.

Oval Foramen and Oval Fossa

The oval foramen normally closes functionally at birth. Anatomic closure occurs by the third month and results from tissue proliferation and adhesion of the septum primum to the left margin of the septum secundum. The septum primum forms the floor of the oval fossa (Fig. 13-52). The inferior edge of the septum secundum forms a rounded fold, the border of the oval fossa (L. *limbus fossae ovalis*), which marks the former boundary of the oval foramen. There is often a lunate impression on the left side of the interatrial septum, which indicates the former site of the oval foramen.

Ductus Arteriosus and Ligamentum Arteriosum

Functional closure of the DA is usually completed within the first few days after birth (Fig. 13-53*A*). Anatomic closure of the DA and formation of the ligamentum arteriosum normally occurs by the 12th postnatal week (see Fig. 13-53*C*). This short, thick ligament extends from the left pulmonary artery to the arch of the aorta.

PATENT DUCTUS ARTERIOSUS

PDA, a common anomaly, is two to three times more frequent in females than in males (see Fig. 13-53*B*). The reason for this preponderance is not known.

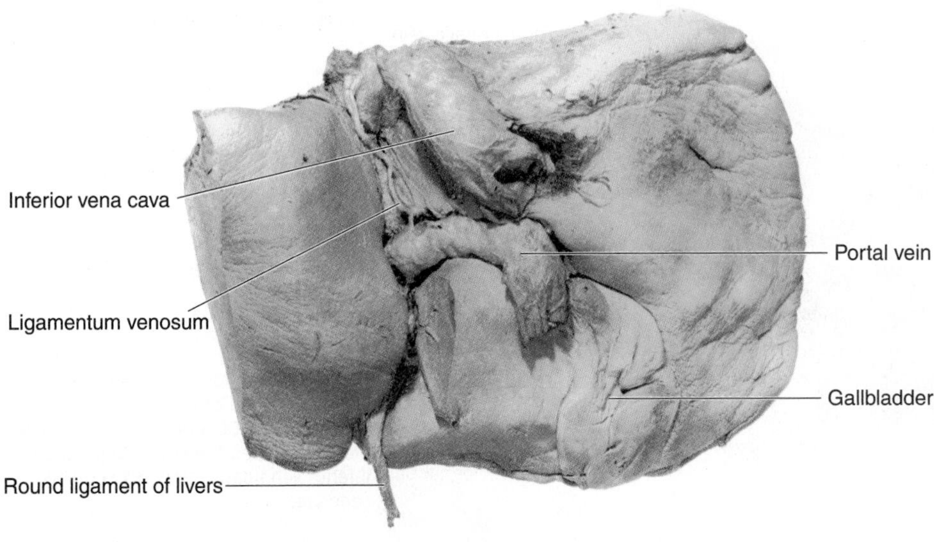

Figure 13-51. Dissection of the visceral surface of an adult liver. Note that the umbilical vein is represented by the round ligament of the liver and the ductus venosus by the ligamentum venosum.

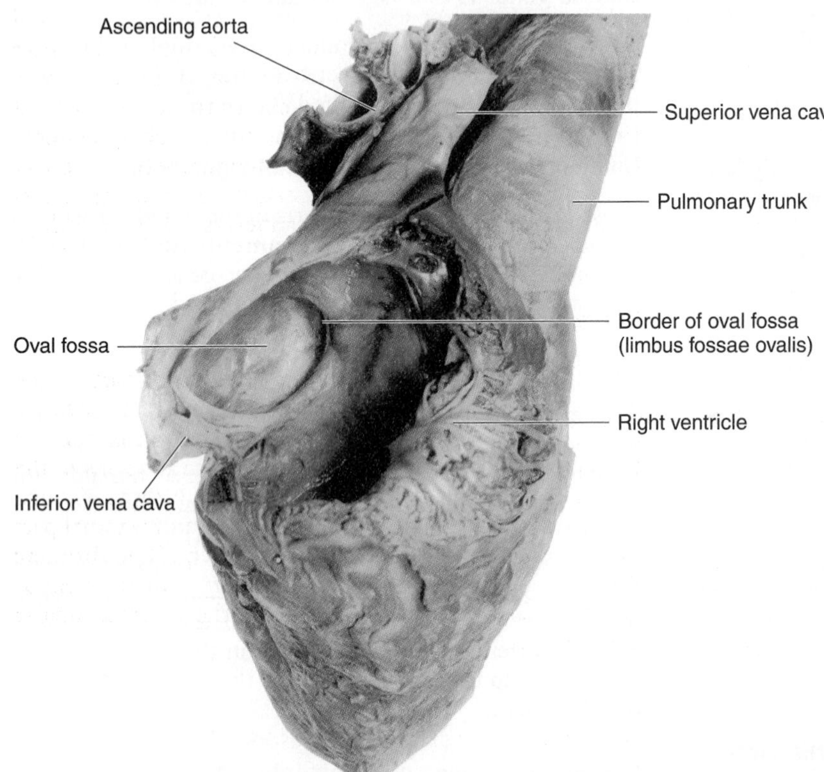

Figure 13-52. Dissection of the right atrial aspect of the interatrial septum of an adult heart. Observe the oval fossa and the border of the oval fossa. The floor of the oval fossa is formed by the septum primum, whereas the border of the fossa is formed by the free edge of the septum secundum. Aeration of the lungs at birth is associated with a dramatic decrease in pulmonary vascular resistance and a marked increase in pulmonary flow. Because of the increased pulmonary blood flow, the pressure in the left atrium is increased above that in the right atrium. This increased left atrial pressure closes the oval foramen by pressing the valve of the oval foramen against the septum secundum. This forms the oval fossa, a landmark of the interatrial septum.

Functional closure of the DA usually occurs soon after birth; however, if it remains patent, aortic blood is shunted into the pulmonary trunk. It has been suggested that persistent patency of the DA may result from failure of TGF-β induction after birth. PDA is the most common congenital anomaly associated with maternal rubella infection during early pregnancy. Premature infants and infants born at high altitude may have a PDA; the patency is the result of hypoxia and immaturity. Virtually all infants whose birth weight is less than 1750 g have a PDA in the first 24 hours of postnatal life. A PDA that persists in a full-term infant is a pathologic entity. Surgical closure by ligation and division is the usual treatment of the DA.

The **embryologic basis of PDA** is failure of the DA to involute after birth and form the ligamentum arteriosum. Failure of contraction of the muscular wall of the DA after birth is the primary cause of patency. There is some evidence that the low oxygen content of the blood in newborn infants with respiratory distress syndrome can adversely affect

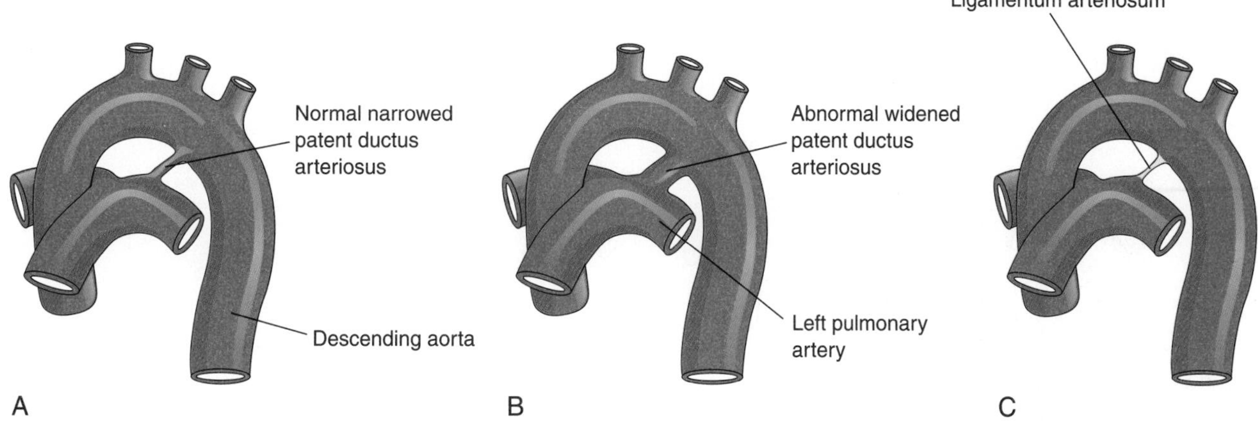

FIGURE 13-53. Closure of the ductus arteriosus (DA). **A,** The DA of a newborn infant. **B,** Abnormal patent DA in a 6-month-old infant. **C,** The ligamentum arteriosum in a 6-month-old infant.

closure of the DA; for example, PDA commonly occurs in small premature infants with respiratory difficulties associated with a deficiency of surfactant.

PDA may occur as an isolated anomaly or in association with cardiac defects. Large differences between aortic and pulmonary blood pressures can cause a heavy flow of blood through the DA, thereby preventing normal constriction. Such pressure differences may be caused by coarctation of the aorta (see Fig. 13-41*C*), TGA (see Fig. 13-32), or pulmonary stenosis and atresia (see Fig. 13-34).

DEVELOPMENT OF THE LYMPHATIC SYSTEM

The lymphatic system begins to develop at the end of the sixth week, approximately 2 weeks after the primordia of the cardiovascular system are recognizable. Lymphatic vessels develop in a manner similar to that previously described for blood vessels (see Chapter 4) and make connections with the venous system. The early lymphatic capillaries join each other to form a network of lymphatics (Fig. 13-54*A*).

Development of Lymph Sacs and Lymphatic Ducts

There are *six primary lymph sacs* present at the end of the embryonic period (see Fig. 13-54*A*):

- *Two jugular lymph sacs* near the junction of the subclavian veins with the anterior cardinal veins (the future internal jugular veins)
- *Two iliac lymph sacs* near the junction of the iliac veins with the posterior cardinal veins
- *One retroperitoneal lymph sac* in the root of the mesentery on the posterior abdominal wall
- *One chyle cistern* (L. *cisterna chyli*) located dorsal to the retroperitoneal lymph sac

Lymphatic vessels soon connect to the lymph sacs and pass along main veins; to the head, neck, and upper limbs from the jugular lymph sacs; to the lower trunk and lower limbs from the iliac lymph sacs; and to the primordial gut from the retroperitoneal lymph sac and the **chyle cistern.** Two large channels (right and left thoracic ducts) connect the jugular lymph sacs with this cistern. Soon a large anastomosis forms between these channels (see Fig. 13-54*B*).

Thoracic Duct

The thoracic duct develops from the caudal part of the right thoracic duct, the anastomosis between the left and right thoracic ducts, and the cranial part of the left thoracic duct. As a result, there are many variations in the origin, course, and termination of the adult thoracic duct. The **right lymphatic duct** is derived from the cranial part of the right thoracic duct (see Fig. 13-54*C*). The **thoracic duct** and right lymphatic duct connect with the venous system at the venous angle between the internal jugular and subclavian veins.

Development of the Lymph Nodes

Except for the superior part of the chyle cistern, the lymph sacs are transformed into groups of lymph nodes during the early fetal period. Mesenchymal cells invade each lymph sac and break up its cavity into a network of lymphatic channels—the primordia of the **lymph sinuses.** Other mesenchymal cells give rise to the capsule and connective tissue framework of the lymph nodes.

Development of the Lymphocytes

The lymphocytes are derived originally from stem cells in the umbilical vesicle (yolk sac) mesenchyme and later from the liver and spleen. These early lymphocytes eventually enter the bone marrow, where they divide to form

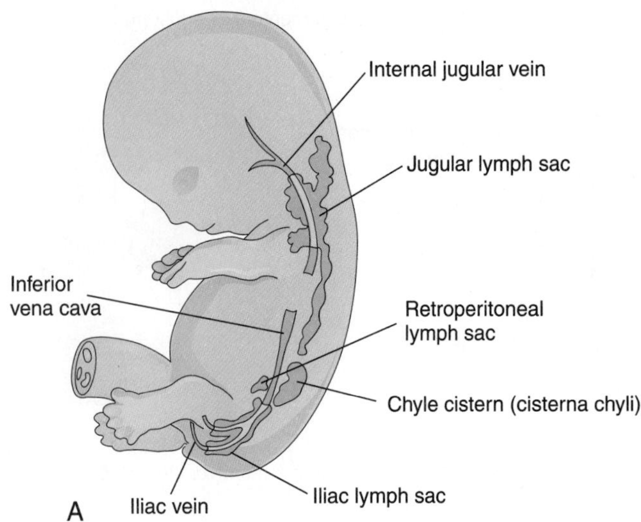

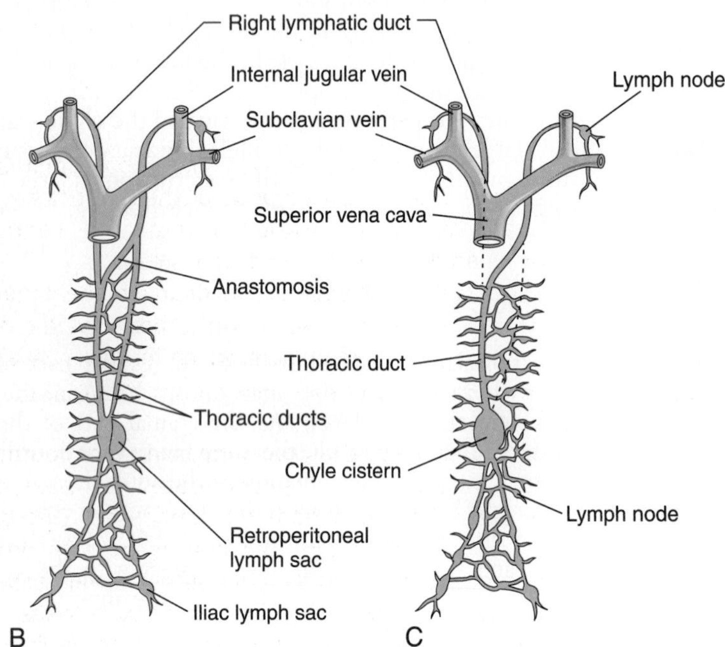

FIGURE 13-54. Development of the lymphatic system. **A,** Left side of a $7^1/_2$-week embryo showing the primary lymph sacs. **B,** Ventral view of the lymphatic system at 9 weeks showing the paired thoracic ducts. **C,** Later in the fetal period, illustrating formation of the thoracic duct and right lymphatic duct.

lymphoblasts. The lymphocytes that appear in lymph nodes before birth are derived from the *thymus*, a derivative of the third pair of pharyngeal pouches (see Chapter 9). Small lymphocytes leave the thymus and circulate to other lymphoid organs. Later, some mesenchymal cells in the lymph nodes also differentiate into lymphocytes. Lymph nodules do not appear in the lymph nodes until just before and/or after birth.

Development of the Spleen and Tonsils

The **spleen** develops from an aggregation of mesenchymal cells in the dorsal mesogastrium (see Chapter 11).

The **palatine tonsils** develop from the second pair of pharyngeal pouches and nearby mesenchyme. The **tubal tonsils** develop from aggregations of lymph nodules around the pharyngeal openings of the pharyngotympanic tubes. The **pharyngeal tonsils** (adenoids) develop from an aggregation of lymph nodules in the wall of the nasopharynx. The **lingual tonsil** develops from an aggregation of lymph nodules in the root of the tongue. Lymph nodules also develop in the mucosa of the respiratory and digestive systems.

ANOMALIES OF THE LYMPHATIC SYSTEM

Congenital anomalies of the lymphatic system are uncommon. There may be diffuse swelling of a part of the body—**congenital lymphedema**. This condition

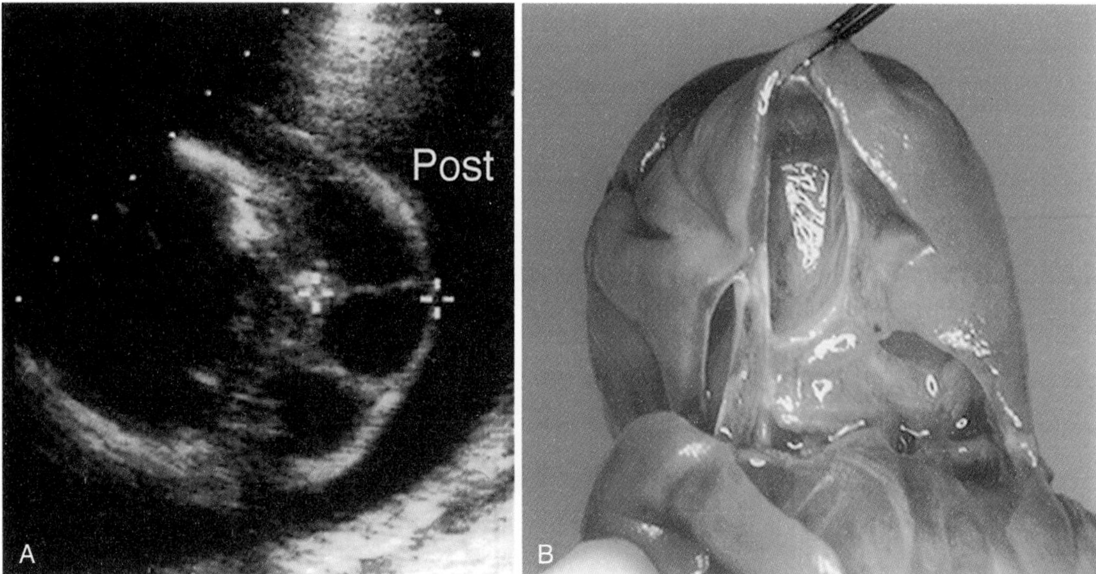

FIGURE 13-55. Cystic hygroma. **A,** Transverse axial sonogram of the neck in a fetus with a large cystic hygroma. **B,** Photograph of a neck dissection. Cystic hygroma was demonstrated from this cross-sectional view of the posterior fetal neck at 18.5 weeks' gestation. The lesion was characterized by multiple, septated cystic areas within the mass itself as shown in the pathology specimen (**B**). Post, posterior. (Courtesy of Wesley Lee, MD, Division of Fetal Imaging, William Beaumont Hospital, Royal Oak, MI.)

may result from dilation of primordial lymphatic channels or from congenital hypoplasia of lymphatic vessels. More rarely, diffuse cystic dilation of lymphatic channels involves widespread portions of the body. In **cystic hygroma**, large swellings usually appear in the inferolateral part of the neck and consist of large single or multilocular, fluid-filled cavities (Fig. 13-55). Hygromas may be present at birth, but they often enlarge and become evident during infancy. Most hygromas appear to be derived from abnormal transformation of the jugular lymph sacs. Hygromas are believed to arise from parts of a jugular lymph sac that are pinched off or from lymphatic spaces that fail to establish connections with the main lymphatic channels.

SUMMARY OF THE CARDIOVASCULAR SYSTEM

- The cardiovascular system begins to develop at the end of the third week, and the heart starts to beat at the beginning of the fourth week. Mesenchymal cells derived from splanchnic mesoderm proliferate and form isolated cell clusters, which soon develop into heart tubes that join to form the primordial vascular system. Splanchnic mesoderm surrounding the heart tube forms the primordial myocardium.
- The **heart primordium** consists of four chambers: the bulbus cordis, ventricle, atrium, and sinus venosus.
- The TA (primordium of ascending aorta and pulmonary trunk) is continuous caudally with the bulbus cordis, which becomes part of the ventricles. As the heart grows, it bends to the right and soon acquires the general external appearance of the adult heart. The heart becomes partitioned into four chambers between the fourth and seventh weeks.
- Three systems of paired veins drain into the primordial heart: the vitelline system, which becomes the portal system; the cardinal veins, which form the caval system; and the umbilical system, which involutes after birth.
- As the pharyngeal arches form during the fourth and fifth weeks, they are penetrated by pharyngeal arteries that arise from the aortic sac. During the sixth to eighth weeks, the pharyngeal arch arteries are transformed into the adult arterial arrangement of the carotid, subclavian, and pulmonary arteries.
- The critical period of heart development is from day 20 to day 50 after fertilization. Numerous events occur during cardiac development, and deviation from the normal pattern at any time may produce one or more congenital heart defects. Because partitioning of the primordial heart results from complex cellular and molecular processes, defects of the cardiac septa are relatively common, particularly ventricular septal defects (VSDs). Some congenital anomalies result from abnormal transformation of the pharyngeal arch arteries into the adult arterial pattern (e.g., the right sixth pharyngeal arch artery).
- Because the lungs are nonfunctional during prenatal life, the fetal cardiovascular system is structurally designed so that the blood is oxygenated in the placenta and most of it bypasses the lungs. The modifications that establish the postnatal circulatory pattern at birth are not abrupt, but extend into infancy.

Failure of these changes in the circulatory system to occur at birth results in two of the most common congenital anomalies of the heart and great vessels: patent oval foramen and PDA.

- The lymphatic system begins to develop late in the sixth week in close association with the venous system. Six primary lymph sacs develop, which later become interconnected by lymphatic vessels. Lymph nodes develop along the network of lymphatic vessels; lymph nodules do not appear until just before or after birth.

CLINICALLY ORIENTED PROBLEMS

CASE 13-1

A pediatrician detected a cardiac defect in an infant, and he explained to the baby's mother that this is a common birth defect.

- What is the most common type of congenital cardiac defect?
- What percentage of congenital heart disease results from this defect?
- Discuss blood flow in infants with this defect.
- What problems would the infant likely encounter if the cardiac defect were large?

CASE 13-2

A female infant was born normally after a pregnancy complicated by a rubella infection during the first trimester of pregnancy. She had congenital cataracts and congenital heart disease. A radiograph of the infant's chest at 3 weeks showed generalized cardiac enlargement with some increase in pulmonary vascularity.

- What congenital cardiovascular anomaly is commonly associated with maternal rubella during early pregnancy?
- What probably caused the cardiac enlargement?

CASE 13-3

A newborn infant was referred to a pediatrician because of the blue color of his skin (cyanosis). An ultrasound examination was ordered to confirm the preliminary diagnosis of tetralogy of Fallot.

- In the tetralogy of Fallot, there are four cardiac abnormalities. What are they?
- What is one of the most obvious signs of the tetralogy of Fallot?
- What radiographic technique might be used to confirm a tentative diagnosis of this type of CHD?
- What do you think would be the main aim of therapy in these cases?

CASE 13-4

A male infant was born after a full-term normal pregnancy. Severe generalized cyanosis was observed on the first day. A chest radiograph revealed a slightly enlarged heart with a narrow base and increased pulmonary vascularity. A clinical diagnosis of transformation of the great arteries (TGA) was made.

- What radiographic technique would likely be used to verify the diagnosis?
- What would this technique reveal in the present case?
- How was the infant able to survive after birth with this severe congenital anomaly of the great arteries?

CASE 13-5

During an autopsy on a 72-year-old man who died from chronic heart failure, it was observed that his heart was very large and that the pulmonary artery and its main branches were dilated. Opening the heart revealed a very large atrial septal defect.

- What type of atrial septal defect was probably present?
- Where would the defect likely be located?
- Explain why the pulmonary artery and its main branches were dilated.

Discussion of these problems appears at the back of the book.

References and Suggested Reading

Alfred J: Genes at the heart of DiGeorge. Nature Rev Genet 2:240, 2001.

Amato JJ, Douglas WI, Desai U, et al: Ectopia cordis. Chest Surg Clin North Am 10:297, 2000.

American Academy of Pediatrics (Task Force on Sudden Infant Death Syndrome): The changing concept of sudden infant death syndrome: Diagnostic coding shifts, controversies regarding the sleeping environment and new variables to consider reducing risk. Pediatrics 116:1245, 2005.

Anderson RH, Brown NA, Moorman AFM: Development and structures of the venous pole of the heart. Dev Dyn 235:2, 2006.

Anderson RH, Webb S, Brown NA: Clinical anatomy of the atrial septum with reference to its developmental components. Clin Anat 12:362, 1999.

Andrews RE, Simpson JM, Sharland GK, et al: Outcome after preterm delivery of infants antenatally diagnosed with congenital heart disease. J Pediatr 148:213, 2006.

Bernstein E: The cardiovascular system. In Behrman RE, Kliegman RM, Jenson HB (eds): Nelson Textbook of Pediatrics, 17th ed. Philadelphia, WB Saunders, 2004.

Brickner ME, Hillis LD, Lange RA: Congenital heart disease in adults. N Engl J Med 342:256, 334, 2000.

Brown MD, Wernovsky G, Mussatto KA, Berger S: Long-term and developmental outcomes of children with complex congenital heart disease. Clin Perinatol 32:1043, 2005.

Cohen MS, Frommelt MA: Does fetal diagnosis make a difference? Clin Perinatol 32:877, 2005.

Conte G, Pellegrini A: On the development of the coronary arteries in human embryos, stages 13–19. Anat Embryol 169:209, 1984.

Forouhar AS, Liebling M, Hickerson A, et al: The embryonic vertebrate heart tube is a dynamic suction pump. Science 312:751, 2006.

Goldmuntz E: The epidemiology and genetics of congenital heart disease. Clin Perinatol 28:1, 2001.

Gruber PJ: Cardiac development: New concepts. Clin Perinatol 32:845, 2005.

Hardy KM, Mjaatvedt CH, Antin PB: Hot hearts in the Sonoran Desert: The 11th Weinstein Cardiovascular Development Conference in Tucson. Dev Dyn 235:170, 2006.

Harris BS, Spruill L, Edmonson AM, et al: Differentiation of cardiac Purkinje fibers requires precise spatiotemporal regulation of Nkx2-5 expression. Dev Dyn 235:38, 2006.
Harvey NL, Oliver G: Choose your fate: Artery, vein or lymphatic vessel ? Curr Opin Genet Dev 14:499, 2004.
Harvey RP: Seeking a regulatory roadmap for heart morphogenesis. Cell Dev Biol 10:99, 1999.
Harvey RP, Rosenthal N: Heart Development. Orlando, Academic Press, 1999.
Hauser M: Congenital anomalies of the coronary arteries. Heart 91:1240, 2005.
Jirásek JE: An Atlas of Human Prenatal Developmental Mechanics. Anatomy and Staging. London and New York, Taylor & Francis, 2004.
Kiserud T: The ductus venosus. Semin Perinatol 25:11, 2001.
Le Douarin NM, Kalcheim C: The Neural Crest, 2nd ed. Cambridge, Cambridge University Press, 1999.
Lin AE, Pierpont ME (eds): Heart development and the genetic aspects of cardiovascular malformations. Am J Med Genet 97:235, 2000.
Lu CW, Wang JK, Chang CI, et al: Noninvasive diagnosis of aortic coarctations in neonates with patent ductus arteriosus. J Pediatr 148:217, 2006.
Moore KL, Dalley AF: Clinically Oriented Anatomy, 5th ed. Baltimore, Williams & Wilkins, 2006.
Olson EN: The path to the heart and the road not taken. Science 291:2327, 2001.
O'Rahilly R: The timing and sequence of events in human cardiogenesis. Acta Anat 79:70, 1971.
Pelech AN, Broeckel U: Toward the etiologies of congenital heart diseases. Clin Perinatol 32:825, 2005.
Pierpont MEM, Markwald RR, Lin AE: Genetic aspects of atrioventricular septal defects. Am J Med Genet 97:289–296, 2000.
Roman BL, Weinstein BM: Building the vertebrate vasculature: Research is going swimmingly. BioEssays 22:882, 2000.
Rothenberg EV: Stepwise specification of lymphocyte developmental lineages. Curr Opin Genet Dev 10:370, 2000.
Shima DT, Mailhos C: Vascular developmental biology: Getting nervous. Curr Opin Genet Dev 10:536, 2000.
Silverman NH, Schmidt KG: Ultrasound evaluation of the fetal heart. In Callen PW (ed): Ultrasonography in Obstetrics and Gynecology, 4th ed. Philadelphia, WB Saunders, 2000.
Simpson LL: Screening for congenital heart disease. Obstet Gynecol Clin North Am 31:51, 2004.
Srivastava D: Making or breaking the heart: From lineage determination to morphogenesis. Cell 126:1037, 2006.
Srivastava D, Olson EN: A genetic blueprint for cardiac development. Nature 407:221, 2000.
Szwast A, Rychik J: Current concepts in fetal cardiovascular disease. Clin Perinatol 32:857, 2005.
Tomanek RJ, Zheng W, Peters KG, et al: Multiple growth factors regulate coronary embryonic vasculogenesis. Dev Dyn 221:264, 2001.
Vaughan CJ, Basson CT: Molecular determinants of atrial and ventricular septal defects and patent ductus arteriosus. Am J Med Genet 97:304, 2000.
Watanabe M, Schaefer KS: Cardiac embryology. In Martin RJ, Fanaroff AA, Walsh MC (eds): Fanaroff and Martin's Neonatal-Perinatal Medicine. Diseases of the Fetus and Infant, 8th ed. Philadelphia, Mosby, 2006.
Weese-Mayer DE, Berry-Kravis EM, Zhou L, et al: Sudden infant death syndrome: Case-control frequency differences at genes pertinent to early autonomic nervous system embryologic development. Pediatr Res 56:321, 2004.
Yan M, Sinning AR: Retinoic acid administration is associated with changes in the extracellular matrix and cardiac mesenchyme within the endocardial cushion. Anat Rec 263:53, 2001.
Yutzey KE, Kirby ML: Wherefore heart thou? Embryonic origins of cardiogenic mesoderm. Dev Dyn 223:307, 2002.
Zahka KG, Erenberg F: Congenital defects. In Martin RJ, Fanaroff AA, Walsh MC (eds): Fanaroff and Martin's Neonatal-Perinatal Medicine. Diseases of the Fetus and Infant, 8th ed. Philadelphia, Mosby, 2006.
Zavos PM: Stem cells and cellular therapy: Potential treatment for cardiovascular diseases. Int J Cardiol 107:1, 2006

14

The Skeletal System

Development of Bone and Cartilage 339
- Histogenesis of Cartilage 339
- Histogenesis of Bone 339
- Intramembranous Ossification 339
- Endochondral Ossification 339

Development of Joints 342
- Fibrous Joints 344
- Cartilaginous Joints 344
- Synovial Joints 344

Development of the Axial Skeleton 344
- Development of the Vertebral Column 344
- Development of the Ribs 346
- Development of the Sternum 347
- Development of the Cranium 347
- Newborn Cranium 347
- Postnatal Growth of the Cranium 348

Development of the Appendicular Skeleton 353

Summary of the Skeletal System 355

Clinically Oriented Problems 356

As the notochord and neural tube form, the intraembryonic mesoderm lateral to these structures thickens to form two longitudinal columns of **paraxial mesoderm** (Fig. 14-1*A* and *B*). Toward the end of the third week, these dorsolateral columns located in the trunk become segmented into blocks of mesoderm—the **somites** (see Fig. 14-1*C*). Externally the somites appear as beadlike elevations along the dorsolateral surface of the embryo (see Chapter 5). Each somite differentiates into two parts (see Fig. 14-1*D* and *E*):

- The ventromedial part is the **sclerotome**; its cells form the vertebrae and ribs.
- The dorsolateral part is the **dermomyotome**; cells from its myotome region form myoblasts (primordial muscle cells), and those from its dermatome region form the dermis (fibroblasts).

DEVELOPMENT OF BONE AND CARTILAGE

Mesodermal cells give rise to **mesenchyme—**a meshwork of loosely organized embryonic connective tissue. Bones first appear as condensations of mesenchymal cells that form bone models. *Condensation* marks the beginning of selective gene activity, which precedes cell differentiation (Figs. 14-2 and 14-3). Most flat bones develop in mesenchyme within preexisting membranous sheaths; this type of osteogenesis is called **intramembranous bone formation**. Mesenchymal models of most limb bones are transformed into cartilage bone models, which later become ossified by **endochondral bone formation.**

Bone morphogenetic proteins (BMP-5 and BMP-7), the growth factor Gdf5, members of the transforming growth factor β (TGF-β) superfamily, and other signaling molecules have been implicated as *endogenous regulators of chondrogenesis and skeletal development.*

Histogenesis of Cartilage

Cartilage develops from mesenchyme and first appears in embryos during the fifth week. In areas where cartilage is to develop, the mesenchyme condenses to form **chondrification centers**. The mesenchymal cells differentiate into **chondroblasts** that secrete collagenous fibrils and the ground substance (extracellular matrix). Subsequently, collagenous and/or elastic fibers are deposited in the intercellular substance or matrix. Three types of cartilage are distinguished according to the type of matrix that is formed:

- **Hyaline cartilage**, the most widely distributed type (e.g., in joints)
- **Fibrocartilage** (e.g., in intervertebral discs)
- **Elastic cartilage** (e.g., in auricle of ear)

Histogenesis of Bone

Bone primarily develops in two types of connective tissue, mesenchyme and cartilage, but can also develop in other connective tissues. Like cartilage, bone consists of cells and an organic intercellular substance—the **bone matrix**—that comprises collagen fibrils embedded in an amorphous component. Studies of the cellular and molecular events during embryonic bone formation suggest that osteogenesis and chondrogenesis are programmed early in development and are independent events under the influence of vascular events (see Chapter 21).

Intramembranous Ossification

This type of bone formation occurs in mesenchyme that has formed a membranous sheath (Fig. 14-4), hence, the name intramembranous ossification. The mesenchyme condenses and becomes highly vascular; some cells differentiate into **osteoblasts** (bone-forming cells) and begin to deposit unmineralized matrix—**osteoid.** Calcium phosphate is then deposited in the osteoid tissue as it is organized into bone. Bone osteoblasts are trapped in the matrix and become **osteocytes.** At first, new bone has no organized pattern. Spicules of bone soon become organized and coalesce into lamellae (layers). **Concentric lamellae** develop around blood vessels, forming **osteons** (haversian systems). Some osteoblasts remain at the periphery of the developing bone and continue to lay down lamellae, forming plates of compact bone on the surfaces. Between the surface plates, the intervening bone remains spiculated or spongy. This spongy environment is somewhat accentuated by the action of cells—**osteoclasts**—that reabsorb bone. Osteoclasts are multinucleated cells with a hematopoietic origin. In the interstices of spongy bone, the mesenchyme differentiates into **bone marrow**. During fetal and postnatal life, there is continuous remodeling of bone by the coordinated action of osteoclasts and osteoblasts.

Endochondral Ossification

Endochondral ossification (cartilaginous bone formation) is a type of bone formation that occurs in preexisting cartilaginous models (Fig. 14-5*A* to *E*). In a long bone, for example, the **primary center of ossification** appears in the **diaphysis**—the part of a long bone between its ends—that forms the shaft of the bone. At this center of ossification, chondrocytes (cartilage cells) increase in size (hypertrophy), the matrix becomes calcified, and the cells die. Concurrently, a thin layer of bone is deposited under the **perichondrium** surrounding the diaphysis; thus, the perichondrium becomes the **periosteum.** Invasion by vascular connective tissue from blood vessels surrounding the periosteum also breaks up the cartilage. Some invading cells differentiate into **hemopoietic cells,** blood cells, of the bone marrow. This process continues toward the **epiphyses** (ends of the bone). The spicules of bone are remodeled by the action of osteoclasts and osteoblasts.

Lengthening of long bones occurs at the **diaphysial-epiphysial junction**. The lengthening of bone depends on the epiphysial cartilage plates (growth plates), whose chondrocytes proliferate and participate in endochondral bone formation. Cartilage cells in the **diaphysial-**

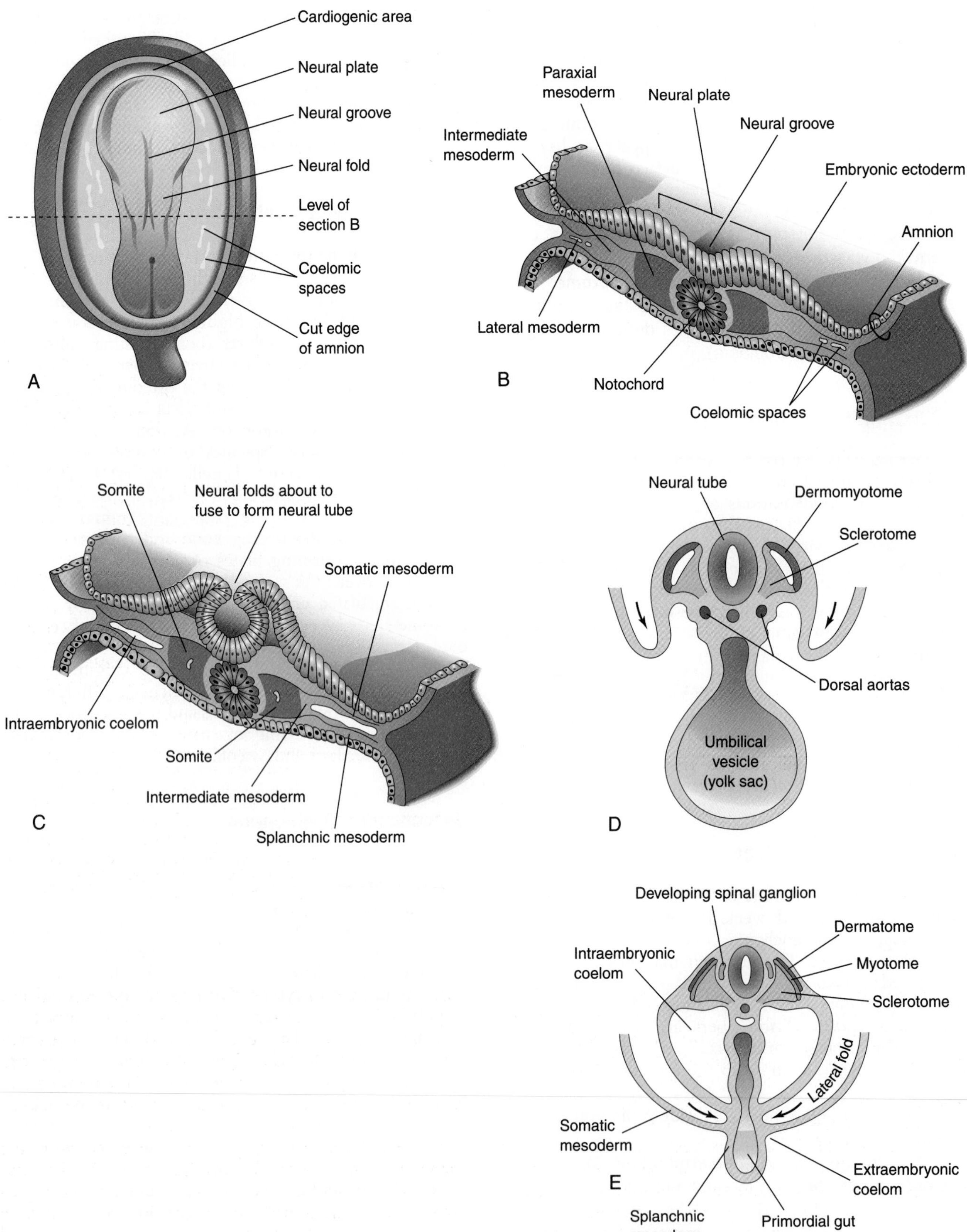

FIGURE 14-1. Illustrations of the formation and early differentiation of somites. **A,** Dorsal view of an embryo of approximately 18 days. **B,** Transverse section of the embryo shown in **A** illustrating the paraxial mesoderm from which the somites are derived. **C,** Transverse section of an embryo of approximately 22 days showing the appearance of the early somites. Note that the neural folds are about to fuse to form the neural tube. **D,** Transverse section of an embryo of approximately 24 days showing folding of the embryo in the horizontal plane (*arrows*). The dermomyotome region of the somite gives rise to the dermatome and myotome. **E,** Transverse section of an embryo of approximately 26 days showing the dermatome, myotome, and sclerotome regions of a somite.

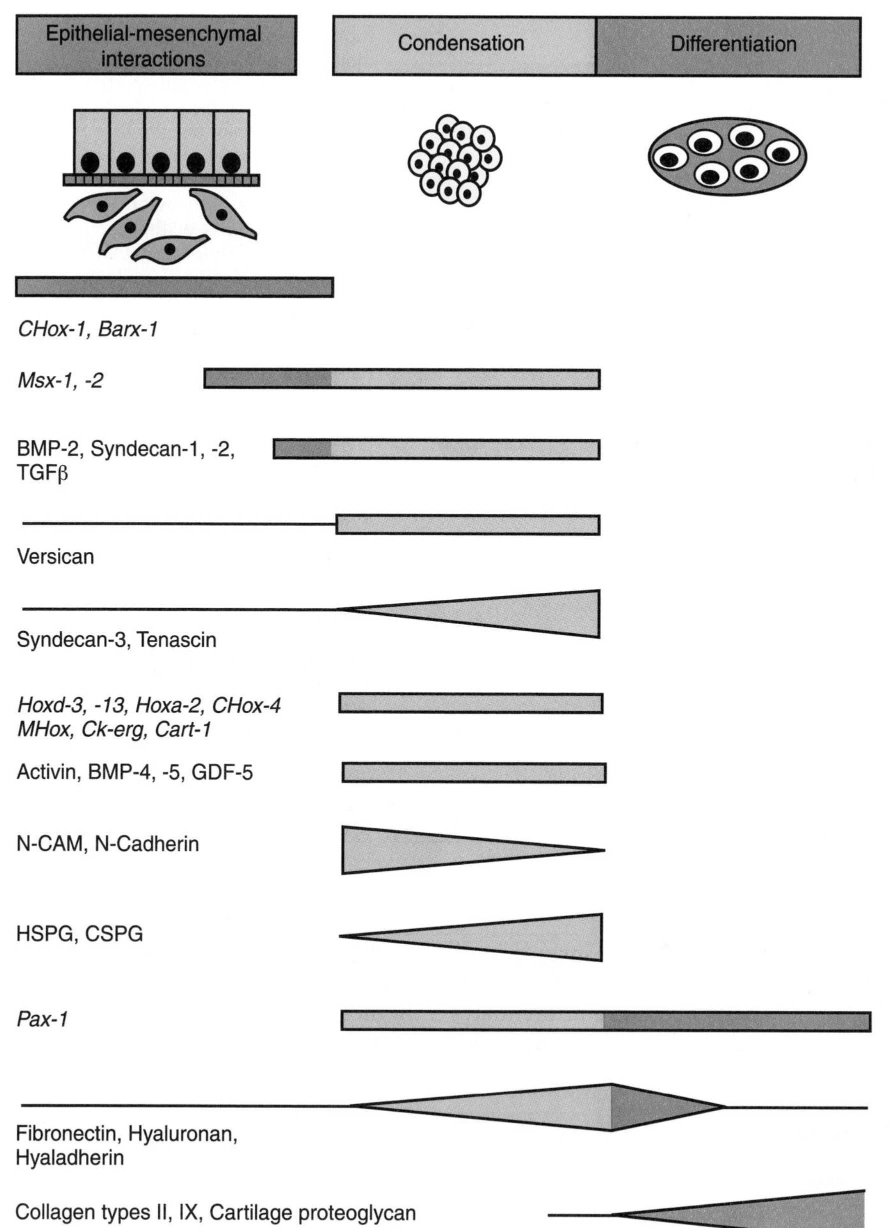

FIGURE 14-2. A summary of the molecules known to be associated with the three major phases of chondrogenesis in the craniofacial skeleton. The three phases are precondensation, characterized by epithelial-mesenchymal interactions (brown); condensation (yellow); and differentiation (blue). The precondensation phase is characterized by expression of *Hox* genes (*CHox-1* [*Hoxa 4*], *Barx-1*), Msx-1, -2, the growth factors bone morphogenetic protein [BMP]-2 and[transforming growth factor β [TGF-β], and syndecan-1. Versican, syndecan-3, and tenascin, which are present in low concentrations precondensation, are up-regulated at condensation. Other *Hox* genes and transcription factors (*Hoxd-3*, *-13*, *Hoxa-2*, Cdxa [*Chox-4*], *Mhox*, *Ck-erg*, and *Cart-1*) and other growth factors (activin, BMP-4, -5, and GDF-5) are expressed at condensation. The cell adhesion molecules neural cell adhesion molecule (N-CAM) and N-cadherin also appear with condensation but are down-regulated during condensation. Heparan sulfate and chondroitin sulfate proteoglycans appear at condensation and are up-regulated during condensation. The transcriptional factor *Pax-1* is present during and after condensation. Extracellular matrix molecules such as fibronectin, hyaluronan, and hyaladherin increase during condensation (yellow) but are down-regulated thereafter (blue). Collagen types II and IX and cartilage proteoglycan appear postcondensation, although mRNAs for the collagens and for the core protein of the proteoglycan are up-regulated during condensation. (From Hall BK, Miyake T: Divide, accumulate, differentiate: cell condensation in skeletal development revisited. Int J Dev Biol 39:881, 1995. See this publication for more details.)

epiphysial region proliferate by mitosis. Toward the diaphysis, the cartilage cells hypertrophy and the matrix becomes calcified. Spicules are isolated from each other by vascular invasion from the **medullary (marrow) cavity**. Bone is deposited on these spicules by osteoblasts; resorption of this bone keeps the spongy bone masses relatively constant in length and enlarges the medullary cavity.

Ossification of limb bones begins at the end of the embryonic period and thereafter makes demands on the maternal supply of calcium and phosphorus. Pregnant women are therefore advised to maintain an adequate intake of these elements to preserve healthy bones and teeth. At birth, the diaphyses are largely ossified, but most of the epiphyses are still cartilaginous. **Secondary ossification centers** appear in the epiphyses in most bones during the first few years after birth. The epiphysial cartilage cells hypertrophy, and there is invasion by vascular connective tissue. Ossification spreads radially, and only the articular cartilage and a transverse plate of cartilage, the **epiphysial cartilage plate**, remain cartilaginous (see Fig. 14-5*E*). Upon completion of growth, this plate is replaced by spongy bone; the epiphyses and diaphysis are united, and no further elongation of the bone occurs.

In most bones, the epiphyses have fused with the diaphysis by the age of 20 years. Growth in the diameter of a bone results from deposition of bone at the periosteum and from resorption on the internal medullary surface. The rate of deposition and resorption is balanced to regulate the thickness of the compact bone and the size of the medullary cavity. The internal reorganization of bone continues throughout life.

The development of irregular bones is similar to that of the epiphyses of long bones. Ossification begins centrally

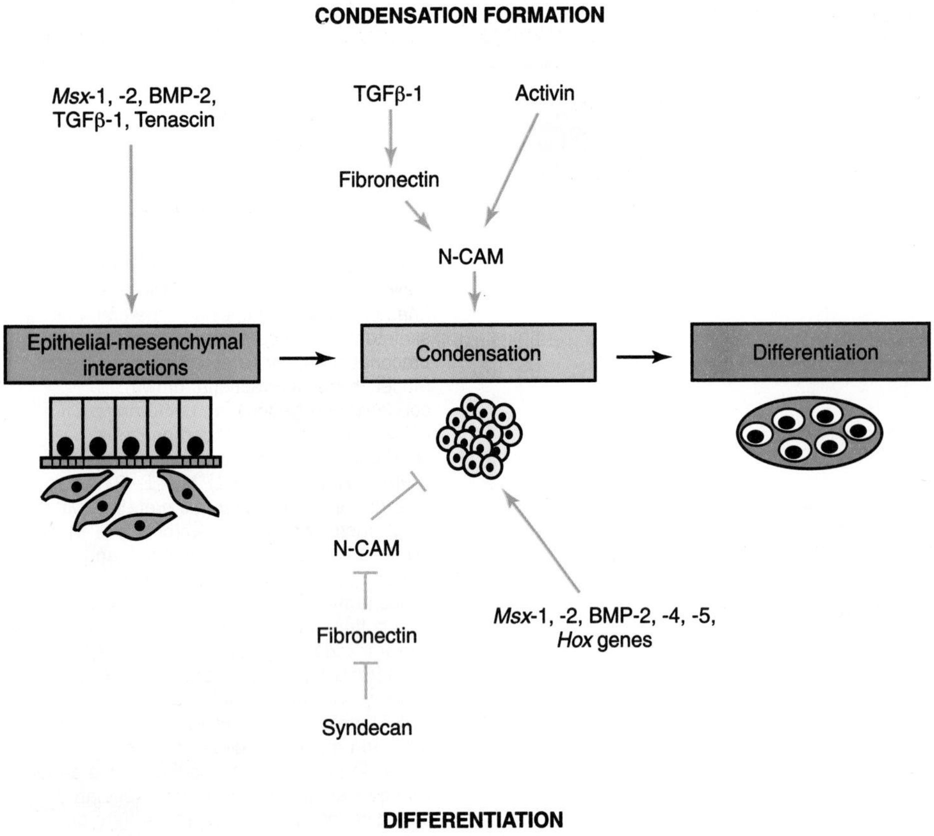

CONDENSATION FORMATION

Msx-1, -2, BMP-2, TGFβ-1, Tenascin

TGFβ-1

Activin

Fibronectin

N-CAM

Epithelial-mesenchymal interactions

Condensation

Differentiation

N-CAM

Fibronectin

Syndecan

Msx-1, -2, BMP-2, -4, -5, *Hox* genes

DIFFERENTIATION

FIGURE 14-3. A summary of the molecular pathways leading to condensation formation and to differentiation of prechondrogenic cells in the three major phases of chondrogenesis shown in Figure 14-2. Condensation is initiated by *Msx-1* and *Msx-2* genes, growth factors, and tenascin regulating epithelial-mesenchymal interactions that in turn control condensation. Transforming growth factor β_1 (TGF-β_1), by up-regulating fibronectin, and activin, by direct action, stimulate accumulation of neural cell adhesion molecule (N-CAM) and so promote condensation. Transition from condensation to overt cell differentiation is mediated negatively by suppression of further condensation and positively by direct enhancement of differentiation. Syndecan, by inhibiting fibronectin, breaks the link to N-CAM and so terminates condensation formation. Cessation of activin synthesis has the same effect. A number of *Hox* and *Msx* genes and bone morphogenetic proteins (BMP)-2, -4, and -5 enhance differentiation directly by acting on condensed cells. (From Hall BK, Miyake T: Divide, accumulate, differentiate: cell condensation in skeletal development revisited. Int J Dev Biol 39:881, 1995. See this publication for more details.)

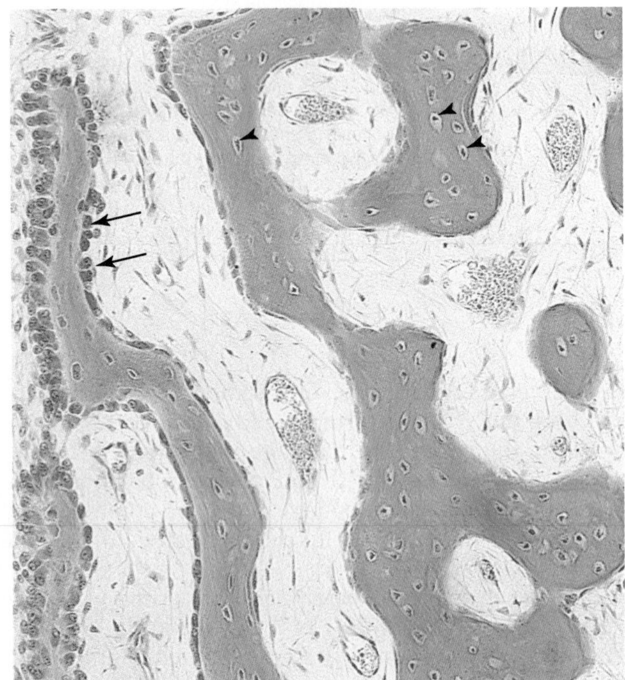

FIGURE 14-4. Light micrograph of intramembranous ossification (×132). Trabeculae of bone are being formed by osteoblasts lining their surface (*arrows*). Observe osteocytes trapped in lacunae (*arrowheads*) and that primordial osteons are beginning to form. The osteons (canals) contain blood capillaries. (From Gartner LP, Hiatt JL: Color Textbook of Histology, 2nd ed. Philadelphia, WB Saunders, 2001.)

and spreads in all directions. In addition to membranous and endochondral ossification, **chondroid tissue**, which also differentiates from mesenchyme, is now recognized as an important factor for skeletal growth.

RICKETS

Rickets is a disease that occurs in children who have a vitamin D deficiency. This vitamin is required for calcium absorption by the intestine. The resulting calcium deficiency causes disturbances of ossification of the epiphysial cartilage plates (i.e., they are not adequately mineralized), and there is disorientation of cells at the metaphysis. The limbs are shortened and deformed, with severe bowing of the limb bones.

DEVELOPMENT OF JOINTS

Joints begin to develop with the appearance of the **interzonal mesenchyme** during the sixth week, and by the end of the eighth week, they resemble adult joints (Fig. 14-6). Joints are classified as fibrous joints, cartilaginous joints, and synovial joints. Joints with little or no movement are classified according to the type of material holding the bones together, for example, the bones involved in fibrous joints are joined by fibrous tissue.

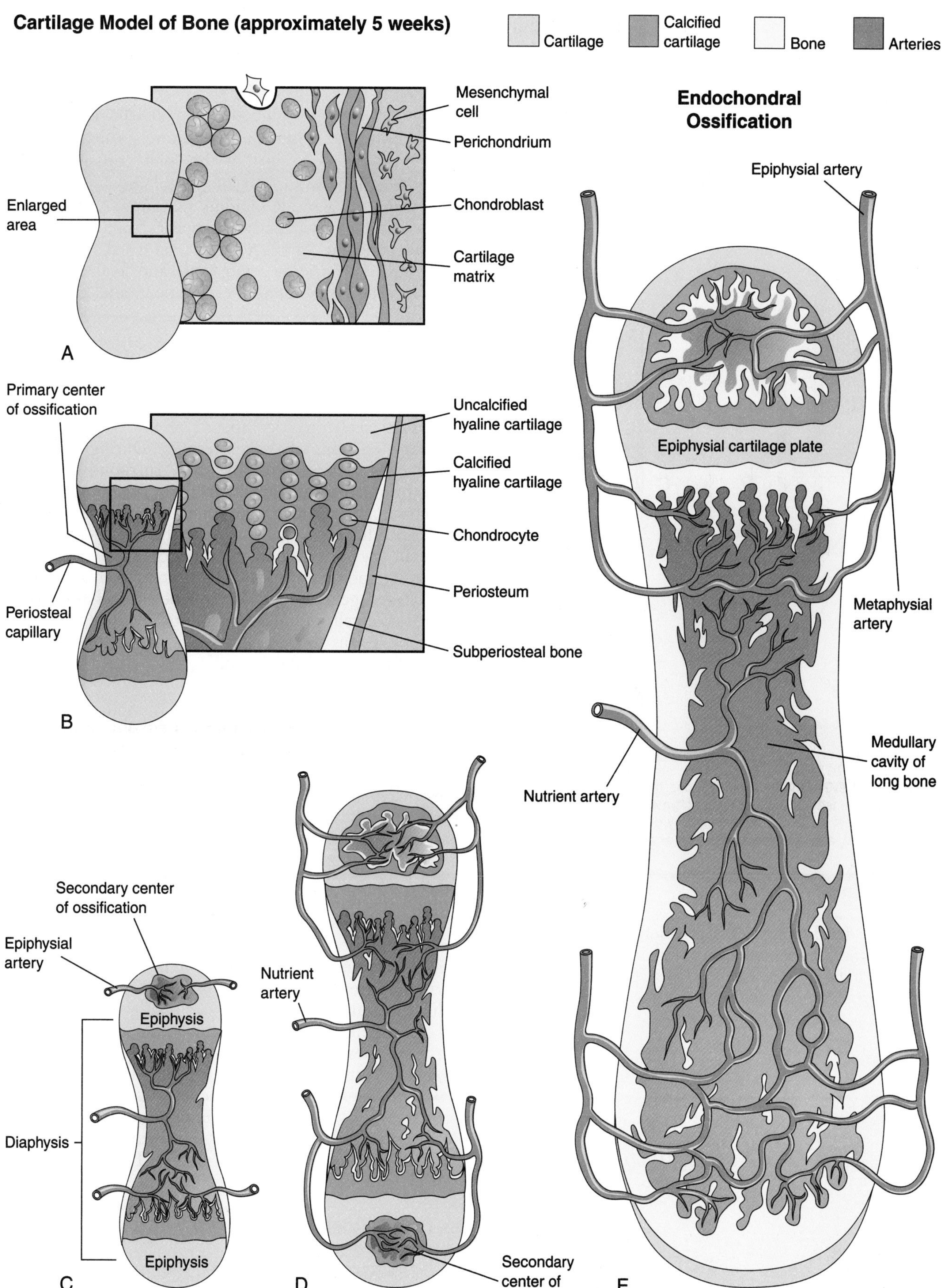

FIGURE 14-5. **A** to **E,** Schematic longitudinal sections illustrating endochondral (intracartilaginous) ossification in a developing long bone.

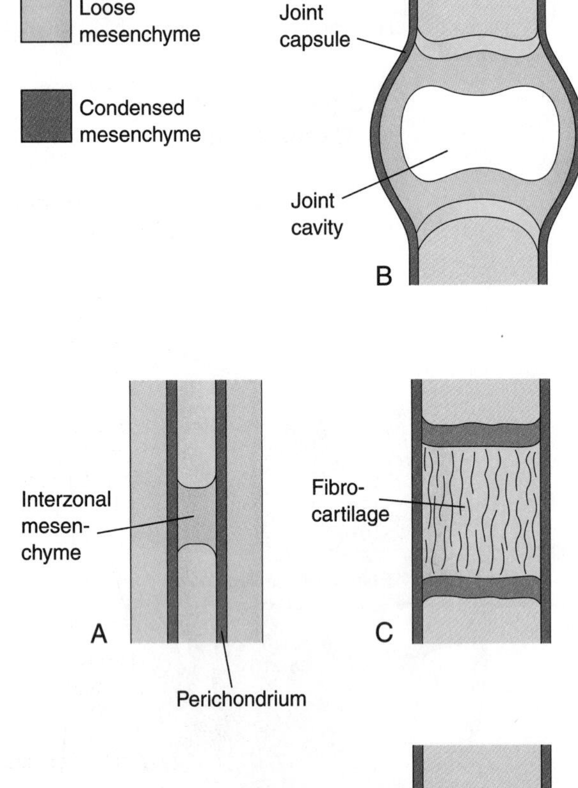

FIGURE 14-6. Development of joints during the sixth and seventh weeks. **A,** Condensed interzonal mesenchyme in the gap between the developing bones. This primordial joint may differentiate into a synovial joint (**B**), a cartilaginous joint (**C**), or a fibrous joint (**D**).

Fibrous Joints

During the development of fibrous joints, the **interzonal mesenchyme** between the developing bones differentiates into dense fibrous tissue (see Fig. 14-6*D*), for example, the sutures of the cranium are fibrous joints.

Cartilaginous Joints

During the development of cartilaginous joints, the interzonal mesenchyme between the developing bones differentiates into **hyaline cartilage** (e.g., the costochondral joints) or **fibrocartilage** (e.g., the pubic symphysis) (see Fig. 14-6*C*).

Synovial Joints

During the development of synovial joints (e.g., the knee joint), the interzonal mesenchyme between the developing bones differentiates as follows (see Fig. 14-6*B*):

- Peripherally it forms the capsular and other ligaments.
- Centrally it disappears, and the resulting space becomes the **joint cavity** or synovial cavity.
- Where it lines the joint capsule and articular surfaces, it forms the **synovial membrane** (which secretes synovial fluid), a part of the joint capsule (fibrous capsule lined with synovial membrane)

Probably as a result of joint movements, the mesenchymal cells subsequently disappear from the surfaces of the articular cartilages. An abnormal intrauterine environment restricting embryonic and fetal movements may interfere with limb development and cause joint fixation.

DEVELOPMENT OF THE AXIAL SKELETON

The axial skeleton is composed of the cranium (skull), vertebral column, ribs, and sternum. During the fourth week, cells in the sclerotomes now surround the neural tube (primordium of spinal cord) and the notochord, the structure about which the primordia of the vertebrae develop. This positional change of the sclerotomal cells is effected by differential growth of the surrounding structures and not by active migration of sclerotomal cells. The *Pax-1* gene, which is expressed in all prospective sclerotomal cells of epithelial somites in chick and mouse embryos, seems to play an essential role in the development of the vertebral column.

Development of the Vertebral Column

During the precartilaginous or mesenchymal stage, mesenchymal cells from the **sclerotomes** are found in three main areas (Fig. 14-7*A*): around the notochord, surrounding the neural tube, and in the body wall. In a frontal section of a 4-week embryo, the sclerotomes appear as paired condensations of mesenchymal cells around the notochord (see Fig. 14-7*B*). Each sclerotome consists of loosely arranged cells cranially and densely packed cells caudally. Some densely packed cells move cranially, opposite the center of the myotome, where they form the **intervertebral (IV) disc** (see Fig. 14-7*C* and *D*). The remaining densely packed cells fuse with the loosely arranged cells of the immediately caudal sclerotome to form the mesenchymal **centrum**, the primordium of the body of a vertebra. Thus, each centrum develops from two adjacent sclerotomes and becomes an intersegmental structure. The nerves now lie in close relationship to the intervertebral discs, and the **intersegmental arteries** lie on each side of the vertebral bodies. In the thorax, the dorsal intersegmental arteries become the **intercostal arteries.**

The notochord degenerates and disappears where it is surrounded by the developing vertebral bodies. Between the vertebrae, the **notochord** expands to form the gelatinous center of the intervertebral disc—the **nucleus pulposus** (see Fig. 14-7*D*). This nucleus is later surrounded by circularly arranged fibers that form the **anulus fibrosus.**

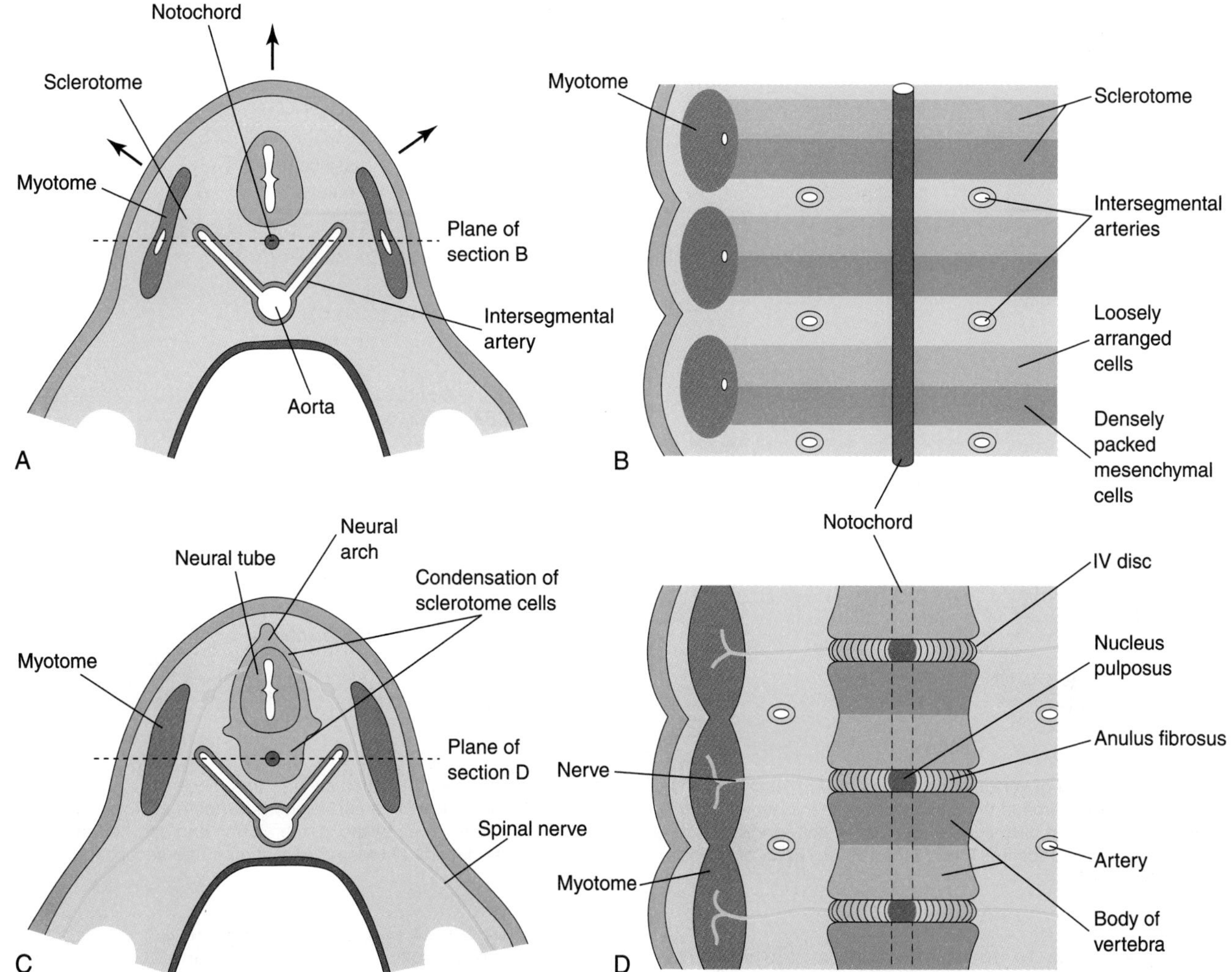

FIGURE 14-7. **A,** Transverse section through a 4-week embryo. The *arrows* indicate the dorsal growth of the neural tube and the simultaneous dorsolateral movement of the somite remnant, leaving behind a trail of sclerotomal cells. **B,** Diagrammatic frontal section of this embryo showing that the condensation of sclerotomal cells around the notochord consists of a cranial area of loosely packed cells and a caudal area of densely packed cells. **C,** Transverse section through a 5-week embryo showing the condensation of sclerotomal cells around the notochord and neural tube, which forms a mesenchymal vertebra. **D,** Diagrammatic frontal section illustrating that the vertebral body forms from the cranial and caudal halves of two successive sclerotomal masses. The intersegmental arteries now cross the bodies of the vertebrae, and the spinal nerves lie between the vertebrae. The notochord is degenerating except in the region of the intervertebral disc, where it forms the nucleus pulposus.

The nucleus pulposus and anulus fibrosus together constitute the intervertebral disc. The mesenchymal cells, surrounding the neural tube, form the **neural arch** (Fig. 14-7*C*). The mesenchymal cells in the body wall form the costal processes that form ribs in the thoracic region.

CHORDOMA

Remnants of the notochord may persist and give rise to a **chordoma**. Approximately one third of these slow-growing malignant tumors occur at the base of the cranium and extend to the nasopharynx. Cordomas infiltrate bone and are difficult to remove. Few patients survive longer than 5 years. Chordomas also develop in the lumbosacral region.

Cartilaginous Stage of Vertebral Development

During the sixth week, chondrification centers appear in each mesenchymal vertebra (Fig. 14-8*A* and *B*). The two centers in each centrum fuse at the end of the embryonic period to form a cartilaginous centrum. Concomitantly, the centers in the neural arches fuse with each other and the centrum. The spinous and transverse processes develop from extensions of chondrification centers in the neural arch. Chondrification spreads until a cartilaginous vertebral column is formed.

Bony Stage of Vertebral Development

Ossification of typical vertebrae begins during the embryonic period and usually ends by the 25th year. There are two primary ossification centers, ventral and dorsal, for the centrum (see Fig. 14-8*C*). These primary ossification

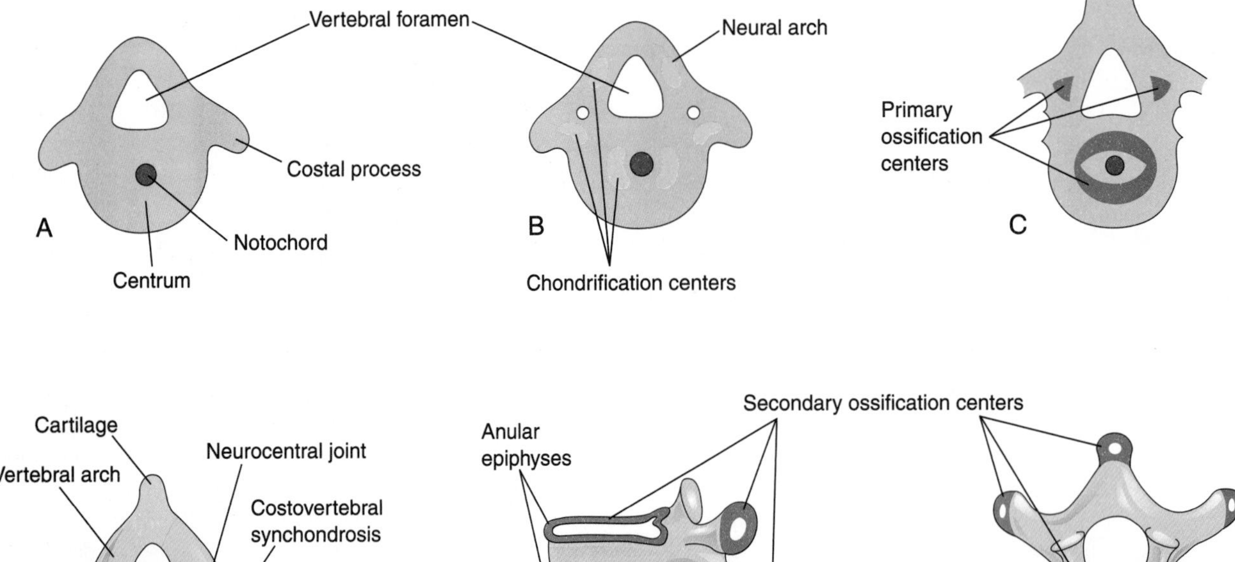

FIGURE 14-8. Stages of vertebral development. **A,** Mesenchymal vertebra at 5 weeks. **B,** Chondrification centers in a mesenchymal vertebra at 6 weeks. The neural arch is the primordium of the vertebral arch. **C,** Primary ossification centers in a cartilaginous vertebra at 7 weeks. **D,** Thoracic vertebra at birth consisting of three bony parts. Note the cartilage between the halves of the vertebral arch and between the arch and the centrum (neurocentral joint). **E** and **F,** Two views of a typical thoracic vertebra at puberty showing the location of the secondary centers of ossification.

centers soon fuse to form one center. Three primary centers are present by the end of the embryonic period: one in the centrum and one in each half of the neural arch.

Ossification becomes evident in the **neural arches** during the eighth week. At birth, each vertebra consists of three bony parts connected by cartilage (see Fig. 14-8*D*). The bony halves of the **vertebral arch** usually fuse during the first 3 to 5 years. The arches first unite in the lumbar region, and union progresses cranially. The vertebral arch articulates with the **centrum** at cartilaginous neurocentral joints, which permit the vertebral arches to grow as the spinal cord enlarges. These joints disappear when the vertebral arch fuses with the centrum during the third to sixth years. Five **secondary ossification centers** appear in the vertebrae after puberty:

- One for the tip of the spinous process
- One for the tip of each transverse process
- Two anular epiphyses, one on the superior and one on the inferior rim of the vertebral body (see Fig. 14-8*E* and *F*).

The **vertebral body** is a composite of the anular epiphyses and the mass of bone between them. The vertebral body includes the centrum, parts of the vertebral arch, and the facets for the heads of the ribs. All secondary centers unite with the rest of the vertebra at approximately 25 years of age. Exceptions to the typical ossification of vertebrae occur in the atlas or C1 vertebra, axis or C2 vertebra, C7 vertebra, lumbar vertebrae, sacrum, and coccyx. Minor developmental anomalies of the vertebrae are common, but in most cases are of little clinical importance.

VARIATION IN THE NUMBER OF VERTEBRAE

Most people have 7 cervical, 12 thoracic, 5 lumbar, and 5 sacral vertebrae. A few have one or two additional vertebrae or one fewer. To determine the number of vertebrae, it is necessary to examine the entire vertebral column because an apparent extra (or absent) vertebra in one segment of the column may be compensated for by an absent (or extra) vertebra in an adjacent segment; for example, 11 thoracic-type vertebrae with 6 lumbar-type vertebrae.

Development of the Ribs

The ribs develop from the mesenchymal **costal processes** of the thoracic vertebrae (see Fig. 14-8*A*). They become cartilaginous during the embryonic period and ossify during the fetal period. The original site of union of the costal processes with the vertebra is replaced by costovertebral synovial joints (see Fig. 14-8*D*). Seven pairs of ribs (1–7)—**true ribs**—attach through their own cartilages to the sternum. Five pairs of ribs (8–12)—**false ribs**—attach to the sternum through the cartilage of another rib or ribs. The last two pairs of ribs (11 and 12)—**floating ribs**—do not attach to the sternum.

Development of the Sternum

A pair of vertical mesenchymal bands, **sternal bars**, develop ventrolaterally in the body wall. Chondrification occurs in these bars as they move medially. They fuse craniocaudally in the median plane to form cartilaginous models of the manubrium, sternebrae (segments of the sternal body), and xiphoid process. Centers of ossification appear craniocaudally in the sternum before birth, except that for the xiphoid process, which appears during childhood.

Development of the Cranium

The cranium (skull) develops from mesenchyme around the developing brain. The cranium consists of:

- The **neurocranium**, a protective case for the brain
- The **viscerocranium**, the skeleton of the face

Cartilaginous Neurocranium

Initially, the cartilaginous neurocranium or **chondrocranium** consists of the cartilaginous base of the developing cranium, which forms by fusion of several cartilages (Fig. 14-9*A* to *D*). Later, endochondral ossification of the chondrocranium forms the bones in the base of the cranium. The ossification pattern of these bones has a definite sequence, beginning with the occipital bone, body of sphenoid, and ethmoid bone.

The **parachordal cartilage**, or basal plate, forms around the cranial end of the notochord (see Fig. 14-9*A*) and fuses with the cartilages derived from the sclerotome regions of the occipital somites. This cartilaginous mass contributes to the **base of the occipital bone**; later, extensions grow around the cranial end of the spinal cord and form the boundaries of the foramen magnum (see Fig. 14-9*C*).

The **hypophysial cartilage** forms around the developing pituitary gland (Latin, *hypophysis cerebri*) and fuses to form the body of the sphenoid bone. The trabeculae cranii fuse to form the body of the ethmoid bone, and the ala orbitalis forms the lesser wing of the sphenoid bone. **Otic capsules** develop around the otic vesicles, the primordia of the internal ears (see Chapter 18), and form the petrous and mastoid parts of the temporal bone. **Nasal capsules** develop around the nasal sacs (see Chapter 9) and contribute to the formation of the ethmoid bone.

Membranous Neurocranium

Intramembranous ossification occurs in the mesenchyme at the sides and top of the brain, forming the **calvaria** (cranial vault). During fetal life, the flat bones of the calvaria are separated by dense connective tissue membranes that form fibrous joints, the **sutures** (Fig. 14-10). Six large fibrous areas—**fontanelles**—are present where several sutures meet. The softness of the bones and their loose connections at the sutures enable the calvaria to undergo changes of shape during birth, called molding. During **molding of the fetal cranium** (adaptation of fetal head to the pelvic cavity during birth), the frontal bones become flat, the occipital bone is drawn out, and one parietal bone slightly overrides the other one. Within a few days after birth, the shape of the calvaria returns to normal.

Cartilaginous Viscerocranium

Most mesenchyme in the head region is derived from the neural crest. **Neural crest cells** migrate into the pharyngeal arches and form the bones and connective tissue of **craniofacial structures**. Homeobox (*Hox*) genes regulate the migration and subsequent differentiation of the neural crest cells, which are crucial for the complex patterning of the head and face. These parts of the fetal cranium are derived from the cartilaginous skeleton of the first two pairs of pharyngeal arches (see Chapter 9).

- The dorsal end of the first pharyngeal arch cartilage forms two middle ear bones, the malleus and incus.
- The dorsal end of the second pharyngeal arch cartilage forms the stapes of the middle ear and the styloid process of the temporal bone. Its ventral end ossifies to form the lesser horn (Latin, *cornu*) and superior part of the body of the hyoid bone.
- The third, fourth, and sixth pharyngeal arch cartilages form only in the ventral parts of the arches. The third arch cartilages give rise to the greater horns and the inferior part of the body of the hyoid bone.
- The fourth pharyngeal arch cartilages fuse to form the laryngeal cartilages, except for the epiglottis (see Chapter 9).

Membranous Viscerocranium

Intramembranous ossification occurs in the maxillary prominence of the first pharyngeal arch (see Chapter 8) and subsequently forms the squamous temporal, maxillary, and zygomatic bones. The squamous temporal bones become part of the neurocranium. The mesenchyme in the mandibular prominence of the first pharyngeal arch condenses around its cartilage and undergoes intramembranous ossification to form the mandible. Some endochondral ossification occurs in the median plane of the chin and in the mandibular condyle.

Newborn Cranium

After recovering from molding, the newborn's cranium is rather round and its bones are thin. Like the fetal cranium (see Fig. 14-10), it is large in proportion to the rest of the skeleton, and the face is relatively small compared with the calvaria. The small facial region of the cranium results from the small size of the jaws, virtual absence of paranasal (air) sinuses, and underdevelopment of the facial bones.

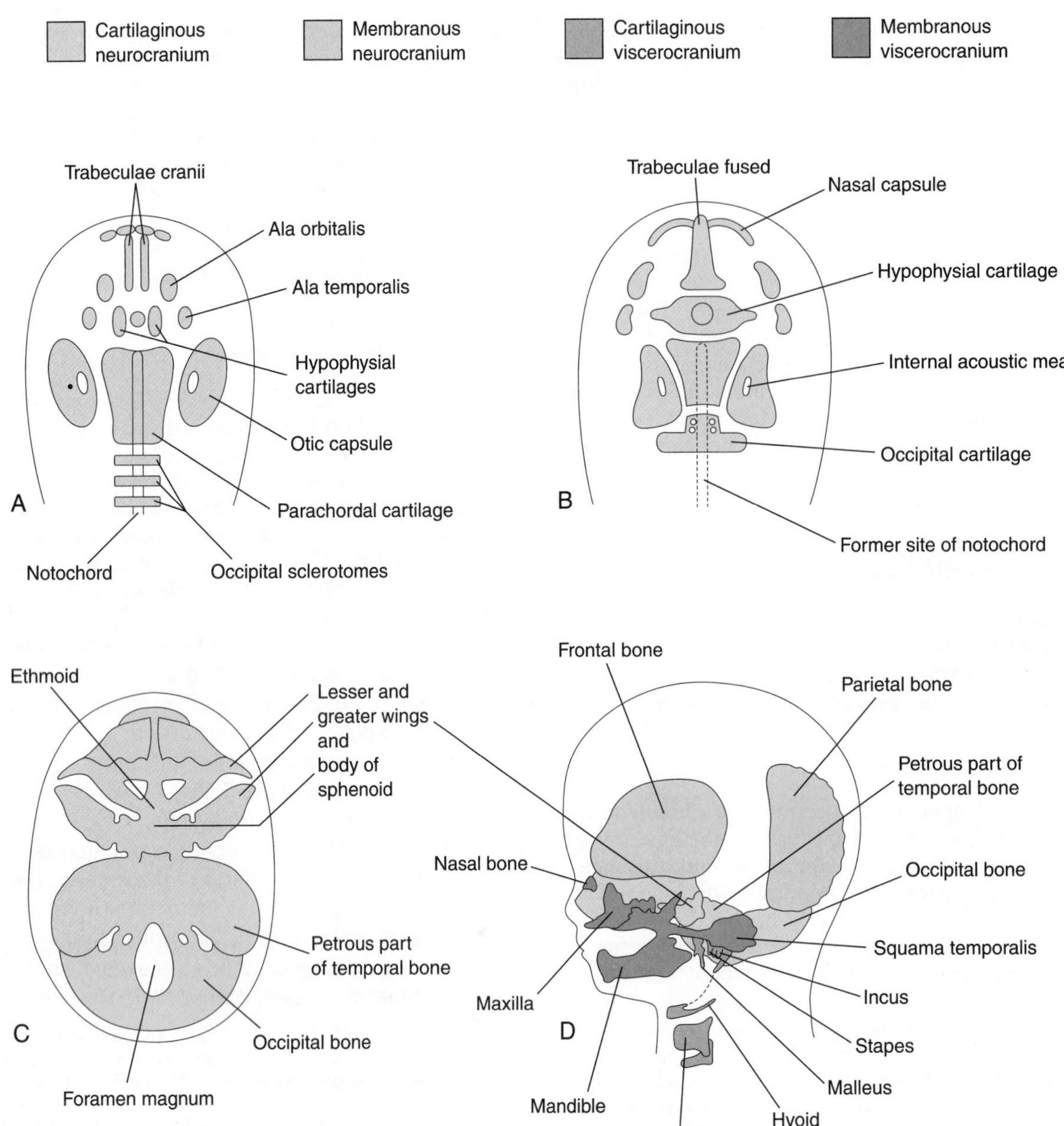

FIGURE 14-9. Stages in the development of the cranium: **A** to **C**, Views of the base of the developing cranium (viewed superiorly). **D**, A lateral view. **A**, At 6 weeks showing the various cartilages that will fuse to form the chondrocranium. **B**, At 7 weeks, after fusion of some of the paired cartilages. **C**, At 12 weeks showing the cartilaginous base of the cranium or chondrocranium formed by the fusion of various cartilages. **D**, At 20 weeks indicating the derivation of the bones of the fetal cranium.

Postnatal Growth of the Cranium

The fibrous sutures of the newborn's calvaria permit the brain to enlarge during infancy and childhood. The increase in the size of the calvaria is greatest during the first 2 years, the period of most rapid postnatal growth of the brain. The calvaria normally increases in capacity until approximately 16 years of age. After this, it usually increases slightly in size for 3 to 4 years because of thickening of its bones. There is also rapid growth of the face and jaws, coinciding with eruption of the primary (deciduous) teeth. These facial changes are more marked after the secondary (permanent) teeth erupt (see Chapter 19). There is concurrent enlargement of the frontal and facial regions, associated with the increase in the size of the **paranasal sinuses** (e.g., frontal and ethmoid sinuses). Most paranasal sinuses are rudimentary or absent at birth. Growth of these sinuses is important in altering the shape of the face and in adding resonance to the voice.

KLIPPEL-FEIL SYNDROME

The main features of this syndrome are shortness of the neck, low hairline, and restricted neck movements. In most cases, the number of cervical

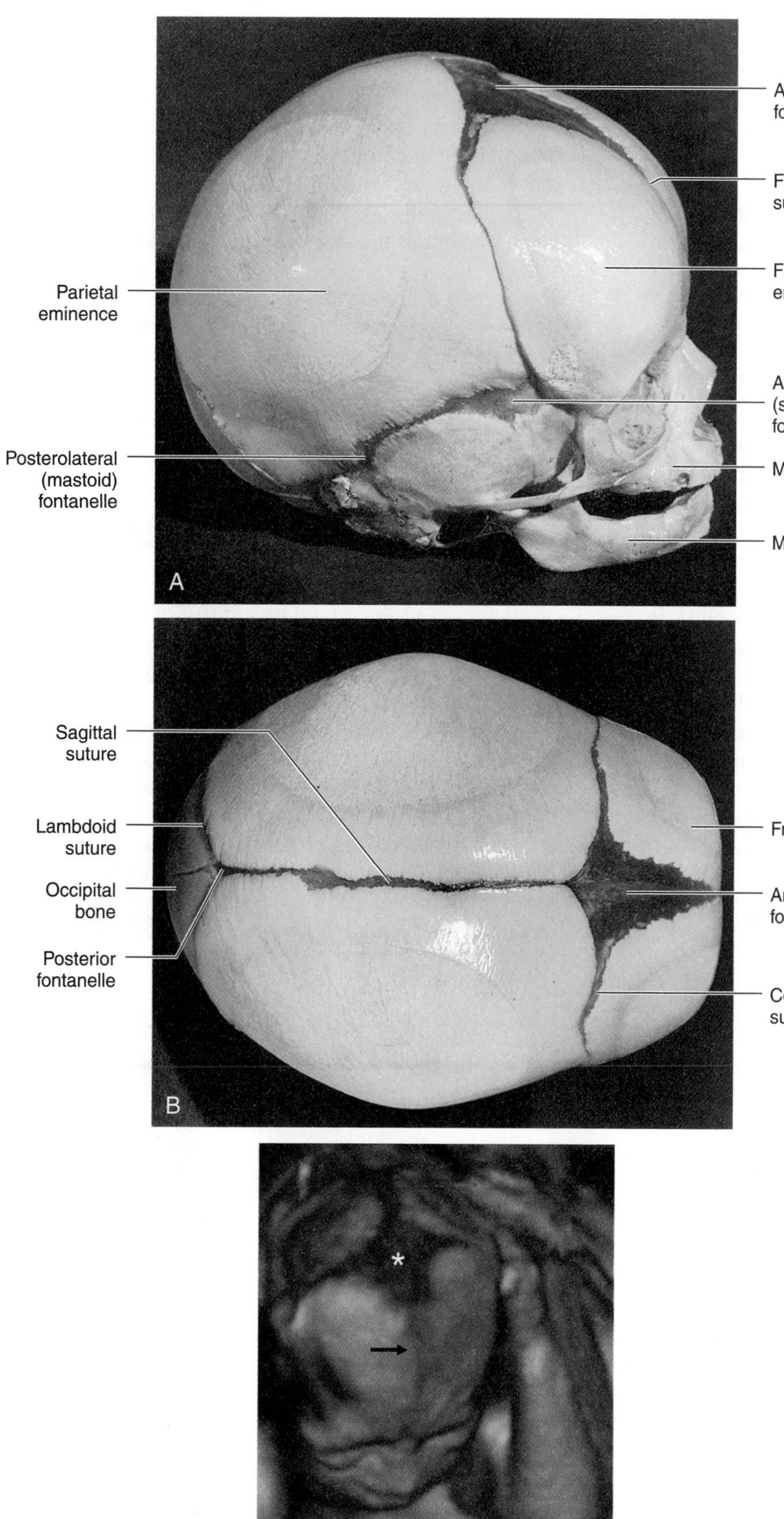

FIGURE 14-10. A fetal cranium showing the bones, fontanelles, and sutures. **A,** Lateral view. **B,** Superior view. The posterior and anterolateral fontanelles disappear because of growth of surrounding bones, within 2 or 3 months after birth, but they remain as sutures for several years. The posterolateral fontanelles disappear in a similar manner by the end of the first year and the anterior fontanelle by the end of the second year. The halves of the frontal bone normally begin to fuse during the second year, and the frontal suture is usually obliterated by the eighth year. The other sutures disappear during adult life, but the times when the sutures close are subject to wide variations. **C,** Three-dimensional ultrasound rendering of the fetal head at 22 weeks (gestational age). Note the anterior fontanelle (*) and the frontal suture (*arrow*). The coronal and sagittal sutures are also shown. (**C,** Courtesy of Dr. G. J. Reid, Department of Obstetrics, Gynecology and Reproductive Sciences, University of Manitoba, Women's Hospital, Winnipeg, Manitoba, Canada.)

vertebral bodies is fewer than normal. In some cases, there is a lack of segmentation of several elements of the cervical region of the vertebral column. The number of cervical nerve roots may be normal but they are small, as are the intervertebral foramina. Individuals with this syndrome are often otherwise normal, but the association of this anomaly with other congenital anomalies is not uncommon.

Spina Bifida

Failure of the halves of the embryonic neural vertebral arch to fuse results in a major defect—spina bifida (see Fig. 17-12). The incidence of this vertebral defect ranges from 0.04% to 0.15%, and it occurs more frequently in girls than boys. Most cases of spina bifida (80%) are "open" and covered by a thin membrane.

A "closed" spina bifida or **spina bifida occulta** is covered by a thick membrane or skin. This defect of the vertebral arch is a consequence of failure of the halves of the neural arch to fuse. Spina bifida occulta is commonly observed in radiographs of the cervical, lumbar, and sacral regions. Frequently only one vertebra is affected. Spina bifida occulta is a relatively minor, insignificant anomaly of the vertebral column that usually causes no clinical symptoms. It can be diagnosed in utero by sonography. Spina bifida occulta of the first sacral vertebra occurs in approximately 20% of vertebral columns that are examined radiographically. The spinal cord and spinal nerves are usually normal and neurologic symptoms are commonly absent. The skin over the bifid vertebral arch is intact, and there may be no external evidence of the vertebral defect. Sometimes the anomaly is indicated by a dimple or a tuft of hair. In approximately 3% of normal adults, there is spina bifida occulta of the atlas. At other cervical levels, this condition is rare and, when present, it is sometimes accompanied by other abnormalities of the cervical region of the vertebral column.

Spina bifida cystica, a severe type of spina bifida involving the spinal cord and meninges, is discussed in Chapter 17. Neurologic symptoms are present in these cases.

Accessory Ribs

Accessory ribs, usually rudimentary, result from the development of the costal processes of cervical or lumbar vertebrae (Fig. 14-11*A*). These processes usually form ribs only in the thoracic region. The most common type of accessory rib is a **lumbar rib**, but it usually causes no problems. A **cervical rib** occurs in 0.5% to 1% of individuals. A cervical rib is attached to the seventh cervical vertebra and may be unilateral or bilateral. Pressure of a cervical rib on the brachial plexus of nerves, located partly in the neck and partly in the axilla, or the subclavian artery often produces neurovascular symptoms (e.g., paralysis and anesthesia of the upper limb).

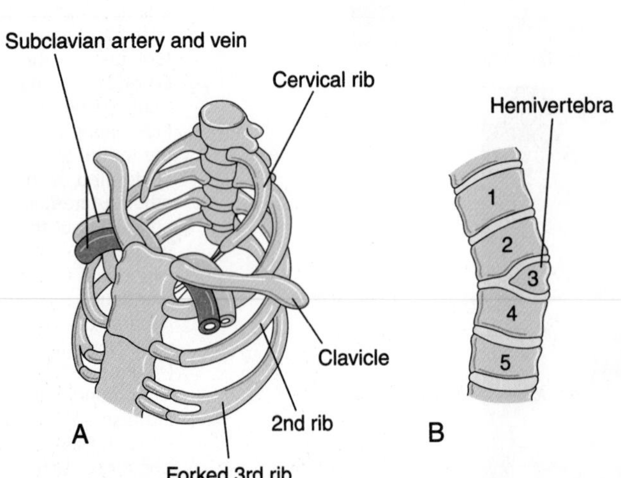

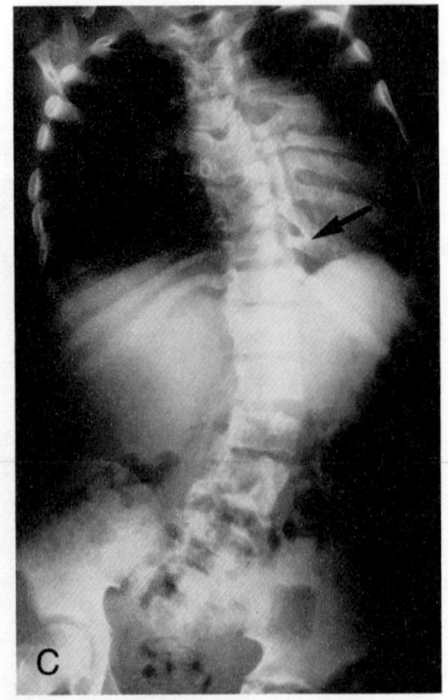

FIGURE 14-11. Vertebral and rib abnormalities. **A,** Cervical and forked ribs. Observe that the left cervical rib has a fibrous band that passes posterior to the subclavian vessels and attaches to the manubrium of the sternum. **B,** Anterior view of the vertebral column showing a hemivertebra. The right half of the third thoracic vertebra is absent. Note the associated lateral curvature (scoliosis) of the vertebral column. **C,** Radiograph of a child with the kyphoscoliotic deformity of the lumbar region of the vertebral column showing multiple anomalies of the vertebrae and ribs. Note the fused ribs (*arrow*). (Courtesy of Dr. Prem S. Sahni, formerly of the Department of Radiology, Children's Hospital, Winnipeg, Manitoba, Canada.)

Fused Ribs

Fusion of ribs occasionally occurs posteriorly when two or more ribs arise from a single vertebra (see Fig. 14-11*C*). Fused ribs are often associated with a hemivertebra.

Hemivertebra

In normal circumstances, the developing vertebral bodies have two chondrification centers that soon unite. A hemivertebra results from failure of one of the chondrification centers to appear and subsequent failure of half of the vertebra to form (see Fig. 14-11*B*). These vertebral defects produce **scoliosis** (lateral curvature) of the vertebral column (see Fig. 14-11*C*). There are other causes of scoliosis (e.g., myopathic scoliosis resulting from weakness of the spinal muscles).

Rachischisis

The term rachischisis (cleft vertebral column) refers to the vertebral abnormalities in a complex group of anomalies (**axial dysraphic disorders**) that primarily affect axial structures (Fig. 14-12). In these infants, the neural folds fail to fuse, either because of faulty induction by the underlying notochord or from the action of teratogenic agents on the neuroepithelial cells in the neural folds. The neural and vertebral defects may be extensive or be restricted to a small area.

Anomalies of the Sternum

A concave depression of the lower sternum—**pes excavatum**—is the most common thoracic wall defect seen by pediatricians. It is probably due to overgrowth of the costal cartilages, which displaces the lower sternum posteriorly. Minor sternal clefts (e.g., a notch or foramen in the xiphoid process) are common and are of no clinical concern. A sternal foramen of varying size and form occurs occasionally at the junction of the third and fourth sternebrae (segments of primordial sternum). This insignificant foramen is the result of incomplete fusion of the cartilaginous sternal bars during the embryonic period.

Cranial Anomalies

These abnormalities range from major defects that are incompatible with life (Fig. 14-12*B*) to those that are minor and insignificant. With large defects, there is often herniation of the meninges and/or brain (see Chapter 17).

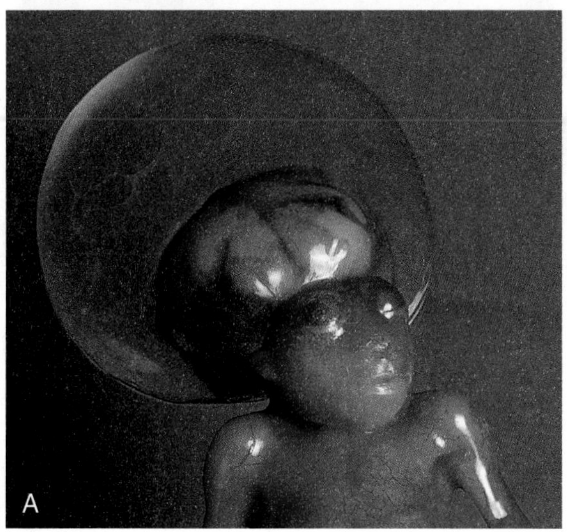

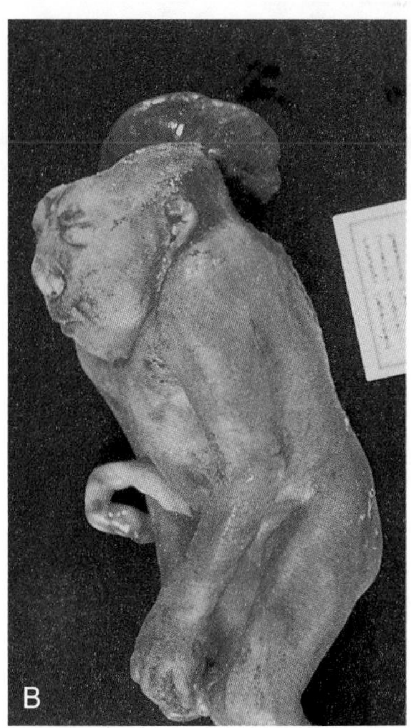

FIGURE 14-12. **A,** A second-trimester fetus with holoacrania or complete absence of the cranium (acrania). Note the cystlike structure surrounding the intact fetal brain. **B,** Lateral view of a newborn infant with acrania and meroencephaly (partial absence of the brain), as well as rachischisis—extensive clefts in vertebral arches of the vertebral column (not clearly visible). (Courtesy of A.E. Chudley, MD, Section of Genetics and Metabolism, Department of Pediatrics and Child Health, University of Manitoba, Children's Hospital, Winnipeg, Manitoba, Canada.)

Acrania

In this condition, the calvaria is absent and extensive defects of the vertebral column are often present (see Fig. 14-12). Acrania associated with **meroencephaly** or **anencephaly** (partial absence of the brain) occurs approximately once in 1000 births and is incompatible with life. Meroencephaly results from failure of the cranial end of the neural tube to close during the fourth week. This anomaly causes subsequent failure of the calvaria to form (see Fig. 14-12*B*).

Craniosynostosis

Prenatal closure of the cranial sutures results in the most severe abnormalities. The cause of craniosynostosis is unclear. Homeobox gene *Msx2* and *Alx4* mutations have been implicated in cases of craniosynostosis and other cranial defects. A recent epidemiologic study of maternal drug use found a strong association between anticonvulsant use during early pregnancy and infant craniosynostosis. These abnormalities are much more common in males than in females and are often associated with other skeletal anomalies. The type of deformed cranium produced depends on which sutures close prematurely. If the sagittal suture closes early, the cranium becomes long, narrow, and wedge shaped—**scaphocephaly** (Fig. 14-13A and *B*). This type of cranial deformity constitutes about half the cases of craniosynostosis. Another 30% of cases involve premature closure of the coronal suture, which results in a high, tower-like cranium—**brachycephaly** (see Fig. 14-13*C*). If the coronal suture closes prematurely on one side only, the cranium is twisted and asymmetrical—**plagiocephaly**. Premature

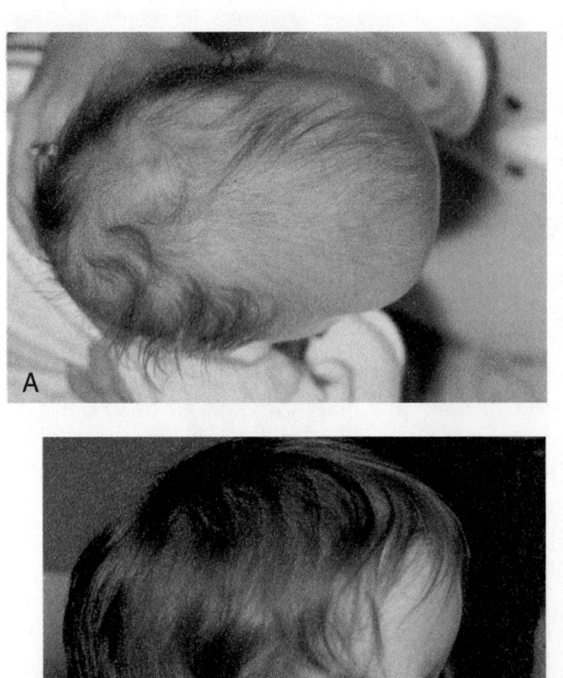

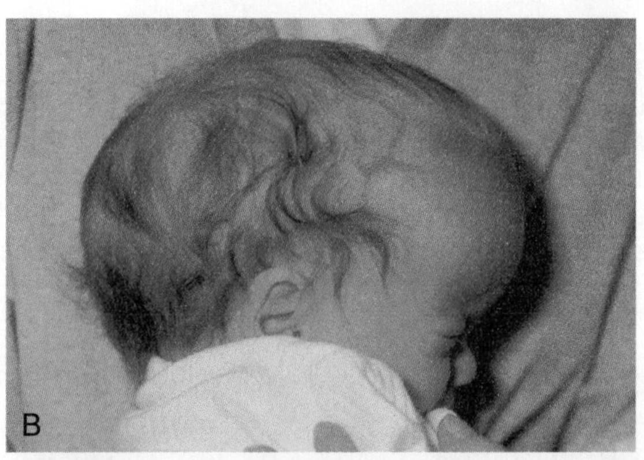

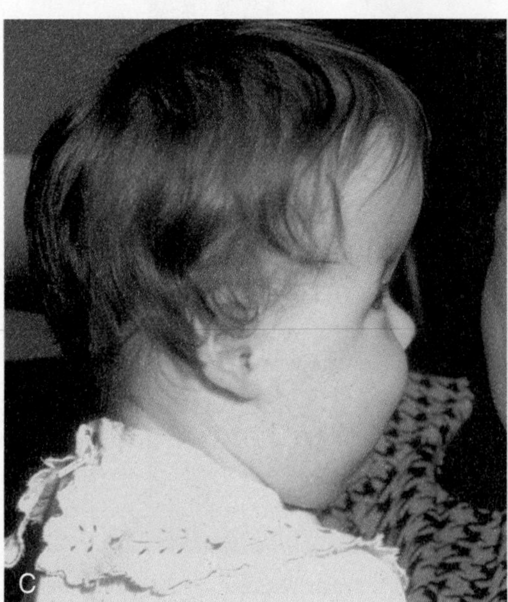

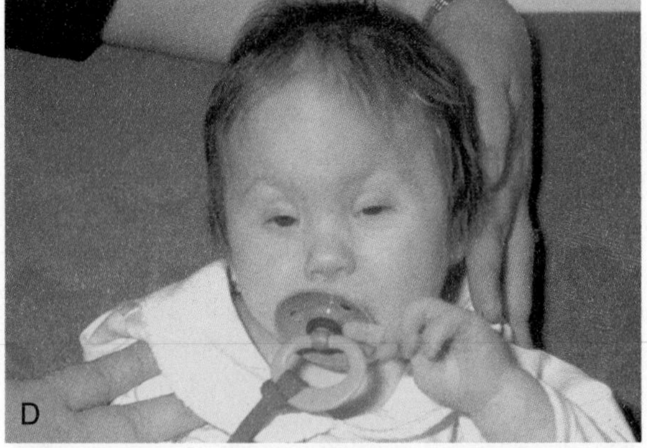

FIGURE 14-13. Craniosynostosis. **A** and **B,** An infant with **scaphocephaly.** This condition results from premature closure (synostosis) of the sagittal suture. Note the elongated, wedge-shaped cranium seen from above (**A**) and the side (**B**). **C,** An infant with bilateral premature closure of the coronal suture (**brachycephaly**). Note the high, markedly elevated forehead. **D,** An infant with premature closure of the frontal suture (**trigonocephaly**). Note the hypertelorism and prominent midline ridging of the forehead. (Courtesy of Dr. John A. Jane, Sr., David D. Weaver Professor of Neurosurgery, Department of Neurological Surgery, University of Virginia Health System, Charlottesville, VA.)

closure of the frontal (metopic) suture results in a deformity of the frontal bone and other anomalies—**trigonocephaly** (see Fig. 14-13*D*).

Microcephaly

Infants with this anomaly are born with a normal-sized or slightly small calvaria. The fontanelles close during early infancy, and the other sutures close during the first year. However, this anomaly is not caused by premature closure of sutures. Microcephaly is the result of abnormal development of the central nervous system in which the brain and, consequently, the cranium fail to grow. Generally, microcephalics are severely mentally retarded. This anomaly is also illustrated and discussed in Chapter 17.

Anomalies at the Craniovertebral Junction

Congenital abnormalities at the craniovertebral junction are present in approximately 1% of newborn infants, but they may not produce symptoms until adult life. The following are examples of these anomalies: **basilar invagination** (superior displacement of bone around the foramen magnum), **assimilation of the atlas** (nonsegmentation at the junction of the atlas and occipital bone), **atlantoaxial dislocation**, Arnold-Chiari malformation (see Chapter 17), and a separate dens (failure of the centers in the dens to fuse with the centrum of the axis).

DEVELOPMENT OF THE APPENDICULAR SKELETON

The appendicular skeleton consists of the pectoral and pelvic girdles and the limb bones. Mesenchymal bones form during the fifth week as condensations of mesenchyme appear in the limb buds (Fig. 14-14*A* to *C*). During the sixth week, the **mesenchymal bone models** in the limbs undergo chondrification to form **hyaline cartilage bone models** (see Fig. 14-14*D* and *E*). The clavicle initially develops by intramembranous ossification, and it later forms growth cartilages at both ends. The models of the pectoral girdle and upper limb bones appear slightly before those of the pelvic girdle and lower limb bones; the bone models appear in a proximodistal sequence. Patterning in the developing limbs is regulated by homeobox-containing (*Hox*) *genes* (see Chapter 21).

Ossification begins in the long bones by the eighth week and initially occurs in the diaphyses of the bones from **primary ossification centers** (see Fig. 14-5). By 12 weeks, primary ossification centers have appeared in nearly all bones of the limbs (Fig. 14-15). The clavicles begin to ossify before any other bones in the body. The femora are the next bones to show traces of ossification. The first indication of the primary center of ossification in the cartilaginous model of a long bone is visible near the center of the future shaft (diaphysis). Primary centers appear at different times in different bones, but most of them appear between the 7th and 12th weeks. Virtually all primary centers of ossification are present at birth.

The **secondary ossification centers** of the bones at the knee are the first to appear in utero. The secondary centers for the distal end of the femur and the proximal end of the tibia usually appear during the last month of intrauterine life. Consequently, these secondary centers are usually present at birth; however, most secondary centers of ossification appear after birth. The part of a bone ossified from a secondary center is the **epiphysis**. The bone formed from the primary center in the diaphysis does not fuse with that formed from the secondary centers in the epiphyses until the bone grows to its adult length. This delay enables lengthening of the bone to continue until the final size is reached. During bone growth, a plate of cartilage known as the **epiphysial cartilage plate** intervenes between the diaphysis and the epiphysis (see Fig. 14-5). The epiphysial plate is eventually replaced by bone development on each of its two sides, diaphysial and epiphysial. When this occurs, growth of the bone ceases.

Bone Age

Bone age is a good index of general maturation. Determination of the number, size, and fusion of epiphysial centers from radiographs is a commonly used method. A radiologist determines the bone age of a person by assessing the ossification centers using two criteria:

- The time of appearance of calcified material in the diaphysis and/or the epiphysis is specific for each diaphysis and epiphysis and for each bone and sex.
- The disappearance of the dark line representing the epiphysial cartilage plate indicates that the epiphysis has fused with the diaphysis.

Fusion of the diaphesial-epiphysial centers, which occurs at specific times for each epiphysis, happens 1 to 2 years earlier in females than in males. In the fetus, ultrasonography is used for the evaluation and measurement of bones as well as for determination of fertilization age.

Generalized Skeletal Malformations

Achondroplasia is the common cause of dwarfism—*shortness of stature* (see Chapter 20). It occurs approximately once in 15,000 births. The limbs become bowed and short (Fig. 14-16) because of disturbance of endochondral ossification at the epiphysial cartilage plates, particularly of long

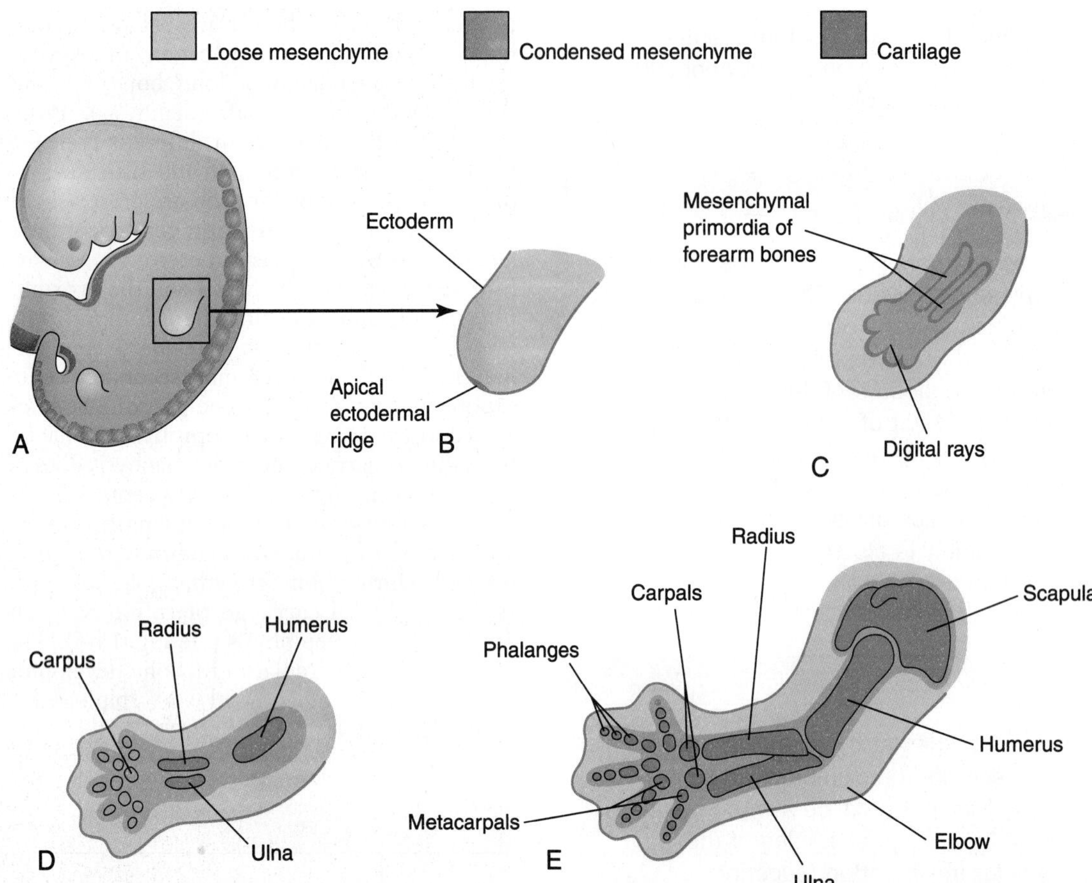

FIGURE 14-14. **A,** An embryo at approximately 28 days showing the early appearance of the limb buds. **B,** Longitudinal section through an upper limb bud showing the apical ectodermal ridge, which has an inductive influence on the mesenchyme in the limb bud. This ridge promotes growth of the mesenchyme and appears to give it the ability to form specific cartilaginous elements. **C,** Similar sketch of an upper limb bud at approximately 33 days showing the mesenchymal primordia of the forearm bones. The digital rays are mesenchymal condensations that undergo chondrification and ossification to form the bones of the hand. **D,** Upper limb at 6 weeks showing the cartilage models of the bones. **E,** Later in the sixth week showing the completed cartilaginous models of the bones of the upper limb.

bones, during fetal life. The trunk is usually short, and the head is enlarged with a bulging forehead and "scooped-out" nose (flat nasal bridge). Achondroplasia is an autosomal dominant disorder, and approximately 80% of cases arise from new mutations; the rate increases with paternal age. The majority of cases are due to a point mutation (f.1,11,12) in the *FGFR3* gene, which results in magnification of the normal inhibiting effect of endochondral ossification, specifically in the zone of chondrocyte proliferation. This results in shortened bone but does not affect periosteal bone growth.

Thanatophoric dysplasia is the most common type of lethal skeletal dysplasia. It occurs approximately once in 20,000 births, and the affected infants die within minutes or days of respiratory failure. This lethal disorder is associated with mutations in the fibroblast growth factor receptor 3.

HYPERPITUITARISM

Congenital infantile hyperpituitarism, which causes an infant to grow at an abnormally rapid rate, is rare. This may result in **gigantism** (excessive height and body proportions) or **acromegaly** in the adult (enlargement of soft tissues, visceral organs, and bones of face, hands, and feet [acral bones-limb bones]). Both gigantism and acromegaly result from an excessive secretion of growth hormone.

HYPOTHYROIDISM AND CRETINISM

A severe deficiency of fetal thyroid hormone production results in **cretinism**, a condition characterized by growth retardation, mental deficiency, skeletal abnormalities, and auditory and

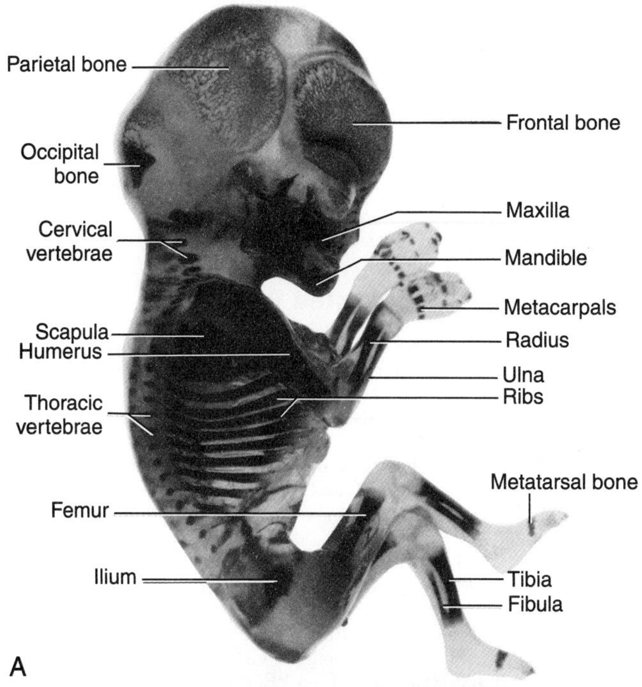

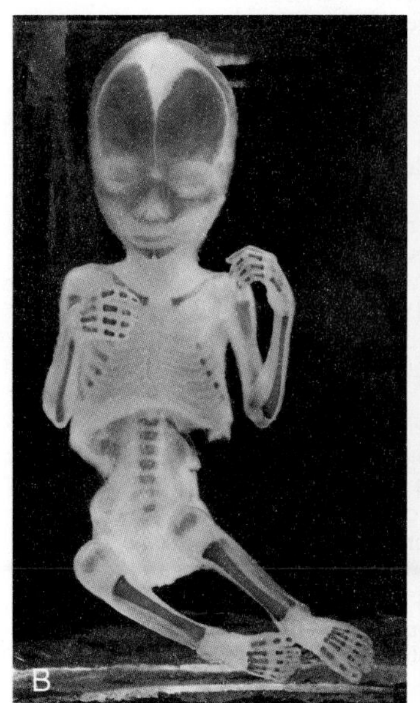

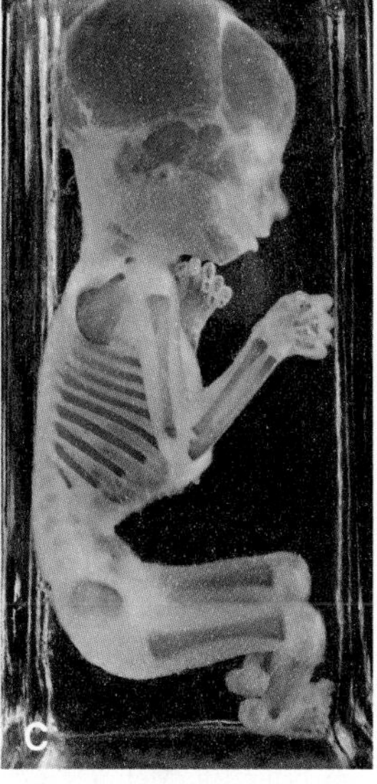

FIGURE 14-15. Alizarin-stained and cleared human fetuses. **A,** A 12-week fetus. Observe the degree of progression of ossification from the primary centers of ossification, which is endochondral in the appendicular and axial parts of the skeleton except for most of the cranial bones (i.e., those that form the cranial vault). Observe that the carpus and tarsus are wholly cartilaginous at this stage, as are the epiphyses of all long bones. **B** and **C,** An approximately 20-week fetus. (**A,** Courtesy of Dr. Gary Geddes, Lake Oswego, OR. **B** and **C,** Courtesy of Dr. David Bolender, Department of Cell Biology, Neurobiology, and Anatomy, Medical College of Wisconsin, Milwaukee, WI.)

neurologic disorders. Bone age appears as less than chronologic age because epiphysial development is delayed. Cretinism is very rare except in areas where there is a lack of iodine in the soil and water. Agenesis of the thyroid gland also results in cretinism.

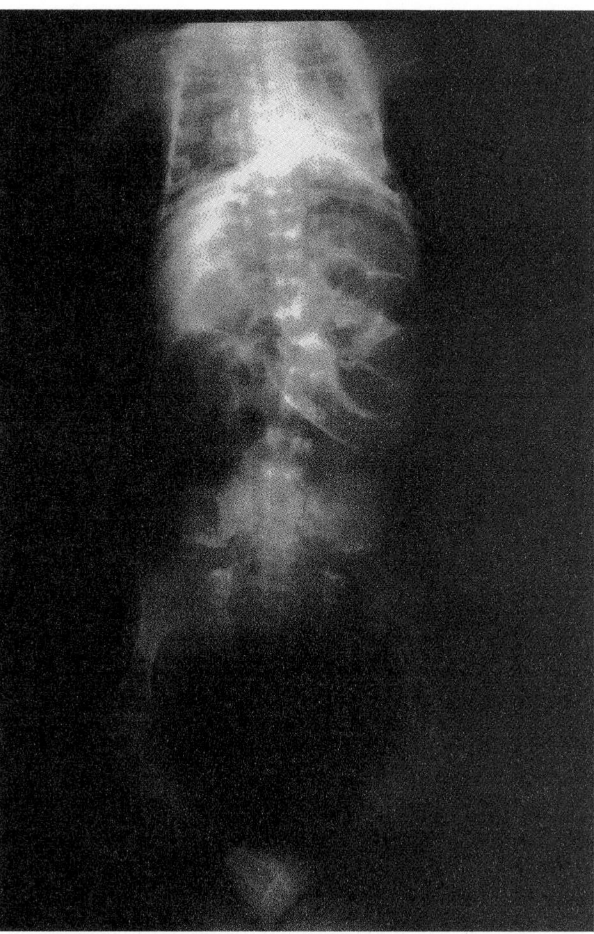

FIGURE 14-16. Radiograph of the skeletal system of a 2-year old-child with achondroplasia. Note the shortening of the humerus and femur with metaphysis flaring. (Courtesy of Dr. Prem S. Sahni, formerly of the Department of Radiology, Children's Hospital, Winnipeg, Manitoba, Canada.)

SUMMARY OF THE SKELETAL SYSTEM

- The skeletal system develops from mesenchyme, derived from mesoderm and the neural crest. In most bones, such as the long bones in the limbs, the condensed mesenchyme undergoes chondrification to form cartilage bone models. Ossification centers appear in these models by the end of the embryonic period, and the bones ossify later by endochondral ossification. Some bones, the flat bones of the cranium, for example, develop by intramembranous ossification.
- The vertebral column and ribs develop from mesenchymal cells derived from the sclerotomes of the somites. Each vertebra is formed by fusion of a condensation of the caudal half of one pair of sclerotomes with the cranial half of the subjacent pair of sclerotomes.
- The developing cranium consists of a neurocranium and a viscerocranium, each of which has membranous and cartilaginous components. The neurocranium forms the calvaria. The viscerocranium forms the skeleton of the face.

- The appendicular skeleton develops from endochondral ossification of the cartilaginous bone models, which form from mesenchyme in the developing limbs.
- Joints are classified as fibrous joints, cartilaginous joints, and synovial joints. They develop from interzonal mesenchyme between the primordia of bones. In a **fibrous joint**, the intervening mesenchyme differentiates into dense fibrous connective tissue. In a **cartilaginous joint**, the mesenchyme between the bones differentiates into cartilage. In a **synovial joint**, a synovial cavity is formed within the intervening mesenchyme by breakdown of the cells. Mesenchyme also gives rise to the synovial membrane, capsule, and ligaments of the joint.

CLINICALLY ORIENTED PROBLEMS

CASE 14-1

A newborn infant presented with a lesion in his lower back, which was thought to be a vertebral arch defect.

- What is the most common congenital anomaly of the vertebral column?
- Where is the defect usually located?
- Does this congenital anomaly usually cause symptoms (e.g., back problems)?

CASE 14-2

A young girl presented with pain in her upper limb, which worsened when she lifted heavy objects. After a radiographic examination, the physician told her parents that she had an accessory rib in her neck.

- Occasionally rudimentary ribs are associated with the seventh cervical vertebra and the first lumbar vertebra. Are these accessory ribs of clinical importance?
- What is the embryologic basis of accessory ribs?

CASE 14-3

The mother of a girl with a "crooked spine" was told that her daughter had scoliosis.

- What vertebral defect can produce scoliosis?
- Define this condition.
- What is the embryologic basis of the vertebral defect?

CASE 14-4

A boy presented with a long, thin head. His mother was concerned that her son might become mentally retarded.

- What is meant by the term craniosynostosis?
- What results from this developmental abnormality?
- Give a common example and describe it.

CASE 14-5

A child presented with characteristics of the Klippel-Feil syndrome.

- What are the main features of this condition?
- What vertebral anomalies are usually present?

Discussion of these problems appears at the back of the book.

References and Suggested Reading

Alvarez J, Horton J, Sohn P, et al: The perichondrium plays an important role in mediating the effects of TGF-1β on endochondral bone formation. Dev Dyn 221:311, 2001.

Brooks CGD, de Vries BBA: Skeletal dysplasias. Arch Dis Child 79:285, 1998.

Cohen AR: Disorders in head size and shape. In Martin RJ, Fanaroff AA, Walsh MC (eds): Fanaroff and Martin's Neonatal-Perinatal Medicine. Diseases of the Fetus and Infant, 8th ed. Philadelphia, Mosby, 2006.

Cohen MM Jr, MacLean RE (eds): Craniosynostosis: Diagnosis, Evaluation, and Management, 2nd ed. New York, Oxford University Press, 2000.

Erlebacher A, Filvaroff EH, Gitelman SE, et al: Toward a molecular understanding of skeletal development. Cell 80:371, 1995.

Franz-Odendaal TA, Hall, BK, Witten PE: Buried alive: How osteoblasts become osteocytes. Dev Dyn 235:176, 2006.

Gartner LP, Hiatt JL: Color Textbook of Histology, 2nd ed. Philadelphia, WB Saunders, 2001.

Hall BK: Bones and Cartilage: Developmental Skeletal Biology. Philadelphia, Elsevier, 2005.

Jirásek JE: An Atlas of Human Prenatal Developmental Mechanics. Anatomy and Staging, London and New York, Taylor & Francis, 2004.

Kalcheim C, Ben-Yair R: Cell rearrangements during development of the somite and its derivatives. Curr Opin Genet Dev 15:371, 2005.

Källén B, Robert-Gnansia E: Maternal drug use, fertility problems, and infant craniostenosis. Cleft Palate Craniofac J 42:589, 2005.

Long F, Schipani E, Asahara H, et al: The CREB family of activators is required for endochondral bone development. Development 128:541, 2001.

Mahony BS: Ultrasound evaluation of the fetal musculoskeletal system. In Callen PW (ed): Ultrasonography in Obstetrics and Gynecology, 4th ed. Philadelphia, WB Saunders, 2000.

Marsh J: Set down in bone. BioEssays 22:402, 2000.

Müller F, O'Rahilly R: The human chondrocranium at the end of the embryonic period, proper, with particular reference to the nervous system. Am J Anat 159:33, 1980.

Muragaki Y, Mundlos S, Upton J, Oslen BR: Altered growth and branching patterns in synpolydactyly caused by mutations in *Hoxd-13*. Science 272:548, 1996.

Nussbaum RL, McInnes RR, Willard HF: Thompson & Thompson Genetics in Medicine, 6th ed. Philadelphia, WB Saunders, 2005.

O'Rahilly R, Müller F, Meyer DB: The human vertebral column at the end of the embryonic period proper. 3. The thoracolumbar region. J Anat 168:81, 1990.

O'Rahilly R, Müller F, Meyer DB: The human vertebral column at the end of the embryonic period proper. 4. The thoracolumbar region. J Anat 168:95, 1990.

Sasaki T, Ito Y, Bringas P, et al: TGFß-mediated FGF signaling is crucial for regulating cranial neural crest cell proliferation during frontal bone development. Development 133:371, 2006.

Slack JMW: Essential Developmental Biology, 2nd ed. Oxford, Blackwell Publishing, 2006.

Sperber GH: Craniofacial Development. Hamilton, BC Decker, 2001.

Wagner EF, Karsenty G: Genetic control of skeletal development. Curr Opin Genet Dev 11:527, 2001.

15

The Muscular System

Development of Skeletal Muscle 358
- Myotomes 358
- Pharyngeal Arch Muscles 358
- Ocular Muscles 358
- Tongue Muscles 359
- Limb Muscles 359

Development of Smooth Muscle 360

Development of Cardiac Muscle 360

Summary of the Muscular System 362

Clinically Oriented Problems 363

The muscular system develops from **mesoderm**, except for the muscles of the iris, which develop from **neuroectoderm**, and the muscles of the esophagus, which are believed to develop by transdifferentiation from smooth muscle. **Myoblasts** (embryonic muscle cells) are derived from **mesenchyme** (embryonic connective tissue). MyoD, a member of the family of myogenic regulatory factors, activates transcription of muscle-specific genes and is considered an important regulatory gene for the induction of myogenic differentiation. The **induction of myogenesis** in mesenchymal cells by MyoD is dependent on their degree of mesenchymal cell differentiation. Much of the mesenchyme in the head is derived from the **neural crest** (see Chapters 4 and 5), particularly the tissues derived from the pharyngeal arches (see Chapter 9); however, the original mesenchyme in these arches gives rise to the musculature of the face and neck (see Table 9-1).

DEVELOPMENT OF SKELETAL MUSCLE

Limb muscles develop by **epitheliomesenchymal transformation** from myogenic precursor cells. Studies show that **myogenic precursor cells** originate from the somatic mesoderm and also from the ventral **dermomyotome of somites** in response to molecular signals from nearby tissues (Figs. 15-1 and 15-2).

The first indication of **myogenesis** (muscle formation) is the elongation of the nuclei and cell bodies of mesenchymal cells as they differentiate into myoblasts. Soon these **primordial muscle cells** fuse to form elongated, multinucleated, cylindrical structures—**myotubes**. At the molecular level, these events are preceded by gene activation and expression of the MyoD family of muscle-specific basic helix-loop-helix transcription factors (MyoD, myogenin, Myf-5, and myogenic regulatory factor 4) in the precursor myogenic cells. It has been suggested that signaling molecules (Shh, from the ventral neural tube and notochord, and others from the dorsal neural tube (Wnts, bone morphogenetic protein [BMP]-4) and overlying ectoderm (Wnts, BMP-4) regulate the beginning of myogenesis and the induction of the myotome (Fig. 15-3). Further muscle growth in the fetus results from the ongoing fusion of myoblasts and myotubes.

During or after fusion of the myoblasts, **myofilaments** develop in the cytoplasm of the myotubes. Other organelles characteristic of striated muscle cells, such as **myofibrils**, also form. Because muscle cells are long and narrow, they are usually called muscle fibers. As the myotubes develop, they become invested with external laminae, which segregate them from the surrounding connective tissue. Fibroblasts produce the perimysium and epimysium layers of the fibrous sheath of the muscle; the **endomysium** is formed by the external lamina, and reticular fibers.

Most skeletal muscles develop before birth, and almost all remaining ones are formed by the end of the first year. The increase in the size of a muscle after the first year results from an increase in the diameter of the fibers because of the formation of more myofilaments. Muscles increase in length and width to grow with the skeleton. Their ultimate size depends on the amount of exercise that is performed. Not all embryonic muscle fibers persist; many of them fail to establish themselves as necessary units of the muscle and soon degenerate.

Myotomes

Each typical myotome part of a somite divides into a dorsal **epaxial division** and a ventral **hypaxial division** (see Fig. 15-1*B*). Every developing spinal nerve also divides and sends a branch to each myotome division, the dorsal primary ramus supplying the epaxial division and the ventral primary ramus, the hypaxial division. The myoblasts that form the skeletal muscles of the trunk are derived from mesenchyme in the myotome regions of the somites (see Fig. 15-1). Some muscles, e.g., the intercostal muscles, remain segmentally arranged like the somites, but most myoblasts migrate away from the myotome and form nonsegmented muscles.

Gene targeting studies in the mouse embryo suggest that *MyoD* and *Myf-5* genes are essential for the development of the hypaxial and epaxial muscles, respectively. Both genes are involved in the development of the abdominal and intercostal muscles.

Derivatives of Epaxial Divisions of Myotomes

Myoblasts from hypaxial divisions of the myotomes form the extensor muscles of the neck and vertebral column (Fig. 15-4). The embryonic extensor muscles derived from the sacral and coccygeal myotomes degenerate; their adult derivatives are the dorsal sacrococcygeal ligaments.

Derivatives of Hypaxial Divisions of Myotomes

Myoblasts from these divisions of the cervical myotomes form the scalene, prevertebral, geniohyoid, and infrahyoid muscles (see Fig. 15-4). The thoracic myotomes form the lateral and ventral flexor muscles of the vertebral column, and the lumbar myotomes form the quadratus lumborum muscle. The sacrococcygeal myotomes form the muscles of the pelvic diaphragm and probably the striated muscles of the anus and sex organs.

Pharyngeal Arch Muscles

The myoblasts from the pharyngeal arches form the muscles of mastication, facial expression, pharynx, and larynx as described in Chapter 9. These muscles are innervated by pharyngeal arch nerves.

Ocular Muscles

The origin of the extrinsic eye muscles is unclear, but they may be derived from mesenchymal cells near the prechordal plate (see Figs. 15-1 and 15-4). The mesenchyme in this area is thought to give rise to three preotic myotomes. Myoblasts differentiate from mesenchymal cells derived from these myotomes. Groups of myoblasts, each supplied by its own nerve (cranial nerve [CN] III, CN IV, or CN VI), form the extrinsic muscles of the eye.

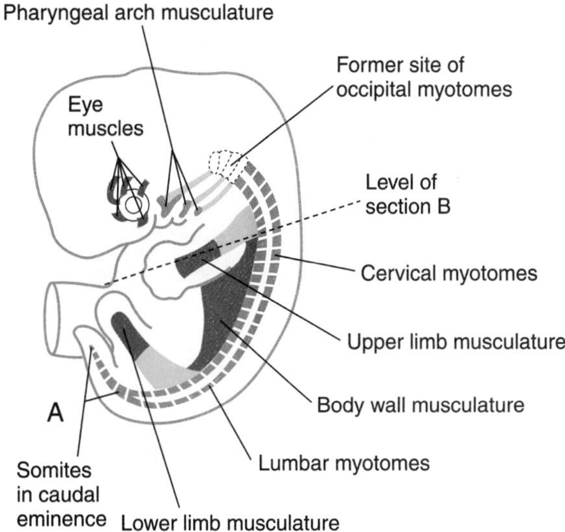

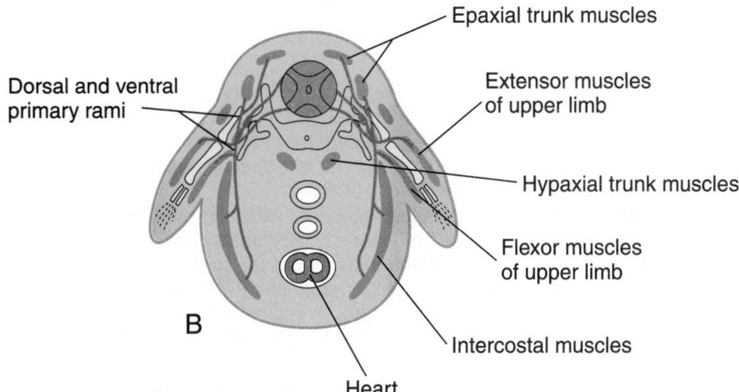

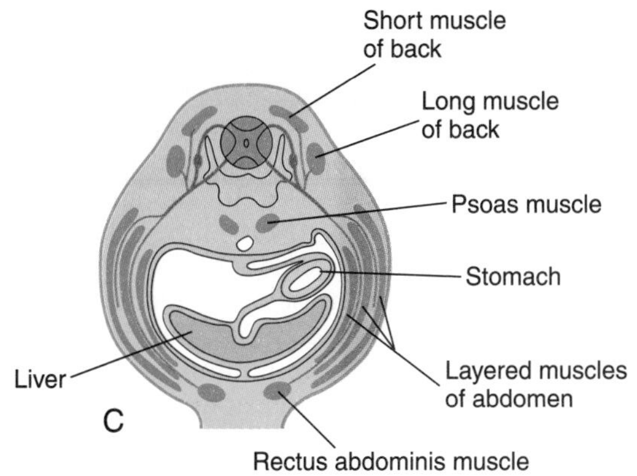

FIGURE 15-1. **A,** Sketch of an embryo (approximately 41 days) showing the myotomes and developing muscular system. **B,** Transverse section of the embryo illustrating the epaxial and hypaxial derivatives of a myotome. **C,** Similar section of a 7-week embryo showing the muscle layers formed from the myotomes.

Tongue Muscles

Initially there are four *occipital (postotic) myotomes*; the first pair disappears. Myoblasts from the remaining myotomes form the tongue muscles, which are innervated by the hypoglossal nerve (CN XII).

Limb Muscles

The musculature of the limbs develops from myoblasts surrounding the developing bones (see Fig. 15-1). Grafting and gene targeting studies in birds and mammals have demonstrated that the precursor myogenic cells in the limb buds originate from the somites. These cells are first located in the ventral part of the dermomyotome and are epithelial in nature (see Fig. 14-1*D*). After **epithelio-mesenchymal transformation**, the cells then migrate into the primordium of the limb. Molecular signals from the neural tube and notochord induce Pax-3 and Myf-5 in the somites. Pax-3 regulates the expression of c-met in the limb bud (a migratory peptide growth factor), which regulates migration of the precursor myogenic cells.

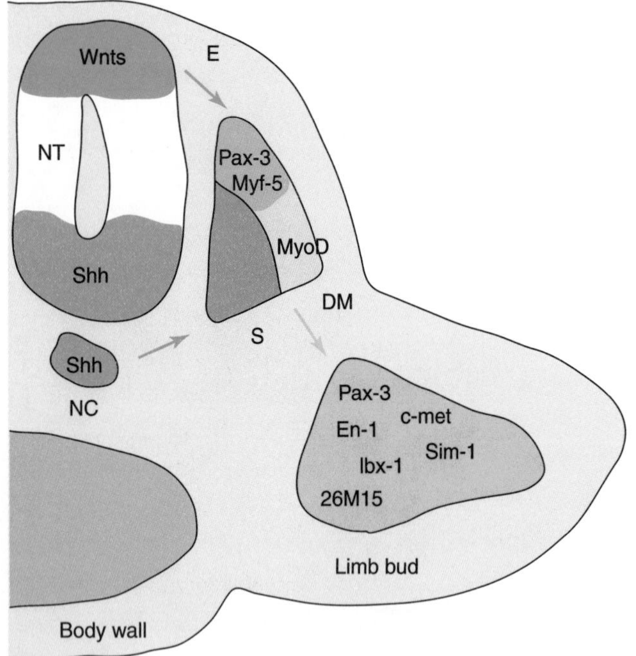

FIGURE 15-2. A model for molecular interactions during myogenesis. Shh and Wnts, produced by the neural tube (NT) and notochord (NC), induce Pax-3 and Myf-5 in the somites. Either of them can activate the initiation of MyoD transcription and myogenesis. Surface ectoderm (E) is also capable of inducing Myf-5 and MyoD. In addition, Pax-3 regulates the expression of c-met, necessary for the migratory ability of myogenic precursor cells, that also express: En-1, Sim-1, Ibx-1 and 26M15. DM, dermamyotome; S, sclerotome. (From Kablar B, Rudnicki MA: Skeletal muscle development in the mouse embryo. Histol Histopathol 15:649, 2000.)

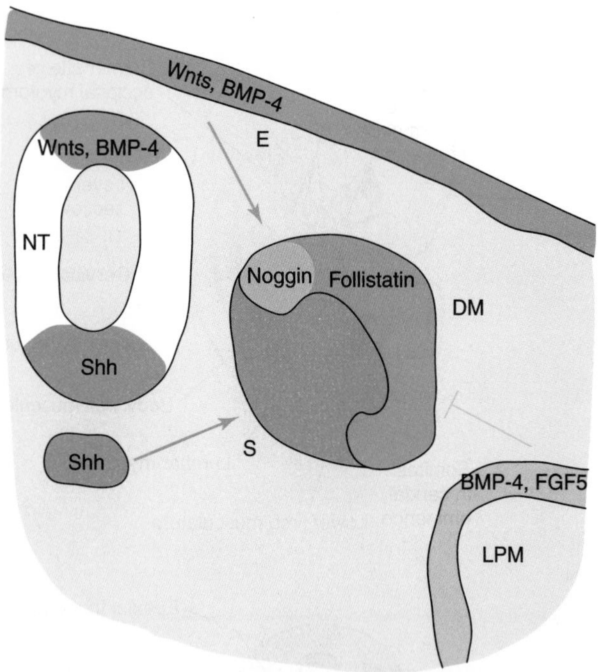

FIGURE 15-3. Embryonic structures and myogenesis. The current view suggests that the dorsal neural tube (NT) and the overlying non-neural ectoderm (E) are sources of signaling molecules belonging to the family of Wnt secreted proteins and bone morphogenetic protein (BMP)-4, whereas the notochord (NC) and the ventral neural tube (green) are sources of the Shh. They positively regulate the onset of myogenesis and the induction of the myotome. By contrast, the lateral plate mesoderm (LPM) produces BMP-4 and FGF5 (fibroblast growth factor 5), negatively regulating muscle terminal differentiation in the lateral part of the myotome lineage. Response to the BMP-4 signal may be mediated by its binding proteins noggin and follistatin. DM, dermamyotome; S, sclerotome. (From Kablar B, Rudnicki MA: Skeletal muscle development in the mouse embryo. Histol Histopathol 15:649, 2000.)

DEVELOPMENT OF SMOOTH MUSCLE

Smooth muscle fibers differentiate from **splanchnic mesenchyme** surrounding the endoderm of the primordial gut and its derivatives (see Fig. 15-1). The somatic mesoderm provides smooth muscle in the walls of many blood and lymphatic vessels. The muscles of the iris (sphincter and dilator pupillae) and the myoepithelial cells in mammary and sweat glands are thought to be derived from mesenchymal cells that originate from ectoderm.

The first sign of differentiation of smooth muscle is the development of elongated nuclei in spindle-shaped myoblasts. During early development, additional myoblasts continue to differentiate from mesenchymal cells but do not fuse as in skeletal muscle; they remain mononucleated. During later development, division of existing myoblasts gradually replaces the differentiation of new myoblasts in the production of new smooth muscle tissue. As smooth muscle cells differentiate, filamentous but nonsarcomeric contractile elements develop in their cytoplasm, and the external surface of each cell acquires a surrounding external lamina. As smooth muscle fibers develop into sheets or bundles, they receive autonomic innervation. Muscle cells and fibroblasts synthesize and lay down collagenous, elastic, and reticular fibers.

DEVELOPMENT OF CARDIAC MUSCLE

Cardiac muscle develops from the lateral splanchnic mesoderm, which gives rise to the mesenchyme surrounding the developing heart tube (see Chapter 13). **Cardiac myoblasts** differentiate from the primordial myocardium. Heart muscle is recognizable in the fourth week and likely develops through expression of cardiac-specific genes. Immunohistochemical studies have revealed a spatial distribution of tissue-specific antigens (myosin heavy chain isoforms) in the embryonic heart between the fourth and eighth weeks. **Cardiac muscle fibers** arise by differentiation and growth of single cells, unlike striated skeletal muscle fibers, which develop by fusion of cells. Growth of cardiac muscle fibers results from the formation of new myofilaments. The myoblasts adhere to each other as in developing skeletal muscle, but the intervening cell membranes do not disintegrate; these areas of adhesion give rise to **intercalated discs**. Late in the embryonic period, special bundles of muscle cells develop with relatively few myofibrils and relatively larger diameters than typical cardiac muscle fibers. These atypical cardiac muscle cells—**Purkinje fibers**—form the conducting system of the heart (see Chapter 13).

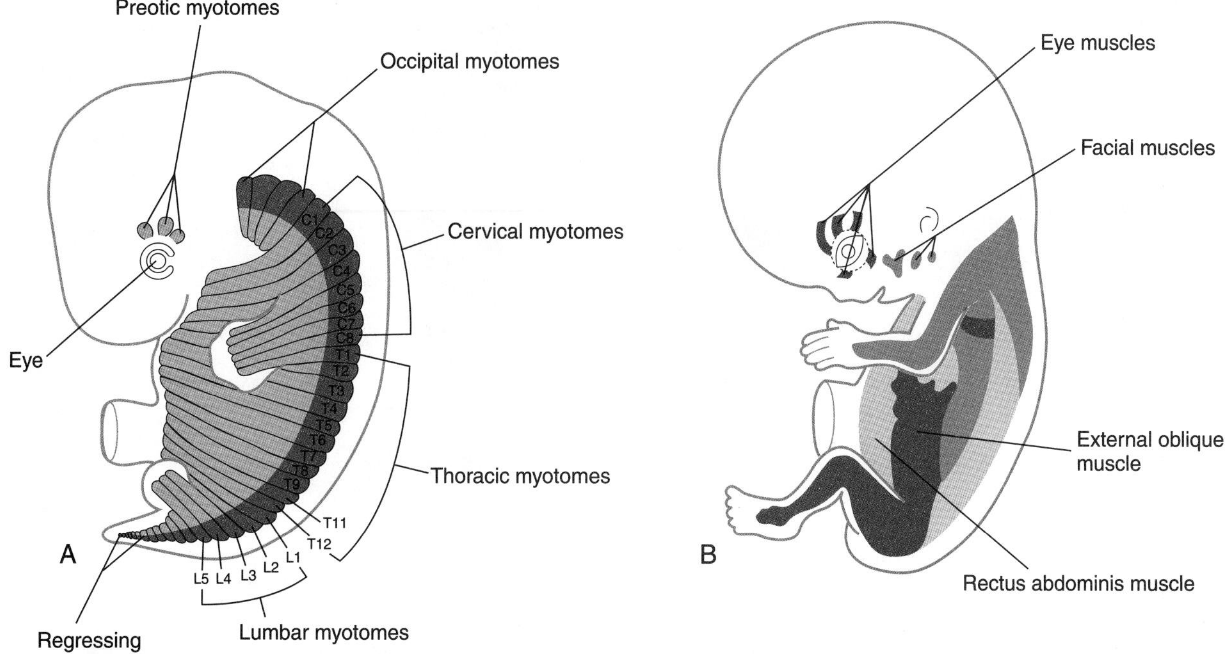

FIGURE 15-4. Illustrations of the developing muscular system. **A,** A 6-week embryo showing the myotome regions of the somites that give rise to skeletal muscles. **B,** An 8-week embryo showing the developing trunk and limb musculature.

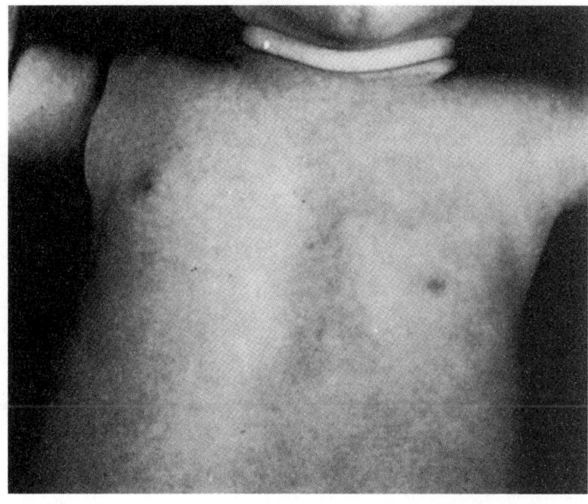

FIGURE 15-5. The thorax of an infant with congenital absence of the left pectoralis major muscle. Note the absence of the anterior axillary fold on the left and the low location of the left nipple. (From Behrman RE, Kliegman RM, Arvin AM [eds]: Nelson Textbook of Pediatrics, 15th ed. Philadelphia, WB Saunders, 1996.)

ANOMALIES OF MUSCLES

Absence of one or more of the skeletal muscles is more common than is generally recognized; common examples are the sternocostal head of the pectoralis major (Fig. 15-5), the palmaris longus, trapezius, serratus anterior, and quadratus femoris. Usually only a single muscle is absent on one side of the body, or only part of the muscle fails to develop. Occasionally the same muscle or muscles may be absent on both sides of the body. Absence of the pectoralis major, often its sternal part, is usually associated with syndactyly (fusion of digits). These anomalies are part of **Poland syndrome**. Absence of the pectoralis major is occasionally associated with absence of the mammary gland in the breast and/or hypoplasia of the nipple.

In rare instances, failure of normal muscle development and growth may be widespread, leading to immobility of multiple joints—**arthrogryposis multiplex congenita** (Fig. 15-6). Persons with this congenital syndrome have congenital stiffness of one or more joints associated with hypoplasia of the associated muscles. The causes encompass both neurogenic and primary myopathic diseases. The involved muscles are replaced partially or completely by fat and fibrous tissue.

Some muscular anomalies, such as **congenital absence of the diaphragm**, cause difficulty in breathing, which is usually associated with incomplete expansion of the lungs or part of a lung (**pulmonary atelectasis**) and pneumonitis (pneumonia). Absence of muscles of the anterior abdominal wall may be associated with severe gastrointestinal and genitourinary anomalies, for example, **exstrophy of the bladder** (see Chapter 12). Occasionally individuals with congenital absence of a muscle develop **muscular dystrophy** in later life. The most common association of this type is between congenital absence of the pectoralis major muscle and the Landouzy-Dejerine facioscapulohumeral form

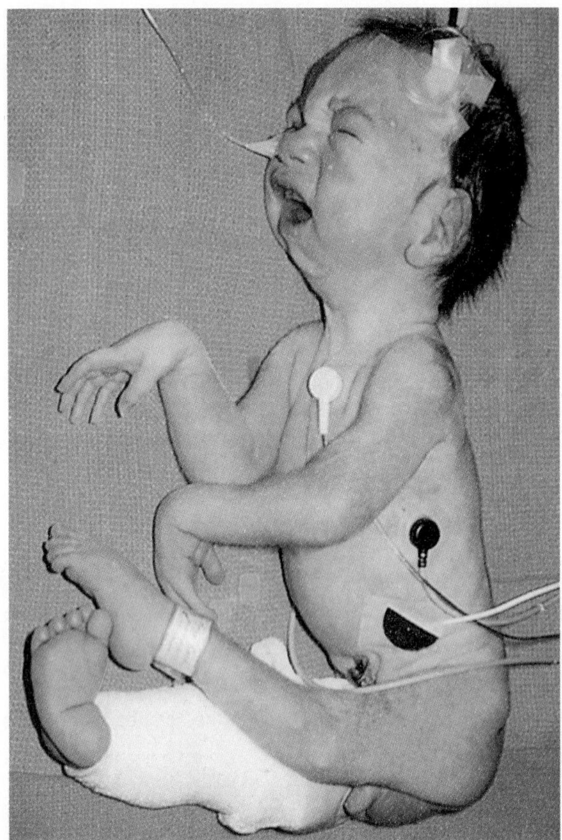

FIGURE 15-6. Neonate with multiple joint contractures: arthrogryposis. (Courtesy of A.E. Chudley, MD, Section of Genetics and Metabolism, Department of Pediatrics and Child Health, Children's Hospital and University of Manitoba, Winnipeg, Manitoba, Canada.)

of muscular dystrophy. Both muscle development and muscle repair have distinctive dependence on expression of muscle regulatory genes.

VARIATIONS IN MUSCLES

All muscles are subject to a certain amount of variation, but some are affected more often than others. Certain muscles are functionally vestigial (rudimentary), such as those of the external ear and scalp. Some muscles present in other primates appear in only some humans (e.g., the sternalis muscle, a band sometimes found parallel to the sternum). Variations in the form, position, and attachments of muscles are common and are usually functionally insignificant.

CONGENITAL TORTICOLLIS

Some cases of torticollis (wryneck) result from tearing of fibers of the sternocleidomastoid muscle during childbirth. Bleeding into the muscle occurs in a localized area, forming a **hematoma** (a small collection of blood). Later a solid mass develops because of necrosis (death) of muscle fibers and fibrosis (formation of fibrous tissue). Shortening of the muscle usually follows, which causes lateral bending of the head to the affected side and a slight turning away of the head from the side of the short muscle (Fig. 15-7). Although birth trauma is commonly considered as a cause of congenital torticollis, the fact that the condition has been observed in infants delivered by cesarean section suggests that there are other causes as well.

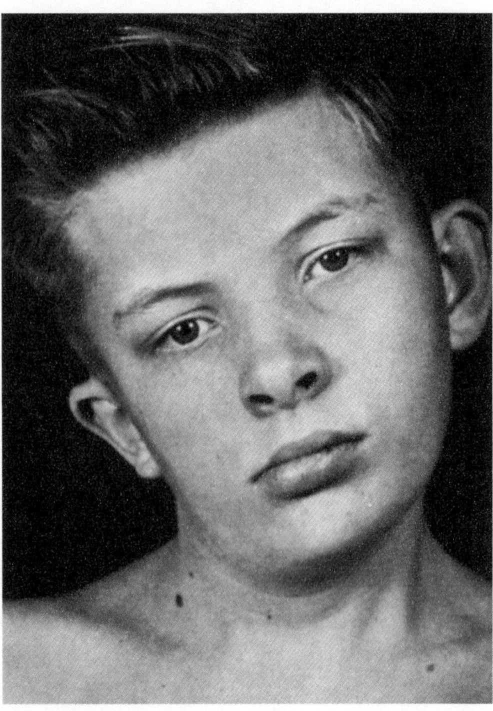

FIGURE 15-7. The head and neck of a 12-year-old boy with congenital torticollis (wryneck). Shortening of the right sternocleidomastoid muscle has caused tilting of the head to the right and turning of the chin to the left. There is also asymmetrical development of the face and cranium. (From Behrman RE, Vaughan VC III: Nelson Textbook of Pediatrics, 13th ed. Philadelphia, WB Saunders, 1987.)

ACCESSORY MUSCLES

Accessory muscles occasionally develop; for example, an accessory soleus muscle is present in approximately 6% of people. It has been suggested that the primordium of the soleus muscle undergoes early splitting to form an accessory soleus. In some cases, accessory muscles are clinically significant.

SUMMARY OF THE MUSCULAR SYSTEM

- Skeletal muscle is derived from the myotome regions of somites.

- Some head and neck muscles are derived from pharyngeal arch mesenchyme.
- The limb muscles develop from myogenic precursor cells surrounding bones in the limbs.
- Cardiac muscle and most smooth muscle are derived from splanchnic mesoderm.
- Absence or variation of some muscles is common and is usually of little consequence.

CLINICALLY ORIENTED PROBLEMS

CASE 15-1

An infant presented with absence of the left anterior axillary fold. In addition, the left nipple was much lower than usual.

- Absence of which muscle probably caused these unusual observations?
- What syndrome would you suspect may be present?
- For what features would you look?
- Would the infant be likely to suffer any disability if absence of this muscle was the only anomaly present?

CASE 15-2

A medical student was concerned when she learned that she had only one palmaris longus muscle.

- Is this a common occurrence?
- What is its incidence?
- Does the absence of this muscle cause a disability?

CASE 15-3

The parents of a 4-year-old girl observed that she always held her head slightly tilted to the right side and that one of her neck muscles was more prominent than the others. The clinical history revealed that her delivery had been a breech birth, one in which the buttocks presented.

- Name the muscle that was likely prominent.
- Did it pull the child's head to the right side?
- What is this deformity called?
- What probably caused the muscle shortening that resulted in this condition?

CASE 15-4

A newborn infant presented with an abdominal wall defect. Failure of striated muscle to develop in the median plane of the anterior abdominal wall is associated with the formation of a severe congenital anomaly of the urinary system.

- What is this anomaly called?
- What is the probable embryologic basis of the failure of muscle to form in this infant?

Discussion of these problems appears at the back of the book.

References and Suggested Reading

Arnold HH, Braun T: Genetics of muscle determination and development. Curr Top Dev Biol 48:129, 2000.
Birchmeier C, Brohmann H: Genes that control the development of migrating muscle precursor cells. Curr Opin Cell Biol 12:725, 2000.
Brand-Saberi B, Müller TS, Wilting J, et al: Scatter factor/hepatocyte growth factor (SG/HGF) induces emigration of myogenic cells at interlimb level in vivo. Dev Biol 179:303, 1996.
Buckingham M: Skeletal muscle formation in vertebrates. Curr Opin Genet Dev 11:440, 2001.
Budorick NE: The fetal musculoskeletal system. In Callen PW (ed): Ultrasonography in Obstetrics and Gynecology, 4th ed. Philadelphia, WB Saunders, 2000.
Cheng JCY, Tang SP, Chen MWN, et al: The clinical presentation and outcome of treatment of congenital muscular torticollis in infants—a study of 1,086 cases. J Pediatr Surg 35:1091, 2000.
Dubowitz V: Muscle Disorders in Childhood, 2nd ed. Philadelphia, WB Saunders, 1995.
Friday BB, Horsley V, Pavlath GK: Calcineurin activity is required for the initiation of skeletal muscle differentiation. J Cell Biol 149:657, 2000.
Gasser RF: The development of the facial muscle in man. Am J Anat 120:357, 1967.
Jirásek JE: An Atlas of Human Prenatal Developmental Mechanics. Anatomy and Staging, London and New York, Taylor & Francis, 2004.
Kablar B, Krastel K, Ying C, et al: MyoD and Myf-5 differentially regulate the development of limb versus trunk skeletal muscle. Development 124:4729, 1997.
Kablar B, Krastel K, Ying C, et al: Myogenic determination occurs independently in somites and limb buds. Dev Biol 206:219, 1999.
Kablar B, Rudnicki MA: Skeletal muscle development in the mouse embryo. Histol Histopathol 15:649, 2000.
Kablar B, Tajbakhsh S, Rudnick MA: Transdifferentiation of esophageal smooth muscle is myogenic bHLH factor-dependent. Development 127:1627, 2000.
Kalcheim C, Ben-Yair R: Cell rearrangements during development of the somite and its derivatives. Curr Opin Genet Dev 15:371, 2005.
Moore KL, Dalley AF: Clinically Oriented Anatomy, 5th ed. Baltimore, Williams & Wilkins, 2006.
Noden DM: Vertebrate craniofacial development—the relation between ontogenetic process and morphological outcome. Brain Behav Evol 38:190, 1991.
O'Rahilly R, Gardner E: The timing and sequence of events in the development of the limbs of the human embryo. Anat Embryol 148:1, 1975.
Ordahl CP, Williams BA, Denetclaw W: Determination and morphogenesis in myogenic progenitor cells: An experimental embryological approach. Curr Topics Dev Biol 48:19, 2000.
Perry RL, Rudnick MA: Molecular mechanisms regulating myogenic determination and differentiation. Front Biosci 5:D750, 2000.
Sabourin LA, Rudnicki MA: The molecular regulation of myogenesis. Clin Genet 57:16, 2000.
Sarnat HB: Neuromuscular disorders. In Behrman RE, Kliegman Jenson HB (eds): Nelson Textbook of Pediatrics, 17th ed. Philadelphia, Elsevier/Saunders, 2004.
Uusitalo M, Kivela T: Development of cytoskeleton in neuroectodermally derived epithelial and muscle cells of human eye. Invest Ophthalmol Vis Sci 36:2584, 1995.
Williams BA, Ordahl CP: Fate restriction of limb muscle precursor cells precedes high-level expression of MyoD family member genes. Development 127:2523, 2000.

16 The Limbs

Early Stages of Limb Development 365

Final Stages of Limb Development 366

Cutaneous Innervation of Limbs 368

Blood Supply to the Limbs 371

Anomalies of the Limbs 372

Summary of Limb Development 377

Clinically Oriented Problems 379

EARLY STAGES OF LIMB DEVELOPMENT

Limb development begins with the activation of a group of mesenchymal cells in the lateral mesoderm. Homeobox genes regulate patterning in the formation of the limbs. The **limb buds** form deep to a thick band of ectoderm (AER). Toward the end of the fourth week, the limb buds first appear as elevations of the ventrolateral body wall (Figs. 16-1*A* and 16-2). The upper limb buds are visible by day 26 or 27, and the lower limb buds appear 1 or 2 days later. Each limb bud consists of a mass of mesenchyme covered by ectoderm. The mesenchyme is derived from the somatic layer of lateral mesoderm.

The limb buds elongate by proliferation of the mesenchyme. The upper limb buds appear disproportionately low on the embryo's trunk because of the early development of the cranial half of the embryo. The earliest stages of limb development are alike for the upper and lower

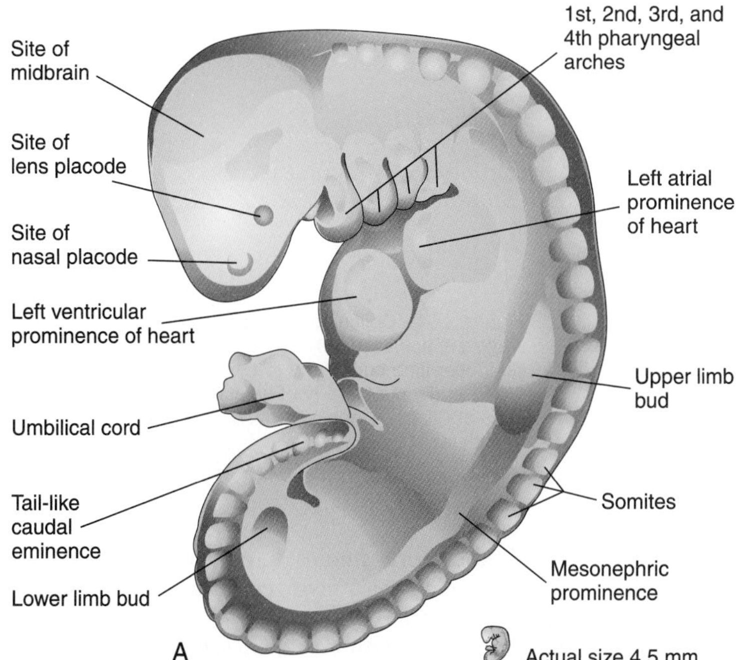

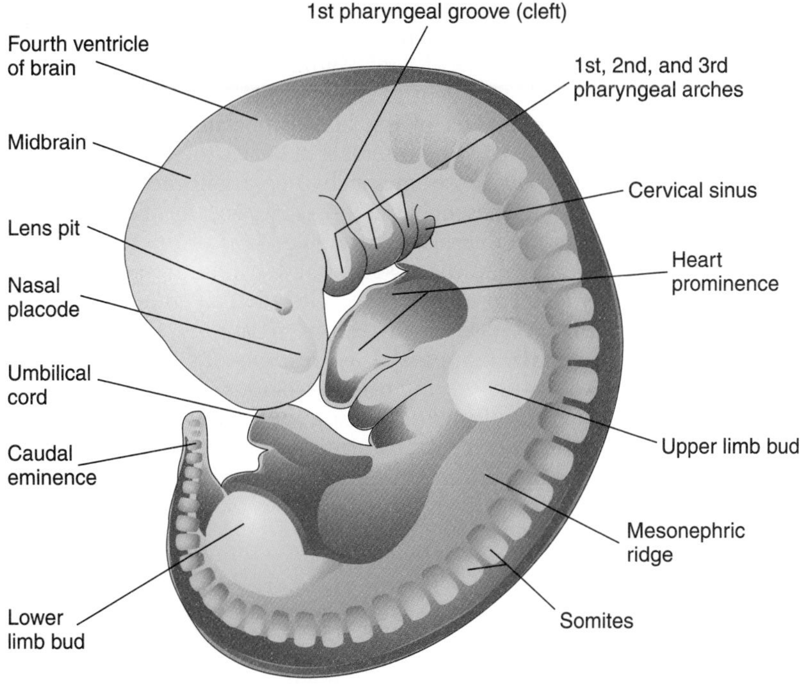

FIGURE 16-1. **A,** Lateral view of a human embryo at Carnegie stage 13, approximately 28 days. The upper limb buds appear as swellings on the ventrolateral body wall. The lower limb buds are not as well developed. **B,** Lateral view of an embryo at Carnegie stage 14, approximately 32 days. The upper limb buds are paddle shaped and the lower limb buds are flipper-like. (Modified from Nishimura H, Semba R, Tanimura T, Tanaka O: Prenatal Development of the Human with Special Reference to Craniofacial Structures: An Atlas. Washington, DC, National Institutes of Health, 1977.)

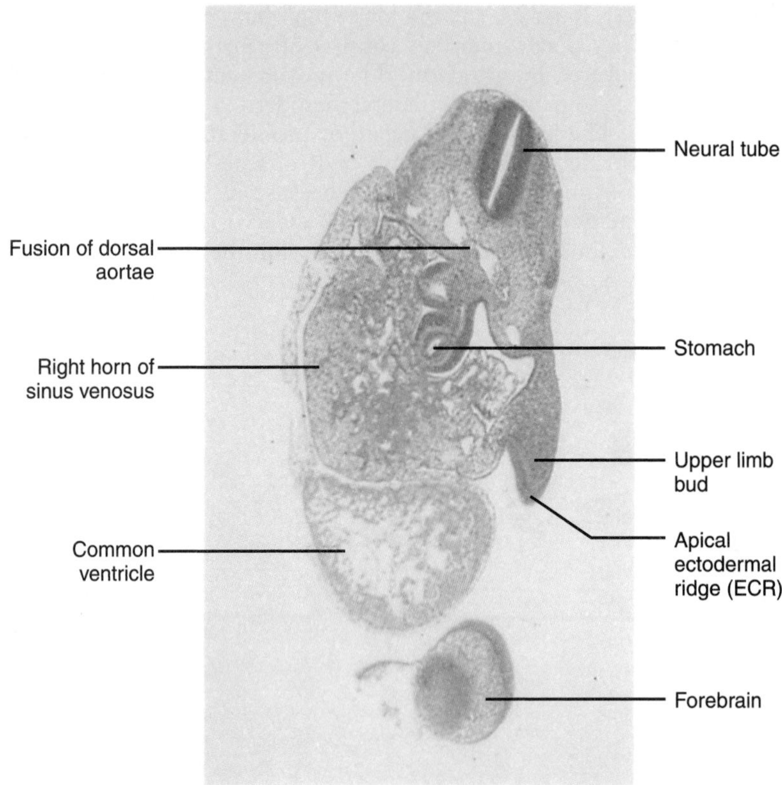

FIGURE 16-2. Oblique section of an embryo at Carnegie stage 13, approximately 28 days. Observe the flipper-like upper limb bud lateral to the embryonic heart and the ECR. (From Moore KL, Persaud TVN, Shiota K: Color Atlas of Clinical Embryology, 2nd ed. Philadelphia, WB Saunders, 2000.)

limbs (see Figs. 16-1*B* and 16-4). Because of their form and function, there are many distinct differences between the development of the hand and foot. The **upper limb buds** develop opposite the caudal cervical segments, and the **lower limb buds** form opposite the lumbar and upper sacral segments.

At the apex of each limb bud, the ectoderm thickens to form an **apical ectodermal ridge** (AER). The AER, a multilayered epithelial structure (see Fig. 16-2), is induced by the underlying mesenchyme. Bone morphogenetic protein signaling is required for its formation. *The AER exerts an inductive influence on the limb mesenchyme that initiates growth and development of the limbs in a proximodistal axis.* Experimental studies show that expression of endogenous fibroblast growth factors and *T-box* genes (*tbx-4* and *tbx-5*) in the AER are essential for this process. Mesenchymal cells aggregate at the posterior margin of the limb bud to form the **zone of polarizing activity**. Fibroblast growth factors from the AER activate the zone of polarizing activity, which causes expression of the sonic hedgehog (*Shh*) genes. It has been suggested that Shh secretions (**morphogens**) control the patterning of the limb along the anterior-posterior axis.

Expression of Wnt7 from the dorsal epidermis of the limb bud and engrailed-1 (EN-1) from the ventral aspect are involved in specifying the dorsal-ventral axis. The AER itself is maintained by inductive signals from Shh and Wnt7. The mesenchyme adjacent to the AER consists of undifferentiated, rapidly proliferating cells, whereas mesenchymal cells proximal to it differentiate into blood vessels and cartilage bone models. The distal ends of the limb buds flatten into paddle-like hand- and footplates (Fig. 16-3). Laboratory studies have shown that endogenous retinoic acid is also involved in limb development and pattern formation.

By the end of the sixth week, mesenchymal tissue in the **handplates** has condensed to form **digital rays** (Figs. 16-3 and 16-4*A* to *C*). These mesenchymal condensations outline the pattern of the digits or fingers. During the seventh week, similar condensations of mesenchyme form digital rays and toes in the **footplates** (see Fig. 16-4*G* to *I*). At the tip of each digital ray, a part of the AER induces development of the mesenchyme into the mesenchymal primordia of the bones (phalanges) in the digits (see Fig. 16-6). The intervals between the digital rays are occupied by loose mesenchyme. Soon the intervening regions of mesenchyme break down, forming notches between the digital rays (see Figs. 16-3, 16-4*D* and *J*, and 16-5*A* to *D*). As the tissue breakdown progresses, separate digits (fingers and toes) are formed by the end of the eighth week (see Fig. 16-4*E*, *F*, *K*, and *L*). **Programmed cell death** (apoptosis) is responsible for the tissue breakdown in the interdigital regions, and it is probably mediated by **bone morphogenetic proteins**, signaling molecules of the transforming growth factor β superfamily. Blocking these cellular and molecular events could account for syndactyly or webbing of the fingers or toes (see Fig. 16-14*C*).

FINAL STAGES OF LIMB DEVELOPMENT

As the limbs elongate, mesenchymal models of the bones are formed by cellular aggregations (see Fig. 16-7*B*).

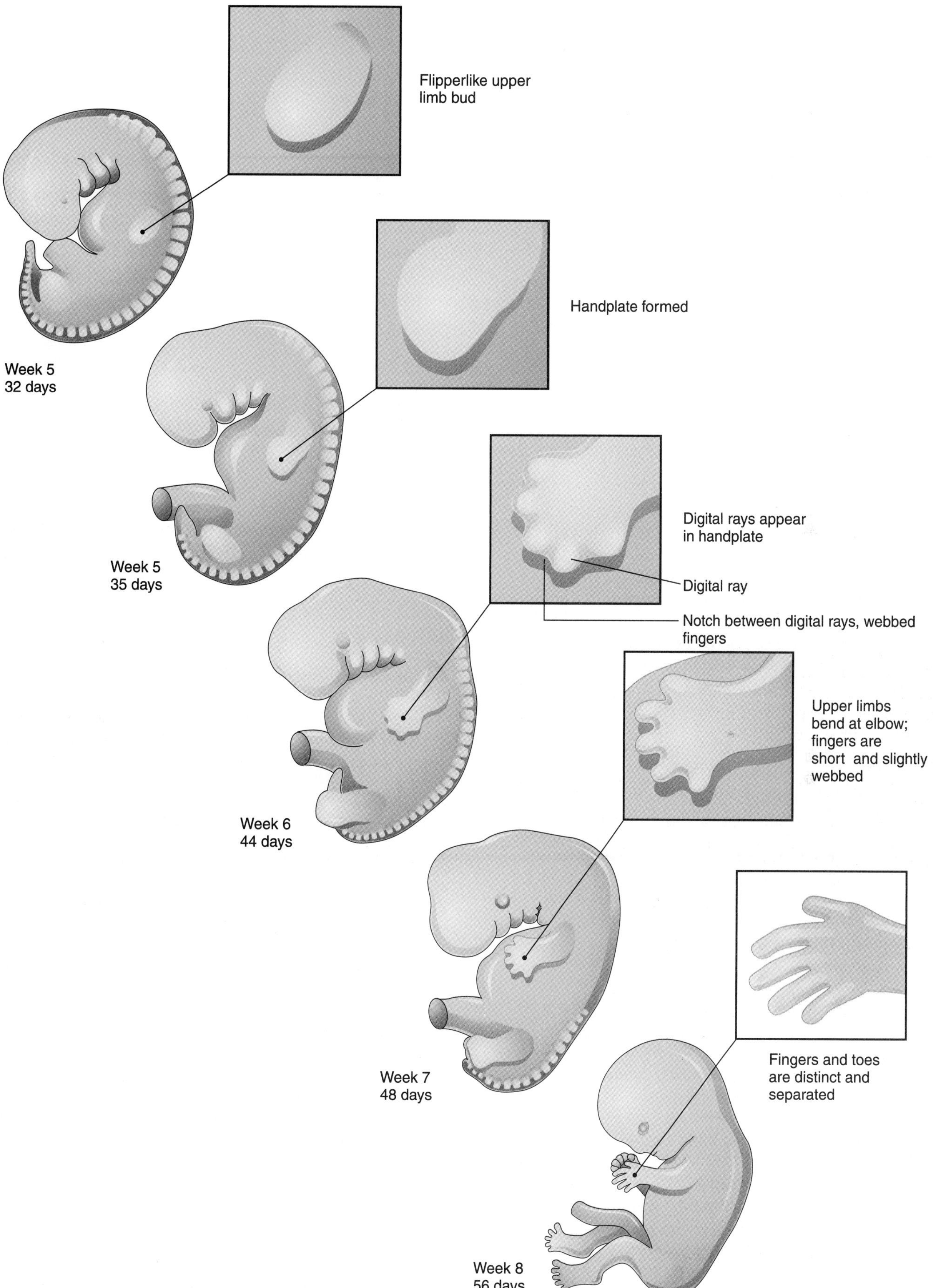

FIGURE 16-3. Illustrations of embryonic development of the limbs (32–56 days). Note that development of the upper limbs precedes that of the lower limbs.

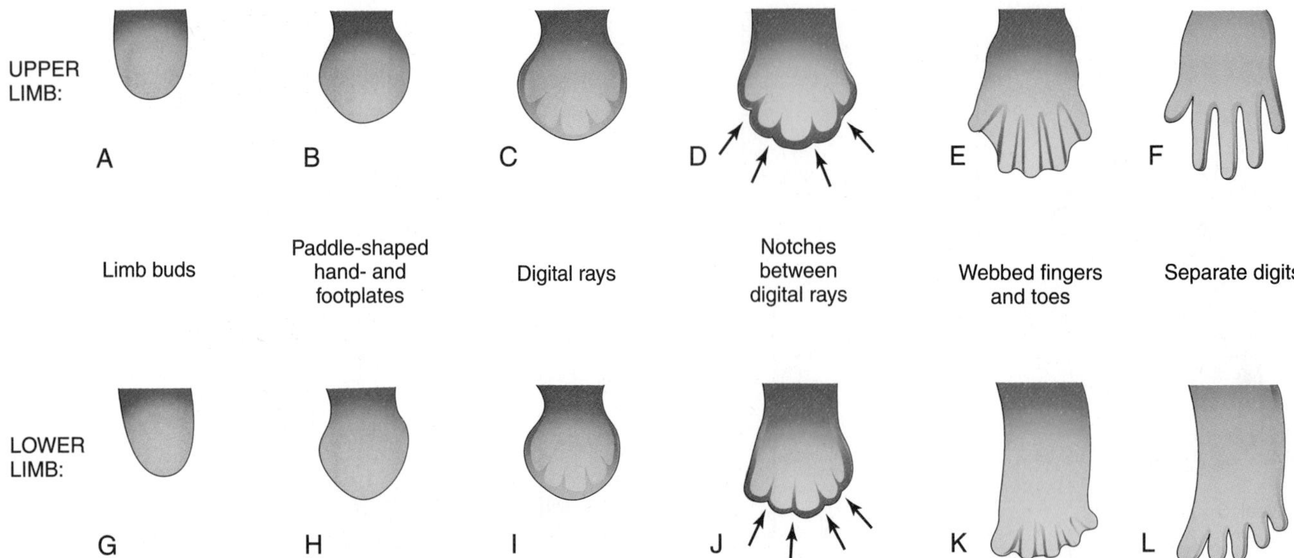

FIGURE 16-4. Illustrations of the development of the hands and feet between the fourth and eighth weeks. The early stages of limb development are alike, except that development of the hands precedes that of the feet by a day or so. **A,** At 27 days. **B,** At 32 days. **C,** At 41 days. **D,** At 46 days. **E,** At 50 days. **F,** At 52 days. **G,** At 28 days. **H,** At 36 days. **I,** At 46 days. **J,** At 49 days. **K,** At 52 days. **L,** At 56 days. The *arrows* in **D** and **J** indicate the tissue breakdown processes the separate the fingers and toes.

Chondrification centers appear in the fifth week. By the end of the sixth week, the entire limb skeleton is cartilaginous (Figs. 16-6*A* to *D* and 16-7*C* and *D*).

Osteogenesis of long bones begins in the seventh week from primary ossification centers in the middle of the cartilaginous models of the long bones. **Ossification centers** are present in all long bones by the 12th week (see Chapter 14). Ossification of the carpal (wrist) bones only begins during the first year after birth.

From the **dermomyotome regions of the somites,** myogenic precursor cells also migrate into the limb buds and later differentiate into **myoblasts,** precursors of muscle cells. As the long bones form, the myoblasts aggregate and form a large muscle mass in each limb bud (see Fig. 16-1). In general, this muscle mass separates into dorsal (extensor) and ventral (flexor) components. The mesenchyme in the limb bud also gives rise to ligaments and blood vessels (see Fig. 16-6). The cervical and lumbosacral myotomes contribute to the muscles of the pectoral and pelvic girdles, respectively.

Early in the seventh week, the limbs extend ventrally. Originally the flexor aspect of the limbs is ventral and the extensor aspect dorsal, and the preaxial and postaxial borders are cranial and caudal, respectively (see Fig. 16-10*A* and *D*). The developing upper and lower limbs rotate in opposite directions and to different degrees (Figs. 16-8 and 16-9):

- The *upper limbs rotate laterally* through 90 degrees on their longitudinal axes; thus, the future elbows come to point dorsally and the extensor muscles lie on the lateral and posterior aspects of the limb.
- The *lower limbs rotate medially* through almost 90 degrees; thus, the future knees come to face ventrally and the extensor muscles lie on the anterior aspect of the lower limb.

Developmentally, the radius and the tibia are homologous bones, as are the ulna and fibula, just as the thumb and great toe are homologous digits. **Synovial joints** appear at the beginning of the fetal period, coinciding with functional differentiation of the limb muscles and their innervation.

Cutaneous Innervation of Limbs

There is a strong relationship between the growth and rotation of the limbs and the cutaneous segmental nerve supply of the limbs. **Motor axons** arising from the spinal cord enter the limb buds during the fifth week and grow into the dorsal and ventral muscle masses. **Sensory axons** enter the limb buds after the motor axons and use them for guidance. **Neural crest cells**, the precursors of Schwann cells, surround the motor and sensory nerve fibers in the limbs and form the neurilemmal and myelin sheaths (see Chapter 17).

During the fifth week, peripheral nerves grow from the developing **limb plexuses** (brachial and lumbosacral) into the mesenchyme of the limb (Fig. 16-10*B* and *E*). The spinal nerves are distributed in segmental bands, supplying both dorsal and ventral surfaces of the limb. A **dermatome** is the area of skin supplied by a single spinal nerve and its spinal ganglion; however, cutaneous nerve areas and dermatomes show considerable overlapping. As the limbs elongate, the cutaneous distribution of the spinal nerves migrates along the limbs and no longer reaches the surface in the distal part of the limbs. Although the original **dermatomal pattern** changes during growth of the limbs, an orderly sequence of distribution can still be recognized in the adult (see Fig. 16-10*C* and *F*). In the upper limb, observe that the areas supplied by C5 and C6 adjoin the areas supplied by T2, T1, and C8, but the overlap between them is minimal at the ventral axial line.

A **cutaneous nerve area** is the area of skin supplied by a peripheral nerve. If the dorsal root supplying the area is

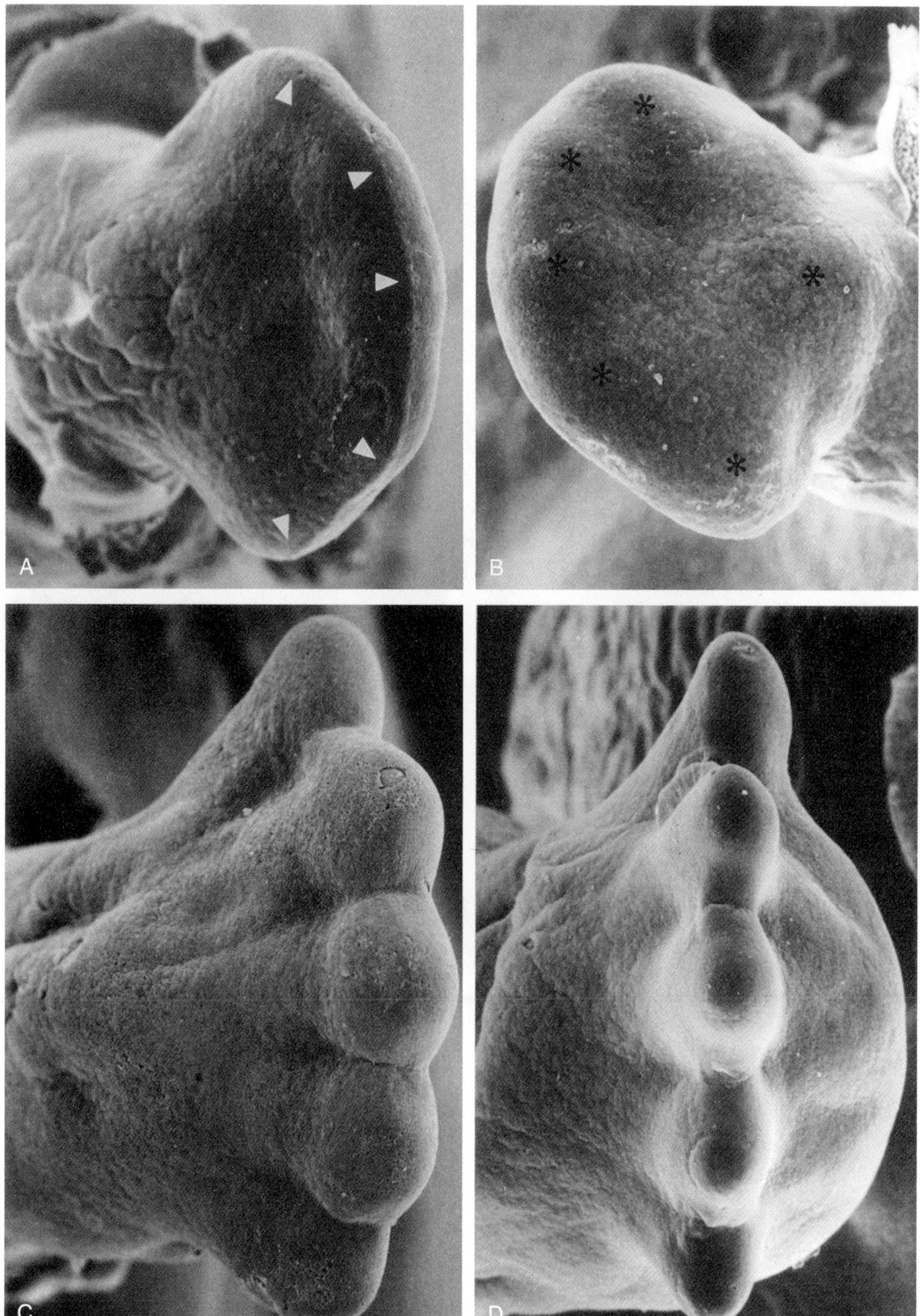

FIGURE 16-5. Scanning electron micrographs. Dorsal (**A**) and plantar (**B**) views of the right foot of a human embryo, Carnegie stage 19 (approximately 48 days). The toe buds (*arrowheads* in **A**) and the heel cushion and metatarsal tactile elevation (*asterisks* in **B**) have just appeared. Dorsal (**C**) and distal (**D**) views of the right foot of human embryos, Carnegie stage 22 (approximately 55 days). The tips of the toes are separated and interdigital degeneration has begun. Note the dorsiflexion of the metatarsus and toes (**C**) as well as the thickened heel cushion (**D**). (From Hinrichsen KV, Jacob HJ, Jacob M, et al: Principles of ontogenesis of leg and foot in man. Ann Anat 176:121, 1994.)

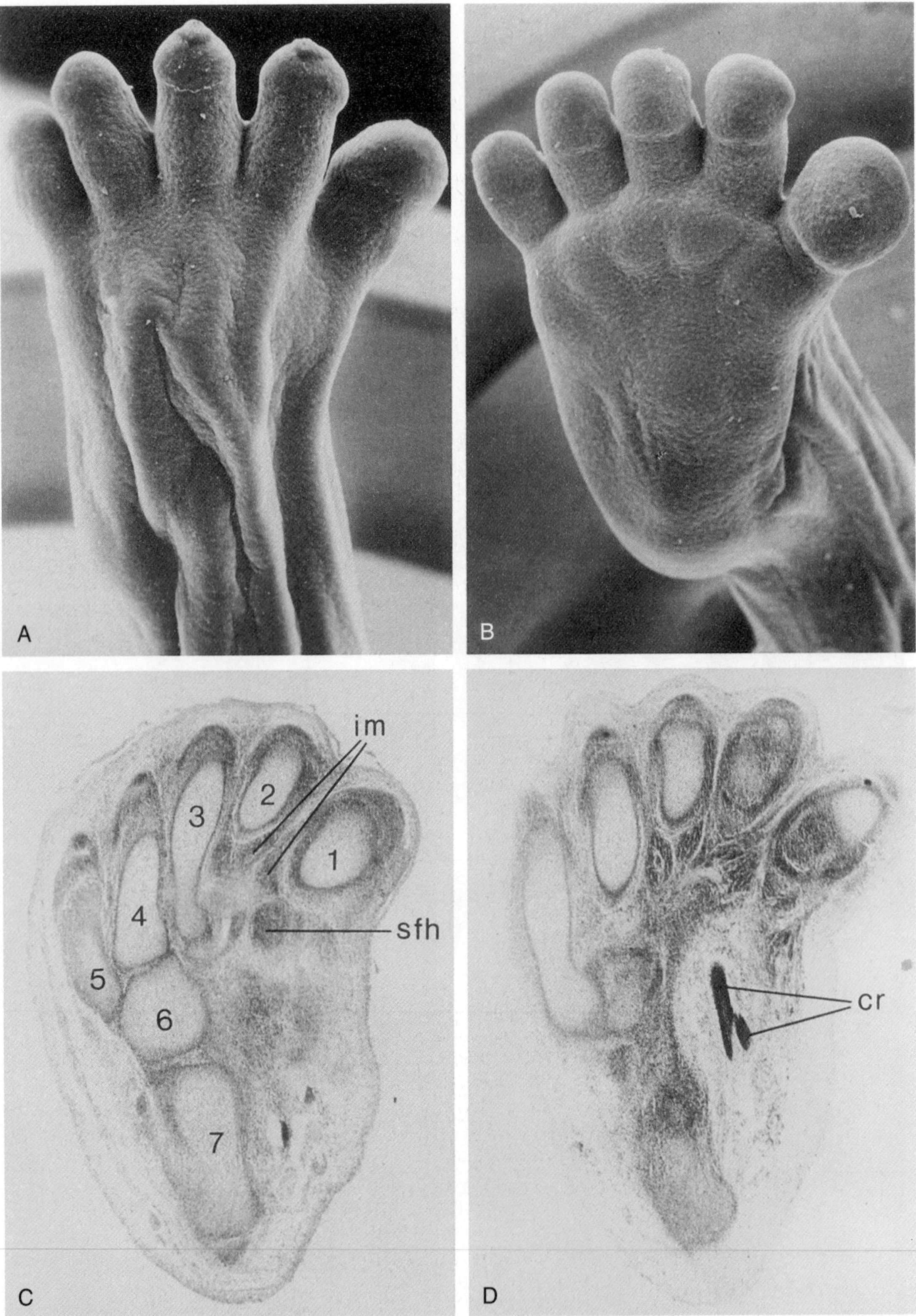

FIGURE 16-6. **A** and **B,** Scanning electron micrographs. **A,** Dorsal view of right foot of human embryo at 8 weeks. **B,** Plantar view of the left foot of this embryo. Although supinated, dorsiflexion of the foot is distinct. **C** and **D,** Paraffin sections of the tarsus and metatarsus of a young human fetus, stained with hematoxylin and eosin. 1–5, metatarsal cartilages; 6, cubital cartilage; 7, calcaneus. The separation of the interosseous muscles (im) and short flexor muscles of the big toe (sfh) is clearly seen. The plantar crossing (cr) of the tendons of the long flexors of the digits and hallux is shown in **D**. (From Hinrichsen KV, Jacob HJ, Jacob M, et al: Principles of ontogenesis of leg and foot in man. Ann Anat 176:121, 1994.)

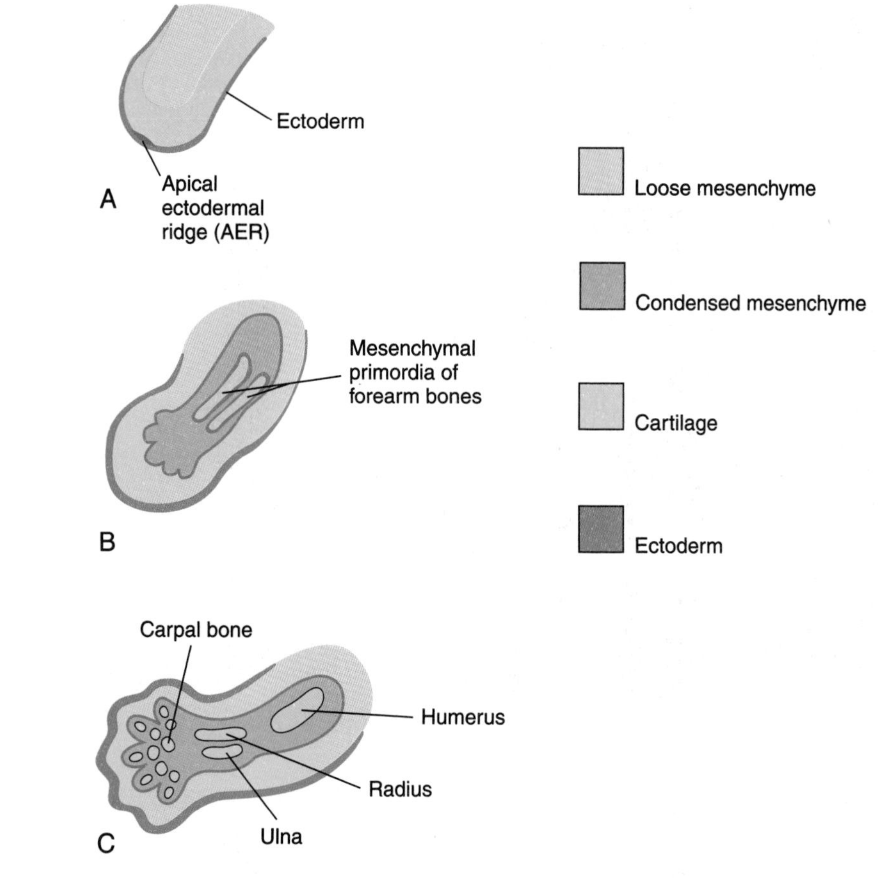

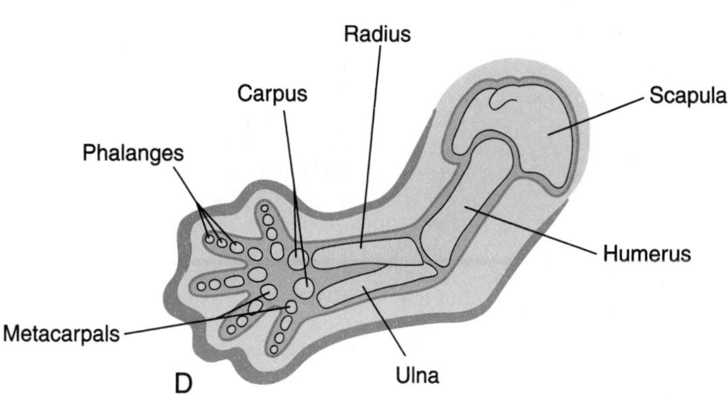

FIGURE 16-7. Schematic longitudinal sections of the upper limb of human embryos showing development of the cartilaginous bones. **A,** At 28 days. **B,** At 44 days. **C,** At 48 days. **D,** At 56 days.

cut, the dermatomal patterns indicate that there may be a slight deficit in the area indicated. Because there is overlapping of dermatomes, a particular area of skin is not exclusively innervated by a single segmental nerve. The limb dermatomes may be traced progressively down the lateral aspect of the upper limb and back up its medial aspect. A comparable distribution of dermatomes occurs in the lower limbs, which may be traced down the ventral aspect and then up the dorsal aspect of the lower limbs. When the limbs descend, they carry their nerves with them; this explains the oblique course of the nerves arising from the brachial and lumbosacral plexuses.

Blood Supply to the Limbs

The limb buds are supplied by branches of the **intersegmental arteries** (Fig. 16-11*A*), which arise from the aorta and form a fine capillary network throughout the mesenchyme. The primordial vascular pattern consists of a **primary axial artery** and its branches (see Fig. 16-11*B*), which drain into a peripheral marginal sinus. Blood in the **marginal sinus** drains into a peripheral vein. The vascular patterns change as the limbs develop, chiefly by **angiogenesis** (sprouting from existing vessels). The new vessels coalesce with other sprouts to form new vessels. The

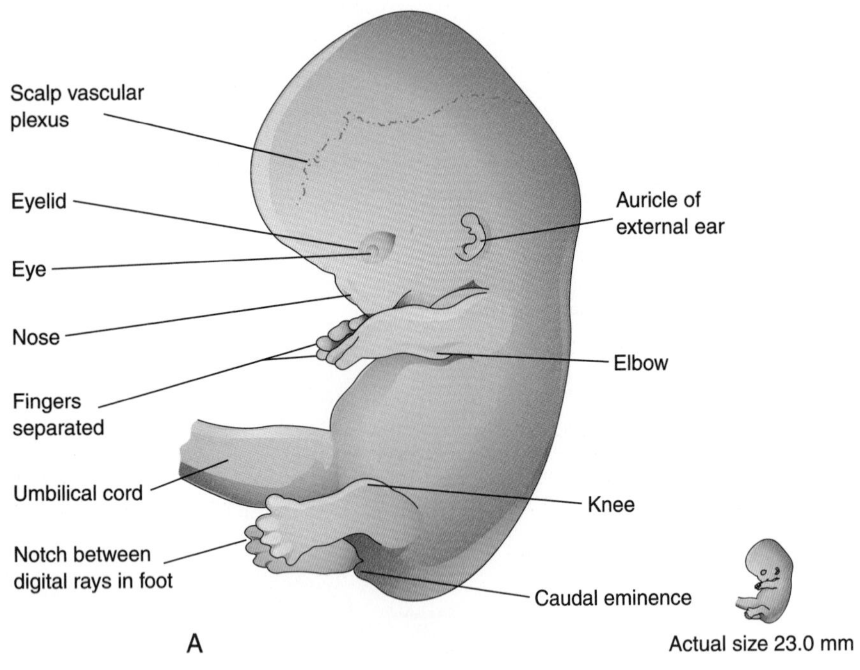

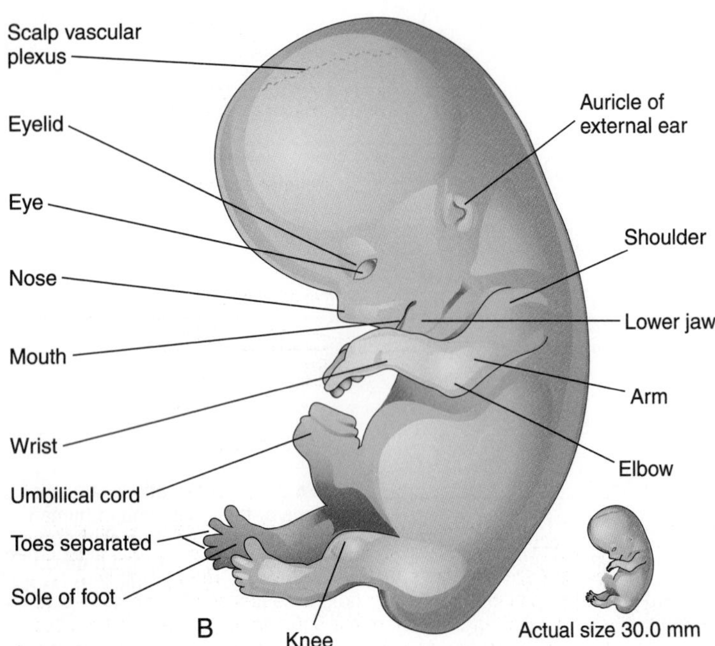

FIGURE 16-8. **A,** Lateral view of an embryo at Carnegie stage 21, approximately 52 days. The fingers are separated and the toes are beginning to separate. Note that the feet are fan shaped. **B,** Lateral view of an embryo at Carnegie stage 23, approximately 56 days. All regions of the limbs are apparent and the digits of the hands and feet are separated. (Modified from Nishimura H, Semba R, Tanimura T, Tanaka O: Prenatal Development of the Human with Special Reference to Craniofacial Structures: An Atlas. Washington, DC, National Institutes of Health, 1977.)

primary axial artery becomes the **brachial artery** in the arm and the **common interosseous artery** in the forearm, which has anterior and posterior interosseous branches. The ulnar and radial arteries are terminal branches of the brachial artery. As the digits (fingers) form, the marginal sinus breaks up and the final venous pattern, represented by the basilic and cephalic veins and their tributaries, develops. In the thigh, the primary axial artery is represented by the **deep artery of the thigh** (Latin, *profunda femoris artery*). In the leg, the primary axial artery is represented by the anterior and posterior **tibial arteries**.

ANOMALIES OF THE LIMBS

Minor limb anomalies are relatively common and can usually be corrected surgically. Although these anomalies are usually of no serious medical consequence, they may serve as indicators of more serious anomalies and may be part of a recognizable pattern of birth defects.

The most **critical period of limb development** is from 24 to 36 days after fertilization. This statement is based on clinical studies of infants exposed to **thalidomide**, a potent human teratogen, during the embryonic period. Exposure to this teratogen before day 33 may cause severe limb

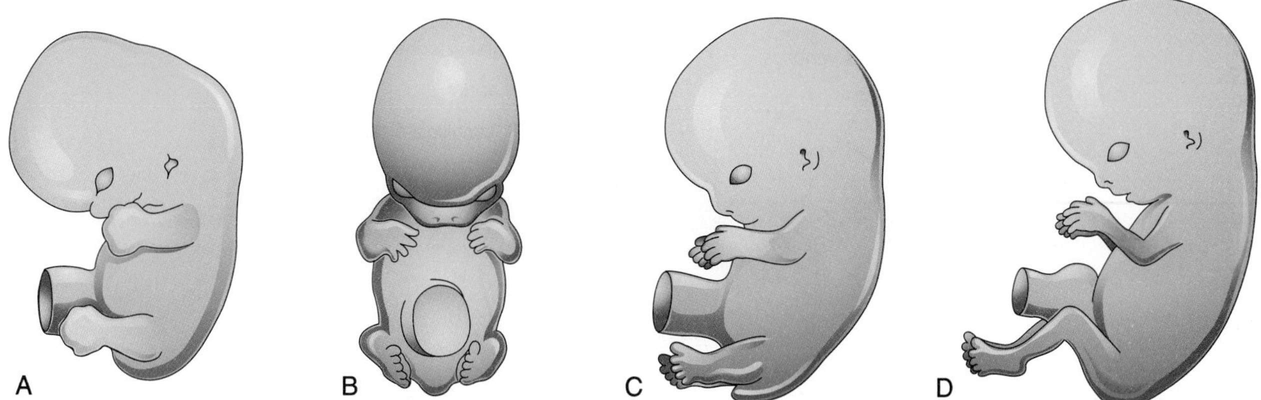

FIGURE 16-9. Illustrations of positional changes of the developing limbs of human embryos. **A,** Approximately 48 days, showing the limbs extending ventrally and the hand- and footplates facing each other. **B,** Approximately 51 days, showing the upper limbs bent at the elbows and the hands curved over the thorax. **C,** Approximately 54 days, showing the soles of the feet facing medially. **D,** Approximately 56 days. Note that the elbows now point caudally and the knees cranially.

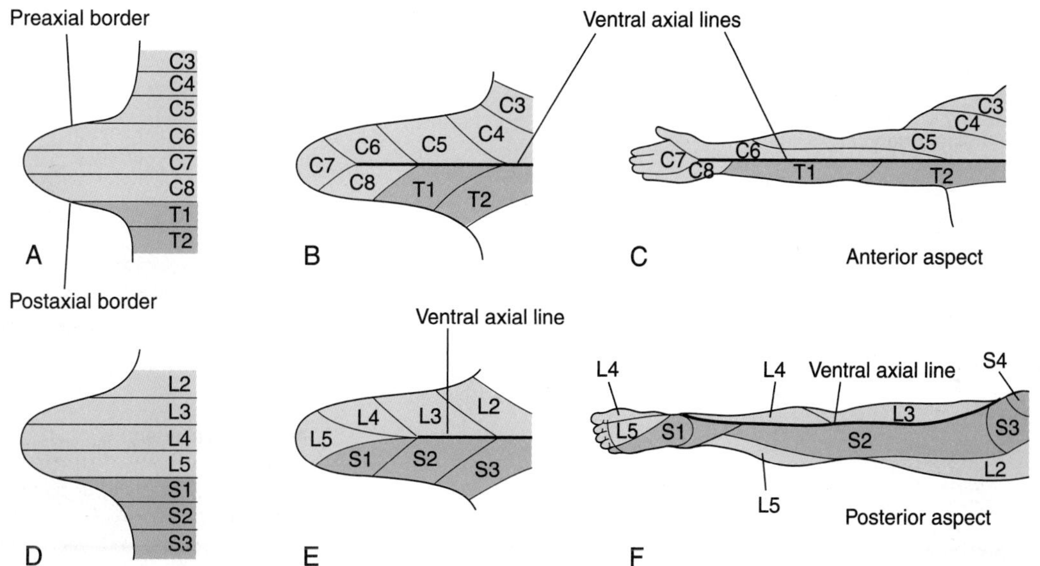

FIGURE 16-10. Illustrations of the development of the dermatomal patterns of the limbs. The axial lines indicate where there is no sensory overlap. **A** and **D,** Ventral aspect of the limb buds early in the fifth week. At this stage, the dermatomal patterns show the primordial segmental arrangement. **B** and **E,** Similar views later in the fifth week showing the modified arrangement of dermatomes. **C** and **F,** The dermatomal patterns in the adult upper and lower limbs. The primordial dermatomal pattern has disappeared but an orderly sequence of dermatomes can still be recognized. **F,** Note that most of the original ventral surface of the lower limb lies on the back of the adult limb. This results from the medial rotation of the lower limb that occurs toward the end of the embryonic period. In the upper limb, the ventral axial line extends along the anterior surface of the arm and forearm. In the lower limb, the ventral axial line extends along the medial side of the thigh and knee to the posteromedial aspect of the leg to the heel.

defects, such as **amelia,** the absence of limbs (Fig. 16-12*A*). Consequently, a teratogen that could cause amelia of the limbs or parts of them must act before 36 days, the end of the critical period of limb development. Many severe limb anomalies occurred from 1957 to 1962 as a result of maternal ingestion of thalidomide. This drug, widely used as a sedative and antinauseant, was withdrawn from the market in December 1961. Since that time, similar limb anomalies have rarely been observed. Because thalidomide is now used for the treatment of leprosy and several other disorders, it must be emphasized that thalidomide is absolutely contraindicated in women of child-bearing age.

Major limb anomalies appear approximately twice in 1000 newborns. Most of these defects are caused by genetic factors (see Fig. 16-14). *Molecular studies* have implicated gene mutation (*Hox* gene, *BMP*, *Shh*, *Wnt7*, *En-1*, and others) in some cases of limb defects. Several unrelated congenital anomalies of the lower limb were found to be associated with a similar aberrant arterial pattern, which might be of some importance in the pathogenesis of these defects.

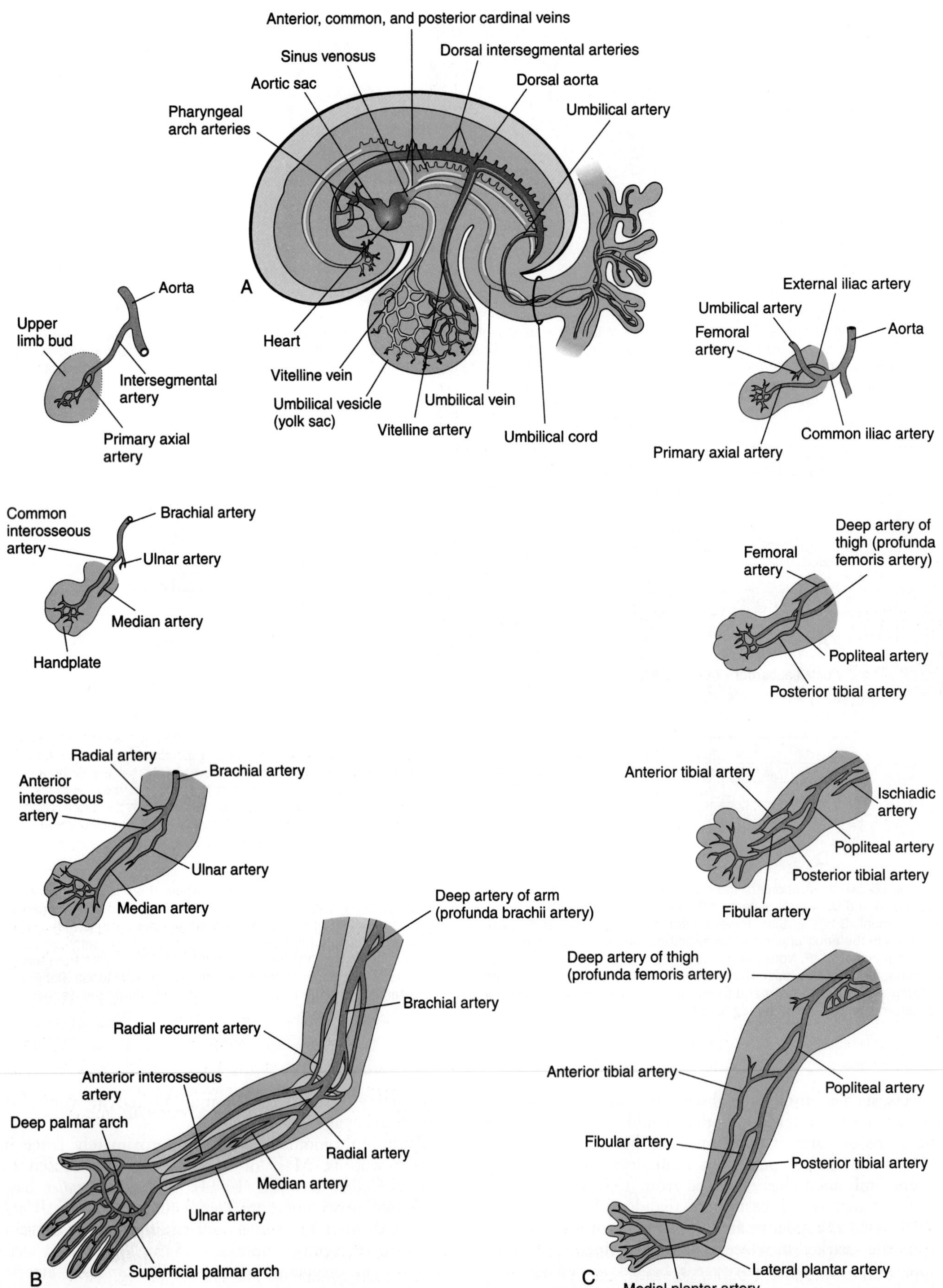

FIGURE 16-11. Development of limb arteries. **A,** Sketch of the primordial cardiovascular system in a 4-week embryo, approximately 26 days. **B,** Development of arteries in the upper limb. **C,** Development of arteries in the lower limb.

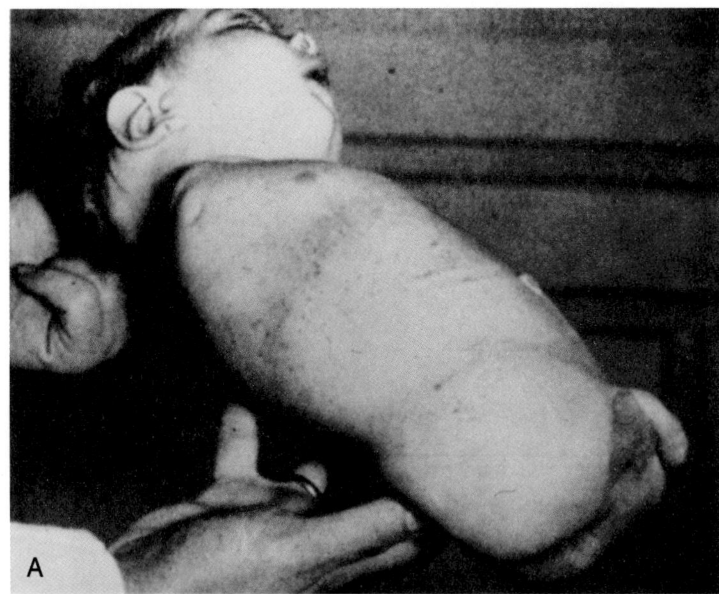

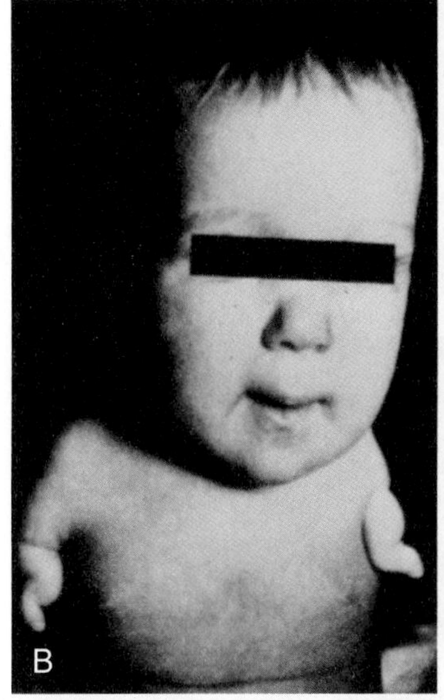

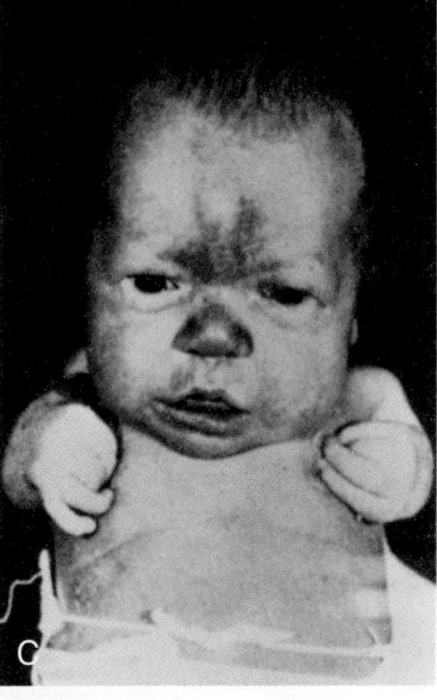

FIGURE 16-12. Limb anomalies caused by maternal ingestion of thalidomide. **A,** Quadruple amelia: absence of upper and lower limbs. **B,** Meromelia of the upper limbs: the limbs are represented by rudimentary stumps. **C,** Meromelia with the rudimentary upper limbs attached directly to the trunk. (From Lenz W, Knapp K: Foetal malformation due to thalidomide. Geriatr Med Monthly 7:253, 1962.)

Limb Anomalies

There are two main types of limb anomalies:

- Amelia, absence of a limb (Figs. 16-12*A* and 16-13*A*)
- Meromelia (Greek, *meros*, part, and *melos*, limb), absence of part of a limb (see Figs. 16-12*B* and *C* and 16-13).

Causes of Limb Anomalies

Anomalies or defects of the limbs originate at different stages of development. Suppression of limb bud development during the early part of the fourth week results in absence of the limbs, **amelia** (see Figs. 16-12*A* and 16-13*A*). Arrest or disturbance of differentiation or growth of the limbs during the fifth week results in various types of **meromelia** (see Figs. 16-12*B* and *C* and 16-13*B* and *C*). Like other congenital anomalies, limb defects are caused by:

- Genetic factors, e.g., chromosomal abnormalities associated with trisomy 18 (see Chapter 20)
- Mutant genes as in brachydactyly or osteogenesis imperfecta, a severe limb defect with fractures occurring before birth
- Environmental factors, e.g., teratogens such as thalidomide
- A combination of genetic and environmental factors (*multifactorial inheritance*), e.g., congenital dislocation of the hip
- Vascular disruption and ischemia, e.g., limb reduction defects

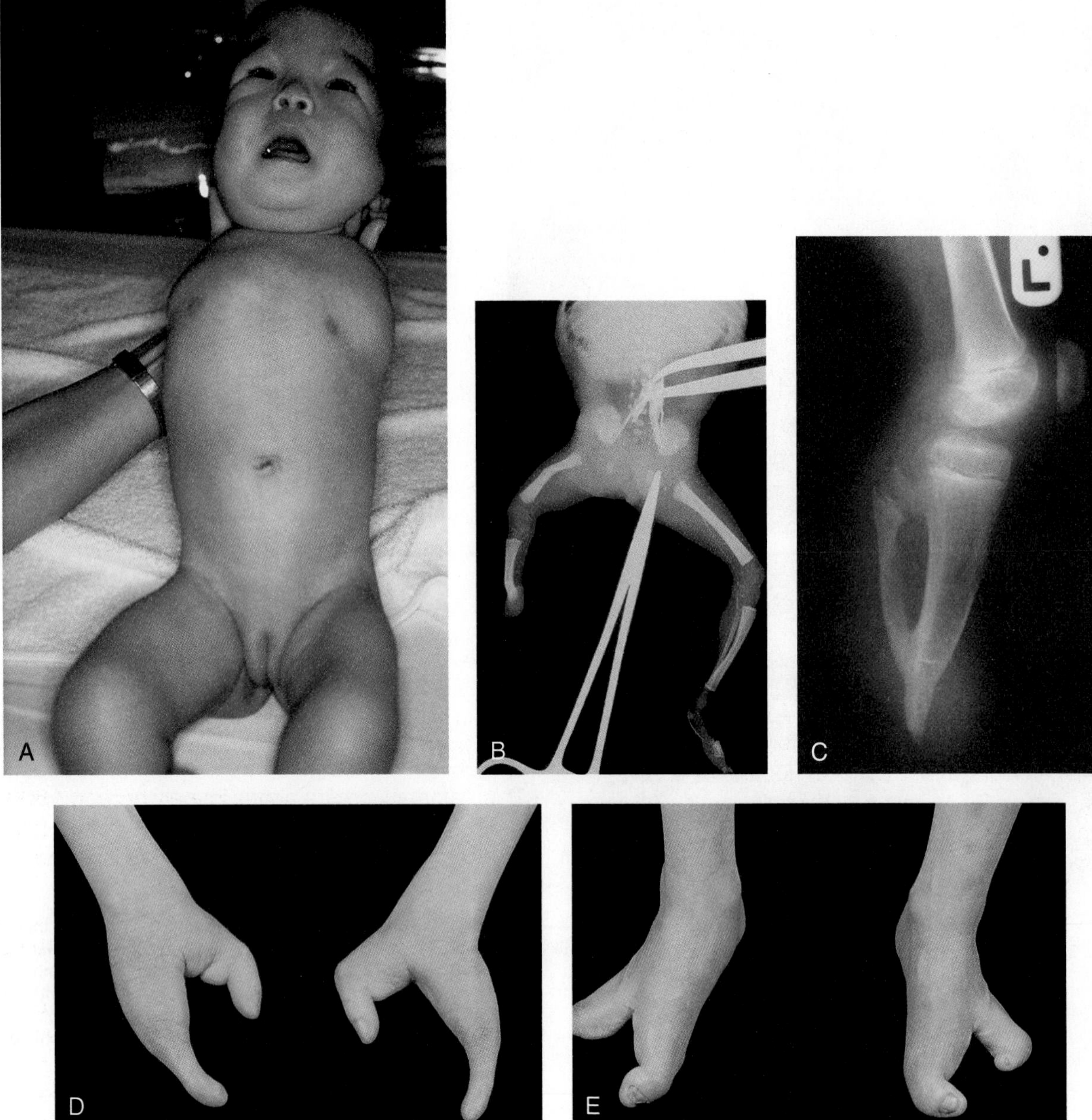

FIGURE 16-13. Various types of limb defects. **A,** Infant with amelia, complete absence of the upper limb. **B,** Radiograph of a female fetus showing absence of the right fibula. Note also that the right leg is shortened and the femur and tibia are bowed and hypoplastic. **C,** Radiograph showing partial absence and fusion of the lower ends of the tibia and fibula in a 5-year-old child. **D,** Absence of the central digits of the hands, resulting in a cleft hand. **E,** Absence of the second to fourth toes, resulting in a cleft foot. (**A,** Courtesy of Dr. Y. Suzuki, Achi, Japan. **B,** Courtesy of Dr. Joseph R. Siebert, Children's Hospital and Regional Medical Center, Seattle, WA. **C,** Courtesy of Dr. Prem S. Sahni, formerly of the Department of Radiology, Children's Hospital, Winnipeg, Manitoba, Canada. **D** and **E,** Courtesy of A.E. Chudley, MD, Section of Genetics and Metabolism, Department of Pediatrics and Child Health, University of Manitoba, Winnipeg, Manitoba, Canada.)

Experimental studies support the suggestion that mechanical influences during intrauterine development may cause some limb defects. A reduced quantity of amniotic fluid (*oligohydramnios*) is commonly associated with limb deformations; however, the significance of in utero mechanical influences on congenital postural deformation is still open to question.

CLEFT HAND AND CLEFT FOOT

In **lobster-claw deformities**, there is absence of one or more central digits, resulting from failure of development of one or more digital rays (see Fig. 16-13*D* and *E*). The hand or foot is divided into two parts that oppose each other like lobster claws.

Congenital Absence of the Radius

The radius is partially or completely absent. The hand deviates laterally (radially), and the ulna bows with the concavity on the lateral side of the forearm. This anomaly results from failure of the mesenchymal primordium of the radius to form during the fifth week of development. Absence of the radius is usually caused by genetic factors.

Brachydactyly

Shortness of the digits (fingers or toes) is the result of reduction in the length of the phalanges. This anomaly is usually inherited as a dominant trait and is often associated with shortness of stature.

Polydactyly

The term **supernumerary digits** refers to the presence of more than the usual number of fingers or toes (Figs. 16-14*A* and *B*). Often the extra digit is incompletely formed and lacks normal muscular development. If the hand is affected, the extra digit is most commonly medial or lateral rather than central. In the foot, the extra toe is usually on the lateral side. Polydactyly is inherited as a dominant trait.

Syndactyly

Syndactyly is the most common anomaly of the hand or foot. **Cutaneous syndactyly** (simple webbing between digits) is the most common limb anomaly. It is more frequent in the foot than in the hand (see Fig. 16-14*C* and *D*). Cutaneous syndactyly results from failure of the webs to degenerate between two or more digits. **Osseous syndactyly** (fusion of the bones—*synostosis*) occurs when the notches between the digital rays fail to develop; as a result, separation of the digits does not occur. Syndactyly is most frequently observed between the third and fourth fingers and between the second and third toes. It is inherited as a simple dominant or simple recessive trait. A case of synpolydactyly (syndactyly and polydactyly), caused by mutations in the NH2-terminal, non-DNA binding part of *HoxD13*, has been reported.

Congenital Clubfoot

Any deformity of the foot involving the talus (ankle bone) is called talipes or clubfoot. **Talipes equinovarus** is the most common type. Clubfoot is a relatively common anomaly, occurring approximately once in 1000 births. It is characterized by an abnormal position of the foot that prevents normal weight bearing. The sole of the foot is turned medially and the foot is inverted (Fig. 16-15). Clubfoot is bilateral in approximately 50% of cases, and it occurs approximately twice as frequently in males. The cause of clubfoot is uncertain. Although it is commonly stated that clubfoot results from abnormal positioning or restricted movement of the fetus's lower limbs in utero, the evidence of this deformation is inconclusive. Clubfoot appears to follow a **multifactorial pattern of inheritance**; hence, any intrauterine position that results in abnormal positioning of the feet may cause clubfeet if the fetus is genetically predispositioned to this deformity.

Congenital Dislocation of the Hip

This deformity occurs approximately once in 1500 newborn infants and is more common in females than in males. The joint capsule is very relaxed at birth, and there is underdevelopment of the acetabulum of the hip bone and the head of femur. Dislocation almost always occurs after birth. There are two causative factors:

- **Abnormal development of the acetabulum** occurs in approximately 15% of infants with congenital dislocation of the hip, which is common after breech deliveries, suggesting that breech posture during the terminal months of pregnancy may result in abnormal development of the acetabulum and the head of femur.
- **Generalized joint laxity** is often a dominantly inherited condition that appears to be associated with congenital dislocation of the hip, which follows a multifactorial pattern of inheritance.

SUMMARY OF LIMB DEVELOPMENT

- **Limb buds** appear toward the end of the fourth week as slight elevations of the ventrolateral body wall. The upper limb buds develop approximately 2 days before the lower limb buds. The tissues of the limb buds are derived from two main sources: mesoderm and ectoderm.
- The **AER** exerts an inductive influence on the limb mesenchyme, promoting growth and development of

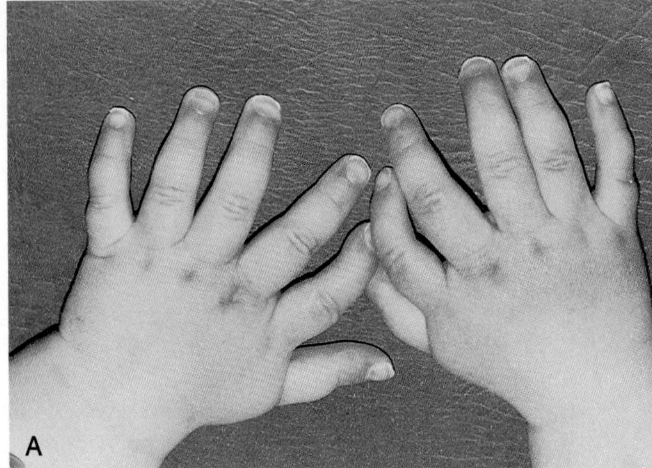

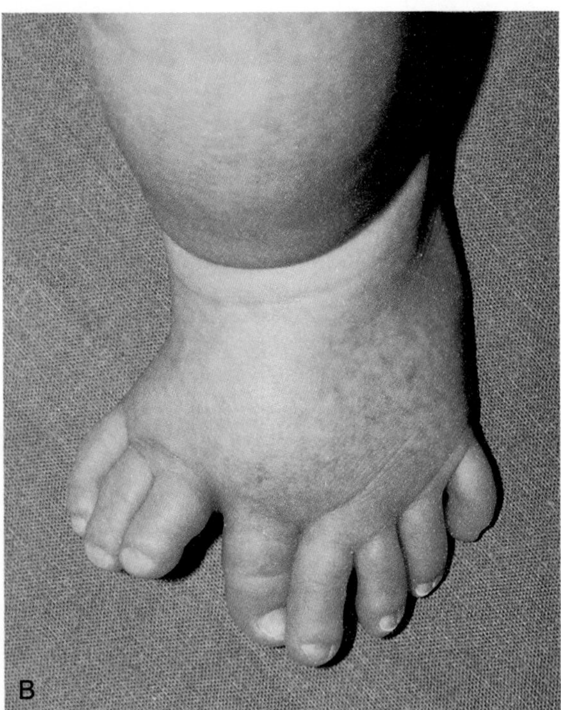

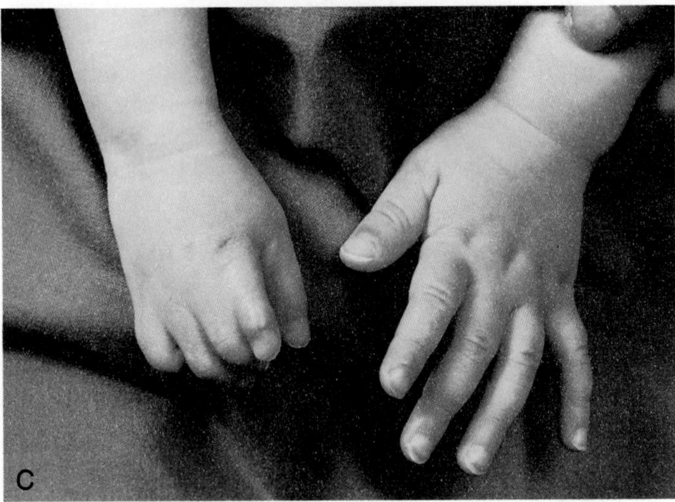

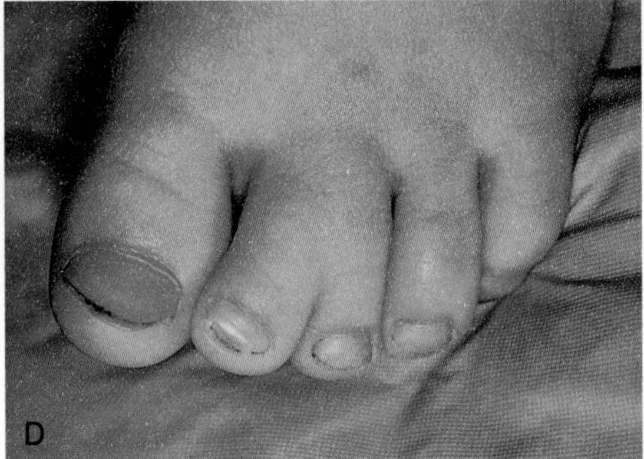

FIGURE 16-14. Various types of digital anomalies. Polydactyly of the hands (**A**), and foot (**B**). This condition results from formation of one or more extra digital rays during the embryonic period. Various forms of syndactyly involving the fingers (**C**), and toes (**D**). Cutaneous syndactyly (**C**) is the most common form of this condition and is probably due to incomplete programmed cell death (apoptosis) in the tissues between the digital rays during embryonic life. **D,** Syndactyly of the second and third toes. (Courtesy of A.E. Chudley, MD, Section of Genetics and Metabolism, Department of Pediatrics and Child Health, Children's Hospital and University of Manitoba, Winnipeg, Manitoba, Canada.)

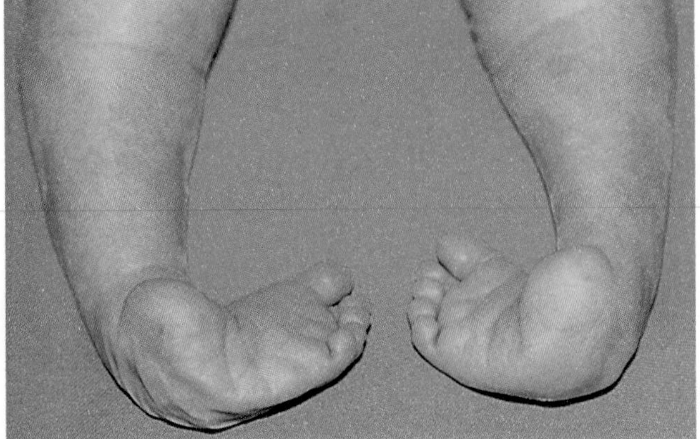

FIGURE 16-15. Neonate with bilateral talipes equinovarus (clubfeet). Observe the hyperextension and incurving of the feet. (Courtesy of A.E. Chudley, MD, Section of Genetics and Metabolism, Department of Pediatrics and Child Health, Children's Hospital and University of Manitoba, Winnipeg, Manitoba, Canada.)

the limbs. The limb buds elongate by proliferation of the mesenchyme within them. **Apoptosis** (programmed cell death) is an important mechanism in limb development, for example, in the formation of the notches between the digital rays.

- Limb muscles are derived from mesenchyme (**myogenic precursor cells**) originating in the somites. The muscle-forming cells (**myoblasts**) form dorsal and ventral muscle masses. Nerves grow into the limb buds after the muscle masses have formed. Most blood vessels of the limb buds arise as buds from the intersegmental arteries and drain into the cardinal veins.
- Initially, the developing limbs are directed caudally; later they project ventrally, and finally, they rotate on their longitudinal axes. The upper and lower limbs rotate in opposite directions and to different degrees.

- The majority of limb anomalies are caused by genetic factors; however, many limb defects probably result from an interaction of genetic and environmental factors (**multifactorial inheritance**).

CLINICALLY ORIENTED PROBLEMS

CASE 16-1

A mother consulted her pediatrician after noticing that when her 11-month-old daughter began to stand independently, her legs seemed to be of different lengths.

- Do more female infants have congenital dislocation of the hip than male infants?
- Are the hip joints of these infants usually dislocated at birth?
- What are the probable causes of congenital dislocation of the hip?

CASE 16-2

A male infant was born with limb defects. His mother said that one of her relatives had a similar defect.

- Are limb anomalies similar to those caused by the drug thalidomide common?
- What was the characteristic malformation syndrome produced by thalidomide?
- Name the limb and other defects commonly associated with the thalidomide syndrome.

CASE 16-3

A newborn infant was born with clubfeet. The physician explained that this was a common type of anomaly.

- What is the most common type of clubfoot?
- How common is it?
- Describe the feet of infants born with this anomaly.

CASE 16-4

A baby was born with syndactyly (webbing between her fingers). The doctor stated this minor defect could be easily corrected surgically.

- Is syndactyly common?
- Does it occur more often in the hands than in the feet?
- What is the embryologic basis of syndactyly?

Discussion of these problems appears at the back of the book.

References and Suggested Reading

Ambler CA, Nowicki JL, Burke AC, et al: Assembly of trunk and limb blood vessels involves extensive migration and vasculogenesis of somite-derived angioblasts. Dev Biol 234:352, 2001.

Brook WJ, Diaz-Benjumea FJ, Cohen SM: Organizing spatial pattern in limb development. Ann Rev Cell Dev Biol 12:161, 1996.

Cohn MJ, Patel K, Krumlauf R, et al: Hox 9 genes and vertebrate limb specification. Nature 387:97, 1997.

Cooperman DR, Thompson GH: Congenital abnormalities of the upper and lower extremities and spine. In Martin RJ, Fanaroff AA, Walsh MC (eds): Fanaroff and Martin's Neonatal-Perinatal Medicine. Diseases of the Fetus and Infant, 8th ed. Philadelphia, Mosby, 2006.

Dahn RD, Fallon JF: Limiting outgrowth: BMPs as negative regulators in limb development. BioEssays 21:721, 1999.

Hall BK: Bones and Cartilage: Developmental Skeletal Biology. Philadelphia, Elsevier, 2005.

Hinrichsen KV, Jacob HJ, Jacob M, et al: Principles of ontogenesis of leg and foot in man. Ann Anat 176:121, 1994.

Kabak S, Boizow L: Organogenese des Extremitätenskeletts und der Extremitätengelenke beim Menschenembryo. Anat Anz 170:349, 1990.

Logan M: Finger or toe: the molecular basis of limb identity. Development 130:6401, 2003.

Maldjian C, Hofkin S, Bonakdarpour A, et al: Abnormalities of the pediatric foot. Acad Radiol 6:191, 1999.

Marini JC, Gerber NL: Osteogenesis imperfecta. JAMA 277:746, 1997.

Martin GR: The roles of FGFs in the early development of vertebrate limbs. Genes Dev 12:1571, 1998.

Moore KL, Dalley AF: Clinically Oriented Anatomy, 5th ed. Baltimore, Williams & Wilkins, 2006.

Muragaki Y, Mundlos S, Upton J, Olsen BR: Altered growth and branching patterns in synpolydactyly caused by mutations in HoxD13. Science 272:548, 1996.

O'Rahilly R, Müller F: Developmental Stages in Human Embryos. Washington, DC, Carnegie Institution of Washington, 1987.

Revest J-M, Spencer-Dene B, Kerr K, et al: Fibroblast growth factor receptor 2-IIIb acts upstream of Shh and Fgf4 and is required for limb bud maintenance but not for the induction of Fgf8, Fgf10, Msx1, or Bmp4. Dev Biol 231:47, 2001.

Riddle RD, Tabin CJ: How limbs develop. Sci Am 280:74, 1999.

Robertson WW Jr, Corbett D: Congenital clubfoot. Clin Orthop 338:14–18, 1997.

Slack JMW: Essential Developmental Biology, 2nd ed. Oxford, Blackwell Publishing, 2006.

Van Allen MI: Structural anomalies resulting from vascular disruption. Pediatr Clin North Am 39:255, 1992.

Van Heest AE: Congenital disorders of the hand and upper extremity. Pediatr Clin North Am 43:1113, 1996.

Zuniga A: Globalisation reaches gene regulation: The case for vertebrate limb development. Curr Opin Genet Dev 15:403, 2005.

17

The Nervous System

Origin of the Nervous System 381

Development of the Spinal Cord 381
- Development of the Spinal Ganglia 383
- Development of the Spinal Meninges 384
- Positional Changes of the Spinal Cord 384
- Myelination of Nerve Fibers 386
- Congenital Anomalies of the Spinal Cord 386

Development of the Brain 392
- Brain Flexures 392
- Hindbrain 393
- Choroid Plexuses and Cerebrospinal Fluid (CSF) 398
- Midbrain 398
- Forebrain 399

Congenital Anomalies of the Brain 404

Development of the Peripheral Nervous System 413
- Spinal Nerves 414
- Cranial Nerves 414

Development of the Autonomic Nervous System 416
- Sympathetic Nervous System 416
- Parasympathetic Nervous System 416

Summary of the Nervous System 416

Clinically Oriented Problems 417

The nervous system consists of three main parts:

- The **central nervous system** (CNS), which includes the brain and spinal cord
- The **peripheral nervous system** (PNS), which includes neurons outside the CNS and cranial and spinal nerves that connect the brain and spinal cord with peripheral structures
- The **autonomic nervous system** (ANS), which has parts in both the CNS and PNS and consists of neurons that innervate smooth muscle, cardiac muscle, glandular epithelium, or combinations of these tissues

ORIGIN OF THE NERVOUS SYSTEM

The nervous system develops from the **neural plate** (Fig. 17-1*A*), a thickened area of embryonic ectoderm. It is the notochord and paraxial mesenchyme that induce the overlying ectoderm to differentiate into the neural plate. Signaling molecules involve members of the transforming growth factor β family, Shh, and BMPs. Formation of the neural folds, neural tube, and neural crest from the neural plate is illustrated in Figures 17-1*B* to *F* and 17-2.

- The neural tube differentiates into the CNS, consisting of the brain and spinal cord.
- The neural crest gives rise to cells that form most of the PNS and ANS, consisting of cranial, spinal, and autonomic ganglia, and many other structures.

Neurulation—formation of the neural plate and neural tube—begins during stage 10 of development (22–23 days) in the region of the fourth to sixth pairs of somites. At this stage, the cranial two thirds of the neural plate and tube, as far caudal as the fourth pair of somites, represent the future brain, and the caudal one third of the neural plate and tube represents the future spinal cord. Fusion of the neural folds and formation of the **neural tube** proceeds in cranial and caudal directions until only small areas of the tube remain open at both ends (Fig. 17-3*A* and *B*). Here the lumen of the neural tube—**neural canal**—communicates freely with the amniotic cavity (see Fig. 17-3*C*). The cranial opening, the **rostral neuropore**, closes on approximately the 25th day and the **caudal neuropore** 2 days later (see Fig. 17-3*D*). *Closure of the neuropores* coincides with the establishment of a blood vascular circulation for the neural tube. The walls of the neural tube thicken to form the brain and the spinal cord (Fig. 17-4). The neural canal forms the ventricular system of the brain and the central canal of the spinal cord.

NONCLOSURE OF THE NEURAL TUBE

The current hypothesis is that there are multiple, possibly five, closure sites involved in the formation of the neural tube. Failure of closure of site 1 results in spina bifida cystica; meroencephaly (anencephaly) results from failure of closure of site 2; craniorachischisis results from failure of sites 2, 4, and 1 to close; and site 3 nonfusion is rare. Descriptions of these neural tube defects (NTDs) are given later. It has been suggested that the most caudal region may have a fifth closure site from the second lumbar vertebra to the second sacral vertebra and that closure inferior to the second sacral vertebra is by secondary neurulation. Epidemiologic analysis of infants born with NTDs supports the concept that there is multisite closure sites of the neural tube in humans.

DEVELOPMENT OF THE SPINAL CORD

The neural tube caudal to the fourth pair of somites develops into the spinal cord (Figs. 17-4 and 17-5). The lateral walls of the neural tube thicken, gradually reducing the size of the **neural canal** until only a minute **central canal** of the spinal cord is present at 9 to 10 weeks (see Fig. 17-5*C*). Initially, the wall of the neural tube is composed of a thick, pseudostratified, columnar neuroepithelium (see Fig. 17-5*D*). These neuroepithelial cells constitute the **ventricular zone** (ependymal layer), which gives rise to all neurons and macroglial cells (macroglia) in the spinal cord (Figs. 17-5*E* and 17-6). Macroglial cells are the larger members of the neuroglial family of cells, which includes astrocytes and oligodendrocytes. Soon a **marginal zone** composed of the outer parts of the neuroepithelial cells becomes recognizable (see Fig. 17-5*E*). This zone gradually becomes the white matter (substance) of the spinal cord as axons grow into it from nerve cell bodies in the spinal cord, spinal ganglia, and brain. Some dividing neuroepithelial cells in the ventricular zone differentiate into primordial neurons—**neuroblasts**. These embryonic cells form an **intermediate zone** (mantle layer) between the ventricular and marginal zones. Neuroblasts become neurons as they develop cytoplasmic processes (see Fig. 17-6).

The primordial supporting cells of the central nervous system—**glioblasts** (spongioblasts)—differentiate from neuroepithelial cells, mainly after neuroblast formation has ceased. The glioblasts migrate from the ventricular zone into the intermediate and marginal zones. Some glioblasts become astroblasts and later **astrocytes**, whereas others become oligodendroblasts and eventually **oligodendrocytes** (see Fig. 17-6). When the neuroepithelial cells cease producing neuroblasts and glioblasts, they differentiate into ependymal cells, which form the **ependyma** (ependymal epithelium) lining the central canal of the spinal cord. Sonic hedgehog signaling controls the proliferation, survival, and patterning of neuroepithelial progenitor cells by regulating Gli transcription factors (see Fig. 17-2).

Microglial cells (microglia), which are scattered throughout the gray and white matter, are small cells that are derived from **mesenchymal cells** (see Fig. 17-6). Microglial cells invade the CNS rather late in the fetal period after it has been penetrated by blood vessels. Microglia originate in the bone marrow and are part of the mononuclear phagocytic cell population.

Proliferation and differentiation of neuroepithelial cells in the developing spinal cord produce thick walls and thin

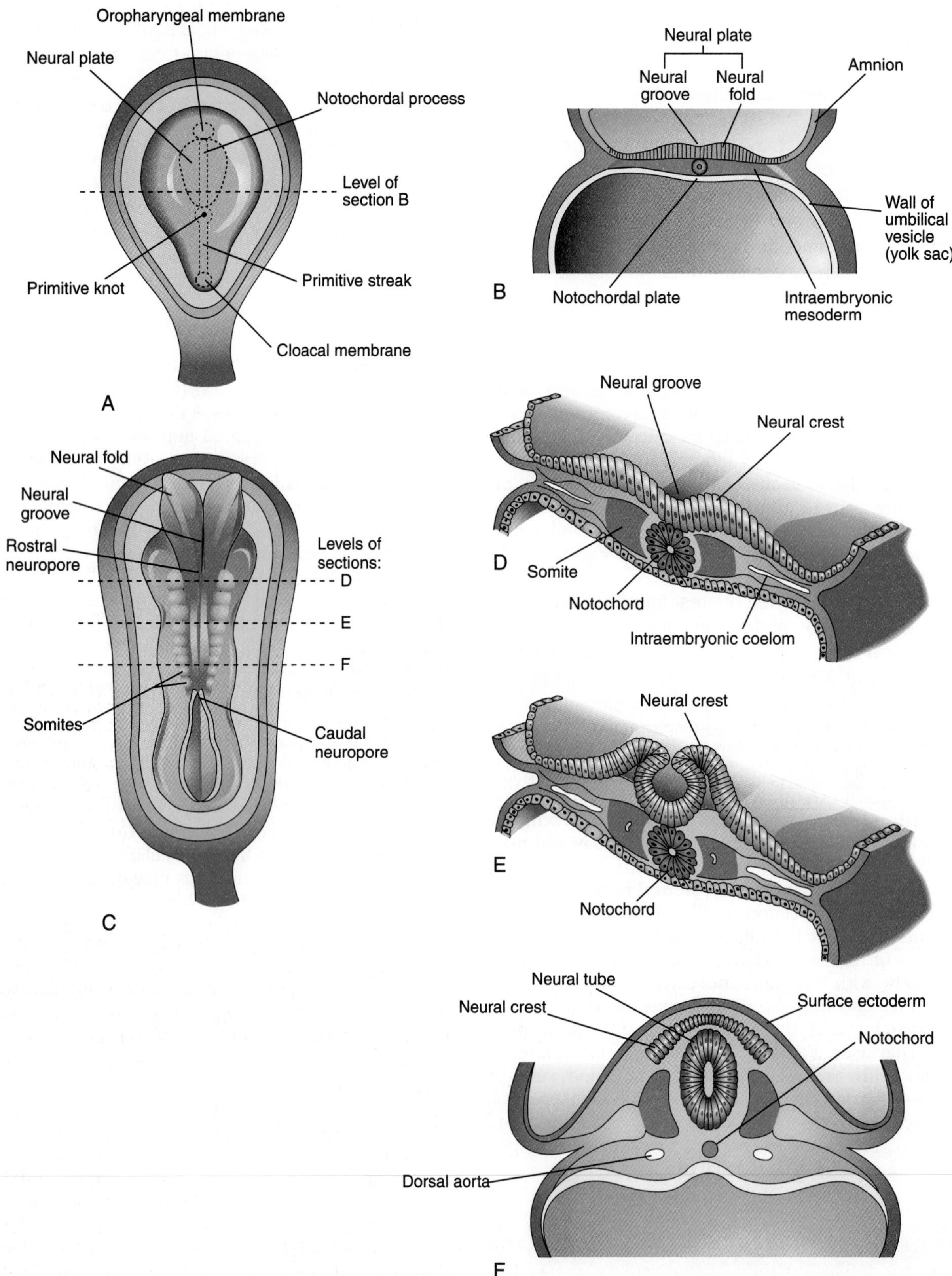

FIGURE 17-1. Illustrations of the neural plate and folding of it to form the neural tube. **A,** Dorsal view of an embryo of approximately 17 days, exposed by removing the amnion. **B,** Transverse section of the embryo showing the neural plate and early development of the neural groove and neural folds. **C,** Dorsal view of an embryo of approximately 22 days. The neural folds have fused opposite the fourth to sixth somites, but are spread apart at both ends. **D** to **F,** Transverse sections of this embryo at the levels shown in **C** illustrating formation of the neural tube and its detachment from the surface ectoderm (primordium of epidermis). Note that some neuroectodermal cells are not included in the neural tube, but remain between it and the surface ectoderm as the neural crest.

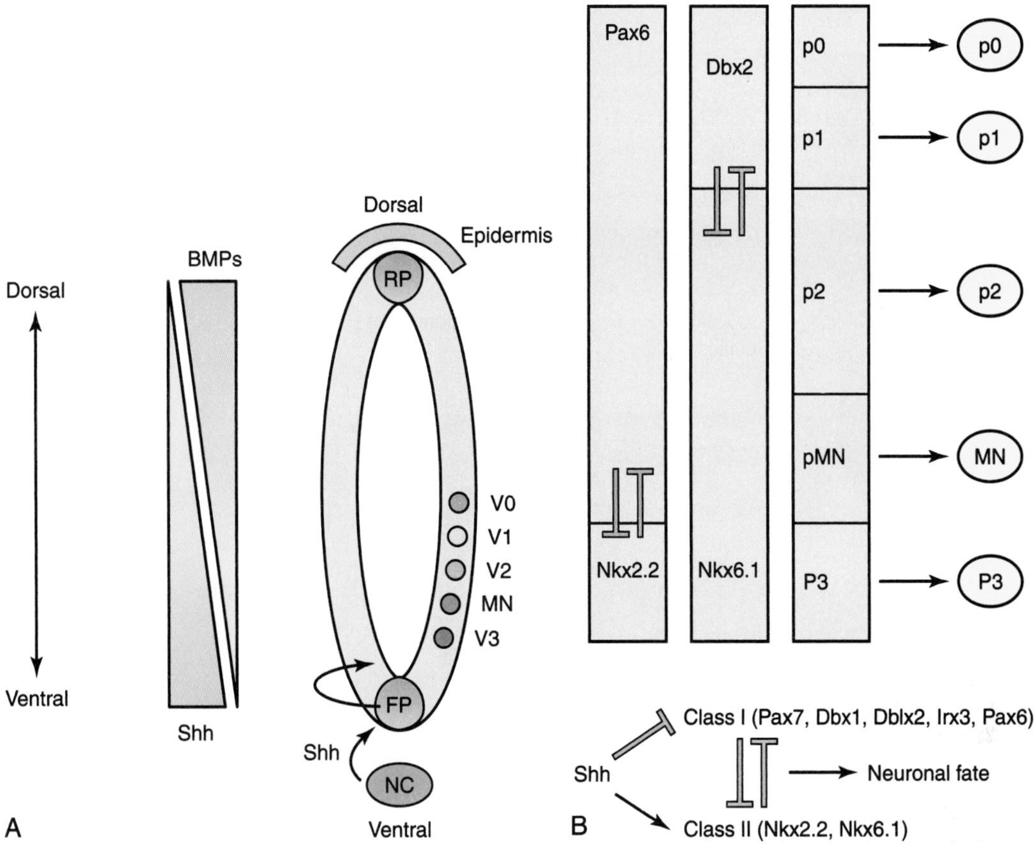

FIGURE 17-2. Morphogens and transcription factors specify the fate of progenitors in the ventral neural tube. **A,** Sonic hedgehog (Shh) is secreted by the notochord (NC) and the floorplate (FP) of the neural tube in a ventral to dorsal gradient. Similarly, bone morphogenetic proteins (BMPs), members of the transforming growth factor β superfamily, are secreted by the roofplate (RP) of the neural tube and the overlying epidermis, in a dorsal to ventral gradient. These opposing morphogen gradients determine dorsal-ventral cell fates. **B,** Shh concentration gradients define the ventral expression domains of class I (repressed) and class II (activated) homeobox transcription factors. Reciprocal negative interactions assist to establish boundaries of gene expression in the embryonic ventral spinal cord. p, progenitor; MN, motor neuron; V, ventral interneuron. (Courtesy of Dr. David Eisenstat, Department of Human Anatomy and Cell Science, and Dr. Jeffrey T. Wigle, Department of Biochemistry and Medical Genetics, University of Manitoba, Winnipeg, Manitoba, Canada. Adapted from Jessel TM: Neuronal specification in the spinal cord: inductive signals and transcription codes. Nat Rev Genet 1:20, 2000.)

roof- and floor-plates (see Fig. 17-5*B*). Differential thickening of the lateral walls of the spinal cord soon produces a shallow longitudinal groove on each side—the **sulcus limitans** (Figs. 17-5*B* and 17-7). This groove separates the dorsal part, the **alar plate** (lamina), from the ventral part, the **basal plate** (lamina). The alar and basal plates produce longitudinal bulges extending through most of the length of the developing spinal cord. This regional separation is of fundamental importance because the alar and basal plates are later associated with afferent and efferent functions, respectively.

Cell bodies in the alar plates form the dorsal gray columns that extend the length of the spinal cord. In transverse sections of the cord, these columns are the **dorsal gray horns**. Neurons in these columns constitute afferent nuclei, and groups of these nuclei form the dorsal gray columns. As the alar plates enlarge, the dorsal median septum forms. Cell bodies in the basal plates form the ventral and lateral gray columns. In transverse sections of the spinal cord, these columns are the **ventral gray horns** and **lateral gray horns**, respectively (see Fig. 5-7*C*). Axons of ventral horn cells grow out of the spinal cord and form the ventral roots of the spinal nerves. As the basal plates enlarge, they bulge ventrally on each side of the median plane. As this occurs, the **ventral median septum** forms, and a deep longitudinal groove—the **ventral median fissure**—develops on the ventral surface of the spinal cord.

Development of the Spinal Ganglia

The unipolar neurons in the **spinal ganglia** (dorsal root ganglia) are derived from **neural crest cells** (Figs. 17-8 and 17-9). The axons of cells in the spinal ganglia are at first bipolar, but the two processes soon unite in a T-shaped fashion. Both processes of spinal ganglion cells have the structural characteristics of axons, but the peripheral process is a dendrite in that there is conduction toward the cell body. The peripheral processes of **spinal ganglion cells** pass in the spinal nerves to sensory endings in somatic or visceral structures (see Fig. 17-8). The central processes enter the spinal cord and constitute the **dorsal roots of spinal nerves**.

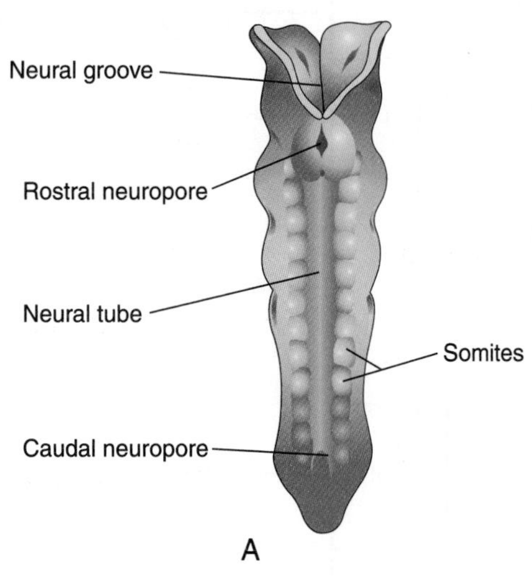

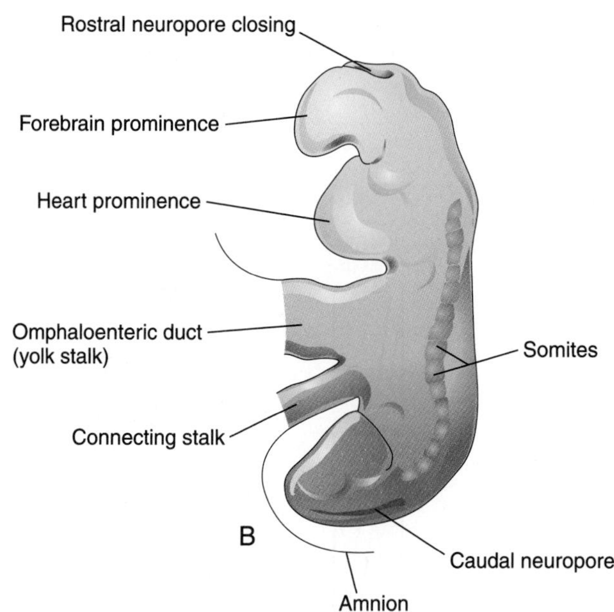

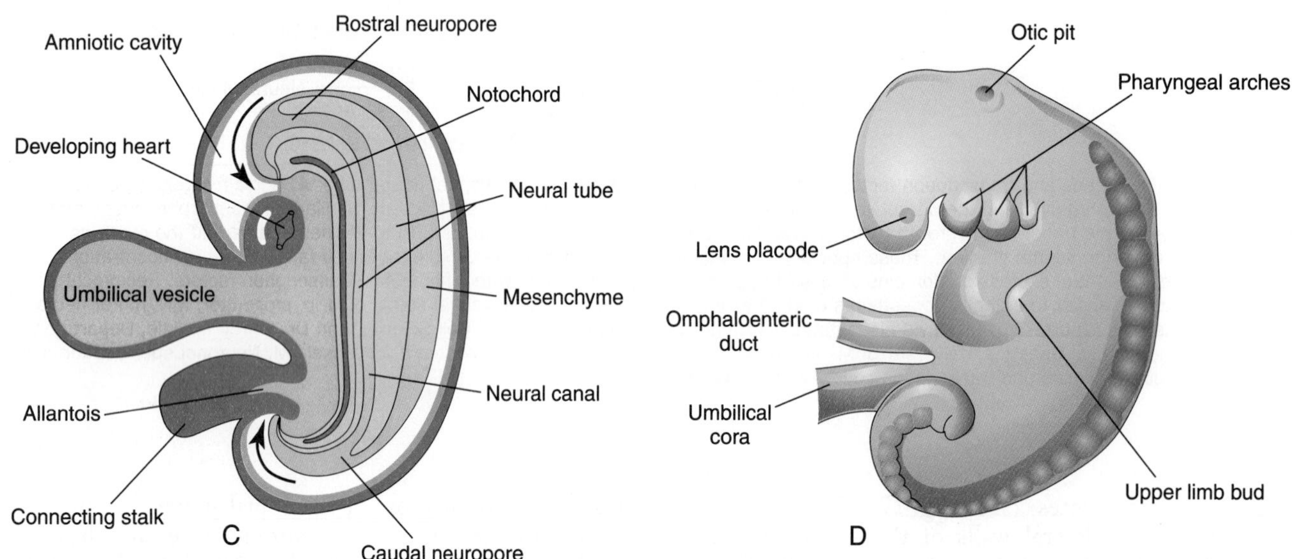

FIGURE 17-3. **A,** Dorsal view of an embryo of approximately 23 days showing fusion of the neural folds, forming the neural tube. **B,** Lateral view of an embryo of approximately 24 days showing the forebrain prominence and closing of the rostral neuropore. **C,** Diagrammatic sagittal section of the embryo showing the transitory communication of the neural canal with the amniotic cavity (*arrows*). **D,** Lateral view of an embryo of approximately 27 days. Note that the neuropores shown in **B** are closed.

Development of the Spinal Meninges

The mesenchyme surrounding the neural tube (see Fig. 17-3*C*) condenses to form a membrane called the **primordial meninx** or **meninges**. The external layer of this membrane thickens to form the **dura mater** (Fig. 17-10). The internal layer the pia-arachnoid, composed of pia mater and arachnoid mater (**leptomeninges**), is derived from neural crest cells. Fluid-filled spaces appear within the leptomeninges that soon coalesce to form the **subarachnoid space**. The origin of the pia mater and arachnoid from a single layer is indicated in the adult by **arachnoid trabeculae**—numerous delicate strands of connective tissue that pass between the pia and arachnoid. Cerebrospinal fluid (CSF) begins to form during the fifth week.

Positional Changes of the Spinal Cord

The spinal cord in the embryo extends the entire length of the vertebral canal (see Fig. 17-10*A*). The spinal nerves pass through the intervertebral foramina opposite their levels of origin. Because the vertebral column and dura mater grow more rapidly than the spinal cord, this positional relationship to the spinal nerves does not persist. The caudal end of the spinal cord gradually comes

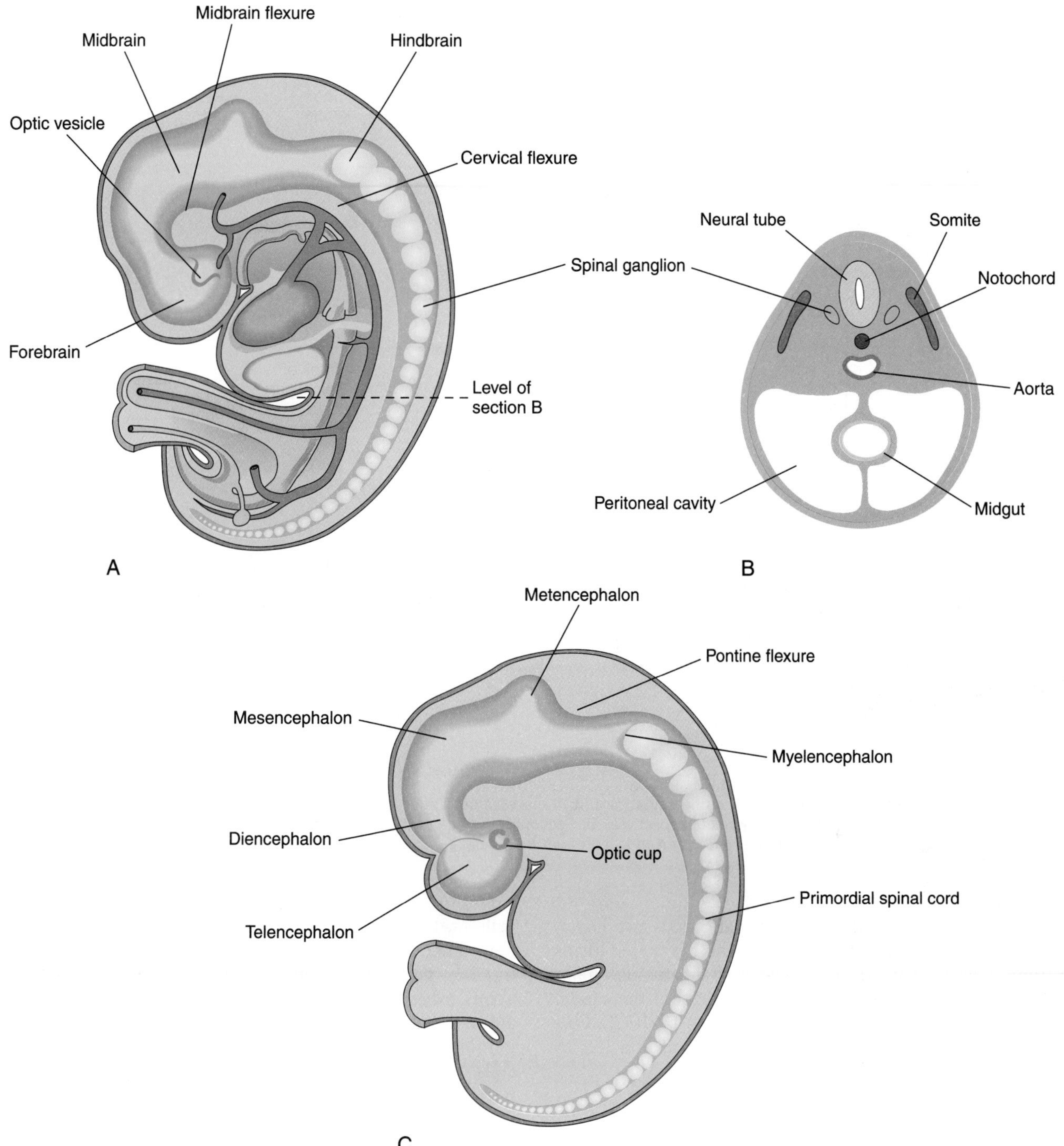

FIGURE 17-4. **A,** Schematic lateral view of an embryo of approximately 28 days showing the three primary brain vesicles: forebrain, midbrain, and hindbrain. Two flexures demarcate the primary divisions of the brain. **B,** Transverse section of this embryo showing the neural tube that will develop into the spinal cord in this region. The spinal ganglia derived from the neural crest are also shown. **C,** Schematic lateral view of the central nervous system of a 6-week embryo showing the secondary brain vesicles and pontine flexure. The flexure occurs as the brain grows rapidly.

to lie at relatively higher levels. In a 6-month-old fetus, it lies at the level of the first sacral vertebra (see Fig. 17-10*B*). The **spinal cord in the newborn** terminates at the level of the second or third lumbar vertebra (see Fig. 17-10*C*). The **spinal cord in the adult** usually terminates at the inferior border of the first lumbar vertebra (see Fig. 17-10*D*). This is an average level because the caudal end of the spinal cord may be as superior as the 12th thoracic vertebra or as inferior as the third lumbar vertebra. As a result, the spinal nerve roots, especially those of the lumbar and sacral segments, run obliquely from the spinal cord to the corresponding level of the vertebral column. The nerve roots inferior to the end of the cord—the **medullary cone** (Latin [L]. *conus medullaris*)—form a bundle of spinal nerve roots, the **cauda equina** (L. horse's tail). Although the dura mater and arachnoid mater usually

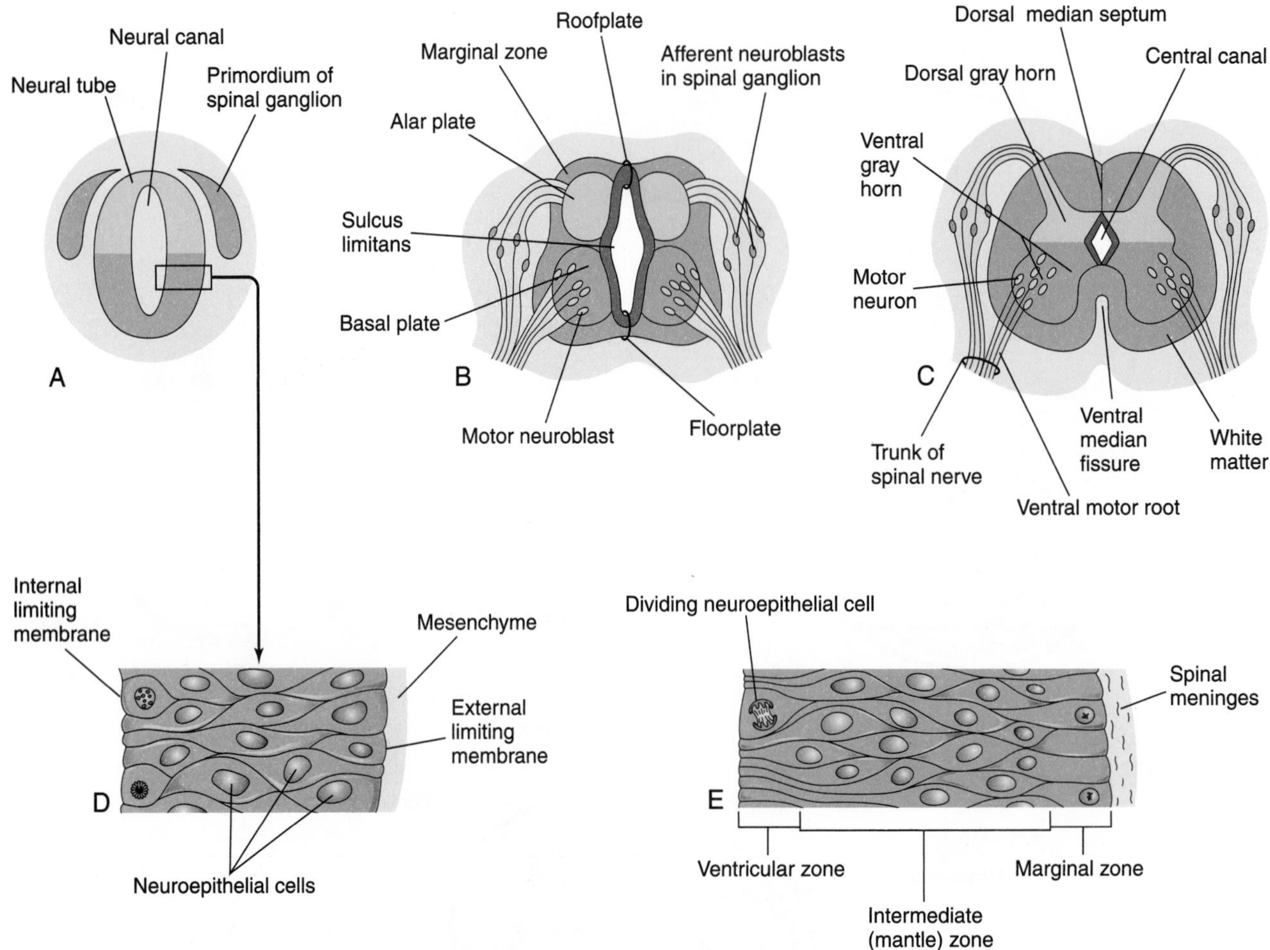

FIGURE 17-5. Illustrations of the development of the spinal cord. **A,** Transverse section of the neural tube of an embryo of approximately 23 days. **B** and **C,** Similar sections at 6 and 9 weeks, respectively. **D,** Section of the wall of the neural tube shown in **A**. **E,** Section of the wall of the developing spinal cord showing its three zones. In **A** to **C,** note that the neural canal of the neural tube is converted into the central canal of the spinal cord.

end at S2 vertebra in adults, the pia mater does not. Distal to the caudal end of the spinal cord, the pia mater forms a long fibrous thread, the **terminal filum** (L. *filum terminale*), which indicates the original level of the caudal end of the embryonic spinal cord (see Fig. 17-10*C*). This thread extends from the medullary cone and attaches to the periosteum of the first coccygeal vertebra.

Myelination of Nerve Fibers

Myelin sheaths surrounding nerve fibers within the spinal cord begin to form during the late fetal period and continue to form during the first postnatal year. **Myelin basic proteins**, a family of related polypeptide isoforms, are essential in myelination. In general, fiber tracts become myelinated at approximately the time they become functional. Motor roots are myelinated before sensory roots. The myelin sheaths surrounding nerve fibers within the spinal cord are formed by **oligodendrocytes**. The plasma membranes of these cells wrap around the axon, forming a number of layers (Fig. 17-11*F* to *H*). The myelin sheaths around the axons of peripheral nerve fibers are formed by the plasma membranes of **neurolemma cells** (Schwann cells), which are analogous to oligodendrocytes. These neuroglial cells are derived from neural crest cells that migrate peripherally and wrap themselves around the axons of somatic motor neurons and preganglionic autonomic motor neurons as they pass out of the central nervous system (see Figs. 17-8 and 17-11*A* to *E*). These cells also wrap themselves around both the central and peripheral processes of somatic and visceral sensory neurons, as well as around the axons of postsynaptic autonomic motor neurons. Beginning at approximately 20 weeks, peripheral nerve fibers have a whitish appearance, resulting from the deposition of myelin.

Congenital Anomalies of the Spinal Cord

Most congenital anomalies of the spinal cord result from defective closure of the neural tube during the fourth week. These **NTDs** affect the tissues overlying the spinal cord: meninges, vertebral arches, muscles, and skin (Fig. 17-12B to D). Anomalies involving the embryonic neural arches are referred to as **spina bifida**. This term denotes nonfusion of the primordial halves of the embryonic **neural arches**, which is common to all types of

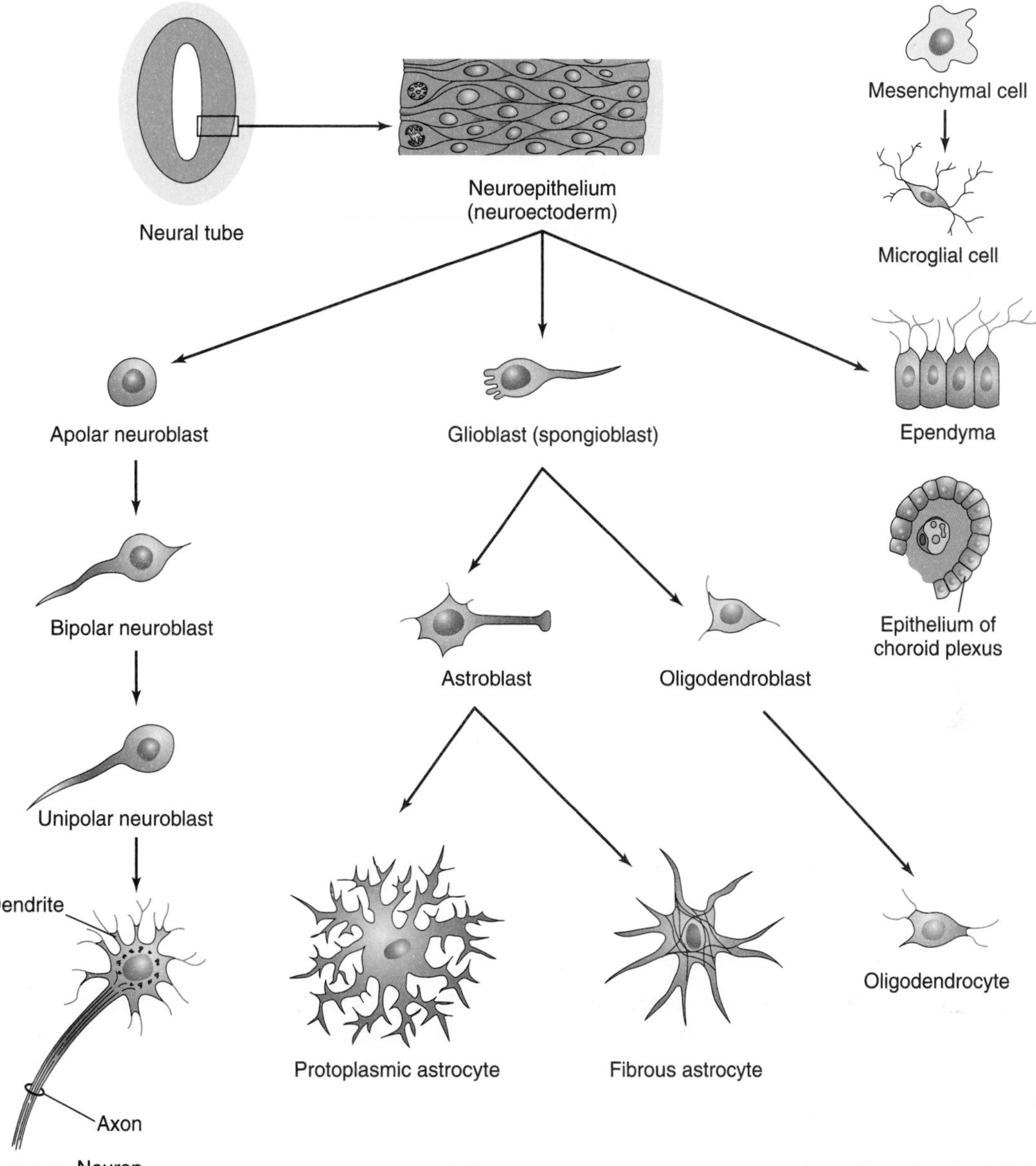

FIGURE 17-6. Histogenesis of cells in the central nervous system. After further development, the multipolar neuroblast (*lower left*) becomes a nerve cell or neuron. Neuroepithelial cells give rise to all neurons and macroglial cells. Microglial cells are derived from mesenchymal cells that invade the developing nervous system with the blood vessels.

spina bifida. Severe anomalies also involve the spinal cord and meninges. Spina bifida ranges from clinically significant types to minor anomalies that are functionally unimportant.

SPINAL DERMAL SINUS

A posterior skin dimple in the median plane of the sacral region of the back may be associated with a spinal dermal sinus (Fig. 17-13). The dimple indicates the region of closure of the caudal neuropore at the end of the fourth week; therefore, the dimple represents the last place of separation between the surface ectoderm and the neural tube. In some cases, the dimple is connected with the dura mater by a fibrous cord.

SPINA BIFIDA OCCULTA

This defect in the vertebral arch is the result of failure of the embryonic halves of the arch to grow normally and fuse in the median plane (see Fig. 17-12*A*). Spina bifida occulta occurs in the L5 or S1 vertebra in approximately 10% of otherwise normal people. In its most minor form, the only

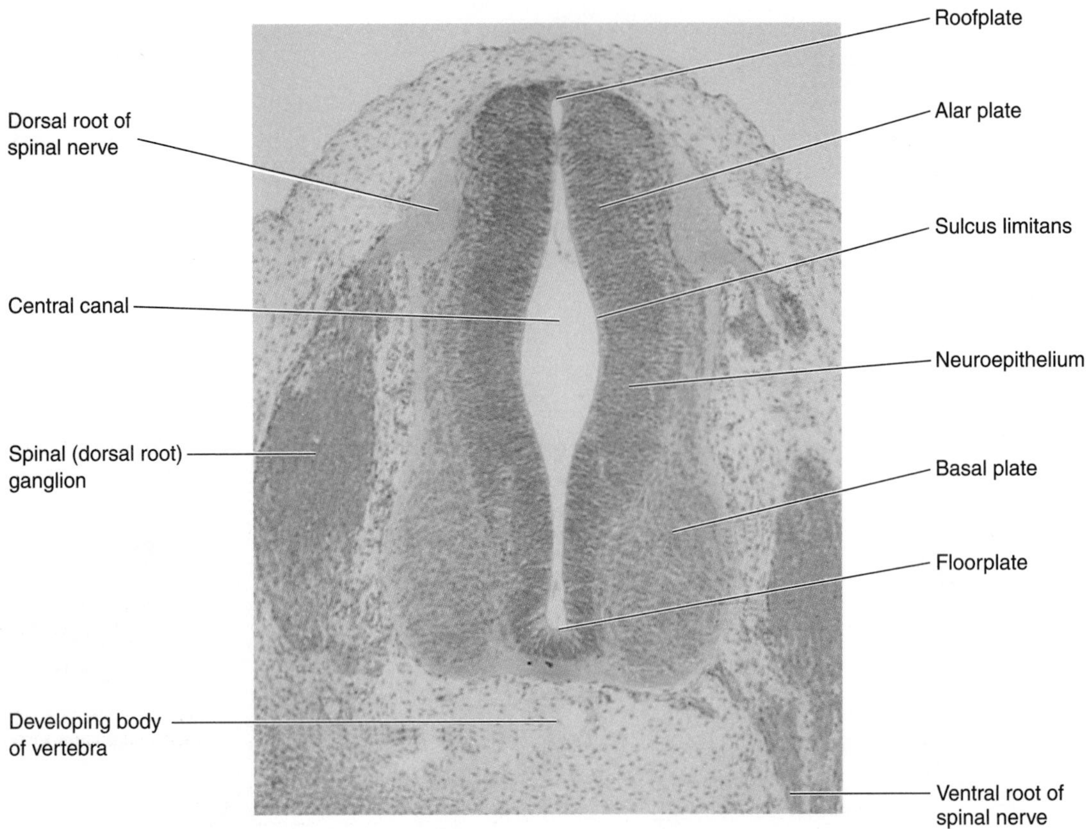

FIGURE 17-7. Transverse section of an embryo (×100) at Carnegie stage 16 at approximately 40 days. The ventral root of the spinal nerve is composed of nerve fibers arising from neuroblasts in the basal plate (developing ventral horn of spinal cord), whereas the dorsal root is formed by nerve processes arising from neuroblasts in the spinal ganglion. (From Moore KL, Persaud TVN, Shiota K: Color Atlas of Clinical Embryology, 2nd ed. Philadelphia, WB Saunders, 2000.)

evidence of its presence may be a small dimple with a tuft of hair arising from it (Fig. 17-14). Spina bifida occulta usually produces no clinical symptoms. A small percentage of affected infants have functionally significant defects of the underlying spinal cord and dorsal roots.

SPINA BIFIDA CYSTICA

Severe types of spina bifida, involving protrusion of the spinal cord and/or meninges through the defects in the vertebral arches, are referred to collectively as **spina bifida cystica** because of the cystlike sac that is associated with these anomalies (Figs. 17-12*B* to *D*, 17-15, and 17-16). Spina bifida cystica occurs approximately once in every 1000 births.

When the sac contains meninges and CSF, the anomaly is called **spina bifida with meningocele** (see Fig. 17-12*B*). The spinal cord and spinal roots are in their normal position, but there may be spinal cord abnormalities. If the spinal cord and/or nerve roots are included in the sac, the anomaly is called **spina bifida with meningomyelocele** (see Figs. 17-12*C*, 17-16, and 17-17).

Spina bifida cystica shows considerable geographic variation in incidence. In the British Isles, for example, the incidence varies from 4.2 per 1000 newborn infants in South Wales to 1.5 per 1000 in southeastern England. Severe cases of spina bifida with meningomyelocele involving several vertebrae are often associated with partial absence of the brain—**meroencephaly** (see Figs. 17-13 and 17-19). Spina bifida cystica shows varying degrees of neurologic deficit, depending on the position and extent of the lesion. There is usually a corresponding dermatome loss of sensation along with complete or partial skeletal muscle paralysis. The level of the lesion determines the area of **anesthesia** (area of skin without sensation) and the muscles affected. **Sphincter paralysis** (bladder and/or anal sphincters) is common with **lumbosacral meningomyeloceles** (see Figs. 17-15 to 17-17). There is almost invariably a **saddle anesthesia** when the sphincters are involved, i.e., loss of sensation in the body region that would contact the saddle during horseback riding.

Spina bifida cystica and/or meroencephaly is strongly suspected in utero when there is a **high level of alpha fetoprotein** (AFP) in the amniotic fluid

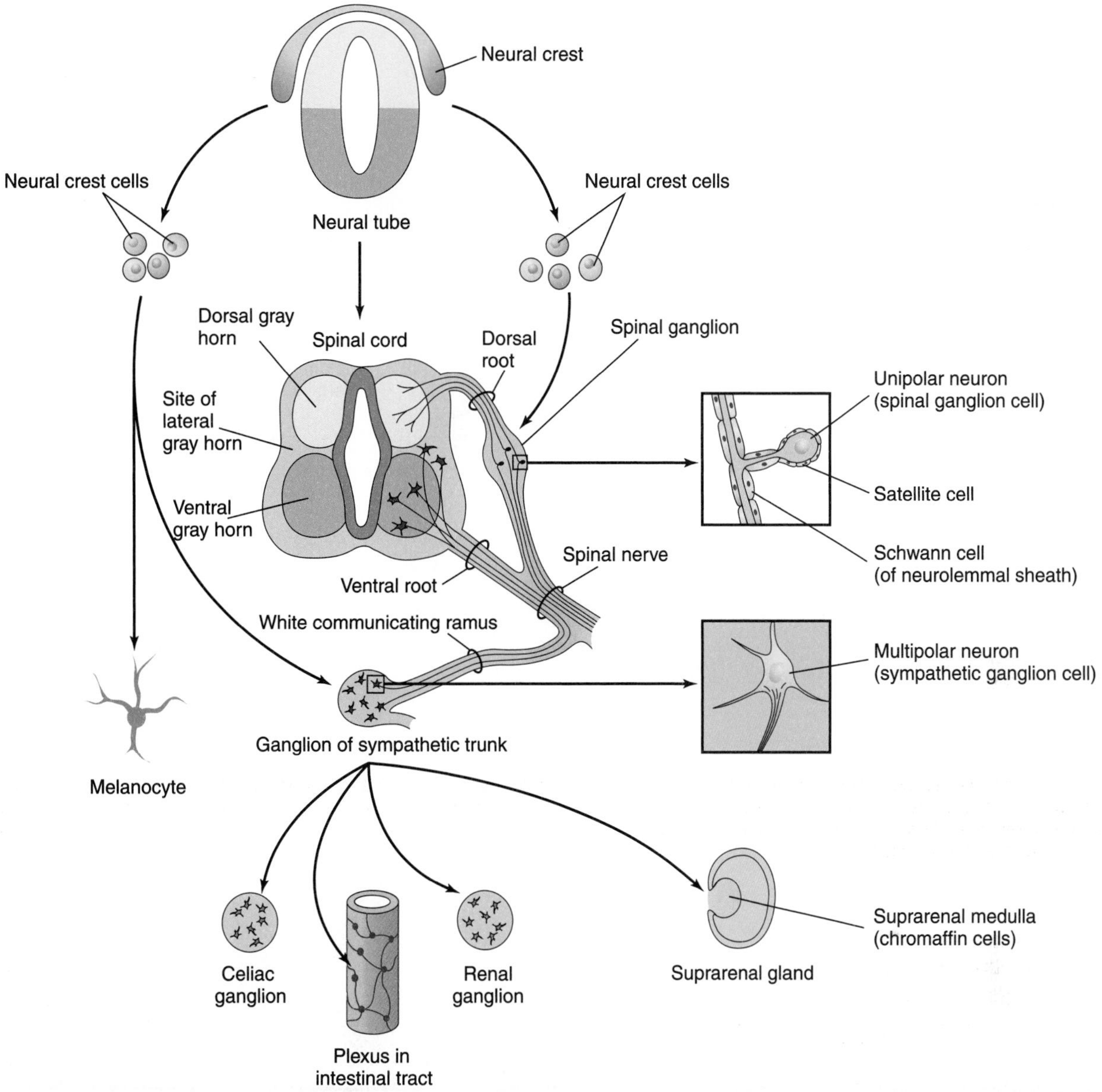

Neural crest
Neural crest cells
Neural tube
Neural crest cells
Dorsal gray horn
Spinal cord
Dorsal root
Spinal ganglion
Site of lateral gray horn
Ventral gray horn
Unipolar neuron (spinal ganglion cell)
Satellite cell
Schwann cell (of neurolemmal sheath)
Spinal nerve
Ventral root
White communicating ramus
Multipolar neuron (sympathetic ganglion cell)
Ganglion of sympathetic trunk
Melanocyte
Celiac ganglion
Renal ganglion
Suprarenal gland
Suprarenal medulla (chromaffin cells)
Plexus in intestinal tract

FIGURE 17-8. Diagrams showing some derivatives of the neural crest. Neural crest cells also differentiate into the cells in the afferent ganglia of cranial nerves and many other structures (see Chapter 5). The formation of a spinal nerve is also illustrated.

A
B
C
D
Neural crest cell
Bipolar neuroblasts
Unipolar afferent neuron

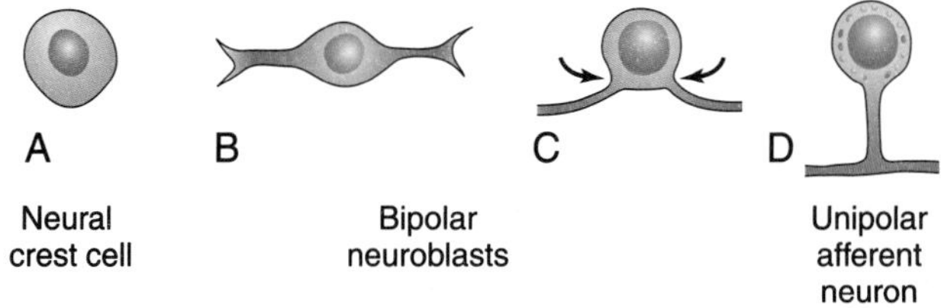

FIGURE 17-9. **A** to **D,** Diagrams of successive stages in the differentiation of a neural crest cell into a unipolar afferent neuron in a spinal ganglion.

(see Chapter 6). AFP may also be elevated in the maternal blood serum. Amniocentesis is usually performed on pregnant women with high levels of serum AFP for the determination of the AFP level in the amniotic fluid. An ultrasound scan may reveal the presence of an NTD that has resulted in spina bifida cystica. The fetal vertebral column can be detected by ultrasound at 10 to 12 weeks' gestation (8–10 weeks after conception), and, if present, spina bifida cystica is sometimes visible as a cystic mass adjacent to the affected area of the vertebral column.

MENINGOMYELOCELE AND MENINGOCELES

Meningomyelocele is a severe type of spinal bifida cystica that is often associated with a marked neurologic deficit inferior to the level of the

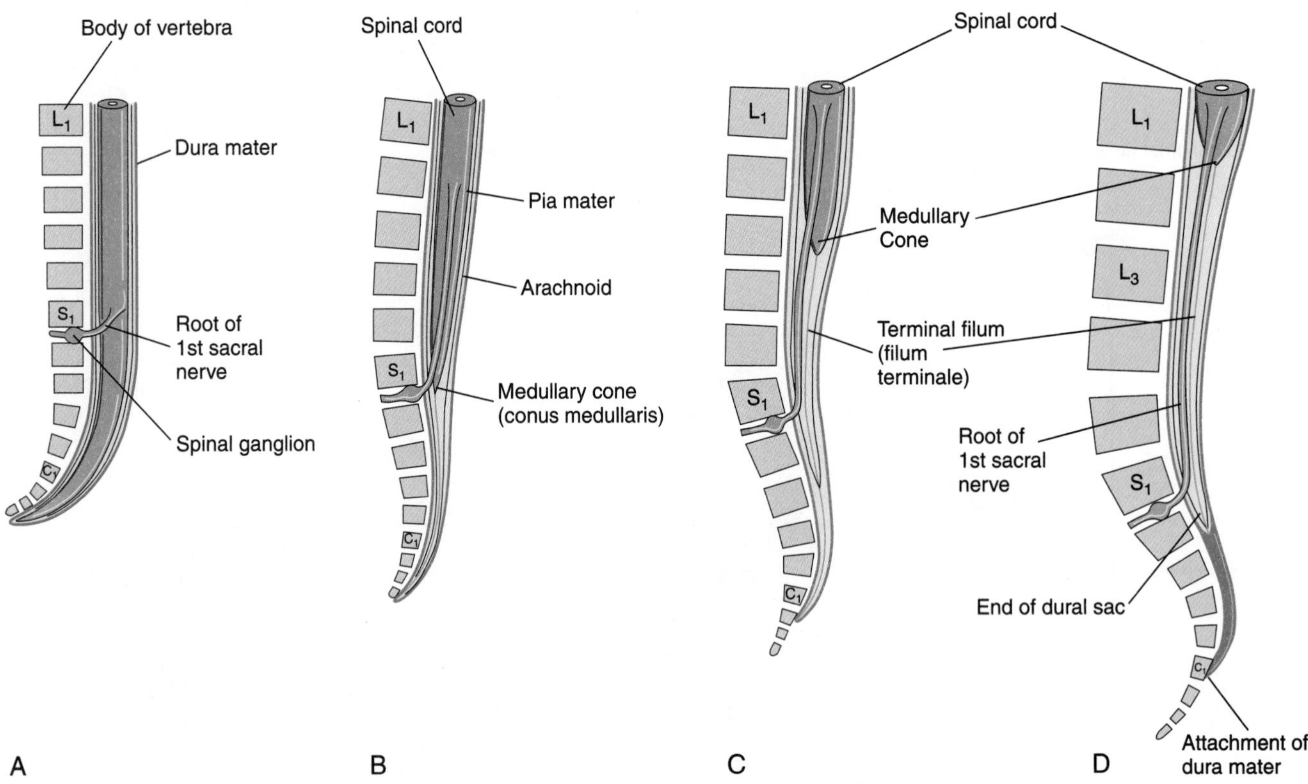

FIGURE 17-10. Diagrams showing the position of the caudal end of the spinal cord in relation to the vertebral column and meninges at various stages of development. The increasing inclination of the root of the first sacral nerve is also illustrated. **A,** At 8 weeks. **B,** At 24 weeks. **C,** Newborn. **D,** Adult.

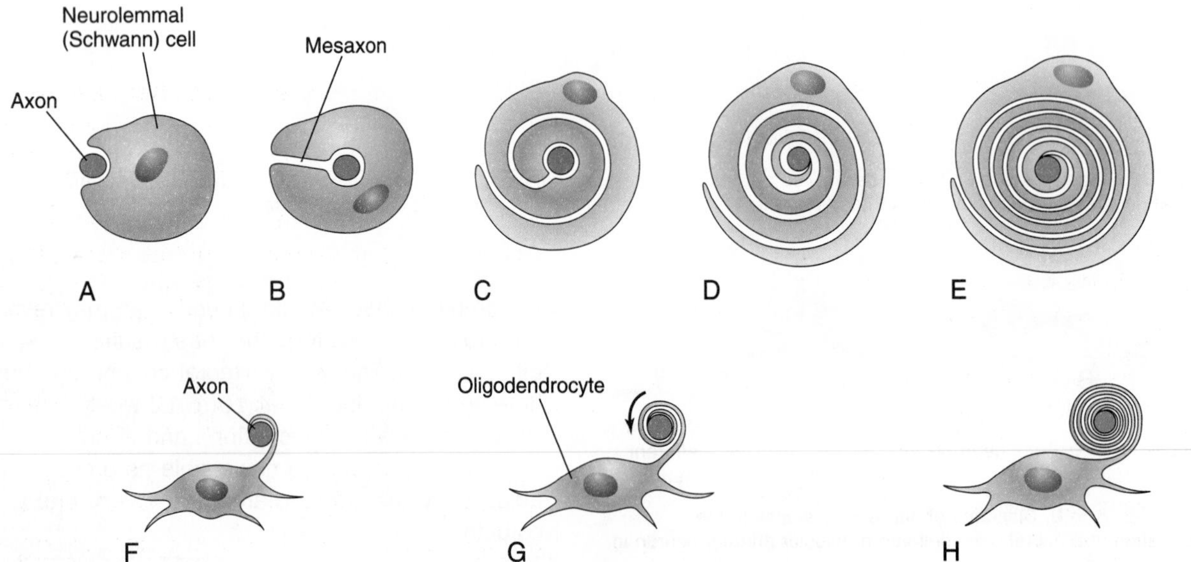

FIGURE 17-11. Diagrammatic sketches illustrating myelination of nerve fibers. **A** to **E,** Successive stages in the myelination of an axon of a peripheral nerve fiber by a neurolemmal cell. The axon first indents the cell; the cell then rotates around the axon as the mesaxon (site of invagination) elongates. The cytoplasm between the layers of the cell membrane gradually condenses. Cytoplasm remains on the inside of the sheath between the myelin and axon. **F** to **H,** Successive stages in the myelination of a nerve fiber in the central nervous system by an oligodendrocyte. A process of the neuroglial cell wraps itself around an axon, and the intervening layers of cytoplasm move to the body of the cell.

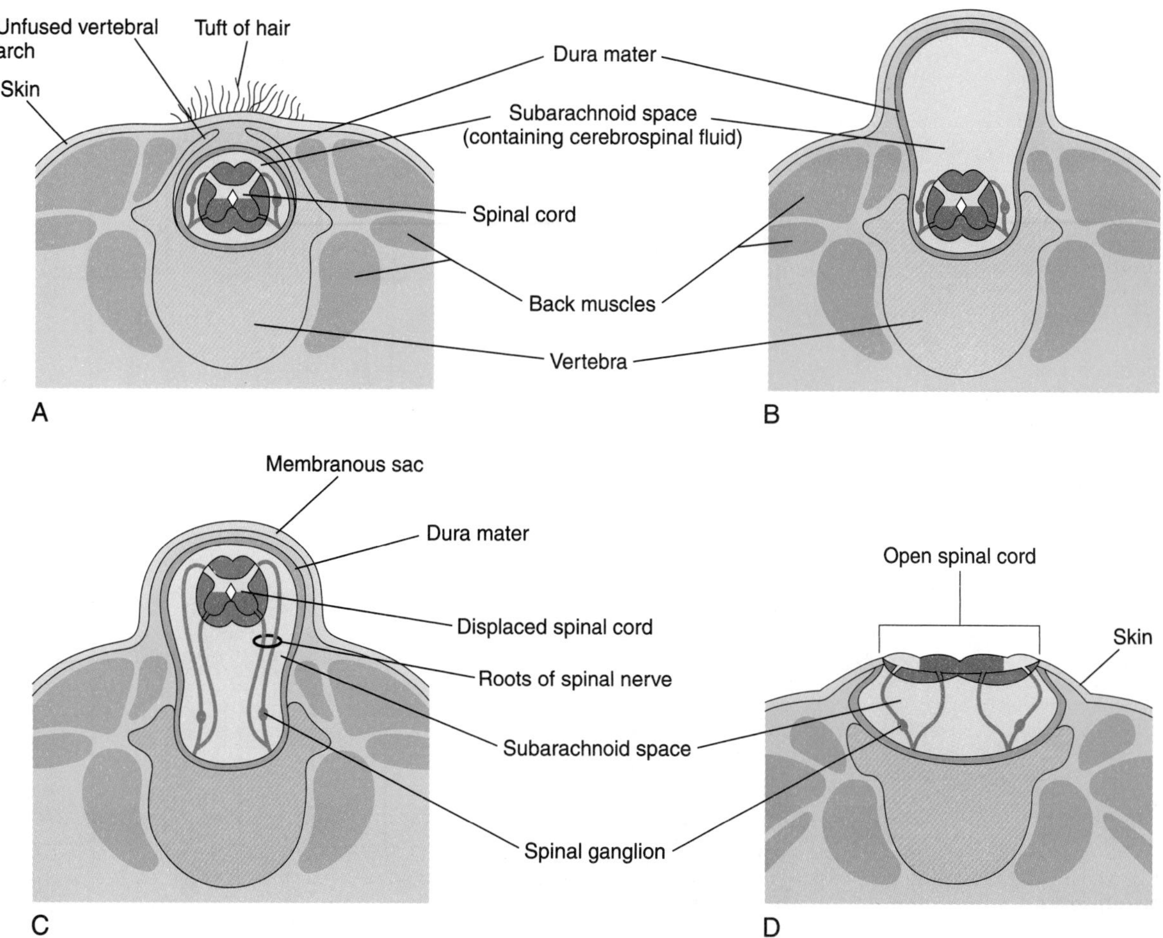

FIGURE 17-12. Diagrammatic sketches illustrating various types of spina bifida and the commonly associated anomalies of the vertebral arch, spinal cord, and meninges. **A,** Spina bifida occulta. Observe the unfused vertebral arch. **B,** Spina bifida with meningocele. **C,** Spina bifida with meningomyelocele. **D,** Spina bifida with myeloschisis. The types illustrated in **B** to **D** are referred to collectively as spina bifida cystica because of the cystlike sac associated with them.

protruding sac. This deficit occurs because nervous tissue is incorporated in the wall of the sac, impairing development of nerve fibers. **Meningomyeloceles** may be covered by skin or a thin, easily ruptured membrane (see Figs. 17-15*A*, 17-16, and 17-17).

Spina bifida with meningomyelocele is a more common and a much more severe anomaly than spina bifida with meningocele. These NTDs may occur anywhere along the vertebral column, but they are most common in the lumbar and sacral region (see Fig. 17-19). Some cases of meningomyelocele are associated with **craniolacunia** (defective development of the calvaria). This results in depressed nonossified areas on the inner surfaces of the flat bones of the calvaria.

MYELOSCHISIS

This is the most severe type of spina bifida (see Figs. 17-12*D* and 17-13). In these cases, the spinal cord in the affected area is open because the neural folds failed to fuse (Gr. *schisis*, a cleaving). As a result, the spinal cord is represented by a flattened mass of nervous tissue. Spina bifida with myeloschisis may result from an NTD that is caused by a local overgrowth of the neural plate (Fig. 17-18). As a result, the caudal neuropore fails to close at the end of the fourth week.

ETIOLOGY OF NEURAL TUBE DEFECTS

Nutritional and environmental factors undoubtedly play a role in the production of NTDs. Epidemiologic studies have shown that folic acid supplements taken before conception and continued for at least 3 months during pregnancy reduce the incidence of NTDs. As a result, the U.S. Public Health Service recommended in 1992 that "all women of childbearing age who are capable of becoming pregnant should consume 0.4 mg, 400 μg, of folic acid daily." Certain drugs increase the risk of

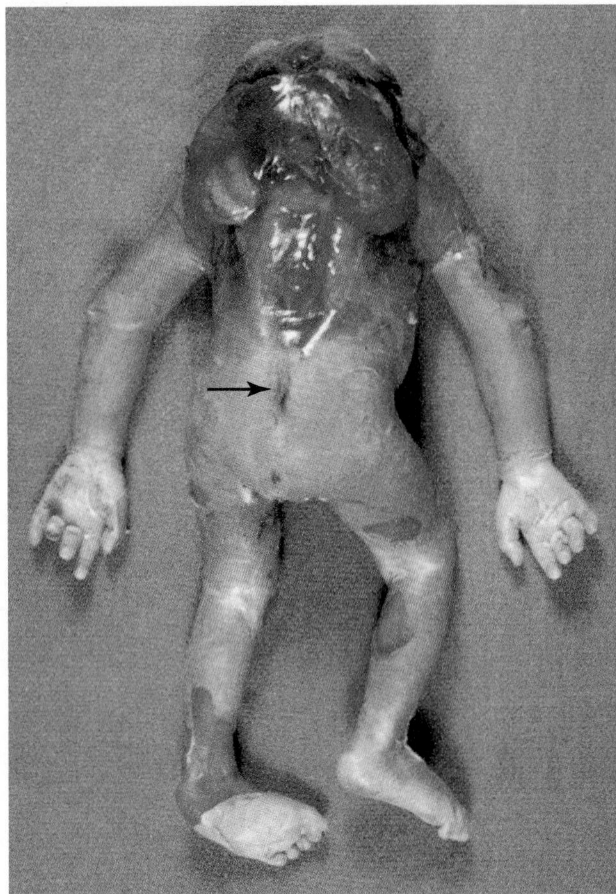

FIGURE 17-13. A fetus at 20 weeks' gestation with severe neural tube defects, including acrania, cerebral regression (meroencephaly [anencephaly]), iniencephaly (enlargement of foramen magnum), and a sacral dimple (*arrow*). (Courtesy of Dr. Marc Del Bigio, Department of Pathology [Neuropathology], University of Manitoba, Winnipeg, Manitoba, Canada.)

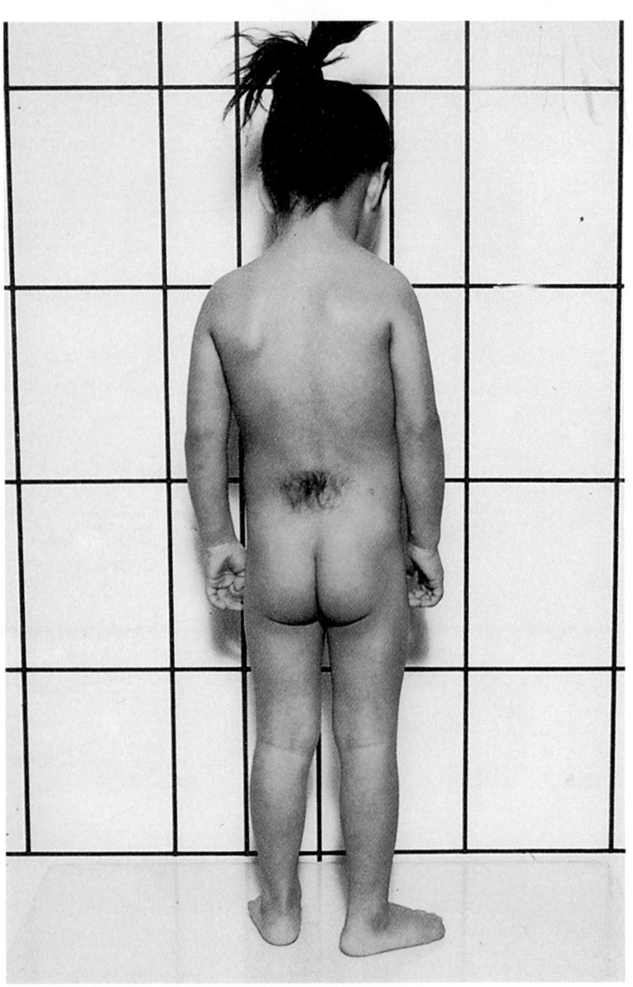

FIGURE 17-14. A female child with a hairy patch in the lumbosacral region indicating the site of a spina bifida occulta. (Courtesy of A.E. Chudley, MD, Section of Genetics and Metabolism, Department of Pediatrics and Child Health, Children's Hospital and University of Manitoba, Winnipeg, Manitoba, Canada.)

meningomyelocele (e.g., valproic acid). This anticonvulsant drug causes NTDs in 1% to 2% of pregnancies if given during early pregnancy (fourth week of development) when the neural folds are fusing (Fig. 17-19). Pregnant animals exposed to hyperthermia or high levels of vitamin A produce offspring with NTDs.

DEVELOPMENT OF THE BRAIN

The **neural tube** cranial to the fourth pair of somites develops into the brain. Fusion of the neural folds in the cranial region and closure of the rostral neuropore form three primary brain vesicles from which the brain develops (Fig. 17-20). The three **primary brain vesicles** form:

- The forebrain (prosencephalon)
- The midbrain (mesencephalon)
- The hindbrain (rhombencephalon)

During the fifth week, the forebrain partly divides into two **secondary brain vesicles**, the *telencephalon* and *diencephalon*; the midbrain does not divide; the hindbrain partly divides into the *metencephalon* and *myelencephalon*; consequently, there are five secondary brain vesicles.

Brain Flexures

During the fourth week, the embryonic brain grows rapidly and bends ventrally with the head fold. This produces the **midbrain flexure** in the midbrain region and the **cervical flexure** at the junction of the hindbrain and spinal cord (Fig. 17-21*A*). Later, unequal growth of the brain between these flexures produces the **pontine flexure** in the opposite direction. This flexure results in thinning of the roof of the hindbrain.

Initially, the primordial brain has the same basic structure as the developing spinal cord; however, the brain flexures produce considerable variation in the outline of transverse sections at different levels of the brain and in the position of the gray and white matter (substance). The **sulcus limitans** extends cranially to the junction of the midbrain and forebrain, and the alar and basal plates are recognizable only in the midbrain and hindbrain (Fig. 17-5*C*).

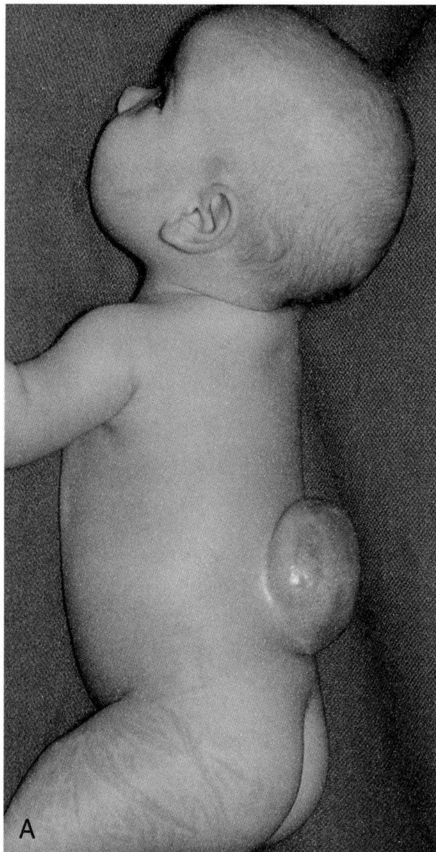

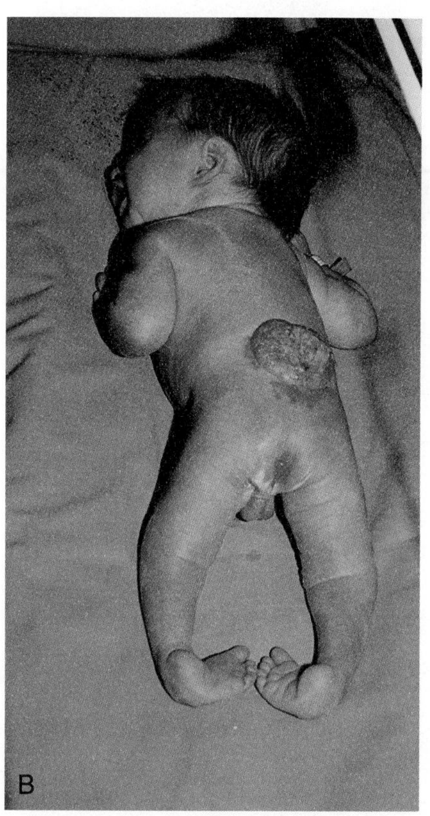

FIGURE 17-15. Infants with spina bifida cystica. **A,** Spina bifida with meningomyelocele in the lumbar region. **B,** Spina bifida with myeloschisis in the lumbar region. Note the nerve involvement has affected the lower limbs. (Courtesy of the late Dr. Dwight Parkinson, Department of Surgery and Department of Human Anatomy and Cell Science, University of Manitoba, Winnipeg, Manitoba, Canada.)

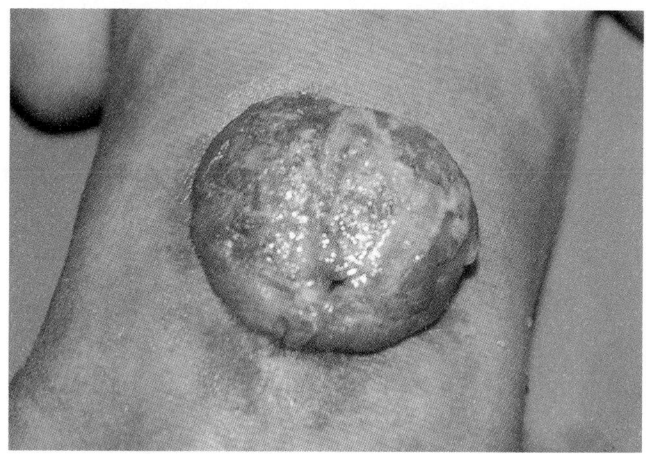

FIGURE 17-16. The back of a newborn with a large lumbar meningomyelocele. The neural tube defect is covered with a thin membrane. (Courtesy of A.E. Chudley, MD, Section of Genetics and Metabolism, Department of Pediatrics and Child Health, Children's Hospital and University of Manitoba, Winnipeg, Manitoba, Canada.)

Hindbrain

The *cervical flexure* demarcates the hindbrain from the spinal cord (see Fig. 17-21*A*). Later, this junction is arbitrarily defined as the level of the superior rootlet of the first cervical nerve, which is located roughly at the foramen magnum. The *pontine flexure*, located in the future pontine region, divides the hindbrain into caudal (myelencephalon) and rostral (metencephalon) parts. The **myelencephalon** becomes the **medulla oblongata** (often called the medulla), and the **metencephalon** becomes the **pons** and **cerebellum**. The cavity of the hindbrain becomes the **fourth ventricle** and the **central canal** in the medulla.

Myelencephalon

The caudal part of the myelencephalon (closed part of medulla) resembles the spinal cord, both developmentally and structurally (see Fig. 17-21*B*). The **neural canal** of the neural tube forms the small *central canal* of the myelencephalon. Unlike those of the spinal cord, neuroblasts from the alar plates in the myelencephalon migrate into the marginal zone and form isolated areas of gray matter—the **gracile nuclei** medially and the **cuneate nuclei** laterally. These nuclei are associated with correspondingly named tracts that enter the medulla from the spinal cord. The ventral area of the medulla contains a pair of fiber bundles—the **pyramids**— that consist of corticospinal fibers descending from the developing cerebral cortex.

The rostral part of the myelencephalon ("open" part of medulla) is wide and rather flat, especially opposite the pontine flexure (see Fig. 17-21*C* and *D*). The pontine

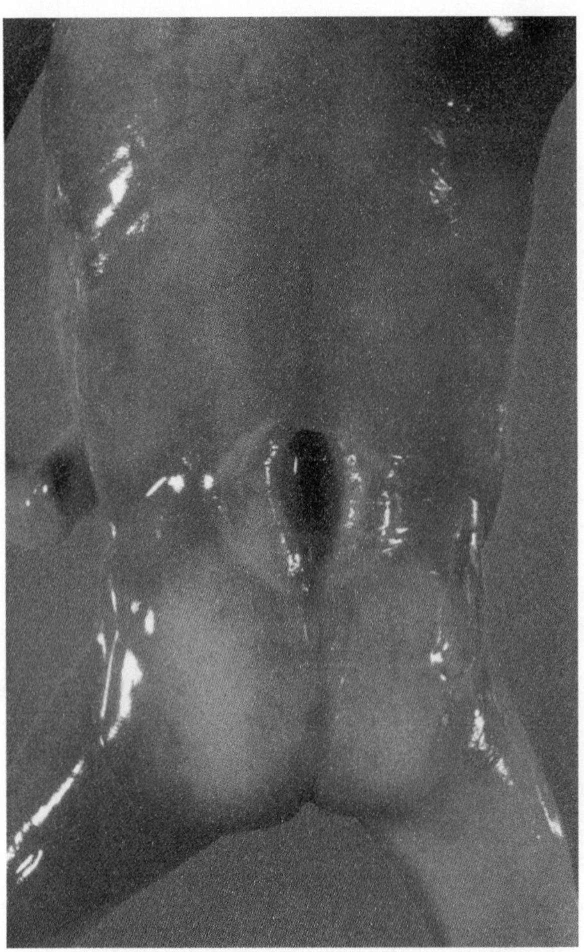

FIGURE 17-17. A 19-week female fetus showing an open spinal defect in the lumbosacral region (spina bifida with myeloschisis). (Courtesy of Dr. Joseph R. Siebert, Children's Hospital and Regional Medical Center, Seattle, Washington.)

flexure causes the lateral walls of the medulla to move laterally like the pages of an open book. As a result, its **roofplate** is stretched and greatly thinned. In addition, the cavity of this part of the myelencephalon (part of future fourth ventricle) becomes somewhat rhomboidal (diamond shaped). As the walls of the medulla move laterally, the alar plates come to lie lateral to the basal plates. As the positions of the plates change, the motor nuclei generally develop medial to the sensory nuclei (see Fig. 17-21*C*).

Neuroblasts in the basal plates of the medulla, like those in the spinal cord, develop into motor neurons. In the medulla, the neuroblasts form nuclei (groups of nerve cells) and organize into three cell columns on each side (see Fig. 17-21*D*). From medial to lateral, they are:

- The general somatic efferent, represented by neurons of the hypoglossal nerve
- The special visceral efferent, represented by neurons innervating muscles derived from the pharyngeal arches (see Chapter 9)
- The general visceral efferent, represented by some neurons of the vagus and glossopharyngeal nerves

Neuroblasts in the alar plates of the medulla form neurons that are arranged in four columns on each side. From medial to lateral, they are:

- The general visceral afferent receiving impulses from the viscera
- The special visceral afferent receiving taste fibers
- The general somatic afferent receiving impulses from the surface of the head
- The special somatic afferent receiving impulses from the ear

Some neuroblasts from the alar plates migrate ventrally and form the neurons in the **olivary nuclei** (see Fig. 17-21*C* and *D*).

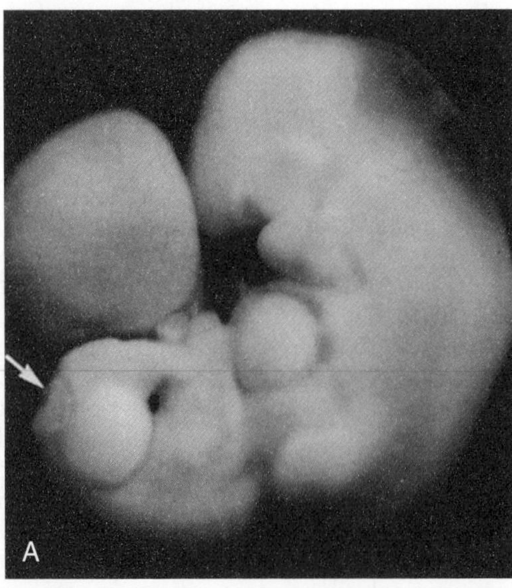

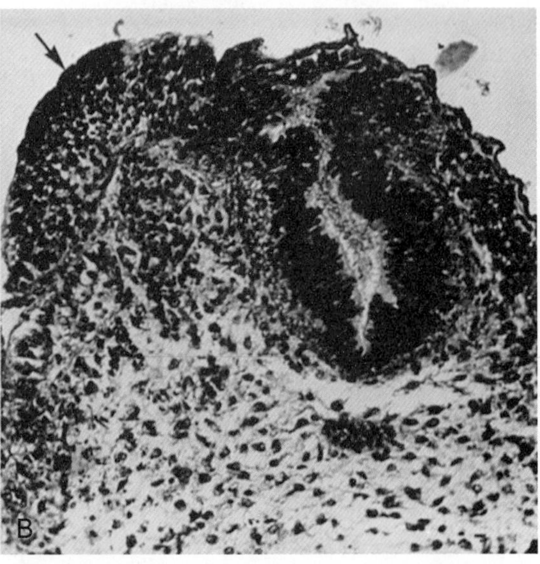

FIGURE 17-18. **A,** An embryo of approximately 30 days. The *white arrow* indicates the site of the neural tube defect (NTD) resulting from failure of closure of the caudal neuropore. Normally this neuropore is closed by day 28. **B,** Photomicrograph of a transverse section through the NTD. The *black arrow* indicates an abnormal fold of neural tissue extending over the left side of the embryo. It appears that this overgrown neural fold has prevented closure of the neural tube. (From Lemire RJ, Shepard TH, Alvord JE Jr: Caudal myeloschisis (lumbo-sacral spina bifida cystica) in a five millimeter (horizon XIV) human embryo. Anat Rec 152:9, 1965.)

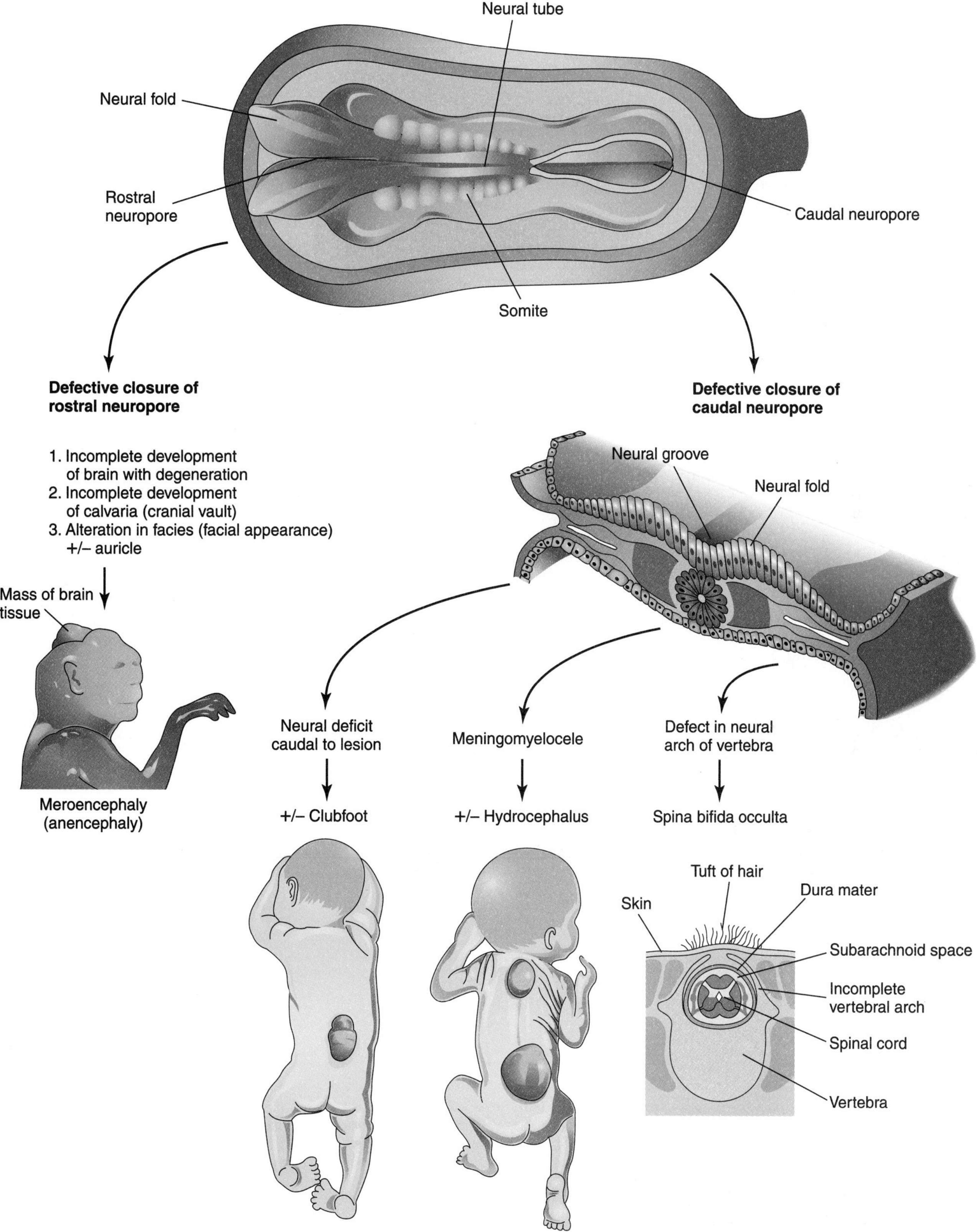

FIGURE 17-19. Schematic illustrations explaining the embryologic basis of neural tube defects. Meroencephaly, partial absence of brain, results from defective closure of the rostral neuropore, and meningomyelocele results from defective closure of the caudal neuropore. (Modified from Jones KL: Smith's Recognizable Patterns of Human Malformations, 4th ed. Philadelphia, WB Saunders, 1988.)

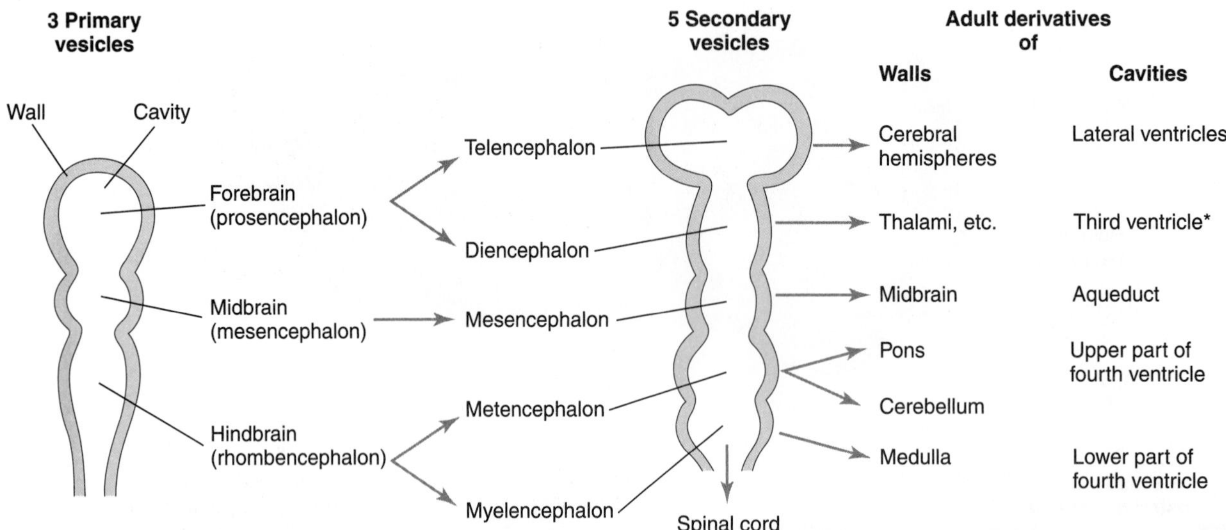

FIGURE 17-20. Diagrammatic sketches of the brain vesicles indicating the adult derivatives of their walls and cavities. *The rostral part of the third ventricle forms from the cavity of the telencephalon; most of this ventricle is derived from the cavity of the diencephalon.

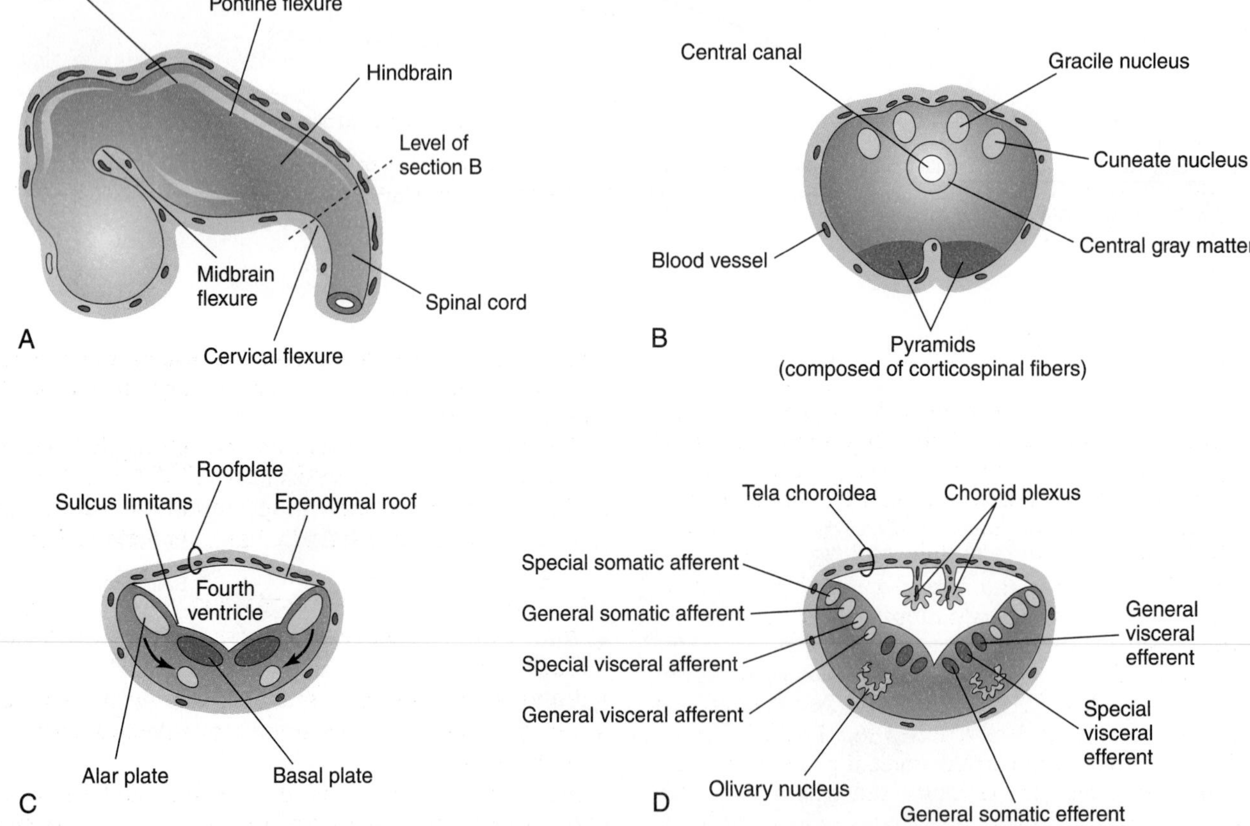

FIGURE 17-21. **A,** Sketch of the developing brain at the end of the fifth week showing the three primary divisions of the brain and the brain flexures. **B,** Transverse section of the caudal part of the myelencephalon (developing closed part of the medulla). **C** and **D,** Similar sections of the rostral part of the myelencephalon (developing open part of the medulla) showing the position and successive stages of differentiation of the alar and basal plates. The arrows in **C** show the pathway taken by neuroblasts from the alar plates to form the olivary nuclei.

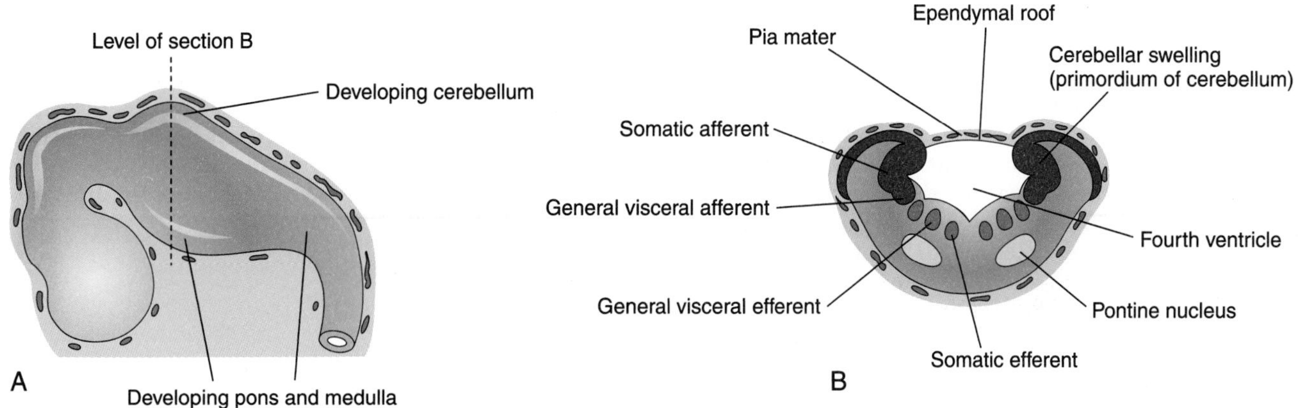

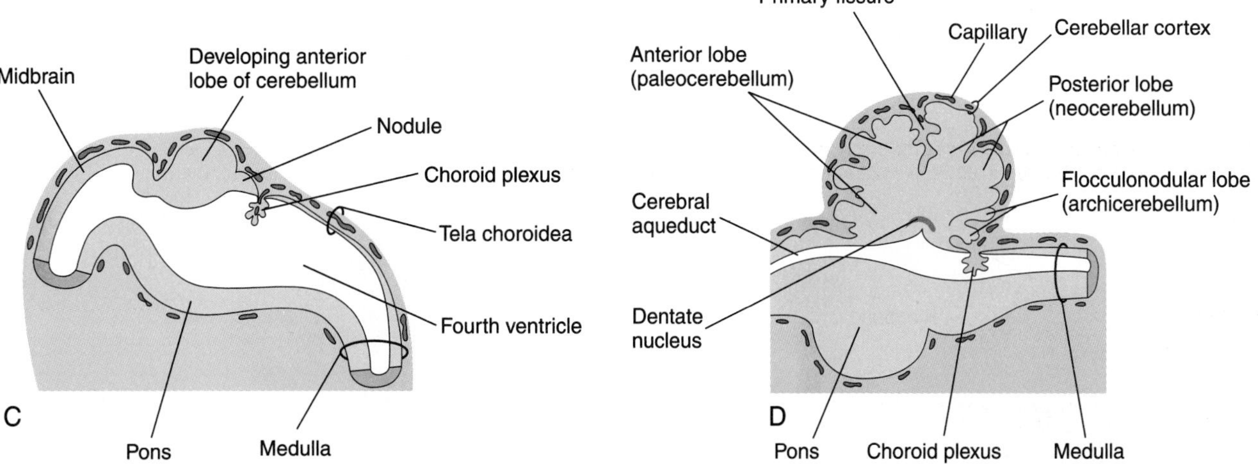

FIGURE 17-22. **A,** Sketch of the developing brain at the end of the fifth week. **B,** Transverse section of the metencephalon (developing pons and cerebellum) showing the derivatives of the alar and basal plates. **C** and **D,** Sagittal sections of the hindbrain at 6 and 17 weeks, respectively, showing successive stages in the development of the pons and cerebellum.

Metencephalon

The walls of the metencephalon form the **pons** and **cerebellum**, and the cavity of the metencephalon forms the *superior part of the fourth ventricle* (Fig. 17-22*A*). As in the rostral part of the myelencephalon, the pontine flexure causes divergence of the lateral walls of the pons, which spreads the gray matter in the floor of the fourth ventricle (see Fig. 17-22*B*). As in the myelencephalon, neuroblasts in each basal plate develop into motor nuclei and organize into three columns on each side.

The **cerebellum** develops from thickenings of dorsal parts of the alar plates. Initially, the **cerebellar swellings** project into the fourth ventricle (see Fig. 17-22*B*). As the swellings enlarge and fuse in the median plane, they overgrow the rostral half of the fourth ventricle and overlap the pons and medulla (Fig. 17-22*D*). Some neuroblasts in the intermediate zone of the alar plates migrate to the marginal zone and differentiate into the neurons of the **cerebellar cortex**. Other neuroblasts from these plates give rise to the central nuclei, the largest of which is the **dentate nucleus** (see Fig. 17-22*D*). Cells from the alar plates also give rise to the **pontine nuclei**, the cochlear and vestibular nuclei, and the sensory nuclei of the trigeminal nerve.

The structure of the cerebellum reflects its phylogenetic (evolutionary) development (see Fig. 17-22*C* and *D*):

- The **archicerebellum** (flocculonodular lobe), the oldest part phylogenetically, has connections with the vestibular apparatus.
- The **paleocerebellum** (vermis and anterior lobe), of more recent development, is associated with sensory data from the limbs.
- The **neocerebellum** (posterior lobe), the newest part phylogenetically, is concerned with selective control of limb movements.

Nerve fibers connecting the cerebral and cerebellar cortices with the spinal cord pass through the marginal layer of the ventral region of the metencephalon. This region of the **brainstem** is called the **pons** (L. bridge) because of the robust band of nerve fibers that crosses the median plane and forms a bulky ridge on its anterior and lateral aspects.

Choroid Plexuses and Cerebrospinal Fluid (CSF)

The thin ependymal roof of the fourth ventricle is covered externally by pia mater, derived from mesenchyme associated with the hindbrain (see Fig. 17-22*C* and *D*). This vascular membrane, together with the ependymal roof, forms the **tela choroidea of the fourth ventricle**. Because of the active proliferation of the pia mater, the tela choroidea invaginates the fourth ventricle, where it differentiates into the **choroid plexus** (infoldings of choroidal arteries of the pia mater). Similar plexuses develop in the roof of the third ventricle and in the medial walls of the lateral ventricles. The choroid plexuses secrete ventricular fluid, which becomes **CSF** when additions are made to it from the surfaces of the brain and spinal cord and from the pia-arachnoid layer of the meninges. The thin roof of the fourth ventricle evaginates in three locations. These outpouchings rupture to form openings, **median** and **lateral apertures** (also called the foramen of Magendie and foramina of Luschka, respectively), which permit the CSF to enter the subarachnoid space from the fourth ventricle. The main site of absorption of CSF into the venous system is through the **arachnoid villi**, which are protrusions of the arachnoid mater into the **dural venous sinuses** (large venous channels between the layers of the dura mater). The arachnoid villi consist of a thin, cellular layer derived from the epithelium of the arachnoid and the endothelium of the sinus.

Midbrain

The midbrain (mesencephalon) undergoes less change than any other part of the developing brain (Fig. 17-23*A*), except for the caudal part of the hindbrain. The *neural canal* narrows and becomes the **cerebral aqueduct** (see Fig. 17-22*D*), a channel that connects the third and fourth ventricles. Neuroblasts migrate from the alar plates of the midbrain into the **tectum** (roof) and aggregate to form four large groups of neurons, the paired **superior**

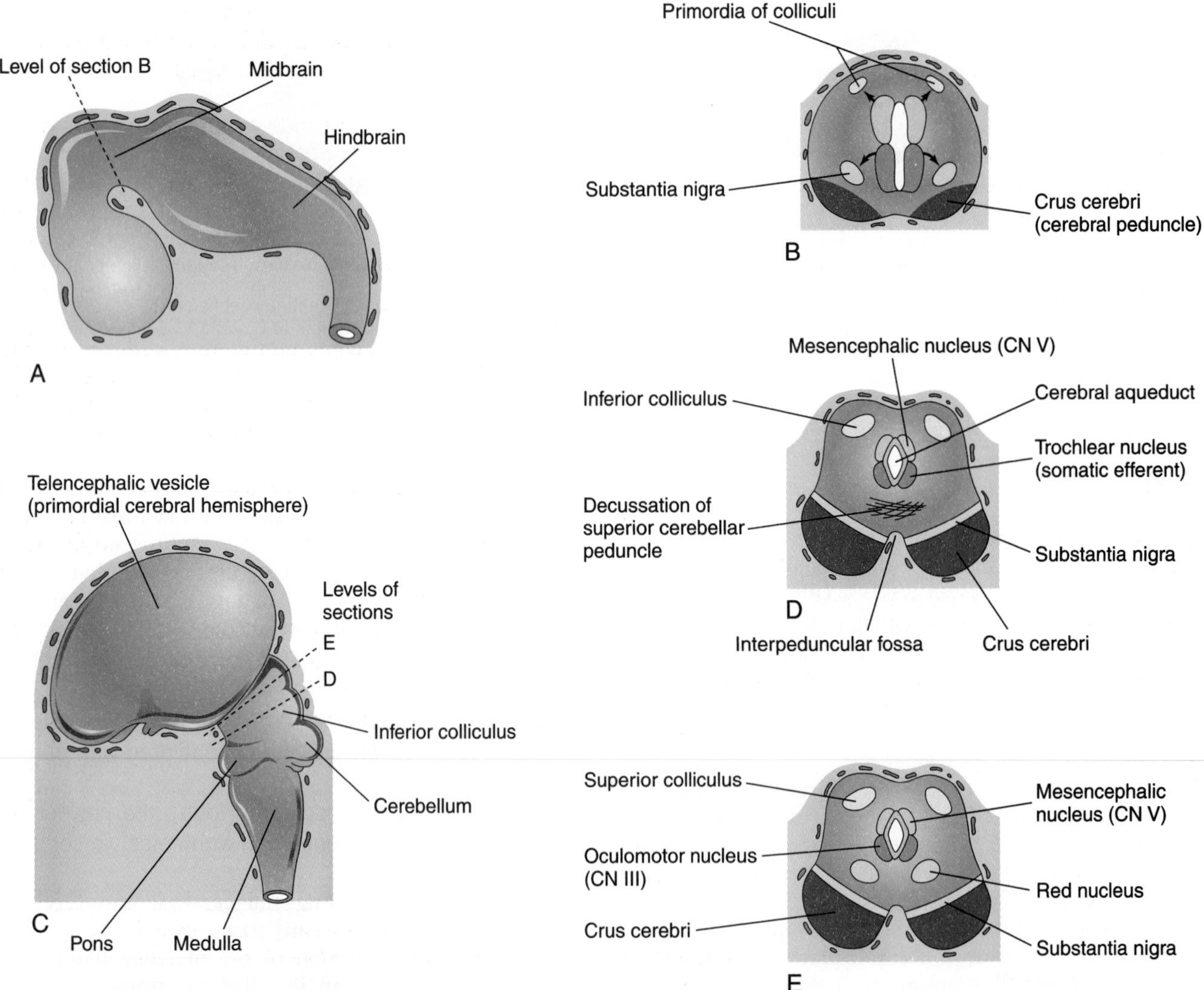

FIGURE 17-23. **A,** Sketch of the developing brain at the end of the fifth week. **B,** Transverse section of the developing midbrain showing the early migration of cells from the basal and alar plates. **C,** Sketch of the developing brain at 11 weeks. **D** and **E,** Transverse sections of the developing midbrain at the level of the inferior and superior colliculi, respectively. CN, cranial nerve.

and inferior colliculi (see Fig. 17-23*A* and *B*), which are concerned with visual and auditory reflexes, respectively. Neuroblasts from the basal plates may give rise to groups of neurons in the **tegmentum of midbrain** (red nuclei, nuclei of third and fourth cranial nerves (CNs), and the reticular nuclei). The **substantia nigra**, a broad layer of gray matter adjacent to the cerebral peduncle (see Fig. 17-23*D* and *E*), may also differentiate from the basal plate, but some authorities believe that it is derived from cells in the alar plate that migrate ventrally. Fibers growing from the cerebrum form the stemlike **cerebral peduncles** anteriorly (see Fig. 17-23*B*). The cerebral peduncles become progressively more prominent as more descending fiber groups (corticopontine, corticobulbar, and corticospinal) pass through the developing midbrain on their way to the **brainstem** and spinal cord.

Forebrain

As closure of the rostral neuropore occurs, two lateral outgrowths—**optic vesicles**—appear (Fig. 17-4*A*), one on each side of the forebrain. The optic vesicles are the *primordia of the retinae and optic nerves* (see Chapter 18). A second pair of diverticula, the **telencephalic vesicles**, soon arise more dorsally and rostrally (see Fig. 17-23*C*). They are the *primordia of the cerebral hemispheres*, and their cavities become the **lateral ventricles** (see Fig. 17-28*B*). The rostral or anterior part of the forebrain, including the primordia of the **cerebral hemispheres**, is the telencephalon, and the caudal or posterior part of the forebrain is the diencephalon. The cavities of the telencephalon and diencephalon contribute to the formation of the **third ventricle**, although the cavity of the diencephalon contributes more.

Diencephalon

Three swellings develop in the lateral walls of the third ventricle, which later become the *thalamus*, *hypothalamus*, and the *epithalamus* (see Fig. 17-24*C* to *E*). The thalamus is separated from the epithalamus by the **epithalamic sulcus** and from the hypothalamus by the **hypothalamic sulcus**. The latter sulcus is not a continuation of the sulcus limitans into the forebrain and does not, like the sulcus limitans, divide sensory and motor areas.

The **thalamus** develops rapidly on each side and bulges into the cavity of the third ventricle, reducing it to a narrow cleft. The thalami meet and fuse in the midline in approximately 70% of brains, forming a bridge of gray matter across the third ventricle—the **interthalamic adhesion**.

The **hypothalamus** arises by proliferation of neuroblasts in the intermediate zone of the diencephalic walls, ventral to the hypothalamic sulci. Later, a number of nuclei concerned with endocrine activities and homeostasis develop. A pair of nuclei, the **mammillary bodies**, form pea-sized swellings on the ventral surface of the hypothalamus (see Fig. 17-24*C*).

The **epithalamus** develops from the roof and dorsal portion of the lateral wall of the diencephalon. Initially, the epithalamic swellings are large, but later they become relatively small.

The **pineal gland** (pineal body) develops as a median diverticulum of the caudal part of the roof of the diencephalon (see Fig. 17-24*C* and *D*). Proliferation of cells in its walls soon converts it into a solid cone-shaped gland.

The **pituitary gland** (L. *hypophysis*) is ectodermal in origin (Fig. 17-25 and Table 17-1). It develops from two sources:

- An upgrowth from the ectodermal roof of the stomodeum, the **hypophysial diverticulum** (Rathke's pouch)
- A downgrowth from the neuroectoderm of the diencephalon, the **neurohypophysial diverticulum**

This double origin explains why the pituitary gland is composed of two completely different types of tissue:

- The **adenohypophysis** (glandular part) or anterior lobe arises from oral ectoderm.
- The **neurohypophysis** (nervous part) or posterior lobe originates from neuroectoderm.

By the third week, the **hypophysial diverticulum** projects from the roof of the stomodeum and lies adjacent to the floor (ventral wall) of the diencephalon (see Fig. 17-25*C*). By the fifth week this diverticulum has elongated and become constricted at its attachment to the oral epithelium, giving it a nipple-like appearance (see Fig. 17-25*C*). By this stage, it has come into contact with the **infundibulum** (derived from the neurohypophysial diverticulum), a ventral downgrowth of the diencephalon (see Figs. 17-24 and 17-25). The stalk of the hypophysial diverticulum regresses.

The parts of the pituitary gland that develop from the ectoderm of the stomodeum—*pars anterior, pars intermedia, and pars tuberalis*—form the **adenohypophysis** (see Table 17-1). The stalk of the hypophysial diverticulum passes between the chondrification centers of the developing presphenoid and basisphenoid bones of the cranium (see Fig. 17-25*E*). During the sixth week, the connection of the diverticulum with the oral cavity degenerates and disappears (see Fig. 17-25*D* and *E*).

Cells of the anterior wall of the hypophysial diverticulum proliferate and give rise to the **pars anterior** of the pituitary gland. Later, an extension, the **pars tuberalis**,

TABLE 17-1. Derivation and Terminology of Pituitary Gland

Origin		Derivative	Parts	Lobe
Oral Ectoderm (Hypophysial diverticulum from roof of stomodeum)	→	Adenohypophysis (glandular portion)	Pars anterior Pars tuberalis	Anterior lobe
			Pars intermedia	
Neuroectoderm (Neurohypophysial diverticulum from floor of diencephalon)	→	Neurohypophysis (nervous portion)	Pars nervosa Infundibular stem Median eminence	Posterior lobe

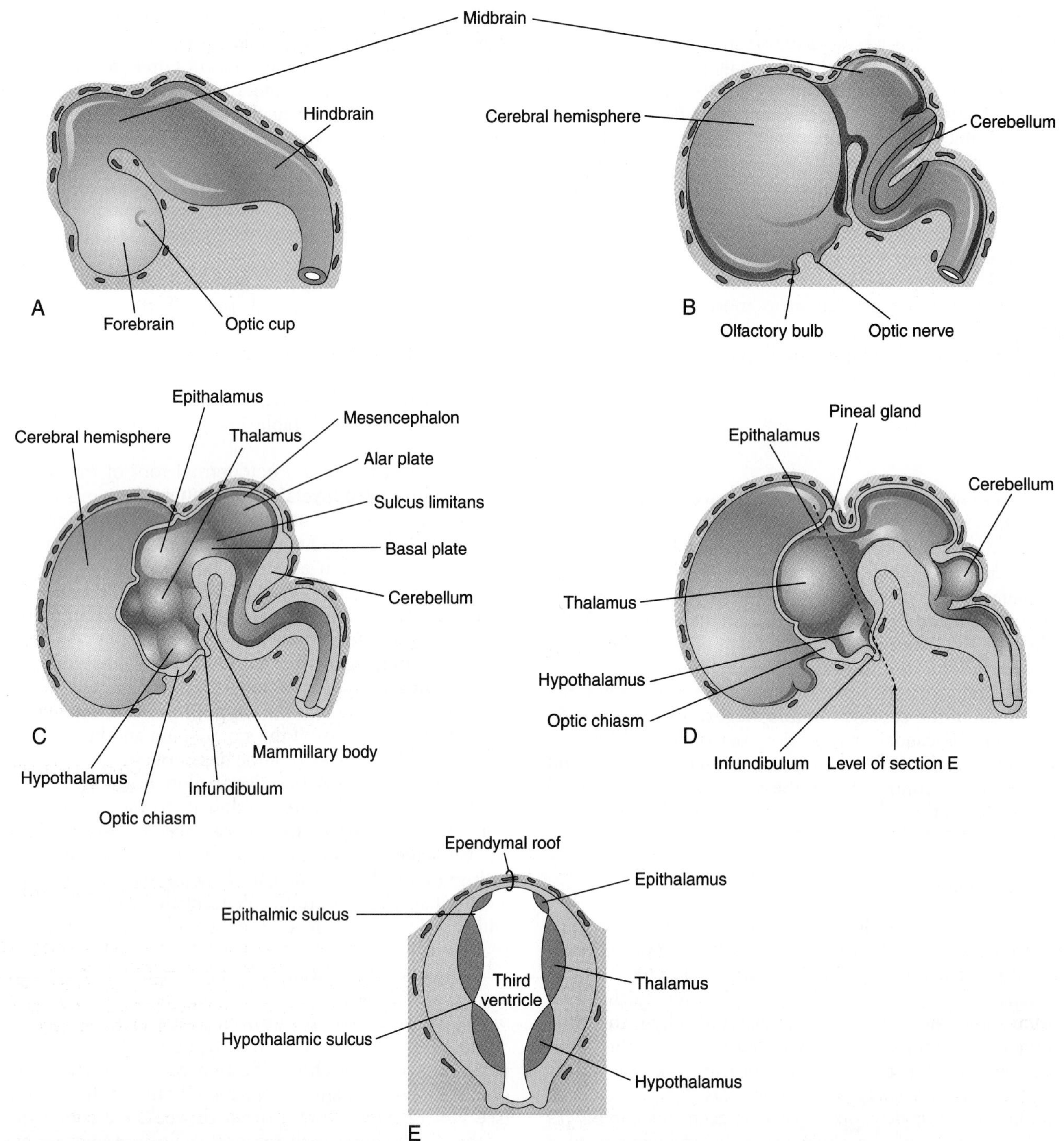

FIGURE 17-24. **A,** External view of the brain at the end of the fifth week. **B,** Similar view at 7 weeks. **C,** Median section of this brain showing the medial surface of the forebrain and midbrain. **D,** Similar section at 8 weeks. **E,** Transverse section of the diencephalon showing the epithalamus dorsally, the thalamus laterally, and the hypothalamus ventrally.

grows around the **infundibular stem** (see Fig. 17-25*E*). The extensive proliferation of the anterior wall of the hypophysial diverticulum reduces its lumen to a narrow cleft (see Fig. 17-25*E*). This residual cleft is usually not recognizable in the adult pituitary gland, but it may be represented by a zone of cysts. Cells in the posterior wall of the hypophysial pouch do not proliferate; they give rise to the thin, poorly defined **pars intermedia** (see Fig. 17-25*F*).

The part of the pituitary gland that develops from the neuroectoderm of the **infundibulum** of the diencephalon is the **neurohypophysis** (see Table 17-1). The infundibulum gives rise to the **median eminence**, **infundibular stem**, and **pars nervosa**. Initially, the walls of the infundibulum are thin, but the distal end of the infundibulum soon becomes solid as the neuroepithelial cells proliferate. These cells later differentiate into **pituicytes**, the primary cells of the posterior lobe of the pituitary gland, which are

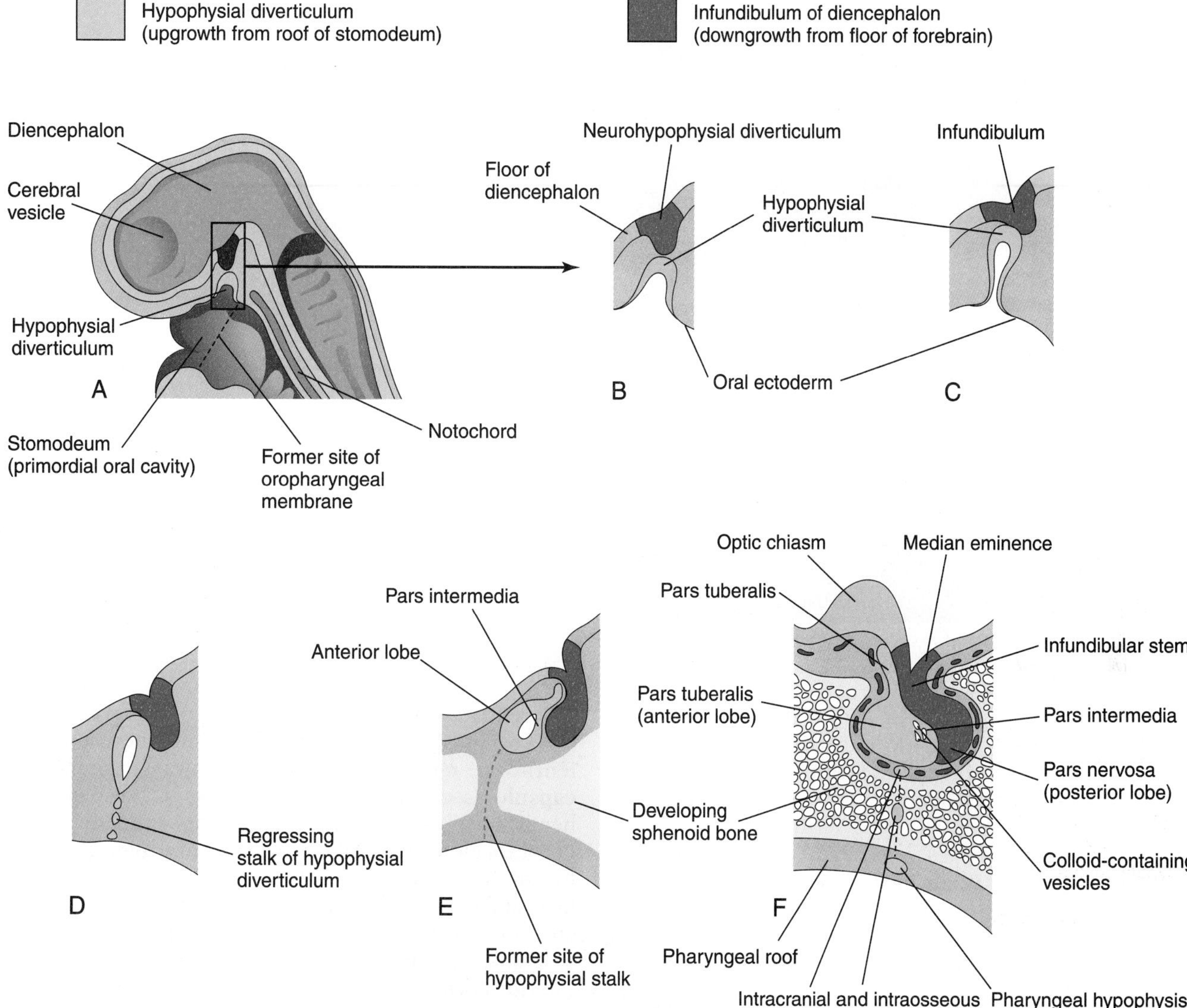

FIGURE 17-25. Diagrammatic sketches illustrating the development of the pituitary gland. **A,** Sagittal section of the cranial end of an embryo of approximately 36 days showing the hypophysial diverticulum, an upgrowth from the stomodeum, and the neurohypophysial diverticulum, a downgrowth from the forebrain. **B** to **D,** Successive stages of the developing pituitary gland. By 8 weeks, the diverticulum loses its connection with the oral cavity and is in close contact with the infundibulum and the posterior lobe (neurohypophysis) of the pituitary gland. **E** and **F,** Later stages showing proliferation of the anterior wall of the hypophysial diverticulum to form the anterior lobe (adenohypophysis) of the pituitary gland.

closely related to neuroglial cells. Nerve fibers grow into the pars nervosa from the hypothalamic area, to which the infundibular stem is attached.

PHARYNGEAL HYPOPHYSIS AND CRANIOPHARYNGIOMA

A remnant of the stalk of the hypophysial diverticulum may persist and form a **pharyngeal hypophysis** in the roof of the oropharynx (see Fig. 17-25*F*). Rarely, masses of anterior lobe tissue develop outside the capsule of the pituitary gland, within the sella turcica of the sphenoid bone. A remnant of the hypophysial diverticulum, the **basipharyngeal canal,** is visible in sections of the newborn sphenoid bone in approximately 1% of cases. It can also be identified in a small number of radiographs of crania of newborn infants (usually those with cranial anomalies). Occasionally a **craniopharyngioma** develops in the pharynx or in the basisphenoid (posterior part of sphenoid) from remnants of the stalk of the hypophysial diverticulum (Fig. 17-26), but most often they form in and/or superior to the sella turcica.

Telencephalon

The telencephalon consists of a median part and two lateral diverticula, the **cerebral vesicles** (see Fig. 17-25*A*). These vesicles are the primordia of the **cerebral**

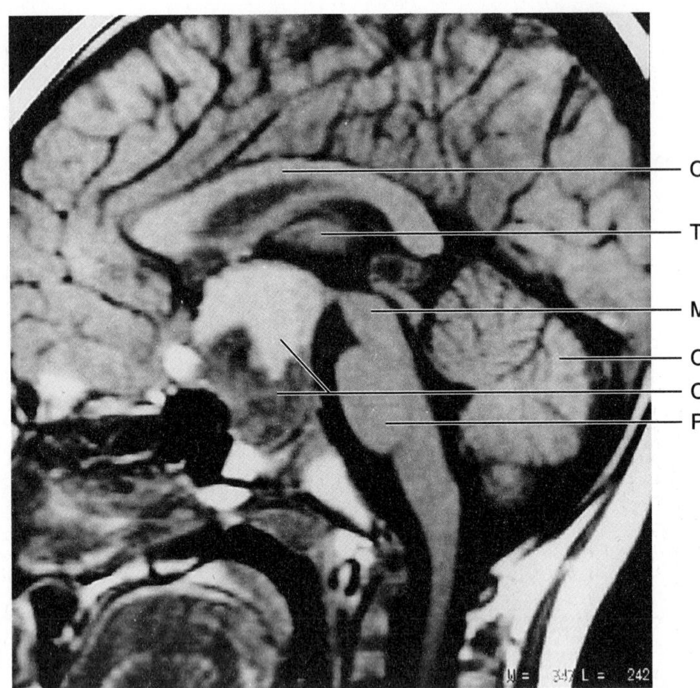

FIGURE 17-26. Sagittal magnetic resonance image of a 4-year-old boy who presented with a headache and optic atrophy. A large mass (4 cm) occupies an enlarged sella turcica, expanding inferiorly into the sphenoid bone and superiorly into the suprasellar cistern. A craniopharyngioma was confirmed by surgery. The inferior half of the mass is solid and appears dark, whereas the superior half is cystic and appears brighter. (Courtesy of Dr. Gerald S. Smyser, Altru Health System, Grand Forks, ND.)

hemispheres (see Figs. 17-24*B* and 17-25*A*). The cavity of the median portion of the telencephalon forms the extreme anterior part of the third ventricle (Fig. 17-27). At first, the cerebral hemispheres are in wide communication with the cavity of the third ventricle through the **interventricular foramina** (Figs. 17-27 and 17-28*B*). Along the **choroid fissure**, part of the medial wall of the developing cerebral hemisphere (see Fig. 17-30*A*), becomes very thin. Initially, this thin ependymal portion lies in the roof of the hemisphere and is continuous with the ependymal roof of the third ventricle (see Fig. 17-28*A*). The **choroid plexus of the lateral ventricle** later forms at this site (Figs. 17-27 and 17-29).

As the cerebral hemispheres expand, they cover successively the diencephalon, midbrain, and hindbrain. The hemispheres eventually meet each other in the midline, flattening their medial surfaces. The mesenchyme trapped in the longitudinal fissure between them gives rise to the **cerebral falx** (L. *falx cerebri*), a median fold of dura mater. The **corpus striatum** appears during the sixth week as a prominent swelling in the floor of each cerebral hemisphere (see Fig. 17-29*B*). The floor of each hemisphere expands more slowly than its thin cortical walls because it contains the rather large corpus striatum; consequently, the cerebral hemispheres become C shaped (Fig. 17-30).

The growth and curvature of the hemispheres also affect the shape of the lateral ventricles. They become roughly C-shaped cavities filled with CSF. The caudal end of each cerebral hemisphere turns ventrally and then rostrally, forming the temporal lobe; in so doing, it carries the lateral ventricle (forming its **temporal horn**) and choroid fissure with it (see Fig. 17-30). Here, the thin medial wall of the hemisphere is invaginated along the choroid fissure by vascular pia mater to form the *choroid plexus of the temporal horn* (see Fig. 17-29*B*). As the cerebral cortex differentiates, fibers passing to and from it pass through the corpus striatum and divide it into the caudate and lentiform nuclei. This fiber pathway—the **internal capsule** (see Fig. 17-29C)—becomes C shaped as the hemisphere assumes this form. The **caudate nucleus** becomes elongated and C shaped, conforming to the outline of the lateral ventricle (see Fig. 17-30). Its pear-shaped head and elongated body lie in the floor of the frontal horn and body of the lateral ventricle, whereas its tail makes a U-shaped turn to gain the roof of the temporal or inferior horn.

Cerebral Commissures

As the cerebral cortex develops, groups of nerve fibers—**commissures**—connect corresponding areas of the cerebral hemispheres with one another (see Fig. 17-29). The most important of these commissures cross in the **lamina terminalis**, the rostral (anterior) end of the forebrain. This lamina extends from the roof plate of the diencephalon to the *optic chiasm* (the decussation or crossing of the fibers of the optic nerve). The lamina is the natural pathway from one hemisphere to the other. The first commissures to form, the *anterior commissure* and *hippocampal commissure*, are small fiber bundles that connect phylogenetically older parts of the brain. The **anterior commissure** connects the olfactory bulb and related areas of one hemisphere with those of the opposite side. The **hippocampal commissure** connects the hippocampal formations.

The largest cerebral commissure is the **corpus callosum** (see Fig. 17-29*A*), connecting neocortical areas. The corpus callosum initially lies in the lamina terminalis, but fibers are added to it as the cortex enlarges; as a result, it gradually extends beyond the lamina terminalis. The rest of the **lamina terminalis** lies between the corpus callosum

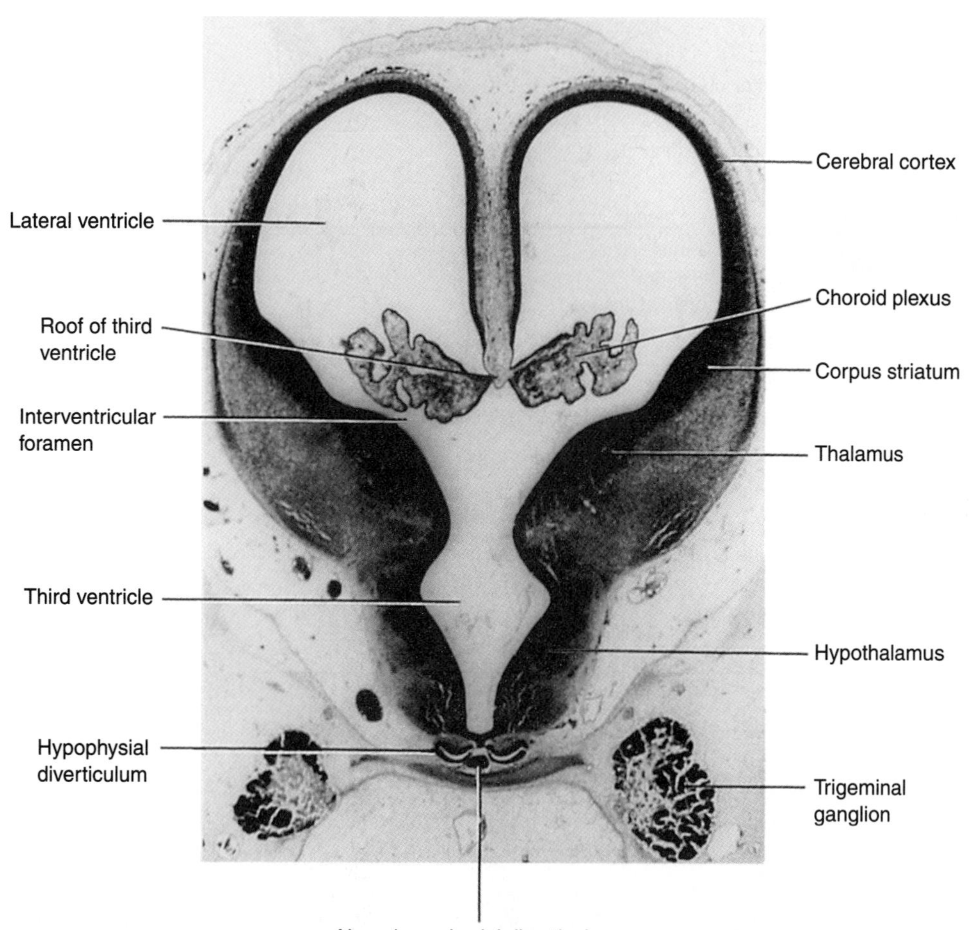

FIGURE 17-27. Photomicrograph of a transverse section through the diencephalon and cerebral vesicles of a human embryo (approximately 50 days) at the level of the interventricular foramina (×20). The choroid fissure is located at the junction of the choroid plexus and the medial wall of the lateral ventricle. (Courtesy of Professor Jean Hay [retired], Department of Anatomy, University of Manitoba, Winnipeg, Manitoba, Canada.)

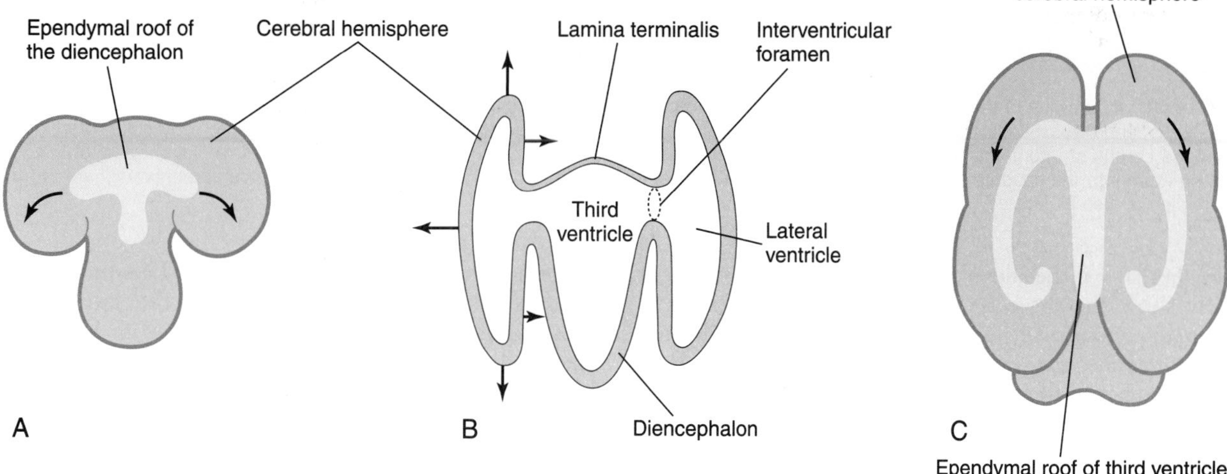

FIGURE 17-28. **A,** Sketch of the dorsal surface of the forebrain indicating how the ependymal roof of the diencephalon is carried out to the dorsomedial surface of the cerebral hemispheres. **B,** Diagrammatic section of the forebrain showing how the developing cerebral hemispheres grow from the lateral walls of the forebrain and expand in all directions until they cover the diencephalon. The *arrows* indicate some directions in which the hemispheres expand. The rostral wall of the forebrain, the lamina terminalis, is very thin. **C,** Sketch of the forebrain showing how the ependymal roof is finally carried into the temporal lobes as a result of the C-shaped growth pattern of the cerebral hemispheres.

and the fornix. It becomes stretched to form the thin *septum pellucidum*, a thin plate of brain tissue.

At birth, the corpus callosum extends over the roof of the diencephalon. The optic chiasm (L., Greek [Gr], *chiasma*), which develops in the ventral part of the lamina terminalis (see Fig. 17-29*A*), consists of fibers from the medial halves of the retinae, which cross to join the optic tract of the opposite side.

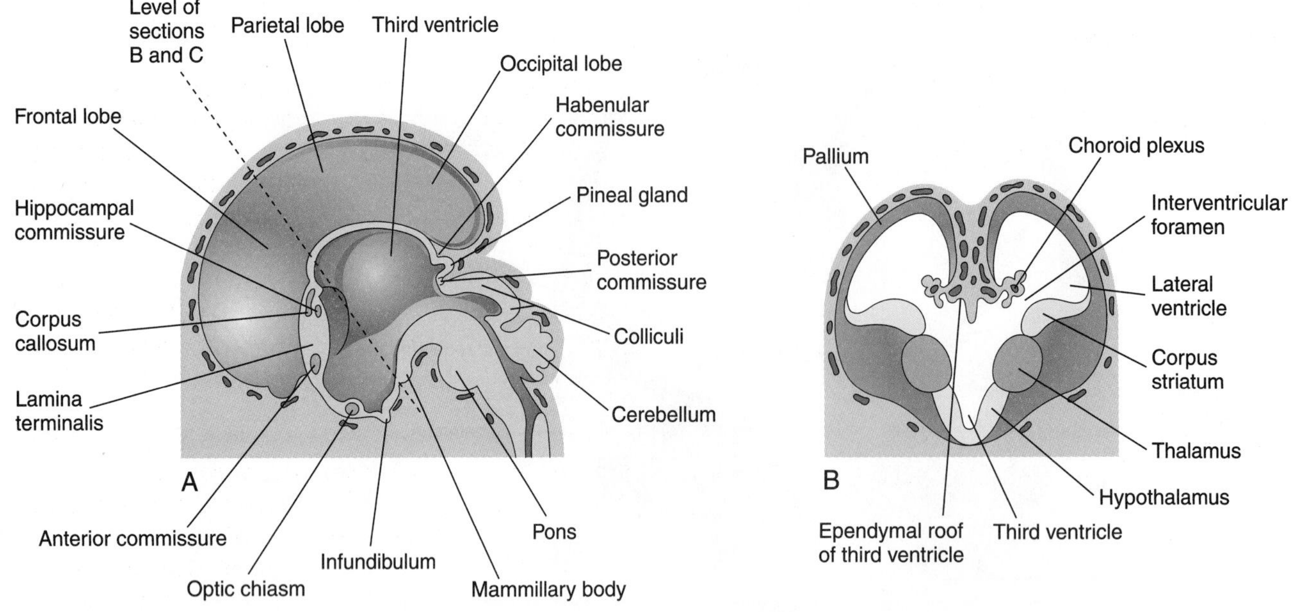

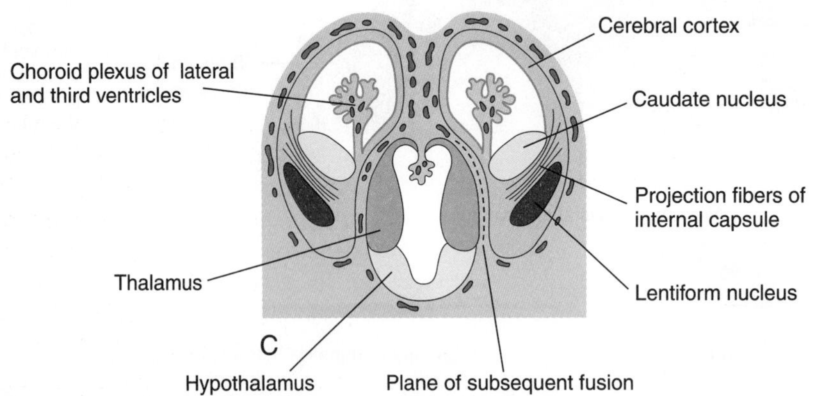

FIGURE 17-29. **A,** Drawing of the medial surface of the forebrain of a 10-week embryo showing the diencephalic derivatives, the main commissures, and the expanding cerebral hemispheres. **B,** Transverse section of the forebrain at the level of the interventricular foramina showing the corpus striatum and choroid plexuses of the lateral ventricles. **C,** Similar section at approximately 11 weeks showing division of the corpus striatum into the caudate and lentiform nuclei by the internal capsule. The developing relationship of the cerebral hemispheres to the diencephalon is also illustrated.

The walls of the developing cerebral hemispheres initially show the three typical zones of the neural tube (*ventricular*, *intermediate*, and *marginal*); later a fourth one, the *subventricular zone*, appears. Cells of the intermediate zone migrate into the marginal zone and give rise to the cortical layers. The gray matter is thus located peripherally, and axons from its cell bodies pass centrally to form the large volume of white matter—the **medullary center**.

Initially, the surface of the cerebral hemispheres is smooth (Fig. 17-31*A*); however, as growth proceeds, sulci (grooves or furrows between the gyri) and gyri (tortuous convolutions) develop (see Figs. 17-31*B* and *C*). The gyri are caused by infolding of the cerebral cortex. The sulci and gyri permit a considerable increase in the surface area of the cerebral cortex without requiring an extensive increase in cranial size (Fig. 17-32*B* and *C*). As each cerebral hemisphere grows, the cortex covering the external surface of the corpus striatum grows relatively slowly and is soon overgrown (see Fig. 17-31*D*). This buried cortex, hidden from view in the depths of the **lateral sulcus** (fissure) of the cerebral hemisphere (see Fig. 17-32), is the **insula** (L. *island*).

CONGENITAL ANOMALIES OF THE BRAIN

Because of the complexity of its embryologic history, abnormal development of the brain is common (approximately three per 1000 births). Most major congenital anomalies of the brain, such as **meroencephaly** (anencephaly) and meningoencephalocele, result from *defective closure of the rostral neuropore* (NTDs) during the fourth week (Fig. 17-33*C*) and involve the overlying tissues (meninges and calvaria). The factors causing NTDs are genetic, nutritional, and/or environmental in nature. Congenital anomalies of the brain can be caused by

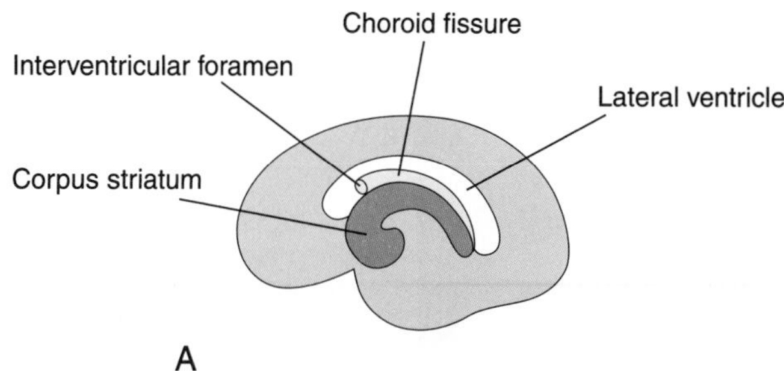

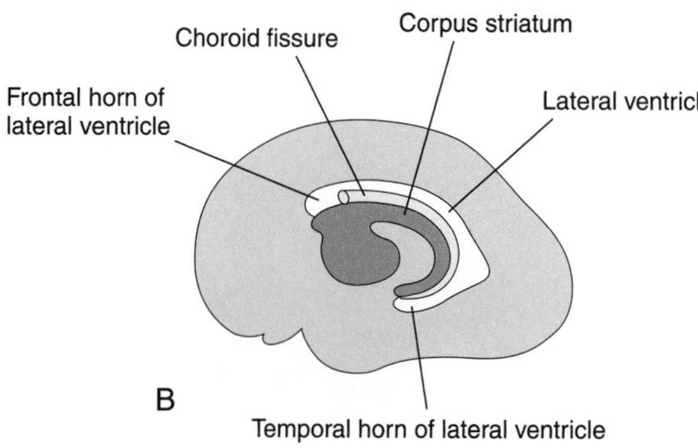

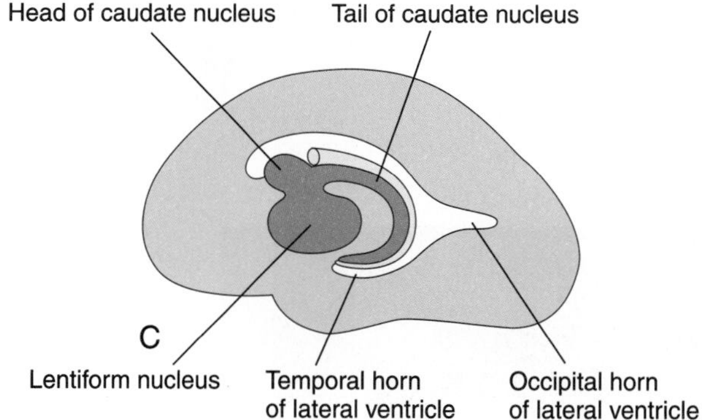

FIGURE 17-30. Schematic diagrams of the medial surface of the developing right cerebral hemisphere showing the development of the lateral ventricle, choroid fissure, and corpus striatum. **A,** At 13 weeks. **B,** At 21 weeks. **C,** At 32 weeks.

alterations in the morphogenesis or the histogenesis of the nervous tissue or can result from developmental failures occurring in associated structures (notochord, somites, mesenchyme, and cranium). **Abnormal histogenesis of the cerebral cortex** can result in seizures (Fig. 17-34) and various types of mental retardation. Subnormal intellectual development may result from exposure of the embryo/fetus during the 8- to 16-week period to certain viruses and high levels of radiation (see Chapter 20). Prenatal factors (e.g., risk factors include maternal infection or thyroid disorder, Rh factor incompatibility, some hereditary and genetic conditions) result in the majority of cases of **cerebral palsy**; however, this central motor deficit may result from events during birth (perinatal). In other cases, the deficit may occur postnatally (e.g., risk factors include severe neonatal jaundice).

CRANIUM BIFIDUM

Defects in the formation of the cranium (cranium bifidum) are often associated with congenital anomalies of the brain and/or meninges. Defects of the cranium are usually in the median plane of the calvaria (see Fig. 17-33*A*). The defect is often in the squamous part of the occipital bone and may include the posterior part of the foramen magnum. When the defect is small, usually only the meninges herniate and the anomaly is a **cranial meningocele**, or cranium bifidum with meningocele (see Fig. 17-33*B*).

Cranium bifidum associated with herniation of the brain and/or its meninges occurs approximately once in every 2000 births. When the cranial defect is large, the meninges and part of the brain herniate, forming a **meningoencephalocele** (see Figs. 17-33*C* and 17-35). If the protruding brain contains part of the ventricular system, the anomaly is a **meningohydroencephalocele** (see Fig. 17-33*D*).

EXENCEPHALY AND MEROENCEPHALY

Meroencephaly (anencephaly) is a severe anomaly of the brain that results from failure of the rostral neuropore to close during the fourth week. As a result, the forebrain primordium is abnormal and development of the calvaria is defective (see Figs. 17-19, 17-36, and 17-37). Most of the embryo's brain is exposed or extruding from the cranium—**exencephaly**. Because of the abnormal structure and vascularization of the embryonic exencephalic brain, the nervous tissue undergoes degeneration. The remains of the brain appear as a spongy, vascular mass consisting mostly of hindbrain structures. Although this NTD is often called **anencephaly** (Gr. *an*, without, + *enkephalos*, brain), a rudimentary brainstem and functioning neural tissue are always present in living infants. For this reason, meroencephaly (Gr. *meros*, part) is the better term for this anomaly.

Meroencephaly is a common lethal anomaly, occurring at least once in every 1000 births. It is two to four times more common in females than in males. It is always associated with **acrania** (absence of the calvaria) and may be associated with **rachischisis** when defective neural tube closure is extensive (see Figs. 17-13 and 17-37). Meroencephaly is the most common serious anomaly seen in stillborn fetuses. Infants with this severe NTD may survive after birth, but only for a short period. Meroencephaly is suspected in utero when there is an elevated level of AFP in the amniotic fluid (see Chapter 6). Meroencephaly can

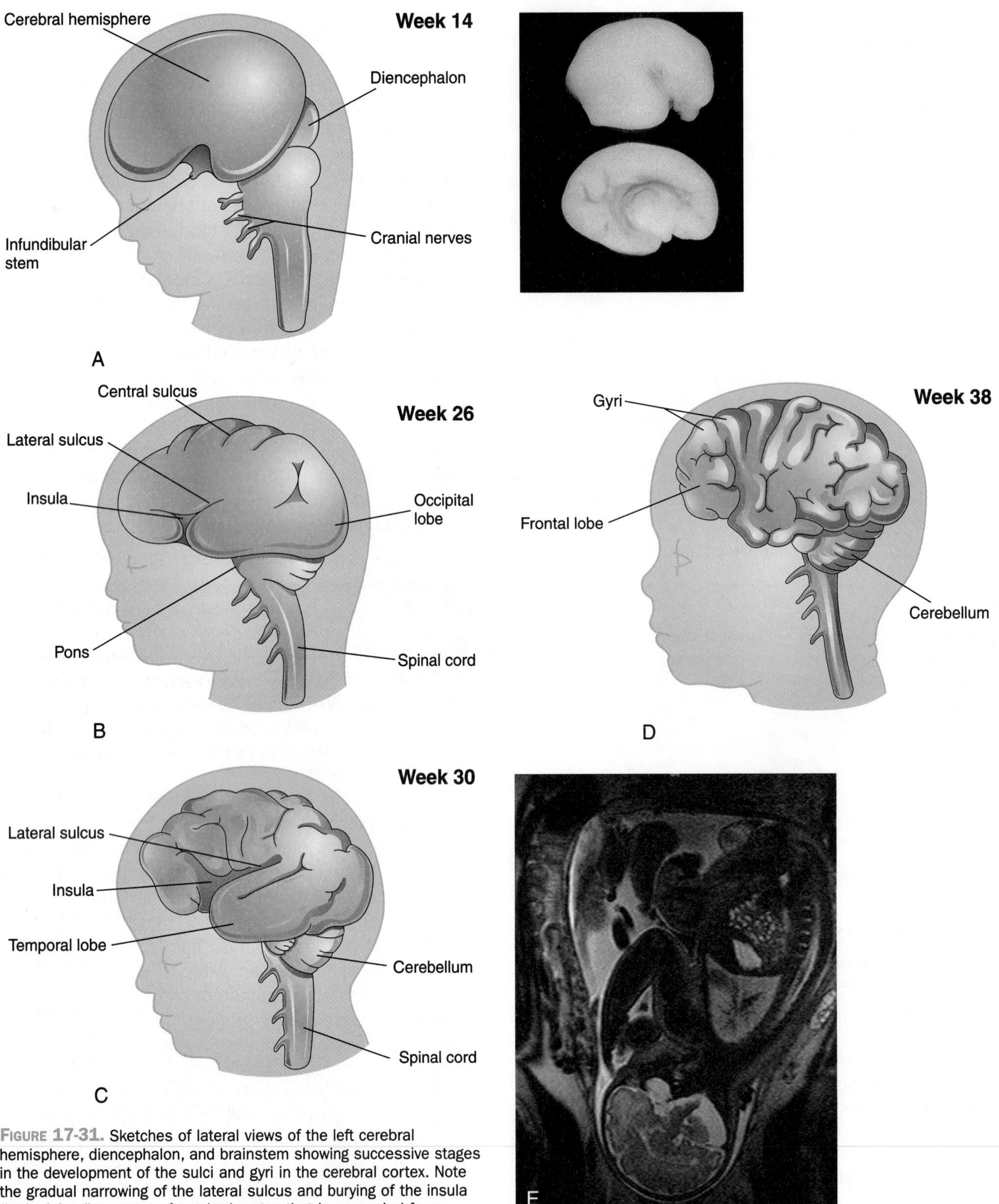

FIGURE 17-31. Sketches of lateral views of the left cerebral hemisphere, diencephalon, and brainstem showing successive stages in the development of the sulci and gyri in the cerebral cortex. Note the gradual narrowing of the lateral sulcus and burying of the insula (Latin, island), an area of cerebral cortex that is concealed from surface view. Note that the surface of the cerebral hemispheres grows rapidly during the fetal period, forming many gyri (convolutions), which are separated by many sulci (grooves). **A,** At 14 weeks. **B,** At 26 weeks. **C,** At 30 weeks. **D,** At 38 weeks. **E,** Magnetic resonance image (MRI) of a pregnant woman showing a mature fetus. Observe the brain and spinal cord. **Inset,** The smooth lateral (top) and medial (bottom) surfaces of a human fetal brain (14 weeks). (**Inset,** Courtesy of Dr. Marc Del Bigio, Department of Pathology [Neuropathology], University of Manitoba, Winnipeg, Manitoba, Canada. **E,** Courtesy of Dr. Stuart C. Morrison, Division of Radiology [Pediatric Radiology], The Children's Hospital, Cleveland, Ohio.)

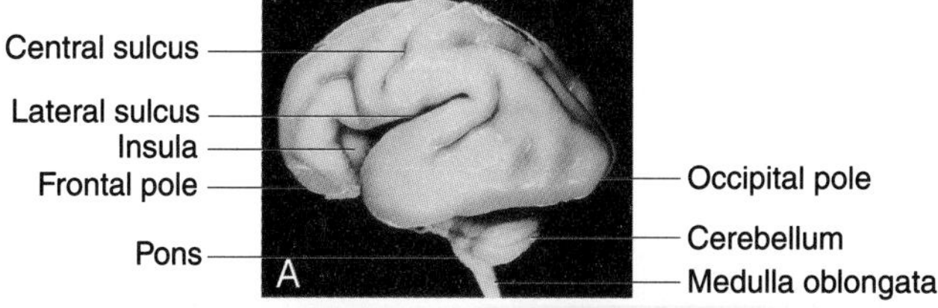

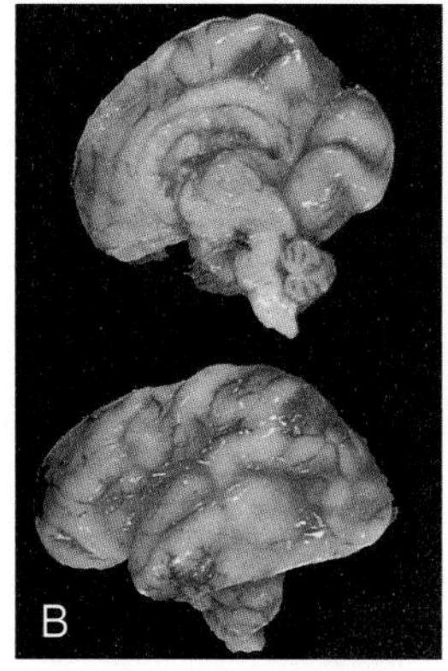

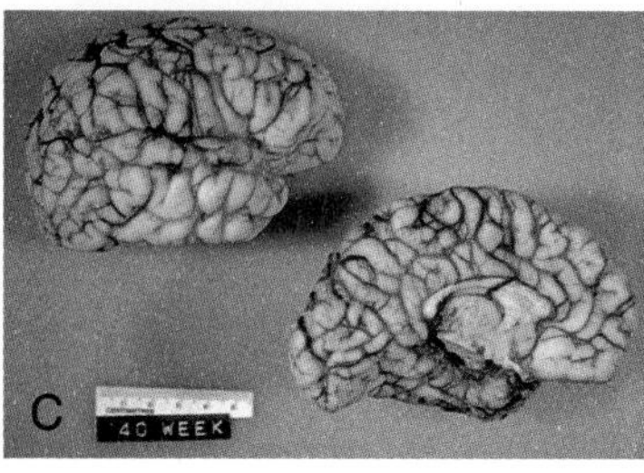

FIGURE 17-32. **A,** Lateral view of the brain of a stillborn fetus (25 weeks). **B,** The medial (top) and lateral (bottom) surfaces of the fetal brain (week 25). **C,** The lateral (top) and medial (bottom) surfaces of the fetal brain (week 38). Note that as the brain enlarges, the gyral pattern of the cerebral hemispheres becomes more complex; compare with Figure 17-31. (**A,** From Nishimura H, Semba R, Tanimura T, Tanaka O: Prenatal Development of the Human with Special Reference to Craniofacial Structures: An Atlas. U.S. Department of Health, Education, and Welfare, National Institutes of Health, Bethesda, 1977. **B** and **C,** Courtesy of Dr. Marc Del Bigio, Department of Pathology [Neuropathology], University of Manitoba, Winnipeg, Manitoba, Canada.)

be easily diagnosed by ultrasonography and MRI (see Fig. 17-37), fetoscopy, and radiography because extensive parts of the brain and calvaria are absent.

Meroencephaly usually has a multifactorial inheritance. An excess of amniotic fluid (*polyhydramnios*) is often associated with meroencephaly, possibly because the fetus lacks the neural control for swallowing amniotic fluid; thus, the fluid does not pass into the intestines for absorption and subsequent transfer to the placenta for disposal.

MICROCEPHALY

In this uncommon condition, the calvaria and brain are small, but the face is normal size (Fig. 17-38). These infants are grossly mentally retarded because the brain is underdeveloped. Microcephaly is the result of microencephaly because growth of the calvaria is largely the result of pressure from the growing brain.

The cause of microcephaly is often uncertain. Some cases appear to be genetic in origin (autosomal recessive), and others are caused by environmental factors. Exposure to large amounts of ionizing radiation, infectious agents (e.g., cytomegalovirus, rubella virus, and *Toxoplasma gondii* [see Chapter 20]), and certain drugs (maternal alcohol abuse) during the fetal period are contributing factors in some cases.

Microcephaly can be detected in utero by ultrasound scans carried out over the period of gestation. A small head may result from **premature synostosis** (osseous union) of all the cranial sutures (see Chapter 14); however, the calvaria is thin with exaggerated convolutional markings.

AGENESIS OF THE CORPUS CALLOSUM

In this condition, there is a complete or partial **absence of the corpus callosum**, the main neocortical commissure of the cerebral hemispheres (Fig. 17-39*A* and *B*). The condition may be asymptomatic, but seizures and mental deficiency are common. A published paper reported that in two sisters with agenesis of the corpus callosum, the only symptoms were seizures, recurrent in one but only occasional and minor in the other. Their IQs were average. Agenesis of the corpus callosum is associated with more than 50 different human congenital syndromes.

HYDROCEPHALUS

Significant **enlargement of the head** usually results from an imbalance between the production and absorption of CSF; as a result, there is an excess of CSF in the ventricular system of the brain (Fig. 17-40). Hydrocephalus results from impaired circulation and absorption of CSF and, in rare cases, from increased production of CSF by a **choroid plexus adenoma**. Impaired circulation of CSF often results from **congenital aqueductal stenosis** (see Figs. 17-40 and 17-41). The cerebral aqueduct is narrow or consists of several minute channels. In a few cases, aqueductal stenosis is transmitted by an X-linked recessive trait, but most cases appear to result from a fetal viral infection (e.g., cytomegalovirus or *Toxoplasma gondii* [see Chapter 20]) or prematurity associated with intraventricular hemorrhage. Blood in the subarachnoid space may cause obliteration of the cisterns or arachnoid villi.

Blockage of CSF circulation results in dilation of the ventricles proximal to the obstruction, internal

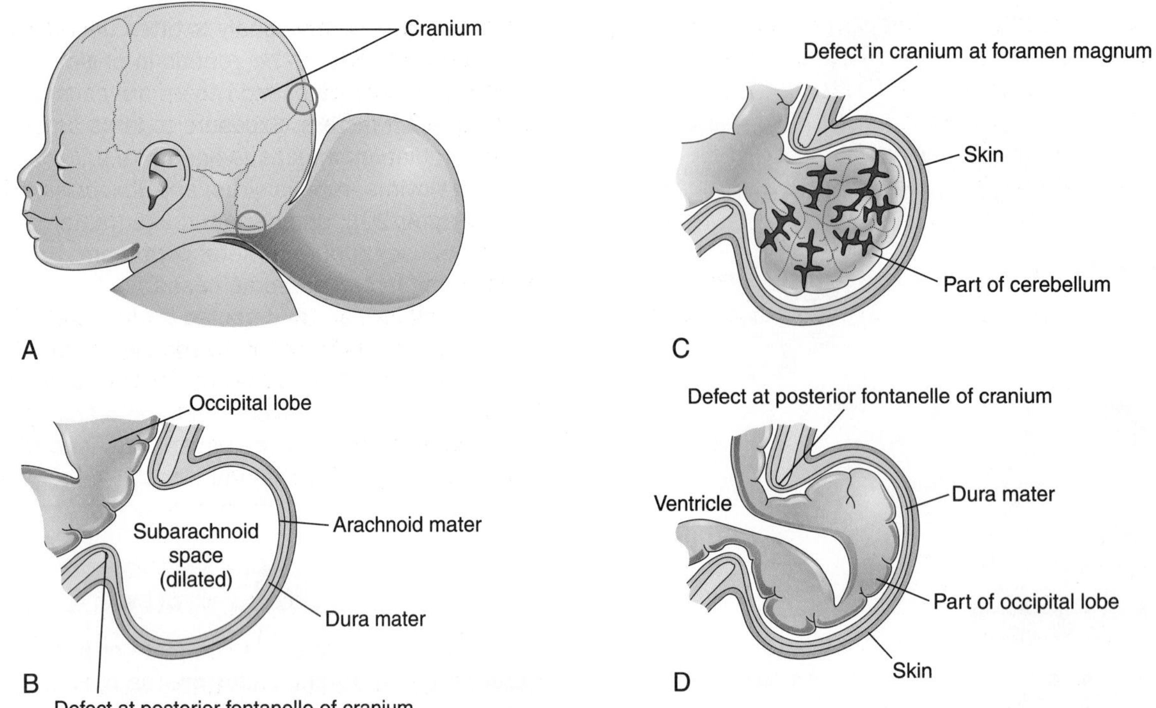

FIGURE 17-33. Schematic drawings illustrating cranium bifidum (bony defect in cranium) and various types of herniation of the brain and/or meninges. **A,** Sketch of the head of a newborn infant with a large protrusion from the occipital region of the cranium. The *upper red circle* indicates a cranial defect at the posterior fontanelle. The *lower red circle* indicates a cranial defect near the foramen magnum. **B,** Meningocele consisting of a protrusion of the cranial meninges that is filled with cerebrospinal fluid (CSF). **C,** Meningoencephalocele consisting of a protrusion of part of the cerebellum that is covered by meninges and skin. **D,** Meningohydroencephalocele consisting of a protrusion of part of the occipital lobe that contains part of the posterior horn of a lateral ventricle.

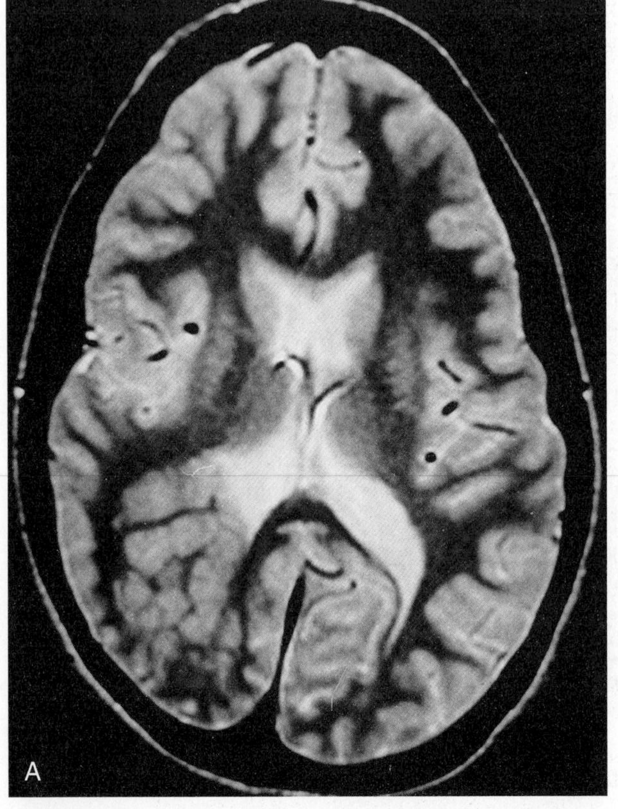

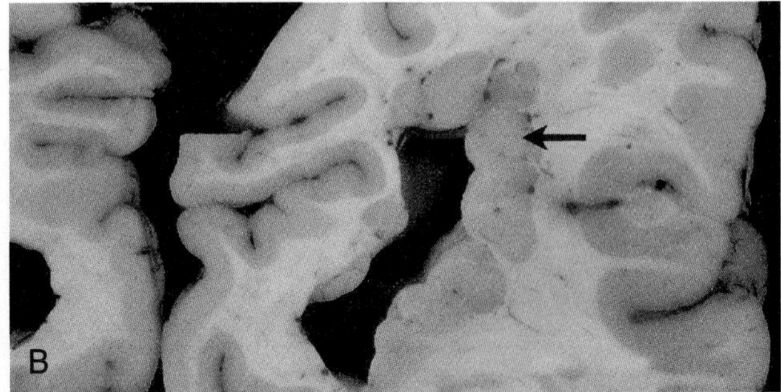

FIGURE 17-34. **A,** Focal heterotopic cerebral cortex. Magnetic resonance image of a 19-year-old woman with seizures showing a focal heterotopic cortex of the right parietal lobe, indenting the right lateral ventricle; note the lack of organized cortex at the overlying surface of the brain. Heterotopic cortex is the result of an arrest of centrifugal migration of neuroblasts along the radial processes of glial cells. **B,** A coronal section of an adult brain with periventricular heterotopia (*arrow*) in the parietal cerebrum. The lobulated gray matter structures along the ventricle represent cells that failed to migrate but nevertheless differentiated into neurons. (**A,** Courtesy of Dr. Gerald Smyser, Altru Health System, Grand Forks, ND. **B,** Courtesy of Dr. Marc R. Del Bigio, Department of Pathology [Neuropathology], University of Manitoba, Winnipeg, Manitoba, Canada.)

accumulation of CSF, and pressure on the cerebral hemispheres (see Fig. 17-41). This squeezes the brain between the ventricular fluid and the cranium. In infants, the internal pressure results in an accelerated rate of expansion of the brain and cranium because most of the fibrous sutures are not fused. Hydrocephalus usually refers to **obstructive or noncommunicating hydrocephalus**, in which all or part of the ventricular system is enlarged. All ventricles are enlarged if the apertures of the fourth ventricle or the subarachnoid spaces are blocked, whereas the lateral and third ventricles are dilated when only the **cerebral aqueduct** is obstructed (see Fig. 17-41). Obstruction of an interventricular foramen can produce dilation of one ventricle.

Hydrocephalus resulting from obliteration of the subarachnoid cisterns or malfunction of the arachnoid villi is called **nonobstructive or communicating hydrocephalus**. Although hydrocephalus may be associated with spina bifida cystica, enlargement of the head may not be obvious at birth. Hydrocephalus often produces thinning of the bones of the calvaria, prominence of the forehead, atrophy of the cerebral cortex and white matter (see Fig. 17-40*B* and *C*), and compression of the basal ganglia and diencephalon.

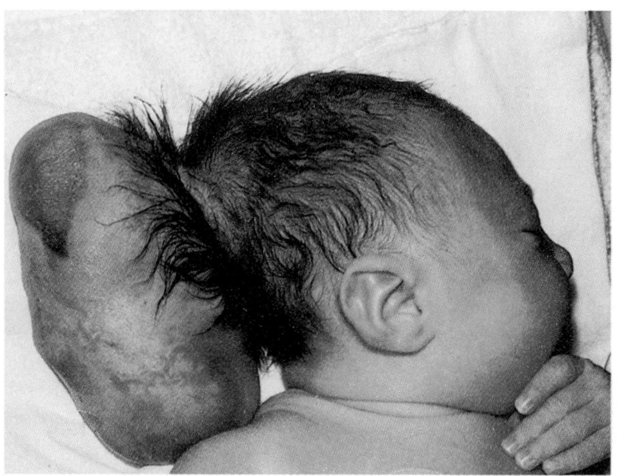

FIGURE 17-35. An infant with a large meningoencephalocele in the occipital area. (Courtesy of A.E. Chudley, MD, Section of Genetics and Metabolism, Department of Pediatrics and Child Health, Children's Hospital and University of Manitoba, Winnipeg, Manitoba, Canada.)

HOLOPROSENCEPHALY

Genetic and environmental factors have been implicated in this severe and relatively common developmental defect (Fig. 17-42). Maternal diabetes and teratogens, such as high doses of alcohol, can destroy embryonic cells in the median plane of the embryonic disc during the third week, producing a wide range of birth defects resulting from defective formation of the forebrain. The infants have a small forebrain, and the lateral ventricles often merge to form one large ventricle.

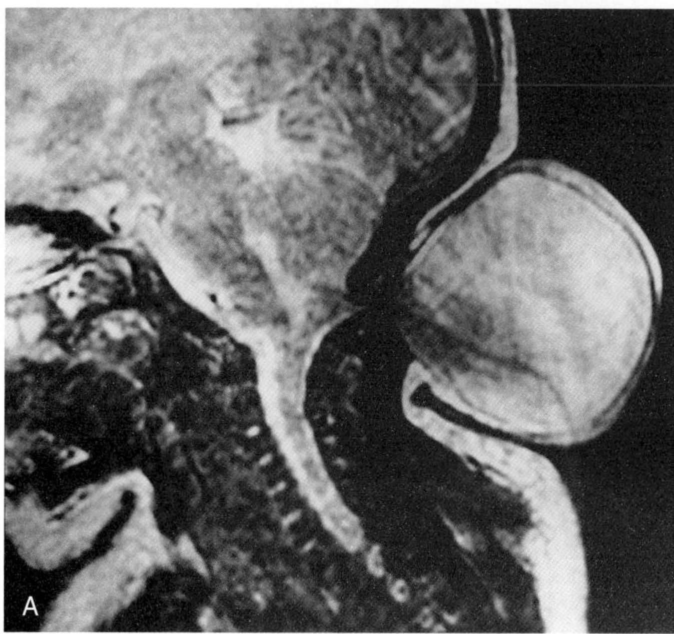

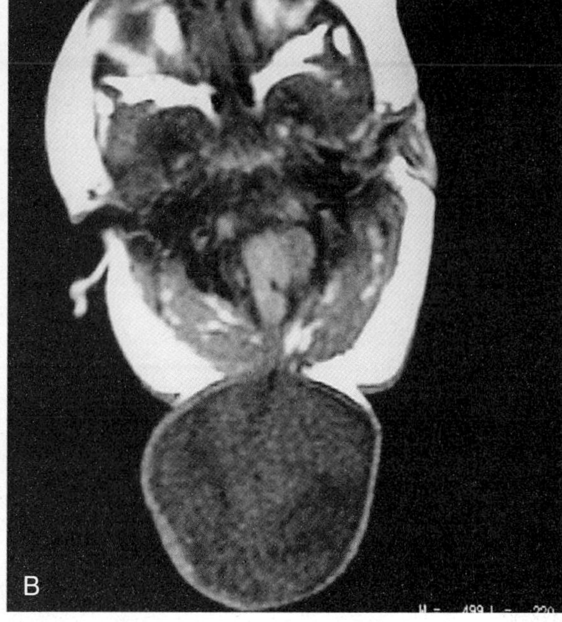

FIGURE 17-36. Magnetic resonance images (MRIs) of a 1-day-old infant. **A,** Sagittal MRI taken so that the cerebrospinal fluid (CSF) is bright. The image is blurred because of movement of the infant. **B,** Axial image located at the cranial defect near the foramen magnum and taken so that CSF appears dark. (Compare with Figure 17-33*C*.) (Courtesy of Dr. Gerald S. Smyser, Altru Health System, Grand Forks, ND.)

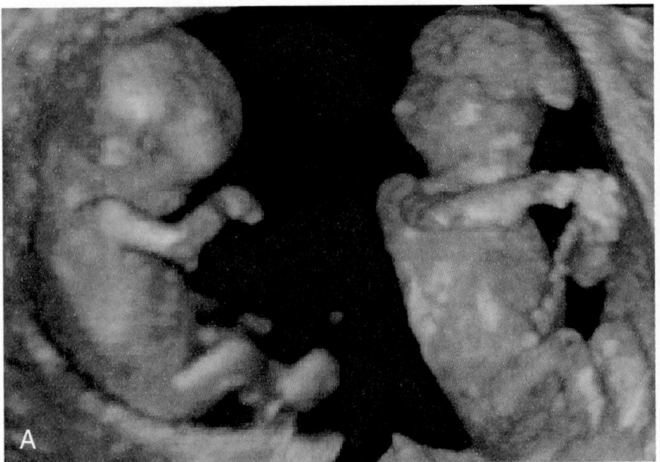

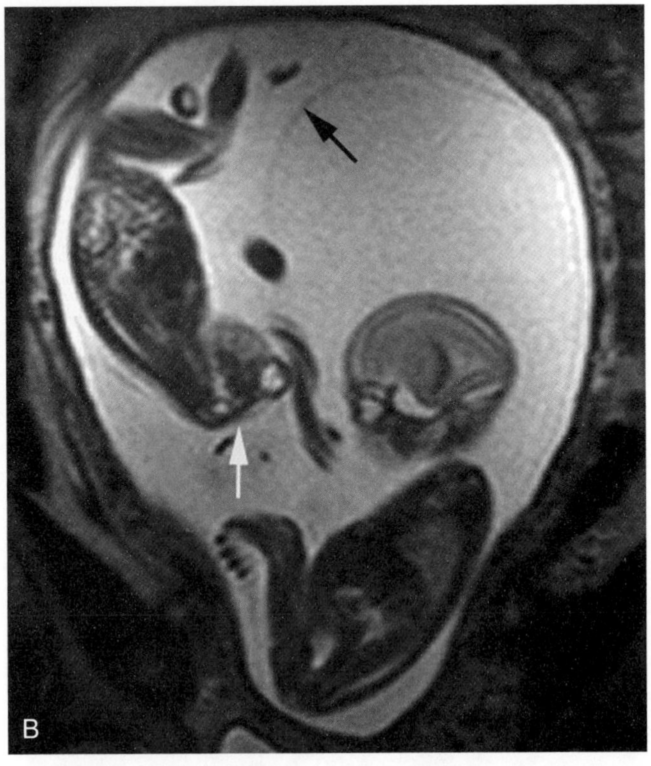

FIGURE 17-37. **A,** Sonogram of a normal fetus at 12 weeks' gestation (*left*) and a fetus at 14 weeks' gestation showing acrania and meroencephaly (*right*). **B,** Magnetic resonance image (MRI) of diamniotic-monochorionic twins, one with meroencephaly. Note the absent calvarium (*white arrow*) of the abnormal twin and the amnion of the normal twin (*black arrow*). (**A,** From Pooh RK, Pooh KH: Transvaginal 3D and Doppler ultrasonography of the fetal brain. Semin Perinatol 25:38, 2001. **B,** Courtesy of Deborah Levine, MD, Director of Obstetric and Gynecologic Ultrasound, Beth Israel Deaconess Medical Center, Boston, MA.)

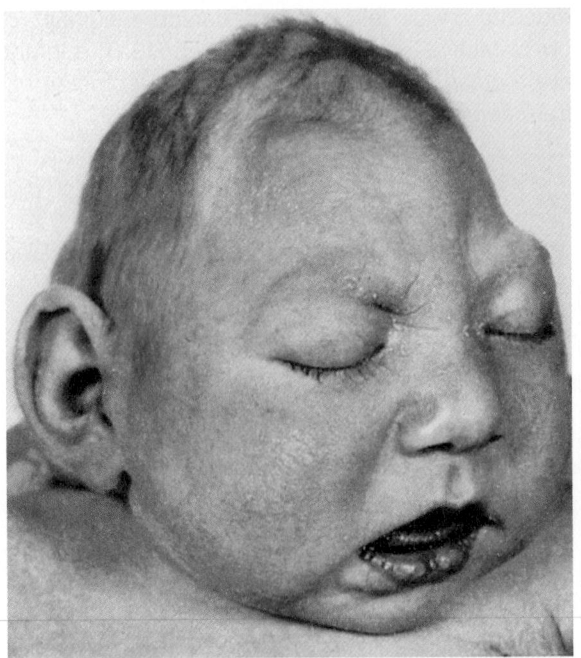

FIGURE 17-38. An infant with microcephaly showing the typical normal-sized face and small calvaria. (From Laurence KM, Weeks R: Abnormalities of the central nervous system. In Norman AP [ed]: Congenital Abnormalities in Infancy, 2nd ed. Cambridge, MA, Blackwell Scientific, 1971. Courtesy of Blackwell Scientific Publications.)

Defects in forebrain development often cause facial anomalies resulting from a reduction in tissue in the frontonasal prominence (see Chapter 9). **Holoprosencephaly** is often indicated when the eyes are abnormally close together (*hypotelorism*). Molecular studies have led to the identification of several holoprosencephaly-related genes, including sonic hedgehog (Shh).

HYDRANENCEPHALY

In this extremely rare anomaly (Fig. 17-43), the cerebral hemispheres are absent or represented by membranous sacs with remnants of the cerebral cortex dispersed over the membranes. The brainstem (midbrain, pons, and medulla) is relatively intact. These infants generally appear normal at birth; however, the head grows excessively after birth because of the accumulation of CSF. A **ventriculoperitoneal shunt** is usually made to prevent further enlargement of the calvaria. Mental development fails to occur, and there is little or no cognitive development. The cause of this unusual, severe anomaly is uncertain; however, there is evidence that it may be the result of an early obstruction of blood flow to the areas supplied by the internal carotid arteries.

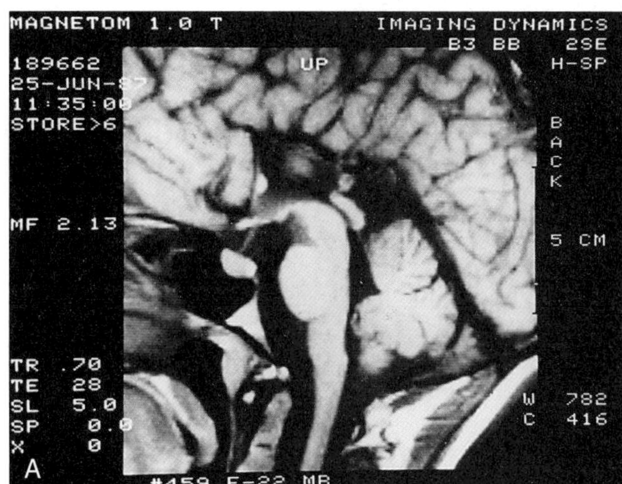

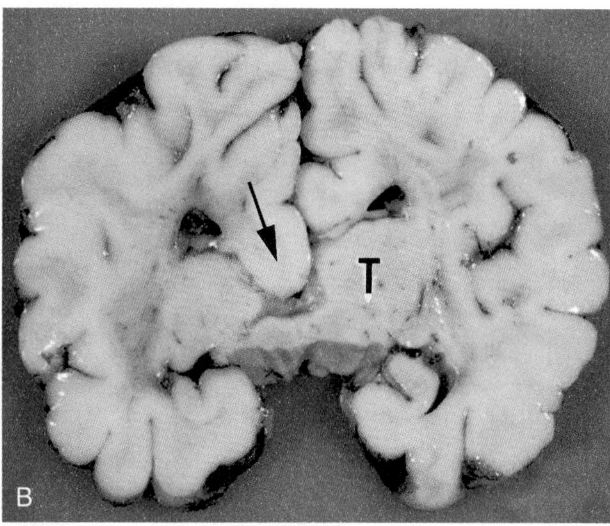

FIGURE 17-39. **A,** Sagittal magnetic resonance imaging of the brain of a 22-year-old woman with normal mentation and motor function. There is complete absence of the corpus callosum. **B,** A coronal slice through a child's brain showing agenesis of the corpus callosum, which would normally cross the midline to connect the two cerebral hemispheres. Note the thalamus (T) and the downward displacement of the cingulum into the lateral and third ventricles (*arrow*). (**A,** Courtesy of Dr. Gerald S. Smyser, Altru Health System, Grand Forks, ND. **B,** Courtesy of Dr. Marc R. Del Bigio, Department of Pathology [Neuropathology], University of Manitoba, Winnipeg, Manitoba, Canada.)

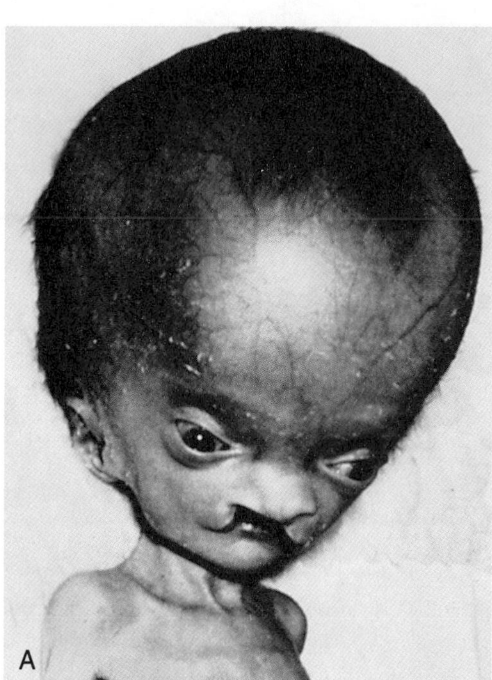

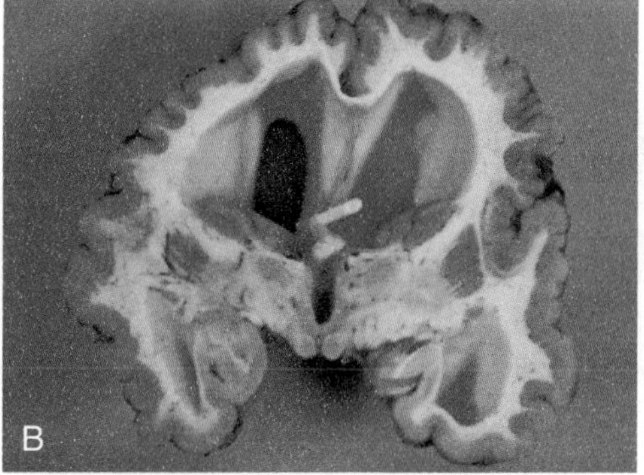

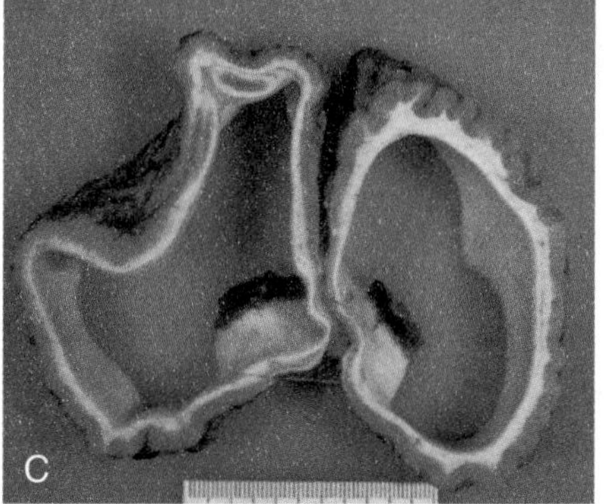

FIGURE 17-40. **A,** An infant with hydrocephalus and bilateral cleft palate. **B** and **C,** The brain of a 10-year-old child who had developed hydrocephalus in utero as a result of aqueductal stenosis. The thin white matter is well myelinated. A shunt tube meant to treat the hydrocephalus lies in the frontal horn of the ventricle. (Courtesy of Dr. Marc R. Del Bigio, Department of Pathology [Neuropathology], University of Manitoba, Winnipeg, Manitoba, Canada.)

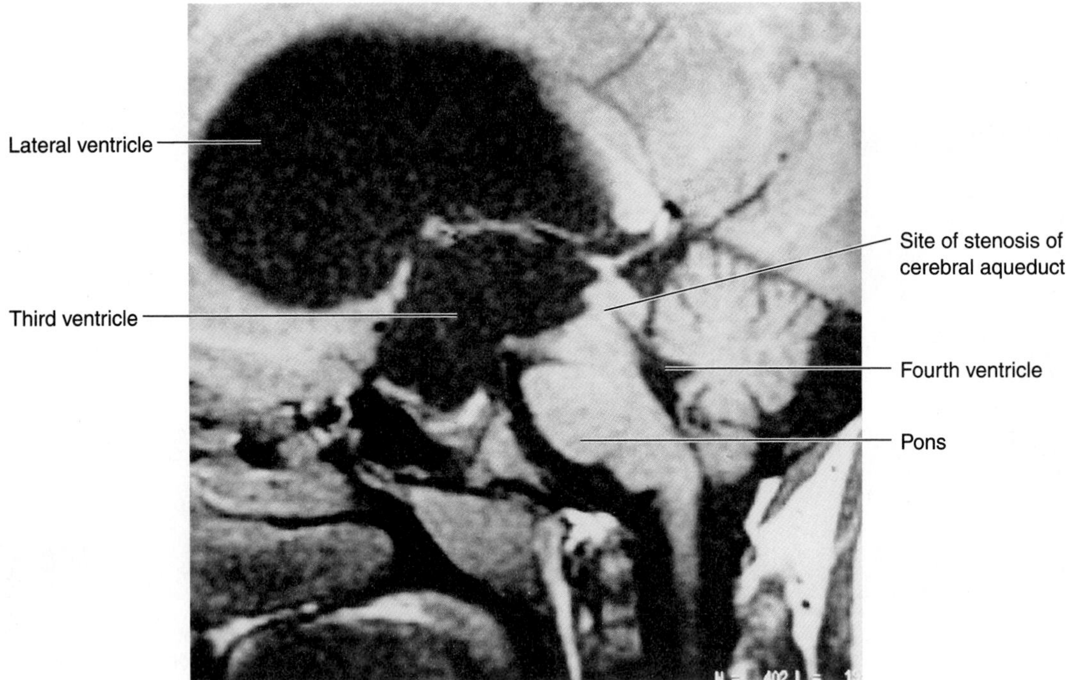

FIGURE 17-41. Congenital stenosis of the cerebral aqueduct. This sagittal magnetic resonance image of a 9-month-old infant with a large head shows very large lateral and third ventricles. The cerebrospinal fluid (CSF) appears dark in these images. The cerebral aqueduct appears as a dark line of fluid ventral to the tectum of the midbrain. The cranial end of the aqueduct is stenotic (narrow), which results in the absence of dark CSF. (Courtesy of Dr. Gerald S. Smyser, Altru Health System, Grand Forks, ND.)

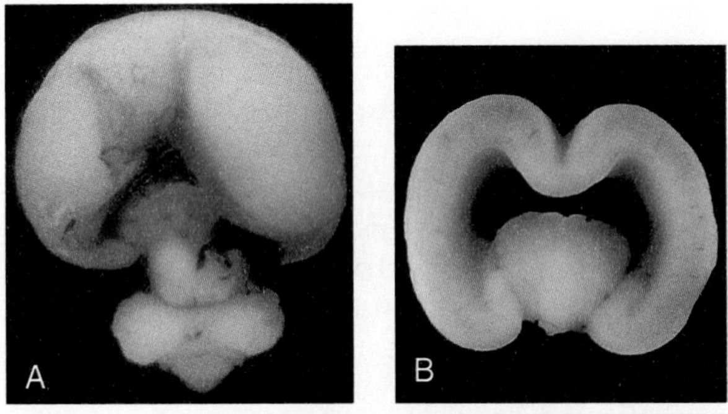

FIGURE 17-42. A frontal view of an intact (**A**), and coronally sectioned (**B**) fetal brain 21 weeks' gestation with holoprosencephaly. This defect is due to failure of cleavage of the prosencephalon (rostral neural tube) into right and left cerebral hemispheres, telencephalon and diencephalon, and into olfactory bulbs and optic tracts. (Courtesy of Dr. Marc R. Del Bigio, Department of Pathology [Neuropathology], University of Manitoba, Winnipeg, Manitoba, Canada).

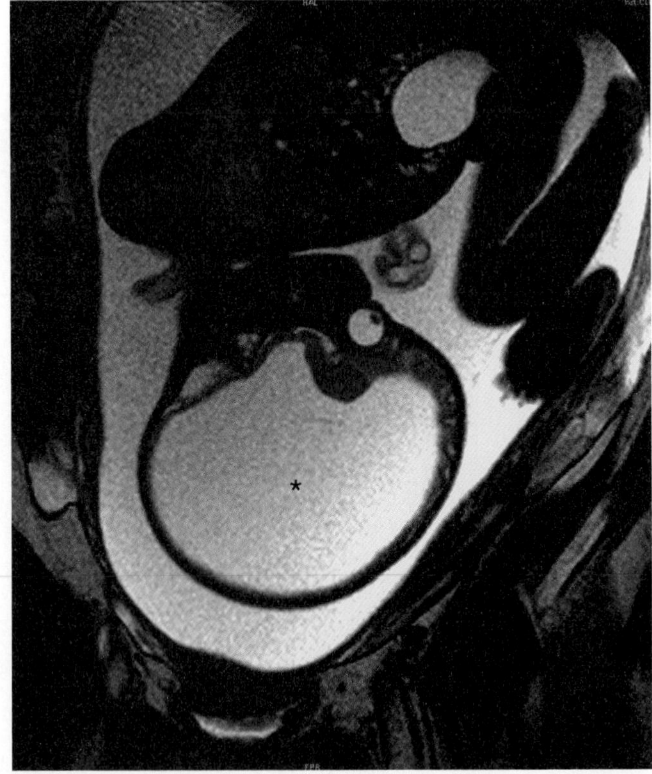

FIGURE 17-43. Magnetic resonance image of a fetus with massive hydrocephaly (*). Note the greatly reduced cerebral and displaced cerebral hemispheres and cerebellum. (Courtesy of Dr. Stuart C. Morrison, Division of Radiology [Pediatric Radiology], The Children's Hospital, Cleveland, Ohio.)

ARNOLD-CHIARI MALFORMATION

This is the most common congenital anomaly involving the cerebellum (Fig. 17-44). It is a tonguelike projection of the medulla and inferior displacement of the vermis of the cerebellum through the foramen magnum into the vertebral canal. The anomaly results in a type of communicating hydrocephalus in which there is interference with the absorption of CSF; as a result, the entire ventricular system is

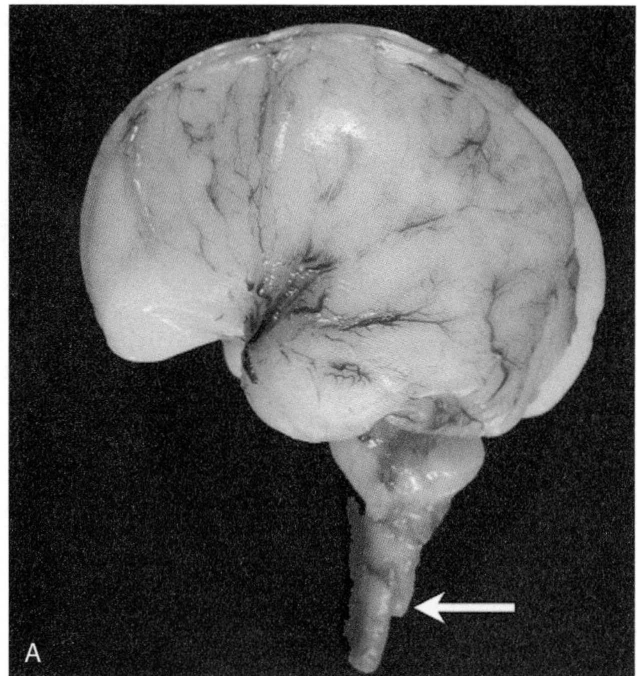

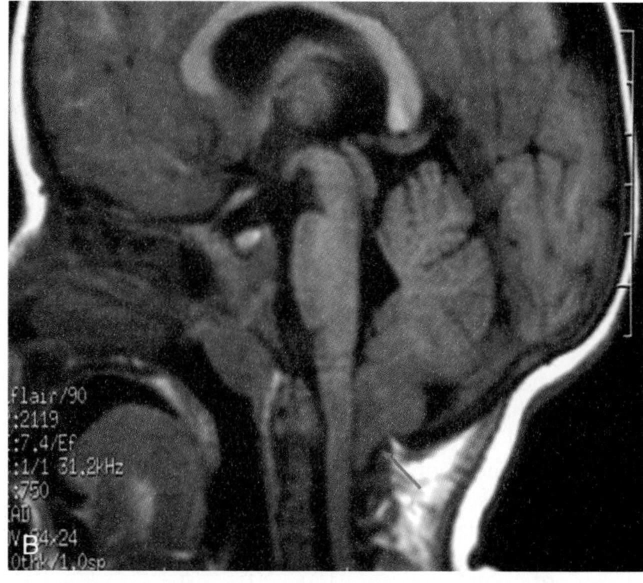

FIGURE 17-44. **A,** An Arnold-Chiari type II malformation in a 23-week gestational age fetus. In situ exposure of the hindbrain reveals cerebellar tissue (*arrow*) well below the foramen magnum. **B,** Magnetic resonance image of a child with Arnold-Chiari type I malformation. Note the cerebellar tonsils lie inferior to the foramen magnum (*red arrow*). (**A,** Courtesy of Dr. Marc R. Del Bigio, Department of Pathology [Neuropathology], University of Manitoba, Winnipeg, Manitoba, Canada. **B,** Courtesy of Dr. R. Shane Tubbs and Dr. W. Jerry Oakes, Children's Hospital Birmingham, Birmingham, Alabama.)

distended. The **Arnold-Chiari malformation** occurs once in every 1000 births and is frequently associated with spina bifida with meningomyelocele, spina bifida with myeloschisis, and hydrocephaly. The cause of the Arnold-Chiari malformation is uncertain; however, the posterior cranial fossa is abnormally small in these infants.

MENTAL RETARDATION

Congenital impairment of intelligence may result from various genetically determined conditions (e.g., Down syndrome). Mental retardation may also result from the action of a mutant gene or from a chromosomal abnormality (e.g., an extra chromosome 13, 17, or 21). Chromosomal abnormalities and mental deficiency are discussed in Chapter 20.

Maternal alcohol abuse is the most common cause of mental retardation. The 8- to 16-week period of human development is also the period of greatest sensitivity for fetal brain damage resulting from large doses of radiation. By the end of the 16th week, most neuronal proliferation and cell migration to the cerebral cortex are completed. Cell depletion of sufficient degree in the cerebral cortex results in severe mental retardation. Therapeutic abortion may be recommended when exposure exceeds 10,000 mrad. Disorders of protein, carbohydrate, or fat metabolism may also cause mental retardation. Maternal and fetal infections (e.g., syphilis, rubella virus, toxoplasmosis, and cytomegalovirus) and cretinism are commonly associated with mental retardation. *Retarded mental development* throughout the postnatal growth period can result from birth injuries, toxins (e.g., lead), cerebral infections (e.g., meningitis), cerebral trauma from head injuries, and poisoning.

DEVELOPMENT OF THE PERIPHERAL NERVOUS SYSTEM

The PNS consists of cranial, spinal, and visceral nerves and cranial, spinal, and autonomic ganglia. The PNS develops from various sources, mostly from the neural crest. All sensory cells (somatic and visceral) of the PNS are derived from **neural crest cells**. The cell bodies of these sensory cells are located outside the CNS. With the exception of the cells in the spiral ganglion of the cochlea and the vestibular ganglion of CN VIII (vestibulocochlear nerve), all peripheral sensory cells are at first bipolar. Later, the two processes unite to form a single process with peripheral and central components resulting in a unipolar type of neuron (see Fig. 17-9*D*). The peripheral process terminates in a sensory ending, whereas the central process enters the spinal cord or brain (see Fig. 17-8). The sensory cells in the ganglion of CN VIII remain bipolar.

The cell body of each afferent neuron is closely invested by a capsule of modified Schwann cells—**satellite cells** (see Fig. 17-8), which are derived from neural crest cells. This capsule is continuous with the **neurolemmal sheath** of Schwann cells that surrounds the axons of afferent neurons. External to the satellite cells is a layer of connective tissue that is continuous with the endoneurial sheath of the nerve fibers. This connective tissue and the endoneurial sheath are derived from mesenchyme.

Neural crest cells in the developing brain migrate to form sensory ganglia only in relation to the trigeminal (CN V), facial (CN VII), vestibulocochlear (CN VIII), glossopharyngeal (CN IX), and vagus (CN X) nerves. Neural crest cells also differentiate into multipolar neurons of the autonomic ganglia (see Fig. 17-8), including ganglia of the sympathetic trunks that lie along the sides of the vertebral bodies; collateral, or prevertebral, ganglia in plexuses of the thorax and abdomen (e.g., the cardiac, celiac, and mesenteric plexuses); and parasympathetic, or terminal, ganglia in or near the viscera (e.g., the submucosal or Meissner's plexus). Cells of the paraganglia—**chromaffin cells**—are also derived from the neural crest. The term paraganglia includes several widely scattered groups of cells that are similar in many ways to medullary cells of the suprarenal glands. The cell groups largely lie retroperitoneally, often in association with sympathetic ganglia. The carotid and aortic bodies also have small islands of chromaffin cells associated with them. These widely scattered groups of cells constitute the **chromaffin system**. Neural crest cells also give rise to melanoblasts (the precursors of the melanocytes) and cells of the medulla of the suprarenal gland.

Spinal Nerves

Motor nerve fibers arising from the spinal cord begin to appear at the end of the fourth week (see Figs. 17-4, 17-7, and 17-8). The nerve fibers arise from cells in the basal plates of the developing spinal cord and emerge as a continuous series of rootlets along its ventrolateral surface. The fibers destined for a particular developing muscle group become arranged in a bundle, forming a **ventral nerve root**. The nerve fibers of the **dorsal nerve root** are formed by axons derived from neural crest cells that migrate to the dorsolateral aspect of the spinal cord, where they differentiate into the cells of the **spinal ganglion** (see Figs. 17-8 and 17-9). The central processes of neurons in the spinal ganglion form a single bundle that grows into the spinal cord, opposite the apex of the dorsal horn of gray matter (see Fig. 17-5*B* and *C*). The distal processes of spinal ganglion cells grow toward the ventral nerve root and eventually join it to form a spinal nerve. Immediately after being formed, a mixed spinal nerve divides into dorsal and ventral primary rami (L. branches). The **dorsal primary ramus**, the smaller division, innervates the dorsal axial musculature (see Fig. 15-1), vertebrae, posterior intervertebral joints, and part of the skin of the back. The **ventral primary ramus**, the major division of each spinal nerve, contributes to the innervation of the limbs and ventrolateral parts of the body wall. The major **nerve plexuses** (cervical, brachial, and lumbosacral) are formed by ventral primary rami.

As each limb bud develops, the nerves from the spinal cord segments opposite to the bud elongate and grow into the limb. The nerve fibers are distributed to its muscles, which differentiate from myogenic cells that originate from the somites (see Chapter 15). The skin of the developing limbs is also innervated in a segmental manner. Early in development, successive ventral primary rami are joined by connecting loops of nerve fibers, especially those supplying the limbs (e.g., the **brachial plexus**). The dorsal division of the trunks of these plexuses supplies the extensor muscles and the extensor surface of the limbs; the ventral divisions of the trunks supply the flexor muscles and the flexor surface. The dermatomes and cutaneous innervation of the limbs are described in Chapter 16.

Cranial Nerves

Twelve pairs of cranial nerves form during the fifth and sixth weeks. They are classified into three groups, according to their embryologic origins.

Somatic Efferent Cranial Nerves

The trochlear (CN IV), abducent (CN VI), hypoglossal (CN XII), and the greater part of the oculomotor (CN III) nerves are homologous with the ventral roots of spinal nerves (Fig. 17-45). The cells of origin of these nerves are located in the somatic efferent column (derived from the basal plates) of the **brainstem**. Their axons are distributed to muscles derived from the head myotomes (preotic and occipital; see Fig. 15-4).

The **hypoglossal nerve (CN XII)** resembles a spinal nerve more than do the other somatic efferent CNs. CN XII develops by the fusion of the ventral root fibers of three or four occipital nerves (see Fig. 17-45*A*). Sensory roots, corresponding to the dorsal roots of spinal nerves, are absent. The somatic motor fibers originate from the hypoglossal nucleus, consisting of motor cells resembling those of the ventral horn of the spinal cord. These fibers leave the ventrolateral wall of the medulla in several groups, the hypoglossal nerve roots, which converge to form the common trunk of CN XII (see Fig. 17-45*B*). They grow rostrally and eventually innervate the muscles of the tongue, which are thought to be derived from occipital myotomes (see Fig. 15-4). With development of the neck, the hypoglossal nerve comes to lie at a progressively higher level.

The **abducent nerve (CN VI)** arises from nerve cells in the basal plates of the metencephalon. It passes from its ventral surface to the posterior of the three preotic myotomes from which the lateral rectus muscle of the eye is thought to originate.

The **trochlear nerve (CN IV)** arises from nerve cells in the somatic efferent column in the posterior part of the midbrain. Although a motor nerve, it emerges from the brainstem dorsally and passes ventrally to supply the superior oblique muscle of the eye.

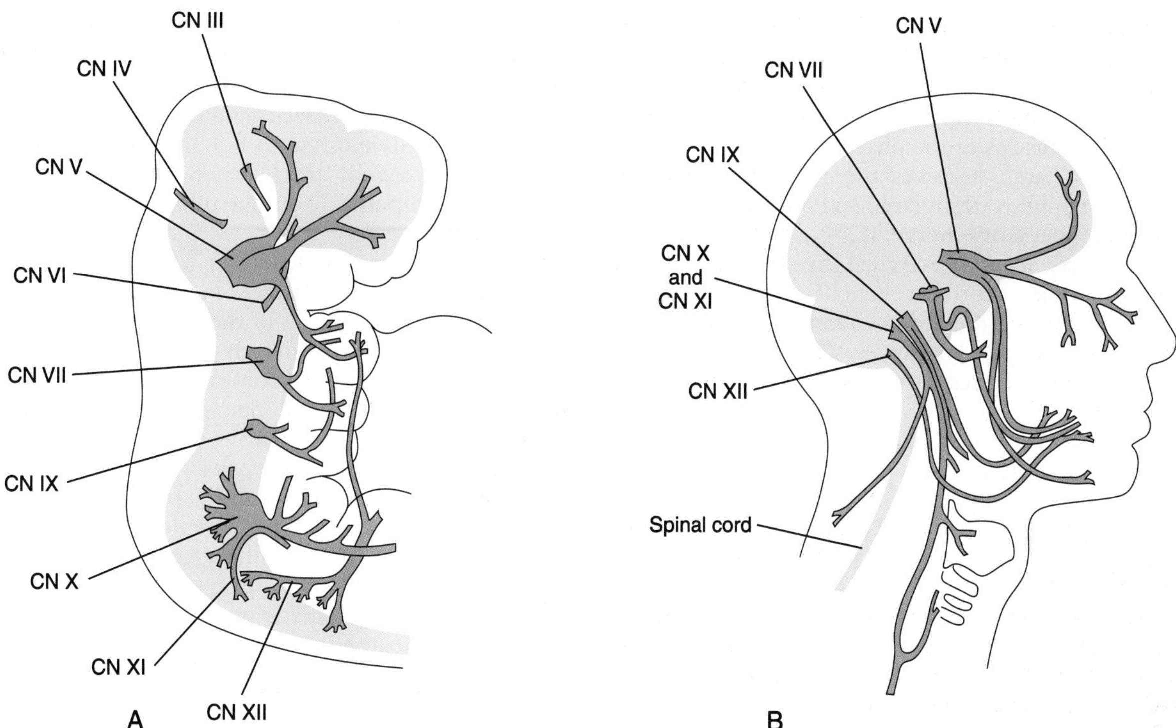

FIGURE 17-45. **A,** Schematic drawing of a 5-week embryo showing the distribution of most of the cranial nerves, especially those supplying the pharyngeal arches. **B,** Schematic drawing of the head and neck of an adult showing the general distribution of most of the cranial nerves.

The **oculomotor nerve (CN III)** supplies most of the muscles of the eye (i.e., the superior, inferior, and medial recti and inferior oblique muscles), which are derived from the first preotic myotomes.

Nerves of Pharyngeal Arches

CNs V, VII, IX, and X supply the embryonic pharyngeal arches; thus, the structures that develop from these arches are innervated by these CNs (see Fig. 17-45*A* and Table 9-1).

The **trigeminal nerve (CN V)** is the nerve of the first pharyngeal arch, but it has an ophthalmic division that is not a pharyngeal arch component. CN V is chiefly sensory and is the principal sensory nerve for the head. The large **trigeminal ganglion** lies beside the rostral end of the pons, and its cells are derived from the most anterior part of the neural crest. The central processes of cells in this ganglion form the large sensory root of CN V, which enters the lateral portion of the pons. The peripheral processes of cells in this ganglion separate into three large divisions (ophthalmic, maxillary, and mandibular nerves). Their sensory fibers supply the skin of the face as well as the lining of the mouth and nose (see Fig. 9-7). The motor fibers of CN V arise from cells in the most anterior part of the special visceral efferent column in the metencephalon. The motor nucleus of CN V lies at the mid-level of the pons. The fibers leave the pons at the site of the entering sensory fibers and pass to the muscles of mastication and to other muscles that develop in the mandibular prominence of the first pharyngeal arch (see Table 9-1). The mesencephalic nucleus of CN V differentiates from cells in the midbrain that extend rostrally from the metencephalon.

The **facial nerve (CN VII)** is the nerve of the second pharyngeal arch. It consists mostly of motor fibers that arise principally from a nuclear group in the special visceral efferent column in the caudal part of the pons. These fibers are distributed to the muscles of facial expression and to other muscles that develop in the mesenchyme of the second pharyngeal arch (see Table 9-1). The small general visceral efferent component of CN VII terminates in the peripheral autonomic ganglia of the head. The sensory fibers of CN VII arise from the cells of the geniculate ganglion. The central processes of these cells enter the pons, and the peripheral processes pass to the greater superficial petrosal nerve and, via the chorda tympani nerve, to the taste buds in the anterior two thirds of the tongue.

The **glossopharyngeal nerve (CN IX)** is the nerve of the third pharyngeal arch. Its motor fibers arise from the special and, to a lesser extent, general visceral efferent columns of the anterior part of the myelencephalon. CN IX forms from several rootlets that arise from the medulla just caudal to the developing internal ear. All the fibers from the special visceral efferent column are distributed to the stylopharyngeus muscle, which is derived from mesenchyme in the third pharyngeal arch (see Table 9-1). The general efferent fibers are distributed to the otic ganglion, from which postganglionic fibers pass to the parotid and posterior lingual glands. The sensory fibers of CN IX are distributed as general sensory and special visceral afferent fibers (taste fibers) to the posterior part of the tongue.

The **vagus nerve (CN X)** is formed by fusion of the nerves of the fourth and sixth pharyngeal arches (see Table 9-1). It has large visceral efferent and visceral afferent components that are distributed to the heart, foregut and its derivatives, and to a large part of the midgut. The nerve of the fourth pharyngeal arch becomes the superior laryngeal nerve, which supplies the cricothyroid muscle and constrictor muscles of the pharynx. The nerve of the sixth pharyngeal arch becomes the recurrent laryngeal nerve, which supplies various laryngeal muscles.

The **spinal accessory nerve (CN XI)** emerges as a series of rootlets from the cranial five or six cervical segments of the spinal cord (see Fig. 17-45). The fibers of the traditional cranial root are now considered to be part of CN X (Lachman and colleagues, 2002). The fibers of the CN X supply the sternocleidomastoid and trapezius muscles.

Special Sensory Nerves

The **olfactory nerve (CN I)** arises from the olfactory organ. The olfactory **receptor neurons** differentiate from cells in the epithelial lining of the primordial nasal sac. The central processes of the bipolar olfactory neurons are collected into bundles to form approximately 20 olfactory nerves around which the cribriform plate of the ethmoid bone develops. These unmyelinated nerve fibers end in the **olfactory bulb.**

The **optic nerve (CN II)** is formed by more than a million nerve fibers that grow into the brain from neuroblasts in the primordial retina. Because the retina develops from the evaginated wall of the forebrain, the optic nerve actually represents a fiber tract of the brain. Development of the optic nerve is described in Chapter 18.

The **vestibulocochlear nerve (CN VIII)** consists of two kinds of sensory fiber in two bundles; these fibers are known as the vestibular and cochlear nerves. The **vestibular nerve** originates in the semicircular ducts, and the **cochlear nerve** proceeds from the cochlear duct, in which the **spiral organ** (of Corti) develops. The bipolar neurons of the vestibular nerve have their cell bodies in the **vestibular ganglion.** The central processes of these cells terminate in the vestibular nuclei in the floor of the fourth ventricle. The bipolar neurons of the cochlear nerve have their cell bodies in the **spiral ganglion.** The central processes of these cells end in the ventral and dorsal cochlear nuclei in the medulla.

DEVELOPMENT OF THE AUTONOMIC NERVOUS SYSTEM

Functionally, the autonomic system can be divided into sympathetic (thoracolumbar) and parasympathetic (craniosacral) parts.

Sympathetic Nervous System

During the fifth week, **neural crest cells** in the thoracic region migrate along each side of the spinal cord, where they form paired cellular masses (ganglia) dorsolateral to the aorta (see Fig. 17-8). All these segmentally arranged **sympathetic ganglia** are connected in a bilateral chain by longitudinal nerve fibers. These ganglionated cords—**sympathetic trunks**—are located on each side of the vertebral bodies. Some neural crest cells migrate ventral to the aorta and form neurons in the **preaortic ganglia**, such as the celiac and mesenteric ganglia (see Fig. 17-8). Other neural crest cells migrate to the area of the heart, lungs, and gastrointestinal tract, where they form terminal ganglia in **sympathetic organ plexuses**, located near or within these organs.

After the sympathetic trunks have formed, axons of sympathetic neurons, located in the **intermediolateral cell column** (lateral horn) of the thoracolumbar segments of the spinal cord, pass through the ventral root of a spinal nerve and a **white ramus communicans** (communicating branch) to a paravertebral ganglion (see Fig. 17-8). Here they may synapse with neurons or ascend or descend in the sympathetic trunk to synapse at other levels. Other presynaptic fibers pass through the **paravertebral ganglia** without synapsing, forming splanchnic nerves to the viscera. The postsynaptic fibers course through a **gray communicating branch** (gray ramus communicans), passing from a sympathetic ganglion into a spinal nerve; hence, the sympathetic trunks are composed of ascending and descending fibers.

Parasympathetic Nervous System

The **presynaptic parasympathetic fibers** arise from neurons in nuclei of the brainstem and in the sacral region of the spinal cord. The fibers from the brainstem leave through the oculomotor (CN III), facial (CN VII), glossopharyngeal (CN IX), and vagus (CN X) nerves. The **postsynaptic neurons** are located in peripheral ganglia or in plexuses near or within the structure being innervated (e.g., the pupil of the eye and salivary glands).

SUMMARY OF THE NERVOUS SYSTEM

- The CNS develops from a dorsal thickening of ectoderm—the **neural plate,** which appears around the middle of the third week. The neural plate is induced by the underlying notochord and paraxial mesenchyme.
- The neural plate becomes infolded to form a **neural groove** that has neural folds on each side. When the **neural folds** begin to fuse to form the neural tube beginning during the fourth week, some neuroectodermal cells are not included in it, but remain between the neural tube and surface ectoderm as the **neural crest.**
- The cranial end of the neural tube forms the brain, the primordia of which are the forebrain, midbrain, and hindbrain. The **forebrain** gives rise to the **cerebral hemispheres** and **diencephalon**. The embryonic **midbrain** becomes the adult midbrain, and the **hindbrain** gives rise to the **pons**, **cerebellum**, and **medulla oblongata**. The remainder of the neural tube becomes the spinal cord.
- The **neural canal**, the lumen of the neural tube, becomes the **ventricles of the brain** and the **central**

canal of the spinal cord. The walls of the neural tube thicken by proliferation of its neuroepithelial cells. These cells give rise to all nerve and macroglial cells in the CNS. The microglia differentiate from mesenchymal cells that enter the CNS with the blood vessels.

- The **pituitary gland** develops from two completely different parts: an ectodermal upgrowth from the stomodeum, the **hypophysial diverticulum** that forms the **adenohypophysis**, and a neuroectodermal downgrowth from the diencephalon, the **neurohypophysial bud** that forms the **neurohypophysis**.
- Cells in the cranial, spinal, and autonomic ganglia are derived from **neural crest cells** that originate in the neural crest. **Schwann cells**, which myelinate the axons external to the spinal cord, also arise from neural crest cells. Similarly, most of the ANS and all chromaffin tissue, including the suprarenal medulla, develop from neural crest cells.
- **Congenital anomalies of the CNS** are common (approximately three per 1000 births). Defects in the closure of the neural tube (**NTDs**) account for most severe anomalies (e.g., spinal bifida cystica). Some anomalies of the CNS are caused by genetic factors (e.g., numerical chromosomal abnormalities such as trisomy 21); others result from environmental factors such as infectious agents, drugs, and metabolic disease. Most CNS anomalies are caused by a combination of genetic and environmental factors (**multifactorial inheritance**).
- Gross congenital anomalies (e.g., **meroencephaly** [anencephaly]) are incompatible with life. Other severe anomalies (e.g., spina bifida with meningomyelocele) cause functional disability (e.g., muscle paralysis in the lower limbs).
- There are two main types of hydrocephalus: **obstructive or noncommunicating hydrocephalus** (blockage of CSF flow in the ventricular system) and **nonobstructive or communicating hydrocephalus** (blockage of CSF flow in the subarachnoid space). In most cases, congenital hydrocephalus is associated with spina bifida with meningomyelocele.
- **Mental retardation** may result from chromosomal abnormalities occurring during gametogenesis, from metabolic disorders, maternal alcohol abuse, or infections occurring during prenatal life. Various postnatal conditions (e.g., cerebral infection or trauma) may also cause abnormal mental development.

CLINICALLY ORIENTED PROBLEMS

Case 17-1

A pregnant woman developed polyhydramnios over the course of a few days (acute polyhydramnios). After an ultrasound examination, a radiologist reported that the fetus had acrania and meroencephaly.

- How soon can meroencephaly (anencephaly) be detected by ultrasound scanning?
- Why is polyhydramnios associated with meroencephaly?
- What other techniques could be used to confirm the diagnosis of meroencephaly?

Case 17-2

A male infant was born with a large lumbar meningomyelocele that was covered with a thin membranous sac. Within a few days, the sac ulcerated and began to leak. A marked neurologic deficit was detected inferior to the level of the sac.

- What is the embryological basis of this anomaly?
- What is the basis of the neurological deficit?
- What structures would likely be affected?

Case 17-3

A computed tomography (CT) scan of an infant with an enlarged head showed dilation of the lateral and third ventricles.

- What is this condition called?
- Where would the blockage most likely be to produce this abnormal dilation of the ventricles?
- Is this condition usually recognizable before birth?
- How do you think this condition might be treated surgically?

Case 17-4

An infant was born with an abnormally large head.

- Is an enlarged head in an infant synonymous with hydrocephalus?
- What condition is usually associated with an abnormally small head?
- Is growth of the cranium dependent on growth of the brain?
- What environmental factors are known to cause microencephaly?

Case 17-5

A radiologist reported that a child's cerebral ventricles were dilated posteriorly and that the lateral ventricles were widely separated by a dilated third ventricle. Agenesis of the corpus callosum was diagnosed.

- What is the common symptom associated with agenesis of the corpus callosum?
- Are some patients asymptomatic?
- What is the basis of the dilated third ventricle?

Discussion of these problems appears at the back of the book.

References and Suggested Reading

Barkovich AJ, Kuzniecky RI, Jackson GD, et al: A developmental and genetic classification for malformations of cortical development. Neurology 65:1773, 2005.

Bell JE: The pathology of central nervous system defects in human fetuses of different gestational ages. In Persaud TVN (ed): Advances in the Study of Birth Defects, Vol 7. Central Nervous System and Craniofacial Malformations. New York, Alan R. Liss, 1982.

Botto LD, Lisi A, Robert-Gnansia E, et al: International retrospective cohort study of neural tube defects in relation to folic acid recommendations: Are the recommendations working? BMJ 330:571, 2005.

Cayuso J, Ulloa F, Cox B, et al: The sonic hedgehog pathway independently controls the patterning, proliferation and survival of neuroepithelial cells by regulating Gli activity. Development 133:517, 2006.

Evans OB, Hutchins JB: Development of the nervous system. In Haines DE (ed): Fundamental Neuroscience, 2nd ed. New York, Churchill Livingstone, 2002.

Ever L, Gaiano N: Radial “glial” progenitors: neurogenesis and signaling. Curr Opin Neurobiol 15: 29, 2005.

Gasser RF: Evidence that some events of mammalian embryogenesis can result from differential growth, making migration unnecessary. Anat Rec B New Anat 289:53, 2006.

Gressens P, Hüppi PS: Normal and abnormal brain development. In Martin RJ, Fanaroff AA, Walsh MC (eds): Fanaroff and Martin’s Neonatal-Perinatal Medicine. Diseases of the Fetus and Infant, 8th ed. Philadelphia, Mosby, 2006.

Guillemont F, Molnar Z, Tarabykin V, Stoykova A: Molecular mechanisms of cortical differentiation. Eur J Neurosci 23:857, 2006.

Harland R: Neural induction. Curr Opin Genet Dev 10:357, 2000.

Howard B, Chen Y, Zecevic N: Cortical progenitor cells in the developing human telencephalon. Glia 53:57, 2006.

Jirásek JE: An Atlas of Human Prenatal Developmental Mechanics. Anatomy and Staging. London and New York, Taylor & Francis, 2004.

Johnston MV, Kinsman S: Congenital anomalies of the central nervous system. In Behrman RE, Kliegman RM, Jenson HB (eds): Nelson Textbook of Pediatrics, 17th ed. Philadelphia, WB Saunders, 2004.

Kollias SS, Ball WS, Prenger EC: Review of the embryologic development of the pituitary gland and report of a case of hypophyseal duplication detected by MRI. Neuroradiology 37:3, 1995.

Lachman N, Acland RD, Rosse C: Anatomical evidence for the absence of a morphologically distinct cranial root of the accessory nerve in man. Clin Anat 15:4, 2002.

LeDouarin N, Kalcheim C: The Neural Crest, 2nd ed. Cambridge, UK, Cambridge University Press, 1999.

Moore KL, Dalley AF: Clinically Oriented Anatomy, 5th ed. Baltimore, Williams & Wilkins, 2006.

Müller F, O’Rahilly R: The development of the human brain from a closed neural tube at stage 13. Anat Embryol (Berl) 177:203–224, 1988.

Nakatsu T, Uwabe C, Shiota K: Neural tube closure in humans initiates at multiple sites: Evidence from human embryos and implications for the pathogenesis of neural tube defects. Anat Embryol 201:455, 2000.

Noden DM: Spatial integration among cells forming the cranial peripheral neurons. J Neurobiol 24:248, 1993.

O’Rahilly R, Müller F: Embryonic Human Brain. An Atlas of Developmental Stages, 2nd ed. New York, Wiley-Liss, 1999.

Pevny L, Placzek M: SOX genes and neural progenitor identity. Curr Opin Neurobiol 15:7, 2005.

Pooh KH: Transvaginal 3D and Doppler ultrasonography of the fetal brain. Semin Perinatol 25:38, 2001.

Ren T, Anderson A, Shen W-B, et al: Imaging, anatomical, and molecular analysis of callosal formation in the developing human fetal brain. Anat Rec A Discov Mol Cell Evol Biol 288:191, 2006.

Slack JMW: Essential Developmental Biology, 2nd ed. Oxford, Blackwell Publishing, 2006.

Turnpenny L, Cameron IT, Spalluto CM, et al: Human embryonic germ cells for future neuronal replacement therapy. Brain Res Bull 68:76, 2005.

Van Dyke DC, Stumbo PJ, Berg MJ, Niebyl JR: Folic acid and prevention of birth defects. Dev Med Child Neurol 44:426, 2002.

Yao G, Chen XN, Flores-Sarnat L, et al: Deletion of chromosome 21 disturbs human brain morphogenesis. Genet Med 8:1, 2006.

Zhu X, Lin CR, Prefontaine GG, et al: Genetic control of pituitary development and hypopituitarism. Curr Opin Genet Dev 15:332, 2005.

18

The Eye and Ear

Development of Eye and Related Structures 420
Development of the Retina 420
Development of the Ciliary Body 425
Development of the Iris 425
Development of the Lens 427
Development of the Aqueous Chambers 428
Development of the Cornea 429
Development of the Choroid and Sclera 429
Development of the Eyelids 429
Development of the Lacrimal Glands 430
Development of the Ear 430
Development of the Internal Ear 431
Development of the Middle Ear 433
Development of the External Ear 433
Summary of the Development of the Eye 437
Summary of the Development of the Ear 437
Clinically Oriented Problems 437

DEVELOPMENT OF EYE AND RELATED STRUCTURES

Early eye development results from a series of inductive signals. The eyes are derived from four sources:

- The neuroectoderm of the forebrain
- The surface ectoderm of the head
- The mesoderm between the above layers
- Neural crest cells

The **neuroectoderm** of the forebrain differentiates into the retina, the posterior layers of the iris, and the optic nerve. The **surface ectoderm** forms the lens of the eye and the corneal epithelium. The **mesoderm** between the neuroectoderm and surface ectoderm gives rise to the fibrous and vascular coats of the eye. Mesenchyme is derived from mesoderm. Neural crest cells migrate into the mesenchyme from the neural crest and differentiate into the choroid, sclera, and corneal endothelium. Homeobox-containing genes, including the transcription regulator Pax6, fibroblast growth factors, and other inducing factors play an important role in the molecular development of the eye (see Chapter 21).

Eye development is first evident at the beginning of the fourth week. **Optic grooves** (Latin [L]. *sulci*) appear in the neural folds at the cranial end of the embryo (Fig. 18-1*A* and *B*). As the neural folds fuse to form the forebrain, the optic grooves evaginate to form hollow diverticula—**optic vesicles**—that project from the wall of the forebrain into the adjacent mesenchyme (see Fig. 18-1*C*). The cavities of the optic vesicles are continuous with the cavity of the forebrain. Formation of the optic vesicles is induced by the mesenchyme adjacent to the developing brain, probably through a chemical mediator. As the optic vesicles grow, their distal ends expand and their connections with the forebrain constrict to form hollow **optic stalks** (see Fig. 18-1*D*).

The optic vesicles soon come in contact with the surface ectoderm. Concurrently, the surface ectoderm adjacent to the vesicles thickens to form **lens placodes**, the primordia of the lenses (see Fig. 18-1*C*). Formation of lens placodes is induced by the optic vesicles after the surface ectoderm has been conditioned by the underlying mesenchyme. An inductive message passes from the optic vesicles, stimulating the surface ectodermal cells to form the **lens primordia.** The lens placodes invaginate as they sink deep to the surface ectoderm, forming **lens pits** (Figs. 18-1*D* and 18-2). The edges of the pits approach each other and fuse to form spherical **lens vesicles** (see Figs. 18-1*F* and *H*), which soon lose their connection with the surface ectoderm. Development of the lenses from the lens vesicles is described after formation of the eyeball is discussed.

As the lens vesicles are developing, the optic vesicles invaginate to form double-walled **optic cups** (see Figs. 18-1*H* and 18-2). The opening of each cup is large at first, but its rim infolds around the lens (Fig. 18-3*A*). By this stage, the lens vesicles have lost their connection with the surface ectoderm and have entered the cavities of the optic cups (Fig. 18-4). Linear grooves—**retinal fissures** (optic fissures) —develop on the ventral surface of the optic cups and along the optic stalks (see Figs. 18-1*E* to *H* and 18-3*A* to *D*). The fissures contain vascular mesenchyme from which the hyaloid blood vessels develop. The **hyaloid artery**, a branch of the ophthalmic artery, supplies the inner layer of the optic cup, the lens vesicle, and the mesenchyme in the **cavity of the optic cup** (see Figs. 18-1*H* and 18-3). The **hyaloid vein** returns blood from these structures. As the edges of the retinal fissure fuse, the hyaloid vessels are enclosed within the **primordial optic nerve** (see Fig. 18-3*C* to *F*). Distal parts of the hyaloid vessels eventually degenerate, but proximal parts persist as the **central artery** and **vein of the retina** (see Fig. 18-8*D*).

Development of the Retina

The retina develops from the walls of the *optic cup*, an outgrowth of the forebrain (see Figs. 18-1 and 18-2). The outer, thinner layer of the optic cup becomes the retinal pigment epithelium (**pigmented layer of retina**), and the inner, thicker layer differentiates into the neural retina (**neural layer of retina**).

During the embryonic and early fetal periods, the two retinal layers are separated by an **intraretinal space** (see Fig. 18-4), which is the original cavity of the optic cup. Before birth, this space gradually disappears as the two layers of the retina fuse (see Fig. 18-8*D*), but this fusion is not firm; hence, when an adult eyeball is dissected, the neural layer is often separated from the pigment layer. Because the optic cup is an outgrowth of the forebrain, the layers of the optic cup are continuous with the wall of the brain (see Fig. 18-1*H*).

Under the influence of the developing lens, the inner layer of the optic cup proliferates to form a thick **neuroepithelium** (see Fig. 18-4). Subsequently, the cells of this layer differentiate into the **neural retina**, the light-sensitive region of the optic part of the retina. This region contains photoreceptors (rods and cones) and the cell bodies of neurons (e.g., bipolar and ganglion cells). Fibroblast growth factor signaling regulates retinal ganglion cell differentiation. Because the optic vesicle invaginates as it forms the optic cup, the neural retina is "inverted," that is, light-sensitive parts of the photoreceptor cells are adjacent to the retinal pigment epithelium. As a result, light must pass through the thickest part of the retina before reaching the receptors; however, because the retina overall is thin and transparent, it does not form a barrier to light. The axons of ganglion cells in the superficial layer of the neural retina grow proximally in the wall of the **optic stalk** to the brain (see Figs. 18-3 and 18-4). As a result, the cavity of the optic stalk is gradually obliterated as the axons of the many ganglion cells form the **optic nerve** (see Fig. 18-3*F*).

Myelination of optic nerve fibers is incomplete at birth. After the eyes have been exposed to light for approximately 10 weeks, myelination is complete, but the process normally stops short of the **optic disc,** where the optic nerve enters the eyeball. Normal newborn infants can see, but not too well; they respond to changes in illumination and are able to fixate points of contrast. Visual acuity has been estimated to be in the range of 20/400. At 2 weeks of age, the infants show a more sustained interest in large objects.

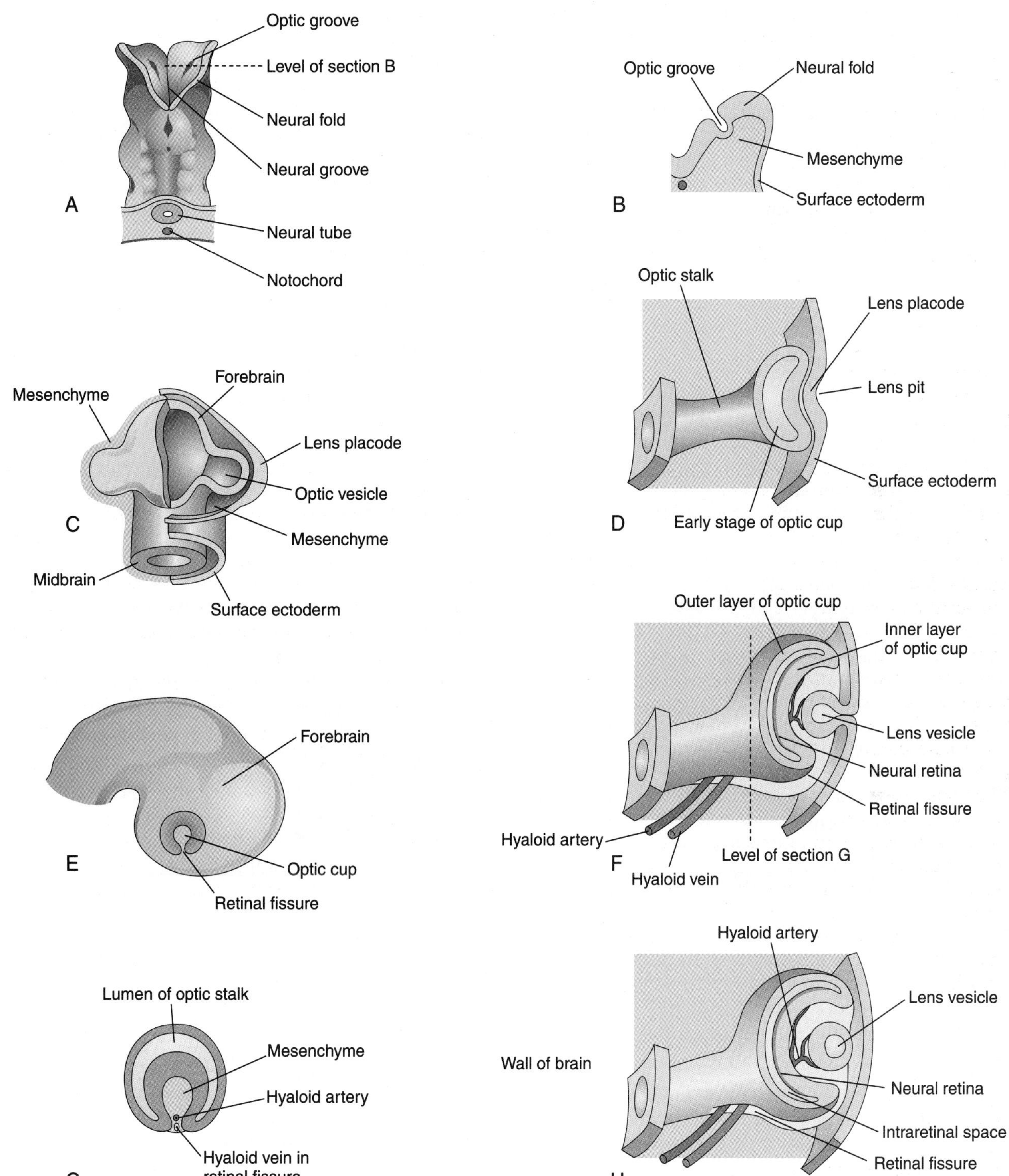

FIGURE 18-1. Illustrations of the early stages of eye development. **A,** Dorsal view of the cranial end of an embryo of approximately 22 days showing the optic grooves, the first indication of eye development. **B,** Transverse section of a neural fold showing the optic groove in it. **C,** Schematic drawing of the forebrain of an embryo of approximately 28 days showing its covering layers of mesenchyme and surface ectoderm. **D, F,** and **H,** Schematic sections of the developing eye illustrating successive stages in the development of the optic cup and lens vesicle. **E,** Lateral view of the brain of an embryo of approximately 32 days showing the external appearance of the optic cup. **G,** Transverse section of the optic stalk showing the retinal fissure and its contents. Note that the edges of the retinal fissure are growing together, thereby completing the optic cup and enclosing the central artery and vein of the retina in the optic stalk and cup.

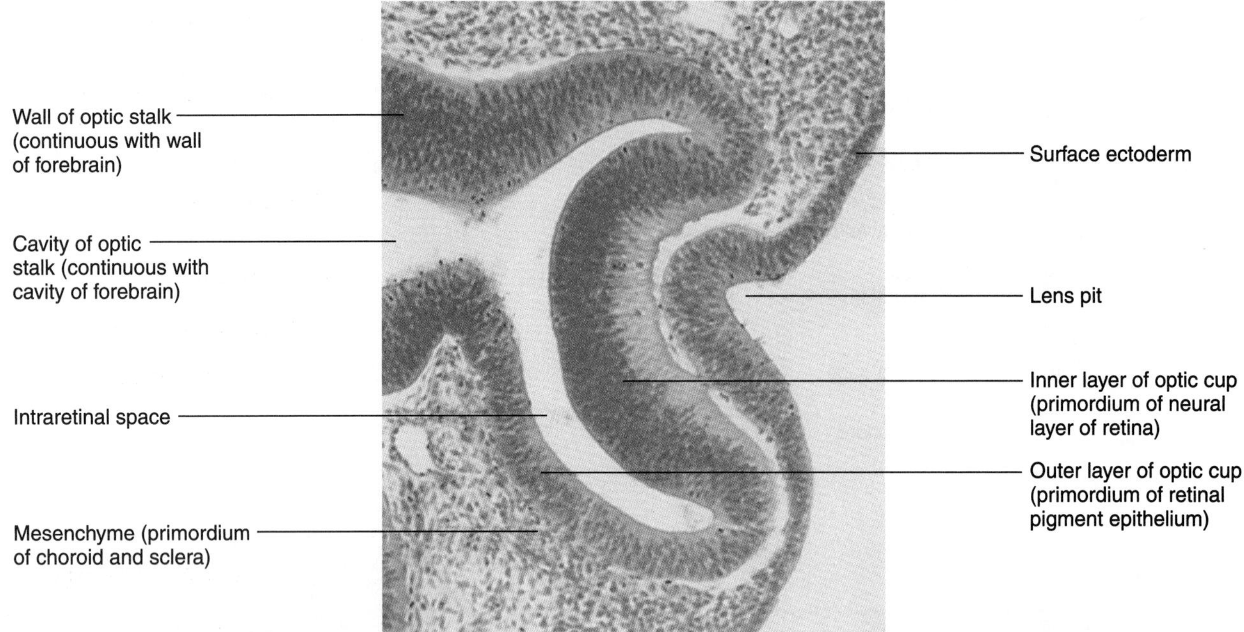

FIGURE 18-2. Photomicrograph of a sagittal section of the eye of an embryo (×200) at Carnegie stage 14, approximately 32 days. Observe the primordium of the lens (invaginated lens placode), the walls of the optic cup (primordium of retina), and the optic stalk (primordium of optic nerve). (From Moore KL, Persaud TVN, Shiota K: Color Atlas of Clinical Embryology, 2nd ed. Philadelphia, WB Saunders, 2000.)

CONGENITAL ANOMALIES OF THE EYE

The type and severity of congenital eye anomalies depend on the embryonic stage during which development is disrupted. Several environmental teratogens cause congenital eye defects (see Chapter 20). Most common eye anomalies result from defects in closure of the retinal fissure.

Coloboma of the Retina

This defect is characterized by a localized gap in the retina, usually inferior to the optic disc. The defect is bilateral in most cases. A typical coloboma of the retina results from defective closure of the retinal fissure.

Coloboma of the Iris

Coloboma is a defect in the inferior sector of the iris or a notch in the pupillary margin, giving the pupil a keyhole appearance (see Fig. 18-9). The defect may be limited to the iris or it may extend deeper and involve the ciliary body and retina. *A typical coloboma of the iris results from failure of closure of the retinal fissure during the sixth week.* The defect may be caused by environmental factors. A simple coloboma is frequently hereditary and is transmitted as an autosomal dominant characteristic.

Congenital Detachment of the Retina

Congenital detachment of the retina occurs when the inner and outer layers of the optic cup fail to fuse during the fetal period to form the retina and obliterate the intraretinal space (see Figs. 18-3 and 18-8). The separation of the neural and pigmented layers of the retina may be partial or complete. Retinal detachment may result from unequal rates of growth of the two retinal layers; as a result, the layers of the optic cup are not in perfect apposition. Sometimes the layers of the optic cup appear to have fused and separated later; such secondary detachments usually occur in association with other anomalies of the eye and head.

Knowledge about eye development makes it clear that when there is a detached retina, it is not a detachment of the entire retina because the retinal pigment epithelium remains firmly attached to the choroid. The detachment is at the site of adherence of the outer and inner layers of the optic cup. Although separated from the retinal pigment epithelium, the neural retina retains its blood supply (central artery of retina), derived from the embryonic hyaloid artery.

Postnatally, the retinal pigmented epithelium normally becomes fixed to the choroid, but its attachment to the neural retina is not firm; hence, a detached retina may follow a blow to the eyeball, as may occur during a boxing match. As a result, fluid accumulates between the layers and vision is impaired.

Cyclopia

In this very rare anomaly, the eyes are partially or completely fused, forming a single **median eye**

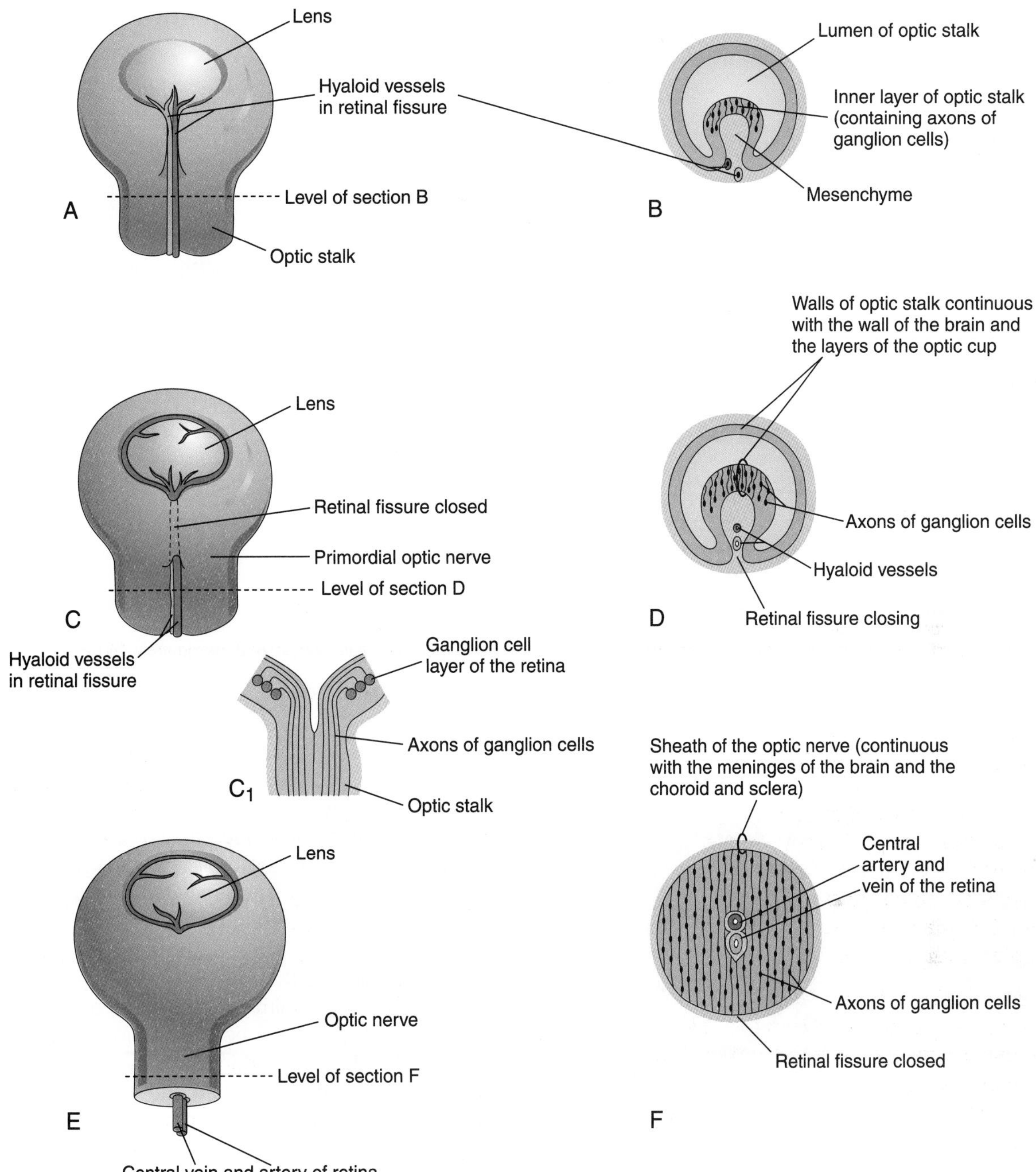

FIGURE 18-3. Illustrations of the closure of the retinal fissure and formation of the optic nerve. **A, C,** and **E,** Views of the inferior surface of the optic cup and stalk showing progressive stages in the closure of the retinal fissure. **C_1,** Schematic sketch of a longitudinal section of a part of the optic cup and stalk showing axons of ganglion cells of the retina growing through the optic stalk to the brain. **B, D,** and **F,** Transverse sections of the optic stalk showing successive stages in closure of the retinal fissure and formation of the optic nerve. The retinal fissure normally closes during the sixth week. Defects in closure of the fissure result in coloboma of the iris and/or retina. Note that the lumen of the optic stalk is gradually obliterated as axons of ganglion cells accumulate in the inner layer of the optic stalk as the optic nerve forms.

enclosed in a single orbit (Fig. 18-5). There is usually a tubular nose (**proboscis**) superior to the eye. **Cyclopia** (single eye) and **synophthalmia** (fusion of eyes) represent a spectrum of ocular defects in which the eyes are partially or completely fused. These severe eye anomalies are associated with other craniocerebral defects that are incompatible with life. Cyclopia appears to result from severe suppression of midline cerebral structures—**holoprosencephaly** (see Chapter 17)—that develop from the cranial part of the neural plate. Cyclopia is transmitted by recessive inheritance.

Microphthalmia

Congenital microphthalmia is a heterogeneous group of eye anomalies. The eye may be very small with

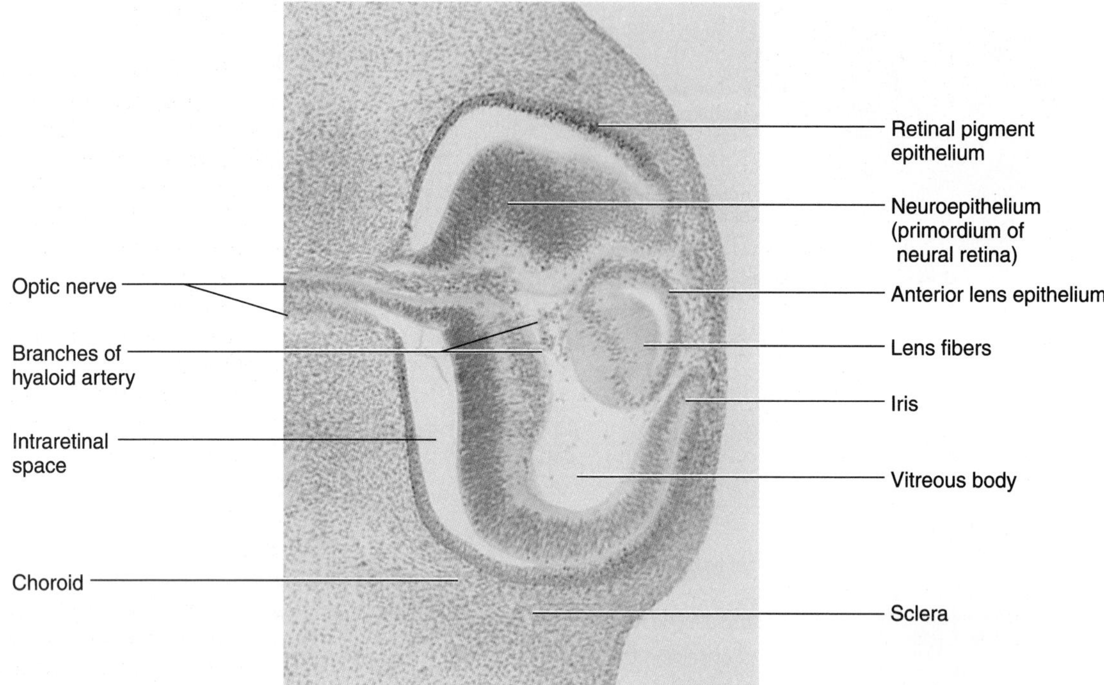

FIGURE 18-4. Photomicrograph of a sagittal section of the eye of an embryo (×100) at Carnegie stage 18, approximately 44 days. Observe that it is the posterior wall of the lens vesicle that forms the lens fibers. The anterior wall does not change appreciably as it becomes the anterior lens epithelium. (From Nishimura H [ed]: Atlas of Human Prenatal Histology. Tokyo, Igaku-Shoin, 1983.)

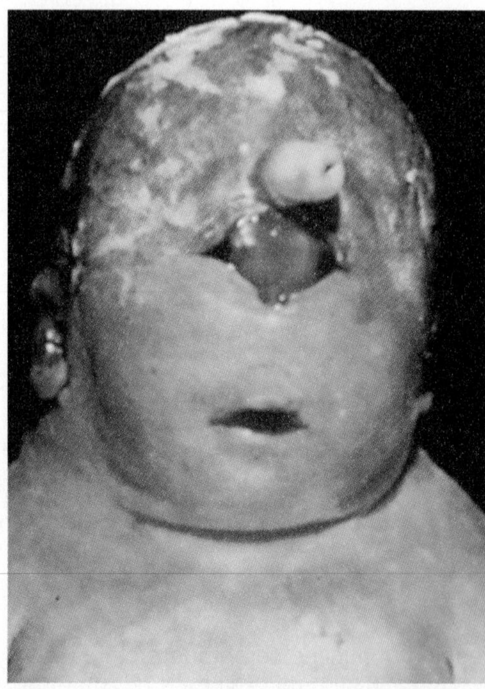

FIGURE 18-5. Male newborn infant with cyclopia (synophthalmia). Cyclopia (fusion of eyes) is a severe, uncommon anomaly of the face and eye associated with a proboscis-like appendage superior to the eye. Several facial bones are absent, e.g., nasal bones and ethmoids. The white substance covering his head is vernix caseosa—a fatty protective covering. (Courtesy of Dr. Susan Phillips, Department of Pathology, Health Sciences Centre, Winnipeg, Manitoba, Canada.)

other ocular defects or it may be a normal-appearing rudimentary eye. The affected side of the face is underdeveloped and the orbit is small. Microphthalmia may be associated with other congenital anomalies (e.g., a facial cleft; see Chapter 9) and be part of a syndrome (e.g., trisomy 13; see Chapter 20).

Severe microphthalmia results from arrested development of the eye before or shortly after the optic vesicle has formed in the fourth week. The eye is essentially underdeveloped and the lens does not form. If the interference with development occurs before the retinal fissure closes in the sixth week, the eye is larger, but the microphthalmos is associated with gross ocular defects. When eye development is arrested in the eighth week or during the early fetal period, simple microphthalmos results (small eye with minor ocular abnormalities). Some cases of microphthalmos are inherited. The hereditary pattern may be autosomal dominant, autosomal recessive, or X linked. Most cases of simple microphthalmia are caused by **infectious agents** (e.g., rubella virus, *Toxoplasma gondii*, and herpes simplex virus) that cross the placental membrane during the late embryonic and early fetal periods.

Anophthalmia

Anophthalmia denotes congenital absence of the eye, which is rare. The eyelids form, but no eyeball

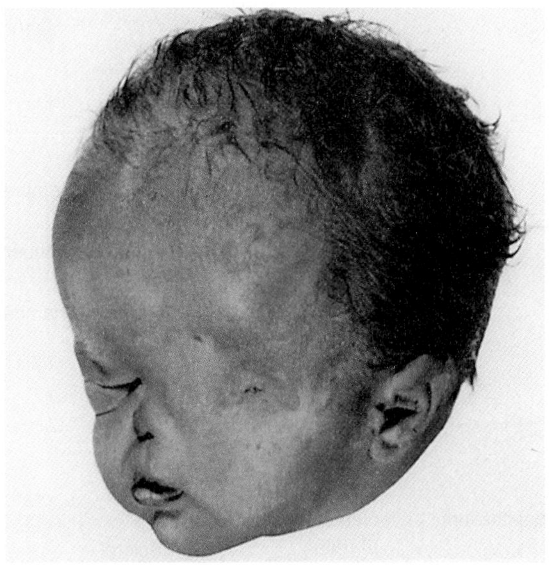

FIGURE 18-6. Photograph of the head of an infant with anophthalmia (congenital absence of most eye tissues) and a single nostril. The eyelids are formed but are mostly fused.

develops (Fig. 18-6). This severe defect is usually accompanied by other severe craniocerebral anomalies. In **primary anophthalmos**, eye development is arrested early in the fourth week and results from failure of the optic vesicle to form. In **secondary anophthalmos**, development of the forebrain is suppressed and absence of the eye or eyes is one of several associated anomalies.

Development of the Ciliary Body

The ciliary body is a wedge-shaped extension of the choroid. Its medial surface projects toward the lens, forming **ciliary processes** (see Fig. 18-8). The pigmented portion of the ciliary epithelium is derived from the outer layer of the optic cup and is continuous with the retinal pigment epithelium (Figs. 18-7 and 18-8*D*). The non-pigmented portion of the ciliary epithelium represents the anterior prolongation of the neural retina in which no neural elements develop. The **ciliary muscle**—the smooth muscle of the ciliary body that is responsible for focusing the lens—and the connective tissue in the ciliary body develop from mesenchyme located at the edge of the optic cup in the region between the anterior scleral condensation and the ciliary pigment epithelium.

Development of the Iris

The iris develops from the rim of the optic cup, which grows inward and partially covers the lens (see Figs. 18-7 and 18-8). The two layers of the optic cup remain thin in this area. The epithelium of the iris represents both layers of the optic cup; it is continuous with the double-layered epithelium of the ciliary body and with the retinal pigment epithelium and neural retina. The connective tissue framework (stroma) of the iris is derived from neural crest cells that migrate into the iris. The **dilator pupillae** and **sphincter pupillae** muscles of the iris are derived from **neuroectoderm of the optic cup**. They appear to arise from the anterior epithelial cells of the iris. These smooth muscles result from a transformation of epithelial cells into smooth muscle cells.

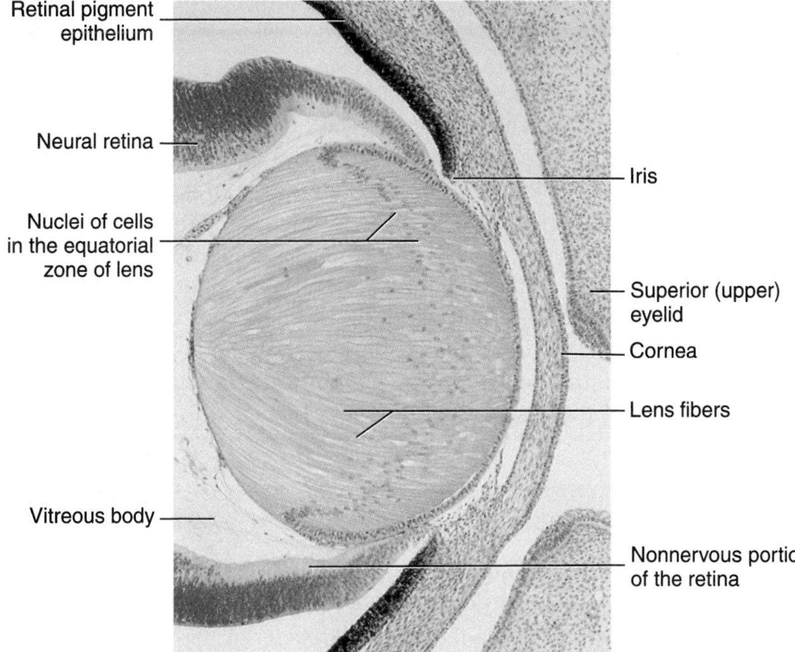

FIGURE 18-7. Sagittal section of part of the developing eye of an embryo (×280) at Carnegie stage 23, approximately 56 days. The lens fibers have elongated and obliterated the cavity of the lens vesicle. Note that the inner layer of the optic cup has thickened to form the primordial neural retina and that the outer layer is heavily pigmented (retinal pigment epithelium). (From Moore KL, Persaud TVN, Shiota K: Color Atlas of Clinical Embryology, 2nd ed. Philadelphia, WB Saunders, 2000.)

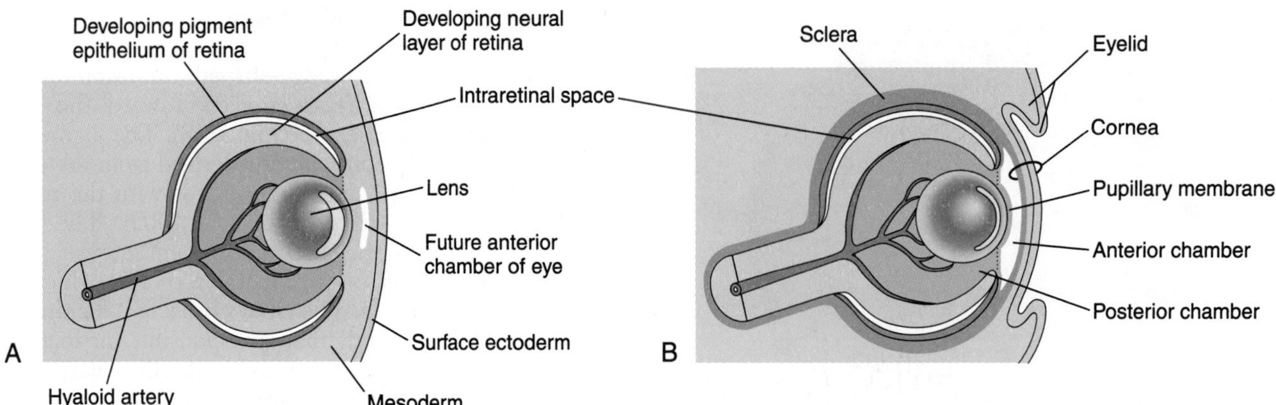

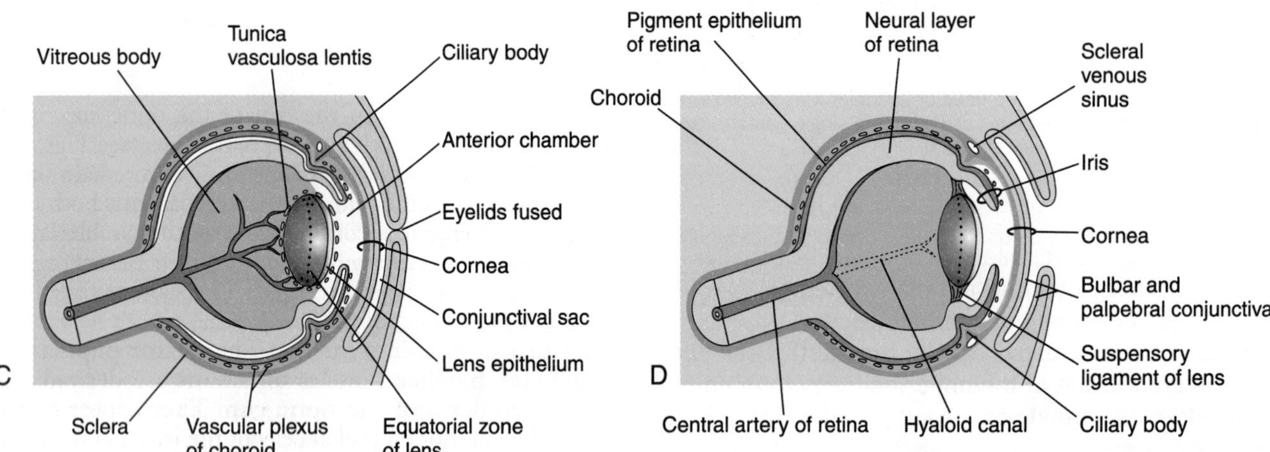

FIGURE 18-8. Diagrammatic drawings of sagittal sections of the eye showing successive developmental stages of the lens, retina, iris, and cornea development. **A,** At 5 weeks. **B,** At 6 weeks. **C,** At 20 weeks. **D,** Newborn. Note that the layers of the optic cup fuse to form the retinal pigment epithelium and neural retina and that they extend anteriorly as the double epithelium of the ciliary body and its iris. The retina and optic nerve are formed from the optic cup and optic stalk (outgrowths of brain). At birth, the eye is approximately three fourths of adult size. Most growth occurs during the first year. After puberty, growth of the eye is negligible.

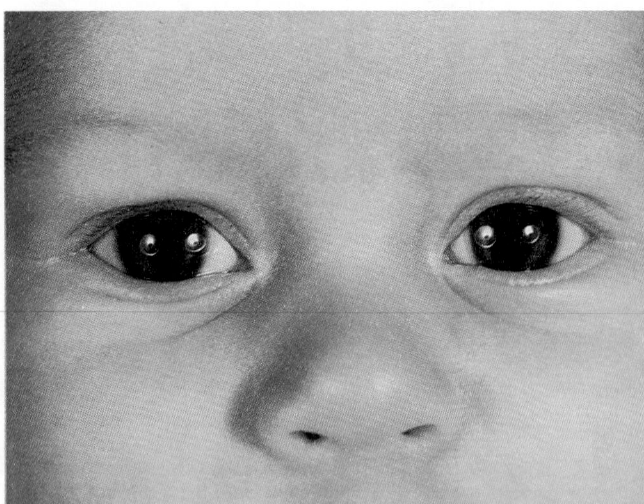

FIGURE 18-9. Bilateral coloboma of iris. Observe the defect in the inferior part of the iris (at the 6 o'clock position). (Courtesy of A.E. Chudley, MD, Section of Genetics and Metabolism, Department of Pediatrics and Child Health, Children's Hospital, University of Manitoba, Winnipeg, Manitoba, Canada.)

COLOR OF THE IRIS

The iris is typically light blue or gray in most newborn infants. The iris acquires its definitive color as pigmentation occurs during the first 6 to 10 months. The concentration and distribution of pigment-containing cells—**chromatophores**—in the loose vascular connective tissue of the iris determine eye color. If the melanin pigment is confined to the pigmented epithelium on the posterior surface of the iris, the iris appears blue. If melanin is also distributed throughout the stroma (supporting tissue) of the iris, the eye appears brown.

CONGENITAL ANIRIDIA

In this rare anomaly, there is almost complete absence of the iris. This defect results from an arrest of development at the rim of the optic cup during the eighth week. The anomaly may be associated with glaucoma and other eye abnormalities. Aniridia may be familial, the transmission being dominant or sporadic. In humans, mutation of the *Pax6* gene results in aniridia.

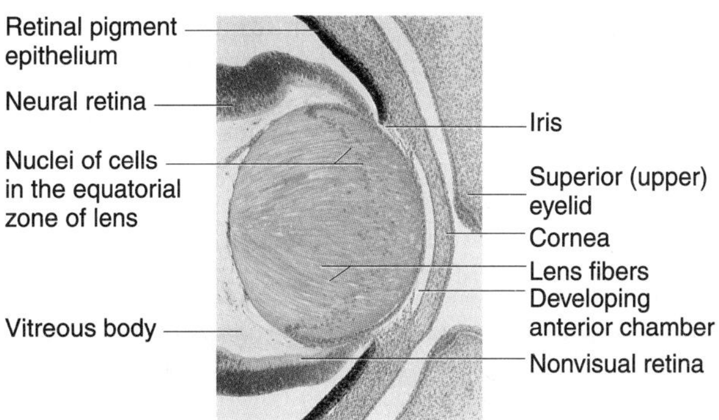

FIGURE 18-11. Photomicrograph of a portion of the developing eye of the embryo shown in Figure 18-10. Observe that the lens fibers have elongated and obliterated the cavity of the lens vesicle. Note that the inner layer of the optic cup has thickened greatly to form the neural retina and that the outer layer is heavily pigmented (retinal pigment epithelium). (From Moore KL, Persaud TVN, Shiota K: Color Atlas of Clinical Embryology, 2nd ed. Philadelphia, WB Saunders, 2000.)

Development of the Lens

The lens develops from the **lens vesicle**, a derivative of the surface ectoderm (see Fig. 18-1). The anterior wall of this vesicle, composed of cuboidal epithelium, becomes the subcapsular **lens epithelium** (see Fig. 18-8*C*). The nuclei of the tall columnar cells forming the posterior wall of the lens vesicle undergo dissolution. These cells lengthen considerably to form highly transparent epithelial cells, the **primary lens fibers**. As these fibers grow, they gradually obliterate the cavity of the lens vesicle (see Figs. 18-8*A* to *C* and 18-10).

The rim of the lens is known as the **equatorial zone** because it is located midway between the anterior and posterior poles of the lens (Fig. 18-11). The cells in the equatorial zone are cuboidal; as they elongate, they lose their nuclei and become **secondary lens fibers**. These new lens fibers are added to the external sides of the primary lens fibers. Although secondary lens fibers continue to form during adulthood and the lens increases in diameter, the primary lens fibers must last a lifetime.

The developing lens is supplied with blood by the distal part of the **hyaloid artery** (see Figs. 18-4 and 18-8); however, it becomes avascular in the fetal period when this part of the artery degenerates. Thereafter, the lens depends on diffusion from the aqueous humor in the **anterior chamber of the eye**, which bathes its anterior surface, and from the vitreous humor in other parts. The developing lens is invested by a vascular mesenchymal layer, the **tunica vasculosa lentis**. The anterior part of this capsule is the **pupillary membrane** (see Fig. 18-8*B*). The part of the hyaloid artery that supplies the tunica vasculosa lentis disappears during the late fetal period. As a result, the tunica vasculosa lentis and pupillary membrane degenerate (Fig. 18-8*C* and *D*); however, the **lens capsule** produced by the anterior lens epithelium and the lens fibers persists. The lens capsule represents a greatly thickened basement membrane and has a lamellar structure because of its development. The former site of the hyaloid artery is indicated by the **hyaloid canal** in the vitreous body (see Fig. 18-8*D*), which is usually inconspicuous in the living eye.

The **vitreous body** forms within the cavity of the optic cup (see Fig. 18-8*C*). It is composed of **vitreous humor**, an avascular mass of transparent, gel-like, intercellular substance. The **primary vitreous humor** is derived from

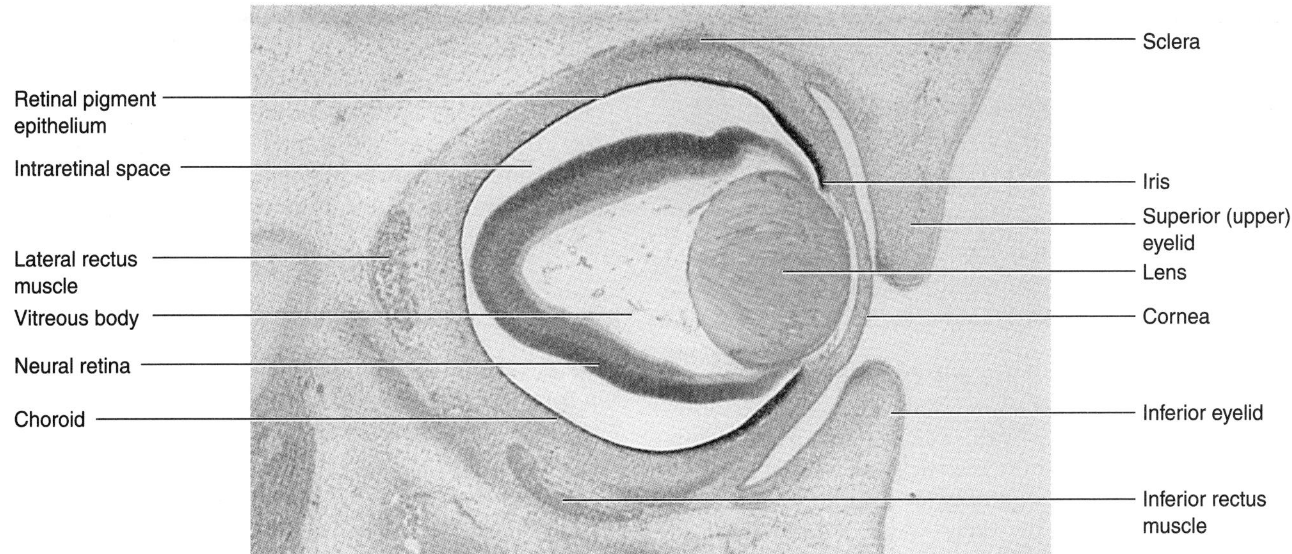

FIGURE 18-10. Photomicrograph of a sagittal section of the eye of an embryo (×50) at Carnegie stage 23, approximately 56 days. Observe the developing neural retina and retinal pigment epithelium. The intraretinal space normally disappears as these two layers of the retina fuse. (From Moore KL, Persaud TVN, Shiota K: Color Atlas of Clinical Embryology, 2nd ed. Philadelphia, WB Saunders, 2000.)

mesenchymal cells of neural crest origin. The primary vitreous humor does not increase but it is surrounded by a gelatinous **secondary vitreous humor**, the origin of which is uncertain. However, it is generally believed to arise from the inner layer of the optic cup. The secondary vitreous humor consists of primitive hyalocytes (vitreous cells), collagenous material, and traces of hyaluronic acid.

Persistent Pupillary Membrane

Remnants of the pupillary membrane, which covers the anterior surface of the lens during the embryonic period (see Fig. 18-8*B*), may persist as weblike strands of connective tissue or vascular arcades over the pupil in newborns, especially in premature infants. This tissue seldom interferes with vision and tends to atrophy. Very rarely the entire pupillary membrane persists, giving rise to **congenital atresia of the pupil**; surgery is needed in some cases to provide an adequate pupil.

Persistence of the Hyaloid Artery

The distal part of the hyaloid artery normally degenerates as its proximal part becomes the central artery of the retina. If the distal part of the hyaloid artery persists, it may appear as a freely moving, nonfunctional vessel or as a wormlike structure projecting from the optic disc. Sometimes the hyaloid artery remnant may appear as a fine strand traversing the vitreous body. In other cases, a remnant of the artery may form a cyst. In unusual cases, the entire distal part of the artery persists and extends from the optic disc through the vitreous body to the lens. In most of these unusual cases, the eye is microphthalmic (very small).

Congenital Aphakia

Absence of the lens is extremely rare and results from failure of the lens placode to form during the fourth week. Congenital aphakia could also result from failure of lens induction by the optic vesicle.

Development of the Aqueous Chambers

The **anterior chamber of the eye** develops from a cleft-like space that forms in the mesenchyme located between the developing lens and cornea (see Figs. 18-4, 18-8, and 18-11). The mesenchyme superficial to this space forms the substantia propria of the cornea and the mesothelium of the anterior chamber. After the lens is established, it induces the surface ectoderm to develop into the epithelium of the cornea and conjunctiva.

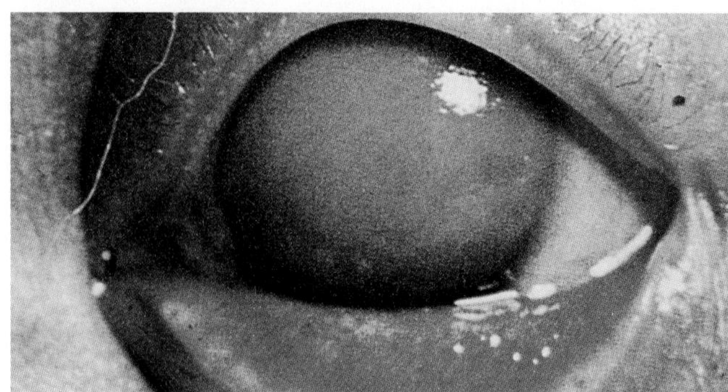

FIGURE 18-12. Severe congenital glaucoma resulting from the effects of an infection of the rubella virus. Observe the dense corneal haze, enlarged corneal diameter, and deep anterior chamber. (Courtesy of Dr. Daniel I. Weiss, Department of Ophthalmology, New York University College of Medicine. From Cooper LA, Green RH, Krugman S, et al: Neonatal thrombocytopenic purpura and other manifestations of rubella contracted in utero. Am J Dis Child 110:416, 1965. Copyright 1965. American Medical Association.)

The **posterior chamber of the eye** develops from a space that forms in the mesenchyme posterior to the developing iris and anterior to the developing lens. When the pupillary membrane disappears and the pupil forms (see Fig. 18-8*C* and *D*), the anterior and posterior chambers of the eye are able to communicate with each other through a circumferential **scleral venous sinus** (L. *sinus venosus sclerae*). This vascular structure encircling the anterior chamber is the outflow site of aqueous humor from the anterior chamber of the eye to the venous system.

Congenital Glaucoma

Abnormal elevation of intraocular pressure in newborn infants usually results from abnormal development of the drainage mechanism of the aqueous humor during the fetal period (Fig. 18-12). *Intraocular tension* rises because of an imbalance between the production of aqueous humor and its outflow. This imbalance may result from abnormal development of the *scleral venous sinus* (see Fig. 18-8*D*). Congenital glaucoma is genetically heterogeneous, but the condition may result from a rubella infection during early pregnancy (see Chapter 20).

Congenital Cataracts

In this condition, the lens is opaque and frequently appears grayish white. Without treatment, blindness results. Many lens opacities are inherited, dominant transmission being more common than recessive or sex-linked transmission. Some congenital cataracts are caused by teratogenic agents, particularly the **rubella virus** (Fig. 18-13), that affect early development of the lenses. The lenses are

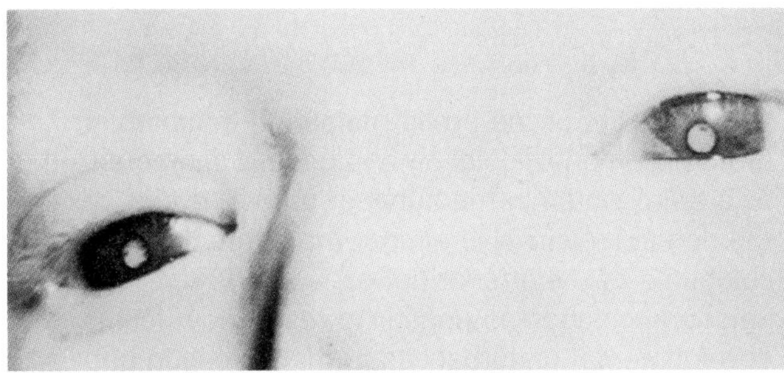

FIGURE 18-13. Bilateral congenital cataracts resulting from the teratogenic effects of the rubella virus. (Courtesy of Dr. Richard Bargy, Department of Ophthalmology, Cornell-New York Hospital, New York, New York.)

vulnerable to rubella virus between the fourth and seventh weeks, when primary lens fibers are forming.

Cataract and other ocular abnormalities caused by the rubella virus could be completely prevented if immunity to rubella were conferred on all women of reproductive age. Physical agents, such as **radiation**, can also damage the lens and produce cataracts. Another cause of cataract is an enzymatic deficiency—**congenital galactosemia**. These cataracts are not present at birth, but may appear as early as the second week after birth. Because of the enzyme deficiency, large amounts of galactose from milk accumulate in the infant's blood and tissues, causing injury to the lens and resulting in cataract formation.

Treatment of cataracts requires surgery, typically at a very early age (younger than 4 months), to remove the damaged lens. In most cases, corrective eyewear is required, although some studies have shown that artificial intraocular lenses may be safely implanted. More than 70% of patients with bilateral congenital cataracts can attain reasonable visual acuity. Extended treatment with refractive correction and additional surgery may be required.

Development of the Cornea

The cornea is induced by the lens vesicle. The inductive influence results in transformation of the surface ectoderm into the transparent, multilayered avascular cornea, the part of the fibrous tunic of the eye that bulges out of the orbit.

The cornea is formed from three sources:

- The external corneal epithelium, derived from **surface ectoderm**
- The **mesenchyme**, derived from mesoderm, which is continuous with the developing sclera
- **Neural crest cells** that migrate from the lip of the optic cup and differentiate into the corneal endothelium

EDEMA OF THE OPTIC DISC

The optic nerve is surrounded by three sheaths that evaginated with the optic vesicle and stalk; consequently, they are continuous with the meninges of the brain.

- The outer dural sheath from the dura mater is thick and fibrous and blends with the sclera.
- The intermediate sheath from the arachnoid mater is thin.
- The inner sheath from the pia mater is vascular and closely invests the optic nerve and central vessels of the retina as far as the optic disc.
- Cerebrospinal fluid is present in the subarachnoid space between the intermediate and inner sheaths of the optic nerve.

The relationship of the sheaths of the optic nerve to the meninges of the brain and the subarachnoid space is important clinically. An increase in CSF pressure (often resulting from increased intracranial pressure) slows venous return from the retina, causing **papilledema** (fluid accumulation) of the optic disc. This occurs because the retinal vessels are covered by pia mater and lie in the extension of the subarachnoid space that surrounds the optic nerve.

Development of the Choroid and Sclera

The mesenchyme surrounding the optic cup (largely of neural crest origin) reacts to the inductive influence of the retinal pigment epithelium by differentiating into an inner vascular layer, the **choroid**, and an outer fibrous layer, the **sclera** (see Fig. 18-8*C*). The sclera develops from a condensation of mesenchyme external to the choroid and is continuous with the stroma (supporting tissue) of the cornea. Toward the rim of the optic cup, the choroid becomes modified to form the cores of the **ciliary processes**, consisting chiefly of capillaries supported by delicate connective tissue. The first **choroidal blood vessels** appear during the 15th week; by the 23rd week, arteries and veins can be easily distinguished.

Development of the Eyelids

The eyelids develop during the sixth week from **neural crest cell mesenchyme** and from two cutaneous folds of ectoderm that grow over the cornea (see Fig. 18-8*B*). The eyelids adhere to one another by the beginning of the 10th week and remain adherent until the 26th to the 28th week (see Fig. 18-8*C*). While the eyelids are adherent, there is a closed **conjunctival sac** anterior to the cornea. As the eyelids open, the **bulbar conjunctiva** is reflected over the anterior part of the sclera and the surface epithelium of the cornea (see Fig. 18-8*D*). The **palpebral conjunctiva** lines the inner surface of the eyelids.

The **eyelashes** and **glands** in the eyelids are derived from the surface ectoderm in a manner similar to that described for other parts of the integument (see Chapter 19). The connective tissue and **tarsal plates** develop from mesenchyme in the developing eyelids. The orbicularis oculi muscle is derived from mesenchyme in the second pharyngeal arch (see Chapter 9) and is supplied by its nerve (CN VII).

CONGENITAL PTOSIS OF THE EYELID

Drooping of the superior (upper) eyelids at birth is relatively common (Fig. 18-14). **Ptosis** (blepharoptosis) may result from failure of normal development of the **levator palpebrae superioris** muscle. Congenital ptosis may more rarely result from prenatal injury or dystrophy of the superior division of the **oculomotor nerve** (CN III), which supplies this muscle. If ptosis is associated with inability to move the eyeball superiorly, there is also failure of the superior rectus muscle of the eyeball to develop normally. Congenital ptosis may be transmitted as an autosomal dominant trait. Congenital ptosis is also associated with several syndromes.

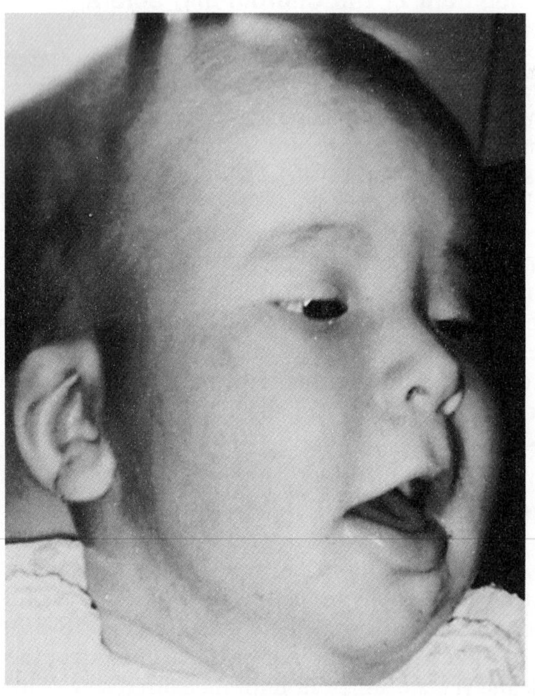

FIGURE 18-14. Child with congenital bilateral ptosis. Drooping of the superior eyelids usually results from abnormal development or failure of development of the levator palpebrae superioris, the muscle that elevates the eyelid. In bilateral cases, as here, the infant contracts the frontalis muscle of the forehead in an attempt to raise the eyelids. (From Avery ME, Taeusch HW Jr: Schaffer's Diseases of the Newborn, 5th ed. Philadelphia, WB Saunders, 1984.)

COLOBOMA OF THE EYELID

Large defects of the eyelid (**palpebral colobomas**) are uncommon. A coloboma is usually characterized by a small notch in the superior (upper) eyelid, but the defect may involve almost the entire lid. A coloboma of the inferior (lower) eyelid is rare. Palpebral colobomas appear to result from local developmental disturbances in the formation and growth of the eyelids.

CRYPTOPHTHALMOS

Cryptophthalmos (L. *kryptos*, hidden) results from congenital absence of the eyelids; as a result, skin covers the eye. The eyeball is small and defective, and the cornea and conjunctiva usually do not develop. Fundamentally, the defect means absence of the palpebral fissure (slit) between eyelids; usually there is varying absence of eyelashes and eyebrows and other eye defects. Cryptophthalmos is an autosomal recessive condition that is usually part of the *cryptophthalmos syndrome*.

Development of the Lacrimal Glands

At the superolateral angles of the orbits, the lacrimal glands develop from a number of solid buds from the surface ectoderm. The buds branch and become canalized to form the **nasolacrimal ducts**. The lacrimal glands are small at birth and do not function fully until approximately 6 weeks; hence, the newborn infant does not produce tears when it cries. Tears are often not present with crying until 1 to 3 months.

DEVELOPMENT OF THE EAR

The ear is composed of three anatomic parts:

- The *external ear*, consisting of the auricle (pinna), the external acoustic meatus, and the external layer of the tympanic membrane (eardrum)
- The *middle ear*, consisting of three small auditory ossicles (ear bones), and the internal layer of the tympanic membrane, which is connected to the oval window of the internal ear by the ossicles
- The *internal ear*, consisting of the vestibulocochlear organ, which is concerned with both hearing and balance

The external and middle parts of the ear are concerned with the transference of sound waves to the internal ear, which converts the waves into nerve impulses and registers changes in equilibrium.

Development of the Internal Ear

The internal ear is the first of the three parts of the ear to develop. Early in the fourth week, a thickening of surface ectoderm, the **otic placode**, appears on each side of the myelencephalon, the caudal part of the hindbrain (Fig. 18-15*A* and *B*). Inductive signals from the paraxial mesoderm and notochord stimulate the surface ectoderm to form the placodes. Each otic placode soon invaginates and sinks deep to the surface ectoderm into the underlying mesenchyme. In so doing, it forms an **otic pit** (see Fig. 18-15*C* and *D*). The edges of the otic pit soon come together and fuse to form an **otic vesicle**—the *primordium of the membranous labyrinth* (Figs. 18-15*E* to *G* and 18-16). The otic vesicle then loses its connection with the surface ectoderm, and a diverticulum grows from the vesicle and elongates to form the **endolymphatic duct** and **sac** (Fig. 18-17*A* to *E*). Two regions of the otic vesicle are recognizable:

- A dorsal **utricular part**, from which the small endolymphatic duct, utricle, and semicircular ducts arise
- A ventral **saccular part**, which gives rise to the saccule and cochlear duct

Three disclike diverticula grow out from the utricular part of the **primordial membranous labyrinth**. Soon the central parts of these diverticula fuse and disappear (see Fig. 18-17*B* to *E*). The peripheral unfused parts of the diverticula become the **semicircular ducts**, which are attached to the utricle and are later enclosed in the semicircular canals of the bony labyrinth. Localized dilatations, the **ampullae**, develop at one end of each semicircular duct. Specialized receptor areas—**cristae ampullares**—differentiate in the ampullae and in the utricle and saccule (maculae utriculi and sacculi).

From the ventral saccular part of the otic vesicle, a tubular diverticulum—the **cochlear duct**—grows and coils to form the **membranous cochlea** (see Fig. 18-17*C* to *E*). A connection of the cochlea with the saccule, the **ductus reuniens**, soon forms. The **spiral organ** (of Corti) differentiates from cells in the wall of the cochlear duct (see Fig. 18-17*F* to *I*). Ganglion cells of the vestibulocochlear nerve (cranial nerve [CN] VIII) migrate along the coils of the membranous cochlea and form the **spiral ganglion** (of cochlea). Nerve processes extend from this ganglion to the spiral organ, where they terminate on the **hair cells**. The cells in the spiral ganglion retain their embryonic bipolar condition.

Inductive influences from the otic vesicle stimulate the mesenchyme around the otic vesicle to condense and differentiate into a **cartilaginous otic capsule** (see Fig. 18-17*F*). The transforming growth factor β_1 may play a role in modulating epithelial-mesenchymal interaction in

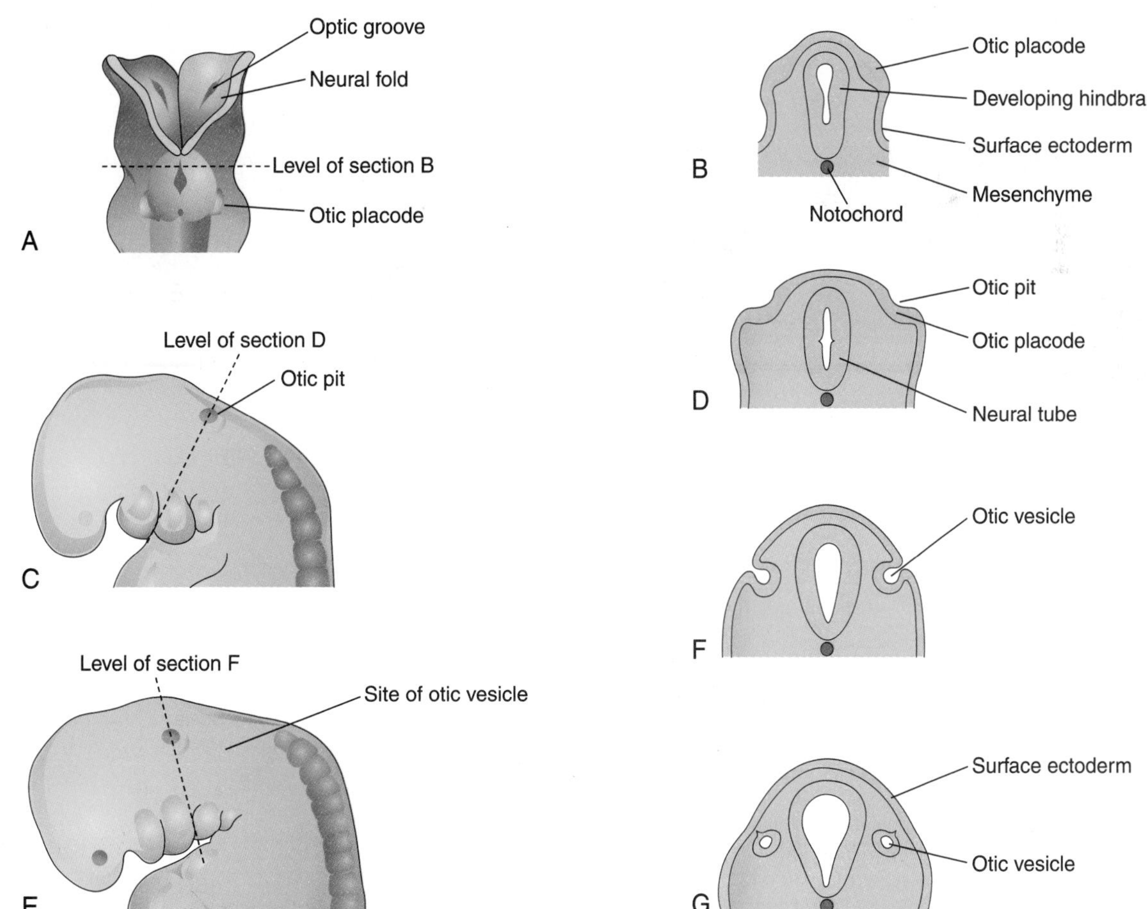

FIGURE 18-15. Drawings illustrating early development of the internal ear. **A,** Dorsal view of a 4-week embryo (approximately 22 days) showing the otic placodes. **B, D, F,** and **G,** Schematic coronal sections illustrating successive stages in the development of otic vesicles. **C** and **E,** Lateral views of the cranial region of embryos, approximately 24 and 28 days, respectively.

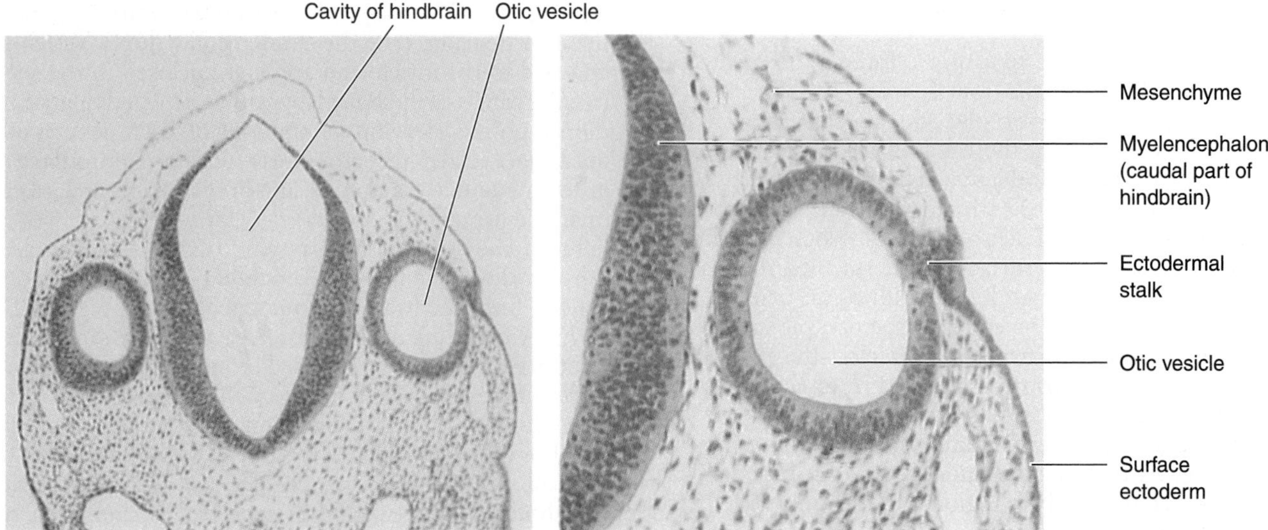

FIGURE 18-16. *Left,* Photomicrograph of a transverse section of an embryo (×55) at Carnegie stage 12, approximately 26 days. Observe the otic vesicles, the primordia of the membranous labyrinths, which give rise to the internal ears. *Right,* Higher magnification of the right otic vesicle (×120). Note the ectodermal stalk, which is still attached to the remnant of the otic placode. The otic vesicle will soon lose its connection with the surface ectoderm (primordium of epidermis). (From Nishimura H [ed]: Atlas of Human Prenatal Histology. Tokyo, Igaku-Shoin, 1983.)

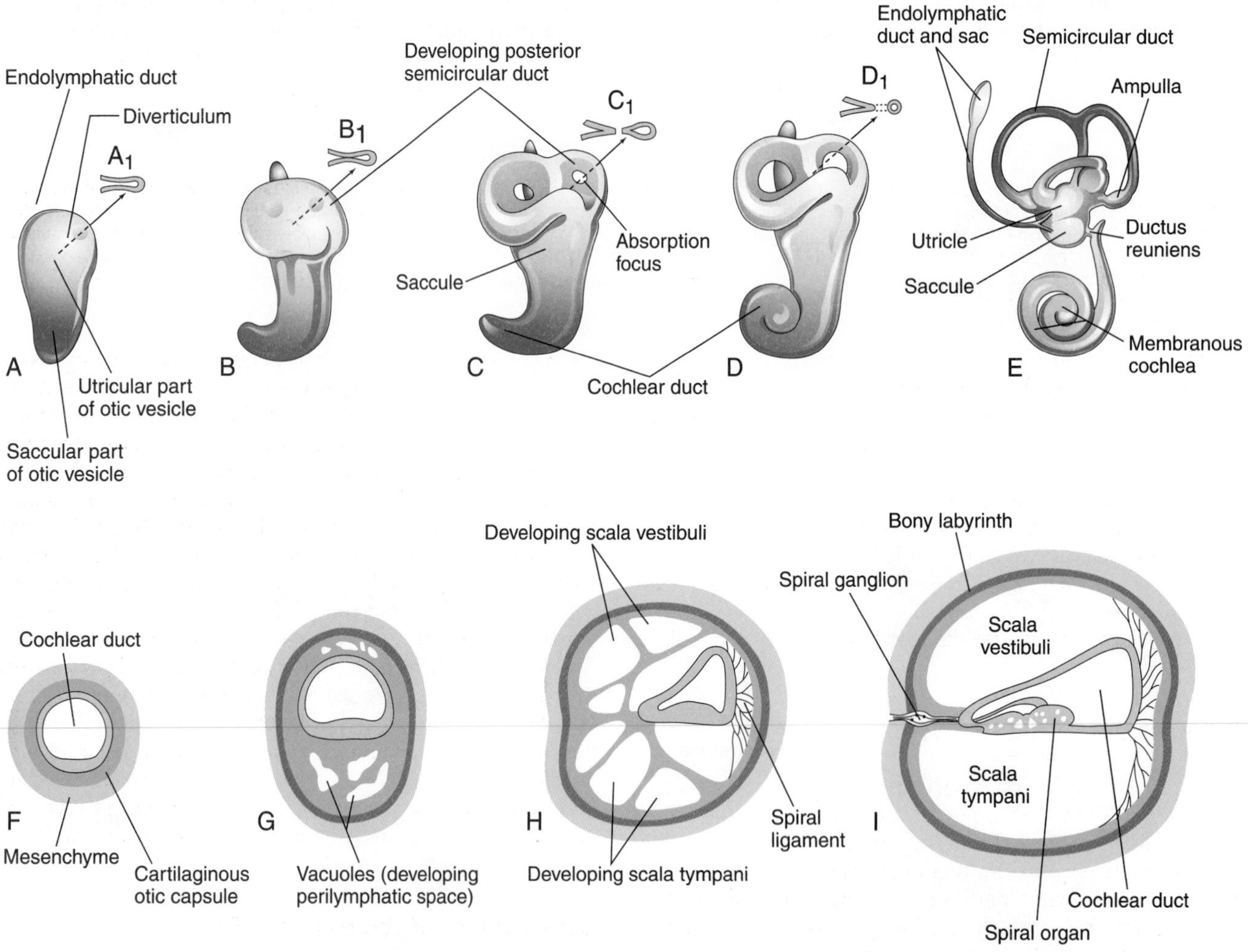

FIGURE 18-17. Drawings of the otic vesicle showing the development of the membranous and bony labyrinths of the internal ear. **A** to **E,** Lateral views showing successive stages in the development of the otic vesicle into the membranous labyrinth from the fifth to eighth weeks. **A** to **D,** Diagrammatic sketches illustrating the development of a semicircular duct. **F** to **I,** Sections through the cochlear duct showing successive stages in the development of the spiral organ and the perilymphatic space from the 8th to the 20th weeks.

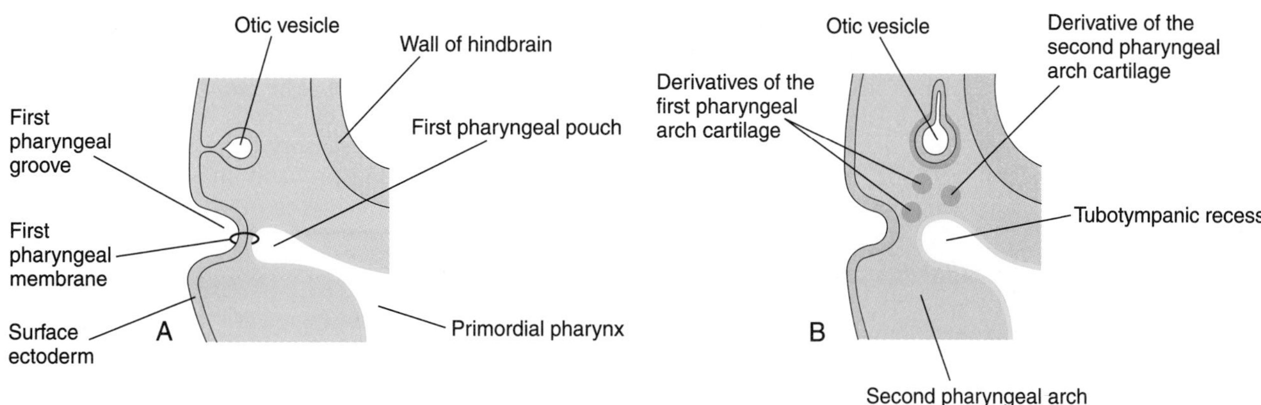

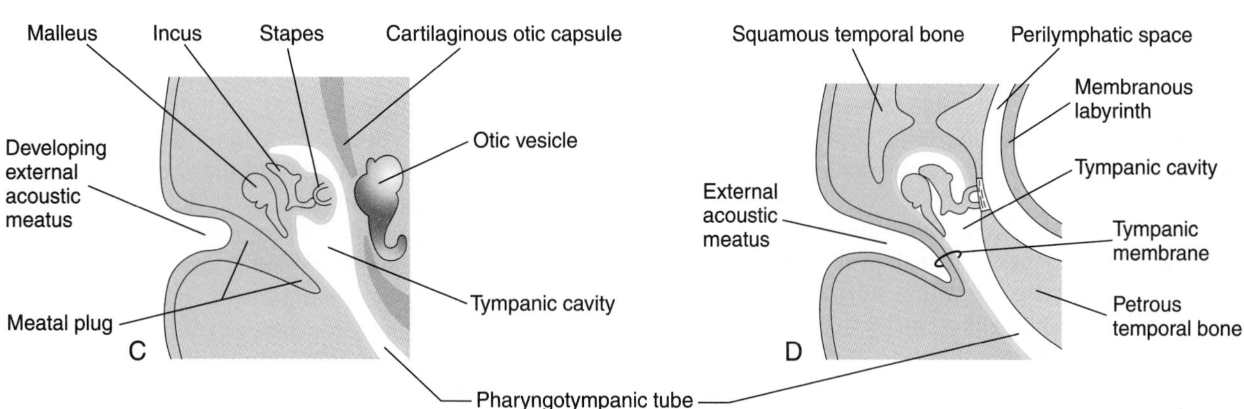

FIGURE 18-18. Schematic drawings illustrating development of the external and middle ear. Observe the relationship of these parts of the ear to the otic vesicle, the primordium of the internal ear. **A,** At 4 weeks, illustrating the relation of the otic vesicle to the pharyngeal apparatus. **B,** At 5 weeks, showing the tubotympanic recess and pharyngeal arch cartilages. **C,** Later stage showing the tubotympanic recess (future tympanic cavity and mastoid antrum) beginning to envelop the ossicles. **D,** Final stage of ear development showing the relationship of the middle ear to the perilymphatic space and the external acoustic meatus. Note that the tympanic membrane develops from three germ layers: surface ectoderm, mesenchyme, and endoderm of the tubotympanic recess.

the internal ear and in directing the formation of the otic capsule. As the **membranous labyrinth** enlarges, vacuoles appear in the cartilaginous otic capsule and soon coalesce to form the **perilymphatic space**. The membranous labyrinth is now suspended in **perilymph** (fluid in perilymphatic space). The perilymphatic space related to the cochlear duct develops two divisions, the **scala tympani** and **scala vestibuli** (see Fig. 18-17*H* and *I*). The cartilaginous otic capsule later ossifies to form the **bony labyrinth** of the internal ear. The internal ear reaches its adult size and shape by the middle of the fetal period (20–22 weeks).

Development of the Middle Ear

Development of the **tubotympanic recess** (Fig. 18-18*B*) from the first pharyngeal pouch is described in Chapter 9. The proximal part of the tubotympanic recess forms the **pharyngotympanic tube** (auditory tube). The distal part of the recess expands and becomes the **tympanic cavity** (see Fig. 18-18*C*), which gradually envelops the small bones of the middle ear—**auditory ossicles** (malleus, incus, and stapes), their tendons and ligaments, and the chorda tympani nerve. Development of the ossicles is described in Chapter 9. These structures receive a more or less complete epithelial investment. It has been suggested that, in addition to apoptosis in the middle ear, an epithelium-type organizer located at the tip of the tubotympanic recess probably plays a role in the early development of the middle ear and tympanic membrane.

During the late fetal period, expansion of the tympanic cavity gives rise to the **mastoid antrum**, located in the petromastoid part of the temporal bone. The mastoid antrum is almost adult size at birth; however, no mastoid cells are present in newborn infants. By 2 years of age, the mastoid cells are well developed and produce conical projections of the temporal bones, the **mastoid processes**. The middle ear continues to grow through puberty. The **tensor tympani muscle**, attached to the malleus, is derived from mesenchyme in the first pharyngeal arch and is innervated by CN V, the nerve of this arch. The **stapedius muscle** is derived from the second pharyngeal arch and is supplied by CN VII, the nerve of this arch.

Development of the External Ear

The **external acoustic meatus**, the passage of the external ear leading to the tympanic membrane, develops from the dorsal part of the first pharyngeal groove. The ectodermal cells at the bottom of this funnel-shaped tube proliferate to form a solid epithelial plate, the **meatal plug** (see Fig. 18-18*C*). Late in the fetal period, the central cells of this plug degenerate, forming a cavity that becomes the internal part of the external acoustic meatus (see Fig. 18-18*D*). The external acoustic meatus, relatively short at birth, attains its adult length in approximately the ninth year.

The primordium of the **tympanic membrane** is the first **pharyngeal membrane**, which forms the external surface of the tympanic membrane. In the embryo, the pharyngeal membrane separates the first pharyngeal groove from the first pharyngeal pouch (see Fig. 18-18*A*). As development proceeds, mesenchyme grows between the two parts of the pharyngeal membrane and differentiates into the collagenic fibers in the tympanic membrane.

To summarize, the tympanic membrane develops from three sources:

- Ectoderm of the first pharyngeal groove
- Endoderm of the tubotympanic recess, a derivative of the first pharyngeal pouch
- Mesenchyme of the first and second pharyngeal arches

The **auricle** (pinna), which projects from the side of the head, develops from mesenchymal proliferations in the first and second pharyngeal arches—**auricular hillocks**—surrounding the first pharyngeal groove (Fig. 18-19*A*). As the auricle grows, the contribution by the first arch is reduced (see Fig. 18-19*B* to *D*). The **lobule** (earlobe) is the last part of the auricle to develop. The auricles begin to develop at the base of the neck (see Fig. 18-19*A* and *B*). As the mandible develops, the auricles assume their normal position at the side of the head (see Fig. 18-19*D*).

The parts of the auricle derived from the first pharyngeal arch are supplied by its nerve, the mandibular branch of the **trigeminal nerve**; the parts derived from the second arch are supplied by cutaneous branches of the cervical plexus, especially the **lesser occipital** and **greater auricular nerves**. The *facial nerve* of the second pharyngeal arch has few cutaneous branches; some of its fibers contribute to the sensory innervation of the skin in the mastoid region and probably in small areas on both aspects of the auricle.

Congenital Deafness

Because formation of the internal ear is independent of development of the middle and external ears, congenital impairment of hearing may be the result of maldevelopment of the sound-conducting apparatus of the middle and external ears or of the neurosensory structures of the internal ear. Approximately three in every 1000 newborns have significant hearing loss, of which there are many subtypes. Most types of congenital deafness are caused by genetic factors, and many of the genes responsible have been identified. Mutations in the *GJB2* gene are responsible for approximately 50% of nonsyndromic recessive hearing loss. Congenital deafness may be associated with several other head and neck anomalies as a part of the first arch syndrome (see Chapter 9). Abnormalities of the malleus and incus are often associated with this syndrome. A **rubella infection** during the critical period of development of the internal ear, particularly the seventh and eighth weeks, can cause maldevelopment of the spiral organ and deafness. **Congenital fixation of the stapes** results in

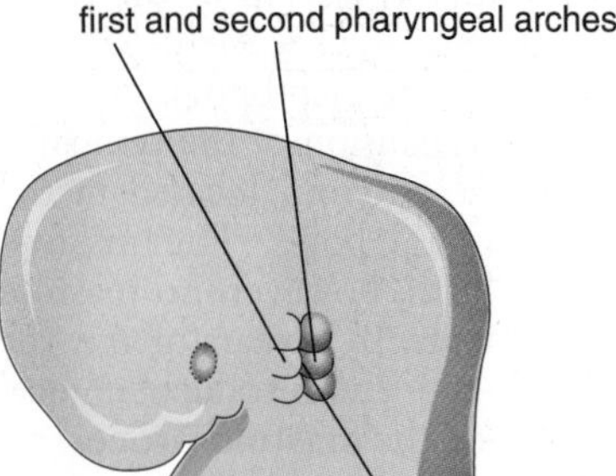

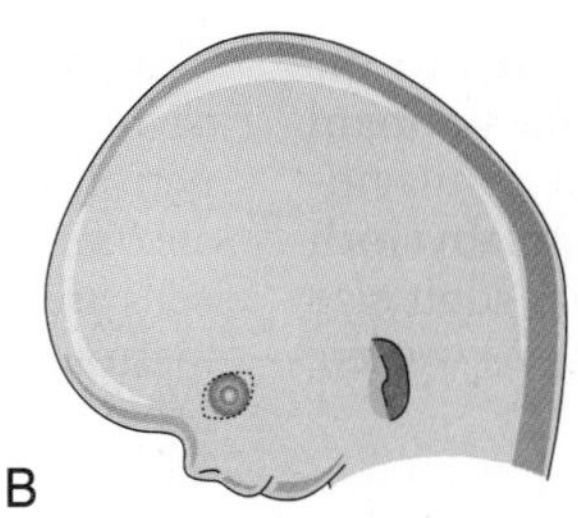

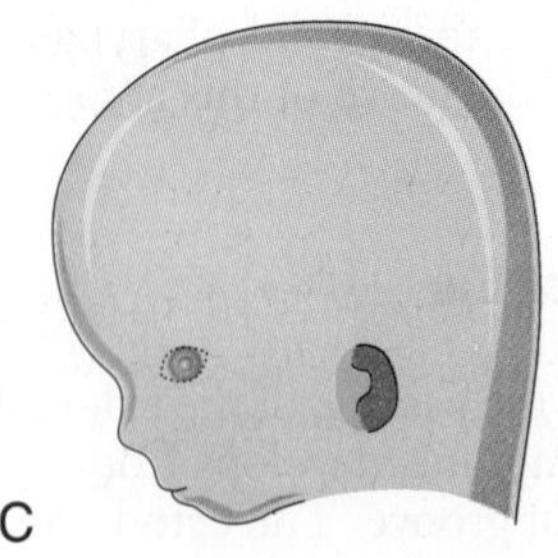

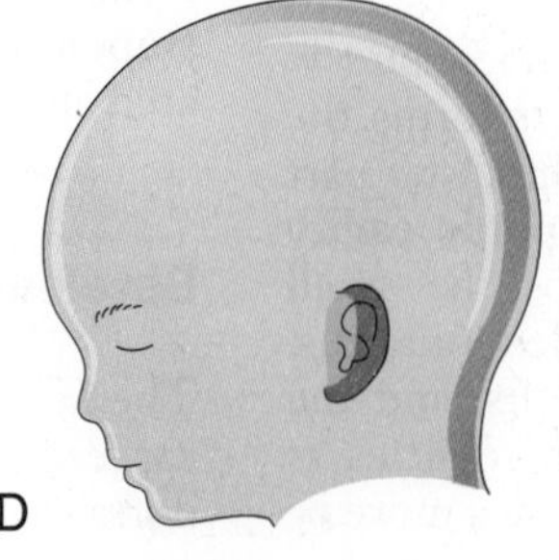

FIGURE 18-19. Illustrations of the development of the auricle, the part of the external ear not contained within the head. **A,** At 6 weeks. Note that three auricular hillocks are located on the first pharyngeal arch and three on the second arch. **B,** At 8 weeks. **C,** At 10 weeks. **D,** At 32 weeks. As the mandible and teeth develop, the auricles move from the superior neck region to the side of the head.

conductive deafness in an otherwise normal ear. Failure of differentiation of the anular ligament, which attaches the base of the stapes to the oval window (fenestra vestibuli), results in fixation of the stapes to the bony labyrinth.

Auricular Abnormalities

Severe anomalies of the external ear are rare, but minor deformities are common. There is a wide variation in the shape of the auricle. Almost any minor auricular defect may occasionally be found as a usual feature in a particular family. Minor anomalies of the auricles may serve as indicators of a specific pattern of congenital anomalies. For example, the auricles are often abnormal in shape and low-set in infants with chromosomal syndromes (Fig. 18-20) such as trisomy 18 and in infants affected by maternal ingestion of certain drugs (e.g., trimethadione).

Auricular Appendages

Auricular appendages (skin tags) are common and may result from the development of accessory auricular hillocks (Fig. 18-21). The appendages usually appear anterior to the auricle, more often unilaterally than bilaterally. The appendages, often with narrow pedicles, consist of skin but may contain some cartilage.

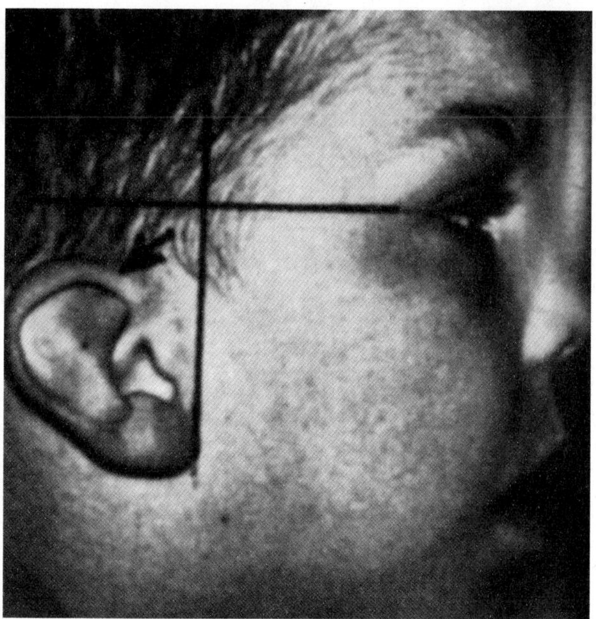

FIGURE 18-20. Low-set slanted ear. This designation is made when the margin of the auricle or helix (*arrow*) meets the cranium at a level inferior to the horizontal plane through the corner of the eye. (From Jones KL: Smith's Recognizable Patterns of Human Malformation, 5th ed. Philadelphia, WB Saunders, 1996.)

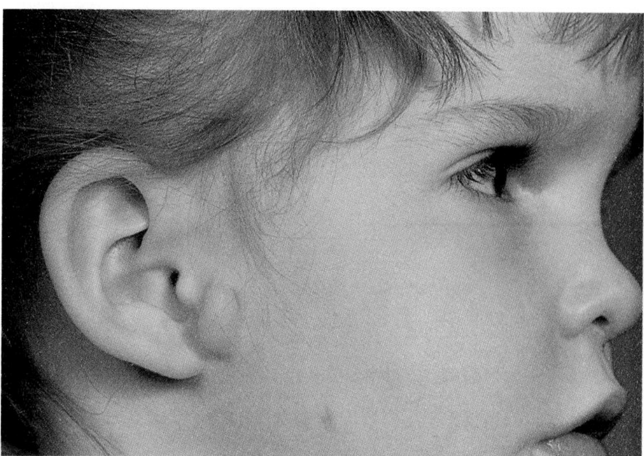

FIGURE 18-21. A child with a preauricular tag or skin tag. (Courtesy of A.E. Chudley, MD, Section of Genetics and Metabolism, Department of Pediatrics and Child Health, University of Manitoba, Children's Hospital, Winnipeg, Manitoba, Canada.)

Absence of the Auricle

Anotia (absence of the auricle) is rare but is commonly associated with the first pharyngeal arch syndrome (see Chapter 9). **Anotia** results from failure of mesenchymal proliferation.

Microtia

Microtia (a small or rudimentary auricle) results from suppressed mesenchymal proliferation (Fig. 18-22). This anomaly often serves as an indicator of associated anomalies, such as an atresia of the external acoustic meatus and middle ear anomalies.

Preauricular Sinuses and Fistulas

Pitlike cutaneous depressions or shallow sinuses are occasionally located in a triangular area anterior to the auricle (Fig. 18-23). The sinuses are usually narrow tubes or shallow pits that have pinpoint external openings. Some sinuses contain a vestigial cartilaginous mass. **Preauricular sinuses** may be associated with internal anomalies, such as deafness and kidney malformations. The embryologic basis of auricular sinuses is uncertain, but some are related to abnormal mesenchymal proliferation and defective closure of the dorsal part of the first pharyngeal groove. Most of this pharyngeal groove normally disappears as the external acoustic meatus forms. Other auricular sinuses appear to represent ectodermal folds that are sequestered during formation of the auricle. Preauricular sinuses are familial and frequently bilateral. They are asymptomatic and have only minor cosmetic importance; however, they often develop serious infections. **Auricular fistulas** (narrow canals) connecting the preauricular skin with the tympanic cavity or the tonsillar sinus (fossa) (see Fig. 9-10*F*) are extremely rare.

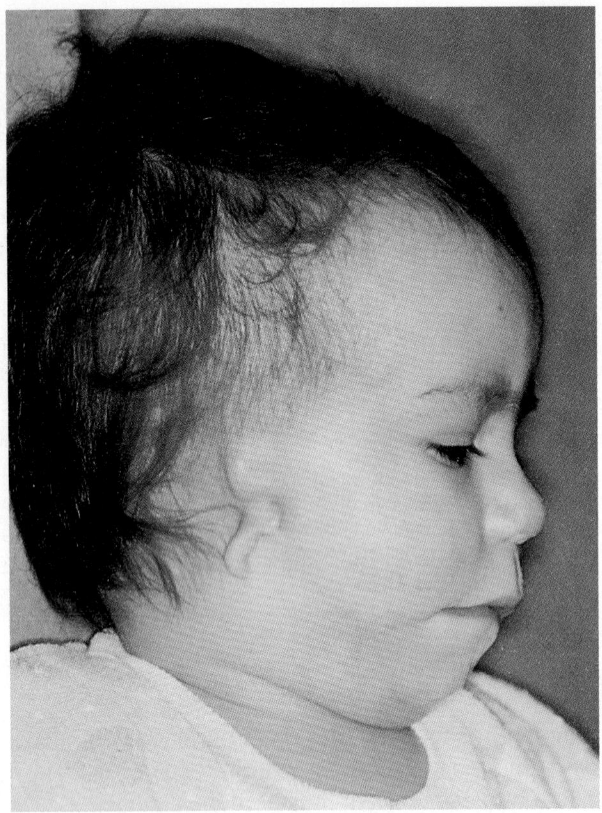

FIGURE 18-22. Child with a rudimentary auricle (microtia). She also has several other congenital anomalies. (Courtesy of A.E. Chudley, MD, Section of Genetics and Metabolism, Department of Pediatrics and Child Health, Children's Hospital, University of Manitoba, Winnipeg, Manitoba, Canada.)

Atresia of the External Acoustic Meatus

Atresia (blockage) of this canal results from failure of the meatal plug to canalize (see Fig. 18-18C). Usually the deep part of the meatus is open, but the superficial part is blocked by bone or fibrous tissue. Most cases are associated with the *first arch syndrome* (see Chapter 9). Often abnormal development of both the first and second pharyngeal arches is involved. The auricle is also usually severely affected and anomalies of the middle and/or internal ear are sometimes present. Atresia of the external acoustic meatus can occur bilaterally or unilaterally and usually results from autosomal dominant inheritance.

Absence of the External Acoustic Meatus

Absence of the external acoustic meatus is rare; usually the auricle is normal (Fig. 18-24). This anomaly results from failure of inward expansion of the first pharyngeal groove and failure of the meatal plug to disappear (see Fig. 18-18C).

Congenital Cholesteatoma

This is a rest of epithelial cells (fragment of embryonic tissue that is retained after birth). The rest appears as a white cystlike structure medial to or within the tympanic membrane. The rest probably consists of cells from the meatal plug that were displaced during its canalization (see Fig. 18-18C). It has been suggested that congenital cholesteatoma may originate from an epidermoid formation that normally involutes by 33 weeks' gestation.

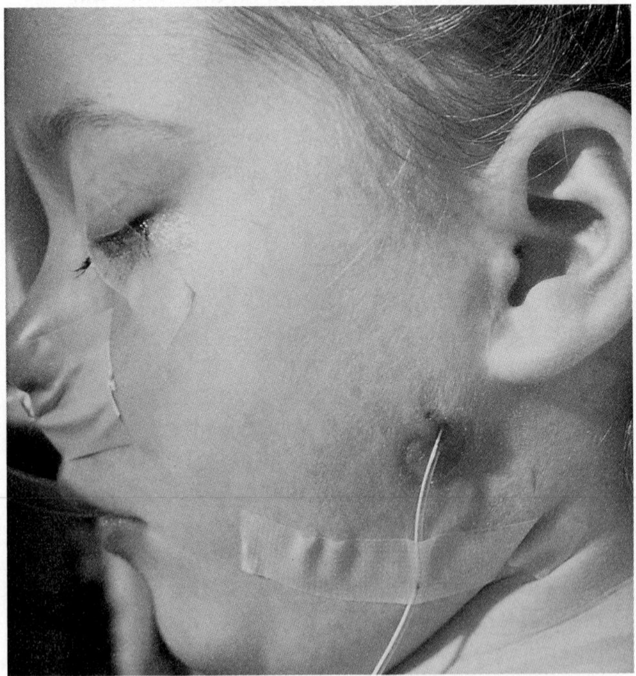

FIGURE 18-23. A child with an auricular fistula relating to the first pharyngeal arch. Note the external orifice of the fistula below the auricle and the upward direction of the catheter (sinus tract) toward the external acoustic meatus. (Courtesy of Dr. Pierre Soucy, Division of Paediatric General Surgery, Children's Hospital of Eastern Ontario, Ottawa, Ontario, Canada.)

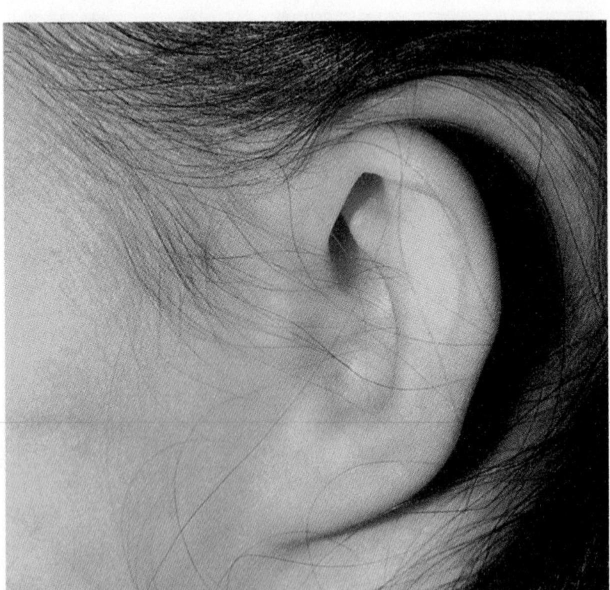

FIGURE 18-24. A child with no external acoustic meatus; however, the auricle is normal. A computed tomography scan revealed normal middle and internal ear structures. (Courtesy of A.E. Chudley, MD, Section of Genetics and Metabolism, Department of Pediatrics and Child Health, Children's Hospital, University of Manitoba, Winnipeg, Manitoba, Canada.)

SUMMARY OF THE DEVELOPMENT OF THE EYE

The first indication of the eye is the **optic groove**, which forms at the beginning of the fourth week. The groove deepens to form a hollow optic vesicle that projects from the forebrain. The **optic vesicle** contacts the surface ectoderm and induces development of the **lens placode**, the primordial lens.

- As the lens placode invaginates to form a **lens pit** and **lens vesicle**, the optic vesicle invaginates to form an **optic cup**. The retina forms from the two layers of the optic cup.
- The retina, optic nerve fibers, muscles of the iris, and epithelium of the iris and ciliary body are derived from the **neuroectoderm** of the forebrain. The sphincter and dilator muscles of the iris develop from the ectoderm at the rim of the optic cup. The surface ectoderm gives rise to the **lens** and the epithelium of the lacrimal glands, eyelids, conjunctiva, and cornea. The mesenchyme gives rise to the eye muscles, except those of the iris, and to all connective and vascular tissues of the cornea, iris, ciliary body, choroid, and sclera.
- The eye is sensitive to the teratogenic effects of **infectious agents** (e.g., cytomegalovirus and rubella virus); see Chapter 20. **Defects of sight** may result from infection of tissues and organs by certain microorganisms during the fetal period (e.g., rubella virus and *Treponema pallidum*, the microorganism that causes syphilis). Most ocular anomalies are caused by defective closure of the retinal fissure during the sixth week (e.g., coloboma of the iris). Congenital cataract and glaucoma may result from intrauterine infections, but most congenital cataracts are inherited.

SUMMARY OF THE DEVELOPMENT OF THE EAR

- The **otic vesicle** develops from the surface ectoderm during the fourth week. The vesicle develops into the **membranous labyrinth** of the internal ear.
- The otic vesicle divides into a *dorsal utricular part*, which gives rise to the **utricle**, **semicircular ducts**, and **endolymphatic duct**, and a *ventral saccular part*, which gives rise to the **saccule** and **cochlear duct**. The cochlear duct gives rise to the **spiral organ**.
- The **bony labyrinth** develops from the mesenchyme adjacent to the membranous labyrinth. The epithelium lining the tympanic cavity, mastoid antrum, and pharyngotympanic tube is derived from the endoderm of the **tubotympanic recess**, which develops from the first pharyngeal pouch. The **auditory ossicles** develop from the dorsal ends of the cartilages in the first two pharyngeal arches. The epithelium of the **external acoustic meatus** develops from the ectoderm of the first pharyngeal groove.
- The **tympanic membrane** is derived from three sources: endoderm of the first pharyngeal pouch, ectoderm of the first pharyngeal groove, and mesenchyme between the above layers.
- The **auricle** develops from the fusion of six **auricular hillocks,** which form from mesenchymal prominences around the margins of the first pharyngeal groove.
- Congenital deafness may result from abnormal development of the membranous labyrinth and/or bony labyrinth, as well as from abnormalities of the auditory ossicles. **Recessive inheritance** is the most common cause of congenital deafness, but a **rubella virus infection** near the end of the embryonic period is a major environmental factor known to cause abnormal development of the spiral organ and defective hearing.
- There are many minor anomalies of the auricle; however, some of them may alert the clinician to the possible presence of associated major anomalies (e.g., defects of middle ear). Low-set, severely malformed ears are often associated with **chromosomal abnormalities**, particularly trisomy 13 and trisomy 18.

CLINICALLY ORIENTED PROBLEMS

CASE 18-1

An infant was born blind and deaf with congenital heart disease. The mother had had a severe viral infection early in her pregnancy.

- Considering the congenital anomalies present, name the virus that was probably involved.
- What is the common congenital cardiovascular lesion found in infants whose mothers have this infection early in pregnancy?
- Is the history of a rash during the first trimester an essential factor in the development of embryonic disease (embryopathy)?

CASE 18-2

An infant was born with bilateral ptosis.

- What is the probable embryologic basis of this condition?
- Are hereditary factors involved?
- Injury to what nerve could also cause congenital ptosis?

CASE 18-3

An infant has small, multiple calcifications in the brain, microcephaly, and microphthalmia. The mother was known to have a fondness for very rare meat.

- What protozoon might be involved?
- What is the embryologic basis of the infant's congenital anomalies?
- What advice might the doctor give the mother concerning future pregnancies?

CASE 18-4

A mentally deficient female infant had low-set, malformed ears; a prominent occiput; and rocker-bottom feet. A chromosomal abnormality was suspected.

- What type of chromosomal aberration was probably present?
- What is the usual cause of this abnormality?
- How long would the infant likely survive?

CASE 18-5

An infant was born with partial detachment of the retina in one eye. The eye was microphthalmic, and there was persistence of the distal end of the hyaloid artery.

- What is the embryologic basis of congenital detachment of the retina?
- What is the usual fate of the hyaloid artery?

Discussion of problems appears at the back of the book.

References and Suggested Reading

Barald KF, Kelley MW: From placodes to polarization. New tunes in inner ear development. Development 131:4119, 2004.

Barishak YR: Embryology of the Eye and Its Adnexa, 2nd ed. Basel, Karger, 2001.

Bauer PW, MacDonald CB, Melhem ER: Congenital inner ear malformation. Am J Otol 19:669, 1998.

Blazer S, Zimmer EZ, Mezer E, Bronshtein M: Early and late onset fetal microphthalmia. Am J Obstet Gynecol 194:1354, 2006.

Carlson BM: Human Embryology and Developmental Biology, 3rd ed. St. Louis, Mosby-Year Book, 2004.

FitzPatrick DR, van Heyningen V: Developmental eye disorders. Curr Opin Genet Dev 15:348, 2005.

Gartner LP, Hiatt JL: Color Textbook of Histology, 2nd ed. Philadelphia, WB Saunders, 2001.

Haddad J Jr: The ear. In Behrman RE, Kliegman RM, Jenson HB (eds): Nelson Textbook of Pediatrics, 17th ed. Philadelphia, Elsevier/Saunders, 2004.

Jones KL: Smith's Recognizable Patterns of Human Malformation, 6th ed. Philadelphia, WB Saunders, 2005.

Kozmik Z: Pax genes in eye development and evolution. Curr Opin Genet Dev 15:430, 2005.

Litsiou A, Hanson S, Streit A: A balance of FGF, BMP and WNT signalling positions the future placode territory in the head. Development 132:4051, 2005.

Mallo M: Formation of the middle ear: Recent progress on the developmental and molecular mechanisms. Dev Biol 231:410, 2001.

Marles SL, Greenberg CR, Persaud TVN, et al: A new familial syndrome of unilateral upper eyelid coloboma, aberrant anterior hairline pattern and anal anomalies in Manitoba Indians. Am J Med Genet 42:793, 1992.

Maroon H, Walshe J, Mahmood R, et al: Fgf3 and Fgf8 are required together for formation of the otic placode and vesicle. Development 129:2099, 2002.

McAvoy JW, Chamberlain CG, Delongh RV, et al: Lens development. Eye 13:425, 1999.

McCabe KL, McGuire C, Reh TA: Pea expression is regulated by FGF signaling in developing retina. Dev Dyn 235:327, 2006.

Moore KL, Dalley AF: Clinically Oriented Anatomy, 5th ed. Baltimore, Williams & Wilkins, 2006.

Olitsky SE, Nelson LB: Disorders of the eye. In Behrman RE, Kliegman RM, Jenson HB (eds): Nelson Textbook of Pediatrics, 17th ed. Philadelphia, Elsevier/Saunders, 2004.

O'Rahilly R: The early development of the otic vesicle in staged human embryos. J Embryol Exp Morphol 11:741, 1963.

O'Rahilly R: The prenatal development of the human eye. Exp Eye Res 21:93, 1975.

Porter CJW, Tan SW: Congenital auricular anomalies: Topographic anatomy, embryology, classification, and treatment strategies. Plast Reconstr Surg 115:1701, 2005.

Rinkwitz S, Bober E, Baker R: Development of the vertebrate inner ear. Ann N Y Acad Sci 942:1, 2001.

Rodriguez-Vázquez JF: Development of the stapes and associated structures in human embryos. J Anat 207:165, 2005.

Sellheyer K: Development of the choroid and related structures. Eye 4:255, 1990.

Sevel D, Isaacs R: A re-evaluation of corneal development. Trans Am Ophthalmol Soc 86:178, 1989.

Toriello HV, Reardon W, Gorlin RJ: Hereditary Hearing Loss and its Syndromes, 2nd ed. Oxford, UK, Oxford University Press, 2004.

Wilson RS, Char F: Drug-induced ocular malformations. In Persaud TVN (ed): Advances in the Study of Birth Defects. Vol. 7: Central Nervous System and Craniofacial Malformations. New York, Alan R. Liss, 1982.

Wright KW: Embryology and eye development. In Wright KW (ed): Textbook of Ophthalmology. Baltimore, Williams & Wilkins, 1997.

19

The Integumentary System

Development of Skin and Skin Appendages 440
- Epidermis 440
- Dermis 441
- Glands of the Skin 441
- Development of Hairs 447
- Development of Nails 448
- Development of Teeth 448

Summary of the Integumentary System 455

Clinically Oriented Problems 456

The integumentary system consists of the skin and its appendages: sweat glands, nails, hairs, sebaceous glands, and arrector muscles of hairs (arrector pili muscles). The system also includes the mammary glands and teeth. At the external orifices, the digestive tract, for example, the mucous membrane and integument (Latin [L]. covering) or skin are continuous.

DEVELOPMENT OF SKIN AND SKIN APPENDAGES

The skin, the outer integument or protective covering of the body, is a complex organ system and is the body's largest organ. The skin consists of two layers that are derived from surface ectoderm and its underlying mesenchyme (Fig. 19-1).

- The epidermis is a superficial epithelial tissue that is derived from surface ectoderm.
- The dermis is a deeper layer composed of dense, irregularly arranged connective tissue that is derived from mesenchyme. This meshwork of embryonic connective tissue or mesenchyme, derived from mesoderm, forms the connective tissues in the dermis.

Ectodermal (epidermal)/mesenchymal (dermal) interactions involve mutual inductive mechanisms. Skin structures vary from one part of the body to another. For example, the skin of the eyelids is thin and soft and has fine hairs, whereas the skin of the eyebrows is thick and has coarse hairs. The embryonic skin at 4 to 5 weeks consists of a single layer of surface ectoderm overlying the mesoderm (see Fig. 19-1*A*).

Epidermis

During the first and second trimesters of pregnancy, epidermal growth occurs in stages and results in an increase in epidermal thickness. The primordium of the epidermis is the layer of surface ectodermal cells (see Fig. 19-1*A*). These cells proliferate and form a layer of squamous epithelium, the **periderm**, and a basal (germinative) layer (see Fig. 19-1*B*). The cells of the periderm continually undergo keratinization and desquamation and are replaced by cells arising from the basal layer. The exfoliated peridermal cells form part of the white greasy substance—**vernix caseosa**—that covers the fetal skin. Later, the vernix (L. varnish) contains **sebum**, the secretion from **sebaceous glands** (Fig. 19-3). The vernix protects the developing skin from constant exposure to amniotic fluid, with its high urine content, during the fetal period. In addition, the greasy vernix facilitates birth of the fetus.

The basal layer of the epidermis becomes the **stratum germinativum** (see Fig. 19-1*D*), which produces new cells that are displaced into the more superficial layers. By 11 weeks, cells from the stratum germinativum have formed an intermediate layer (see Fig. 19-1*C*). Replacement of peridermal cells continues until approximately the 21st week; thereafter, the periderm disappears and the **stratum corneum** forms (see Fig. 19-1*D*). Proliferation of cells in the stratum germinativum also forms **epidermal ridges**, which extend into the developing dermis (Figs. 19-1*C* and 19-2). These ridges begin to appear in embryos at 10 weeks and are permanently established by 17 weeks. The epidermal ridges produce grooves on the surface of the palms and the soles, including the digits (fingers and toes). The type of pattern that develops is determined genetically and constitutes the basis for examining fingerprints in criminal investigations and medical genetics. **Abnormal chromosome complements** affect the development of ridge patterns, e.g., infants with Down syndrome have distinctive patterns on their hands and feet that are of diagnostic value.

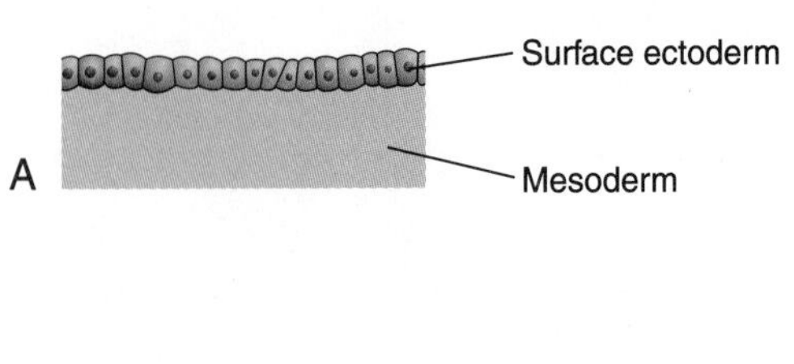

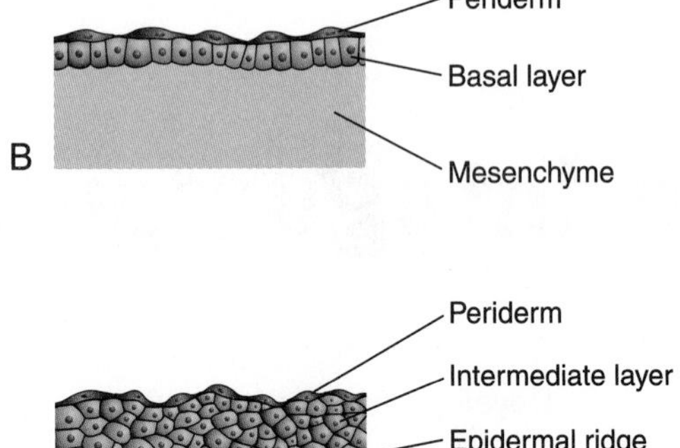

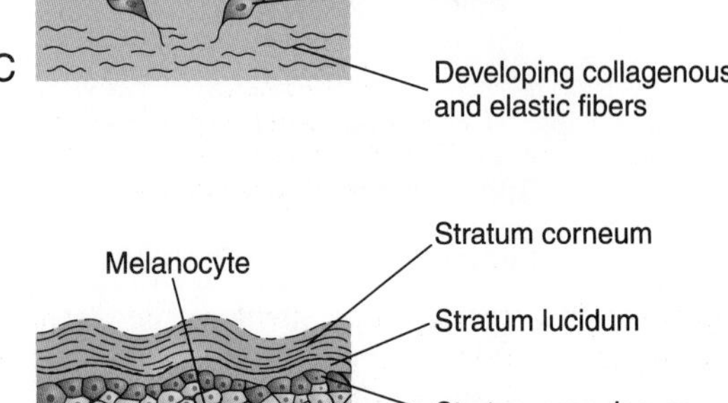

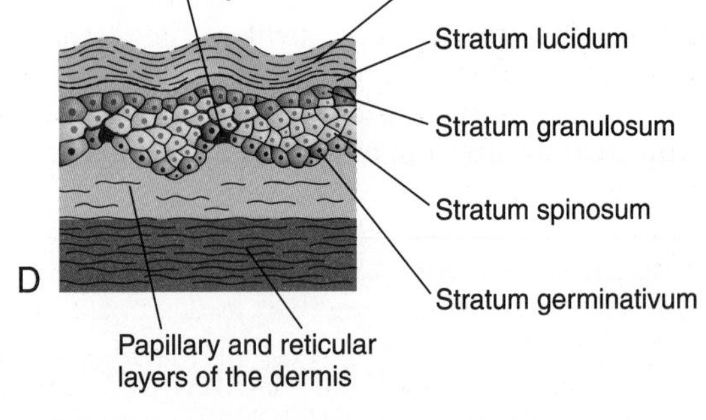

FIGURE 19-1. Illustrations of the successive stages of skin development. **A,** At 4 weeks. **B,** At 7 weeks. **C,** At 11 weeks. The cells of the periderm continually undergo keratinization and desquamation. The exfoliated peridermal cells form part of the vernix caseosa. **D,** Newborn. Note the melanocytes in the basal layer of the epidermis and the way their processes extend between the epidermal cells to supply them with melanin.

Late in the embryonic period, **neural crest cells** migrate into the mesenchyme of the developing dermis and differentiate into **melanoblasts.** Later these cells migrate to the **dermoepidermal junction** and differentiate into **melanocytes** (see Fig. 19-1*D*). The differentiation of

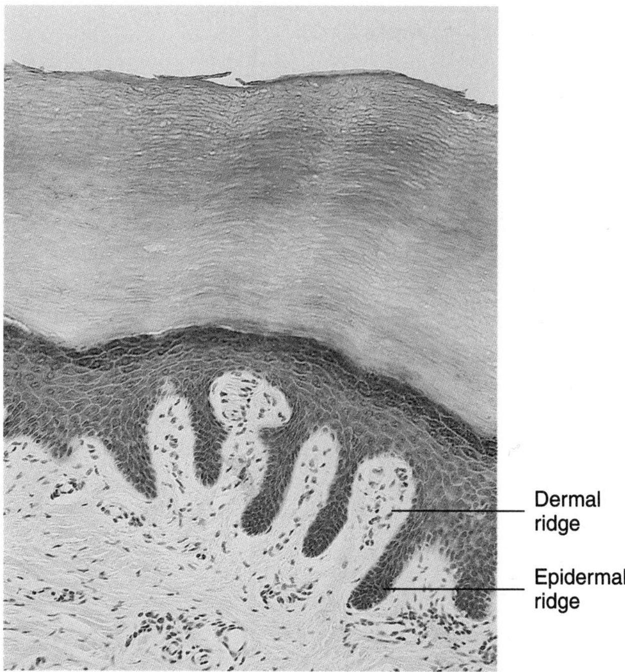

FIGURE 19-2. Light micrograph of thick skin (×132). Observe the epidermis and dermis as well as the dermal ridges interdigitating with the epidermal ridges. (From Gartner LP, Hiatt JL: Color Textbook of Histology, 2nd ed. Philadelphia, WB Saunders, 2001.)

melanoblasts into melanocytes involves the formation of **pigment granules**. Wnt signaling regulates this process. Melanocytes appear in the developing skin at 40 to 50 days, immediately after the migration of neural crest cells. In white races, the cell bodies of melanocytes are usually confined to basal layers of the epidermis; however, their **dendritic processes** extend between the epidermal cells. Only a few melanin-containing cells are normally present in the dermis (see Fig. 19-1*D*). The melanocytes begin producing melanin (Greek [Gr]. *melas*, black) before birth and distribute it to the epidermal cells. Pigment formation can be observed prenatally in the epidermis of dark-skinned races; however, there is little evidence of such activity in light-skinned fetuses. Increased amounts of melanin are produced in response to ultraviolet light. The relative content of melanin inside the melanocytes accounts for the different colors of skin.

The transformation of the surface ectoderm into a multilayered epidermis results from continuing inductive interactions with the dermis. Skin is classified as thick or thin based on the thickness of the epidermis.

- **Thick skin** covers the palms and soles; it lacks hair follicles, arrector muscles of hairs, and sebaceous glands, but it has sweat glands.
- **Thin skin** covers most of the rest of the body; it contains hair follicles, arrector muscles of hairs, sebaceous glands, and sweat glands (see Fig. 19-3).

Dermis

The dermis develops from mesenchyme, which is derived from the mesoderm underlying the surface ectoderm (see Fig. 19-1*A* and *B*). Most of the mesenchyme that differentiates into the connective tissue of the dermis originates from the somatic layer of lateral mesoderm; however, some of it is derived from the dermatomes of the somites (see Chapter 14). By 11 weeks, the mesenchymal cells have begun to produce collagenous and elastic connective tissue fibers (see Fig. 19-1*D*). As the **epidermal ridges** form, the dermis projects into the epidermis, forming **dermal ridges** that interdigitate with the epidermal ridges (see Fig. 19-2). **Capillary loops** (endothelial tubes) develop in some of these ridges and provide nourishment for the epidermis. Sensory nerve endings form in others. The developing afferent nerve fibers apparently play an important role in the spatial and temporal sequence of dermal ridge formation. The development of the dermatomal pattern of innervation of the skin is described in Chapter 16.

The blood vessels in the dermis begin as simple, endothelium-lined structures that differentiate from mesenchyme. As the skin grows, new capillaries grow out from the primordial vessels (**angiogenesis**). Such capillary-like vessels have been observed in the dermis at the end of the fifth week. Some capillaries acquire muscular coats through differentiation of myoblasts developing in the surrounding mesenchyme and become arterioles and arteries. Other capillaries, through which a return flow of blood is established, acquire muscular coats and become venules and veins. As new blood vessels form, some transitory ones disappear. By the end of the first trimester, the major vascular organization of the fetal dermis is established.

Glands of the Skin

Two kinds of glands, sebaceous and sweat glands, are derived from the epidermis and grow into the dermis. The mammary glands develop in a similar manner.

Sebaceous Glands

Most sebaceous glands develop as buds from the sides of developing **epithelial root sheaths** of hair follicles (Fig. 19-3). The glandular buds grow into the surrounding connective tissue and branch to form the primordia of several alveoli and their associated ducts. The central cells of the alveoli break down, forming an oily secretion—**sebum**—that is released into the hair follicle and passes to the surface of the skin, where it mixes with desquamated peridermal cells to form *vernix caseosa*. Sebaceous glands independent of hair follicles (e.g., in the glans penis and labia minora) develop in a similar manner to buds from the epidermis.

Sweat Glands

Eccrine sweat glands are located in the skin throughout most of the body. They develop as epidermal downgrowths (cellular buds) into the underlying mesenchyme (see Fig. 19-3). As the buds elongate, their ends coil to form the primordium of the secretory part of the gland (Fig. 19-4*A* to *C*). The epithelial attachment of the developing gland to the epidermis forms the primordium of the

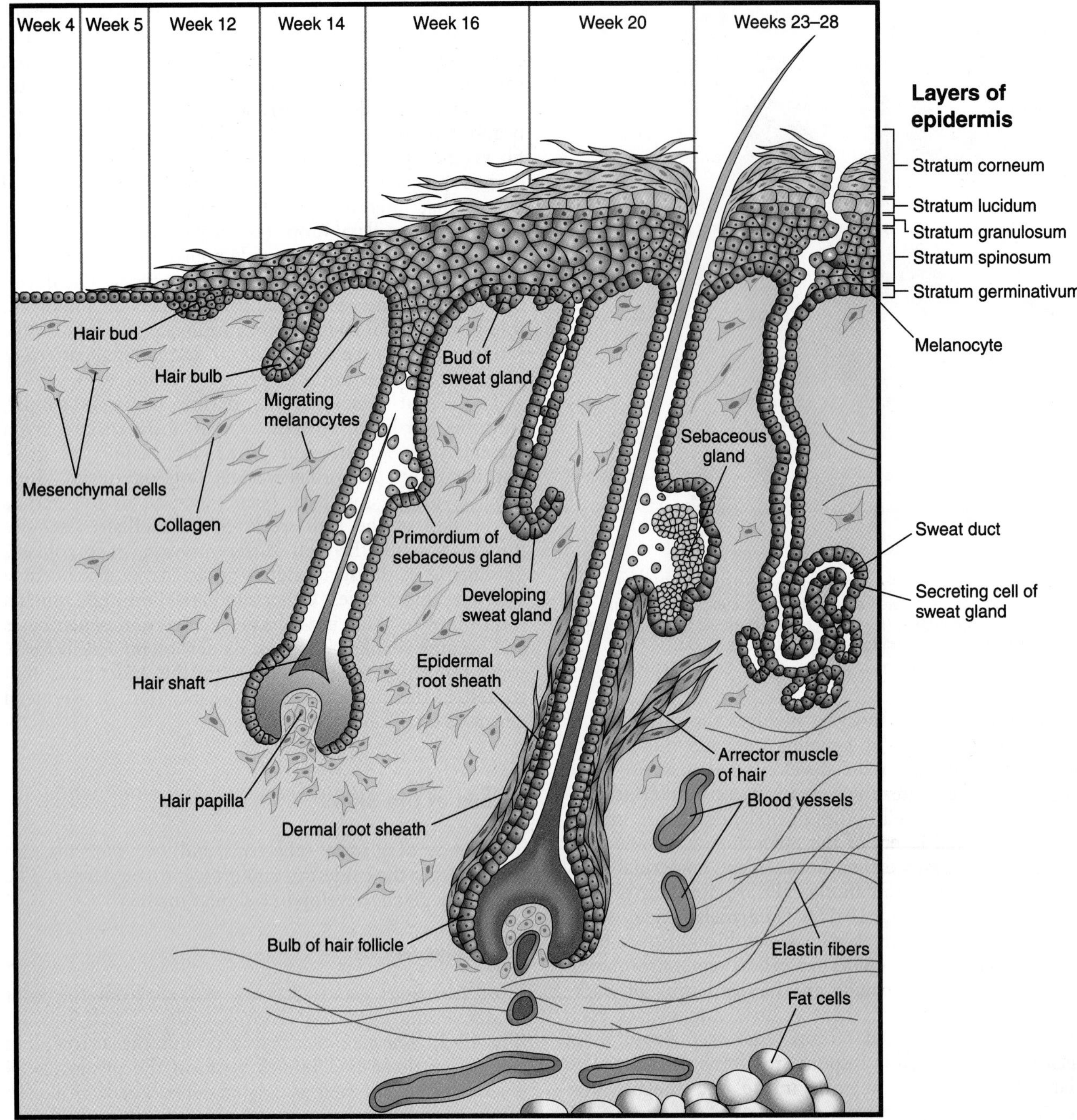

FIGURE 19-3. Drawing of the successive stages in the development of a hair and its associated sebaceous gland and arrector muscle of hair (L. *musculi arrector pili*). Note that the sebaceous gland develops as an outgrowth from the side of the hair follicle.

sweat duct. The central cells of the primordial ducts degenerate, forming a lumen. The peripheral cells of the secretory part of the gland differentiate into myoepithelial and secretory cells (see Fig. 19-4*D*). The myoepithelial cells are thought to be specialized smooth muscle cells that assist in expelling sweat from the glands. Eccrine sweat glands begin to function shortly after birth.

The distribution of the large **apocrine sweat glands** in humans is mostly confined to the axilla, pubic, and perineal regions and areolae of the nipples. They develop from downgrowths of the stratum germinativum of the epidermis that give rise to hair follicles. As a result, the ducts of these glands open, not onto the skin surface as do eccrine sweat glands, but into the upper part of hair follicles superficial to the openings of the sebaceous glands. They begin to secrete during puberty.

DISORDERS OF KERATINIZATION

Ichthyosis (Gr. *ichthys*, fish) is a general term that is applied to a group of skin disorders resulting from excessive keratinization (Fig. 19-5*B*). The skin is

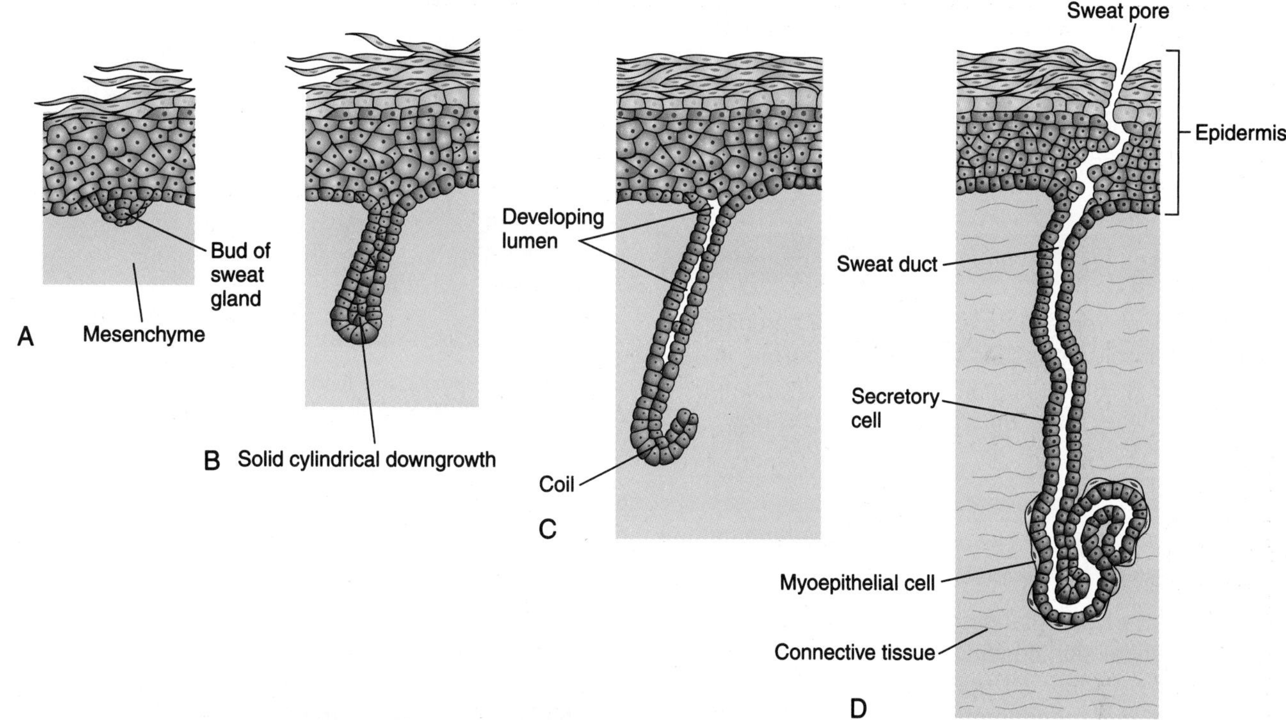

FIGURE 19-4. Illustrations of the successive stages of the development of a sweat gland. **A** and **B,** The cellular buds of the glands develop at approximately 20 weeks as a solid growth of epidermal cells into the mesenchyme. **C,** Its terminal part coils and forms the body of the gland. The central cells degenerate to form the lumen of the gland. **D,** The peripheral cells differentiate into secretory cells and contractile myoepithelial cells.

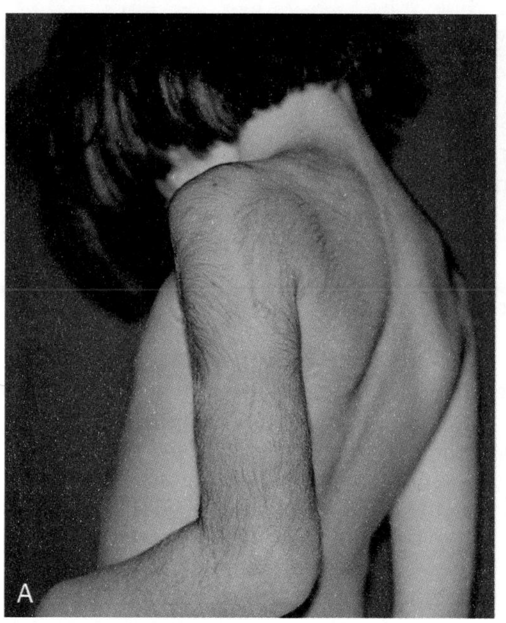

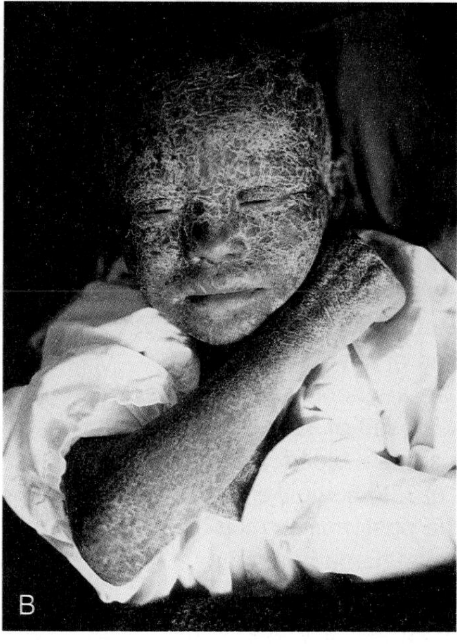

FIGURE 19-5. **A,** A child with congenital hypertrichosis and hyperpigmentation. Note the excessive hairiness on the shoulders and back. **B,** A child with severe keratinization of the skin (ichthyosis) from the time of birth. (**A,** Courtesy of Dr. Mario Joao Branco Ferreira, Servico de Dermatologia, Hospital de Desterro, Lisbon, Portugal. **B,** Courtesy of Dr. Joao Carlos Fernandes Rodrigues, Servico de Dermatologia, Hospital de Desterro, Lisbon, Portugal.)

characterized by dryness and fishskin-like scaling, which may involve the entire body surface. A **harlequin fetus** results from a rare keratinizing disorder that is inherited as an autosomal recessive trait. The skin is markedly thickened, ridged, and cracked. Most affected infants die during the first week of life. A **collodion infant** is covered by a thick, taut membrane that resembles collodion or parchment. This membrane cracks with the first respiratory efforts and begins to fall off in large sheets. Complete shedding may take several weeks, occasionally leaving normal-appearing skin. **Lamellar ichthyosis** is an autosomal recessive disorder. A newborn infant with this condition may first appear to be a collodion baby, but the scaling persists. Growth of hair may be curtailed and development of sweat glands is often impeded. Affected infants often suffer severely in hot weather because of their inability to sweat.

Congenital Ectodermal Dysplasia

This condition represents a group of rare hereditary disorders involving tissues that are ectodermal in origin. The teeth are completely or partially absent. Often the hairs, nails, and skin are also severely affected.

Ectrodactyly-Ectodermal Dysplasia-Clefting Syndrome

Ectrodactyly-ectodermal dysplasia-clefting syndrome is a congenital skin condition that is inherited as an autosomal dominant trait. It involves both ectodermal and mesodermal tissues, consisting of **ectodermal dysplasia** associated with hypopigmentation of skin and hair, scanty hair and eyebrows, absence of eyelashes, nail dystrophy, hypodontia and microdontia, **ectrodactyly**, and cleft lip and palate.

Angiomas of Skin

These vascular anomalies are developmental defects in which some transitory and/or surplus primitive blood or lymphatic vessels persist. Those composed of blood vessels may be mainly arterial, venous, or **cavernous angiomas**, but they are often of a mixed type. Angiomas composed of lymphatics are called **cystic lymphangiomas** or **cystic hygromas** (see Chapter 13). True angiomas are benign tumors of endothelial cells, usually composed of solid or hollow cords; the hollow cords contain blood. **Nevus flammeus** denotes a flat, pink or red, flamelike blotch that often appears on the posterior surface of the neck. A **port-wine stain hemangioma** is a larger and darker angioma than a nevus flammeus and is nearly always anterior or lateral on the face and/or neck (Fig. 19-6). It is sharply demarcated when it is near the median plane, whereas the **common angioma** (pinkish-red blotch) may cross the median plane. A port-wine stain in the area of distribution of the trigeminal nerve is sometimes associated with a similar type of angioma of the meninges of the brain (**Sturge-Weber syndrome**). Hemangiomas are among the most common benign neoplasms found in infants and children.

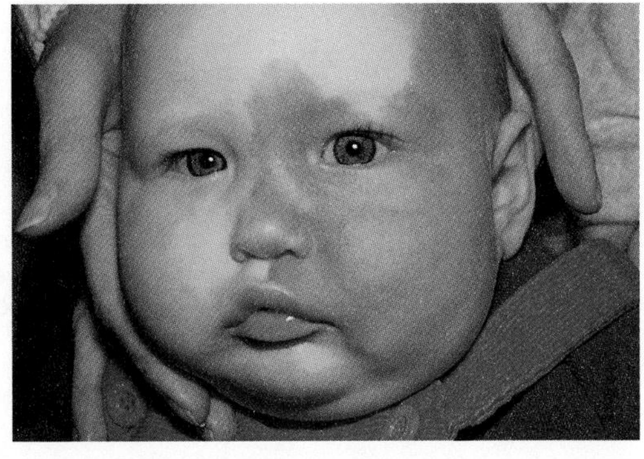

FIGURE 19-6. Hemangioma (port-wine stain) in an infant. (From Dorland's Illustrated Medical Dictionary, 30th ed. Philadelphia, WB Saunders, 2003.)

Albinism

In **generalized albinism**, an autosomal recessive trait, the skin, hairs, and retina lack pigment; however, the iris usually shows some pigmentation. Albinism occurs when the melanocytes fail to produce melanin because of the lack of the enzyme tyrosinase. In *localized albinism*—**piebaldism**—an autosomal dominant trait, there is a lack of melanin in patches of skin and/or hair.

Absence of Skin

In rare cases, small areas of skin fail to form, giving the appearance of ulcers. The area usually heals by scarring unless a skin graft is performed. Absence of patches of skin is most common in the scalp.

Mammary Glands

Mammary glands are a modified and highly specialized type of sweat glands. **Mammary buds** begin to develop during the sixth week as solid downgrowths of the epidermis into the underlying mesenchyme (Fig. 19-7*C*). These changes occur in response to an inductive influence from the mesenchyme. The mammary buds develop as downgrowths from thickened **mammary crests**, which are thickened strips of ectoderm extending from the axillary to the inguinal regions (see Fig. 19-7*A* and *B*). The mammary crests (ridges) appear during the fourth week but normally persist in humans only in the pectoral area, where the breasts develop (see Fig. 19-7*B*). Each primary bud soon gives rise to several secondary mammary buds that develop into lactiferous ducts and their branches (see Fig. 19-7*D* and *E*). Canalization of these buds is induced by placental sex hormones entering the fetal circulation. This process continues until late gestation, and by term, 15 to 19 lactiferous ducts are formed. The fibrous connective tissue and fat of the mammary gland develop from the surrounding mesenchyme.

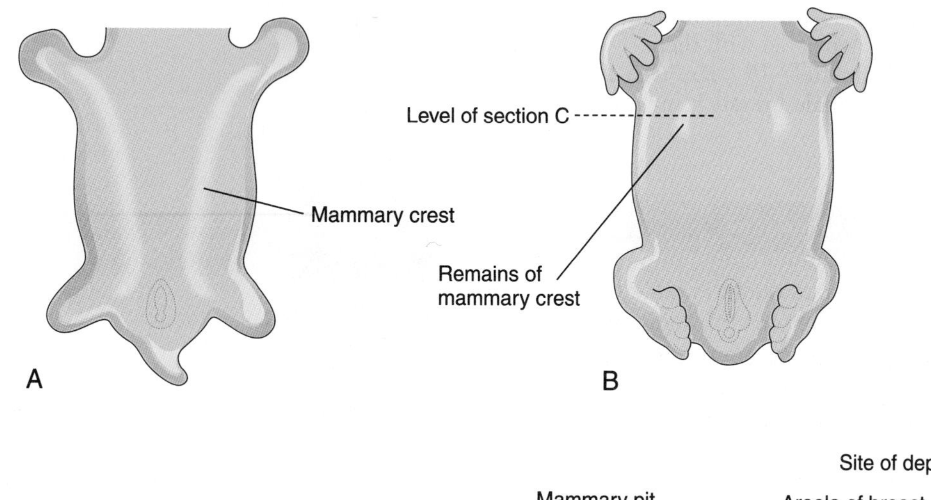

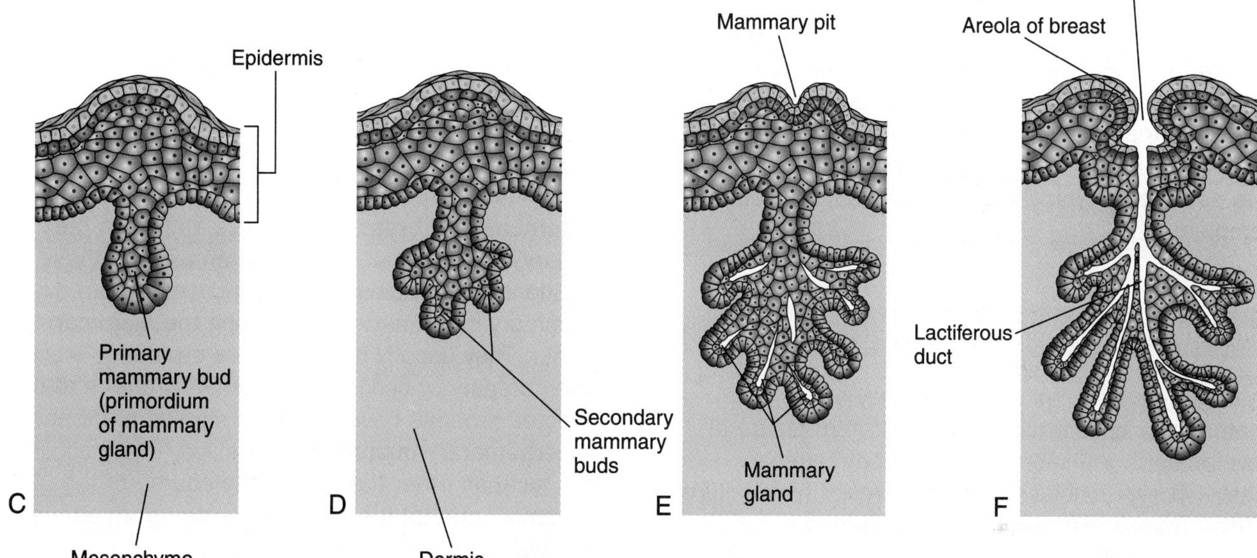

FIGURE 19-7. The development of mammary glands. **A,** Ventral view of an embryo of approximately 28 days showing the mammary crests. **B,** Similar view at 6 weeks showing the remains of these crests. **C,** Transverse section of a mammary crest at the site of a developing mammary gland. **D** to **F,** Similar sections showing successive stages of breast development between the 12th week and birth.

During the late fetal period, the epidermis at the site of origin of the mammary gland becomes depressed, forming a shallow **mammary pit** (see Fig. 19-7*E*). The nipples are poorly formed and depressed in newborn infants. Soon after birth, the **nipples** usually rise from the mammary pits because of proliferation of the surrounding connective tissue of the **areola**, the circular area of skin around the nipple. The smooth muscle fibers of the nipple and areola differentiate from surrounding mesenchymal cells.

The **rudimentary mammary glands** of newborn males and females are identical and are often enlarged. Some secretion, often called "witch's milk," may be produced. These transitory changes are caused by maternal hormones passing through the placental membrane into the fetal circulation. The breasts of newborns contain lactiferous ducts but no alveoli. Before puberty, there is little branching of the ducts. In females, the breasts enlarge rapidly during puberty (Fig. 19-8), mainly because of development

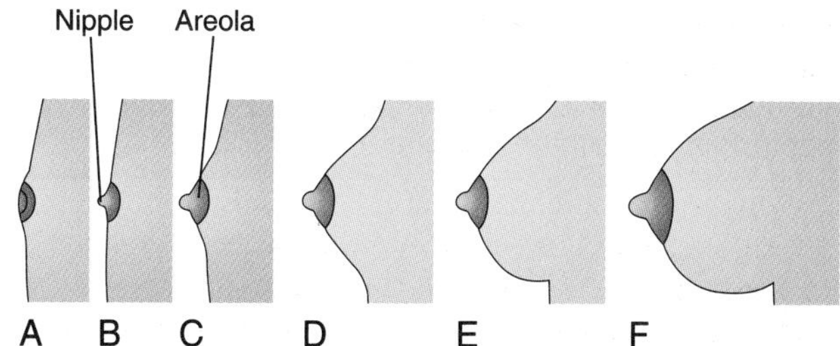

FIGURE 19-8. Sketches of the progressive stages in the postnatal development of the female breast. **A,** Newborn. **B,** Child. **C,** Early puberty. **D,** Late puberty. **E,** Young adult. **F,** Pregnant female. Note that the nipple is inverted at birth (**A**). Normally the nipple elevates during childhood. Failure of this process to occur gives rise to an inverted nipple. At puberty (12–15 years), the breasts of females enlarge because of development of the mammary glands and the increased deposition of fat.

of the mammary glands and the accumulation of the fibrous stroma and fat associated with them. Full development occurs at approximately 19 years (see Fig. 19-8*E*). The lactiferous ducts of male breasts remain rudimentary throughout life.

Gynecomastia

The rudimentary lactiferous ducts in males normally undergo no postnatal development. **Gynecomastia** (Gr. *gyne*, woman + *mastos*, breast) refers to the development of the rudimentary lactiferous ducts in the male mammary tissue. During midpuberty, approximately two thirds of boys develop varying degrees of hyperplasia of the breasts. This subareolar hyperplasia may persist for a few months to 2 years. A decreased ratio of testosterone to estradiol is found in boys with gynecomastia. Approximately 80% of males with **Klinefelter syndrome** have gynecomastia (see Chapter 20). It is associated typically with an XXY chromosome complement.

Absence of Nipples (Athelia) or Breasts (Amastia)

These rare congenital anomalies may occur bilaterally or unilaterally. They result from failure of development or disappearance of the mammary crests. These conditions may also result from failure of mammary buds to form. More common is **hypoplasia of the breast**, often found in association with gonadal agenesis and Turner syndrome (see Chapter 20).

Aplasia of Breast

The breasts of a postpubertal female often differ somewhat in size. Marked differences are regarded as anomalies because both glands are exposed to the same hormones at puberty. In these cases, there is often associated rudimentary development of muscles of the thoracic wall, usually the pectoralis major (see Chapter 15).

Supernumerary Breasts and Nipples

An extra breast (**polymastia**) or nipple (**polythelia**) occurs in approximately 1% of the female population (Fig. 19-9) and is an inheritable condition. An extra breast or nipple usually develops just inferior to the normal breast. **Supernumerary nipples** are also relatively common in males; often they are mistaken for moles (Fig. 19-10). Less commonly, **supernumerary breasts** or nipples appear in the axillary or abdominal regions of females. In these positions, the nipples or breasts develop from extra mammary buds that develop along the mammary crests. They usually become more obvious in women when pregnancy occurs. Approximately one third of affected persons have two extra nipples or breasts. **Supernumerary mammary tissue** very rarely occurs in a location other than along the course of the mammary crests. It probably develops from tissue that was displaced from these crests.

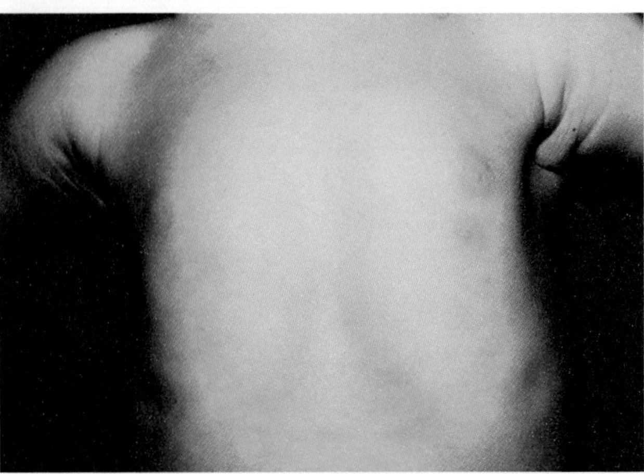

FIGURE 19-9. Female infant with an extra nipple (polythelia) on the left side. (Courtesy of A.E. Chudley, MD, Section of Genetics and Metabolism, Department of Pediatrics and Child Health, Children's Hospital and University of Manitoba, Winnipeg, Manitoba, Canada.)

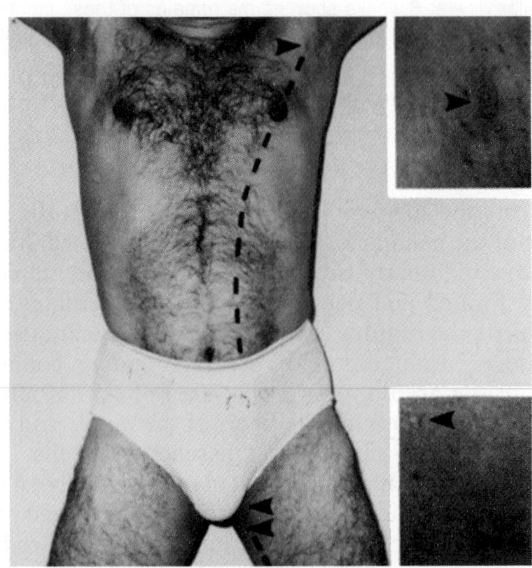

FIGURE 19-10. A man with polythelia (extra nipples) in the axillary and thigh regions. *Insets* are enlargements of the nipples (*arrowheads*). The *broken line* indicates the original position of the left mammary crests, along which the extra nipples developed. (Courtesy of Dr. Kunwar Bhatnagar, Professor of Anatomy, School of Medicine, University of Louisville, Louisville, KY.)

Inverted Nipples

Sometimes the nipples fail to elevate above the skin surface after birth, that is, they remain in their prenatal location (see Figs. 19-7*F* and 19-8*A*). Inverted nipples may make breast-feeding of an infant difficult; however, a number of breast-feeding techniques can be used to reduce this difficulty.

Development of Hairs

Hairs begin to develop early in the fetal period (weeks 9–12), but they do not become easily recognizable until approximately the 20th week (see Fig. 19-3). Hairs are first recognizable on the eyebrows, upper lip, and chin. The hair follicle begins as a proliferation of the stratum germinativum of the epidermis and extends into the underlying dermis (see Fig. 19-3). The **hair buds** soon become club shaped, forming **hair bulbs**. The epithelial cells of the hair bulb constitute the **germinal matrix**, which later produces the hair. The hair bulbs (primordia of hair roots) are soon invaginated by small mesenchymal hair papillae (see Figs. 19-3 and 19-11). The peripheral cells of the developing hair follicles form the **epithelial root sheaths**, and the surrounding mesenchymal cells differentiate into the **dermal root sheaths**. As cells in the germinal matrix proliferate, they are pushed toward the surface, where they become keratinized to form **hair shafts**. The hair grows through the epidermis on the eyebrows and upper lip by the end of the 12th week.

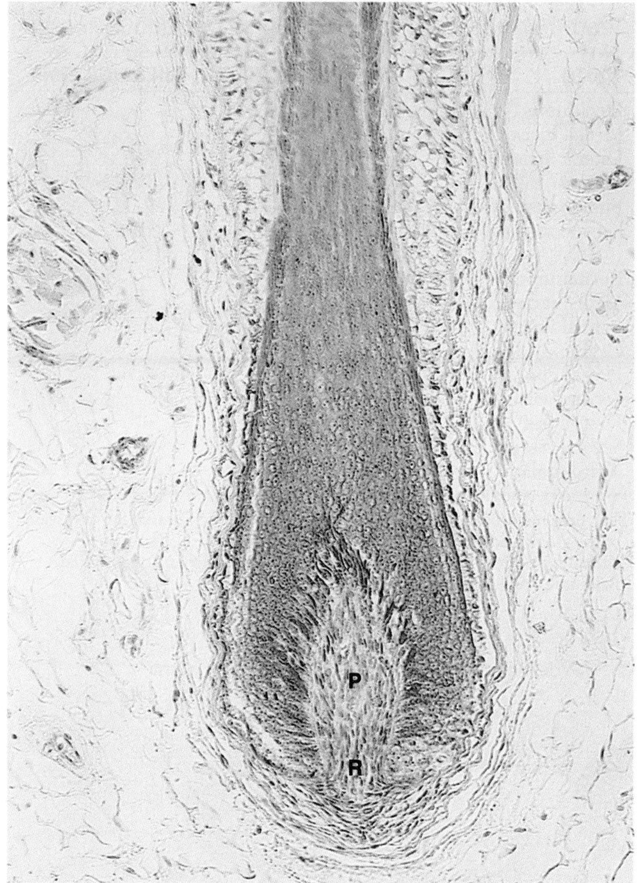

FIGURE 19-11. Light micrograph of a longitudinal section of a hair follicle with its hair root (R) and papilla (P) (×132). (From Gartner LP, Hiatt JL: Color Textbook of Histology, 2nd ed. Philadelphia, WB Saunders, 2001.)

The first hairs that appear—**lanugo** (downy hair)—are fine, soft, and lightly pigmented. Lanugo begins to appear toward the end of week 12 and is plentiful by 17 to 20 weeks. These hairs help to hold the vernix caseosa on the skin. Lanugo is replaced by coarser hairs during the perinatal period. This hair persists over most of the body, except in the axillary and pubic regions, where it is replaced at puberty by even coarser terminal hairs. In males, similar coarse hairs also appear on the face and often on the chest.

Melanoblasts migrate into the hair bulbs and differentiate into **melanocytes**. The melanin produced by these cells is transferred to the hair-forming cells in the germinal matrix several weeks before birth. The relative content of **melanin** accounts for different hair colors. **Arrector muscles of hairs**, small bundles of smooth muscle fibers, differentiate from the mesenchyme surrounding the hair follicle and attach to the dermal root sheath of the hair follicles and the papillary layer of the dermis (see Fig. 19-3). Contractions of the arrector muscles depress the skin over their attachment and elevate the skin around the hair shafts, forming tiny "goose bumps" on the surface of the skin. The arrector muscles are poorly developed in the hairs of the axilla and in certain parts of the face. The hairs forming the eyebrows and the cilia forming the eyelashes have no arrector muscles.

Alopecia

Absence or loss of scalp hair may occur alone or with other abnormalities of the skin and its derivatives. **Congenital alopecia** may be caused by failure of hair follicles to develop, or it may result from follicles producing poor-quality hairs.

Hypertrichosis

Excessive hairiness results from the development of supernumerary hair follicles or from the persistence of lanugo hairs that normally disappear during the perinatal period. It may be localized (e.g., on the shoulders and back) or diffuse (see Fig. 19-5*A*). **Localized hypertrichosis** is often associated with spina bifida occulta.

Pili Torti

In this familial disorder, the hairs are twisted and bent (L. *tortus*, twisted). Other ectodermal defects (e.g., distorted nails) may be associated with this condition. Pili torti is usually first recognized at 2 to 3 years of age.

Development of Nails

Toenails and fingernails begin to develop at the tips of the digits at approximately 10 weeks (Fig. 19-12). Development of **fingernails** precedes that of **toenails** by approximately 4 weeks (see Chapter 6). The primordia of nails appear as thickened areas or nail fields of epidermis at the tip of each digit. Later these **nail fields** migrate onto the dorsal surface, carrying their innervation from the ventral surface. The nail fields are surrounded laterally and proximally by folds of epidermis, the **nail folds**. Cells from the proximal nail fold grow over the nail field and become keratinized to form the **nail plate** (see Fig. 19-12*B*). At first, the developing nail is covered by a narrow band of epidermis, the **eponychium** (cuticle). This later degenerates, exposing the nail, except at its base, where it persists as the **cuticle**. The skin under the free margin of the nail is the **hyponychium**. The fingernails reach the fingertips by approximately 32 weeks; the toenails reach the toetips by approximately 36 weeks. Nails that have not reached the tips of the digits at birth indicate prematurity.

Congenital Anonychia

Absence of nails at birth is extremely rare. Anonychia results from failure of nail fields to form or from failure of the proximal nail folds to form nail plates. The abnormality is permanent. It may be associated with congenital absence or extremely poor development of hairs and with abnormalities of the teeth. Anonychia may be restricted to one or more nails of the digits of the hands and/or feet.

Deformed Nails

This disorder occurs occasionally and may be a manifestation of a generalized skin disease or systemic disease. There are a number of congenital diseases with nail defects.

Development of Teeth

Two sets of teeth normally develop: the primary dentition or **deciduous teeth** and the secondary dentition or **permanent teeth**. Teeth develop from oral ectoderm, mesenchyme, and neural crest cells.

The **enamel** is derived from ectoderm of the oral cavity; all other tissues differentiate from the surrounding mesenchyme and neural crest cells. Experimental evidence suggests that **neural crest cells** are imprinted with morphogenetic information before, or shortly after, they migrate from the neural crest. As the mandible and maxilla grow to accommodate the developing teeth, the shape of the face changes.

Odontogenesis (tooth development) is a property of the oral epithelium. Tooth development is a continuous process involving reciprocal induction between neural crest mesenchyme and the overlying oral epithelium. It is usually divided into stages for descriptive purposes based on the appearance of the developing tooth. The first tooth buds appear in the anterior mandibular region; later, tooth development occurs in the anterior maxillary region and then progresses posteriorly in both jaws. Tooth development continues for years after birth (Table 19-1). The first indication of tooth development occurs early in the sixth

TABLE 19–1. The Order and Usual Time of Eruption of Teeth and the Time of Shedding of Deciduous Teeth

TOOTH	USUAL ERUPTION TIME	SHEDDING TIME
Deciduous		
Medial incisor	6–8 mo	6–7 yr
Lateral incisor	8–10 mo	7–8 yr
Canine	16–20 mo	10–12 yr
First molar	12–16 mo	9–11 yr
Second molar	20–24 mo	10–12 yr
Permanent*		
Medial incisor	7–8 yr	
Lateral incisor	8–9 yr	
Canine	10–12 yr	
First premolar	10–11 yr	
Second premolar	11–12 yr	
First molar	6–7 yr	
Second molar	12 yr	
Third molar	13–25 yr	

*The permanent teeth are not shed. If they are not properly cared for or disease of the gingiva develops, they may have to be extracted.
Modified from Moore KL, Dalley AF: Clinically Oriented Anatomy, 5th ed. Baltimore, Williams & Wilkins, 2006.

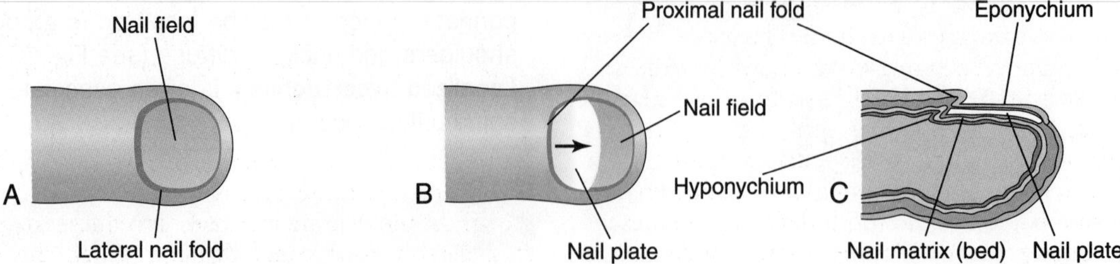

FIGURE 19-12. Successive stages in the development of a fingernail. **A,** The first indication of a nail is a thickening of the epidermis, the nail field, at the tip of the finger. **B,** As the nail plate develops, it slowly grows toward the tip of the finger. **C,** The fingernail reaches the end of the finger by 32 weeks.

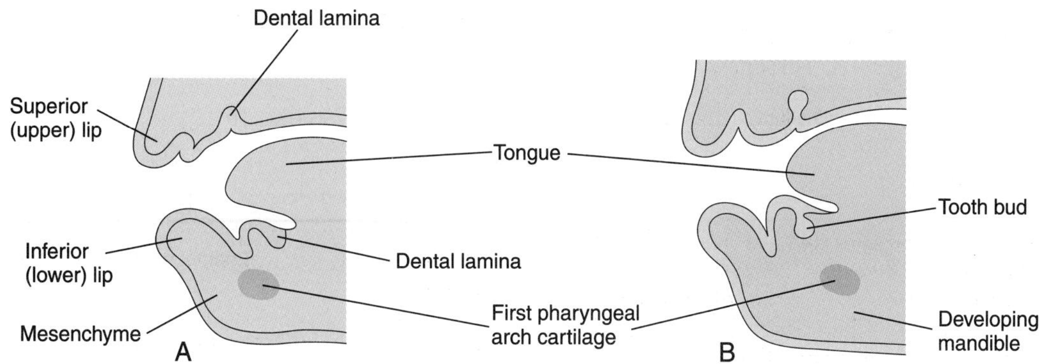

FIGURE 19-13. Sketches of sagittal sections through the developing jaws illustrating early development of the teeth. **A,** Early in the sixth week, showing the dental laminae. **B,** Later in the sixth week, showing tooth buds arising from the laminae.

week of embryonic development as a thickening of the oral epithelium. These U-shaped bands—dental laminae—follow the curves of the primitive jaws (Figs. 19-13*A* and 19-14*A*).

Bud Stage of Tooth Development

Each dental lamina develops 10 centers of proliferation from which swellings—**tooth buds** (tooth germs)—grow into the underlying mesenchyme (see Figs. 19-13*B* and 19-14*B*). These buds develop into the **deciduous teeth** (see Table 19-1). The tooth buds for **permanent teeth** that have deciduous predecessors begin to appear at approximately 10 weeks from deep continuations of the dental lamina (see Fig. 19-14*D*). They develop lingual (toward tongue) to the **deciduous tooth buds**. The permanent molars have no deciduous predecessors and develop as buds from posterior extensions of the **dental laminae** (horizontal bands). The tooth buds for the permanent teeth appear at different times, mostly during the fetal period. The buds for the second and third permanent molars develop after birth. The deciduous teeth have well-developed crowns at birth (see Fig. 19-14*G*), whereas the permanent teeth remain as tooth buds.

Cap Stage of Tooth Development

As each tooth bud is invaginated by mesenchyme—the **primordium of the dental papilla and dental follicle**—the bud becomes cap shaped (Fig. 19-15). The ectodermal part of the developing tooth, the **enamel organ**, eventually produces enamel. The internal part of each cap-shaped tooth, the **dental papilla**, is the primordium of dentine and the dental pulp. Together, the dental papilla and enamel organ form the tooth bud. The *outer cell layer* of the enamel organ is the **outer enamel epithelium**, and the *inner cell layer* lining the papilla is the **inner enamel epithelium** (see Fig. 19-14*D*). The central core of loosely arranged cells between the layers of enamel epithelium is the **enamel reticulum** (stellate reticulum). As the enamel organ and dental papilla of the tooth develop, the mesenchyme surrounding the developing tooth condenses to form the **dental sac** (dental follicle), a vascularized capsular structure (see Fig. 19-14*E*). The dental sac is the primordium of the *cement* and *periodontal ligament*. The **cement** (L. *cementum*) is the bonelike mineralized connective tissue covering the root of the tooth. The **periodontal ligament** is the fibrous connective tissue that surrounds the root of the tooth, attaching it to the alveolar bone (see Fig. 19-14*G*).

Bell Stage of Tooth Development

As the enamel organ differentiates, the developing tooth assumes the shape of a bell (see Figs. 19-14*D* and *E* and 19-15). The mesenchymal cells in the dental papilla adjacent to the internal enamel epithelium differentiate into **odontoblasts**, which produce predentine and deposit it adjacent to the epithelium. Later, the **predentine** calcifies and becomes dentine, the second hardest tissue in the body. As the dentine thickens, the odontoblasts regress toward the center of the dental papilla; however, their fingerlike cytoplasmic processes—**odontoblastic processes** (Tomes processes)—remain embedded in the dentine (see Fig. 19-14*F* and *I*). Enamel is the hardest tissue in the body. It overlies and protects the dentine from being fractured (Fig. 19-16). The color of the translucent enamel is based on the thickness and color of the underlying dentine.

Cells of the *inner enamel epithelium* differentiate into **ameloblasts** under the influence of the odontoblast, which produce enamel in the form of prisms (rods) over the dentine. As the enamel increases, the ameloblasts migrate toward the *outer enamel epithelium*. Enamel and dentine formation begins at the cusp (tip) of the tooth and progresses toward the future root.

The **root of the tooth** begins to develop after dentine and enamel formation are well advanced (Fig. 19-17). The inner and outer enamel epithelia come together in the **neck of the tooth** (cementoenamel junction), where they form a fold, the **epithelial root sheath** (see Fig. 19-14*F*). This sheath grows into the mesenchyme and initiates root formation. The *odontoblasts* adjacent to the epithelial root sheath form dentine that is continuous with that of the crown. As the dentine increases, it reduces the **pulp cavity** to a narrow **root canal** through which the vessels and nerves pass (see Fig. 19-14*H*). The inner cells of the dental sac differentiate into **cementoblasts**, which produce cement that is restricted to the root. Cement is deposited

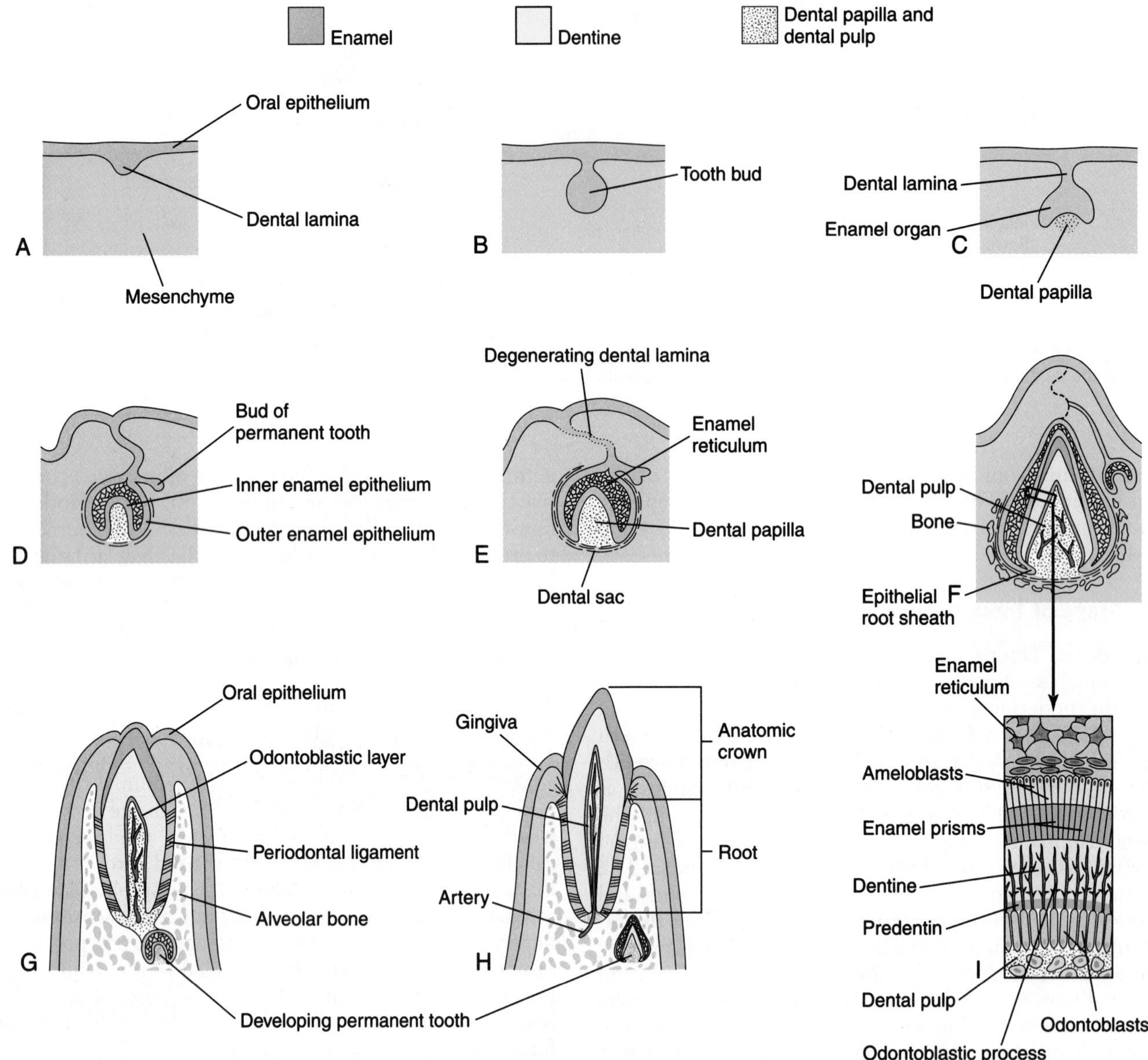

FIGURE 19-14. Schematic drawings of sagittal sections illustrating successive stages in the development and eruption of an incisor tooth. **A,** At 6 weeks, showing the dental lamina. **B,** At 7 weeks, showing the tooth bud developing from the dental lamina. **C,** At 8 weeks, showing the cap stage of tooth development. **D,** At 10 weeks, showing the early bell stage of a deciduous tooth and the bud stage of a permanent tooth. **E,** At 14 weeks, showing the advanced bell stage of tooth development. Note that the connection (dental lamina) of the tooth to the oral epithelium is degenerating. **F,** At 28 weeks, showing the enamel and dentine layers. **G,** At 6 months postnatally, showing early stage of tooth eruption. **H,** At 18 months postnatally, showing a fully erupted deciduous incisor tooth. The permanent incisor tooth now has a well-developed crown. **I,** Section through a developing tooth showing ameloblasts (enamel producers) and odontoblasts (dentine producers).

over the dentine of the root and meets the enamel at the neck of the tooth.

As the teeth develop and the jaws ossify, the outer cells of the dental sac also become active in bone formation. Each tooth soon becomes surrounded by bone, except over its crown. The tooth is held in its **alveolus** (bony socket) by the strong **periodontal ligament**, a derivative of the dental sac (see Fig. 19-14*G* and *H*). The periodontal ligament is located between the cement of the root and the bony alveolus. Some fibers of this ligament are embedded in the cement; other fibers are embedded in the bony wall of the alveolus.

Tooth Eruption

As the **deciduous teeth** develop, they begin a continuous slow movement toward the oral cavity (see Fig. 19-14*G*). The process called **eruption** results in the emergence of the tooth from its developmental position in the jaw to its functional position in the mouth. The **mandibular teeth** usually erupt before the **maxillary teeth**, and girls' teeth usually erupt sooner than boys' teeth. The child's dentition contains **20 deciduous teeth**. As the root of the tooth grows, its crown gradually erupts through the oral epithelium. The part of the oral mucosa around the erupted

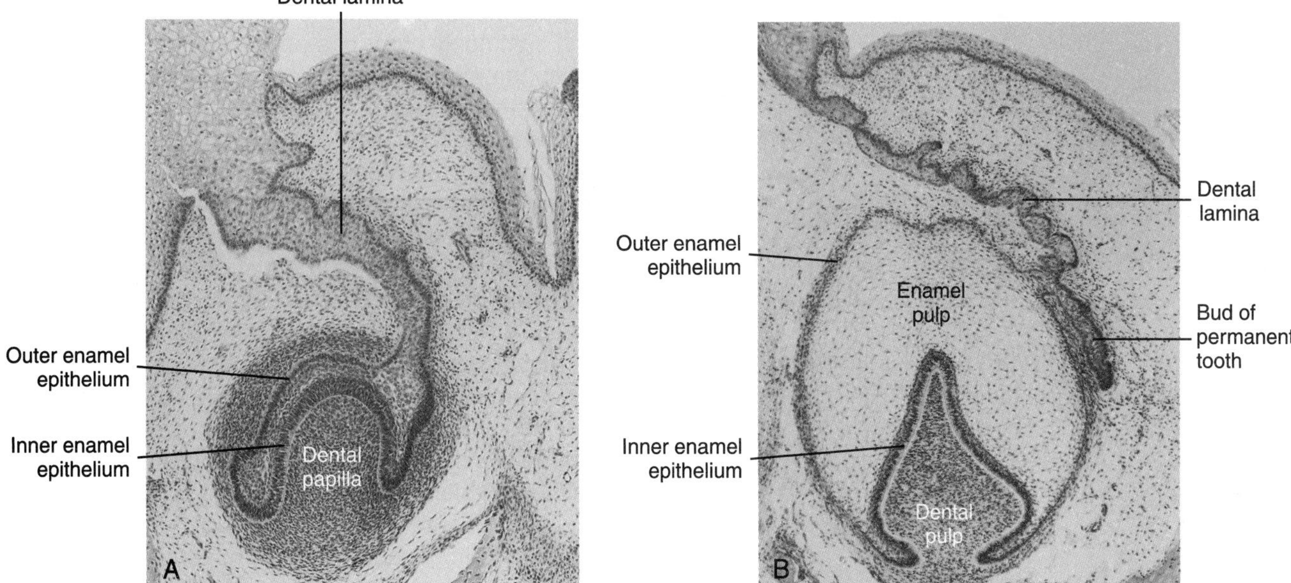

FIGURE 19-15. Photomicrograph of the primordium of a lower incisor tooth. **A,** At 12-week-old fetus (early bell stage). A caplike enamel organ is formed and the dental papilla is developing beneath it. **B,** Primordium of a lower incisor tooth in a 15-week-old fetus (late bell stage). Observe the inner and outer enamel layers, the dental papilla, and bud of the permanent tooth. (From Moore KL, Persaud TVN, Shiota K: Color Atlas of Clinical Embryology, 2nd ed. Philadelphia, WB Saunders, 2000.)

crown becomes the **gingiva** (gum). Usually eruption of the deciduous teeth occurs between the 6th and 24th months after birth (see Table 19-1). The mandibular medial or **central incisor teeth** usually erupt 6 to 8 months after birth, but this process may not begin until 12 or 13 months in some children. Despite this, all 20 deciduous teeth are usually present by the end of the second year in healthy children. Delayed eruption of all teeth may indicate a systemic or nutritional disturbance such as hypopituitarism or hypothyroidism.

The complete permanent dentition consists of 32 teeth. The **permanent teeth** develop in a manner similar to that described for deciduous teeth. As a permanent tooth grows, the root of the corresponding deciduous tooth is gradually resorbed by **osteoclasts** (odontoclasts). Consequently, when the deciduous tooth is shed, it consists only of the crown and the uppermost part of the root. The permanent teeth usually begin to erupt during the sixth year and continue to appear until early adulthood (Fig. 19-18; see Table 19-1). The shape of the face is affected by the development of the paranasal sinuses and the growth of the maxilla and mandible to accommodate the teeth (see Chapter 9). It is the lengthening of the **alveolar processes** (bony sockets supporting the teeth) that results in the increase in the depth of the face during childhood.

NATAL TEETH

Natal teeth are erupted at birth (L. *natus*, birth). There are usually two in the position of the mandibular incisors. Natal teeth are observed in approximately one in 2000 newborn infants. Natal teeth may produce maternal discomfort during breast-feeding. In addition, the infant's tongue may be lacerated or the teeth may detach and be aspirated; for these reasons, natal teeth are sometimes extracted. Because these are prematurely erupting decidual teeth, spacers may be required to prevent overcrowding of the other teeth.

ENAMEL HYPOPLASIA

Defective enamel formation causes pits and/or fissures in the enamel of teeth (Figs. 19-19 and 19-20*A*). These defects result from temporary disturbances of enamel formation. Various factors may injure ameloblasts, the enamel builders (e.g., nutritional deficiency, tetracycline therapy, and infectious diseases such as measles). **Rickets** occurring during the critical in utero period of tooth development (6–12 weeks) is a common cause of enamel hypoplasia. Rickets, a disease in children who are deficient in vitamin D, is characterized by disturbance of ossification of the epiphysial cartilages and disorientation of cells at the metaphysis (see Chapter 14).

VARIATIONS OF TOOTH SHAPE

Abnormally shaped teeth are relatively common (see Figs. 19-19*A* to *G* and 19-20*A* to *E*). Occasionally

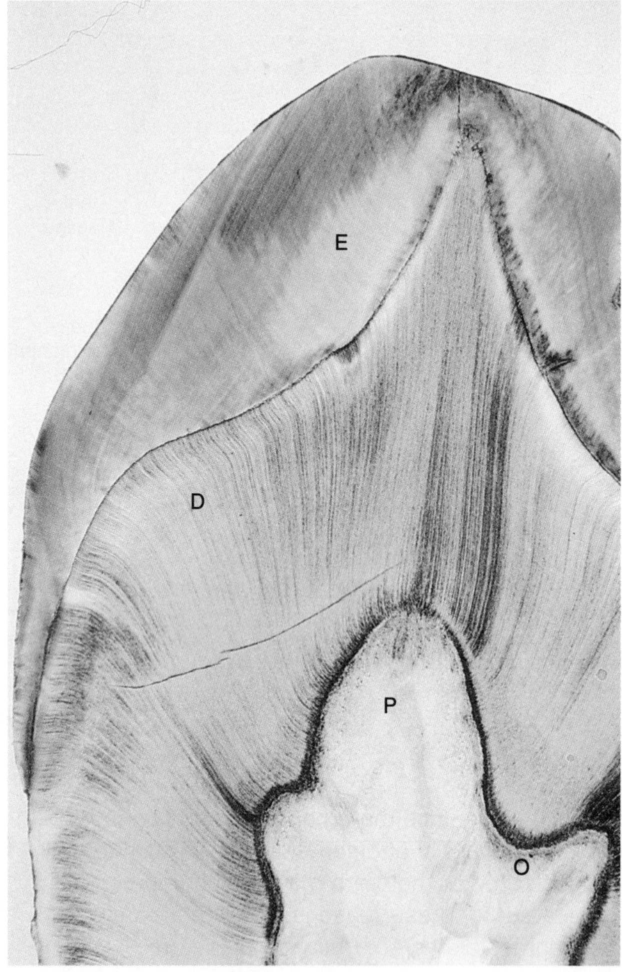

FIGURE 19-16. Photomicrograph of a section of the crown and neck of a tooth (×17). Observe the enamel (E), dentine (D), dental pulp (P), and odontoblasts (O). (From Gartner LP, Hiatt JL: Color Textbook of Histology, 2nd ed. Philadelphia, WB Saunders, 2001.)

there are spherical masses of enamel— **enamel pearls**—on the root of a tooth that is separate from the enamel of the crown. They are formed by **aberrant groups of ameloblasts**. In other cases, the maxillary lateral incisor teeth may have a slender, tapering shape (peg-shaped incisors). **Congenital syphilis** affects the differentiation of the permanent teeth, resulting in screwdriver-shaped incisors, with central notches in their incisive edges. The molars are also affected and are called **mulberry molars** because of their characteristic features.

NUMERICAL ABNORMALITIES

One or more **supernumerary teeth** may develop, or the normal number of teeth may fail to form (see Fig. 19-19). Supernumerary teeth usually develop in the area of the maxillary incisors and can disrupt the position and eruption of normal teeth. The extra teeth commonly erupt posterior to the normal ones (or can remain unerupted) and are asymptomatic in most cases. In **partial anodontia**, one or more teeth are absent; this is often a familial trait. In **total anodontia**, no teeth develop; this is an extremely rare condition. It is usually associated with congenital ectodermal dysplasia.

Occasionally a tooth bud either partially or completely divides into two separate teeth. A partially divided tooth germ is called **gemination.** The result is a **macrodont** or megadont (large teeth) with a common root canal system. If the tooth germ completely divides into two separate teeth, the result is twinning with one additional tooth in the dentition. Fusion of two teeth results in one fewer tooth in the dentition. This condition can be differentiated radiographically from gemination by two separate root canal systems found with fusion.

ABNORMALLY SIZED TEETH

Disturbances during the differentiation of teeth may result in gross alterations of dental morphology, such as macrodontia (large teeth) and microdontia (small teeth).

DENTIGEROUS CYST

A cyst may develop in a mandible, maxilla, or maxillary sinus that contains an unerupted tooth. The dentigerous (tooth-bearing) cyst develops because of cystic degeneration of the enamel reticulum of the enamel organ of an unerupted tooth. Most cysts are deeply situated in the jaw and are associated with misplaced or malformed secondary teeth that have failed to erupt.

AMELOGENESIS IMPERFECTA

Amelogenesis imperfecta is a complex group of at least 14 different clinical entities that involve developmental **aberrations in enamel formation** in the absence of any systemic disorder. This is a **congenital, inherited ectodermal defect** that primarily affects the enamel only. The enamel may be hypoplastic, hypocalcified, or hypomature. Depending on the type of amelogenesis imperfecta, the enamel may be hard or soft, pitted or smooth, and thin or normal in thickness. The incidence of amelogenesis imperfecta ranges from 1 in 700 to 1 in 8000, depending on the population studied.

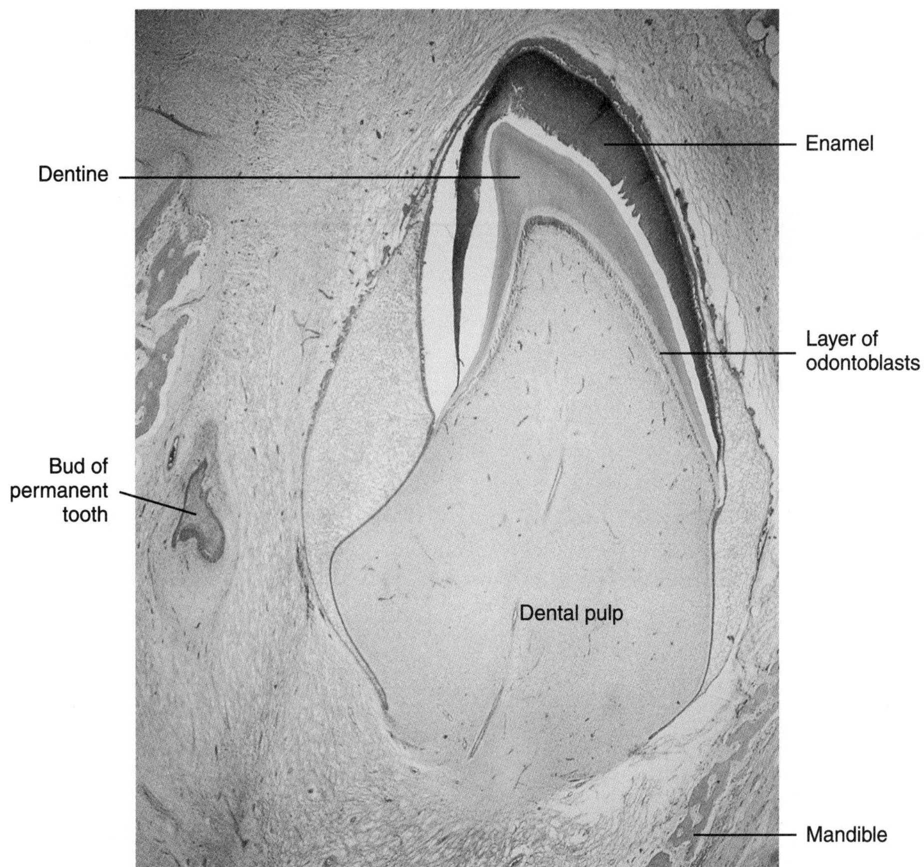

FIGURE 19-17. Photomicrograph of a section of a lower incisor tooth in a term fetus. The enamel and dentine layers and the pulp are clearly demarcated. (From Moore KL, Persaud TVN, Shiota K: Color Atlas of Clinical Embryology, 2nd ed. Philadelphia, WB Saunders, 2000.)

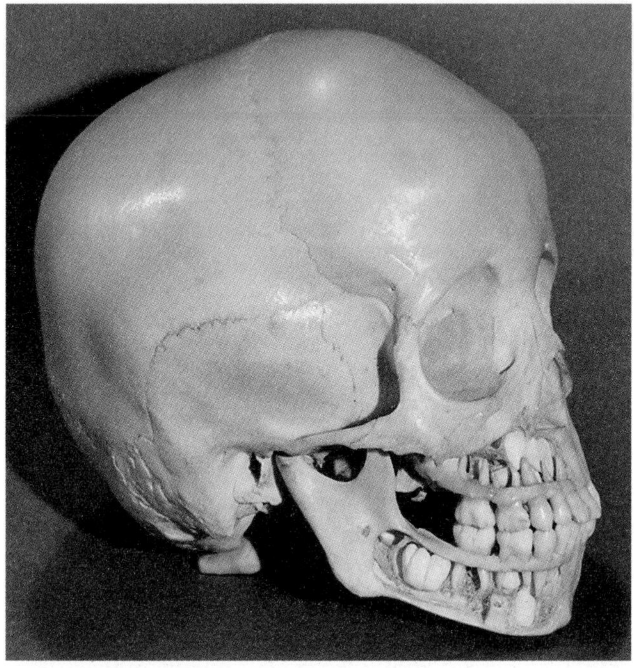

FIGURE 19-18. A 4-year-old child's cranium. Bone has been removed from the mandible to expose the relationship of the developing permanent teeth to the erupted deciduous teeth.

Multiple modes of inheritance patterns are involved. Classification of this condition is based on clinical and radiographic findings as well as mode of inheritance.

DENTINOGENESIS IMPERFECTA

This condition is relatively common in white children (Fig. 19-21). The teeth are brown to gray-blue with an opalescent sheen because the odontoblasts fail to differentiate normally and poorly calcified dentine results. Both deciduous and permanent teeth are usually involved. The enamel tends to wear down rapidly, exposing the dentine. This anomaly is inherited as an autosomal dominant trait with the genetic defect in most cases localized on chromosome 4q.

DISCOLORED TEETH

Foreign substances incorporated into the developing enamel and dentine discolor the teeth. The hemolysis associated with erythroblastosis fetalis or

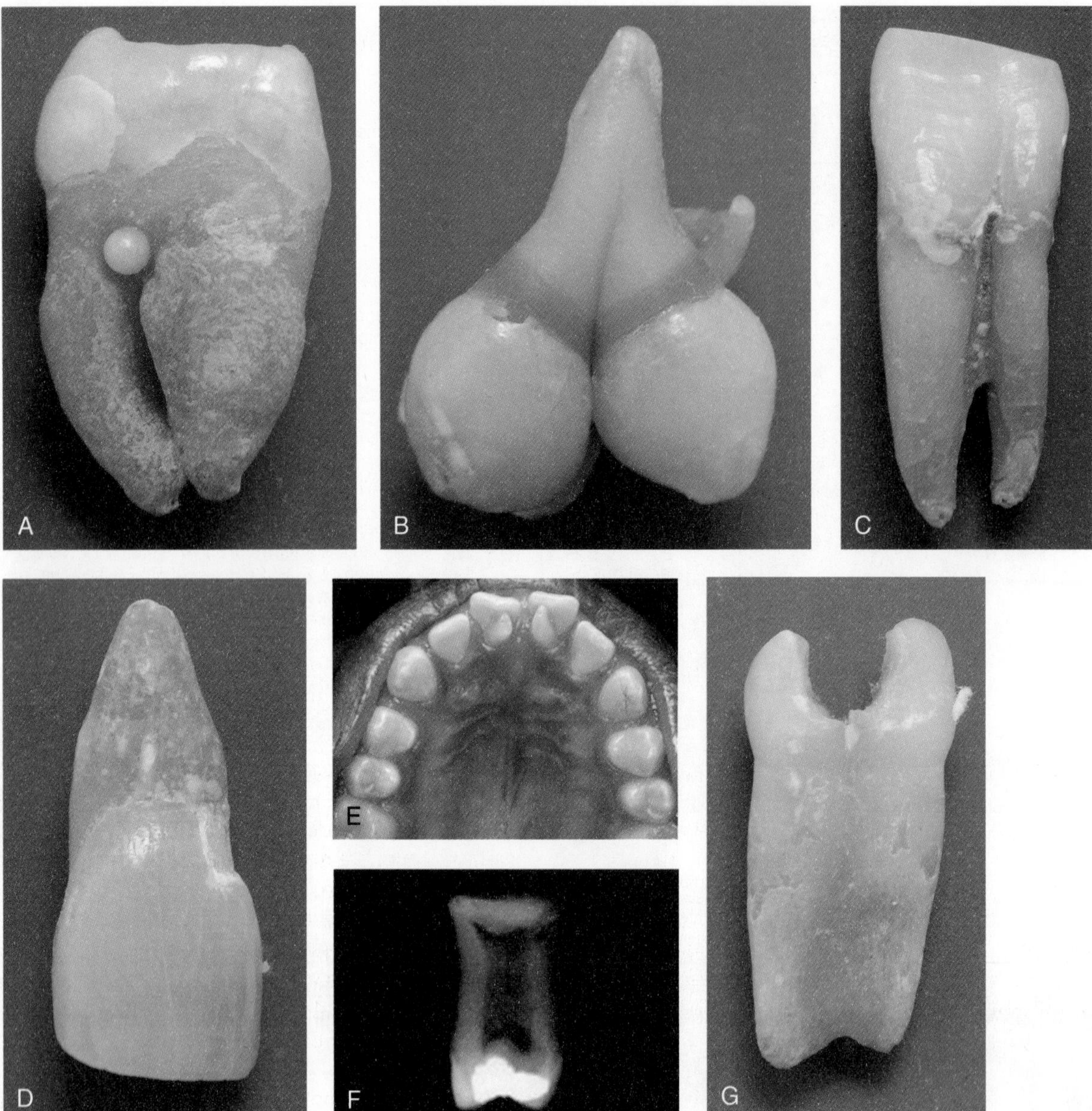

FIGURE 19-19. Some common anomalies of teeth. **A,** Enamel pearl (furcation of a permanent maxillary third molar). **B,** Gemination and tetracycline staining (maxillary third molar). **C,** Fusion (permanent mandibular central and lateral incisors). **D,** Abnormally short root (microdont permanent maxillary central incisor). **E,** Dens invaginatus (talon cusps on the lingual surface of the permanent maxillary central incisor). **F,** Taurodont tooth (radiograph of the mesial surface of the permanent maxillary second molar). **G,** Fusion (primary mandibular central and lateral incisors). (Courtesy of Dr. Blaine Cleghorn, Faculty of Dentistry, Dalhousie University, Halifax, Nova Scotia, Canada.)

hemolytic disease of the newborn (see Chapter 7) may produce blue to black discoloration of the teeth. All **tetracyclines** are extensively incorporated into the teeth. The critical period at risk is from approximately 14 weeks of fetal life to the 10th postnatal month for deciduous teeth and from approximately 14 weeks of fetal life to the eighth postnatal year for permanent teeth. **Tetracycline staining** affects both enamel and dentine because it binds to hydroxyapatite. The brownish-yellow discoloration (mottling) of the teeth, produced by tetracycline, is due to the conversion of tetracycline to a colored by-product under the action of light. The dentine is probably affected more than the enamel because it is more permeable than enamel after tooth mineralization is complete. The enamel is completely formed on all but the third molars by approximately 8 years of age. For this reason, tetracyclines should not be administered to pregnant women or children younger than 8 years of age.

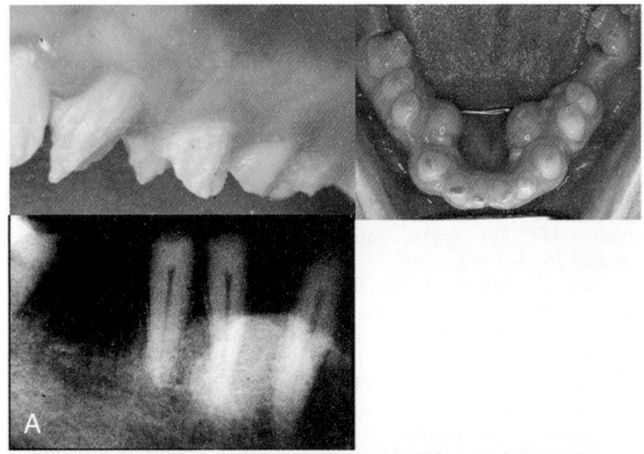

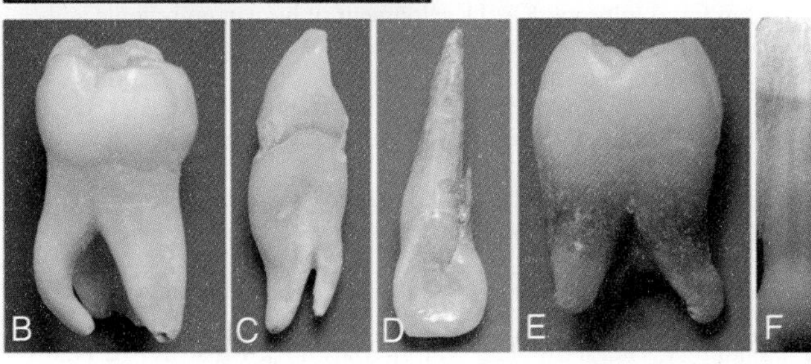

FIGURE 19-20. More common anomalies of teeth. **A,** Amelogenesis imperfecta. **B,** Extra root (mandibular molar). **C,** Extra root (mandibular canine). **D,** Accessory root (maxillary lateral incisor). Extra roots present challenges for root canal therapy and extraction. **E,** Tetracycline staining (root of maxillary third molar). **F,** A midline supernumerary tooth (M, mesiodens) located near the apex of the central incisor. The prevalence of supernumerary teeth is 1% to 3% in the general population (**A** to **E,** Courtesy of Dr. Blaine Cleghorn, Faculty of Dentistry, Dalhousie University, Halifax, Nova Scotia, Canada. **F,** Courtesy of Dr. Steve Ahing, Faculty of Dentistry, University of Manitoba, Winnipeg, Manitoba, Canada.)

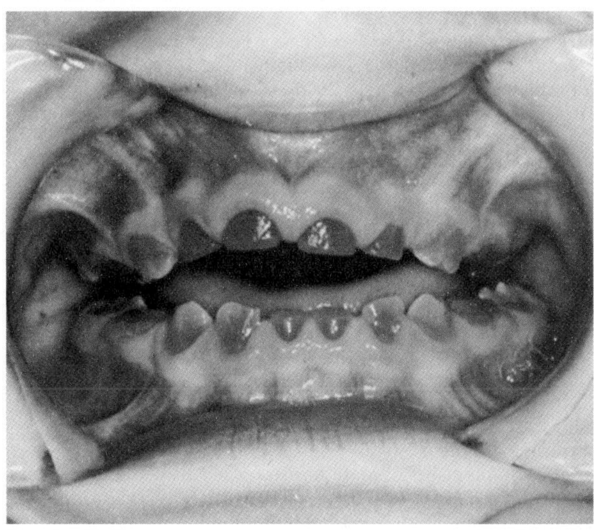

FIGURE 19-21. The teeth of a child with dentinogenesis imperfecta. (From Thompson MW: Genetics in Medicine, 4th ed. Philadelphia, WB Saunders, 1986.)

SUMMARY OF THE INTEGUMENTARY SYSTEM

- The skin and its appendages develop from ectoderm, mesenchyme, and neural crest cells. The epidermis is derived from surface ectoderm. The dermis is derived from mesenchyme. **Melanocytes** are derived from **neural crest cells** that migrate into the epidermis.
- Cast-off cells from the epidermis mix with secretions of sebaceous glands to form the vernix caseosa, a whitish, greasy coating of the skin, which protects the epidermis.
- **Hairs** develop from downgrowths of the epidermis into the dermis. By approximately 20 weeks, the fetus is completely covered with fine, downy hairs—**lanugo**. These hairs are shed before birth or shortly thereafter and are replaced by coarser hairs.
- Most **sebaceous glands** develop as outgrowths from the sides of hair follicles; however, some glands develop as downgrowths of the epidermis into the dermis. **Sweat glands** also develop from epidermal downgrowths into the dermis. **Mammary glands** develop in a similar manner.
- Congenital anomalies of the skin are mainly disorders of keratinization (**ichthyosis**) and pigmentation (**albinism**). Abnormal blood vessel development results in various types of angioma.
- **Nails** may be absent or malformed. Hair may be absent or excessive. **Absence of mammary glands** is extremely rare, but supernumerary breasts (**polymastia**) or nipples (**polythelia**) are relatively common.
- **Teeth** develop from ectoderm, mesoderm, and neural crest cells. The **enamel** is produced by **ameloblasts**, which are derived from the oral ectoderm; all other dental tissues develop from mesenchyme, derived from mesoderm and neural crest cells.
- Common congenital anomalies of teeth are defective formation of enamel and dentine, abnormalities in shape, and variations in number and position.
- **Tetracyclines** are extensively incorporated into the enamel and dentine of developing teeth, producing brownish-yellow discoloration and hypoplasia of the enamel. They should not be prescribed for pregnant women or children younger than 8 years of age.

CLINICALLY ORIENTED PROBLEMS

CASE 19-1

A newborn infant had two erupted mandibular incisor teeth.

- What are these teeth called?
- How common is this anomaly?
- Are they supernumerary teeth?
- What problems and/or danger might be associated with the presence of teeth at birth?

CASE 19-2

The deciduous teeth of an infant had a brownish-yellow color and some hypoplasia of the enamel. The mother recalled that she had been given antibiotics during the second trimester of her pregnancy.

- What is the probable cause of the infant's tooth discoloration?
- Dysfunction of what cells would cause the enamel hypoplasia?
- Would the secondary dentition be discolored?

CASE 19-3

An infant was born with a small, irregularly shaped, light-red blotch on the posterior surface of the neck. It was level with the surrounding skin and blanched when light pressure was applied to it.

- Name this congenital anomaly.
- What do these observations probably indicate?
- Is this condition common?
- Are there other names for this skin anomaly?

CASE 19-4

A newborn infant had a tuft of hair in the lumbosacral region of the back.

- What does this tuft of hair probably indicate?
- Is this condition common?
- Is this anomaly clinically important?

CASE 19-5

The skin of a newborn infant had a collodion type of covering that fissured and exfoliated shortly after birth. Later, lamellar ichthyosis developed.

- Briefly describe this condition.
- Is it common?
- How is it inherited?

Discussion of these problems appears at the back of the book.

References and Suggested Reading

Berkovitz BKB, Holland GR, Moxham B: Oral Anatomy, Histology, and Embryology, 3rd ed. Philadelphia, Mosby, 2005.

Buss PW, Hughes HE, Clarke A: Twenty-four cases of the EEC syndrome: Clinical presentation and management. J Med Genet 32:716, 1995.

Christison-Lagay ER, Fishman SJ: Vascular anomalies. Surg Clin North Am 86:393, 2006.

Cobourne MT: The genetic control of early odontogenesis. Br J Orthod 26:21, 1999.

Darmstadt GL, Sidbury R: The skin. In Behrman RE, Kliegman RM, Jenson HB (eds): Nelson Textbook of Pediatrics, 17th ed. Philadelphia, Elsevier/Saunders, 2004.

Eichenfield LF, Frieden IJ, Esterly NB: Textbook of Neonatal Dermatology. Philadelphia, WB Saunders, 2001.

Gartner LP, Hiatt JL: Color Textbook of Histology, 2nd ed. Philadelphia, WB Saunders, 2001.

Johnson CL, Holbrook KA: Development of human embryonic and fetal dermal vasculature. J Invest Dermatol 93(Suppl):105, 1989.

LeDouran N, Kalcheim C: The Neural Crest, 2nd ed. Cambridge, UK, Cambridge University Press, 1999.

Moore KL, Dalley AF: Clinically Oriented Anatomy, 5th ed. Baltimore, Williams & Wilkins, 2006.

Moore SJ, Munger BL: The early ontogeny of the afferent nerves and papillary ridges in human digital glabrous skin. Dev Brain Res 48:119, 1989.

Müller M, Jasmin JR, Monteil RA, Loubiere R: Embryology of the hair follicle. Early Hum Dev 26:59, 1999.

Narendran V, Hoath SB: The skin. In Martin RJ, Fanaroff AA, Walsh MC (eds): Fanaroff and Martin's Neonatal-Perinatal Medicine. Diseases of the Fetus and Infant, 8th ed. Philadelphia, Mosby, 2006.

Ohazama A, Sharpe PT: TNF signalling in tooth development. Curr Opin Genet Dev 14:513, 2004.

Paller AS, Mancini AJ: Hurwitz Clinical Pediatric Dermatology: A Textbook of Skin Disorders of Childhood and Adolescence, 3rd ed. Philadelphia, WB Saunders, 2006.

Sharpe PT: Homeobox genes in initiation and shape of tooth during development in mammalian embryos. In Teaford MF, Smith MM, Ferguson MW (eds): Development, Function and Evolution of Tooth. Cambridge, UK, Cambridge University Press, 2000.

Smolinski KN: Hemangiomas of infancy: Clinical and biological characteristics. Clin Pediatr 44:747, 2005.

Sperber GH: Craniofacial Development. Hamilton, BC Decker, 2001.

Ten Cate AR: Development of the tooth. In Ten Cate AR (ed): Oral Histology. Development, Structure, and Function, 5th ed. St. Louis, CV Mosby, 1998.

Watts A, Addy MA: Tooth discolouration and staining: A review of the literature. Br Dent J 190:309, 2001.

Wilkins Osborne MP: Breast anatomy and development. In Harris JR (ed): Diseases of the Breast, 2nd ed. Philadelphia, Lippincott Williams & Wilkins, 2000.

Winter GB: Anomalies of tooth formation and eruption. In Welbury RR (ed): Paediatric Dentistry, 2nd ed. Oxford, UK, Oxford University Press, 2001.

Witkop CJ: Amelogenesis imperfecta, dentinogenesis imperfecta, and dentin dysplasia revisited: problems in classification. J Oral Pathol 17:547, 1988.

20 Congenital Anatomic Anomalies or Human Birth Defects

We ought not to set them aside with idle thoughts or idle words about "curiosities" or "chances." Not one of them is without meaning; not one that might not become the beginning of excellent knowledge, if only we could answer the question—why is it rare, or being rare, why did it in this instance happen?

—James Paget, Lancet 2:1017, 1882.

Classification of Birth Defects 458

Teratology: Study of Abnormal Development 458

Anomalies Caused by Genetic Factors 459
- Numerical Chromosomal Abnormalities 459
- Structural Chromosomal Abnormalities 466
- Anomalies Caused by Mutant Genes 469
- Developmental Signaling Pathways 471

Anomalies Caused by Environmental Factors 471
- Principles in Teratogenesis 474
- Human Teratogens 475

Anomalies Caused by Multifactorial Inheritance 484

Summary of Congenital Anatomic Anomalies or Human Birth Defects 484

Clinically Oriented Problems 484

Congenital anatomic anomalies, birth defects, and congenital malformations are terms currently used to describe developmental disorders present at birth. Birth defects are the leading cause of infant mortality and may be structural, functional, metabolic, behavioral, or hereditary.

CLASSIFICATION OF BIRTH DEFECTS

The most widely used reference guide for classifying birth defects is the *International Classification of Diseases* (Medicodes' Hospital and Payer, 1995); however, no single classification has universal appeal. Each is limited, having been designed for a particular purpose. Attempts to classify congenital anatomic anomalies or human birth defects, especially those that result from **errors of morphogenesis** (development of form), reveal the frustration and obvious difficulties in the formulation of concrete proposals that could be used in medical practice. A practical classification system for congenital anomalies that takes into consideration the time at onset of the injury, possible etiology, and pathogenesis is now widely accepted among clinicians.

TERATOLOGY: STUDY OF ABNORMAL DEVELOPMENT

Teratology is the branch of science that studies the causes, mechanisms, and patterns of abnormal development. A fundamental concept in teratology is that certain stages of embryonic development are more vulnerable to disruption than others. Until the 1940s, it was generally believed that human embryos were protected from environmental agents such as drugs and viruses by their extraembryonic/fetal membranes (amnion and chorion) and their mothers' abdominal and uterine walls.

In 1941, the first well-documented cases were reported that an environmental agent (**rubella virus**) could produce severe anatomic anomalies, such as cataracts, cardiac defects, and deafness if the rubella infection was present during the critical period of development of the eyes, heart, and ears. Severe limb anomalies and other developmental disruptions were found in infants of mothers who had consumed a sedative called **thalidomide** during early pregnancy. This discovery, more than six decades ago, focused worldwide attention on the role of drugs in the *etiology (causes) of human birth defects*. It is estimated that 7% to 10% of human anatomic anomalies result from the disruptive actions of drugs, viruses, and other environmental factors.

More than 20% of infant deaths in North America are attributed to birth defects. Major structural anomalies, for example, *spina bifida cystica*, a severe type of vertebral defect in which part of the neural tube fails to fuse, are observed in approximately 3% of newborn infants. Additional anomalies can be detected after birth; thus, the incidence reaches approximately 6% in 2 year olds and 8% in 5 year olds.

The **causes of congenital anatomic anomalies** or birth defects are often divided into:

- **Genetic factors** such as chromosome abnormalities
- **Environmental factors** such as drugs and viruses

However, many common congenital anomalies are caused by **multifactorial inheritance** (genetic and environmental factors acting together in a complex manner).

For 50% to 60% of congenital anomalies, the etiology is unknown (Fig. 20-1). The anomalies may be single or multiple and of major or minor clinical significance. Single minor anomalies are present in approximately 14% of newborns. Anomalies of the external ear, for example, are of no serious medical significance, but they indicate the possible presence of associated major anomalies. For example, the presence of a single umbilical artery alerts the clinician to the possible presence of cardiovascular and renal anomalies. Ninety percent of infants with three or more minor anomalies also have one or more major defects. Of the 3% born with clinically significant congenital anomalies, 0.7% have multiple major defects. Most of these infants die during infancy. Major developmental defects are much more common in early embryos (10%–15%); however, most of them abort spontaneously

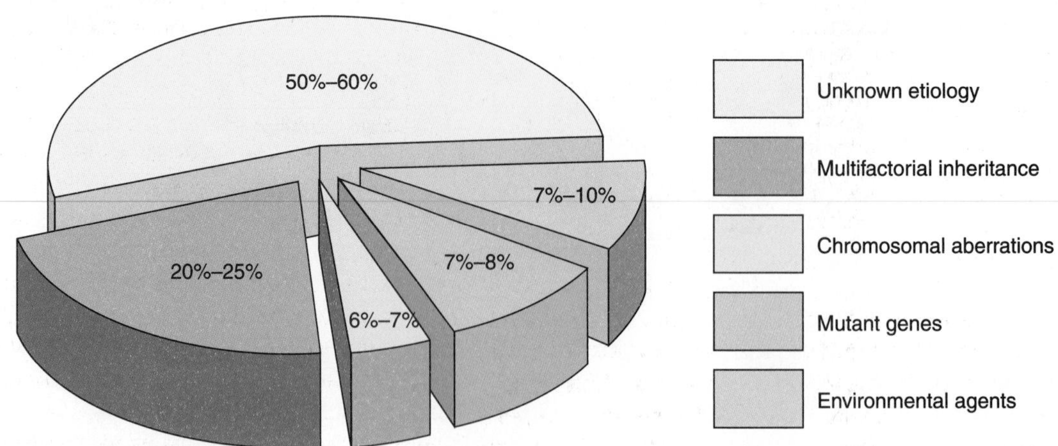

FIGURE 20-1. Graphic illustration of the causes of human congenital anomalies or birth defects. Note that the causes of most anomalies are unknown and that 20% to 25% of them are caused by a combination of genetic and environmental factors (multifactorial inheritance).

during the first 6 weeks. Chromosome abnormalities are present in 50% to 60% of spontaneously aborted embryos.

ANOMALIES CAUSED BY GENETIC FACTORS*

Numerically, genetic factors are the most important causes of congenital anomalies. It has been estimated that they cause approximately one third of all congenital anatomic anomalies (see Fig. 20-1). Nearly 85% of all anomalies have no known causes. Any mechanism as complex as mitosis or meiosis may occasionally malfunction. Chromosomal abnormalities or aberrations are present in 6% to 7% of zygotes (single-cell embryos). Many of these early abnormal embryos never undergo normal cleavage and become blastocysts. In vitro studies of cleaving zygotes less than 5 days old have revealed a high incidence of abnormalities. More than 60% of day 2 cleaving zygotes were found to be abnormal. Many defective zygotes, blastocysts, and 3-week embryos abort spontaneously, and the overall frequency of chromosome abnormalities in these embryos is at least 50%.

Two kinds of change occur in chromosome complements: numerical and structural. The changes may affect the **sex chromosomes** and/or the **autosomes**—chromosomes other than sex chromosomes. In some instances, both kinds of chromosome are affected. Persons with chromosome abnormalities usually have characteristic **phenotypes** (morphologic characteristics), such as the physical characteristics of infants with Down syndrome (see Fig. 20-6). They often look more like other persons with the same chromosome abnormality than their own siblings (brothers or sisters). This characteristic appearance results from genetic imbalance. Genetic factors initiate anomalies by biochemical or other means at the subcellular, cellular, or tissue level. The abnormal mechanisms initiated by the genetic factors may be identical or similar to the causal mechanisms initiated by a teratogen, for example, a drug.

Numerical Chromosomal Abnormalities

In the United States, approximately one in 120 live-born infants has a chromosomal abnormality. Numerical aberrations of chromosomes usually result from **nondisjunction**, an error in cell division in which there is failure of a chromosomal pair or two chromatids of a chromosome to disjoin during mitosis or meiosis. As a result, the chromosomal pair or chromatids pass to one daughter cell and the other daughter cell receives neither (Fig. 20-2). Nondisjunction may occur during maternal or paternal gametogenesis (see Chapter 2). The chromosomes in somatic cells are normally paired; they are called **homologous chromosomes** (homologs). Normal human females have 22 pairs of autosomes plus two X chromosomes, whereas normal males have 22 pairs of autosomes plus one X chromosome and one Y chromosome.

*The authors are grateful to A.E. Chudley, MD, FRCPC, FCCMG, Professor of Pediatrics and Child Health and Head, Section of Genetics and Metabolism, Children's Hospital, Health Sciences Centre, University of Manitoba, Winnipeg, Manitoba, Canada, for assistance with the preparation of this section.

GLOSSARY OF TERATOLOGIC TERMS

A **congenital anatomic anomaly** or birth defect is a structural abnormality of any type; however, *not all variations of development are anomalies*. Anatomic variations are common, for example, bones vary among themselves, not only in their basic shape but in lesser details of surface structure. There are four clinically significant types of congenital anomalies: malformation, disruption, deformation, and dysplasia.

- **Malformation:** A morphologic defect of an organ, part of an organ, or larger region of the body that results from an *intrinsically abnormal developmental process*. Intrinsic implies that the developmental potential of the primordium is abnormal from the beginning, such as a chromosomal abnormality of a gamete at fertilization. Most malformations are considered to be a defect of a *morphogenetic or developmental field* that responds as a coordinated unit to embryonic interaction and results in complex or multiple malformations.
- **Disruption:** A morphologic defect of an organ, part of an organ, or a larger region of the body that *results from the extrinsic breakdown of, or an interference with, an originally normal developmental process*. Thus, morphologic alterations after exposure to **teratogens**—agents such as drugs and viruses—should be considered as disruptions. *A disruption cannot be inherited*, but inherited factors can predispose to and influence the development of a disruption.
- **Deformation:** An abnormal form, shape, or position of a part of the body that *results from mechanical forces*. Intrauterine compression that results from **oligohydramnios**—insufficient amount of amniotic fluid—produces an *equinovarus foot* or *clubfoot* (see Chapter 16), an example of a deformation produced by extrinsic forces. Some central nervous system defects, such as *meningomyelocele*—a severe type of spina bifida—produce intrinsic functional disturbances that also cause fetal deformation.
- **Dysplasia:** An abnormal organization of cells into tissue(s) and its morphologic result(s). Dysplasia is the process and the consequence of **dyshistogenesis** (abnormal tissue formation). All abnormalities relating to histogenesis are therefore classified as dysplasias, e.g., *congenital ectodermal dysplasia* (see Chapter 19). Dysplasia is causally nonspecific and often affects several organs because of the nature of the underlying cellular disturbances.

Other descriptive terms are used to describe infants with multiple anomalies and terms have evolved to express causation and pathogenesis.

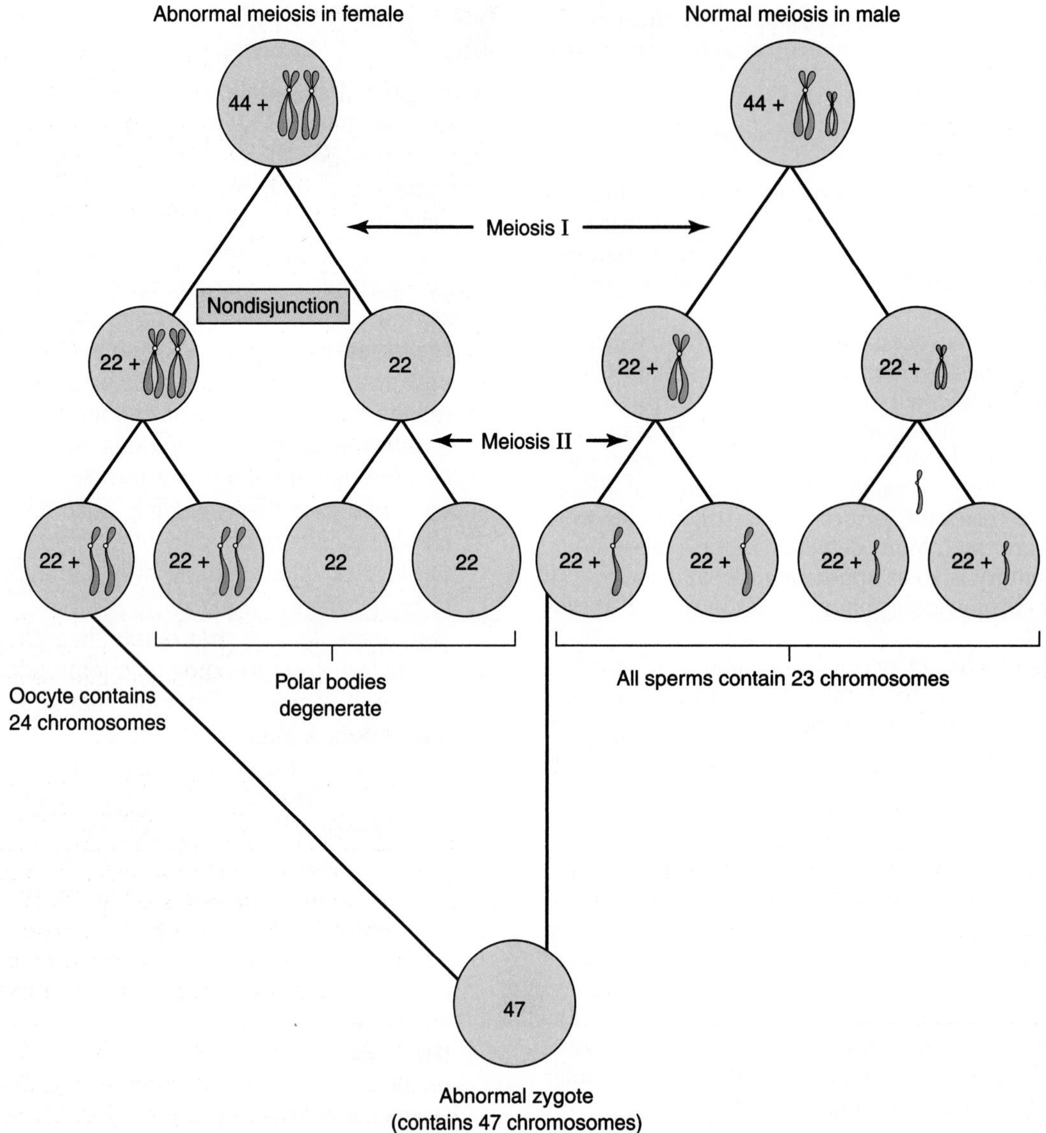

FIGURE 20-2. Diagram showing nondisjunction of chromosomes during the first meiotic division of a primary oocyte resulting in an abnormal oocyte with 24 chromosomes. Subsequent fertilization by a normal sperm produces a zygote with 47 chromosomes—**aneuploidy**—deviation from the human diploid number of 46.

- A *polytopic field defect* is a pattern of anomalies derived from the disturbance of a single developmental field.
- A *sequence* is a pattern of multiple anomalies derived from a single known or presumed structural defect or mechanical factor.
- A *syndrome* is a pattern of multiple anomalies thought to be pathogenetically related and not known to represent a single sequence or a polytopic field defect.
- An *association* is a nonrandom occurrence in two or more individuals of multiple anomalies not known to be a polytopic field defect, sequence, or syndrome.

Whereas a sequence is a pathogenetic and not a causal concept, a syndrome often implies a single cause, such as trisomy 21 (Down syndrome). In both cases, however, the pattern of anomalies is known or considered to be pathogenetically related. In the case of a sequence, the primary initiating factor and cascade of secondary developmental complications are known. For example, the *Potter sequence*, attributed to oligohydramnios, results from either renal agenesis or leakage of amniotic fluid. An association, in contrast, refers to statistically, not pathogenetically or causally, related defects. One or more sequences, syndromes, or field defects may very well constitute an association.

Dysmorphology is an area of clinical genetics that is concerned with the diagnosis and interpretation of patterns of structural defects. Recurrent patterns of birth defects are the hallmarks of syndrome recognition. Identifying these patterns in individuals has resulted in improved understanding of the etiology and pathogenesis of these conditions.

INACTIVATION OF GENES

During embryogenesis, one of the two X chromosomes in female somatic cells is randomly inactivated and appears as a mass of **sex chromatin** (see Chapter 6). Inactivation of genes on one X chromosome in somatic cells of female embryos occurs during implantation. X inactivation is important clinically because it means that each cell from a carrier of an X-linked disease has the mutant gene causing the disease, either on the active X chromosome or on the inactivated X chromosome that is represented by sex chromatin. Uneven X inactivation in monozygotic twins is one reason given for discordance for a variety of congenital anomalies. The genetic basis for discordance is that one twin preferentially expresses the paternal X and the other the maternal X.

ANEUPLOIDY AND POLYPLOIDY

Changes in chromosome number represent either aneuploidy or polyploidy. **Aneuploidy** is any deviation from the human diploid number of 46 chromosomes. An aneuploid is an individual who has a chromosome number that is not an exact multiple of the haploid number of 23 (e.g., 45 or 47). A polyploid is an individual who has a chromosome number that is a multiple of the haploid number of 23 other than the diploid number (e.g., 69; Fig. 20-10). The principal cause of aneuploidy is nondisjunction during cell division (see Fig. 20-2), resulting in an unequal distribution of one pair of homologous chromosomes to the daughter cells. One cell has two chromosomes and the other has neither chromosome of the pair. As a result, the embryo's cells may be hypodiploid (45, X, as in Turner syndrome [Figs. 20-3 to Fig. 20-5]) or hyperdiploid (usually 47, as in trisomy 21 or Down syndrome [Fig. 20-6]). Embryos with **monosomy**—missing a chromosome—usually die. Approximately 99% of embryos lacking a sex chromosome (45, X) abort spontaneously (see Fig. 20-5).

Turner Syndrome

Approximately 1% of monosomy X female embryos survive. The incidence of 45, X or Turner syndrome in newborn females is approximately 1 in 8000 live births. Half of the affected individuals have 45, X; the other half have a variety of abnormalities of a sex chromosome. The phenotype of Turner syndrome is female (Figs. 20-3 and 20-4). Secondary sexual characteristics do not develop in 90% of affected girls, and hormone replacement is required. **Phenotype** refers to the morphologic characteristics of an individual as determined by the genotype and the environment in which it is expressed. The monosomy X chromosome abnormality is the most common cytogenetic abnormality observed in live-born humans and fetuses that abort spontaneously (Fig. 20-5); it accounts for approximately 18% of all abortions caused by chromosome abnormalities. The error in gametogenesis (**nondisjunction**) that causes monosomy X (Turner syndrome), when it can be traced, is in the paternal gamete (sperm) in approximately 75% of cases, that is, it is the paternal X chromosome that is usually missing. The most frequent chromosome constitution in Turner syndrome is 45, X; however, nearly 50% of these people have other karyotypes.

Trisomy of Autosomes

The presence of three chromosome copies in a given chromosome pair is called **trisomy**. Trisomies are the most common abnormalities of chromosome number. The usual cause of this numerical error is **meiotic nondisjunction** of chromosomes (see Fig. 20-2), resulting in a gamete with 24 instead of 23 chromosomes and subsequently in a zygote with 47 chromosomes. Trisomy of the autosomes is associated with three main syndromes (Table 20-1):

- Trisomy 21 or Down syndrome (Fig. 20-6)
- Trisomy 18 or Edwards syndrome (Fig. 20-7)
- Trisomy 13 or Patau syndrome (Fig. 20-8)

Infants with trisomy 13 and trisomy 18 are severely malformed and mentally retarded and usually die early in infancy. More than half of **trisomic embryos** spontaneously abort early. Trisomy of the autosomes occurs with increasing frequency as maternal age increases. For example, trisomy 21 occurs once in approximately 1400 births in mothers ages 20 to 24 years, but once in approximately 25 births in mothers 45 years and older (Table 20-2). *Errors in meiosis occur with increasing maternal age*, and the most common aneuploidy seen in older mothers is trisomy 21. Because of the current trend of increasing maternal age, it has been estimated that by the end of this decade, children born to women older than 34 years will account for 39% of infants with trisomy 21. Translocation or mosaicism occurs in approximately 5% of the affected children. **Mosaicism**, two or more cell types containing different numbers of chromosomes (normal and abnormal), leads to a less severe phenotype and the IQ of the child may be nearly normal.

Trisomy of Sex Chromosomes

Trisomy of the sex chromosomes is a common disorder (Table 20-3); however, because there are no characteristic

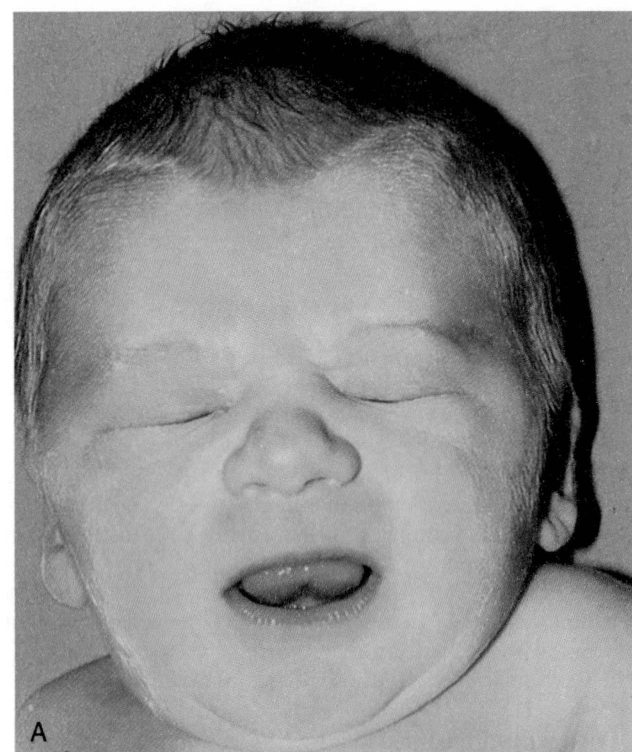

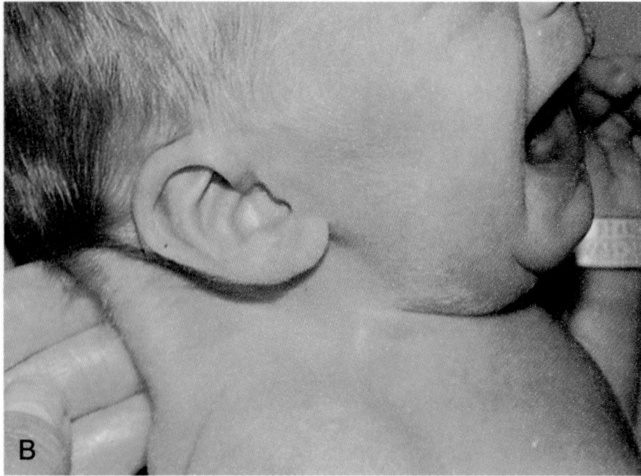

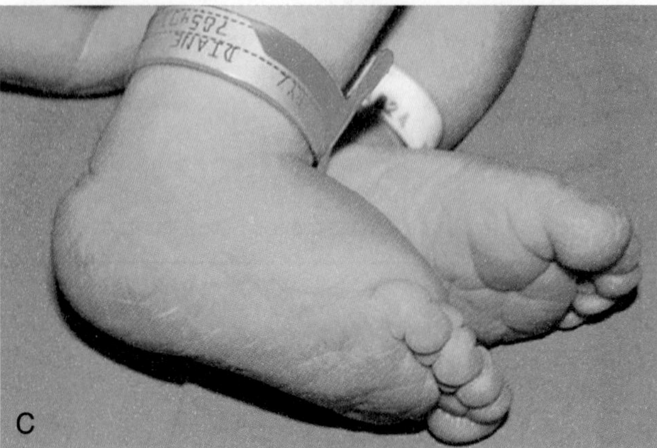

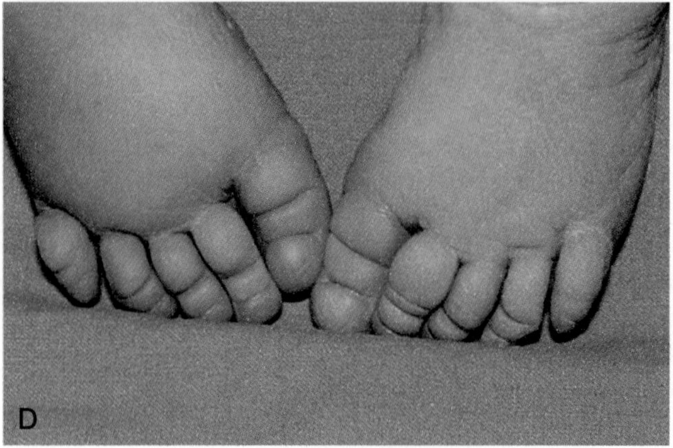

FIGURE 20-3. Female infant with Turner syndrome (45, X). **A,** Face of infant with Turner syndrome. **B,** Lateral view of infant's head and neck showing a short neck, prominent ears, and redundant skin at the back of the neck. These infants have defective gonadal development (*gonadal dysgenesis*). **C,** Infant's feet showing the characteristic lymphedema (puffiness and swelling), a useful diagnostic sign. **D,** Lymphedema of toes, a condition that usually leads to nail underdevelopment (hypoplasia). (Courtesy of A.E. Chudley, MD, Section of Genetics and Metabolism, Department of Pediatrics and Child Health, Children's Hospital, Winnipeg, Manitoba, Canada.)

physical findings in infants or children, this disorder is not usually detected until puberty (Fig. 20-9). Sex chromatin studies were useful in the past for detecting some types of trisomy of the sex chromosomes because two masses of sex chromatin are present in nuclei of XXX females (trisomy X) and nuclei of XXY males (Klinefelter syndrome) contain a mass of sex chromatin (see Chapter 6). Today, diagnosis is best achieved by chromosome (DNA) analysis.

TETRASOMY AND PENTASOMY

Tetrasomy and pentasomy of the sex chromosomes also occur. Persons with these abnormalities have four or five sex chromosomes, respectively; the following chromosome complexes have been reported in females: 48, XXXX and 49, XXXXX; and males: 48, XXXY, 48, XXYY, 49, XXXYY, and 49, XXXXY. The extra sex chromosomes do not accentuate sexual characteristics; however, usually the greater the number of sex chromosomes present, the greater the severity of mental retardation and physical impairment.

MOSAICISM

A person who has at least two cell lines with two or more different genotypes (genetic constitutions) is a **mosaic**. Either the autosomes or sex chromosomes may be involved. Usually the anomalies are less

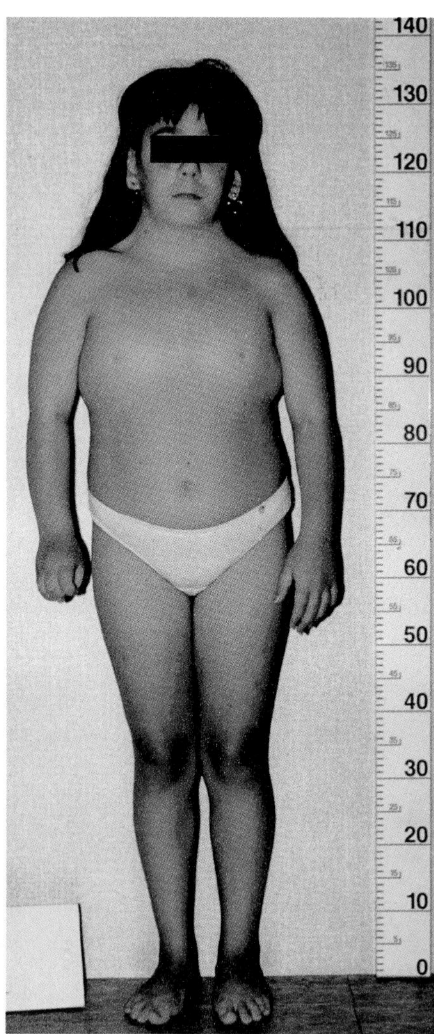

FIGURE 20-4. Turner syndrome in a 14-year-old girl. Note the classic features of the syndrome: short stature, webbed neck, absence of sexual maturation, broad shieldlike chest with widely spaced nipples, and lymphedema of the hands and feet. (Courtesy of Dr. F. Antoniazzi and Dr. V. Fanos, Department of Pediatrics, University of Verona, Verona, Italy.)

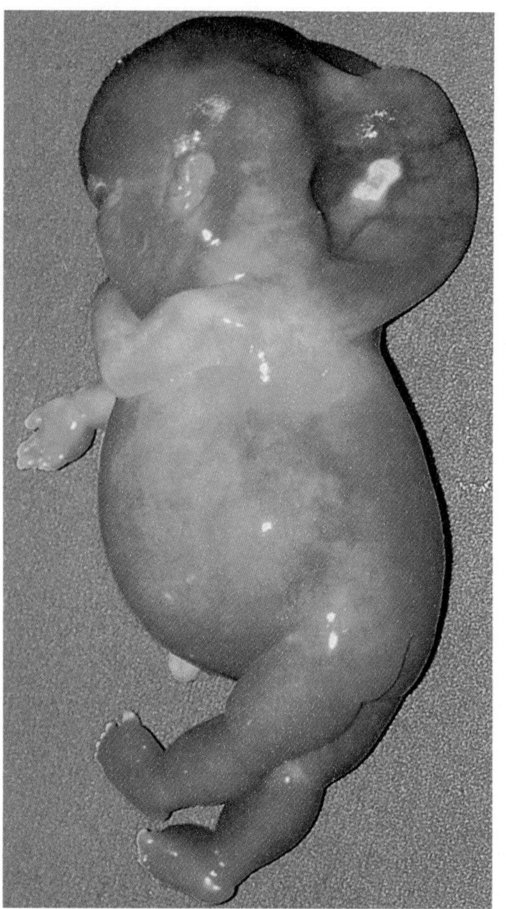

FIGURE 20-5. Female fetus (16 weeks) with Turner syndrome; 99% of fetuses with 45, X karyotype abort spontaneously. Note the excessive accumulation of watery fluid (*hydrops*) and the large *cystic hygroma* (lymphangioma) in the posterior head and cervical region. The hygroma causes the loose neck skin and webbing seen postnatally (see Fig. 20-3*B*). (Courtesy of A.E. Chudley, MD, Section of Genetics and Metabolism, Department of Pediatrics and Child Health, Children's Hospital, Winnipeg, Manitoba, Canada.)

TABLE 20–1. Trisomy of the Autosomes

CHROMOSOMAL ABERRATION/SYNDROME	INCIDENCE	USUAL CLINICAL MANIFESTATIONS
Trisomy 21 or Down syndrome*	1:800	Mental deficiency; brachycephaly, flat nasal bridge; upward slant to palpebral fissures; protruding tongue; simian crease; clinodactyly of fifth digit; congenital heart defects; gastrointestinal tract abnormalities.
Trisomy 18 syndrome†	1:8000	Mental deficiency; growth retardation; prominent occiput; short sternum; ventricular septal defect; micrognathia; low-set malformed ears, flexed digits, hypoplastic nails; rocker-bottom feet.
Trisomy 13 syndrome†	1:12,000	Mental deficiency; severe central nervous system malformations; sloping forehead; malformed ears, scalp defects; microphthalmia; bilateral cleft lip and/or palate; polydactyly; posterior prominence of the heels.

*The importance of this disorder in the overall problem of mental deficiency (retardation) is indicated by the fact that persons with Down syndrome represent 10% to 15% of institutionalized mental defectives. The incidence of trisomy 21 at fertilization is greater than at birth; however, 75% of embryos are spontaneously aborted and at least 20% are stillborn.

†Infants with this syndrome rarely survive beyond 6 months.

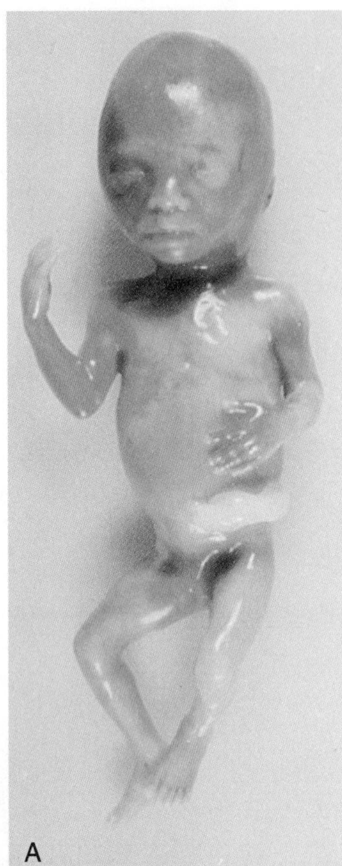

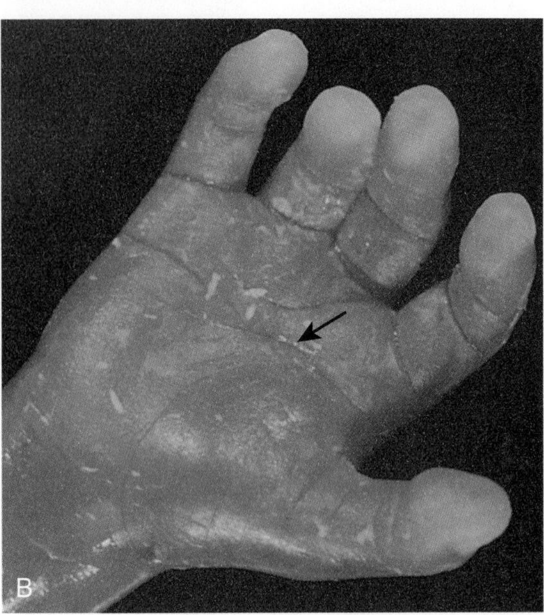

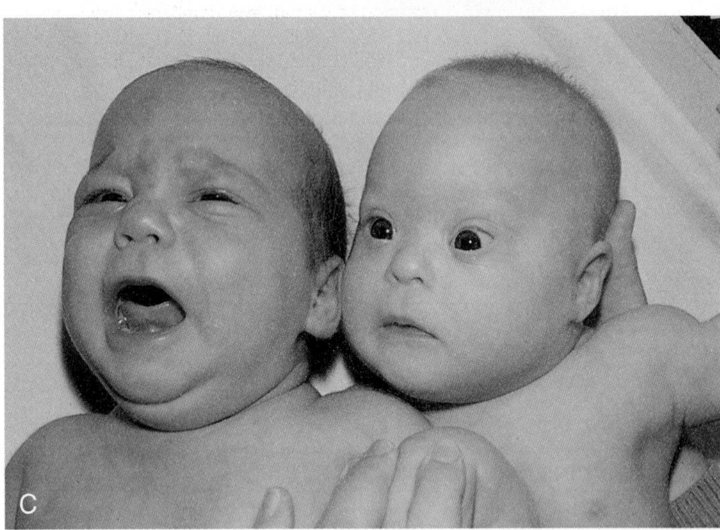

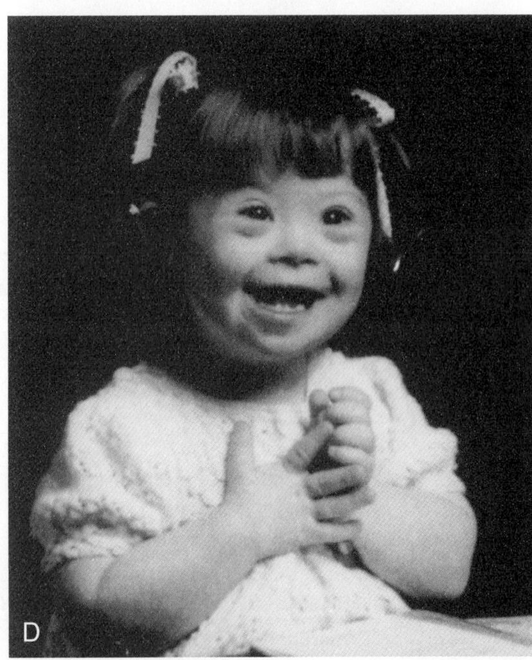

FIGURE 20-6. **A** Anterior view of a female fetus (16.5 weeks) with Down syndrome. **B,** Hand of fetus. Note the single, transverse palmar *flexion crease* (simian crease, *arrow*) and the *clinodactyly* (incurving) of the fifth digit. **C,** Anterior view of the faces of *dizygotic male twins* that are discordant for Down syndrome (trisomy 21). The one on the right is smaller and hypotonic compared with the unaffected twin. The twin on the right developed from a zygote that contained an extra 21 chromosome. Note the characteristic facial features of Down syndrome in this infant: upslanting palpebral fissures, epicanthal folds, and flat nasal bridge. **D,** A 2 1/2-year-old girl with Down syndrome. (**A** and **B,** Courtesy of Dr. D.K. Kalousek, Department of Pathology, University of British Columbia, Vancouver, British Columbia, Canada; **C** and **D,** Courtesy of A.E. Chudley, MD, Section of Genetics and Metabolism, Department of Pediatrics and Child Health, Children's Hospital, Winnipeg, Manitoba, Canada.)

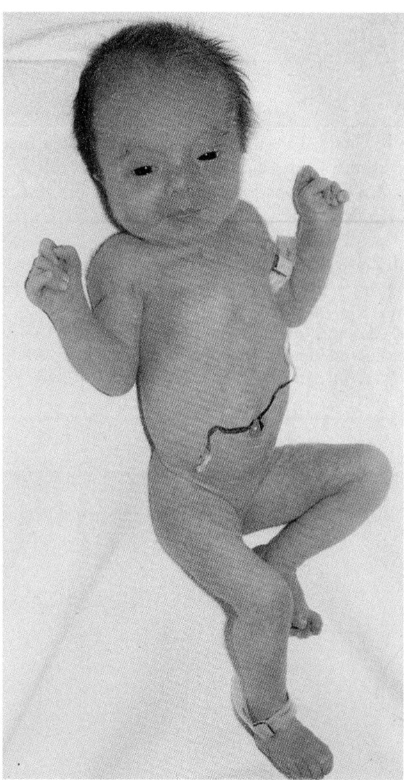

FIGURE 20-7. Female neonate (newborn infant) with trisomy 18. Note the growth retardation, clenched fists with characteristic positioning of the fingers (second and fifth ones overlapping the third and fourth), short sternum, and narrow pelvis. (Courtesy of A.E. Chudley, MD, Section of Genetics and Metabolism, Department of Pediatrics and Child Health, Children's Hospital, Winnipeg, Manitoba, Canada.)

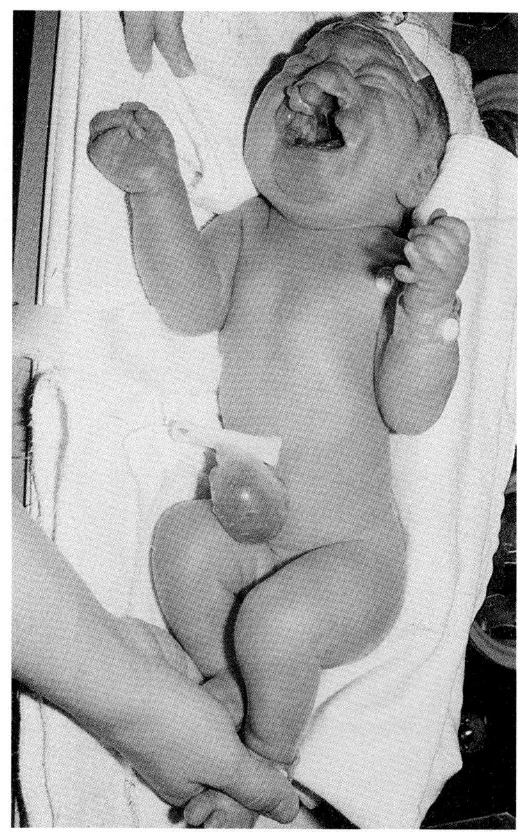

FIGURE 20-8. Female neonate with trisomy 13. Note the bilateral cleft lip, low-set malformed left ear, and polydactyly (extra digits). A small *omphalocele* (herniation of viscera into umbilical cord) is also present. (Courtesy of A.E. Chudley, MD, Section of Genetics and Metabolism, Department of Pediatrics and Child Health, Children's Hospital, Winnipeg, Manitoba, Canada.)

serious than in persons with monosomy or trisomy, e.g., the features of Turner syndrome are not as evident in 45, X/46, XX mosaic females as in the usual 45, X females. **Mosaicism** usually results from nondisjunction during early cleavage of the zygote (see Chapter 2). Mosaicism resulting from loss of a chromosome by anaphase lagging also occurs; the chromosomes separate normally but one of them is delayed in its migration and is eventually lost.

TRIPLOIDY

The most common type of polyploidy is triploidy (69 chromosomes). **Triploid fetuses** have severe intrauterine growth retardation with a disproportionately small trunk (Fig. 20-10). Several other anomalies are common. **Triploidy** could result from the second polar body failing to separate from the oocyte during the second meiotic division (see Chapter 2); but more likely triploidy results when an oocyte is fertilized by two sperms (dispermy) almost simultaneously. Triploidy occurs in approximately 2% of embryos, but most of them abort spontaneously. Triploid fetuses account for approximately 20% of chromosomally abnormal miscarriages. Although triploid fetuses have been born alive, this is exceptional. These infants all died within a few days because of multiple anomalies and low birth weight.

TABLE 20–2. Incidence of Down Syndrome in Newborn Infants

MATERNAL AGE (YEARS)	INCIDENCE
20–24	1:1400
25–29	1:1100
30–34	1:700
35	1:350
37	1:225
39	1:140
41	1:85
43	1:50
45+	1:25

TETRAPLOIDY

Doubling the diploid chromosome number to 92 (tetraploidy) probably occurs during the first cleavage division. Division of this abnormal zygote would

Table 20-3. Trisomy of the Chromosomes

CHROMOSOME COMPLEMENT*	SEX	INCIDENCE†	USUAL CHARACTERISTICS
47, XXX	Female	1:1000	Normal in appearance; usually fertile; 15%–25% are mildly mentally retarded.
47, XXY	Male	1:1000	Klinefelter's syndrome: small testes, hyalinization of seminiferous tubules; aspermatogenesis; often tall with disproportionately long lower limbs. Intelligence is less than in normal siblings. Approximately 40% of these males have gynecomastia (see Fig. 20-9).
47, XYY	Male	1:1000	Normal in appearance; usually tall; often exhibit aggressive behavior.

*The numbers designate the total number of chromosomes including the sex chromosomes shown after the comma.
†Data from Hook EB, Hamerton JL. The frequency of chromosome abnormalities detected in consecutive newborn studies—differences between studies—results by sex and by severity of phenotypic involvement. In Hook EB, Porter IH (eds): Population Cytogenetics: Studies in Humans. New York, Academic Press, 1977. For more information, refer to Nussbaum RL, McInnes RR, Willard HF: Thompson & Thompson Genetics in Medicine, 6th ed (revised reprint). Philadelphia, WB Saunders, 2004.

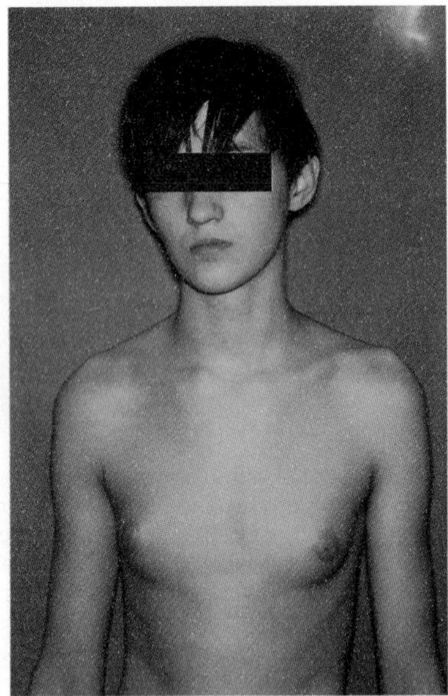

Figure 20-9. Adolescent male with Klinefelter syndrome (XXY trisomy). Note the presence of breasts; approximately 40% of males with this syndrome have *gynecomastia* (development of mammary glands) and small testes. (Courtesy of Children's Hospital, Winnipeg, Manitoba, Canada.)

subsequently result in an embryo with cells containing 92 chromosomes. *Tetraploid embryos abort very early*, and often all that is recovered is an empty chorionic sac, which used to be referred to as a "blighted embryo."

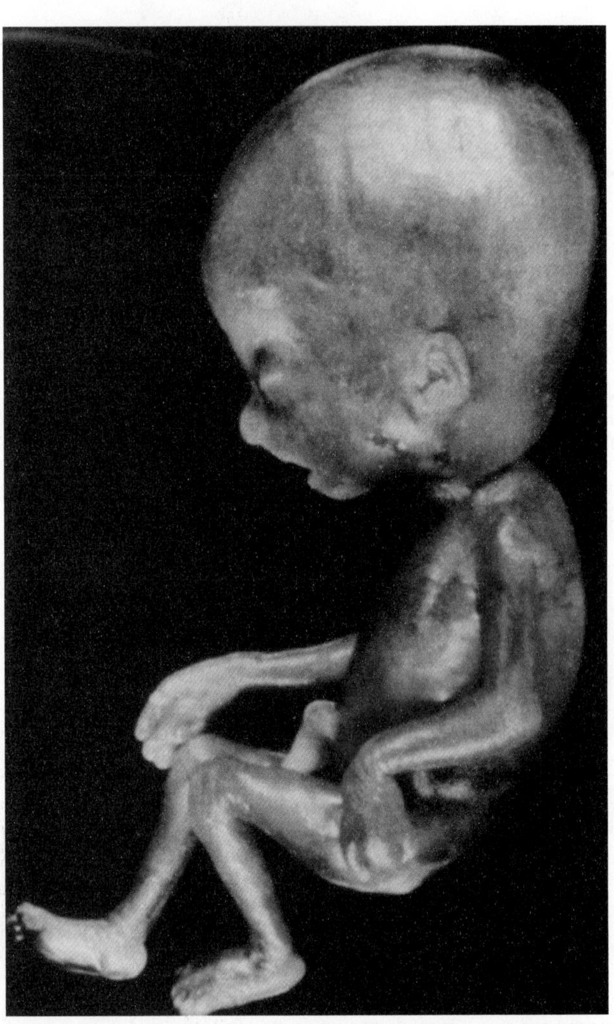

Figure 20-10. Triploid fetus illustrating severe head-to-body disproportion. Triploidy is characterized by a complete extra set of chromosomes. Triploid fetuses account for nearly 20% of chromosomally abnormal miscarriages. (From Crane JP: Ultrasound evaluation of fetal chromosome disorders. In Callen PW [ed]: Ultrasonography in Obstetrics and Gynecology, 3rd ed. Philadelphia, WB Saunders, 1994.)

Structural Chromosomal Abnormalities

Most abnormalities of chromosome structure result from **chromosome breakage** followed by reconstitution in an abnormal combination (Fig. 20-11). Chromosome breakage may be induced by various environmental factors, for example, radiation, drugs, chemicals, and viruses. The resulting type of structural chromosome abnormality depends on what happens to the broken pieces. The only two aberrations of chromosome structure that are likely to be transmitted from parent to child are **structural rearrangements**, such as inversion and translocation.

Translocation

This is the transfer of a piece of one chromosome to a nonhomologous chromosome. If two nonhomologous chromosomes exchange pieces, it is a **reciprocal trans-**

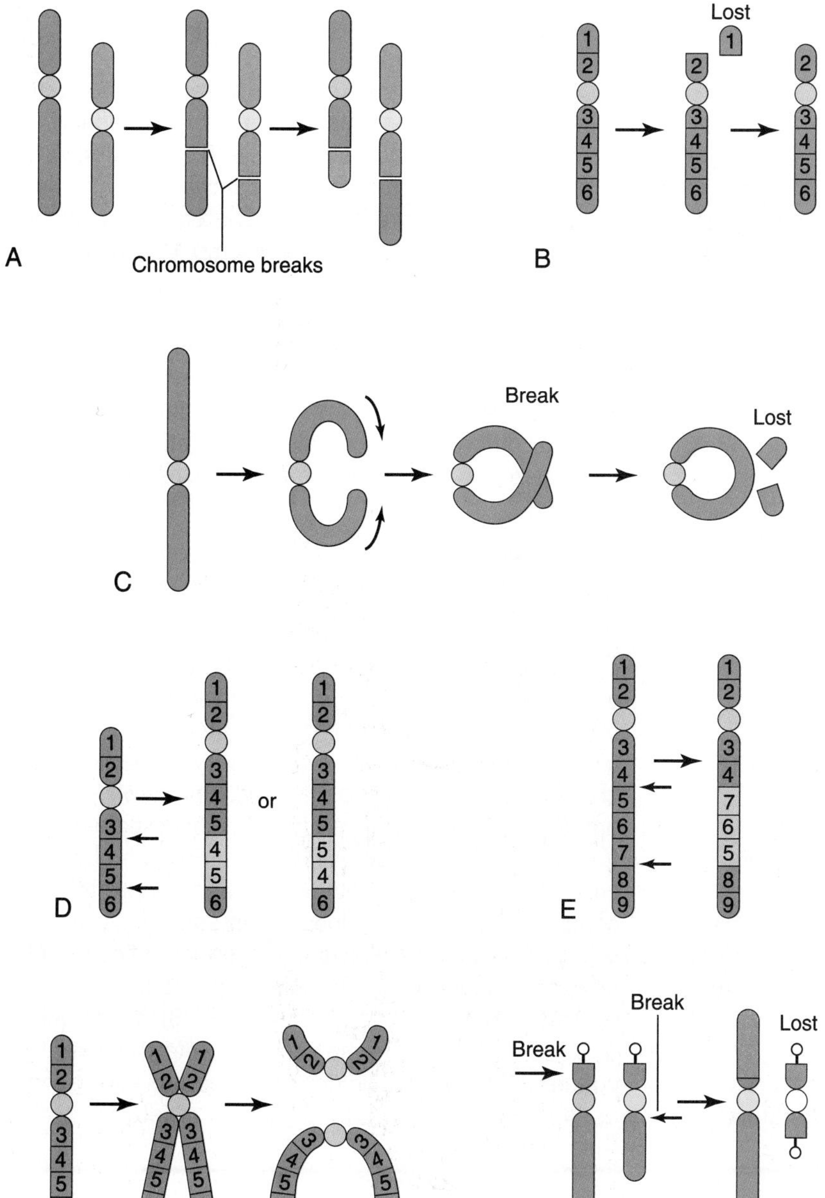

FIGURE 20-11. Diagrams illustrating various structural chromosomal abnormalities. **A,** Reciprocal translocation. **B,** Terminal deletion. **C,** Ring chromosome. **D,** Duplication. **E,** Paracentric inversion. **F,** Isochromosome. **G,** Robertsonian translocation. *Arrows* indicate how the structural abnormalities are produced.

location (see Fig. 20-11*A* and *G*). Translocation does not necessarily cause abnormal development. Persons with a translocation between a number 21 chromosome and a number 14 chromosome, for example (see Fig. 20-11*G*), are phenotypically normal. Such persons are **balanced translocation carriers**. They have a tendency, independent of age, to produce germ cells with an abnormal translocation chromosome. Three percent to 4% of persons with Down syndrome have **translocation trisomies,** that is, the extra 21 chromosome is attached to another chromosome.

Deletion

When a chromosome breaks, part of it may be lost (see Fig. 20-11*B*). A partial terminal deletion from the short arm of chromosome 5 causes the **cri du chat syndrome** (Fig. 20-12). Affected infants have a weak catlike cry, microcephaly (abnormally small head), severe mental deficiency (retardation), and congenital heart disease. A **ring chromosome** is a type of deletion chromosome from which both ends have been lost, and the broken ends have rejoined to form a ring-shaped chromosome (see Fig. 20-11*C*). Ring chromosomes are rare but have been found for all chromosomes. These abnormal chromosomes have been described in persons with Turner syndrome, trisomy 18, and other structural chromosomal abnormalities.

MICRODELETIONS AND MICRODUPLICATIONS

High-resolution banding techniques have allowed detection of very small interstitial and terminal deletions in a number of disorders. An acceptable

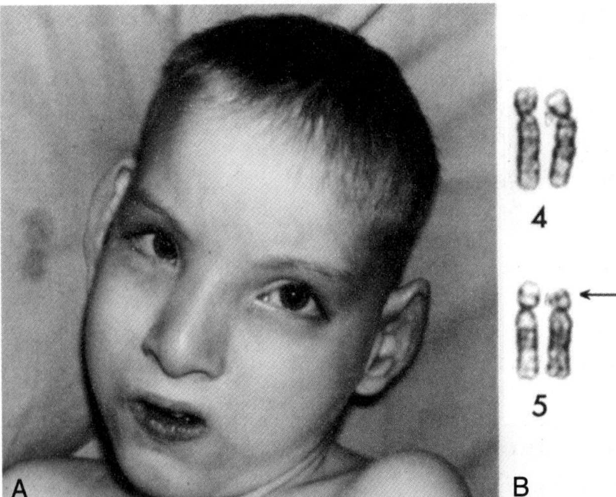

FIGURE 20-12. **A,** Male child with cri du chat syndrome. Note microcephaly and hypertelorism (increased distance between orbits). **B,** Partial karyotype of this child showing a terminal deletion of the short arm (end) of chromosome number 5. The *arrow* indicates the site of the deletion. (**A,** From Gardner EJ: Principles of Genetics, 5th ed. New York, John Wiley & Sons, Inc., 1975. **B,** Courtesy of the late Dr. M. Ray, Department of Human Genetics, University of Manitoba, Winnipeg, Manitoba, Canada.)

resolution of chromosome banding on routine analysis reveals 550 bands per haploid set, whereas high-resolution chromosome banding reveals up to 1300 bands per haploid set. Because the deletions span several contiguous genes, these disorders, as well as those with microduplications, are referred to as **contiguous gene syndromes** (Table 20-4). Two examples are

- **Prader-Willi syndrome** (PWS), a sporadically occurring disorder associated with short stature, mild mental retardation, obesity, hyperphagia (overeating), and hypogonadism (inadequate gonadal function).
- **Angelman syndrome** (AS), characterized by severe mental retardation, microcephaly, brachycephaly (shortness of head), seizures, and ataxic (jerky) movements of the limbs and trunk.

Both PWS and AS are often associated with a visible deletion of band q12 on chromosome 15. The clinical phenotype is determined by the parental origin of the deleted chromosome 15. If the deletion arises in the mother, AS occurs; if passed on by the father, the child exhibits the PWS phenotype. This suggests the phenomenon of **genetic imprinting** whereby differential expression of genetic material is dependent on the sex of the transmitting parent.

MOLECULAR CYTOGENETICS

Several new methods for merging classic cytogenetics with DNA technology have facilitated a more precise definition of chromosome abnormalities, location, or origins, including unbalanced translocations, accessory or marker chromosomes, and gene mapping. One new approach to chromosome identification is based on **fluorescent in situ hybridization** (FISH), whereby chromosome-specific DNA probes can adhere to complementary regions located on specific chromosomes. This allows improved identification of chromosome location and number in metaphase spreads or even in interphase cells. FISH techniques using interphase cells may soon obviate the need to culture cells for specific chromosome analysis, such as in the case of prenatal diagnosis of fetal trisomies.

TABLE 20–4. Examples of Contiguous Gene Syndromes (Microdeletion or Microduplication Syndromes)

SYNDROME	CLINICAL FEATURES	CHROMOSOME FINDINGS	PARENTAL ORIGIN
Prader-Willi	Hypotonia, hypogonadism, obesity with hyperphagia, distinct face, short stature, small hands and feet, mild developmental delay	del 15 q12 (most cases)	Paternal
Angelman's	Microcephaly, macrosomia, ataxia, excessive laughter, seizures, severe mental retardation	del 15 q12 (most cases)	Maternal
Miller-Dieker	Type I lissencephaly, dysmorphic face, seizures, severe developmental delay, cardiac anomalies	del 17 p13.3 (most cases)	Either parent
DiGeorge	Thymic hypoplasia, parathyroid hypoplasia, conotruncal cardiac defects, facial dysmorphism	del 22 q11 (some cases)	Either parent
Velocardiofacial (Shprintzen's)	Palatal defects, hypoplastic alae nasi, long nose, conotruncal cardiac defects, speech delay, learning disorder, schizophrenia-like disorder	del 22 q11 (most cases)	Either parent
Smith-Magenis	Brachycephaly, broad nasal bridge, prominent jaw, short broad hands, speech delay, mental retardation	del 17 p11.2	Either parent
Williams	Short stature; hypercalcemia; cardiac anomalies, especially supravalvular aortic stenosis; characteristic elfin-like face; mental retardation	del 17 q11.23 (most cases)	Either parent
Beckwith-Wiedemann	Macrosomia, macroglossia, omphalocele (some cases), hypoglycemia, hemihypertrophy, transverse ear lobes	dup 11 p15 (some cases)	Paternal

Studies using **subtelomeric FISH probes** in individuals with mental retardation of unknown etiology, with or without birth defects, have identified submicroscopic chromosome deletions or duplications in 5% to 10% of these individuals. Alterations in DNA sequence copy number are present in solid tumors and are found in association with developmental abnormalities and/or mental retardation. **Comparative genomic hybridization** can detect and map these changes in specific regions of the genome. Microarray-based SGH (array comparative genomic hybridization) is now being used to identify genomic rearrangements in individuals who had been previously considered to have mental retardation or multiple birth defects of unknown etiology despite normal test results from traditional chromosome or gene analysis. Thus, these investigations have become important in the routine evaluation of patients with previously unexplained mental retardation.

Duplications

These abnormalities may be represented as a duplicated part of a chromosome, within a chromosome (see Fig. 20-11*D*), attached to a chromosome, or as a separate fragment. Duplications are more common than deletions and are less harmful because there is no loss of genetic material. However, there is often a resulting clinical effect on the phenotype leading to either mental impairment or birth defects in individuals with chromosome duplication. Duplication may involve part of a gene, a whole gene, or a series of genes.

Inversion

This is a chromosomal aberration in which a segment of a chromosome is reversed. Paracentric inversion is confined to a single arm of the chromosome (see Fig. 20-11*E*), whereas pericentric inversion involves both arms and includes the centromere. Carriers of pericentric inversions are at risk of having offspring with abnormalities because of unequal crossing over and malsegregation at meiosis.

Isochromosomes

The abnormality resulting in isochromosomes occurs when the centromere divides transversely instead of longitudinally (see Fig. 20-11*E*). An isochromosome is a chromosome in which one arm is missing and the other duplicated. An isochromosome appears to be the most common structural abnormality of the X chromosome. Persons with this abnormality are often short in stature and have other stigmata of Turner syndrome. These characteristics are related to the loss of an arm of an X chromosome.

Anomalies Caused by Mutant Genes

Seven percent to 8% of congenital anomalies are caused by gene defects (see Fig. 20-1). A **mutation** usually involves a loss or change in the function of a gene and is any permanent, heritable change in the sequence of genomic DNA. Because a random change is unlikely to lead to an improvement in development, most mutations are deleterious and some are lethal.

The **mutation rate** can be increased by a number of environmental agents, such as large doses of radiation. Anomalies resulting from gene mutations are inherited according to mendelian laws; consequently, predictions can be made about the probability of their occurrence in the affected person's children and other relatives. An example of a dominantly inherited congenital anomaly—**achondroplasia** (Fig. 20-13)—results from a G-to-A transition mutation at nucleotide 1138 of the cDNA in the fibroblast growth factor receptor 3 gene on chromosome 4p. Other congenital anomalies, such as, congenital suprarenal (adrenal) hyperplasia (see Fig. 20-18) and microcephaly, are attributed to autosomal recessive inheritance. Autosomal recessive genes manifest themselves only when homozygous; as a consequence, many carriers of these genes (heterozygous persons) remain undetected.

Fragile X syndrome is the most commonly inherited cause of moderate mental retardation (Fig. 20-14). It is one of more than 200 X-linked disorders associated with mental impairment. The fragile X syndrome has a frequency of 1 in 1500 male births and may account for much of the excess of males in the mentally retarded population. The diagnosis can be confirmed by chromosome analysis demonstrating the fragile X chromosome at Xq27.3 or by DNA studies showing an expansion of CGG nucleotides in a specific region of the *FMRI* gene.

Several genetic disorders have been confirmed to be due to **expansion of trinucleotides** in specific genes. Other examples include myotonic dystrophy, Huntington chorea, spinobulbar atrophy (Kennedy syndrome), Friedreich's ataxia, and others. X-linked recessive genes are usually manifest in affected (hemizygous) males and occasionally in carrier (heterozygous) females, for example, fragile X syndrome.

The **human genome** comprises an estimated 30,000 to 40,000 genes per haploid set or 3 billion base pairs. Because of the Human Genome Project and international research collaboration, many disease- and birth defect–causing mutations in genes have been and will continue to be identified. Most genes will be sequenced and their specific function determined. Understanding the cause of birth defects will require a better understanding of gene expression during early development. The majority of genes that are expressed in a cell are expressed in a wide

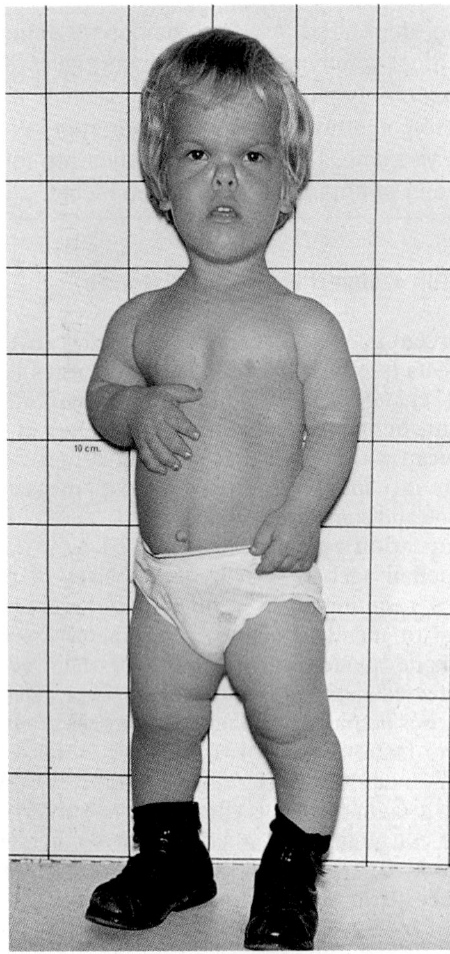

FIGURE 20-13. A boy with achondroplasia showing short stature, short limbs and fingers, normal length of trunk, bowed legs, a relatively large head, prominent forehead, and depressed nasal bridge. (Courtesy of A.E. Chudley, MD, Section of Genetics and Metabolism, Department of Pediatrics and Child Health, Children's Hospital, Winnipeg, Manitoba, Canada.)

variety of cells and are involved in basic cellular metabolic functions such as nucleic acid and protein synthesis, cytoskeleton and organelle biogenesis, and nutrient transport and other cellular mechanisms. These genes are referred to as **housekeeping genes**. The specialty genes are expressed at specific times in specific cells and define the hundreds of different cell types that make up the human organism. An essential aspect of developmental biology is **regulation of gene expression**. Regulation is often achieved by transcription factors that bind to regulatory or promoter elements of specific genes.

Genomic imprinting is an epigenetic process whereby the female and male germlines confer a sex-specific mark on a chromosome subregion, so that only the paternal or maternal allele of a gene is active in the offspring. In other words, the sex of the transmitting parent will influence expression or nonexpression of certain genes in the offspring (see Table 20-4). This is the reason for **PWS** and **AS**, in which case the phenotype is determined by whether the microdeletion is transmitted by the father (PWS) or the mother (AS). In a substantial number of cases of PWS and AS, as well as several other genetic disorders, the condition arises from a phenomenon referred to as **uniparental disomy**. In the situation with PWS and AS, both chromosomes 15s originate from only one parent. PWS occurs when both chromosomes 15s are derived from the mother, and AS occurs when both are paternally derived. The mechanism for this is believed to begin with a trisomic conceptus, followed by a loss of the extra chromosome in an early postzygotic cell division. This results in a "rescued" cell, in which both chromosomes have been derived from one parent. Uniparental disomy has involved several chromosome pairs. Some are associated with adverse clinical outcomes involving chromosome pairs 6 (transient neonatal diabetes mellitus), 7 (Silver-Russel syndrome), and 15 (PWS and AS), whereas others (1 and 22) are not associated with any abnormal phenotypic effect.

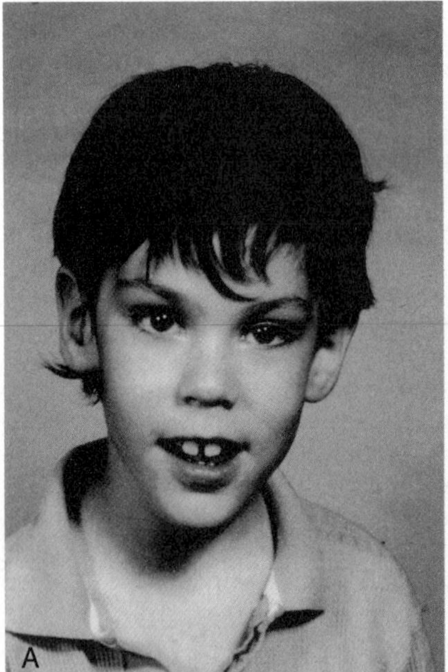

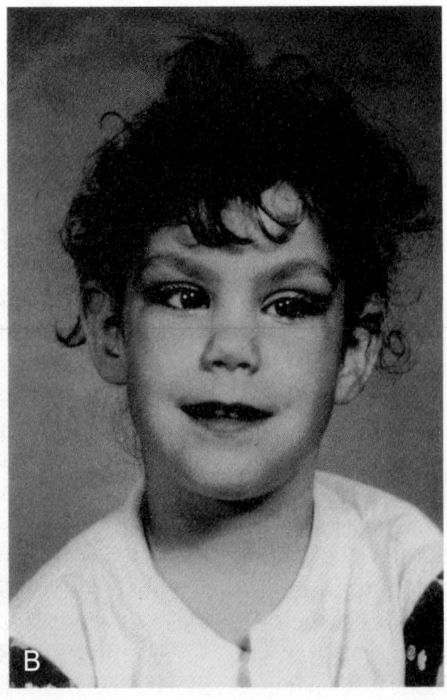

FIGURE 20-14. Siblings with fragile X syndrome. **A,** An 8-year-old mentally deficient (retarded) boy exhibiting a relatively normal appearance with a long face and prominent ears. **B,** His 6-year-old sister also has this syndrome. She has a mild learning disability and similar features of long face and prominent ears. Note the strabismus (crossed right eye). Although an X-linked disorder, sometimes female carriers have expression of the disease. (Courtesy of A.E. Chudley, MD, Section of Genetics and Metabolism, Department of Pediatrics and Child Health, Children's Hospital, Winnipeg, Manitoba, Canada.)

TABLE 20-5. Examples of Disorders in Humans Associated with Homeobox Mutations

NAME	CLINICAL FEATURES	GENE
Waardenburg syndrome (type I)	White forelock, lateral displacement of medial canthi of the eyes, cochlear deafness, heterochromia, tendency to facial clefting, autosomal dominant inheritance	*HuP2* gene in humans, homolog of *Pax3* gene of mouse
Synpolydactyly (type II syndactyly)	Webbing and duplication of fingers, supernumerary metacarpal, autosomal dominant inheritance	*HOX D 13* mutation
Holoprosencephaly (one form)	Incomplete separation of lateral cerebral ventricles, anophthalmia or cyclopia, midline facial hypoplasia or clefts, single maxillary central incisors, hypotelorism, autosomal dominant inheritance with widely variable expression	*HPE 3* (sonic hedgehog) mutation gene that is homologous to the Drosophila segment polarity gene hedgehog
Schizencephaly (type II)	Full-thickness cleft within the cerebral ventricles often leading to seizures, spasticity, and mental retardation	Germline mutation in the *EMX2* homeobox gene, homologous to the mouse EMX2

Homeobox genes are a group of genes found in all vertebrates. They have highly conserved sequences and order. They are involved in early embryonic development and specify identity and spatial arrangements of body segments. Protein products of these genes bind to DNA and form transcriptional factors that regulate gene expression. Disorders associated with some homeobox mutations are described in Table 20-5.

Developmental Signaling Pathways

Normal embryogenesis is regulated by several complex signaling cascades (see Chapter 21). Mutations or alterations in any of these signaling pathways can lead to birth defects. Many signaling pathways are cell autonomous and only alter the differentiation of that particular cell, as seen in proteins produced by HOX A and HOX D gene clusters (in which mutations lead to a variety of limb defects). Other **transcriptional factors** act by influencing the pattern of gene expression of other adjacent cells. These short-range signal controls can act as simple on-off switches (*paracrine signals*); others, termed **morphogens**, elicit many responses depending on their level of expression with other cells.

One such developmental signaling pathway is initiated by the secreted protein called **sonic hedgehog** (Shh) that sets off a chain of events in target cells, resulting in activation and repression of target cells by transcription factors in the Gli family. Perturbations in the regulation of the Shh-Patched-Gli (Shh-Ptch-Gli) pathway leads to several human diseases including some cancers and birth defects.

Shh is expressed in the notochord, the floorplate of the neural tube, the brain, and other regions such as the zone of polarizing activity of the developing limbs, and the gut. Sporadic and inherited mutations in the human *Shh* gene leads to **holoprosencephaly** (see Fig. 17-42), a midline defect of variable severity involving abnormal central nervous system (CNS) septation, facial clefting, single central incisor, hypotelorism, or a single cyclopic eye. Shh protein needs to be processed to an active form and is modified by the addition of a cholesterol moiety. Defects in cholesterol biosynthesis, such as in the autosomal recessively inherited disorder Smith-Lemli-Opitz syndrome, share many features, particularly brain and limb anomalies reminiscent of Shh-pathway diseases. This suggests that Shh signaling may play a key role in several genetic disorders.

The three *Gli* genes identified as transcriptional factors are in the Shh-Ptch-Gli pathway. Mutations in the *Gli3* gene have been implicated in several autosomal dominantly inherited disorders, including Greig cephalopolysyndactyly syndrome (deletions or point mutations); Pallister-Hall syndrome with hypothalamic hamartomas, central or postaxial polydactyly, among other anomalies of the face, brain, and limbs (frameshift or nonsense mutations); simple familial postaxial polydactyly type A and B as well as preaxial polydactyly type IV (nonsense, missense, and frameshift mutations).

A comprehensive, **updated listing of all human genetic disorders and gene loci** can be found on the Internet (Online Mendelian Inheritance in Man [OMIM]): McKusick-Nathans Institute for Genetic Medicine, Johns Hopkins University [Baltimore, MD] and National Center for Biotechnology Information, National Library of Medicine [Bethesda, MD], 2006; www.ncbi.nlm.nih.gov/omim/).

ANOMALIES CAUSED BY ENVIRONMENTAL FACTORS

Although the human embryo is well protected in the uterus, environmental agents—**teratogens**—may cause developmental disruptions after maternal exposure to them (Table 20-6). *A teratogen is any agent that can produce a congenital anomaly or increase the incidence of an anomaly in the population.* **Environmental factors**, such as infection and drugs, may simulate genetic conditions, e.g., when two or more children of normal parents are affected.

The important principle is that "not everything that is familial is genetic." The organs and parts of an embryo are most sensitive to teratogenic agents during periods of rapid differentiation (Fig. 20-15). Environmental factors cause 7% to 10% of congenital anomalies (see Fig. 20-1). Because biochemical differentiation precedes morphologic differentiation, the period during which structures are sensitive to interference by teratogens often precedes the stage of their visible development by a few days.

Teratogens do not appear to be effective in causing anomalies until cellular differentiation has begun; however,

TABLE 20–6. Teratogens Known to Cause Human Congenital Anatomical Anomalies or Birth Defects

AGENTS	MOST COMMON CONGENITAL ANATOMICAL ANOMALIES
Drugs	
Alcohol	Fetal alcohol syndrome (FAS): intrauterine growth restriction (IUGR); mental retardation, microcephaly; ocular anomalies; joint abnormalities; short palpebral fissures
Androgens and high doses of progestogens	Varying degrees of masculinization of female fetuses: ambiguous external genitalia resulting in labial fusion and clitoral hypertrophy
Aminopterin	IUGR; skeletal defects; malformations of the central nervous system (CNS), notably meroencephaly (most of the brain is absent)
Cocaine	IUGR; prematurity; microcephaly; cerebral infarction; urogenital anomalies, neurobehavioral disturbances
Diethystilbestrol	Abnormalities of uterus and vagina; cervical erosion and ridges
Isotretinoin (13-cis-retinoic acid)	Craniofacial abnormalities; neural tube defects (NTDs), such as spina bifida cystica; cardiovascular defects; cleft palate; thymic aplasia
Lithium carbonate	Various anomalies usually involving the heart and great vessels
Methotrexate	Multiple anomalies, especially skeletal, involving the face, cranium, limbs, and vertebral column
Phenytoin (Dilantin)	Fetal hydantoin syndrome: IUGR; microcephaly; mental retardation; ridged frontal suture; inner epicanthal folds; eyelid ptosis; broad depressed nasal bridge; phalangeal hypoplasia
Tetracycline	Stained teeth; hypoplasia of enamel
Thalidomide	Abnormal development of limbs, e.g., meromelia (partial absence) and amelia (complete absence); facial anomalies; systemic anomalies; e.g., cardiac and kidney defects
Trimethadione	Development delay; V-shaped eyebrows; low-set ears; cleft lip and/or palate
Valproic acid	Craniofacial anomalies; NTDs; often hydrocephalus; heart and skeletal defects
Warfarin	Nasal hypoplasia; stippled epiphyses; hypoplastic phalanges; eye anomalies; mental retardation
Chemicals	
Methylmercury	Cerebral atrophy; spasticity; seizures; mental retardation
Polychlorinated biphenyls	IUGR; skin discolorization
Infections	
Cytomegalovirus	Microcephaly; chorioretinitis; sensorineural hearing loss; delayed psychomotor/mental development; hepatosplenomegaly; hydrocephaly; cerebral palsy; brain (periventricular) calcification
Herpes simplex virus	Skin vesicles and scarring; chorioretinitis; hepatomegaly; thrombocytopenia; petechiae; hemolytic anemia; hydranencephaly
Human parvovirus B19	Eye defects; degenerative changes in fetal tissues
Rubella virus	IUGR; postnatal growth retardation; cardiac and great vessel abnormalities; microcephaly; sensorineural deafness; cataract; microphthalmos; glaucoma; pigmented retinopathy; mental retardation; newborn bleeding; hepatosplenomegaly; osteopathy; tooth defects
Toxoplasma gondii	Microcephaly; mental retardation; microphthalmia; hydrocephaly; chorioretinitis; cerebral calcifications; hearing loss; neurologic disturbances
Treponema pallidum	Hydrocephalus; congenital deafness; mental retardation; abnormal teeth and bones
Venezuelan equine encephalitis virus	Microcephaly; microphthalmia; cerebral agenesis; CNS necrosis; hydrocephalus
Varicella virus	Cutaneous scars (dermatome distribution); neurologic anomalies (limb paresis [incomplete paralysis], hydrocephaly, seizures, etc.); cataracts; microphthalmia; Horner syndrome; optic atrophy; nystagmus; chorioretinitis; microcephaly; mental retardation; skeletal anomalies (hypoplasia of limbs, fingers, and toes, etc.); urogenital anomalies
Radiation	
High levels of ionizing radiation	Microcephaly; mental retardation; skeletal anomalies; growth retardation; cataracts

their early actions (e.g., during the first 2 weeks) may cause the death of the embryo. The exact mechanisms by which drugs, chemicals, and other environmental factors disrupt embryonic development and induce abnormalities still remain obscure. Even thalidomide's mechanisms of action on the embryo are a "mystery," and more than 20 hypotheses have been postulated to explain how this hypnotic agent disrupts embryonic development.

Many studies have shown that certain hereditary and environmental influences may adversely affect embryonic development by altering such fundamental processes as the intracellular compartment, surface of the cell, extracellular matrix, and fetal environment. It has been suggested that the initial cellular response may take more than one form (genetic, molecular, biochemical, biophysical), resulting in different sequences of cellular changes (cell death, faulty cellular interaction-induction, reduced biosynthesis of substrates, impaired morphogenetic movements, and mechanical disruption). Eventually these different types of pathologic lesion could possibly lead to the final defect (intrauterine death, developmental anomalies, fetal growth retardation, or functional disturbances) through a common pathway.

Rapid progress in molecular biology is providing more information on the genetic control of differentiation, as well as the cascade of events involved in the expression of homeobox genes and pattern formation. It is reasonable to speculate that disruption of gene activity at any critical stage could lead to a developmental defect. This view is supported by recent experimental studies that showed that exposure of mouse and amphibian embryos to the teratogen **retinoic acid** altered the domain of gene expression and disrupted normal morphogenesis. Researchers are now directing increasing attention to the molecular mechanisms of abnormal development in an attempt to understand better the pathogenesis of congenital anomalies.

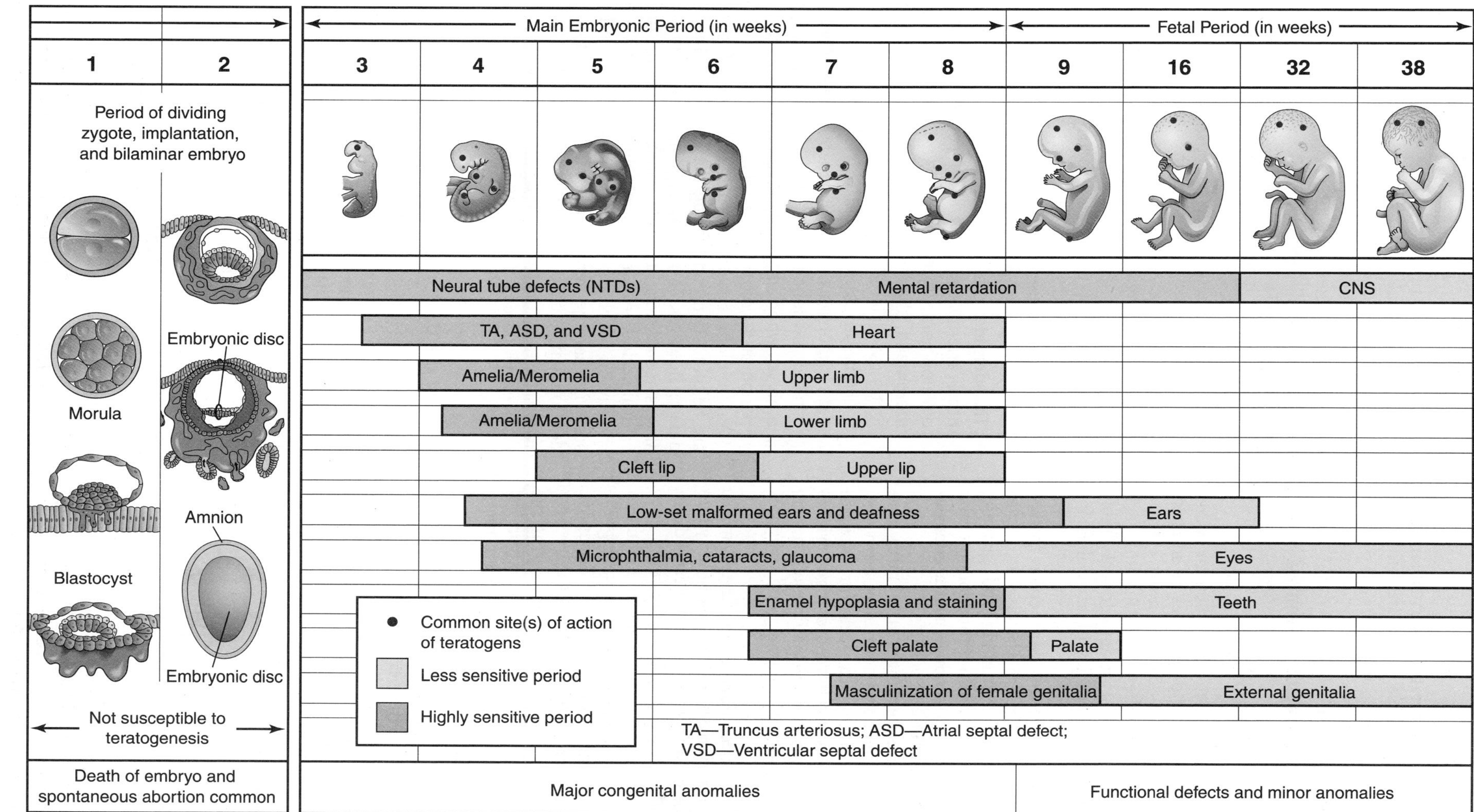

FIGURE 20-15. Schematic illustration of critical periods in human prenatal development. During the first 2 weeks of development, the embryo is usually not susceptible to teratogens; a teratogen either damages all or most of the cells, resulting in death of the embryo, or damages only a few cells, allowing the conceptus to recover and the embryo to develop without birth defects. *Mauve denotes highly sensitive periods* when major defects may be produced (e.g., amelia, absence of limbs, neural tube defects, e.g., spina bifida cystica). Green indicates stages that are less sensitive to teratogens when minor defects may be induced (e.g., hypoplastic thumbs).

Principles in Teratogenesis

When considering the possible teratogenicity of an agent such as a drug or chemical, three important principles must be considered:

- Critical periods of development
- Dose of the drug or chemical
- Genotype (genetic constitution) of the embryo

Critical Periods of Human Development

The stage of development of an embryo when an agent, such as a drug or virus, is present determines its susceptibility to a teratogen (see Fig. 20-15). The **most critical period in development** is when cell division, cell differentiation, and morphogenesis are at their peak. Table 20-7 indicates the relative frequencies of anomalies for certain organs.

The **critical period for brain development** is from 3 to 16 weeks, but its development may be disrupted after this because the brain is differentiating and growing rapidly at birth and continues to do so throughout the first 2 years at least. Teratogens may produce mental retardation during the embryonic and fetal periods.

Tooth development continues long after birth (see Chapter 19); hence, development of permanent teeth may be disrupted by tetracyclines from 18 weeks (prenatal) to 16 years. The skeletal system also has a prolonged critical period of development extending into childhood; hence, the growth of skeletal tissues provides a good gauge of general growth.

Environmental disturbances during the first 2 weeks after fertilization may interfere with cleavage of the zygote and implantation of the blastocyst and/or cause early death and spontaneous abortion of the embryo; however, they are not known to cause congenital anomalies in human embryos (see Fig. 20-15). Teratogens acting during the first 2 weeks either kill the embryo or their disruptive effects are compensated for by powerful regulatory properties of the early embryo. Most development during the first 2 weeks is concerned with the formation of extraembryonic structures such as the amnion, umbilical vesicle (yolk sac), and chorionic sac (see Chapter 3).

Development of the embryo is most easily disrupted when the tissues and organs are forming (Figs. 20-15 and 20-16). During this organogenetic period (see Chapter 5), teratogens may induce major congenital anomalies. If present during the embryonic period, microorganisms often kill the embryo.

Table 20-7. Incidence of Major Anomalies in Human Organs at Birth*

ORGAN	INCIDENCE
Brain	10:1000
Heart	8:1000
Kidneys	4:1000
Limbs	2:1000
All other	6:1000
Total	30:1000

*Data from Connor JM, Ferguson-Smith MA: Essential Medical Genetics, 2nd ed. Oxford, UK, Blackwell Scientific Publications, 1987.

Physiologic defects, for example, minor morphologic anomalies of the external ear, and functional disturbances such as mental retardation are likely to result from disruption of development during the fetal period. Some microorganisms, such as *Toxoplasma gondii*, are known to cause serious congenital anomalies, particularly of the brain and eyes, when they infect the fetus (see Figs. 20-22 and 20-23 and Table 20-6).

Each tissue, organ, and system of an embryo has a critical period during which its development may be disrupted (see Fig. 20-15). The type of congenital anomaly produced depends on which parts, tissues, and organs are most susceptible at the time that the teratogen is active. The following examples illustrate that teratogens may affect different organ systems that are developing at the same time:

- **High levels of radiation** produce anomalies of the CNS (brain and spinal cord) and eyes.
- **Rubella virus** infection causes eye defects (glaucoma and cataracts), deafness, and cardiac anomalies.
- **Thalidomide** is a drug that induces limb defects and other anomalies. Early in the critical period of limb development, it causes severe limb defects such as **meromelia**, absence of part of the upper and/or lower limbs (see Fig. 20-20). Later in the sensitive period, thalidomide causes mild to moderate limb defects, e.g., hypoplasia of radius and ulna. There is no clinical evidence that thalidomide damages the embryo when it is administered after the critical period of development.

Embryologic timetables, such as shown in Figure 20-15, are helpful when considering the cause of a human birth defect; however, it is wrong to assume that anomalies always result from a single event occurring during the critical period or that one can determine from these tables the day on which the anomaly was produced. All one can state is that the teratogen would have had to disrupt development before the end of the critical period of the tissue, part, or organ concerned. The critical period for limb development, for example, is 24 to 36 days after fertilization.

Dose of the Drug or Chemical

Animal research has shown that there is a dose-response relationship for teratogens; however, the dose used in animals to produce anomalies is often at levels much higher than human exposures. Consequently, animal studies are not readily applicable to human pregnancies. For a drug to be considered a human teratogen, a dose-response relationship has to be observed, that is, the greater the exposure during pregnancy, the more severe the phenotypic effect.

Genotype (Genetic Constitution) of the Embryo

There are numerous examples in experimental animals and several suspected cases in humans that show that there are genetic differences in response to a teratogen. **Phenytoin**, for example, is a well-known human teratogen (see Table 20-6). Five percent to 10% of embryos exposed to this anticonvulsant medication develop **fetal hydantoin syndrome** (see Fig. 20-19). Approximately one third of exposed embryos, however, have only some congenital anomalies, and more than half of the embryos are unaffected. It appears, therefore, that the genotype of the embryo determines whether a teratogenic agent will disrupt its development.

Human Teratogens

Awareness that certain agents can disrupt prenatal development offers the opportunity to prevent some congenital anomalies; for example, if women are aware of the harmful effects of drugs such as isotretinoin and alcohol, environmental chemicals (e.g., polychlorinated biphenyls), and some viruses, most of them will not expose their embryos to these teratogenic agents. The general objective of teratogenicity testing of drugs, chemicals, food additives, and pesticides is to identify agents that may be teratogenic during human development and to alert physicians and pregnant women of their possible danger to the embryo/fetus.

Proof of Teratogenicity

To prove that an agent is a teratogen, one must show either that the frequency of anomalies is increased above the spontaneous rate in pregnancies in which the mother is exposed to the agent (**prospective approach**) or that malformed infants have a history of maternal exposure to the agent more often than normal children (**retrospective approach**). Both types of data are difficult to obtain in an unbiased form. Case reports are not convincing unless both the agent and type of anomaly are so uncommon that their association in several cases can be judged not coincidental.

Drug Testing in Animals

Although testing of drugs in pregnant animals is important, the results are of limited value for predicting drug effects in human embryos. Animal experiments can suggest only that similar effects may occur in humans. If a drug or chemical produces teratogenic effects in two or more species, the probability of potential human hazard must be considered to be high; however, the dose of the drug has also to be considered.

Drugs as Teratogens

Drugs vary considerably in their teratogenicity. Some teratogens cause severe disruption of development if administered during the organogenetic period (e.g., thalidomide). Other teratogens cause mental and growth restriction and other anomalies if used excessively throughout development (e.g., alcohol).

The use of prescription and nonprescription drugs during pregnancy is surprisingly high. Forty percent to 90% of pregnant women consume at least one drug during pregnancy. Several studies have indicated that some pregnant women take an average of four drugs, excluding nutritional supplements, and approximately half of these women take them during the first trimester. Drug consumption also tends to be higher during the critical period of development among heavy smokers and drinkers.

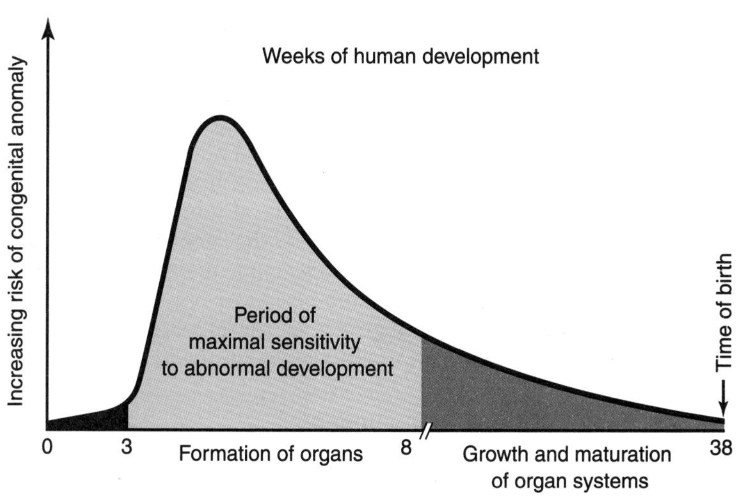

FIGURE 20-16. Schematic illustration showing the increasing risk of birth defects developing during organogenesis.

Despite this, less than 2% of congenital anomalies are caused by drugs and chemicals. Only a few drugs have been positively implicated as human teratogenic agents (see Table 20-6).

Although only 7% to 10% of anomalies are caused by recognizable teratogens (see Fig. 20-1), new agents continue to be identified. It is best for women to avoid using all medication during the first trimester, unless there is a strong medical reason for its use, and then only if it is recognized as reasonably safe for the human embryo. The reason for this caution is that, even though well-controlled studies of certain drugs (e.g., marijuana) have failed to demonstrate a teratogenic risk to human embryos, they do harm the embryo (decreased birth weight).

Cigarette Smoking

Maternal smoking during pregnancy is a well-established cause of **intrauterine growth restriction** (IUGR). Despite warnings that cigarette smoking is harmful to the embryo/fetus, some women continue to smoke during their pregnancies. In heavy cigarette smokers (≥20 per day), premature delivery is twice as frequent as in mothers who do not smoke, and their infants weigh less than normal (see Fig. 6-12). **Low birth weight** (<2000 g) is the chief predictor of infant death. In a case-control study, there was a modest increase in the incidence of infants with conotruncal heart defects and limb deficiencies associated with both maternal and paternal smoking. Moreover, there is some evidence that maternal smoking may cause urinary tract anomalies, behavioral problems, and decreased physical growth. **Nicotine** constricts uterine blood vessels, causing a *decrease in uterine blood flow*, lowering the supply of oxygen and nutrients available to the embryo/fetus from the maternal blood in the intervillous space of the placenta. The resulting deficiency impairs cell growth and may have an adverse effect on mental development. High levels of carboxyhemoglobin, resulting from cigarette smoking, appear in the maternal and fetal blood and may alter the capacity of the blood to transport oxygen. As a result, **chronic fetal hypoxia** (low oxygen levels) may occur and affect fetal growth and development.

Caffeine

Caffeine is the most popular drug in North America because it is present in several widely consumed beverages (e.g., coffee, tea, cola drinks), chocolate products, and some drugs. Caffeine is not known to be a human teratogen; however, there is no assurance that heavy maternal consumption of it is safe for the embryo.

Alcohol

Alcoholism is a drug abuse problem that affects 1% to 2% of women of childbearing age. Both moderate and high levels of alcohol intake during early pregnancy may result in alterations in growth and morphogenesis of the fetus. The greater the intake is, the more severe the signs. Infants born to chronic alcoholic mothers exhibit a specific pattern of defects, including prenatal and postnatal growth deficiency, and mental and other anomalies (Fig. 20-17; see Table 20-6). **Microcephaly**, short palpebral fissures, epicanthal folds, maxillary hypoplasia, short nose, thin upper lip, abnormal palmar creases, joint anomalies, and congenital heart disease are also present in most infants. This pattern of anomalies—**fetal alcohol syndrome** (FAS)—is detected in 1 to 2 infants per 1000 live births. The incidence of FAS is related to the population studied. Clinical experience is often necessary to make an accurate diagnosis of FAS because the physical anomalies in affected children are nonspecific. Nonetheless, the overall pattern of clinical features present is unique, but may vary from subtle to severe.

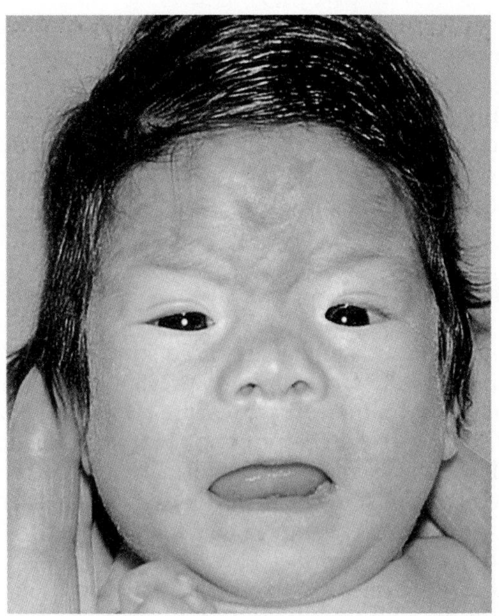

FIGURE 20-17. Fetal alcohol syndrome in an infant. Note the thin upper lip, elongated and poorly formed philtrum (vertical groove in medial part of upper lip), short palpebral fissures, flat nasal bridge, and short nose. (Courtesy of A.E. Chudley, MD, Section of Genetics and Metabolism, Department of Pediatrics and Child Health, Children's Hospital, Winnipeg, Manitoba, Canada.)

Maternal alcohol abuse is now thought to be the most common cause of mental deficiency. Moderate maternal alcohol consumption (1–2 oz of alcohol per day) can result in cognitive impairment and behavioral problems. The term **fetal alcohol effects** was introduced after recognition that many children exposed to alcohol in utero had no external dysmorphic features but had neurodevelopmental impairments. The preferred term for the whole range of prenatal alcohol effects is **fetal alcohol spectrum disorder**. It is estimated that the general population prevalence of fetal alcohol spectrum disorder may be as high as 1%. The susceptible period of brain development spans the major part of gestation; therefore, *the safest advice is total abstinence from alcohol during pregnancy.*

Androgens and Progestogens

The terms *progestogens* and *progestins* are used for substances, natural or synthetic, that induce some or all the biologic changes produced by progesterone, a hormone secreted by the corpus luteum that promotes and maintains a gravid endometrium (see Chapter 7). Some of these substances have androgenic (masculinizing) properties that may affect the female fetus, producing

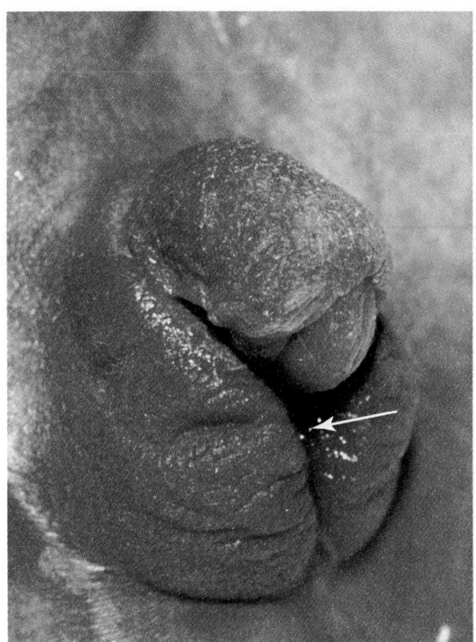

FIGURE 20-18. Masculinized external genitalia of a 46, XX female infant. Observe the enlarged clitoris and fused labia majora. The virilization was caused by excessive androgens produced by the suprarenal (adrenal) glands during the fetal period (congenital adrenal hyperplasia). The *arrow* indicates the opening of the urogenital sinus. (Courtesy of Dr. Heather Dean, MD, Department of Pediatrics and Child Health, University of Manitoba, Winnipeg, Manitoba, Canada.)

masculinization of the external genitalia (Fig. 20-18). The incidence of anomalies varies with the hormone and the dose. Preparations that should be avoided are the progestins, **ethisterone**, and **norethisterone**. From a practical standpoint, the teratogenic risk of these hormones is low. Progestin exposure during the critical period of development is also associated with an increased prevalence of cardiovascular abnormalities, and exposure of male fetuses during this period may double the incidence of **hypospadias** (see Chapter 12). Obviously, the administration of testosterone will also produce masculinizing effects in female fetuses.

Many women use contraceptive hormones—birth control pills. **Oral contraceptives** containing progestogens and estrogens, taken during the early stages of an unrecognized pregnancy, are suspected of being teratogenic agents, but the results of several epidemiologic studies are conflicting. The infants of 13 of 19 mothers who had taken progestogen-estrogen birth control pills during the critical period of development exhibited the **VACTERL syndrome**. The acronym VACTERL stands for **V**ertebral, **A**nal, **C**ardiac, **T**racheal, **E**sophageal, **R**enal, and **L**imb anomalies. As a precaution, use of oral contraceptives should be stopped as soon as pregnancy is suspected or detected because of these possible teratogenic effects.

Diethylstilbestrol (DES) is a human teratogen. Both gross and microscopic congenital abnormalities of the uterus and vagina have been detected in women who were exposed to DES in utero. Three types of lesions were observed: vaginal adenosis, cervical erosions, and transverse vaginal ridges. A number of young women ages 16 to 22 years have developed **adenocarcinoma of the vagina** after a common history of exposure to this synthetic estrogen in utero. However, the probability of cancers developing at this early age in females exposed to DES in utero now appears to be low. The risk of cancer from DES exposure in utero is estimated to be less than 1 in 1000. Males who were exposed to DES in utero, after maternal treatment before the 11th week of gestation, had a higher incidence of genital tract anomalies, including epididymal cysts and hypoplastic (underdeveloped) testes. However, fertility in the men exposed to DES in utero seems to be unaffected.

ANTIBIOTICS

Tetracyclines cross the placental membrane and are deposited in the embryo's bones and teeth at sites of active calcification. As little as 1 g/day of **tetracycline** during the third trimester of pregnancy can produce yellow staining of the deciduous and/or permanent teeth. Tetracycline therapy during the fourth to ninth months of pregnancy may also cause tooth defects (e.g., enamel hypoplasia), yellow to brown discoloration of the teeth, and diminished growth of long bones. Calcification of the permanent teeth begins at birth and, except for the third molars, is complete by 7 to 8 years of age; hence, long-term tetracycline therapy during childhood can affect the permanent teeth.

Deafness has been reported in infants of mothers who have been treated with high doses of **streptomycin** and **dihydrostreptomycin** as antituberculosis agents. More than 30 cases of hearing deficit and eighth cranial nerve damage have been reported in infants exposed to streptomycin derivatives in utero. Penicillin has been used extensively during pregnancy and appears to be harmless to the human embryo and fetus.

ANTICOAGULANTS

All anticoagulants except heparin cross the placental membrane and may cause hemorrhage in the embryo or fetus. **Warfarin** and other **coumarin derivatives** are antagonists of vitamin K. Warfarin is used for the treatment of thromboembolitic disease and in patients with artificial heart valves. **Warfarin is definitely a teratogen.** There are reports of infants with hypoplasia of the nasal cartilage, stippled epiphyses, and various CNS defects whose mothers took this anticoagulant during the critical period of their embryo's development. The period of greatest sensitivity is between 6 and 12 weeks after fertilization, 8 to 14 weeks after the last normal menstrual period. Second- and third-trimester exposure may result in mental retardation, optic atrophy, and microcephaly. **Heparin is not a teratogen.** Furthermore, it does not cross the placental membrane.

ANTICONVULSANTS

Approximately 1 in 200 pregnant women is epileptic and requires treatment with an anticonvulsant. Of the anticonvulsant drugs available, there is strong evidence that **trimethadione** (Tridione) is a teratogen. The main features of the fetal trimethadione syndrome are prenatal and postnatal growth retardation, developmental delay, V-shaped eyebrows, low-set ears, cleft lip and/or palate, and cardiac, genitourinary, and limb defects. *Use of this drug is contraindicated during pregnancy.*

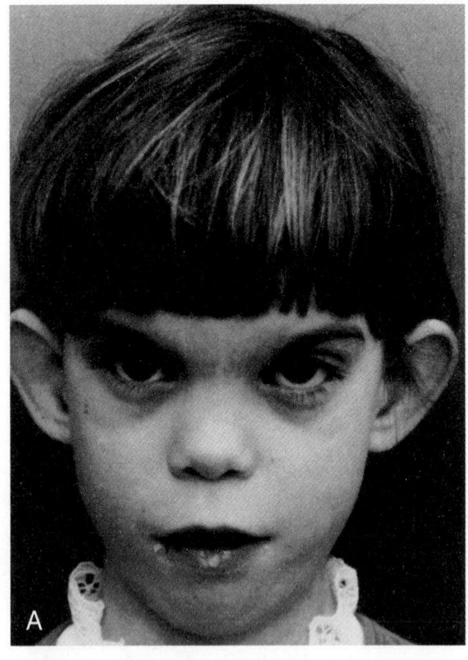

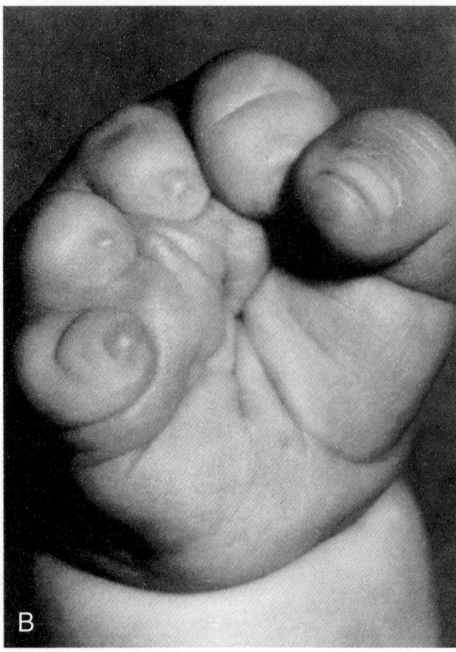

FIGURE 20-19. Fetal hydantoin syndrome in a young girl. **A,** She has a learning disability due to microcephaly and mental retardation. Note the large ears, wide space between the eyes (hypertelorism), epicanthal folds, short nose, and long philtrum. Her mother has epilepsy and ingested Dilantin throughout her pregnancy. **B,** Right hand of infant with severe digital hypoplasia (short fingers) born to a mother who took Dilantin throughout her pregnancy. (**A,** Courtesy of A.E. Chudley, MD, Section of Genetics and Metabolism, Department of Pediatrics and Child Health, Children's Hospital, Winnipeg, Manitoba, Canada. **B,** From Chodirker BN, Chudley AE, Reed MH, Persaud TVN: Am J Med Genet 27:373, © 1987. Reprinted by permission of Wiley-Liss, a division of John Wiley and Sons, Inc.)

Phenytoin (Dilantin, Novophenytoin) is definitely a teratogen (Fig. 20-19). **Fetal hydantoin syndrome** occurs in 5% to 10% of children born to mothers treated with phenytoins or hydantoin anticonvulsants. The usual pattern of anomalies consists of IUGR, microcephaly, mental retardation, ridged frontal suture, inner epicanthal folds, eyelid ptosis, broad depressed nasal bridge, nail and/or distal phalangeal hypoplasia, and hernias.

Valproic acid has been the drug of choice for the management of different types of epilepsy; however, its use in pregnant women has led to a pattern of anomalies consisting of craniofacial, heart, and limb defects. There is also an increased risk of **neural tube defects**. Phenobarbital is considered to be a safe, antiepileptic drug for use during pregnancy. Magnesium sulfate and diazepam are also widely used for seizure prophylaxis; however, more controlled clinical trials are required to establish whether these combinations are free of teratogenic risks.

ANTINAUSEANTS

There has been extensive debate in the lay press and in the courts as to whether Bendectin (a combination of doxylamine succinate and pyridoxine hydrochloride; trade names Debendox, Lenotan, Diclectin) is a human teratogenic drug. Teratologists consider **Bendectin** to be nonteratogenic in humans because large-scale epidemiologic studies of infants have failed to show an increased risk of birth defects after administration of it to pregnant woman.

ANTINEOPLASTIC AGENTS

With the exception of the folic acid antagonist **aminopterin,** few well-documented reports of teratogenic effects are available for assessment. Because the data available on the possible teratogenicity of antineoplastic drugs are inadequate, it is recommended that they should be avoided, especially during the first trimester of pregnancy.

Tumor-inhibiting chemicals are highly teratogenic because these agents inhibit mitosis in rapidly dividing cells. The use of aminopterin during the embryonic period often results in intrauterine death of the embryos, but the 20% to 30% of those that survive are severely malformed. Busulfan and 6-mercaptopurine administered in alternating courses throughout pregnancy have produced multiple severe abnormalities, but neither drug alone appears to cause major anomalies (see Table 20-6). **Methotrexate,** a folic acid antagonist and a derivative of aminopterin, is a *known potent teratogen* that produces major congenital anomalies. It is most often used as a single agent or in combination therapy for neoplastic diseases; however, it may also be indicated in patients with severe rheumatic diseases including rheumatoid arthritis. Multiple skeletal and other congenital anomalies were found in an infant born to a mother who attempted to terminate her pregnancy by taking methotrexate.

CORTICOSTEROIDS

Cortisone causes cleft palate and cardiac defects in susceptible strains of mice and rabbits. Low doses of corticosteroids, including cortisone and hydrocortisone, does not induce cleft palate or any other congenital anomaly in human embryos Because of the risks of fetal bleeding and premature closure of the ductus arteriosus, nonsteroidal anti-inflammatory drugs should not be taken during the last few weeks of pregnancy.

ANGIOTENSIN-CONVERTING ENZYME INHIBITORS

Exposure of the fetus to **angiotensin-converting enzyme inhibitors** as antihypertensive agents causes oligohydramnios, fetal death, hypoplasia of the bones of the calvaria, IUGR, and renal dysfunction. During early pregnancy, the risk to the embryo is apparently less, and there is no indication to terminate a pregnancy. Because of the high incidence of serious perinatal complications, it is recommended that angiotensin-converting enzyme inhibitors not be prescribed during pregnancy.

INSULIN AND HYPOGLYCEMIC DRUGS

Insulin is not teratogenic in human embryos except possibly in maternal insulin coma therapy. Hypoglycemic drugs (e.g., tolbutamide) have been implicated, but evidence of their teratogenicity is weak; consequently, despite their marked teratogenicity in rodents, there is no convincing evidence that oral hypoglycemic agents (particularly sulfonylureas) are teratogenic in human embryos. The incidence of congenital anomalies (e.g., sacral agenesis) is increased two to three times in the offspring of diabetic mothers, and approximately 40% of all perinatal deaths of diabetic infants are the result of congenital anomalies. Women with insulin-dependent diabetes mellitus may significantly decrease their risk of having infants with birth defects by achieving good control of their disease before conception.

RETINOIC ACID (VITAMIN A)

Isotretinoin (13-cis-retinoic acid), which is used for treating severe cystic acne, *is a known human teratogen.* The critical period for exposure appears to be from the third week to the fifth week (5–7 weeks after the LNMP). The risk of spontaneous abortion and birth defects after exposure is high. The most common major anomalies observed are craniofacial dysmorphism (microtia, micrognathia), cleft palate and/or thymic aplasia, cardiovascular anomalies, and neural tube defects. Postnatal longitudinal follow-up of children exposed in utero to **isotretinoin** revealed significant **neuropsychological impairment**.

Vitamin A is a valuable and necessary nutrient during pregnancy, but long-term exposure to large doses is unwise. Pregnant women should avoid high levels of vitamin A because an increased risk of birth defects among the offspring of women who took more than 10,000 IU of vitamin A daily has been reported.

SALICYLATES

There is some evidence that large doses of **acetylsalicylic acid** (ASA) or **aspirin**, the most commonly ingested drug during pregnancy, are potentially harmful to the embryo or fetus. Epidemiologic studies indicate that aspirin is not a teratogenic agent but large doses should be avoided, especially during the first trimester.

THYROID DRUGS

Potassium iodide in cough mixtures and large doses of **radioactive iodine** may cause congenital goiter. Iodides readily cross the placental membrane and interfere with thyroxin production. They may also cause thyroid enlargement and **cretinism** (arrested physical and mental development and dystrophy of bones and soft parts). **Maternal iodine deficiency** may also cause congenital cretinism. Pregnant women have been advised to avoid douches or creams containing povidone-iodine because it is absorbed by the vagina, enters the maternal blood, and may be teratogenic. Propylthiouracil interferes with thyroxin formation in the fetus and may cause goiter. The administration of antithyroid substances for the treatment of maternal thyroid disorders may cause congenital goiter if the mother is given the substances in excess of the amount required to control the disease.

TRANQUILIZERS

Thalidomide is a potent teratogen. This hypnotic agent was once widely used in West Germany and Australia as a tranquilizer and sedative, but no longer is used because of its immunosuppressive properties. The **thalidomide epidemic** started in 1959. It has been estimated that nearly 12,000 infants were born with defects caused by this drug. Because thalidomide was not approved by the U.S. Food and Drug Administration in the United States, relatively few anomalies occurred. The characteristic feature of the thalidomide syndrome is **meromelia**—phocomelia ("seal limbs"), for example (Fig. 20-20),—but the anomalies ranged from amelia (absence of limbs) through intermediate stages of development (rudimentary limbs) to **micromelia** (abnormally small and/or short limbs).

Thalidomide also caused anomalies of other organs, for example, absence of the external and internal ears, hemangioma on the forehead, heart defects, and anomalies of the urinary and alimentary systems. It is well established clinically that the period when thalidomide caused congenital anomalies was 24 to 36 days after fertilization (38–50 days after LNMP). This sensitive period coincides with the critical periods for the development of the affected parts and organs (see Figs. 20-15 and 20-16). Thalidomide is absolutely contraindicated in women of childbearing age.

PSYCHOTROPIC DRUGS

Lithium is the drug of choice for the long-term maintenance of patients with bibolar disorders; however, it has caused congenital anomalies, mainly of the heart and great vessels, in infants born to mothers given the drug

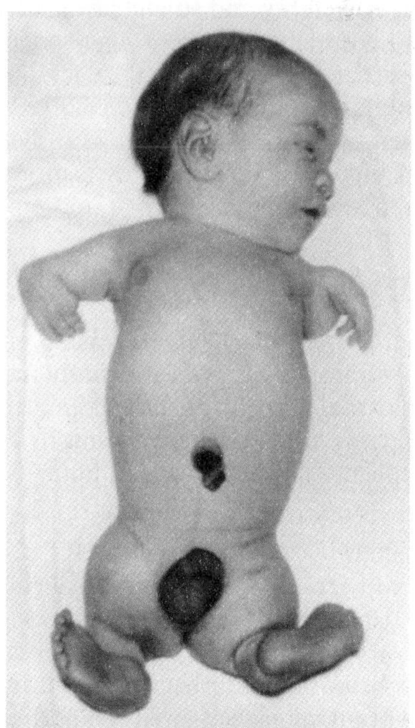

FIGURE 20-20. Newborn male infant showing typically malformed limbs (*meromelia*—limb reduction) caused by thalidomide ingested by his mother during the critical period of limb development. (From Moore KL: Manit Med Rev 43:306, 1963.)

early in pregnancy. Although **lithium carbonate** is a known human teratogen, the U.S. Food and Drug Administration has stated that the agent may be used during pregnancy if "in the opinion of the physician the potential benefits outweigh the possible hazards."

Benzodiazepine derivatives are frequently prescribed for pregnant women. These include **diazepam** and **oxazepam**, which readily cross the placental membrane. The use of these drugs during the first trimester of pregnancy is associated with craniofacial anomalies in the newborn. **Selective serotonin reuptake inhibitors** (SSRIs) are often used to treat depression during pregnancy. Of concern are recent reports warning of an increased risk of atrial and ventricular septal defects and persistent pulmonary hypertension in infants exposed to selective serotonin reuptake inhibitors in utero.

Illicit Drugs

Several currently popular "street drugs" are used for their hallucinogenic properties. There is no evidence that marijuana is a human teratogen; however, there is an indication that marijuana use during the first 2 months of pregnancy affects fetal length and birth weight. In addition, sleep and electroencephalographic patterns in newborns exposed prenatally to marijuana were altered.

Second only to marijuana, **cocaine** is the most widely used illicit drugs among women of childbearing age. Reports dealing with the prenatal effects of cocaine include spontaneous abortion, prematurity, IUGR, microcephaly, cerebral infarction, urogenital anomalies, neurobehavioral disturbances, and neurologic abnormalities.

Methadone, used for the treatment of heroin addiction, is considered to be a "behavioral teratogen," as is heroin. Infants born to narcotic-dependent women maintained on methadone therapy were found to have **CNS dysfunction** and lower birth weights and smaller head circumferences than nonexposed infants. There is also concern about the long-term postnatal developmental effects of methadone. The problem, however, is difficult to resolve because other drugs are often used in combination with methadone, and heavy use of alcohol and cigarettes is prevalent among narcotic-dependent women.

Environmental Chemicals as Teratogens

In recent years, there has been increasing concern about the possible teratogenicity of environmental chemicals, including industrial and agricultural chemicals, pollutants, and food additives. Most of these chemicals have not been positively implicated as teratogens in humans.

Organic Mercury

Infants of mothers whose main diet during pregnancy consists of fish containing abnormally high levels of organic mercury acquire fetal **Minamata disease**, neurologic and behavioral disturbances resembling cerebral palsy. Severe brain damage, mental retardation, and blindness have been detected in infants of mothers who received **methylmercury** in their food. Similar observations have been made in infants whose mothers ate pork that became contaminated when the pigs ate corn grown from seeds sprayed with a mercury-containing fungicide. Methylmercury is a teratogen that causes cerebral atrophy, spasticity, seizures, and mental retardation.

Lead

Abundantly present in the workplace and environment, lead passes through the placental membrane and accumuates in fetal tissues. Prenatal exposure to lead is associated with increased abortions, fetal anomalies, IUGR, and functional deficits. Several reports have indicated that children born to mothers who were exposed to subclinical levels of lead revealed neurobehavioral and psychomotor disturbances.

Polychlorinated Biphenyls

These teratogenic chemicals produce IUGR and skin discoloration. The main dietary source of polychlorinated biphenyls in North America is probably sport fish caught in contaminated waters. In Japan and Taiwan, the teratogenic chemical was detected in contaminated cooking oil.

Infectious Agents as Teratogens

Throughout prenatal life, the embryo and fetus are endangered by a variety of microorganisms. In most cases, the assault is resisted; however, in some cases, abortion or stillbirth occurs, and in others, the infants are born with IUGR, congenital anomalies, or neonatal diseases (see Table 20-6). The microorganisms cross the placental membrane and enter the fetal bloodstream. Because there is a propensity for the CNS to be affected, the fetal blood-brain barrier also apparently offers little resistance to microorganisms.

Rubella (German or Three-Day Measles)

The virus that causes rubella, a communicable disease, is the prime example of an **infective teratogen**. In cases of primary maternal infection during the first trimester of pregnancy, the overall risk of embryonic/fetal infection is approximately 20%. The rubella virus crosses the placental membrane and infects the embryo/fetus. The clinical features of **congenital rubella syndrome** are cataracts, cardiac defects, and deafness; however, the following abnormalities are occasionally observed: mental deficiency, chorioretinitis, glaucoma (Fig. 20-21), microphthalmia, and tooth defects. The earlier in pregnancy the maternal rubella infection occurs, the greater is the danger that the embryo will be malformed.

Most infants have anomalies if the disease occurs during the first 4 to 5 weeks after fertilization. This period includes the most susceptible organogenetic periods of the eye, internal ear, heart, and brain (see Fig. 20-15). The risk of anomalies from rubella infection during the second and third trimesters is low (approximately 10%), but functional defects of the CNS (mental retardation) and internal ear (hearing loss) may result if infection occurs during the late fetal period. There is no evidence of fetal anomalies after the fifth gestational month; however, infections may produce chronic disease and dysfunction of the eye, ear, and CNS.

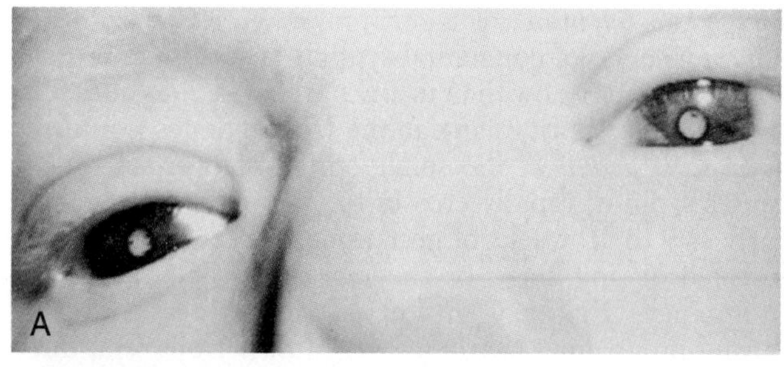

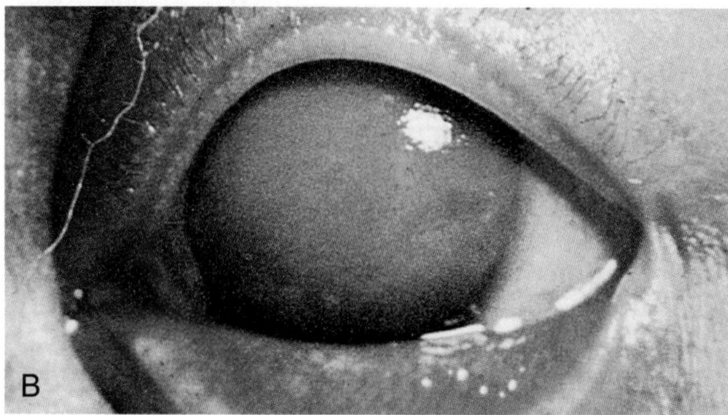

FIGURE 20-21. Congenital eye anomalies caused by infection from the rubella virus. **A,** Bilateral congenital cataracts caused by the rubella virus. Cardiac defects and deafness are other common anomalies. **B,** Severe congenital glaucoma. Observe the dense corneal haze, enlarged corneal diameter, and deep anterior chamber. (**A,** Courtesy of Dr. Richard Bargy, Department of Ophthalmology, Cornell-New York Hospital, New York, NY. **B,** Courtesy of Dr. Daniel I. Weiss, Department of Ophthalmology, New York University College of Medicine, New York, New York. From Cooper LA, Green RH, Krugman S, et al: Neonatal thrombocytopenic purpura and other manifestations of rubella contracted in utero. Am J Dis Child 110:416, 1965. Copyright 1965, American Medical Association.)

CYTOMEGALOVIRUS

Infection with cytomegalovirus (CMV) is the **most common viral infection of the fetus**, occurring in approximately 1% of newborns. Because the disease seems to be fatal when it affects the embryo, it is believed that most pregnancies end in spontaneous abortion when the infection occurs during the first trimester. Newborn infants infected during the early fetal period usually show no clinical signs and are identified through screening programs. CMV infection later in pregnancy may result in severe anomalies: IUGR, microphthalmia, chorioretinitis, blindness, microcephaly, cerebral calcification, mental retardation, deafness, cerebral palsy, and hepatosplenomegaly. Of particular concern are cases of asymptomatic CMV infection, which are often associated with audiologic, neurologic, and neurobehavioral disturbances in infancy.

HERPES SIMPLEX VIRUS

It has been reported that maternal infection with herpes simplex virus in early pregnancy increases the abortion rate by threefold, and infection after the 20th week is associated with a higher rate of prematurity. Infection of the fetus with herpes simplex virus usually occurs very late in pregnancy, probably most often during delivery. The congenital abnormalities that have been observed in newborns included cutaneous lesions and, in some cases, microcephaly, microphthalmia, spasticity, retinal dysplasia, and mental retardation.

VARICELLA (CHICKENPOX)

Varicella and herpes zoster (shingles) are caused by the same virus, **varicella-zoster virus**. There is convincing evidence that maternal varicella infection during the first 4 months of pregnancy causes congenital anomalies: skin scarring, muscle atrophy, hypoplasia of the limb, rudimentary digits, eye and brain damage, and mental retardation. There is a 20% chance of these or other anomalies when the infection occurs during the critical period of development (see Fig. 20-15). After 20 weeks of gestation, there is no proven teratogenic risk.

HUMAN IMMUNODEFICIENCY VIRUS

This retrovirus causes **acquired immunodeficiency syndrome**. There is conflicting information on the fetal effects of in utero infection with human immunodeficiency virus. Some of the congenital anomalies reported are growth failure, microcephaly, and specific craniofacial features. Most cases of transmission of the virus from mother to fetus probably occur at the time of delivery. Breast-feeding increases the risk of transmitting the virus to the newborn. Preventing the transmission of the virus to women and their infants is of obvious importance because of the potential fetal and infantile effects.

TOXOPLASMOSIS

Toxoplasma gondii, an intracellular parasite, occurs widely. It was named after the gondi, a North African rodent in which the organism was first detected. This parasite may be found in the bloodstream, tissues, or reticuloendothelial cells, leukocytes, and epithelial cells.

Maternal infection is usually acquired by:

- Eating raw or poorly cooked meat (usually pork or lamb) containing *Toxoplasma* cysts
- Close contact with infected domestic animals (usually cats) or infected soil

It is thought that the soil and garden vegetables may become contaminated with infected cat feces carrying **oocysts** (the encysted or encapsulated zygote in the life cycle of sporozoan protozoa). Oocysts can also be transported to food by flies and cockroaches.

The *T. gondii organism* crosses the placental membrane and infects the fetus (Figs. 20-22 and 20-23), causing destructive changes in the brain (**intracranial calcifications**) and eyes (**chorioretinitis**) that result in mental deficiency, microcephaly, microphthalmia, and hydrocephaly. Fetal death may follow infection, especially during the early stages of pregnancy. Mothers of congenitally defective infants are often unaware of having had **toxoplasmosis**, the disease caused by the parasitic organism. Because animals (cats, dogs, rabbits, and other domestic and wild animals) may be infected with this parasite, pregnant women should avoid them and the eating of raw or poorly cooked meat from them (e.g., rabbits). In addition, eggs of domestic fowl should be well cooked and unpasteurized milk should be avoided.

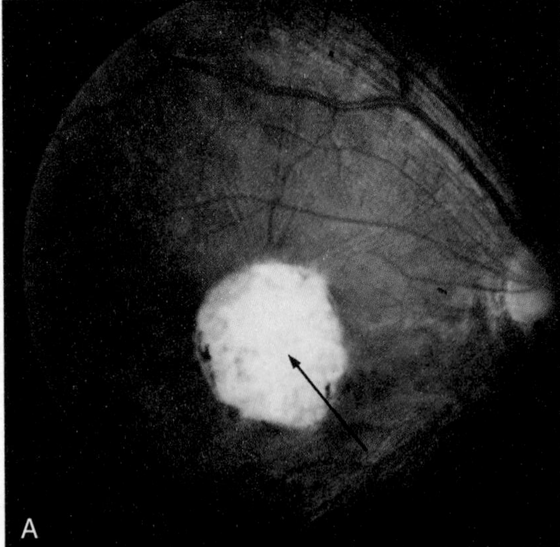

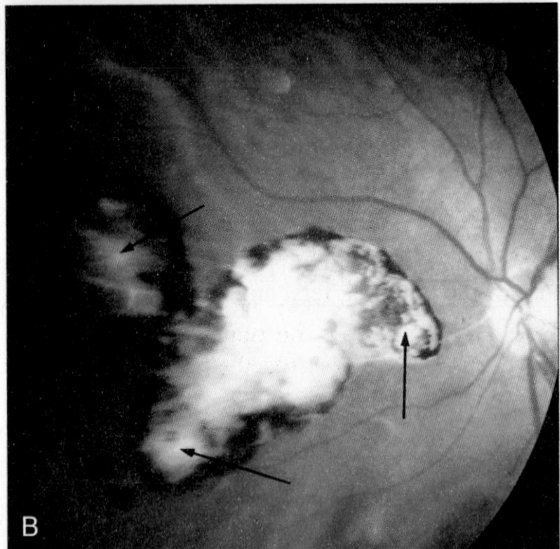

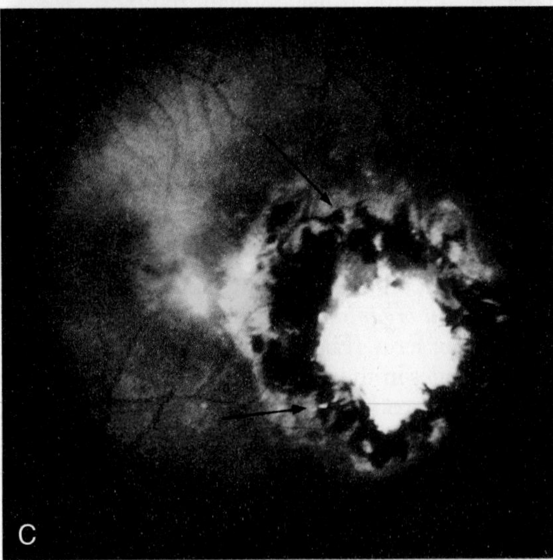

FIGURE 20-22. Chorioretinitis of congenital ocular toxoplasmosis induced by *Toxoplasma* infection. **A,** Necrotizing cicatricial lesion of macula (*arrow*). **B,** Satellite lesion around and adjacent to necrotizing cicatricial main lesion (*arrows*). **C,** Recrudescent lesion adjacent to large necrotizing cicatricial main lesion (*arrows*). (From Yokota K: Congenital anomalies and toxoplasmosis. Congenit Anom (Kyoto) 35:151, 1995.)

CONGENITAL SYPHILIS

The incidence of congenital syphilis is steadily increasing with more cases now than in any of the past 2 decades. One in 10,000 live-born infants in the United States is infected. *Treponema pallidum*, the small, spiral microorganism that causes syphilis, rapidly crosses the placental membrane as early as 9 to 10 weeks of gestation. The fetus can become infected at any stage of the disease or at any stage of pregnancy. **Primary maternal infections** (acquired during pregnancy) nearly always cause serious fetal infection and congenital anomalies; however, adequate treatment of the mother kills the organism, thereby preventing it from crossing the placental membrane and infecting the fetus. **Secondary maternal infections** (acquired before pregnancy) seldom result in fetal disease and anomalies. If the mother is untreated, stillbirths occur in approximately one fourth of cases. Only 20% of all untreated pregnant women will deliver a normal infant at term. **Early fetal manifestations** of untreated maternal syphilis are congenital deafness, abnormal teeth and bones, hydrocephalus, and mental retardation. **Late fetal manifestations** of untreated congenital syphilis are destructive lesions of the palate and nasal septum, dental abnormalities (centrally notched, widely spaced peg-shaped upper central incisors —**Hutchinson teeth**—and abnormal facies (frontal bossing, saddlenose, and poorly developed maxilla).

Radiation as a Teratogen

Exposure to **high levels of ionizing radiation** may injure embryonic cells, resulting in cell death, chromosome injury, and retardation of mental development and physical growth. The severity of the embryonic damage is related to the absorbed dose, the dose rate, and the stage of embryonic or fetal development when the exposure occurs.

In the past, large amounts of ionizing radiation (hundreds to several thousand rads) were given inadvertently to embryos and fetuses of pregnant women who had cancer of the cervix. In all cases, their embryos were severely malformed or killed. Growth retardation, microcephaly, spina bifida cystica (see Chapter 17), pigment changes in the retina, cataracts, cleft palate, skeletal and visceral abnormalities, and mental retardation have been observed in infants who survived after receiving high levels of ionizing radiation. Development of the CNS was nearly always affected.

Observations of Japanese atomic bomb survivors and their children suggest that 8 to 16 weeks after fertilization (10–18 weeks after LNMP) is the period of greatest sensitivity for radiation damage to the brain, resulting in severe mental retardation. By the end of the 16th week, most neuronal proliferation is completed, after which the risk of mental retardation decreases. It is generally accepted that large doses of radiation (>25,000 mrad) are harmful to the developing CNS. Accidental exposure of pregnant women to radiation is a common cause for anxiety.

There is no conclusive proof that human congenital anomalies have been caused by diagnostic levels of radiation. Scattered radiation from a radiographic examination of a region of the body that is not near the uterus

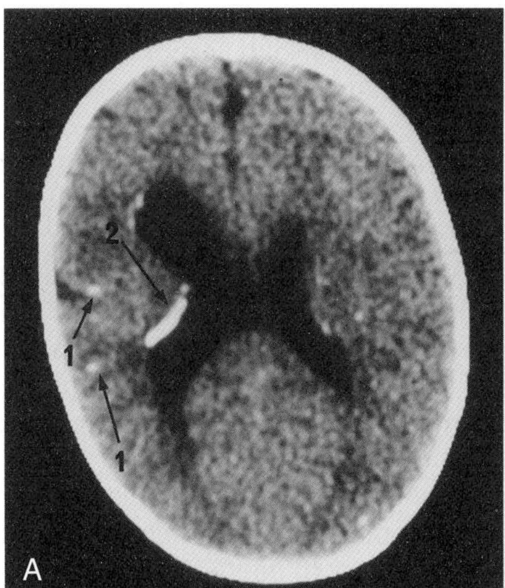

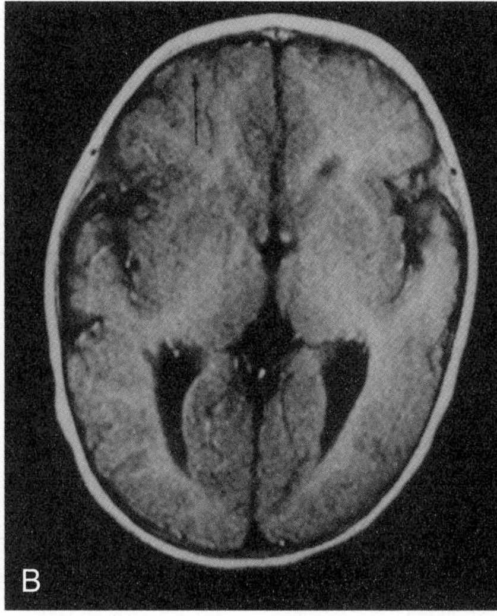

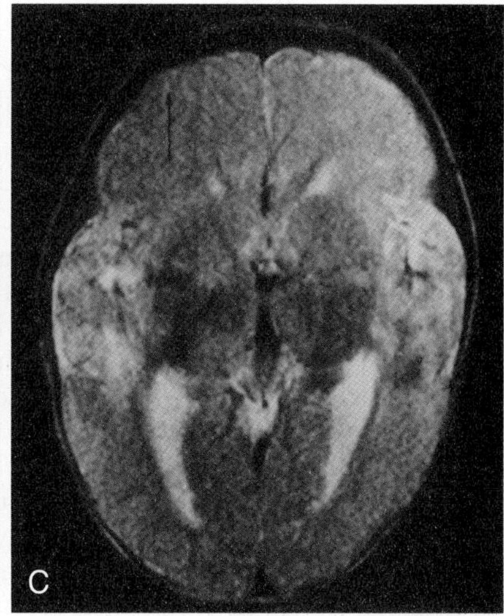

FIGURE 20-23. Congenital cerebral anomalies induced by *Toxoplasma* infection. The diagnostic images were obtained at 2 years and 9 months of age. **A,** Plain computed tomography scan. The lateral ventricles are moderately dilated. Multiple calcified foci are apparent in the brain parenchyma (*arrows 1*) and along the ventricular wall (*arrow 2*). **B,** Magnetic resonance imaging, T1 WI (400/22, 0.5 T). The cortical gyri are widened on the left side and the cortex is thickened in the left frontal lobe (*arrow*) compared with corresponding structure on the right. **C,** Magnetic resonance imaging, T2 WI (2,500/120, 0.5 T). The left frontal lobe shows abnormal hypointensity (*arrow*). (From Yokota K: Congenital anomalies and toxoplasmosis. Congenit Anom (Kyoto) 35:151, 1995.)

(e.g., thorax, sinuses, teeth) produces a dose of only a few millirads, which is not teratogenic to the embryo. For example, a radiograph of the thorax of a pregnant woman in the first trimester results in a whole-body dose to her embryo or fetus of approximately 1 mrad. If the embryonic radiation exposure is 5 rads or less, the radiation risks to the embryo are minuscule; however, it is prudent to be cautious during diagnostic examinations of the pelvic region in pregnant women (radiographic examinations and medical diagnostic tests using radioisotopes) because they result in exposure of the embryo to 0.3 to 2 rads. The recommended limit of maternal exposure of the whole body to radiation from all sources is 500 mrad for the entire gestational period.

ELECTROMAGNETIC FIELDS

There is no evidence that there is an increased risk of IUGR or other developmental defects in human embryos after maternal exposure to low-frequency electromagnetic fields (e.g., electric blankets, video display terminals)

ULTRASONIC WAVES

Ultrasonography is widely used during pregnancy for embryonic/fetal diagnosis and prenatal care. A review of the safety of obstetric ultrasonography indicate that there are no confirmed harmful effects on the fetus from the use of routine diagnostic ultrasound examination.

Maternal Factors as Teratogens

Approximately 4% of pregnant women have diabetes. Poorly controlled diabetes mellitus in the mother, particularly during embryogenesis, is associated with an increased rate of spontaneous miscarriages and a two- to threefold higher incidence of birth defects. Babies of diabetic mothers are usually large (**macrosomia**), with prominent fat pads over the upper back and lower jaw. These infants are at an increased risk for brain anomalies, skeletal defects, sacral agenesis, and congenital heart defects, in addition to neonatal metabolic complications, respiratory distress syndrome, and neurodevelopmental abnormalities.

Phenylketonuria occurs in one per 10,000 infants born in the United States. If untreated, women who are homozygous for **phenylalanine hydroxylase deficiency**—phenylketonuria—and those with **hyperphenylalaninemia** are at a higher risk of having an offspring with microcephaly, cardiac defects, mental retardation, and IUGR. The brain damage and mental retardation can be prevented if the phenylketonuric mother is placed on a phenylalanine-restricted diet before and during the pregnancy.

Mechanical Factors as Teratogens

Amniotic fluid absorbs mechanical pressures, thereby protecting the embryo from most external trauma. A significantly reduced quantity of amniotic fluid (oligohydramnios) may result in mechanically induced deformation of the limbs (see Chapter 7), for example, hyperextension of the knee. Congenital dislocation of the hip and clubfoot may be caused by mechanical forces, particularly in a malformed uterus. Such deformations may be caused by any factor that restricts the mobility of the fetus, thereby causing prolonged compression in an abnormal posture. Intrauterine amputations or other anomalies caused by local constriction during fetal growth may result from **amniotic bands**—rings formed as a result of rupture of the amnion during early pregnancy (see Fig. 7-22).

ANOMALIES CAUSED BY MULTIFACTORIAL INHERITANCE

Many common birth defects (e.g., cleft lip with or without cleft palate) have familial distributions consistent with multifactorial inheritance (see Fig. 20-1). Multifactorial inheritance may be represented by a model in which "liability" to a disorder is a continuous variable determined by a combination of genetic and environmental factors, with a developmental threshold dividing individuals with the anomaly from those without it (Fig. 20-24). Multifactorial traits are often single major anomalies, such as cleft lip, isolated cleft palate, neural tube defects (e.g., meroencephaly, spina bifida cystica), pyloric stenosis, and congenital dislocation of the hip. Some of these anomalies may also occur as part of the phenotype in syndromes determined by single-gene inheritance, chromosome abnormality, or an environmental teratogen. The recurrence risks used for genetic counseling of families having birth defects determined by multifactorial inheritance are empirical risks based on the frequency of the anomaly in the general population and in different categories of relatives. In individual families, such estimates may be inaccurate because they are usually averages for the population rather than precise probabilities for the individual family.

SUMMARY OF CONGENITAL ANATOMIC ANOMALIES OR HUMAN BIRTH DEFECTS

- A congenital anatomic anomaly or birth defect is a structural abnormality of any type that is present at birth. It may be macroscopic or microscopic, on the surface or within the body. There are four clinically significant types of congenital anatomic anomalies: malformation, disruption, deformation, and dysplasia.
- Approximately 3% of live-born infants have an obvious major anomaly. Additional anomalies are detected after birth; thus, the incidence is approximately 6% in 2 year olds and 8% in 5 year olds. Other anomalies (approximately 2%) are detected later (e.g., during surgery, dissection, or autopsy).
- Congenital anomalies may be single or multiple and of minor or major clinical significance. Single minor defects are present in approximately 14% of newborns. These anomalies are of no serious medical consequence; however, they alert the clinician to the possible presence of an associated major anomaly.
- Ninety percent of infants with multiple minor anomalies have one or more associated major anomalies. Of the 3% of infants born with a major congenital anomaly, 0.7% have multiple major anomalies. Major anomalies are more common in early embryos (up to 15%) than they are in newborn infants (up to 3%).
- Some birth defects are caused by genetic factors (chromosome abnormalities and mutant genes). A few congenital abnormalities are caused by environmental factors (infectious agents, environmental chemicals, and drugs); however, most common anomalies result from a complex interaction between genetic and environmental factors. The cause of most congenital anomalies is unknown.
- During the first 2 weeks of development, teratogenic agents usually kill the embryo or have no effect rather than cause congenital anomalies. During the organogenetic period, teratogenic agents disrupt development and may cause major congenital anomalies. During the fetal period, teratogens may produce morphologic and functional abnormalities, particularly of the brain and eyes.

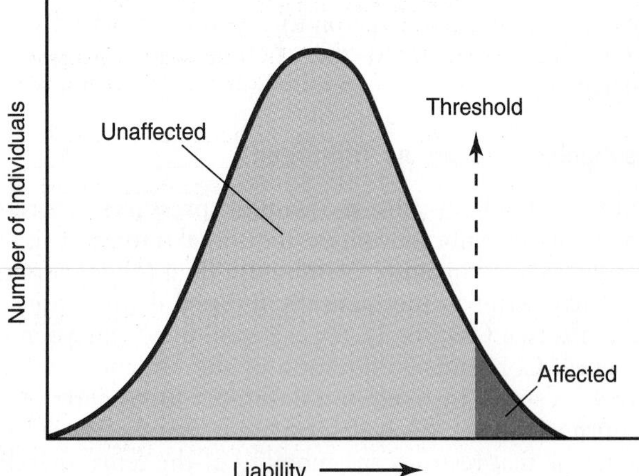

FIGURE 20-24. Multifactorial threshold model. Liability to a trait is distributed normally with a threshold dividing the population into unaffected and affected classes. (From Thompson MW, McInnes RR, Willard HF: Thompson & Thompson Genetics in Medicine, 5th ed. Philadelphia, WB Saunders, 1991.)

CLINICALLY ORIENTED PROBLEMS

CASE 20-1

A physician was concerned about the drugs a woman said she was taking when she first sought medical advice during her pregnancy.

- What percentage of congenital anomalies is caused by drugs, environmental chemicals, and infectious agents?
- Why may it be difficult for physicians to attribute specific congenital anomalies to specific drugs?
- What should pregnant women know about the use of drugs during pregnancy?

CASE 20-2

During a pelvic examination, a 38-year-old woman learned that she was pregnant. The physician was concerned about her age inasmuch as it was her first pregnancy.

- Do women older than the age of 35 have an increased risk of bearing malformed children?
- If a 38-year-old woman becomes pregnant, what prenatal diagnostic tests would likely be performed?

- What genetic abnormality might be detected?
- Can a 44-year-old woman have a normal baby?

CASE 20-3

A pregnant woman asked her physician whether there are any drugs considered safe during early pregnancy.

- Can you name some commonly prescribed drugs that are safe to use?
- What commonly used drugs should be avoided during pregnancy?

CASE 20-4

A 10-year-old girl contracted a rubella infection (German measles) and her mother was worried that the child might develop cataracts and heart defects.

- What would the physician likely tell the mother?

CASE 20-5

A pregnant woman who has two cats that often "spent the night out" was told by a friend that she should avoid close contact with her cats during her pregnancy. She was also told to avoid flies and cockroaches.

- When she consulted her physician, what would she likely be told?

CASE 20-6

The pregnancy of a 28-year-old woman is complicated by diabetes mellitus.

- Does this condition present any risk to the fetus?
- If so, what are the potential risks?

Discussion of these problems appears at the back of the book.

References and Suggested Reading

Bahado-Singh RO, Sutton-Riley J: Biochemical screening for congenital defects. Obstet Gynecol Clin North Am 31:857, 2004.

Baley JE, Toltzis P: Viral infections. In Martin RJ, Fanaroff AA, Walsh MC (eds): Fanaroff and Martin's Neonatal-Perinatal Medicine. Diseases of the Fetus and Infant, 8th ed. Philadelphia, Mosby, 2006.

Bracken MB, Belanger K, Hellenbrand K, et al: Exposure to electromagnetic fields during pregnancy with emphasis on electrically heated beds: association with birth weight and intrauterine growth retardation. Epidemiology 6:263, 1995.

Briggs GG, Freeman RK, Yaffe SJ: Drugs in Pregnancy and Lactation, 7th ed. Baltimore, Williams & Wilkins, 2005.

Canick JA, MacRae AR: Second trimester serum markers. Semin Perinatol 29:203, 2005.

Centers for Disease Control and Prevention: Improved national prevalence estimates for selected major birth defects—United States, 1999–2001 (MMWR 54:1301, 2006). JAMA 295,618, 2006.

Chambers CD, Hernandez-Diaz S, Van Marter LJ, et al: Selective serotonin-reuptake inhibitors and risk of persistent pulmonary hypertension of the newborn. N Engl J Med 354:579, 2006.

Chudley AE, Conry J, Cook JL, et al: Public Health Agency of Canada's National Advisory Committee on Fetal Alcohol Spectrum Disorder. Fetal alcohol spectrum disorder. Canadian guidelines for diagnosis. CMAJ 172(5 Suppl):S1–S21, 2005.

Chudley AE, Hagerman RJ: The fragile X syndrome. J Pediatr 110:821, 1987.

Drugan A, Isada NB, Evans MI: Prenatal diagnosis in the molecular age—indications, procedures, and laboratory techniques. In MacDonald MG, Seshia MMK, Mullett MD (eds): Avery's Neonatology, Pathophysiology & Management of the Newborn, 6th ed. Philadelphia, Lippincott Williams & Wilkins, 2005.

Eberhard-Gran M, Eskild A, Opjordsmoen S: Treating mood disorders during pregnancy: Safety considerations. Drug Saf 28:695, 2005.

EURAP Study Group: Seizure control and treatment in pregnancy. Neurology 66:354, 2006.

Galerneau F, Inzucchi SE: Diabetes mellitus in pregnancy. Obstet Gynecol Clin North Am 31:907, 2004.

Gardner RJM, Sutherland GR: Chromosome Abnormalities and Genetic Counseling, 3rd ed. Oxford, UK, Oxford University Press, 2003.

Goldberg JD: Routine screening for fetal anomalies: expectations. Obstet Gynecol Clin North Am 31:35, 2004.

Hales B: DNA repair disorders causing malformations. Curr Opin Genet Dev 15:234, 2005.

Hall JG: Chromosomal clinical abnormalities. In Behrman RE, Kliegman RM, Jenson HB (eds): Nelson Textbook of Pediatrics, 17th ed. Philadelphia, WB Saunders, 2004.

Holmes LB, Harvey EA, Coull BA, et al: The teratogenicity of anticonvulsant drugs. N Engl J Med 344:1132, 2001.

Hudgins L, Cassidy SB: Congenital anomalies. In Martin RJ, Fanaroff AA, Walsh MC (eds): Fanaroff and Martin's Neonatal-Perinatal Medicine. Diseases of the Fetus and Infant, 8th ed. Philadelphia, Mosby, 2006.

Jones KL: Smith's Recognizable Patterns of Human Malformation, 6th ed. Philadelphia, Elsevier/Saunders, 2005.

Kendrick JS, Merritt RK: Women and smoking: An update for the 1990s. Am J Obstet Gynecol 175:528, 1996.

Kirkilionis AJ, Chudley AE, Gregory CA, et al: Molecular and clinical overlap of Angelman and Prader-Willi syndrome phenotypes. Am J Med Genet 40:454, 1991.

Kriebs JM: Changing the paradigm. HIV in pregnancy. J Perinat Neonat Nurs 20:71, 2006.

Lam PK, Torfs CP: Interaction between maternal smoking and malnutrition in infant risk of gastroschisis. Birth Defects Res A Clin Mol Teratol 76:182, 2006.

Medicodes' Hospital and Payer: International Classification of Diseases, 9th Revision. Clinical Modification, 4th ed., Volumes 1–3. Salt Lake City, Medicode, Inc., 1995.

Mills JL: Depressing observations on the use of selective serotonin-reuptake inhibitors during pregnancy. N Engl J Med 354:636, 2006.

Milunsky A (ed): Genetic Disorders and the Fetus: Diagnosis, Prevention and Treatment, 5th ed. Baltimore, The Johns Hopkins University Press, 2004.

Moore CA, Khoury MJ, Bradley LA: From genetics to genomics: Using gene-based medicine to prevent disease and promote health in children. Semin Perinatol 29:135, 2005.

Newnham JP, Evans SF, Michael CA, et al: Effects of frequent ultrasound during pregnancy: A randomised controlled trial. Lancet 342:887, 1993.

Nicolaides KH: First-trimester screening for chromosomal abnormalities. Semin Perinatol 29:190, 2005.

Nussbaum RL, McInnes RR, Willard HF: Thompson & Thompson Genetics in Medicine, 6th ed. (Revised Reprint). Philadelphia, WB Saunders, 2004.

Persaud TVN: Environmental Causes of Human Birth Defects. Springfield, IL, Charles C Thomas, 1990.

Ralston SJ, Craigo SD: Ultrasound-guided procedures for prenatal diagnosis and therapy. Obstet Gynecol Clin North Am 31:21, 2004.

Reece EA, Eriksson UJ: The pathogenesis of diabetes-associated congenital malformations. Obstet Gynecol Clin North Am 23:29, 1996.

Robertson J, Polifka JE, Avner M, et al: A survey of pregnant women using isotretinoin. Birth Defects Res A Clin Mol Teratol 73:881, 2005.

Roessler E, Belloni E, Gaudenz K, et al: Mutations in the human sonic hedgehog gene cause holoprosencephaly. Nat Genet 14:357, 1996.

Schiller C, Allen PJ: Follow-up of infants prenatally exposed to cocaine. Pediatr Nurs 31:427, 2005.

Schwarz EB, Maselli J, Norton M, Gonzales R: Prescription and teratogenic medications in United States ambulatory practices. Am J Med 118:1240, 2005.

Shepard TH, Fantel AG, Fitzsimmons J: Congenital defect rates among spontaneous abortuses. Twenty years of monitoring. Teratology 39:325, 1989.

Shiota K, Uwabe C, Nishimura H: High prevalence of defective human embryos at the early postimplantation period. Teratology 35:309, 1987.

Slack C, Lurix K, Lewis S, Lichten L: Prenatal genetics. The evolution and future directions of screening and diagnosis. J Perinat Neonat Nurs 20:93, 2006.

Spranger J, Benirschke K, Hall JG, et al: Errors of morphogenesis, concepts and terms. J Pediatr 100:160, 1982.

Wenstrom KD: First-trimester Down syndrome screening: Component analytes and timing for optimal performance. Semin Perinatol 29:195, 2005.

Wilcox AJ, Baird DD, Weinberg CR, et al: Fertility in men exposed prenatally to diethylstilbestrol. N Engl J Med 332:1441, 1995.

21 Common Signaling Pathways Used during Development

Jeffrey T. Wigle and David D. Eisenstat

Morphogens	**488**
Retinoic Acid	**488**
Transforming Growth Factor β/Bone Morphogenetic Protein	**489**
Hedgehog	**489**
Wnt/β-Catenin Pathway	**490**
Notch-Delta Pathway	**491**
Transcription Factors	**491**
Hox/Homeobox Proteins	**492**
Pax Genes	**493**
Basic Helix-Loop-Helix Transcription Factors	**493**
Receptor Tyrosine Kinases	**493**
Common Features	**493**
Regulation of Angiogenesis by Receptor Tyrosine Kinases	**494**
Summary of Common Signaling Pathways Used during Development	**494**

During the process of embryonic development, undifferentiated precursor cells differentiate and organize into the complex structures found in functional adult tissues. This intricate process requires cells to integrate many different cues, both intrinsic and extrinsic, for development to occur properly. These cues control the proliferation, differentiation, and migration of cells to determine the final size and shape of the developing organs. Disruption of these signaling pathways can result in human developmental disorders and birth defects. These key developmental **signaling pathways** are frequently co-opted in the adult by diseases such as cancer.

Given the diverse changes that occur during embryogenesis, it may appear that there should also be a correspondingly diverse set of signaling pathways that regulate these processes. In contrast, the differentiation of many different cell types is regulated through a relatively restricted set of molecular signaling pathways:

- **Morphogens.** These are diffusible molecules that specify which cell type will be generated at a specific anatomic location and direct the migration of cells and their processes to their final destination. These include retinoic acid, transforming growth factor β (TGF-β)/bone morphogenetic proteins (BMPs), and the hedgehog and the Wnt protein families (see Table 21-1 for gene and protein nomenclature).
- **Notch/Delta.** This pathway often specifies which cell fate precursor cells will adopt.
- **Transcription factors.** This set of evolutionarily conserved proteins activates or represses downstream genes that are essential for many different cellular processes. Many transcription factors are members of the homeobox or helix-loop-helix (HLH) families. Their activity can be regulated by all of the other pathways described in this chapter.
- **Receptor tyrosine kinases (RTKs).** Many growth factors signal by binding to and activating membrane-bound RTKs. These kinases are essential for the regulation of cellular proliferation, apoptosis, and migration as well as processes such as the growth of new blood vessels and axonal processes in the nervous system.

MORPHOGENS

Extrinsic signals guide the differentiation and migration of cells during development and thereby dictate the morphology and function of developing tissues (see Chapter 5). Many of these morphogens are found in concentration *gradients* in the embryo, and different morphogens can be expressed in opposing gradients in the dorsal/ventral, anterior/posterior, and medial/lateral axes. The fate of a specific cell can be determined by its location along these gradients. Cells can be attracted or repelled by morphogens depending on the set of receptors expressed on their surface.

Table 21–1. International Nomenclature Standards for Genes and Proteins

Gene	Human	Italics and capitalized	*PAX6*
	Mouse	Italics, first letter capitalized	*Pax6*
Protein	Human	Roman, capitalized	PAX6
	Mouse	Roman, capitalized	PAX6

Retinoic Acid

The anterior (rostral, head)/posterior (caudal, tail), or anteroposterior (AP) axis of the embryo is crucial for determining the correct location for structures such as limbs and for the patterning of the nervous system. For decades, it has been clinically evident that alterations in the level of vitamin A (retinol) in the diet (excessive or insufficient amounts) can lead to the development of congenital malformations (see Chapters 17 and 20). The bioactive form of vitamin A is retinoic acid that is formed by the oxidation of retinol to retinal by *retinol dehydrogenases* and the subsequent oxidation of retinal by *retinal aldehyde dehydrogenase*. Free levels of retinoic acid can be further modulated by cellular retinoic acid binding proteins that sequester retinoic acid. As well, retinoic acid can be actively degraded into inactive metabolites by enzymes such as CYP26 (Fig. 21-1).

Normally, retinoic acid acts to "posteriorize" the body plan. Therefore, either excessive retinoic acid or inhibition of its degradation leads to a truncated body axis where structures have a more posterior nature. In contrast, insufficient retinoic acid or defects in the enzymes such as retinal aldehyde dehydrogenase will lead to a more anteriorized structure. At a molecular level, retinoic acid binds to its receptors inside the cell and activates them. *Retinoic acid receptors* are transcription factors, and therefore their activation will regulate the expression of downstream genes. Crucial targets of retinoic acid receptors in development are the *Hox* genes.

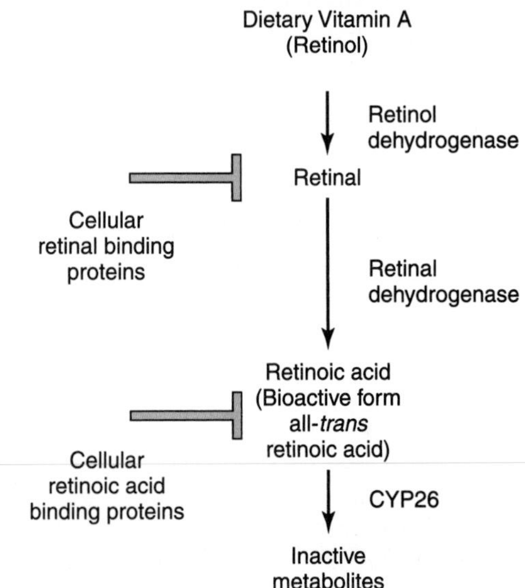

Figure 21-1. Regulation of retinoic acid metabolism and signaling. Dietary retinol (vitamin A) is converted to retinal via the action of retinol dehydrogenases. The concentration of free retinal is controlled by the action of cellular retinal binding proteins. Similarly, retinal is converted to retinoic acid by retinal dehydrogenases, and its free level is modulated by sequestration by cellular retinoic acid binding proteins and degradation by CYP26. The bioactive form of retinoic acid is all-*trans* retinoic acid.

Transforming Growth Factor β/Bone Morphogenetic Protein

Members of the **TGF-β** superfamily include TGF-β, BMPs, activin, and nodal. These molecules contribute to the establishment of dorsoventral patterning, cell fate decisions, and formation of specific organs, including the nervous system, kidneys, skeleton, and blood (see Chapters 5, 16, and 17). In humans, there are three **TGF-β** isoforms (**TGF-β_1**, **TGF-β_2**, and **TGF-β_3**). Binding of these ligands to heterotetrameric (four subunit) complexes, consisting of specific type I (inactive kinase domain) and type II TGF-β receptor subunit (TβR-II) (constitutively active) transmembrane serine-threonine kinase receptors, results in intracellular signaling events (Fig. 21-2). When TGF-β ligands bind to their respective membrane-bound type II receptor, a type I receptor is recruited and transphorylated, and its kinase domain is activated, subsequently phosphorylating intracellular receptor-associated **Smad proteins** (R-Smads). The Smad proteins are a large family of intercellular proteins that are divided into three classes: *receptor-activated* (R-Smads, Smads 1–3, 5, 8), *common-partner* (co-Smads, Smad4), and *inhibitory* Smads (I-Smads, Smad6, Smad7). R-Smad/Smad4 complexes translocate to the nucleus and regulate target gene transcription by interacting with other proteins or as transcription factors by directly binding to DNA. TβR-I activation is a highly regulated process that involves membrane-anchored coreceptors and other receptor-like molecules that can sequester ligands and prevent their binding to respective TβR-II receptors. Dominant negative forms of TβR-II have inactive kinase domains and cannot transphosphorylate TβR-I, thereby blocking downstream signaling events. The diversity of TGF-β ligand, TβR-I and TβR-II, coreceptor, ligand trap, and R-Smad combinations contributes to particular developmental and cell-specific processes, often in combination with other signaling pathways.

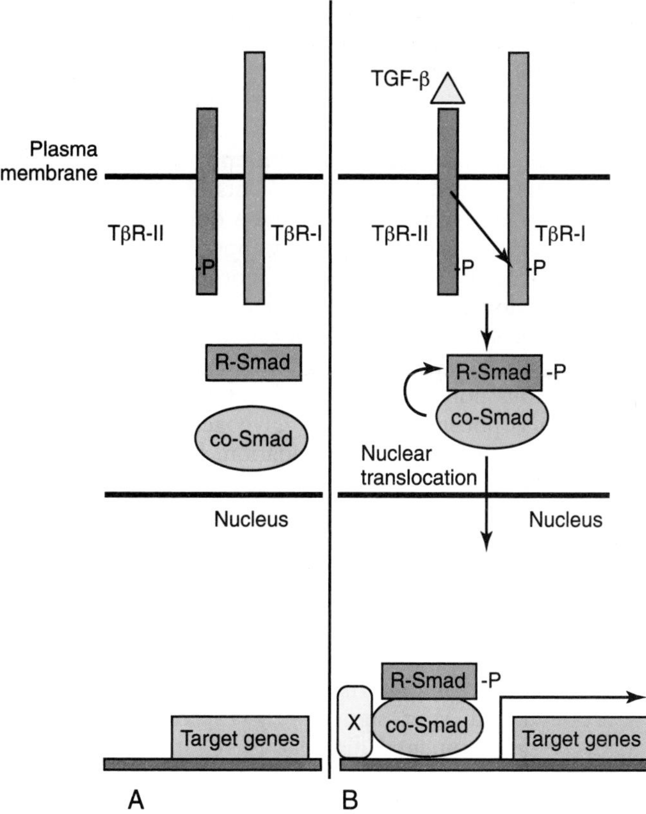

FIGURE 21-2. Transforming growth factor β (TGF-β)/Smad signaling pathway. **A,** The type II TGF-β receptor subunit (TβR-II) is constitutively active. **B,** Upon binding of ligand to TβR-II, a type I receptor subunit is recruited to form a heterodimeric receptor complex and the TβR-I kinase domain is transphosphorylated (-P). Signaling from the activated receptor complex phosphorylates R-Smads, which then bind to a co-Smad, translocate from the cytoplasm to the nucleus, and activate gene transcription with cofactor(s) (X).

Hedgehog

Sonic hedgehog (Shh) was the first mammalian ortholog of the *Drosophila* gene *hedgehog* to be identified. Shh and other related proteins, desert hedgehog and Indian hedgehog, are secreted morphogens critical to early patterning, cell migration, and differentiation of many cell types and organ systems (see Chapter 5). Cells have variable thresholds for response to the secreted Shh signal. The primary receptor for Shh is *Patched* (PTCH in human, PTC family in mouse), a 12-transmembrane domain protein that, in the absence of Shh, inhibits *Smoothened* (Smo), a seven-transmembrane domain G protein–linked protein, and downstream signaling to the nucleus. However, in the presence of Shh, Ptc inhibition is blocked and downstream events follow, including nuclear translocation of **Gli** (*Gli1*, *Gli2*, *Gli3*), with transcriptional activation of target genes, such as *Ptc-1*, *Engrailed*, and others (Fig. 21-3).

The Shh protein is modified post-translationally by the addition of cholesterol and palmitate moieties to the N- and C-termini, respectively. These lipid modifications affect Shh's association with the cell membrane, formation of Shh multimers, and, of significance, affect the movement of Shh, altering its tissue distribution and concentration gradients. One of the best explained activities of Shh activity in vertebrate development is the role of Shh in patterning the *ventral neural tube* (see Chapters 4 and 17). Shh is secreted at high levels by the mesoderm-derived structure, the notochord. The concentration of Shh is highest in the floorplate of the neural tube and lowest in the roofplate, where members of the TGF-β family are highly expressed. The cell fates of four ventral interneuron classes and motor neurons are determined by relative Shh concentrations and by a combinatorial code of homeobox and basic *HLH (bHLH)* genes.

The requirement of Shh pathway signaling for many developmental processes is underscored by the discovery of human mutations of members of the Shh pathway and the corresponding phenotypes of genetically modified mice, in which members of the Shh pathway are either inactivated (loss of function/knockout) or overexpressed (gain of function). Mutations of *SHH* and *PTCH* have been associated with holoprosencephaly, a common congenital brain defect resulting in the fusion of the two cerebral hemispheres, anophthalmia or cyclopia (see Chapter 18) and dorsalization of forebrain structures; this defect in

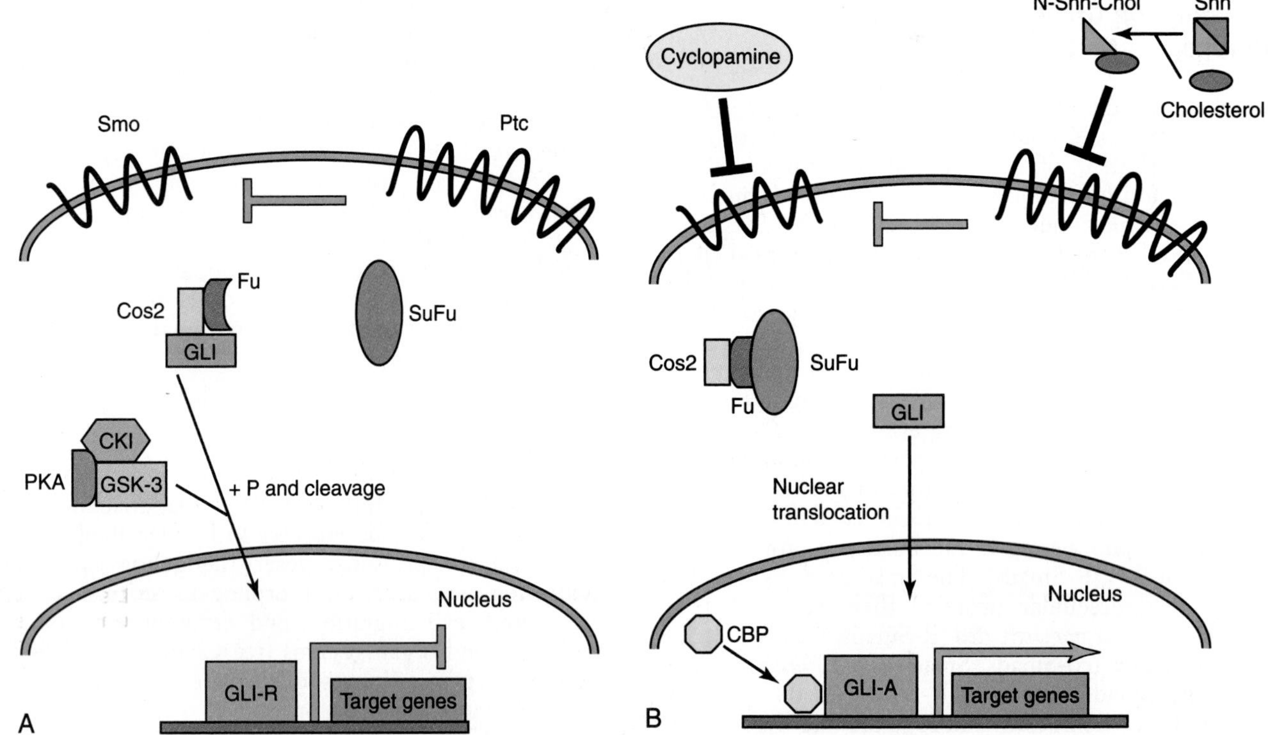

FIGURE 21-3. Sonic hedgehog/Patched signaling pathway. **A,** The Patched (Ptc) receptor inhibits signaling from the Smoothened (Smo) receptor. In a complex with Costal-2 (Cos2) and Fused (Fu), Gli is modified to become a transcriptional repressor, Gli-R. **B,** Sonic hedgehog (Shh) is cleaved and cholesterol is added to its N-terminus. This modified Shh ligand inhibits the Ptc receptor, permitting Smo signaling, and ultimately activated Gli (Gli-A) translocates to the nucleus to activate target genes with CBP. CBP, cyclic AMP binding protein; CKI, casein kinase I; GSK-3, glycogen synthase kinase-3; P, phosphate group; PKA, protein kinase A; SuFu, suppressor of Fused.

sheep can also result from exposure to the teratogen cyclopamine, which disrupts Shh signaling (see Fig. 21-3). Of interest, some patients with severe forms of the inborn error of cholesterol synthesis, the autosomal recessive Smith-Lemli-Opitz syndrome, have holoprosencephaly (see Chapter 20). *GLI3* mutations are associated with autosomal dominant polydactyly syndromes (see Chapter 16), such as Greig's and Pallister-Hall syndromes. Gorlin's syndrome, often due to germline *PTCH* mutations, is a constellation of congenital malformations mostly affecting the epidermis, craniofacial structures (see Chapter 9), and the nervous system. These patients are significantly predisposed to basal cell carcinomas, especially after radiation, and a smaller proportion will develop malignant brain tumors known as medulloblastomas during childhood. Somatic mutations of *PTCH*, *SUFU*, and *SMO* have also been identified in patients with sporadic medulloblastomas not associated with Gorlin's syndrome.

Wnt/β-Catenin Pathway

The **Wnt**-secreted glycoproteins are vertebrate orthologs of the *Drosophila* gene *Wingless*. Similar to the other morphogens previously discussed, the 19 Wnt family members control several processes during development, including establishment of cell polarity, proliferation, apoptosis, cell fate specification, and migration. Wnt signaling is a very complex process and three signaling pathways have been elucidated to date, but only the classic or "canonical" **β-catenin-dependent pathway** is discussed here (Fig. 21-4). Specific Wnts bind to one of 10 Frizzled (Fzd) seven transmembrane domain cell surface receptors, and with low-density lipoprotein receptor–related-protein (LRP5/LRP6) coreceptors, thereby activating downstream intracellular signaling events. β-Catenin plays an integral role in canonical Wnt signaling. In the absence of Wnt binding, in a protein complex with adenomatous polyposis coli (APC) and axin, cytoplasmic β-catenin is phosphorylated by glycogen synthase kinase (GSK-3) and targeted for degradation. In the presence of Wnts, GSK-3 is itself phosphorylated by Dishevelled (Dvl), and thus inactivated; it cannot phosphorylate β-catenin. β-Catenin is stabilized, accumulates in the cytoplasm, and translocates to the nucleus where it activates target gene transcription, in a complex with T-cell factor (TCF) transcription factors. The many β-catenin/TCF target genes include vascular endothelial growth factor (VEGF), c-myc, and matrix metalloproteinases.

Dysregulated Wnt signaling is a prominent feature in many developmental disorders and cancer. A *Frizzled* (*FZD9*) gene is present in the *Williams-Beuren syndrome* deletion region. *LRP5* mutations are found in the *osteoporosis-pseudoglioma syndrome*. *Dvl2* knockout mice have malformations of the cardiac outflow tract, abnormal somite segmentation, and neural tube defects. Similar to the Shh pathway, canonical Wnt pathway mutations (in β-catenin, APC, and *axin1* genes) have been described in children with medulloblastoma. Moreover, somatic *APC* mutations are common (~50%) in adults with sporadic

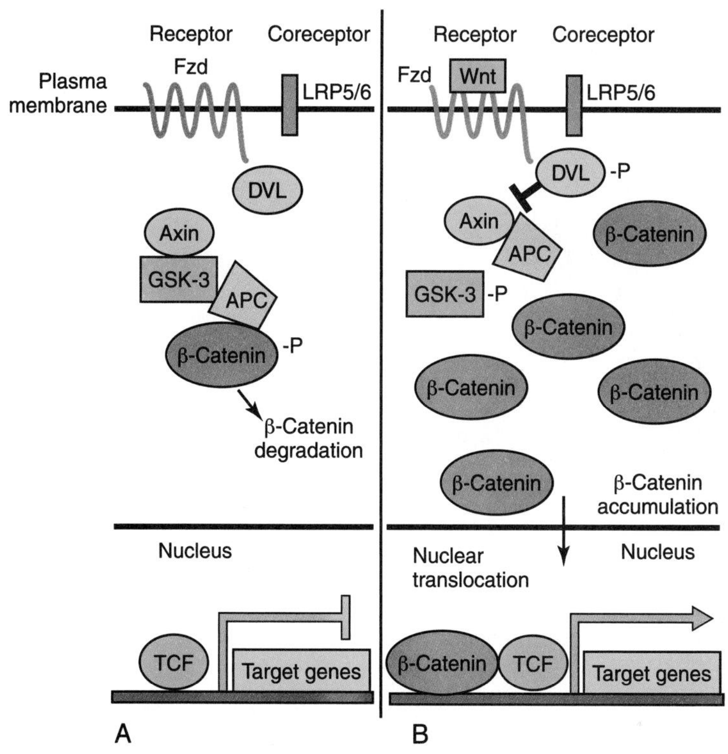

FIGURE 21-4. Wnt/β-catenin canonical signaling pathway. **A,** In the absence of Wnt ligand binding to Frizzled (Fzd) receptor, β-catenin is phosphorylated (-P) by a multiprotein complex and targeted for degradation. Target gene expression is repressed by T-cell factor (TCF). **B,** When Wnt binds to the Fzd receptor, LRP coreceptors are recruited, Dishevelled (DVL) is phosphorylated and β-catenin then accumulates in the cytoplasm. Some β-catenin enters the nucleus to activate target gene transcription. APC, adenomatous polyposis coli; GSK-3, glycogen synthase kinase-3; LRP, lipoprotein receptor–related-protein.

colorectal carcinomas and germline *APC* mutations are a feature of familial adenomatous polyposis and Turcot's syndrome (multiple colorectal adenomas and increased frequency of primary brain tumors).

NOTCH-DELTA PATHWAY

The *Notch signaling pathway* is integral for cell fate determination, including maintenance of stem-cell niches, proliferation, apoptosis, and differentiation. These processes are essential for all aspects of organ development through regulation of lateral and inductive cell-cell signaling. Notch proteins are single transmembrane receptors (Notch 1–4) that interact with membrane-bound *Notch* (see Chapter 5) *ligands* (Delta-like ligands, Dll-1, Dll-3, Dll-4); serrate-like ligands, jagged-1, jagged-2) on adjacent cells (Fig. 21-5). Ligand-receptor binding triggers proteolytic events leading to the release of the *Notch intracellular domain* (NICD). When the NICD translocates to the nucleus, a series of intranuclear events culminates in the induction of expression of hairy-enhancer of split, an HLH transcription factor that maintains the progenitor state by repressing proneural basic *HLH* genes.

The process of **lateral inhibition** ensures that in a population of cells with equivalent developmental potential, there are the correct numbers of two distinct cell types. In the initial cell-cell interaction, the progenitor cell responding to the Notch-ligand Delta, through a negative feedback mechanism, reduces its own expression of Delta, with Notch receptor signaling maintaining the cell as an uncommitted progenitor. However, the adjacent cell maintains Delta expression levels with reduced Notch signaling and differentiation, mediated by, for example, by proneural *HLH* genes. Inductive signaling with other surrounding cells expressing morphogens may overcome the cell's commitment to a neural cell fate (default state) to an alternative glial cell fate. Understanding the function of the Notch-Delta signaling pathway in mammalian development has been assisted by loss-of-function studies in the mouse. Evidence of *JAGGED1* mutations in *Alagille syndrome* (arteriohepatic dysplasia), with liver, kidney, cardiovascular, ocular, and skeletal malformations, and *NOTCH-3* gene mutations in the CADASIL (cerebral autosomal dominant arteriopathy with subcortical infarcts and leukoencephalopathy) adult vascular degenerative disease, with a tendency to early-age onset of strokelike events, support the importance of the Notch signaling pathway in embryonic and postnatal development, respectively.

TRANSCRIPTION FACTORS

Transcription factors belong to a large class of proteins that regulate the expression of many target genes, either through activation or repression mechanisms. Typically, a transcription factor will bind to specific nucleotide sequences in the promoter/enhancer regions of target genes and regulate the rate of transcription of its target genes via interacting with accessory proteins. Recently, it was demonstrated that transcription factors can both activate or repress target gene transcription depending on the cell in which they are expressed, the specific promoter, the chromatin context, and the developmental stage. As well, some transcription factors do not need to bind to DNA to regulate transcription, but may bind to other transcription factors already bound to the promoter DNA thereby regulating transcription. Also, they may bind and sequester other transcription factors from their target genes, thus repressing their transcription.

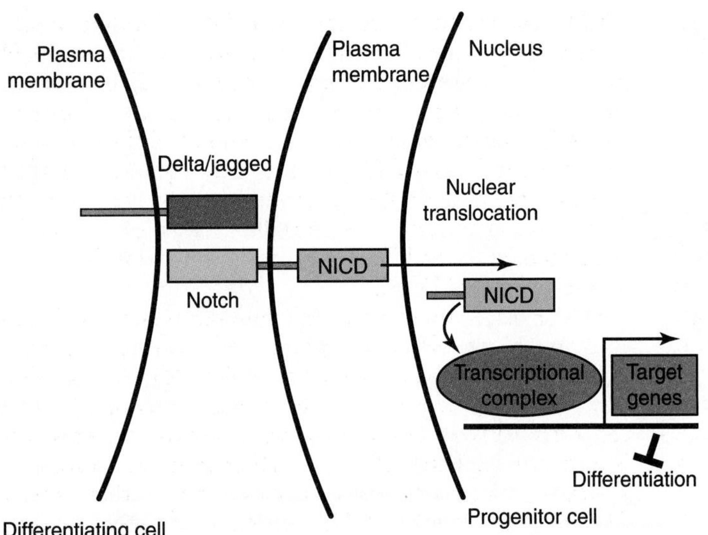

FIGURE 21-5. Notch/Delta signaling pathway. In progenitor cells (*right*), activation of Notch signaling leads to cleavage of the Notch intracellular domain (NICD). NICD translocates to the nucleus, binds to a transcriptional complex, and activates target genes, such as Hes1, that inhibit differentiation. In differentiating cells (*left*), Notch signaling is not active.

Histones are the positively charged nuclear proteins around which genomic DNA is coiled to tightly pack it within the nucleus. Modification of these proteins is a common pathway by which transcription factors regulate the activity of their target promoters. One such modification is *acetylation*. DNA is less tightly bound to acetylated histones, thus allowing for more open access of transcription factors and other proteins to the promoters of their target genes. Histone acetylation status is controlled by genes such as **histone acetyl transferases,** which add acetyl groups, and **histone deacetylases,** which remove acetyl groups. Transcription factors can modify histone acetylation by either recruiting histone acetyl transferases or by recruiting histone deacetylases (Fig. 21-6). Phosphorylation of histones also leads to an opening of the chromatin structure and activation of gene transcription. Disorders of chromatin remodeling include *Rett*, *Rubinstein-Taybi*, and *alpha-thalassemia/X-linked mental retardation* syndromes.

The transcription factor superfamily is composed of many different classes of proteins. In this chapter, we discuss three examples of this diverse family of proteins: Hox/Homeobox, Pax, and bHLH transcription factors.

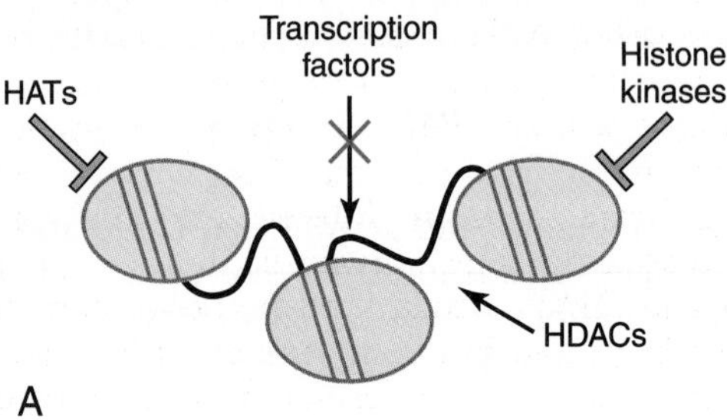

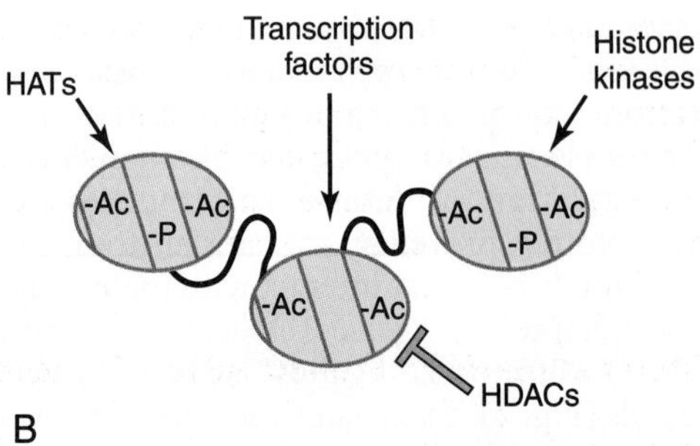

FIGURE 21-6. Histone modifications alter transcriptional properties of chromatin. **A,** In areas of transcriptionally inactive chromatin, the DNA is tightly bound to the histone cores. The histones are not acetylated or phosphorylated. Histone deacetylases (HDACs) are active, whereas histone acetyl transferases (HATs) and histone kinases are inactive. **B,** In areas of transcriptionally active chromatin, the DNA is not as tightly bound to the histone cores. The histone proteins are acetylated (Ac) and phosphorylated (-P). HDACs are inactive, whereas HATs and histone kinases are active.

Hox/Homeobox Proteins

The *Hox* genes were first discovered in the fruit fly, *Drosophila melanogaster*. Mutations in these genes of the HOM-C complex lead to dramatic phenotypes (homeotic transformation) such as the *Antennapedia* gene in which legs instead of antennae sprout from the head. The order of the Hox genes along the AP axis is faithfully reproduced in their organization at the level of the chromosome. In humans, the order of the *Hox* genes along the AP axis and chromosomal location is conserved as well. Defects in *HOXA1* have been shown to impair human neural development, and mutations in *HOXA13* and *HOXD13* result in limb malformations (see Chapter 16).

All the *HOX* genes contain a 180-base pair sequence, the homeobox, which encodes a 60-amino-acid homeodomain composed of three α helices. The third (recognition) helix binds to DNA sites that contain one or more TAAT/ATTA tetranucleotide binding motifs in the promoters of their target genes. The homeodomain is the most conserved region of the protein and is highly conserved across evolution, whereas other regions of the protein are not as well conserved. Mutations in the DNA binding region of the homeobox gene *NKX2.5* are associated with cardiac atrial-septal defects and mutations in *ARX* are associated with the central nervous system malformation syndrome lissencephaly (see Chapter 17).

Pax Genes

The *Pax* genes all contain conserved bipartite DNA binding motifs called the Pax (or paired) domain, and some Pax family members also contain a **homeodomain**. PAX proteins have been shown to both activate and repress transcription of target genes.

The *Drosophila melanogaster* ortholog of *Pax6*, *eyeless*, was shown to be essential for eye development because the homozygous mutant flies had no eyes. In gain-of-function experiments, ectopic expression of *eyeless* led to the formation of additional eyes. In fruit flies, *eyeless* is clearly a master regulator of eye development. Eyeless shares a high degree of sequence conservation with its human ortholog *PAX6*. *PAX6* was shown to be associated with ocular malformations such as aniridia (absence of the iris) and Peter's anomaly. In human eye diseases, the level of *PAX6* expression seems to be crucial as patients with only one functional copy (*haploinsufficiency*) have ocular defects and patients without *PAX6* function are anophthalmic (see Chapter 18). This concept of haploinsufficiency is a recurring theme for many different transcription factors and corresponding human malformations.

PAX3 and *PAX7* encode both homeodomain and Pax DNA binding domains. The human childhood cancer *alveolar rhabdomyosarcoma* results from a **translocation** that results in the formation of a chimeric protein wherein *PAX3* or *PAX7* (including both DNA domains) is fused to the strong activating domains of the Forkhead family transcription factor FOXO1A. The autosomal dominant human disease *Waardenburg's syndrome* type I has been demonstrated to result from mutations in the *PAX3* gene. Patients with this syndrome have hearing deficits, ocular defects (dystopia canthorum), and pigmentation abnormalities best typified by a white forelock.

Basic Helix-Loop-Helix Transcription Factors

The *bHLH* genes are a class of transcription factors that regulate cell fate determination and differentiation in many different tissues during development. At a molecular level, bHLH proteins contain a basic (positively charged) DNA binding region that is followed by two α helices that are separated by a loop. The α helices have a hydrophilic and a hydrophobic side (*amphipathic*). The hydrophobic side of the helix is a motif for protein-protein interactions between different members of the bHLH family. This domain is the most conserved region of the bHLH proteins across different species. bHLH proteins often bind other bHLHs (*heterodimerize*) to regulate transcription. These heterodimers are composed of tissue-specific bHLH proteins bound to ubiquitously expressed bHLH proteins. The powerful prodifferentiation effect of *bHLH* genes can be repressed by several different mechanisms. For example, inhibitor of differentiation (Id) proteins are HLH proteins that lack the basic DNA binding motif. When Id proteins heterodimerize with specific bHLH proteins, they prevent binding of these bHLH proteins to their target gene promoter sequences (called *E-boxes*). Growth factors, which tend to inhibit differentiation, increase the level of Id proteins that sequester bHLH proteins from their target promoters. As well, growth factors can stimulate the phosphorylation of the DNA binding domain of bHLH proteins, which inhibits their ability to bind to DNA.

bHLH genes are crucial for the development of tissues such as muscle (*MyoD/Myogenin*) and neurons (*NeuroD/Neurogenin*) in humans (see Chapter 15). *MyoD* expression was shown to be sufficient to transdifferentiate several different cell lines into muscle cells, demonstrating that it is a master regulator of muscle differentiation. Studies of knockout mice confirmed that *MyoD* and another bHLH *Myf5* are crucial for the differentiation of precursor cells into primitive muscle cells (myoblasts). The differentiation of these myoblasts into fully differentiated muscle cells is controlled by myogenin. Similarly, *Mash1* and *Neurogenin1* are proneural genes that regulate the formation of neuroblasts from the neuroepithelium (see Chapter 17). Mouse models have shown that these genes are crucial for the specification of different subpopulations of precursors in the developing central nervous system. For example, *Mash1* knockout mice had defects in forebrain development, whereas *Neurogenin1* knockout mice had defects in cranial sensory ganglia and ventral spinal cord neurons. Specification of these neuroblasts is regulated by other proneural genes known as *NeuroD* and *Math5*. Muscle and neuronal differentiation (see Chapters 15 and 17) are controlled by a cascade of *bHLH* genes that function at early and at late stages of cellular differentiation. As well, both differentiation pathways are inhibited via signaling through the Notch pathway.

RECEPTOR TYROSINE KINASES

Common Features

Growth factors, such as insulin, epidermal growth factor, nerve growth factor and other neurotrophins, and members of the platelet-derived growth factor family, bind to cell surface transmembrane receptors found on target cells. These receptors, members of the RTK superfamily, have three domains: (1) an extracellular ligand binding domain, (2) a transmembrane domain, and (3) an intracellular kinase domain (Fig. 21-7). These receptors are found as monomers in the quiescent or unbound state, but upon ligand binding, these receptor units dimerize. This process of **dimerization** brings the two intracellular kinase domains into close proximity such that one kinase domain can phosphorylate and activate the other receptor (*transphosphorylation*). Transphosphorylation is required to fully activate the receptors, which then initiate a series of intracellular signaling cascades. The mechanism of transphosphorylation requires both receptor subunits within a dimer to have functional kinase domains for signal transduction to occur. If there is an inactivating mutation

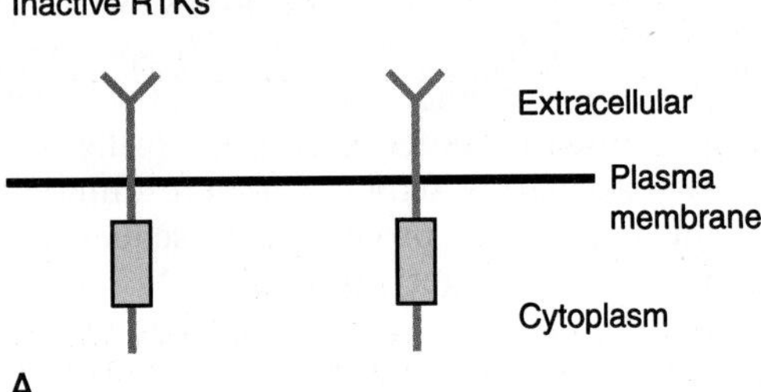

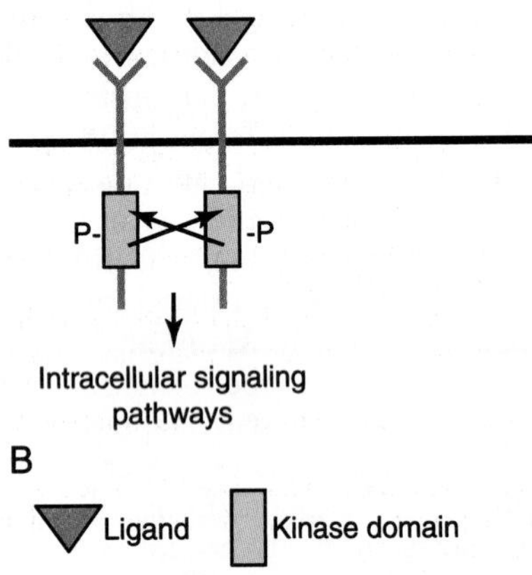

Ligand Kinase domain

FIGURE 21-7. Receptor tyrosine kinase (RTK) signaling. **A,** In the absence of ligand, the receptors are monomers and are inactive. **B,** Upon binding of ligand, the receptors dimerize and transphosphorylation occurs, which activates downstream signaling cascades. P, phosphorylated.

of one receptor subunit's kinase domain, then the functional consequence of this mutation will be to abolish signaling through a heterodimer resulting from the combination of wild-type and mutant receptor subunits (a dominant negative mode of action). Such a mutation in the kinase domain of the VEGF receptor 3 (*VEGFR-3*) results in the autosomal dominantly inherited lymphatic disorder called Milroy disease.

Regulation of Angiogenesis by Receptor Tyrosine Kinases

Growth factors generally promote cellular proliferation, migration, and survival (i.e., are antiapoptotic). Dysregulation of RTKs or their downstream signaling components are frequently found in human cancers. During embryogenesis, signaling through RTKs is crucial for normal development and affects many different processes such as the growth of new blood vessels (see Chapter 4), cellular migration, and neuronal axonal guidance.

Endothelial cells are derived from a progenitor cell (the hemangioblast) that can give rise to both the hematopoietic cell lineage and endothelial cells. The early endothelial cells proliferate and eventually coalesce to form the first primitive blood vessels. This process is termed *vasculogenesis*. After the first blood vessels are formed, they undergo intensive remodeling and maturation into the mature blood vessels in a process called *angiogenesis*. This maturation process involves the recruitment of vascular smooth muscle cells to the vessels that stabilize them. Vasculogenesis and angiogenesis are both dependent on the function of two distinct RTK classes, members of the VEGF and Tie receptor families.

VEGF-A was shown to be essential for endothelial and blood cell development. *VEGF-A* knockout mice fail to develop blood or endothelial cells and die at early embryonic stages. The heterozygous *VEGF-A* mice have severe defects in their vasculature demonstrating that *VEGF-A* gene dose is important (haploinsufficiency). A related molecule, *VEGF-C*, was shown to be crucial for the development of lymphatic endothelial cells. *VEGF-A* signals through two receptors, *VEGFR-1* and *VEGFR-2*, which are expressed by endothelial cells. *VEGF-A* signals predominantly through *VEGFR-2* in order for vasculogenesis to properly occur in the embryo.

The process of angiogenic refinement depends on the function of the angiopoietin/Tie2 signaling pathway. Tie2 is a RTK that is specifically expressed by endothelial cells and angiopoietin 1 and angiopoietin 2 are its ligands that are expressed by the surrounding vascular smooth muscle cells. This represents a paracrine signaling system where receptor and ligand are expressed in adjacent cells. Both the VEGF/VEGFR-2 and angiopoietin/Tie2 signaling pathways are co-opted by tumors to stimulate growth of new blood vessels, which stimulates their growth and metastasis. This demonstrates how normal signaling pathways in the developing human can be reused for disease processes, such as cancer, in the adult.

SUMMARY OF COMMON SIGNALING PATHWAYS USED DURING DEVELOPMENT

- There are marked differences between the various signaling pathways, but they share many *common* features: ligands, membrane-bound receptors and co-receptors, intracellular signaling domains, adapters, and effector molecules.
- Signaling pathways are *co-opted* at various times during development for stem-cell renewal, cell proliferation, migration, apoptosis, and differentiation.
- Pathways have *"default" settings* that result in generation or maintenance of one cell fate rather than another.
- Many genes and signaling pathways are highly conserved throughout evolution. Orthologs of genes critical for invertebrate development (the nematode *Caenorhabditis elegans* and the fruit fly *Drosophila melanogaster*) are found in vertebrates, including the zebrafish, mouse, and human, often as members of multigene families.
- Knowledge of gene function has been acquired by **reverse genetics** using model systems with loss- or gain-of-function transgenic approaches and by **forward genetics** beginning with the description of abnormal phenotypes arising spontaneously in mouse and humans and then subsequent identification of the mutant gene.

- There is evidence of *cross-talk* among pathways. This communication among various signaling pathways facilitates our understanding of the far-reaching consequences of single gene mutations that result in malformation syndromes affecting the development of multiple organ systems or in cancers.

References and Suggested Reading

Abate-Shen C: Deregulated homeobox gene expression in cancer: cause or consequence? Nat Rev Cancer: 2:777, 2002.

Appel B, Eisen JS: Retinoids run rampant: multiple roles during spinal cord and motor neuron development. Neuron 40:461, 2003.

Ausio J, Levin DB, De Amorim GV, Bakker S, Macleod PM: Syndromes of disordered chromatin remodeling. Clin Genet 64:83, 2003.

Bianchi S, Dotti MT, Federico A: Physiology and pathology of Notch signaling system. J Cell Physiol 207:300, 2006.

Charron F, Tessier-Lavigne M: Novel brain wiring functions for classical morphogens: A role as graded positional cues in axon guidance. Development 132:2251, 2005.

Chizhikov VV, Millen KJ: Roof plate-dependent patterning of the vertebrate dorsal central nervous system. Dev Biol 277:287, 2005.

Coultas L, Chawengsaksophak K, Rossant J: Endothelial cells and VEGF in vascular development. Nature 438:937, 2006.

Dellovade T, Romer JT, Curran T, Rubin LJ: The hedgehog pathway and neurological disorders. Annu Rev Neurosci 29:539, 2006.

Eisenberg LM, Eisenberg CA: Wnt signal transduction and the formation of the myocardium. Dev Biol 293:305, 2006.

Gale NW, Yancopoulos GD: Growth factors acting via endothelial cell-specific receptor tyrosine kinases: VEGFs, angiopoietins, and ephrins in vascular development. Genes Dev 13:1055, 1999.

Hooper JE, Scott MP: Communicating with hedgehogs. Nat Rev Mol Cell Biol 6:306, 2005.

Kageyama R, Ohtsuka T, Hatakeyama J, Ohsawa R: Roles of bHLH genes in neural stem cell differentiation. Exp Cell Res 306:343, 2005.

Larsson J, Karlsson S: The role of Smad signaling in hematopoiesis. Oncogene 24:5676, 2005.

Lee JE: Basic helix-loop-helix genes in neural development. Curr Opin Neurobiol 7:13, 1997.

Li F, Chong ZZ, Maiese K: Winding through the WNT pathway during cellular development and demise. Histol Histopathol 21:103, 2006.

Louvi A, Artavanis-Tsakonas S: Notch signaling in vertebrate neural development. Nat Rev Neurosci 7:93, 2006.

Lupo G, Harris WA, Lewis KE: Mechanisms of ventral patterning in the vertebrate nervous system. Nat Rev Neurosci 7:103, 2006.

Marino S: Medulloblastoma: Developmental mechanisms out of control. Trends Mol Med 11:17, 2005.

Marlétaz F, Holland L, Laudet V, Schubert M: Retinoic acid signaling and the evolution of chordates. Int J Biol Sci 2:38, 2006.

Parker MH, Seale P, Rudnicki MA: Looking back to the embryo: Defining transcriptional networks in adult myogenesis. Nat Rev Genet 4:497, 2003.

Pearson JC, Lemons D, McGinnis W: Modulating Hox gene functions during animal body patterning. Nat Rev Genet 6:893, 2005.

Robson EJ, He SJ, Eccles MR: A PANorama of PAX genes in cancer and development. Nat Rev Cancer 6:52, 2006.

Staal FJT, Clevers HC: Wnt signaling and haematopoiesis: A Wnt-Wnt situation. Nat Rev Immunol 5:21, 2005.

Stecca B, Ruiz i Altaba A: Brain as a paradigm of organ growth: Hedgehog-gli signaling in neural stem cells and brain tumors. J Neurobiol 64:476, 2005.

Tian T, Meng AM: Nodal signals pattern vertebrate embryos. Cell Mol Life Sci 63:672, 2006.

Villavicencio EH, Walterhouse DO, Iannaccone PM: The sonic hedgehog-Patched-Gli pathway in human development and disease. Am J Hum Genet 67:1047, 2000.

Wan M, Cao X: BMP signaling in skeletal development. Biochem Biophys Res Commun 328:651, 2005.

Yoon K, Gaiano N: Notch signaling in the mammalian central nervous system: Insights from mouse mutants. Nat Neurosci 8:709, 2005.

Zhu AJ, Scott MP: Incredible journey: How do developmental signals travel through tissue? Genes Dev 18:2985, 2004.

Appendix: Discussion of Clinically Oriented Problems

CHAPTER 1

1. At the beginning of its development, a human embryo is called a zygote. This is an appropriate term because zygotus means united and refers to the union of the oocyte and sperm. The term conceptus refers to all structures that develop from a zygote (e.g., the embryo, amnion, and chorionic sac). The terms, therefore, are not synonymous.
2. The term conceptus is used when referring to an embryo and its extraembryonic membranes, i.e., the products of conception. The term abortus refers to any product or all products of an abortion, that is, the embryo (or fetus) and its membranes, including the placenta. An abortus, therefore, is an aborted conceptus.
3. The development of secondary sexual characteristics occurs, reproductive functions begin, and sexual dimorphism becomes more obvious; consequently, the pubertal changes are not the same in males and females. The ages of presumptive puberty are 12 years in girls and 14 years in boys; however, variations occur.
4. Embryology refers to the study of embryonic development; clinically, it refers to embryonic and fetal development, that is, the study of prenatal development. Teratology refers to the study of abnormal embryonic and fetal development. It is the branch of embryology concerned with congenital anomalies or birth defects and their causes. Embryologic and teratologic studies are applicable to clinical studies because they indicate vulnerable prenatal periods of development.

CHAPTER 2

1. Numerical changes in chromosomes arise chiefly from nondisjunction during a mitotic or meiotic cell division. Most clinically important abnormalities in chromosome number occur during the first meiotic division. Nondisjunction is the failure of double chromatid chromosomes to dissociate during anaphase of cell division. As a result, both chromosomes pass to the same daughter cell and trisomy results. Trisomy 21 (Down syndrome) is the most common numerical chromosomal disorder resulting in congenital anomalies. This syndrome occurs approximately once in every 700 births in women 30 to 34 years of age; however, it is more common in older mothers.
2. A morula with an extra set of chromosomes in its cells is called a triploid embryo. This chromosome abnormality usually results from fertilization of an oocyte by two sperms (dispermy). A fetus could develop from a triploid morula and be born alive; however, this is unusual. Most triploid fetuses abort spontaneously or are stillborn, and most triploid infants die shortly after birth.
3. Blockage of the uterine tubes resulting from infection is a major cause of infertility in women. Because occlusion prevents the oocyte from coming into contact with sperms, fertilization cannot occur. Infertility in men usually results from defects in spermatogenesis. Nondescent of the testes is one cause of aspermatogenesis (failure of sperm formation); however, normally positioned testes may not produce adequate numbers of actively motile sperms.
4. Mosaicism results from nondisjunction of double chromatid chromosomes during early cleavage of a zygote rather than during gametogenesis. As a consequence, the embryo has two cell lines with different chromosome numbers. Persons who develop from these chromosomally abnormal embryos are mosaics. Approximately 1% of persons with Down syndrome are mosaics. They have relatively mild stigmata of the syndrome and are less retarded than usual. Mosaicism can be detected before birth by cytogenetic studies after amniocentesis and chorionic villus sampling (see Chapter 6).
5. Postcoital birth control pills ("morning after pills") may be prescribed in an emergency (e.g., after sexual abuse). Ovarian hormones (estrogen) taken in large doses within 72 hours after sexual intercourse usually prevent implantation of the blastocyst, probably by altering tubal motility, interfering with corpus luteum function, or causing abnormal changes in the endometrium. These hormones prevent implantation, not fertilization. Consequently, they should not be called contraceptive pills. Conception occurs, but the blastocyst does not implant. It would be more appropriate to call them "contraimplantation pills." Because the term *abortion* refers to a premature stoppage of a pregnancy, the term abortion could be applied to such an early termination of pregnancy.
6. Many early embryos are spontaneously aborted. The overall early spontaneous abortion rate is approximately 45%. The common cause of early spontaneous abortion is the presence of chromosomal abnormalities, such as those resulting from nondisjunction, failure of one or more pairs of chromosomes to separate.
7. It has been estimated that between 12% and 25% of couples in North America are infertilie. One third to one half of these cases are due to male infertility. Male infertility may result from endocrine disorders, abnormal spermatogenesis, or blockage of a genital duct. First, Jerry's semen should be evaluated (sperm analysis). The total number, motility, and morphology of the sperms in the ejaculate are assessed in cases of male infertility. A man with fewer than 10 million

sperms per milliliter of semen is likely to be sterile, especially when the specimen of semen contains immotile and morphologically abnormal sperms.

CHAPTER 3

1. Yes, a chest radiograph could be taken because the patient's uterus and ovaries are not directly in the x-ray beam. The only radiation that the ovaries receive would be a negligible, scattered amount. Furthermore, this small amount of radiation would be highly unlikely to damage the products of conception if the patient happened to be pregnant. Most physicians, however, would defer the radiographic examination of the thorax if at all possible, because if the woman had an abnormal child, she might sue the physician, claiming that the x-rays produced the abnormality. A jury may not accept the scientific evidence of the nonteratogenicity of low-dose radiation.
2. Diethylstilbestrol (DES) appears to affect the endometrium by rendering it unprepared for implantation, a process that is regulated by a delicate balance between estrogen and progesterone. The large doses of estrogen would upset this balance. Progesterone makes the endometrium grow thick and succulent so that the blastocyst may become embedded and nourished adequately. DES pills are referred to as "morning after pills" by laypersons. When the media refer to the "abortion pill," they are usually referring to RU486. This drug, developed in France, interferes with implantation of the blastocyst by blocking the production of progesterone by the corpus luteum. A pregnancy can be detected at the end of the second week after fertilization using highly sensitive pregnancy tests. Most tests depend on the presence of an early pregnancy factor in the maternal serum. Early pregnancy can also be detected by ultrasonography.
3. More than 95% of ectopic pregnancies are in the uterine tube, and 60% of them are in the ampulla of the tube. Endovaginal sonography is often used to detect ectopic tubal pregnancies. The surgeon would likely perform a laparoscopic operation to remove the uterine tube containing the conceptus.
4. No, the surgery could not have produced the anomaly of the brain. Exposure of an embryo during the second week of development to the slight trauma that might be associated with abdominal surgery would not cause a congenital anomaly. Furthermore, the anesthetics used during the operation would not induce an anomaly of the brain. Teratogens present during the first 2 weeks of development are not known to induce congenital anomalies.
5. Women older than 40 years of age are more likely to have a baby with congenital anomalies such as Down syndrome; however, women older than 40 may have normal children. Prenatal diagnosis (e.g., using chorionic villi sampling [CVS] or amniocentesis) is now available for women older than 35 years of age. This procedure will tell whether the embryo has severe chromosomal abnormalities (e.g., trisomy 13) that would cause its death shortly after birth. Ultrasound examination of the embryo in utero may also be performed for the detection of certain morphologic anomalies (e.g., anomalies of the limbs and central nervous system). In most cases, the embryo is normal and the pregnancy continues to full term.

CHAPTER 4

1. The hormones in contraceptive (birth control) pills prevent ovulation and development of the luteal (secretory) stage of the menstrual (uterine) cycle. Severe chromosomal abnormalities may have caused the spontaneous abortion. The incidence of chromosomal abnormalities in early abortions is high in women who become pregnant shortly after discontinuing the use of birth control pills. A pronounced increase in polyploidy (cells containing three or more times the haploid number of chromosomes) has been observed in embryos expelled during spontaneous abortions when conception occurred within 2 months after discontinuing oral contraception. Polyploidy is fatal to the developing embryo. This information suggests that it is wise to use some other type of contraception for one or two menstrual cycles before attempting pregnancy after discontinuing oral contraceptives. In the present case, the physician probably told the patient that her abortion was a natural screening process and that it was probably the spontaneous expulsion of an embryo that could not have survived because it likely had severe chromosomal abnormalities. Some women have become pregnant 1 month after discontinuing the use of contraceptive pills and have given birth to normal babies.
2. A highly sensitive radioimmune test would likely indicate that the woman was pregnant. The presence of embryonic and/or chorionic tissue in the endometrial remnants would be an absolute sign of pregnancy. By 5 days after the expected menses (approximately 5 weeks after the last normal menstrual period [LNMP]), the embryo would be in the third week of its development. The blastocyst would be approximately 2 mm in diameter and can be detected with current transvaginal ultrasound techniques.
3. The central nervous system (brain and spinal cord) begins to develop during the third embryonic week. Meroencephaly (anencephaly), in which most of the brain and calvaria are absent, may result from environmental teratogens acting during the third week of development. This severe anomaly of the brain occurs because of failure of the cranial part of the neural tube to develop normally, which usually results from nonclosure of the rostral neuropore.
4. Sacrococcygeal teratomas arise from remnants of the primitive streak. Because cells from the primitive streak are pluripotent, the tumors contain various types of tissue derived from all three germ layers. There is a clear-cut difference in the incidence of these tumors with regard to sex; they are three to four times more frequent in girls than in boys.

5. Endovaginal sonography is an important technique for assessing pregnancy during the third week because the conceptus can be visualized. It is, therefore, possible to determine whether the embryo is developing normally. A negative pregnancy test in the third week does not rule out an ectopic pregnancy because ectopic pregnancies produce human chorionic gonadotrophin at a slower rate than intrauterine pregnancies. This hormone is the basis of pregnancy tests.

CHAPTER 5

1. The physician would likely tell the patient that her embryo was undergoing a critical stage of its development and that it would be safest for her baby if she were to stop smoking and avoid taking any unprescribed medication throughout her pregnancy. The physician would also likely tell her that heavy cigarette smoking is known to cause intrauterine growth restriction (IUGR) and underweight babies and that the incidence of prematurity increases with the number of cigarettes smoked. The physician would also recommend that she not consume alcohol during her pregnancy because of its known teratogenic effects (see fetal alcohol syndrome in Chapter 20).
2. The embryonic period is the most critical period of development because all the main tissues and organs are forming. It is the time when the embryo is most vulnerable to the injurious effects of environmental agents (e.g., large doses of radiation, drugs, and certain viruses).
3. One cannot predict how a drug will affect the human embryo because human and animal embryos may differ in their response to a drug; for example, thalidomide is extremely teratogenic to human embryos but has very little effect on some experimental animals such as rats and mice. Drugs known to be strong teratogens in animals should not be used during human pregnancy, especially during the embryonic period. The germ layers form during gastrulation. All tissues and organs of the embryo develop from the three germ layers: ectoderm, mesoderm, and endoderm. Formation of the primitive streak and notochord are important events during morphogenesis.
4. Information about the starting date of a pregnancy may be unreliable because it depends on the patient's remembering an event (last menses) that occurred 2 or 3 months earlier. In addition, she may have had implantation bleeding (breakthrough bleeding) at the time of her LNMP and may have thought that it was a light menses. Endovaginal sonography is reliable for estimating the probable starting date of a pregnancy and embryonic age.
5. No! To cause severe limb defects a known teratogenic drug would have to act during the critical period of limb development (24–36 days after fertilization). Teratogens interfere with differentiation of tissues and organs, often disrupting or arresting their development. See Chapter 20 for details.

CHAPTER 6

1. Physicians cannot always rely on information about the time of the LNMP provided by their patients, especially in cases in which determination of fertilization age is extremely important, for example, in high-risk pregnancies in which one might wish to induce labor as soon as possible. One can determine with reasonable accuracy the estimated date of confinement or expected date of delivery using diagnostic ultrasonography to estimate the size of the fetal head and abdomen. Normally labor would be induced after 36 to 37 weeks, using hormones (e.g., prostaglandins and oxytocin), unless there is a good reason to do so earlier.
2. CVS would likely be performed for study of the fetus's chromosomes. The most common chromosomal disorder detected in fetuses of women older than 40 years of age is trisomy 21. If the chromosomes of the fetus were normal but congenital abnormalities of the brain or limbs were suspected, ultrasonography would likely be performed. These methods allow one to look for morphologic abnormalities while scanning the entire fetus. The sex of the fetus could be determined by examining the sex chromosomes in cells obtained by CVS. One can often determine fetal sex using ultrasonography. In persons with technical experience, this method can be used to identify the sex (particularly male) with a certainty that approaches 100% after 30 weeks of gestation.
3. There is considerable danger when uncontrolled drugs (over-the-counter drugs) such as aspirin and cough medicine are consumed excessively or indiscriminately by pregnant women. Withdrawal seizures have been reported in infants born to mothers who are heavy drinkers, and fetal alcohol syndrome is present in some of these infants (see Chapter 20). The physician would likely tell the patient not to take any drugs that he or she does not prescribe. He or she might also tell her that drugs that are most detrimental to her fetus are under legal control and that they are dispensed with great care.
4. Many factors (fetal, maternal, and environmental) may reduce the rate of fetal growth (IUGR). Examples of such factors are intrauterine infections, multiple pregnancies, and chromosomal abnormalities (see Chapters 6 and 20). Cigarette smoking, narcotic addiction, and consumption of large amounts of alcohol are also well-established causes of IUGR. A mother interested in the growth and general well-being of her fetus consults her doctor frequently, eats a good-quality diet, and does not use narcotics, smoke, or drink alcohol.
5. Amniocentesis is relatively devoid of risk. The chance of inducing an abortion is estimated to be approximately 0.5%. CVS can also be used for obtaining cells for chromosome study. PUBS refers to percutaneous umbilical cord blood sampling. The needle is inserted into the umbilical vein with the guidance of ultrasonography. Chromosome and hormone studies can be performed on this blood.

6. Neural tube defects are indicated by high levels of alpha fetoprotein (AFP). Diagnostic studies would be done monitoring the levels of AFP. Further studies would be done using ultrasonography. Low levels of AFP may indicate Down syndrome. Chromosome studies would be done to check the chromosome complement of the fetal cells.

CHAPTER 7

1. The common method of estimating the expected date of confinement or estimated date of delivery is to count back 3 months from the first day of the LNMP and then add 1 year and 7 days (Nägele's rule; see Chapter 6). The biparietal diameter of the fetal head could be measured by ultrasonography in a high-risk obstetric patient because this measurement correlates well with fetal age. Foot measurements are also very helpful.
2. Polyhydramnios is the accumulation of an excessive amount of amniotic fluid. When it occurs over the course of a few days, there is an associated high risk of severe fetal anomalies, especially of the central nervous system (e.g., meroencephaly and spina bifida cystica). Fetuses with gross brain defects do not drink the usual amounts of amniotic fluid; hence, the amount of liquid increases. Atresia (blockage) of the esophagus is almost always accompanied by polyhydramnios because the fetus cannot swallow and absorb amniotic fluid. Twinning is also a predisposing cause of polyhydramnios.
3. There is a tendency for twins to "run in families." It appears unlikely that there is a genetic factor in monozygotic (MZ) twinning, but a disposition to dizygotic (DZ) twinning is genetically determined. The frequency of DZ twinning increases sharply with maternal age up to 35 years and then decreases; however, the frequency of MZ twinning is affected very little by the age of the mother. Determination of twin zygosity can usually be made by examining the placenta and fetal membranes. One can later determine zygosity by looking for genetically determined similarities and differences in a twin pair. Differences in genetic markers prove that twins are DZ.
4. A single umbilical artery occurs in approximately 1 of every 200 umbilical cords. This abnormality is accompanied by a 15% to 20% incidence of cardiovascular abnormalities.
5. Two zygotes were fertilized. The resulting blastocysts implanted close together and the placentas fused. The sample of chorionic villi was obtained from the chorionic sac of the female twin. If two chorionic sacs had been observed during ultrasonography, DZ twinning would have been suspected.
6. Amniotic bands form when the amnion tears during pregnancy. The bands surround parts of the embryo's body and produce anomalies such as absence of a hand or deep grooves in a limb; this constitutes **amniotic band syndrome** or the amniotic band disruption complex.

CHAPTER 8

1. A diagnosis of congenital diaphragmatic hernia (CDH) is most likely. The congenital defect in the diaphragm that produces this hernia usually results from the failure of the left pericardioperitoneal canal to close during the sixth week of development; consequently, herniation of abdominal organs into the thorax occurs. This compresses the lungs, especially the left one, and results in respiratory distress. The diagnosis can usually be established by a radiographic or sonographic examination of the chest. The anomaly can also be detected prenatally using ultrasonography. Characteristically, there are air- and/or fluid-filled loops of intestine in the left hemithorax of a newborn infant afflicted with CDH.
2. In the very rare congenital anomaly retrosternal hernia, the intestine may herniate into the pericardial sac, or, conversely, the heart may be displaced into the superior part of the peritoneal cavity. Herniation of the intestine through the sternocostal hiatus causes this condition.
3. CDH occurs approximately once in every 2200 births. A newborn infant in whom a diagnosis of CDH is suspected would immediately be positioned with the head and thorax higher than the abdomen to facilitate the inferior displacement of the abdominal organs from the thorax. After a period of preoperative stabilization, an operation is performed with reduction of the abdominal viscera and closure of the diaphragmatic defect. Mortality rates are approximately 60%. Newborns with CDH often die because of severe respiratory distress from poor development of the lungs.
4. Gastroschisis and epigastric hernias occur in the median plane of the epigastric region. This hernia is uncommon. The defect through which herniation occurs results from failure of the lateral body folds to fuse in this region during the fourth week.

CHAPTER 9

1. The most likely diagnosis is a branchial sinus. When the sinus becomes infected, an intermittent discharge of mucoid material occurs. The material was probably discharged from an external branchial sinus, a remnant of the second pharyngeal groove and/or cervical sinus. Normally, this groove and sinus disappear as the neck forms.
2. The position of the inferior parathyroid glands is variable. They develop in close association with the thymus and are carried caudally with it during its descent through the neck. If the thymus fails to descend to its usual position in the superior mediastinum, one or both inferior parathyroid glands may be located near the bifurcation of the common carotid artery. If an inferior parathyroid gland does not separate from the thymus, it may be carried into the superior mediastinum with the thymus.
3. The patient very likely has a thyroglossal duct cyst that arose from a small remnant of the embryonic

thyroglossal duct. When complete degeneration of this duct does not occur, a cyst may form from it anywhere along the median plane of the neck between the foramen cecum of the tongue and the jugular notch in the manubrium of the sternum. A thyroglossal duct cyst may be confused with an ectopic thyroid gland, such as one that has not descended to its normal position in the neck.

4. Unilateral cleft lip results from failure of the maxillary prominence on the affected side to fuse with the merged medial nasal prominences. Clefting of the maxilla anterior to the incisive fossa results from failure of the lateral palatal process to fuse with the primary palate. Approximately 60% to 80% of persons who have a cleft lip, with or without cleft palate, are males. When both parents are normal and have had one child with a cleft lip, the chance that the next infant will have the same lip anomaly is approximately 4%.
5. There is substantial evidence that anticonvulsant drugs, such as phenytoin or diphenylhydantoin, when given to epileptic women during pregnancy, increase by two- to threefold the incidence of cleft lip and cleft palate when compared with the general population. Cleft lip with cleft palate is caused by many factors, some genetic and others environmental; therefore, this condition has a multifactorial etiology. In most cases, the environmental factor involved is not identifiable.

CHAPTER 10

1. Inability to pass a catheter through the esophagus into the stomach indicates esophageal atresia. Because this anomaly is commonly associated with tracheoesophageal fistula, the pediatrician would suspect this anomaly. A radiographic or sonographic examination would demonstrate the atresia. The presence of this anomaly would be confirmed by imaging the nasogastric tube arrested in the proximal esophageal pouch. If necessary, a small amount of air would be injected to highlight the image. When a certain type of tracheoesophageal fistula (TEF) is present, there would also be air in the stomach that passed to it from a connection between the esophagus and the trachea. A combined radiographic, endoscopic, and surgical approach would usually be used to detect and remove a TEF.
2. An infant with respiratory distress syndrome (RDS) or hyaline membrane disease tries to overcome the ventilatory problem by increasing the rate and depth of respiration. Intercostal, subcostal, sternal retractions, and nasal flaring are prominent signs of respiratory distress. Hyaline membrane disease is a leading cause of RDS and death in live-born, premature infants. A deficiency of pulmonary surfactant is associated with RDS. Glucocorticoid treatment may be given during pregnancy to accelerate fetal lung development and surfactant production.
3. The most common type of TEF connects the trachea with the inferior part of the esophagus. This anomaly is associated with atresia of the esophagus superior to the fistula. A TEF results from incomplete division of the foregut by the tracheoesophageal septum into the esophagus and trachea.
4. In most types of TEF, air passes from the trachea through the TEF into the esophagus and stomach. Pneumonitis (pneumonia) resulting from the aspiration of oral and nasal secretions into the lungs is a serious complication of this anomaly. Giving the baby water or food by mouth is obviously contraindicated in such cases.

CHAPTER 11

1. Complete absence of a lumen (duodenal atresia) usually involves the second (descending) and third (horizontal) parts of the duodenum. The obstruction usually results from incomplete vacuolization of the lumen of the duodenum during the eighth week. The obstruction causes distention of the stomach and proximal duodenum because the fetus swallows amniotic fluid, and the newborn infant swallows air, mucus, and milk. Duodenal atresia is common in infants with Down syndrome, as are other severe congenital anomalies such as anular pancreas, cardiovascular abnormalities, malrotation of the midgut, and anorectal anomalies. Polyhydramnios occurs because the duodenal atresia prevents normal absorption of amniotic fluid from the fetal intestine distal to the obstruction. The fetus swallows amniotic fluid before birth; however, because of duodenal atresia, this fluid cannot pass along the bowel, be absorbed into the fetal circulation, and be transferred across the placental membrane into the mother's circulation from which it enters her urine.
2. The omphaloenteric duct (yolk stalk) normally undergoes complete involution by the 10th week of development, at which time the intestines return to the abdomen. In 2% to 4% of people, a remnant of the omphaloenteric duct persists as a diverticulum of the ileum—Meckel diverticulum—however, only a small number of these anomalies ever become symptomatic. In the present case, the entire omphaloenteric duct persisted so that the diverticulum was connected to the anterior abdominal wall and umbilicus by a sinus tract. This anomaly is rare, and its external opening may be confused with a granuloma (inflammatory lesion) of the stump of the umbilical cord.
3. The fistula was likely connected to the blind end of the rectum. The anomaly—imperforate anus with a rectovaginal fistula—results from failure of the urorectal septum to form a complete separation between the anterior and posterior parts of the urogenital sinus. Because the inferior one third of the vagina forms from the anterior part of the urogenital sinus, it joins the rectum, which forms from the posterior part of the sinus.
4. This anomaly is an omphalocele (exomphalos). A small omphalocele, like the one described here, is sometimes called an umbilical cord hernia; however, it should not

be confused with an umbilical hernia that occurs after birth and is covered by skin. The thin membrane covering the mass in the present case would be composed of peritoneum and amnion. The hernia would be composed of small intestinal loops. Omphalocele occurs when the intestinal loops fail to return to the abdominal cavity from the umbilical cord during the 10th week of fetal life. In the present case, because the hernia is relatively small, the intestine may have entered the abdominal cavity and then herniated later when the rectus muscles did not approach each other close enough to occlude the circular defect in the anterior abdominal wall.

5. The ileum was probably obstructed—ileal atresia. Congenital atresia of the small bowel involves the ileum most frequently; the next most frequently affected region is the duodenum. The jejunum is involved least often. Some meconium (fetal feces) is formed from exfoliated fetal epithelium and mucus in the intestinal lumen and is located distal to the obstructed area (atretic segment). At operation, the atretic ileum would probably appear as a narrow segment connecting the proximal and distal segments of the small bowel. Atresia of the ileum could result from failure of recanalization of the lumen; more likely, the ileal atresia occurred because of a prenatal interruption of the blood supply to the ileum. Sometimes a loop of small bowel becomes twisted, interrupting its blood supply and causing necrosis (death) of the affected segment. The atretic section of bowel usually becomes a fibrous cord connecting the proximal and distal segments of bowel.

CHAPTER 12

1. Double renal pelves and ureters result from the formation of two metanephric diverticula (ureteric buds) on one side of the embryo. Subsequently, the primordia of these structures fuse. Both ureters usually open into the urinary bladder. Occasionally, the extra ureter opens into the urogenital tract inferior to the bladder. This occurs when the accessory ureter is not incorporated into the base of the bladder with the other ureter; instead, the extra ureter is carried caudally with the mesonephric duct and opens with it into the caudal part of the urogenital sinus. Because this part of the urogenital sinus gives rise to the urethra and the epithelium of the vagina, the ectopic (abnormally placed) ureteric orifice may be located in either of these structures, which accounts for the continual dribbling of urine into the vagina. An ectopic ureteral orifice that opens inferior to the bladder results in urinary incontinence because there is no urinary bladder or urethral sphincter between it and the exterior. Normally, the oblique passage of the ureter through the wall of the bladder allows the contraction of the bladder musculature to act like a sphincter for the ureter, controlling the flow of urine from it.
2. Accessory or supernumerary renal arteries are very common. Approximately 25% of kidneys receive two or more branches directly from the aorta; however, more than two is exceptional. Supernumerary arteries enter either through the renal sinus or at the poles of the kidney, usually the inferior pole. Accessory renal arteries, more common on the left side, represent persistent fetal renal arteries that grow out in sequence from the aorta as the kidneys "ascend" from the pelvis to the abdomen. Usually, the inferior vessels degenerate as new ones develop. Supernumerary arteries are approximately twice as common as supernumerary veins. They usually arise at the level of the kidney. The presence of a supernumerary artery is of clinical importance in other circumstances because it may cross the ureteropelvic junction and hinder urine outflow, leading to dilation of the calices and pelvis on the same side (hydronephrosis). Hydronephrotic kidneys frequently become infected (pyelonephritis); infection may lead to destruction of the kidneys.
3. Rudimentary horn pregnancies are very rare; they are clinically important, however, because it is difficult to distinguish between this type of pregnancy and a tubal pregnancy (see text). In the present case, the uterine anomaly was the result of retarded growth of the right paramesonephric duct and incomplete fusion of this duct with its partner during development of the uterus. Most anomalies resulting from incomplete fusion of the paramesonephric ducts do not cause clinical problems; however, a rudimentary horn that does not communicate with the main part of the uterus may cause pain during the menstrual period because of distention of the horn by blood. Because most rudimentary uterine horns are thicker than uterine tubes, a rudimentary horn pregnancy is likely to rupture much later than a tubal pregnancy.
4. Hypospadias of the glans is the term applied to an anomaly in which the urethral orifice is on the ventral surface of the penis near the glans penis. The ventral curving of the penis is called chordee. Hypospadias of the glans results from failure of the urogenital folds on the ventral surface of the developing penis to fuse completely and establish communication with the terminal part of the spongy urethra within the glans penis. Hypospadias may be associated with an inadequate production of androgens by the fetal testes, or there may be resistance to the hormones at the cellular level in the urogenital folds. Hypospadias is thought to have a multifactorial etiology because close relatives of patients with hypospadias are more likely to have the anomaly than the general population. Glanular hypospadias, or hypospadias of the glans, a common anomaly of the urogenital tract, occurs in approximately one in every 300 male infants.
5. This young woman is female, although she has a 46, XY chromosome complement. She has the androgen insensitivity syndrome. Failure of masculinization to occur in these individuals results from a resistance to the action of testosterone at the cellular level in genitalia.
6. The embryologic basis of indirect inguinal hernia is persistence of the processus vaginalis, a fetal outpouching of peritoneum. This fingerlike pouch

evaginates the anterior abdominal wall and forms the inguinal canal. A persistent processus vaginalis predisposes to indirect inguinal hernia by creating a weakness in the anterior abdominal wall and a hernial sac into which abdominal contents may herniate if the intra-abdominal pressure becomes very high (as occurs during straining). The hernial sac would be covered by internal spermatic fascia, cremaster muscle, and cremasteric fascia. For more information about inguinal hernias, see the text.

CHAPTER 13

1. Ventricular septal defect (VSD) is the most common cardiac defect. It occurs in approximately 25% of children with congenital heart disease. Most patients with a large VSD have a massive left-to-right shunt of blood, which causes cyanosis and congestive heart failure.
2. Patent ductus arteriosus (PDA) is the most common cardiovascular anomaly associated with maternal rubella infection during early pregnancy. When the ductus arteriosus is patent in an infant, aortic blood is shunted into the pulmonary artery. One half to two thirds of the left ventricular output may be shunted through the PDA. This extra work for the heart results in cardiac enlargement.
3. The tetrad of cardiac abnormalities present in the tetralogy of Fallot is pulmonary stenosis, VSD, overriding aorta, and right ventricular hypertrophy. Angiocardiography or ultrasonography could be used to reveal the malpositioned aorta (straddling the VSD) and the degree of pulmonary stenosis. Cyanosis occurs because of the shunting of unsaturated blood; however, it may not be present at birth. The main aim of therapy is to improve the oxygenation of the blood in the infant, usually by surgical correction of the pulmonary stenosis and closure of the VSD.
4. Cardiac catheterization and ultrasonography would probably be performed to confirm the diagnosis of transposition of the great arteries. If this anomaly is present, a bolus of contrast material injected into the right ventricle would enter the aorta, whereas contrast material injected into the left ventricle would enter the pulmonary circulation. The infant was able to survive after birth because the ductus arteriosus remains open in these infants, allowing some mixing of blood between the two circulations. In other cases, there is also an atrial septal defect (ASD) or VSD that permits intermixing of blood. Complete transposition of the great arteries is incompatible with life if there are no associated septal defects or a PDA.
5. This would probably be a secundum type of ASD. It would be located in the region of the oval fossa because this is the most common type of clinically significant ASD. Large defects, as in the present case, often extend toward the inferior vena cava. The pulmonary artery and its major branches are dilated because of the increased blood flow through the lungs and the increased pressure within the pulmonary circulation. In these cases, a considerable shunt of oxygenated blood flows from the left atrium to the right atrium. This blood, along with the normal venous return to the right atrium, enters the right ventricle and is pumped to the lungs. Large ASDs may be tolerated for a long time, as in the present case, but progressive dilation of the right ventricle often leads to heart failure.

CHAPTER 14

1. The common congenital anomaly of the vertebral column is spina bifida occulta. This defect of the vertebral arch of the first sacral and/or last lumbar vertebra is present in approximately 10% of people. The defect also occurs in cervical and thoracic vertebrae. The spinal cord and nerves are usually normal, and neurologic symptoms are usually absent. Spina bifida occulta does not cause back problems in most people.
2. A rib associated with the seventh cervical vertebra is of clinical importance because it may compress the subclavian artery and/or brachial plexus, producing symptoms of artery and nerve compression. In most cases, cervical ribs produce no symptoms. These ribs develop from the costal processes of the seventh cervical vertebra. Cervical ribs are present in 0.5% to 1% of people.
3. A hemivertebra can produce a lateral curvature of the vertebral column (scoliosis). A hemivertebra is composed of one half of a body, a pedicle, and a lamina. This anomaly results when the mesenchymal cells from the sclerotomes on one side fail to form the primordium of half of a vertebra. As a result, there are more growth centers on the one side of the vertebral column; this imbalance causes the vertebral column to bend laterally.
4. Craniosynostosis indicates premature closure of one or more of the cranial sutures. This developmental abnormality results in malformations of the cranium. Scaphocephaly, a long narrow cranium, results from premature closure of the sagittal suture. This type of craniosynostosis accounts for approximately 50% of the cases. Brain development is normal in these infants.
5. The features of Klippel-Feil syndrome are short neck, low hairline, and restricted neck movements. In most cases, the number of cervical vertebral bodies is less than normal.

CHAPTER 15

1. Absence of the sternocostal portion of the left pectoralis major muscle is the cause of the abnormal surface features observed. The costal heads of the pectoralis major and pectoralis minor muscles are usually present. Despite its numerous and important actions, absence of all or part of the pectoralis major muscle usually causes no disability; however, the abnormality caused by absence of the anterior axillary

fold is striking, as is the inferior location of the nipple. The actions of other muscles associated with the shoulder joint compensate for the absence of part of the pectoralis major.

2. Approximately 13% of people lack a palmaris longus muscle on one or both sides. Its absence causes no disability.
3. It would be the left sternocleidomastoid muscle that was prominent when tensed. The left one is the unaffected muscle, and it does not pull the child's head to the right side. It is the short, contracted right sternocleidomastoid muscle that tethers the right mastoid process to the right clavicle and sternum; hence, continued growth of the left side of the neck results in tilting and rotation of the head. This relatively common condition—congenital torticollis (wryneck)—may occur because of injury to the muscle during birth. Tearing of some muscle fibers may have occurred, resulting in bleeding into the muscle. Over several weeks, necrosis of some fibers would have occurred, and the blood was replaced by fibrous tissue. This could result in shortening of the muscle and in pulling of the child's head to the side.
4. Absence of striated musculature in the median plane of the anterior abdominal wall of the embryo is associated with exstrophy of the urinary bladder. This severe anomaly is caused by incomplete midline closure of the inferior part of the anterior abdominal wall, and failure of mesenchymal cells to migrate from the somatic mesoderm between the surface ectoderm and the urogenital sinus during the fourth week of development. The absence of mesenchymal cells in the median plane results in failure of striated muscles to develop.

CHAPTER 16

1. The number of female infants with dislocation of the hip is approximately eight times that of male infants. The hip joint is not usually dislocated at birth; however, the acetabulum is underdeveloped. Dislocation of the hip may not become obvious until the infant attempts to stand approximately 12 months after birth. This condition is probably caused by deforming forces acting directly on the hip joint of the fetus.
2. Severe anomalies of the limbs (amelia and meromelia), similar to those produced by thalidomide, are rare and usually have a genetic basis. The thalidomide syndrome consisted of absence of limbs (amelia), gross defects of the limbs (meromelia) such as the hands and feet attached to the trunk by small, irregularly shaped bones, intestinal atresia, and cardiac defects.
3. The most common type of clubfoot is talipes equinovarus, occurring in approximately one of every 1000 newborn infants. In this deformation, the soles of the feet are turned medially and the feet are sharply plantarflexed. The feet are fixed in the tiptoe position, resembling the foot of a horse (Latin. *equinus*, horse).
4. Syndactyly (fusion of digits) is the most common type of limb anomaly. It varies from cutaneous webbing of the digits to synostosis (union of phalanges, the bones of the digits). Syndactyly is more common in the foot than in the hand. This anomaly occurs when separate digital rays fail to form in the fifth week, or the webbing between the developing digits fails to break down between the sixth and eighth weeks. As a consequence, separation of the digits does not occur.

CHAPTER 17

1. Ultrasound scanning of the fetus can detect absence of the calvaria (acrania) as early as 14 weeks (see Fig. 17-37). Fetuses with meroencephaly (absence of part of brain) do not drink the usual amounts of amniotic fluid, presumably because of impairment of the neuromuscular mechanism that controls swallowing. Because fetal urine is excreted into the amniotic fluid at the usual rate, the amount of amniotic fluid increases. Normally, the fetus swallows amniotic fluid, which is absorbed by its intestines and passed to the placenta for elimination through the mother's blood and kidneys. Meroencephaly, often inaccurately called anencephaly (absence of the brain), can be easily and safely detected by a plain radiograph; however, radiographs of the fetus are not usually obtained. Instead, this severe anomaly is usually detected by ultrasonography or amniocentesis. An elevated level of alpha fetoprotein in the amniotic fluid indicates an open neural tube defect, such as acrania with meroencephaly or spina bifida with myeloschisis.
2. A neurologic defect is associated with meningomyelocele because the spinal cord and/or nerve roots are often incorporated into the wall of the protruding sac. This damages the nerves supplying various structures. Paralysis of the lower limbs often occurs, and there may be incontinence of urine and feces resulting from paralysis of the sphincters of the anus and urinary bladder.
3. The condition is called obstructive hydrocephalus. The block would most likely be in the cerebral aqueduct of the midbrain. Obstruction at this site (stenosis or atresia) interferes with or prevents passage of ventricular fluid from the lateral and third ventricles to the fourth ventricle. Hydrocephalus is sometimes recognized before birth; however, most cases are diagnosed in the first few weeks or months after birth. Hydrocephalus can be recognized using ultrasonography of the mother's abdomen during the last trimester. Surgical treatment of hydrocephalus usually consists of shunting the excess ventricular fluid through a plastic tube to another part of the body (e.g., into the bloodstream or peritoneal cavity), from which it will subsequently be excreted by the infant's kidneys.
4. Hydrocephalus is not synonymous with a large head because a large brain (macroencephalon), a subdural hygroma, or a large hematoma can also cause enlargement of the head. Hydrocephalus may or may not enlarge the head. Hydrocephalus ex vacuo causes enlargement of the ventricles resulting from brain

destruction; however, the head is not enlarged. Microencephaly (small brain) is usually associated with microcephaly (small calvaria). Because growth of the cranium is largely dependent on growth of the brain, arrest of brain development can cause microcephaly. During the fetal period, environmental exposure to agents such as cytomegalovirus, *Toxoplasma gondii*, herpes simplex virus, and high-level radiation is known to induce microencephaly and microcephaly. Severe mental retardation may occur as a result of exposure of the embryo/fetus to high levels of radiation during the 8- to 16-week period of development.

5. Agenesis of the corpus callosum, partial or complete, is frequently associated with low intelligence in 70% of cases and seizures in 50% of patients. Some people are asymptomatic and lead normal lives. Agenesis of the corpus callosum may occur as an isolated defect; however, it is often associated with other central nervous system anomalies, such as holoprosencephalies—anomalies resulting from failure of cleavage of the prosencephalon (forebrain). As in the present case, a large third ventricle may be associated with agenesis of the corpus callosum. The large ventricle exists because it is able to rise superior to the roofs of the lateral ventricles when the corpus callosum is absent. The lateral ventricles are usually moderately enlarged.

CHAPTER 18

1. The mother had certainly contracted rubella or German measles during early pregnancy because her infant had the characteristic triad of anomalies resulting from infection of an embryo by the rubella virus. Cataract is common when severe infections occur during the first 6 weeks of pregnancy because the lens vesicle is forming. Congenital cataract is believed to result from invasion of the developing lens by the rubella virus. The most common cardiovascular lesion in infants whose mothers had rubella early in pregnancy is patent ductus arteriosus. Although a history of a rash during the first trimester of pregnancy is helpful for diagnosing the congenital rubella syndrome, embryopathy (embryonic disease) can occur after a subclinical maternal rubella infection (i.e., without a rash).
2. Congenital ptosis (drooping of superior [upper] eyelid) is usually caused by abnormal development or failure of development of the levator palpebrae superioris muscle. Congenital ptosis is usually transmitted by autosomal dominant inheritance; however, injury to the superior branch of the oculomotor nerve (cranial nerve III), which supplies the levator palpebrae superioris muscle, would also cause drooping of the upper eyelid.
3. The protozoon involved was *Toxoplasma gondii*, an intracellular parasite. The congenital anomalies result from invasion of the fetal bloodstream and developing organs by *Toxoplasma* parasites. These parasites disrupt development of the central nervous system, including the eyes, which develop from outgrowths of the brain (optic vesicles). The physician would certainly tell the woman about *Toxoplasma cysts* in meat and advise the woman to cook her meat well, especially if she decided to have more children. He or she would tell the woman that *Toxoplasma oocysts* are often found in cat feces and that it is important to wash her hands carefully after handling a cat or its litter box.
4. The infant had trisomy 18 because the characteristic phenotype of this type of trisomy is present. Low-set, malformed ears associated with severe mental deficiency, prominent occiput, congenital heart defect, and failure to thrive are all suggestive of the trisomy 18 syndrome. This numerical chromosomal abnormality results from nondisjunction of the number 18 chromosome pair during gametogenesis. Its incidence is approximately 1 in 8000 newborn infants. Probably 94% of trisomy 18 fetuses abort spontaneously. Postnatal survival of these infants is poor, with 30% dying within a month of birth; the mean survival time is only 2 months. Less than 10% of these infants survive more than a year.
5. Detachment of the retina is a separation of the two embryonic retinal layers: the neural pigment epithelium derived from the outer layer of the optic cup and the neural retina derived from the inner layer of the cup. The intraretinal space, representing the cavity of the optic vesicle, normally disappears as the retina forms. The proximal part of the hyaloid artery normally persists as the central artery of the retina; however, the distal part of this vessel normally degenerates.

CHAPTER 19

1. Natal teeth (L. *natus*, to be born) occur in approximately 1 in every 2000 newborn infants. There are usually two teeth in the position of the mandibular medial incisors. Natal teeth may be supernumerary ones; however, they are often prematurely erupted primary teeth. If it is established radiographically that they are supernumerary teeth, they would probably be removed so that they would not interfere with the subsequent eruption of the normal primary teeth. Natal teeth may cause maternal discomfort resulting from abrasion or biting of the nipple during nursing. They may also injure the infant's tongue, which, because the mandible is relatively small at birth, lies between the alveolar processes of the jaws.
2. The discoloration of the infant's teeth was likely caused by the administration of tetracycline to the mother during her pregnancy. Tetracyclines become incorporated into the developing enamel and dentine of the teeth and cause discoloration. Dysfunction of ameloblasts resulting from tetracycline therapy causes hypoplasia of the enamel (e.g., pitting). Most likely the secondary dentition would also be affected because enamel formation begins in the permanent teeth before birth (approximately 20 weeks in the incisors).
3. This is an angiomatous anomaly of the skin—a capillary angioma or hemangioma. It is formed by an overgrowth of small blood vessels consisting mostly of

capillaries; however, there are also some arterioles and venules in it. The blotch is red because oxygen is not taken from the blood passing through it. This type of angioma is quite common, and the mother should be assured that this anomaly is of no significance and requires no treatment. It will fade in a few years. Formerly this type of angioma was called a nevus flammeus (flamelike birthmark); however, these names are sometimes applied to other types of angiomas. To avoid confusion, it is better not to use them. Nevus is not a good term because it is derived from a Latin word meaning a mole or birthmark, which may or may not be an angioma.

4. A tuft of hair in the median plane of the back in the lumbosacral region usually indicates the presence of spina bifida occulta. This is the most common developmental anomaly of the vertebrae and is present in L5 and/or L1 in approximately 10% of otherwise normal people. Spina bifida occulta is usually of no clinical significance; however, some infants with this vertebral anomaly may also have a developmental defect of the underlying spinal cord and nerve roots.
5. The superficial layers of the epidermis of infants with lamellar ichthyosis, resulting from excessive keratinization, consist of fishlike, grayish-brown scales that are adherent in the center and raised at the edges. Fortunately, the condition is very rare. It is inherited as an autosomal recessive trait.

CHAPTER 20

1. Seven percent to 10% of congenital anomalies are caused by environmental factors such as drugs and chemicals. It is difficult for clinicians to assign specific defects to specific drugs for the following reasons:
   - The drug may be administered as therapy for an illness that itself may cause the anomaly.
   - The fetal anomaly may cause maternal symptoms that are treated with a drug.
   - The drug may prevent the spontaneous abortion of an already malformed fetus.
   - The drug may be used with another drug that causes the anomaly.

   Women should know that several drugs, for example, cocaine, cause severe anomalies if taken during pregnancy and that these drugs should be avoided.
2. Women older than the age of 35 years are more likely to have a child with Down syndrome or some other chromosomal disorder than are younger women (25–30 years). Nevertheless, most women older than the age of 35 have normal children. The physician caring for a pregnant 40-year-old woman would certainly recommend chorionic villi sampling and/or amniocentesis to determine whether the infant had a chromosomal disorder such as trisomy 21 or trisomy 13. A 44-year-old woman can have a normal baby; however, the chances of having a child with Down syndrome are 1 in 25.
3. Penicillin has been widely used during pregnancy for more than 30 years without any suggestion of teratogenicity. Small doses of aspirin and other salicylates are ingested by most pregnant women, and when they are consumed as directed by a physician, the teratogenic risk is very low. Chronic consumption of large doses of aspirin during early pregnancy may be harmful. Alcohol and other social drugs, such as cocaine, should be avoided.
4. The physician would certainly tell the mother that there was no danger that her child would develop cataracts and cardiac defects because she has German measles. He or she would undoubtedly explain that cataracts often develop in embryos whose mothers contract the disease early in pregnancy. They occur because of the damaging effect the rubella virus has on the developing lens. The physician might say that it is not necessarily bad for a girl to contract German measles before her childbearing years because this attack would probably confer permanent immunity to rubella.
5. Cats may be infected with the parasite *Toxoplasma gondii*. Therefore, it is prudent to avoid contact with the cats and their litter during her pregnancy. Oocysts of these parasites appear in the feces of cats and can be ingested if one is careless in handling the cat's litter. If the woman is pregnant, the parasite can cause severe fetal anomalies of the central nervous system such as mental retardation and blindness.

Index

Page numbers followed by an italic *f* or *t* denote figures or tables, respectively.

A
abdominal circumference, fetal, 98, 99*f*, 102
abdominal pregnancy, 47, 52*f*
abdominal wall defects, 229–231, 232*f*
ventral, alpha-fetoprotein assay for detection of, 105
abducent nerve, formation of, 414
abortion
accidental, definition of, 7
complete, definition of, 7
criminal, definition of, 7
definition of, 7
habitual, definition of, 7
induced, definition of, 7
legally induced, 7
missed, definition of, 7
spontaneous
abnormal embryos and, 39
definition of, 7
early, 49
of embryos, 48–49, 113*f*, 114*f*
multiple pregnancy and, 25
sporadic and recurrent, 48–49
therapeutic, 7
threatened, definition of, 7
abortus, definition of, 7
accessory auricular hillocks, 435, 436*f*
accessory diaphragm, 157
accessory hepatic ducts, 220
accessory lung, 208
accessory muscles, 362
accessory nerve, formation of, 415*f*, 416
accessory pancreatic tissue, 222, 234*f*
accessory placenta, 123–125, 128*f*
accessory renal arteries and veins, 250, 251*f*
accessory ribs, 350
accessory spleen, 224
accessory thymic tissue, 173, 173*f*
accessory thyroid tissue, 175, 176*f*
accidental abortion, definition of, 7
ACE inhibitors, as teratogens, 478–479
acetabulum, abnormal development of, 377
acetylsalicylic acid, fetal effects of, 479
achondroplasia, 355*f*, 470*f*
acini, 179, 222
acoustic meatus, external, 80, 88*f*, 169, 179, 433, 433*f*, 434, 434*f*
absence of, 436, 436*f*
atresia of, 436
acquired immunodeficiency syndrome (AIDS), fetal effects of, 481
acrania, 351*f*, 352, 405, 410*f*
acromegaly, 354
acrosin, and fertilization, 29, 31
acrosome, 19*f*, 20, 29, 30*f*
acrosome reaction, 29, 30*f*
ACTH (adrenocorticotropin)
and adrenal hyperplasia, 262
and labor, 123
active transport, placental, 118
activin(s)
and bone development, 341*f*, 342*f*
as common signaling pathway, 489
activin(s)—cont'd
and digestive system development, 212
and pancreatic development, 222
activin-receptor-like kinase ChALK2, and cardiovascular development, 295
adenocarcinoma, diethylstilbestrol exposure and, 477
adenohypophysis, 399, 399*t*, 401*f*, 417
adenoids. *See* pharyngeal tonsils
adipose tissue, fetal, 101–102, 103
adolescence, definition of, 7
adrenal hyperplasia, congenital (CAH), 262, 263*f*, 274*f*, 283, 477*f*
adrenal (suprarenal) glands, development of, 246*f*, 250*f*, 260
adrenocorticotropin (ACTH)
and adrenal hyperplasia, 262
and labor, 123
adrenogenital syndrome, 262
adulthood, definition of, 7
AFP. *See* Alpha-fetoprotein assay
Africanus, Constantinus, of Salerno, 9
afterbirth, 111, 123, 126*f*
aganglionic megacolon, congenital, 238, 238*f*
age
bone, 353, 355
conceptional, 85
embryonic, 83, 85, 86, 90
estimation of, 80*t*, 86
fertilization, 2, 15, 83
fetal, estimation of, 96, 98, 103*f*
gestational, 15, 96
definition of, 2
estimation of, 83
ultrasound assessment of, 89, 92*f*
maternal
and chromosomal abnormalities, 20, 105, 461, 465*t*
dizygotic twins and, 134
ideal, 21
menstrual, 15
presumptive, of puberty, 496
AIDS, fetal effects of, 481
ala orbitalis, 347, 348*f*
alar plate, 383, 386*f*, 388*f*, 394, 396*f*, 400*f*
ala temporalis, 348*f*
albinism, 444
generalized, 444
localized, 444
alcohol use
and congenital anomalies, 409, 472*t*, 476
and fetal growth, 104, 476
and mental retardation, 413, 417
allantoic cysts, 62, 134, 135*f*
allantois, 60*f*, 61*f*, 62–64, 74*f*, 134, 135*f*
cysts, 134, 135*f*
allograft, placenta as, 121
alopecia, 447
alpha-fetoprotein assay, 105
maternal serum, 389
for neural tube defect detection, 131, 388
alveolar cells, type II, 207
alveolar ducts, 203, 205*f*, 206
alveolar sacs, 206
alveolar period, of lung maturation, 204*f*, 205*f*, 206
alveolar processes, of teeth, 451
alveolocapillary membrane, 204*f*, 206
alveolus (alveoli), pulmonary
definition of, 206
development of, 204*f*, 205*f*, 206
alveolus of teeth, 450
amastia, 446
ambiguous genitalia, 273
amelia, 373, 375, 375*f*, 376, 472*t*, 473*f*
ameloblasts, 449, 450*f*, 451, 452, 455
amelogenesis imperfecta, 452–453, 455*f*
amino acids
in fetal metabolism and growth, 104
transplacental transport of, 119*f*, 120
aminopterin, as teratogen, 472*t*, 478
amnioblasts, 44
amniocentesis
diagnostic, 105
transabdominal, 105
amniochorionic membrane, 112*f*, 115*f*, 116–117
rupture of, 130, 133
amnion, 43*f*, 44, 46*f*, 47*f*, 50*f*, 56*f*, 128, 132*f*
number in twin pregnancies, 137*t*
rupture of, 133, 133*f*
amniotic band disruption complex, 499
amniotic band syndrome, 133, 133*f*
amniotic cavity, 43*f*, 51, 56*f*, 67*f*
formation of, 44–45
amniotic fluid, 128–133
circulation of, 128–130
composition of, 131
disorders of, 130–131 (*See also* Oligohydramnios; Polyhydramnios)
fetal swallowing of, 130
significance of, 131–133
volume of, 128
amniotic sac, 82*f*, 99*f*, 128
ampullae of semicircular duct, 431
ampulla of uterine tube, 22*f*, 26*f*
fertilization in, 31
anal agenesis, 239, 240*f*
with fistula, 239, 240*f*
anal canal, development of, 236–238, 238*f*
anal membrane, 236, 237*f*, 239, 239*f*, 240*f*, 241, 272*f*
anal pit, 212, 212*f*, 235, 236, 237*f*, 240*f*
anal sphincter, external, 236, 288
anal stenosis, 239, 240*f*
anaphase lagging, 465
anastomosis, of placental blood vessels, 135–136
anatomical position, 12–13, 12*f*
anchoring villi, 68, 116*f*, 122
androgen(s)
and masculinization of female fetus, 274
as teratogen, 472*t*, 476–477
androgen insensitivity syndrome, 274–275, 275*f*
androstenedione, 264
anencephaly, 65, 131, 352, 381, 392*f*, 395*f*, 405
aneuploidy, 460*f*, 461
Angelman's syndrome, 468, 468*t*
angioblastic cords, 286, 286*f*
angioblasts, 66
angiogenesis, 66–67, 66*f*, 286–292, 494
angiogenesis factor, 23

angiomas of skin, 444, 455
angiotensin-converting enzyme (ACE) inhibitors, as teratogens, 478–479
animal experiments, 475
aniridia, congenital, 426–427
ankyloglossia, 178, 178*f*
anlage, 2
anocutaneous (white) line, 236
anodontia
  partial, 452
  total, 452
anomalies, congenital. *See* congenital anomalies
anonychia, congenital, 448
anoperineal fistula, 239, 240*f*
anophthalmia, 424–425, 425*f*
  primary, 425
  secondary, 425
anorectal agenesis, 239, 240*f*
  with fistula, 239, 240*f*
anorectal anomalies, 238–240, 238*f*, 239*f*, 240*f*
anorectal atresia, 213
anovulation, 25
anovulatory menstrual cycle, 27
anoxia, fetal, umbilical cord true knots and, 127, 130*f*
anterior, as descriptive term, 12, 12*f*
anterior commissure, 402, 404*f*
antibiotics, as teratogens, 477
antibodies, maternal, transplacental transport of, 119*f*, 120
anticoagulants, as teratogens, 477
anticonvulsants, as teratogens, 392, 475, 477–478
antimüllerian hormone (AMH), 263
antinauseants, as teratogens, 478
antineoplastic agents, as teratogens, 478
antithyroid drugs, as teratogens, 479
antituberculosis agents, as teratogens, 477
antrum, 23, 25*f*
anular epiphyses, 346, 346*f*
anular ligament, failed differentiation of, 435
anular pancreas, 222–223, 224*f*, 241
anulus fibrosus, 344–345, 345*f*
anus
  agenesis of, 239, 240*f*
  ectopic, 239, 240*f*
  imperforate, 222, 239, 239*f*, 240*f*
  membranous atresia of, 239, 239*f*, 240*f*
aorta, 374*f*
  coarctation of, 320–322, 323*f*
    juxtaductal, 320
    postductal, 320, 323*f*
    preductal, 320, 323*f*
  dorsal, 291–292, 319, 324*f*
    persistent, 324, 325*f*
    transformation and adult derivatives of, 321*f*
  semilunar valves of, 306, 308*f*, 317*f*
aortic arches
  circulation through, 296*f*–297*f*
  derivatives of, 321*f*
  fourth pair of, derivatives of, 321*f*
  sixth pair of, derivatives of, 321*f*–322*f*
  third pair of, derivatives of, 321*f*
aortic atresia, 316
aorticopulmonary septal defect, 314
aorticopulmonary septum, 301, 304*f*, 306, 307*f*, 314
aorticopulmonary window defect, 314
aorticoventricular junction, 308*f*
aortic sac, 287*f*, 292, 296*f*–297*f*, 319, 320*f*
  transformation and adult derivatives of, 321*f*
aortic stenosis, 316, 317*f*
aortic vestibule, 304*f*, 306, 307*f*
aortic window, 314
aphakia, congenital, 428
aphonia, with laryngotracheal cleft, 201
apocrine sweat glands, 442
apoptosis
  and cardiovascular development, 295
  endometrial, and implantation, 43
apoptosis-inducing ligands, and placental immunoprotection, 121
appendicular skeleton, development of, 353–355, 354*f*, 355*f*
appendix
  development of, 227–228, 229*f*
  subhepatic, 231, 233*f*
appendix of epipidymis, 248*t*, 268*f*, 270
appendix vesiculosa, 248*t*, 268, 270
applied embryology, 8
aqueductal stenosis, congenital, 407, 411*f*
aqueous chambers of eye, development of, 427*f*, 428
arachnoid mater, 384, 429
arachnoid trabeculae, 384
arachnoid villi, 398, 407, 409
arched collecting tubule, 244, 248*f*, 249*f*
Aristotle (Aristotle of Stagira), 8
Arnheim, Johan Ham van, 10
Arnold-Chiari malformation, 412–413, 413*f*
arrector muscles of hair (arrector pili muscles), 442*f*, 447
arteriocapillary networks, 68
artery (arteries)
  aorta (*See* Aorta; Aortic arches)
  axial, primary, 372, 374*f*
  brachial, 372, 374*f*
  brachiocephalic, 321*f*
  carotid
    common, 318, 321*f*, 322*f*
    external, 318, 321*f*, 322*f*
    internal, 318, 321*f*, 322*f*
  celiac trunk, 148*f*, 212*f*, 214*f*, 222*f*, 292
  central, of retina, 420, 423*f*, 426*f*
  chorionic, 117
  deep, of thigh (profunda fermoris), 372, 374*f*
  endometrial, 44, 115*f*, 116, 116*f*
  femoral, 374*f*
  fibular, 374*f*
  foregut, 148*f*, 214*f*
  great, transposition of, 314–315, 315*f*
  hyaloid, 420, 421*f*, 424*f*
    persistence of, 428
  iliac, 374*f*
    common, 249, 292, 374*f*
    external, 374*f*
    internal, 292, 302*f*, 328*f*, 329*f*
  intercostal, 292, 323*f*, 344
  interosseous, 374*f*
    common, 374*f*
  intersegmental, 321*f*, 324*f*, 326*f*, 344, 345, 374*f*
    dorsal, 67*f*, 287*f*, 344
  ischiadic, 374*f*
  lumbar, 292
  maxillary, 318
  median, 374*f*
  mesenteric
    inferior, 212*f*, 214*f*, 222*f*, 235
    superior, 146, 212*f*, 214*f*, 222*f*, 224
  pharyngeal arch, 163*f*
    double, 324, 324*f*
    fifth, 319
    first, 318
    fourth, 319
    second, 318
    sixth, 319
    third, 318
  plantar, 374*f*
  popliteal, 374*f*
artery (arteries)—cont'd
  pulmonary
    left, 307*f*, 315*f*, 319, 321*f*, 322*f*
    right, 319, 321*f*
  radial, 372, 374*f*
  rectal, 238
    inferior, 238
    superior, 238
  renal, 249, 250, 251*f*
    accessory, 250, 251*f*
  sacral, lateral, 292
  spiral endometrial, 44, 115*f*, 116, 116*f*
  splenic, 224, 225*f*
  stapedial, 318
  subclavian, 319, 321*f*, 322*f*, 323*f*, 325*f*
    right, 319, 321*f*, 322*f*, 324*f*
      anomalous, 324
  tibial, 372, 374*f*
  ulnar, 374*f*
  umbilical, 116*f*, 135*f*, 302*f*, 374*f*
    absence of (SUA), 128, 130*f*
    adult derivatives of, 303*f*
    Doppler velocimetry of, 127–128, 130*f*
    fate of, 292
  vertebral, 292, 327*f*
  vesical, superior, 292, 329*f*, 331
  vitelline, 67*f*, 212*f*, 234*f*, 374*f*
    fate of, 292
arthrogryposis multiplex congenita, 361, 362*f*
arytenoid cartilage, formation of, 165*t*
arytenoid swellings, 198, 200*f*
asphyxia, intrauterine, and surfactant production, 207
aspirin, fetal effects of, 479
assimilation of atlas, 353
assisted in vitro fertilization, 33–35
assisted in vivo fertilization, 35
association, definition of, 460
astroblasts, histogenesis of, 381, 387*f*
astrocytes, histogenesis of, 381, 387*f*
atlantoaxial dislocation, 353
atlas, assimilation of, 353
atomic bomb survivors, birth defect studies in, 482
atrial septal defects, 310–312, 310*f*, 311*f*–313*f*
atrioventricular bundle, 308*f*
atrioventricular canal
  circulation through, 292, 296*f*–298*f*
  development of, 292, 296*f*–299*f*, 300*f*
  partitioning of, 292–293, 298*f*–299*f*
atrioventricular node, 305*f*, 308*f*
atrioventricular septal defect, 313*f*, 314*f*
atrioventricular septum, 299*f*–300*f*
atrioventricular valves, 305*f*, 308*f*
atrium (atria)
  common, 312
  left, formation of, 305*f*
  primordial, 84*f*, 290*f*, 292–293, 293*f*, 296*f*–299*f*, 299*f*–300*f*, 304*f*–305*f*
    partitioning of, 295–297, 299*f*–347*f*, 300*f*
attractants, for sperm, 31
auditory ossicles, 165*f*, 430, 433*f*, 437
auditory (pharyngotympanic) tube, 75, 166, 168*f*, 169*f*, 195
Auerbach plexus, 239
auricle (cardiac), 297, 302*f*, 303*ff*, 304*f*–305*f*
auricle (ear), 372*f*, 434, 434*f*
  absence of, 435
  congenital anomalies of, 435–436, 436*f*
auricular appendages, 435
auricular fistulas, 435, 436*f*
auricular hillocks, 80, 88*f*, 184*f*, 434, 437
  accessory, 435, 436*f*
auricularis muscle, 166*f*
auricular sinuses and cysts, 169
autonomic ganglia, 75, 238, 414

autonomic nervous system, 381, 416
  development of, 416
autosomes, trisomy of, 460*f*, 461
axial artery, primary, 372, 374*f*
axial dysraphic disorders, 351
axial plane, 12*f*, 13
axial skeleton
  congenital anomalies of, 348–355
  development of, 344–348, 345*f*
azygos vein, 288, 289*f*, 290*f*
  lobe of, 207

B
balanced translocation carriers, 467
basal body temperature, ovulation and, 25
basal layer, of endometrium, 21, 22*f*
basal plate, 347, 383, 386*f*, 388*f*, 396*f*
basic helix-loop (bHLH) transcription factor, 493
basilar invagination, 353
basipharyngeal canal, 401
battledore placenta, 125, 127*f*
Bcl-2 proteins, and spermatogenesis, 20
Beckwith-Wiedemann syndrome, 468*t*
bell stage, of tooth development, 449–450, 450*f*
Bendectin, fetal effects of, 478
benzodiazepine derivatives, as teratogens, 480
betamethasone, and fetal lung maturity, 207
bicornuate uterus, 277, 278*f*, 279*f*
  with rudimentary horn, 277, 278*f*
bidiscoid placenta, 123
bifid nose, 192
bifid penis, 277
bifid ureter, 253*f*, 255
bilaminar embryonic disc, 43*f*, 47*f*, 56*f*
  formation of, 43–52
bile duct, 218*f*, 220
bile formation, 220
biliary apparatus, development of, 218–220, 218*f*
biliary atresia, 220–221
bilious emesis, 231
bilirubin, transplacental transport of, 119*f*, 120
biparental inheritance, 33
biparietal diameter (BPD), 98, 105
birth(s)
  multiple, 134–140 (*See also* Twin(s))
  process of, 123–133, 124*f*, 125*f*
birth defects, 458–484. *See also* Congenital anomalies
  causes of, 458, 458*f*
  chromosomal abnormalities and, 458*f*
  classification of, 458
  developmental signaling pathways and, 488
  environmental factors in, 458, 458*f*, 471–484
  genetic factors in, 458*f*, 459–471
  multifactorial inheritance and, 458*f*, 484
  Toxoplasma gondii and, 407, 472*t*, 481
birthmarks, 444, 444*f*
birth weight
  cigarette smoking and, 104, 475
  extremely low, 96
  low, 96, 103
bladder. *See* gallbladder; urinary bladder
blastocyst(s), 3*f*
  definition of, 2
  formation of, 37–38
  implantation of, 28, 48
    inhibition of, 51
    sites of, 45–47, 52*f*
blastocystic cavity, 2, 36, 36*f*, 37*f*, 38*f*
blastoderm, 10
blastogenesis, 28, 37
blastomeres, 2, 35–36, 36*f*
"blighted embryo," 466
blink-startle response, 101
blood, development of, 66*f*, 67
blood-air barrier, 204
blood cells, development of, 66*f*, 67
blood flow. *See* Circulation of blood
blood islands, 66, 66*f*, 286*f*
blood vessels
  anastomosis of fetal, 135–136
  development of, 66–67, 66*f*, 286–292, 289*f*–290*f*, 317–324, 325*f*, 326*f*
body cavities. *See also specific body cavities*
  development of, 146–157
  embryonic, 146–150
    division of, 146–147, 149*f*
bone(s)
  development of, 339–342, 341*f*–343*f*
    intracartilaginous ossification and, 339–342, 343*f*
    intramembranous ossification and, 339, 342*f*
    molecular control of, 339, 341*f*
  histogenesis of, 339
  intramembranous formation of, 339
  shaft of, formation of, 339
bone age, 353, 355
bone marrow, development of, 339
bone matrix, 339
bone morphogenetic proteins (BMPs), 489
  and bone development, 341*f*
  and cardiovascular development, 295
  and gastrulation, 55
  and limb development, 366
bony labyrinth of internal ear, 432*f*, 433
Boveri, Theodor, 11
BPD (biparietal diameter), 98, 105
brachial artery, 374*f*
brachiocephalic artery, 321*f*
brachiocephalic vein, left, 288, 289*f*–290*f*, 297
brachycephaly, 352, 352*f*, 463*t*
brachydactyly, 377
bradykinin, and ductus arteriosus closure, 327
brain
  congenital anomalies of, 405–413
  development of, 392–401, 395*f*–404*f*
    critical period of, 474
brain flexures, 385*f*, 392, 396*f*
brain stem developmental anomaly, and sudden infant death syndrome, 309
brain vesicles
  primary, 385*f*, 392
  secondary, 385*f*, 392
branchial anomalies, 160
branchial apparatus, 160
branchial cysts, 170*f*, 171, 171*f*, 172*f*
branchial fistula, 170*f*, 171, 171*f*
branchial sinuses, 169, 170*f*, 171*f*
  external, 169, 170*f*
  internal, 169, 170*f*
branchial vestiges, 170*f*, 172, 172*f*
branching morphogenesis, 206, 246
branch villi, 68, 116*f*, 117*f*, 118
breasts
  absence of (amastia), 446
  congenital anomalies of, 446
  development of, 444–446, 445*f*
breathing movements, fetal, 206, 207*f*
breech position, 108*f*
broad ligaments, 269, 271*f*
bronchi
  development of, 202–203, 203*f*
  main, 202
  secondary, 203
  segmental, 203
bronchial buds, 147, 150*f*, 200*f*, 202, 202*f*, 203*f*, 246*f*
bronchioles, 203, 204*f*, 205*f*, 206
bronchopulmonary segment, 203, 209
Brown, Louise, 11
brown fat, fetal, 101
buccinator muscle, 166*f*
bud stage, of tooth development, 449, 450*f*
bulbar conjunctiva, 429
bulbar ridges, 301, 304*f*, 305, 307*f*, 308*f*
bulbourethral gland, 28, 29*f*, 248*t*, 268*f*, 269
bulboventricular groove, 296*f*
bulboventricular loop, 292, 294*f*, 296*f*
bulbus cordis, 290*f*, 292, 293*f*, 296*f*
circulation through, 292, 296*f*–298*f*
  partitioning of, 304*f*, 305–306, 307*f*
bundle branches, 308, 308*f*
busulfan, as teratogen, 472*t*, 478

C
caffeine consumption, during pregnancy, 475
CAH. *See* congenital adrenal hyperplasia
calcium, and bone development, 169
calices
  development of, 244, 248*t*
  major, 244, 248*f*
  minor, 244, 248*f*
calvaria, 347–348
  defects of, 352–353, 352*f*
canalicular period, of lung maturation, 203–204, 204*f*, 205*f*
canal of Nuck, 281
cancer
  signaling pathways and, 493, 494
  treatment of, teratogens in, 478, 482
capacitation of sperm, 29, 30*f*
cap stage, of tooth development, 449
capsulin, and spleen development, 224
carbon dioxide, transplacental transport of, 119*f*
carbon monoxide, transplacental transport of, 119*f*, 120
carboxyhemoglobin, cigarette smoking and, 475
cardiac jelly, 292, 293, 293*f*, 294*f*, 296*f*–297*f*
cardiac muscle, development of, 360, 381
cardiac muscle fibers, 360
cardiac myoblasts, 360
cardiac skeleton, 309
cardiac valves, development of, 305*f*, 306–308, 308*f*
cardinal veins, 296*f*–297*f*, 374*f*
  anterior, 287–288, 289*f*–290*f*, 291, 296*f*, 297, 302*f*
  common, 149*f*, 286, 287–288, 289*f*–290*f*, 291–292, 293*f*, 296*f*
  development of, 287–288, 289*f*–290*f*
  posterior, 67*f*, 247*f*, 287–288, 287*f*, 289*f*–290*f*, 296*f*
cardiogenic area, 59, 63*f*, 67
cardiovascular system. *See also specific cardiovascular structures*
  development of, 286–335
    early, 65–67, 292–309
  primordial, 67, 67*f*
Carnegie collection, 10
Carnegie Embryonic Staging System, 80*t*, 86
carotid arteries
  common, 318, 321*f*, 322*f*
  external, 318, 321*f*, 322*f*
  internal, 318, 321*f*, 322*f*
carpus, 354*f*, 371*f*
cartilage
  arytenoid, 165*t*
  bone development in, 339–342, 343*f*
  development of, 339–342
  histogenesis of, 339
  hypophysial, 347, 348*f*

cartilage—cont'd
  parachordal, 347, 348*f*
  pharyngeal arch, derivatives of, 160–162, 165*f*
cartilage matrix, 343*f*
cartilaginous joints, 344, 344*f*
cartilaginous neurocranium, 347, 348*f*
cartilaginous otic capsules, 431, 432*f*, 433, 433*f*
cartilaginous stage, of vertebral development, 345, 346*f*
cartilaginous viscerocranium, 347, 348*f*
cataracts, congenital, 428–429, 429*f*
  rubella virus and, 428–429, 429*f*, 480
cauda equina, 385
caudal, as descriptive term, 12, 12*f*
caudal eminence, 12, 74*f*, 76*f*, 79, 80*t*, 81, 87*f*, 90
caudal neuropore, 79, 80*t*, 81*f*, 82*f*, 83*f*, 339*f*, 381, 384*f*
  defect in closure of, 391, 394*f*
caudal ridges, 147
caudate nucleus, 402, 404*f*, 405*f*
caval system, 335
cavities, body. *See also specific body cavities*
  development of, 146–157
  embryonic
    division of, 146–150
C cells, 169, 195
CDH. *See* Congenital diaphragmatic hernia
cecum
  development of, 226*f*, 227–228, 229*f*
  mobile, 231
  subhepatic, 231, 233*f*
celiac trunk artery, 148*f*, 212*f*, 214*f*, 222*f*, 292
cell adhesion molecules, and bone development, 43, 48, 341*f*, 342*f*
cell contact-mediated interaction, 78*f*
cell cultures, fetal, 106
cell death, programmed. *See* Apoptosis
cell theory, 10
cement, dental, 449
cementoblasts, 449
cementoenamel junction, 449
cementum, 449
centers of growth, 179
central artery and vein of retina, 420, 423*f*, 426*f*
central canal of spinal cord, 381, 386*f*, 388*f*, 396*f*
central incisors, 451, 454*f*, 471
central nervous system. *See* Brain; Spinal cord
central tendon of diaphragm
  development of, 150, 152*f*
  primordial, 73, 147, 149*f*, 150
centromere, 15, 17*f*, 469
centrum, 344, 345–346, 346*f*
cerebellar cortex, 397
cerebellum, 393, 397, 398*f*
cerebral aqueduct, 397*f*, 398, 412*f*
cerebral commissures
  anterior, 402, 404*f*
  hippocampal, 402, 404*f*
  posterior, 402, 404*f*
cerebral cortex, abnormal histogenesis of, 405, 408*f*
cerebral hemispheres
  congenital absence of, 410, 412*f*
  development of, 399, 401–402, 401*f*, 403*f*
cerebral palsy, 405, 481
cerebral peduncles, 398*f*, 399
cerebral vesicles, 4*f*, 80*t*, 401*f*, 403*f*
cerebrospinal fluid
  excessive, in hydrocephalus, 410, 412*f*
  formation of, 384, 398
cervical canal, 21, 22*f*
cervical flexure, 88*f*, 385*f*, 392, 393, 396*f*
cervical myotomes, 358, 359*f*, 361*f*
cervical plexus, 434
cervical pregnancy, 52
cervical ribs, 350, 350*f*
cervical sinus, 79, 87*f*, 160, 169, 170*f*
cervical somites, 153, 153*f*, 246*f*
cervix, 21, 22*f*
CHAOS (congenital high airway obstruction syndrome), 198
cheeks, development of, 182, 184
chemicals, as teratogens, 472*t*
Chiari malformation, 353, 412–413
chickenpox, fetal effects of, 481
childbirth, 123–133, 124*f*, 125*f*
childhood, 7, 8
chimeric models, 11
chin, development of, 182
CHL. *See* Crown-heel length
choanae, 183, 187*f*
  primordial, 183, 187*f*
cholesteatoma, congenital, 436
chondrification centers, 339, 345, 346*f*, 368
chondroblasts, 57, 339, 343*f*
chondrocranium, 347–348, 348*f*
chondrocyte, 339, 343*f*
chondrogenesis, 339, 341*f*, 342*f*
chondroid tissue, 342
chordae tendineae, 301, 305*f*, 308*f*
chorda tympani nerve, 415, 433
chordee, 275–276
chordomas, 62, 345
choriocarcinomas, 67, 122, 123
chorion, 45, 47*f*
  smooth, 111, 112*f*, 114*f*, 115*f*, 116
  villous, 111, 112*f*, 114*f*, 116*f*, 123, 132*f*
chorionic arteries, 117
chorionic cavity, 45, 49*f*, 128*f*
  ultrasound assessment of, 92*f*
chorionic plate, 115, 115*f*, 116*f*, 117, 118
chorionic sac
  development of, 45, 47*f*
  diameter of, ultrasound measurement of, 45, 49*f*, 111, 115*f*
  fusion with decidua, 113
chorionic vessels, 113*f*, 125, 126*f*, 129*f*
chorionic villi
  branch (terminal), 68, 116*f*, 117*f*, 118
  development of, 68, 69*f*
  primary, 45, 47*f*, 48, 49*f*, 68
  secondary, 68, 69*f*, 70
  stem (anchoring), 68, 70, 115, 116*f*, 126*f*
  tertiary, 67, 67*f*
chorionic villus sampling, 83, 106, 106*f*
choroid, development of, 426*f*, 429
choroid fissure, 402, 403*f*, 405*f*
choroid plexus, 396*f*, 398, 402, 403*f*, 404*f*
  development of, 398
chromaffin cells, 389*f*, 414
chromaffin system, 414
chromatid, 15, 17*f*
chromatin patterns, 106
chromatophores, 426
chromosomal abnormalities, 458*f*
  detection of, 106, 131
  in gametes, 21
  maternal age and, 20, 105, 461, 465*t*
  numerical, 417, 459
  parental age and, 20, 105, 461, 465*t*
  and spontaneous abortion, 39, 49
  structural, 466–467, 467*f*
chromosome(s)
  breakage, 466, 467*f*
  crossing over of, 33
  deletion of, 467, 467*f*
  double chromatid, 15, 17*f*, 496
  duplication of, 468*f*, 469
chromosome(s)—cont'd
  haploid number of, 15
  homologous, 15, 459
  inversion of, 467*f*, 468, 469
  microdeletions and microduplications of, 467–468, 468*t*
  nondisjunction of, 35, 459, 460*f*
  ring, 467, 467*f*
  sex (*See* Sex chromosomes)
  single chromatid, 15, 17*f*
  translocation of, 461, 466–467, 467*f*
chromosome studies, 11
chyle cistern, 333, 334*f*, 334*f*
cigarette smoking, fetal effects of, 104, 476
ciliary body, development of, 425, 426*f*
ciliary muscle, 425
ciliary processes, 425, 429
circulation of amniotic fluid, 128–130
circulation of blood
  fetal, 302*f*, 326–327, 328*f*
  fetoplacental, 117, 117*f*
    impaired, and fetal growth, 104
    umbilical cord Doppler velocimetry of, 128
  neonatal, 303*f*, 325
    transitional, 327–330
  placental, 116*f*, 117–118, 117*f*
    maternal, 118
  through primordial heart, 296*f*–298*f*
  uteroplacental
    impaired, and fetal growth, 104
    primordial, 44
    umbilical cord Doppler velocimetry of, 128
circumvallate papillae, 178*f*
cisterna chyli, 333, 334*f*
cleavage of zygote, 35, 36*f*
  definition of, 2
cleavage spindle, 32*f*, 33
cleft face, 192, 192*f*
cleft foot, 376, 376*f*
cleft hand, 376, 376*f*
cleft lip and palate, 188–192, 191*f*, 192*f*
cleft tongue, 179
cleft uvula, 190, 191*f*
cleft vertebral column, 351, 351*f*
climacteric, 27
clitoral urethra, 274
clitoris, development of, 272*f*, 273, 273*f*
cloaca, 73, 76*f*, 214*f*, 235
  partitioning of, 235–236, 237*f*
  persistent, 240*f*
cloacal membrane, 58*f*, 59, 60*f*, 236, 261*f*, 271
cloacal sphincter, 236
clomiphene citrate, for ovulation induction, 25, 33
cloning, 11
closing plug, 3*f*, 44, 44*f*, 46*f*
clubfoot, 377, 378*f*, 459, 483
c-met, and muscle development, 359, 360*f*
coarctation of aorta, 320–322, 323*f*
  juxtaductal, 320
  postductal, 320, 323*f*
  preductal, 320, 323*f*
cocaine use
  and birth defects, 104, 472*t*
  and fetal growth, 480
cochlea, membranous, 431, 432*f*
cochlear duct, 431, 432*f*
cochlear nerve, 416
coelom. *See also specific body cavities*
  extraembryonic, 44*f*, 45, 46*f*, 47*f*, 50*f*, 74*f*, 222*f*, 224
  intraembryonic, 65, 76*f*, 146, 149*f*, 157, 182*f*, 222*f*
coelomic spaces, 44*f*, 45, 63*f*, 65

collecting tubules, 244, 248*f*, 248*t*, 249*f*
collodion baby, 443–444
coloboma
  of eyelid, 430
  of iris, 422, 426*f*
  of retina, 422
colon
  congenitally enlarged (megacolon), 238, 238*f*
  development of, 224–228, 226*f*
  left-sided (nonrotation of midgut), 231, 233*f*
color flow Doppler ultrasound, of umbilical cord, 125
commissures, cerebral
  anterior, 402, 404*f*
  hippocampal, 402, 404*f*
  posterior, 402, 404*f*
common atrium, 312
common ventricle, 313, 366*f*
compaction, 2, 35
compact layer, of endometrium, 21, 27, 38, 46*f*
complement regulatory proteins, and placental immunoprotection, 121
complete abortion, definition of, 7
computed tomography, for fetal assessment, 107
conal growth hypothesis, of transposition of great arteries, 314
conceptional age, 85
conceptus, definition of, 2
condensation, and bone development, 339, 341*f*, 342*f*
conduction system of heart, 308*f*
congenital adrenal hyperplasia (CAH), 262, 263*f*, 274*f*, 283, 477*f*
congenital anomalies, 458–484
  alcohol and, 409, 472*t*, 476
  of anus and rectum, 238–240, 238*f*, 239*f*, 240*f*
  of bladder, 257–260, 259*f*, 260*f*
  of brain, 405–413
  causes of, 458–459, 458*f*
  chromosomal abnormalities and, 458*f*, 459–466
  classification of, 458
  of duodenum, 232
  of ear, 434–436
  environmental factors in, 458*f*, 471–483
  of esophagus, 213
  of eye, 422–427
  of face, 185–194
  genetic mutation and, 459–471
  of genital system, 273–277
  of head and neck, 348, 351*f*, 352–353, 352*f*
  of heart, 309–317
  of hindgut, 238–240
  incidence of major, 474*t*
  of intestines, 219*f*
  of kidneys and ureters, 252–256, 254*f*–257*f*
  of larynx, 198
  of limbs, 375–377
  of lip and palate, 188–192, 191*f*, 192*f*
  of liver, 220–221
  of lungs, 208, 208*f*
  of lymphatic system, 334–335
  of mammary glands, 446
  of midgut, 231–235
  of muscles, 361–362
  of nails, 448
  neurulation abnormalities and, 65
  of pancreas, 222–223
  of pericardium, 147
  of skeleton, 348–355
  of skin, 442–444
  of spinal cord, 386–392
  of spleen, 224
  study of (teratology), 8
  of teeth, 451–454, 455*f*
congenital anomalies—cont'd
  of tongue, 177, 178
  Toxoplasma gondii and, 472*t*, 481, 482*f*
  urachal, 257, 259*f*
  of uterus, 277, 278*f*
  of vagina, 277
  of vena cava, 291
congenital diaphragmatic hernia (CDH), 153–155, 155*f*, 156*f*
  and pulmonary hypoplasia, 208
congenital ectodermal dysplasia, 444
congenital epigastric hernia, 155
congenital heart defects, 309–317
congenital high airway obstruction syndrome (CHAOS), 198
congenital hypoparathyroidism, 173
congenital megacolon, 238, 238*f*
congenital rubella syndrome, 479, 481*f*
conjoined twins, 139, 140*f*, 142*f*, 143*f*
conjunctiva, 428
  bulbar, 429
  palpebral, 426*f*, 429
conjunctival sac, 426*f*, 429
connecting stalk, 3*f*, 43, 45, 47*f*, 50*f*, 56*f*
Constantinus Africanus of Salerno, 9
contiguous gene syndromes, 468, 468*t*
contraceptives, oral
  fetal effects of, 477
  and ovulation, 20, 27
conus arteriosus, 304*f*, 306, 307*f*, 314
conus cordis, 86*f*
copula, 176, 178*f*
cornea, development of, 426*f*, 429
Corner, George W., 104
corniculate cartilage, formation of, 165*t*
coronal plane, 12*f*, 13
corona radiata, 16*f*, 18*f*, 20
  passage of sperm through, 29
coronary sinus, 291*f*, 297, 302*f*, 304*f*–305*f*, 310*f*
  persistent left superior vena cava and, 291
corpora cavernosa clitoridis, 248*t*
corpora cavernosa penis, 248*t*, 273
corpus albicans, 27, 40*f*
corpus callosum, 402–403, 402*f*, 404*f*
  agenesis of, 407, 411*f*
corpus luteum, 24*f*, 25–27, 26*f*, 40*f*, 43
corpus spongiosum penis, 248*t*
corpus striatum, 402, 403*f*, 404, 404*f*
cortex
  cerebral, abnormal histogenesis of, 405, 408*f*
  ovarian, 248*t*, 266*f*
  suprarenal, 248*t*
corticol, and labor, 123
corticosteroids, fetal effects of, 478
corticotropin-releasing hormone (CRH), and labor, 123
cortisone, fetal effects of, 478
cor triloculare biatriatum, 313
costal processes, 345–346, 346*f*
costodiaphragmatic recesses, 152, 152*f*
costovertebral joints, 346–347, 346*f*
coxsackie virus, transplacental transport of, 120
cranial, as descriptive term, 12, 12*f*
cranial meningocele, 405, 408*f*
cranial nerves, 414–415
  formation of, 165*t*
  somatic efferent, 414–415
  special visceral afferent components of, 415
  special visceral efferent (branchial) components of, 162–163
cranial ridges, 147
cranial vault (calvaria), 347, 355*f*
craniofacial anomalies, benzodiazepine derivatives and, 480
craniolacunia, 391
craniopharyngiomas, 401, 402*f*
craniosynostosis, 352–353, 352*f*
craniovertebral junction, anomalies at, 353
cranium, development of, 347–348, 348*f*, 349*f*
cranium bifidum, 405, 408*f*
cremasteric muscle and fascia, 280*f*, 281
cretinism, 354–355, 479
CRH (corticotropin-releasing hormone), and labor, 123
"crib death," 309
Crick, Francis, 11
cricoid cartilage, formation of, 165*t*
cricothyroid muscle, formation of, 162, 165*t*, 166*f*
cri du chat syndrome, 467, 468*f*
criminal abortion, definition of, 7
cristae ampullares, 431
crista terminalis, 297, 298*f*, 301, 302*f*, 304*f*–305*f*
critical periods, of development, 473*f*, 474, 475*f*
CRL. *See* Crown-rump length
crossed renal ectopia, 253*f*, 254, 254*f*
crossing over, of chromosomes, 33
crown-heel length (CHL), 86, 93*f*, 99*f*
crown-rump length (CRL), 2, 80*t*, 86, 93
crura of diaphragm, 151, 152*f*
cryopreservation, of embryos, 35
cryptophthalmos, 430
cryptophthalmos syndrome, 430
cryptorchidism, 276, 281, 282*f*
cumulus oophorus, 23, 25*f*
cuneate nuclei, 393
cuneiform cartilage, formation of, 165*t*
cutaneous nerve area, 368–369
cutaneous syndactyly, 377, 378*f*
cuticle, 448
CVS (chorionic villus sampling), 83, 106, 106*f*
cyanosis, 310, 316
cyanotic heart disease, 314
cyclopia, 424*f*
cyst(s)
  allantoic, 62, 134, 135*f*
  auricular, 169
  branchial, 170*f*, 171, 171*f*, 172*f*
  dentigerous, 452
  Gartner duct, 268*f*, 270
  lingual, congenital, 177
  of lung, congenital, 208, 208*f*
  thyroglossal duct, 174, 175*f*
  urachal, 257, 259*f*
cystic duct, 220
cystic hygroma, 335
cystic kidney disease, 255–256, 257*f*
cytomegalovirus
  as teratogen, 472*t*
  transplacental transport of, 119*f*
cytotrophoblast, 3*f*, 38, 43, 43*f*
cytotrophoblastic shell, 68, 69*f*

D

Darwin, Charles, 11
da Vinci, Leonardo, 9*f*
deafness, 434
decidua, 111
decidua capsularis, 115
decidual cells, 43, 44
decidual reaction, 44
De Conceptu et Generaticne Hominis (Rueff), 9*f*
deep artery of thigh, 374*f*
deformation, definition of, 459
deletion, chromosomal, 467, 467*f*
delivery
  expected date of (EDD), 103
dental sac, 449
dentigerous cyst, 452
dentinogenesis imperfecta, 453
dermal ridges, 441

dermis, development of, 441
dermomyotome, 339, 340*f*
descriptive terminology, 11–13, 12*f*
developmental anatomy, definition of, 7, 8
developmental periods, 2
developmental signaling pathways, 471
dextrocardia, 309, 309*f*
diaphragm
  accessory, 157
  central tendon of
    development of, 150, 152*f*
    primordial, 73, 147, 149*f*, 150
  congenital absence of, 361
  crura of, 151, 152*f*
  development of, 150–153
  eventration of, 154*f*, 155
  innervation of, 153, 153*f*
  positional changes of, 153, 153*f*
  posterolateral defects of, 153–155, 154*f*, 157*f*
  primordial, 151
diaphragmatic hernia, congenital, 156*f*
diaphysis, 339
diazepam, use during pregnancy, 480
diencephalon, 399–400, 403*f*, 406*f*
diethylstilbestrol, 477
  as teratogen, 472*t*
differentiation, 73
  and bone development, 339
digastric muscle, formation of, 165*t*
DiGeorge syndrome, 173, 468*t*
digital rays, 80, 366
dihydrostreptomycin, as teratogen, 477
dilation, 123, 124*f*
dimertization, 493
disruption, definition of, 459
distal, as descriptive term, 12
distal tongue buds, 178*f*
diverticulum
  hepatic, 218
  hypophysial, 399, 401*f*
  ileal, 233–234, 234*f*
  laryngotracheal, 198, 199*f*
  metanephric, 244, 248*f*
  tracheal, 201
dizygotic twins, 136*f*, 137, 137*t*, 141*f*
  maternal age and, 134
Dolly (cloned sheep), 11
dorsal, as descriptive term, 12, 12*f*
dorsal horns, 383
dorsal mesentery
  of esophagus, diaphragm development from, 151, 152*f*
double chromatid chromosomes, 15, 17*f*, 496
double penis, 277
double uterus, 277, 278*f*
Down syndrome, 463*t*, 464*f*, 465*t*
drug(s). *See also specific drugs*
  as teratogens, 472*t*
  testing, in animals, 475
  transplacental transport of, 119*f*, 120
duct(s)
  alveolar, 203, 205*f*, 206
  bile, development of, 218*f*, 220
  cystic, 220
  ejaculatory, 248*t*
  of epididymis, 267
  Gartner, 248*t*
  genital, 265–269
  hepatic, accessory, 220
  lymph
    development of, 334*f*
    right, 334*f*
  mesonephric, 244
    adult derivatives and vestigial remains of, 248*t*
    remnants of, 270
duct(s)—cont'd
  omphaloenteric, 224
  pancreatic, 221–222
  paramesonephric
    adult derivatives and vestigial remains of, 248*t*
    development of, 265
    remnants of, 270
  semicircular, 431
  submandibular, 179
  thoracic, development of, 333, 334*f*
Ductuli efferentes, 248*t*
ductus arteriosus, 302*f*, 321*f*–322*f*
  adult derivatives of, 334*f*
  closure/constriction, 330
    and coarctation of aorta, 323*f*
  patent, 331–333, 334*f*
ductus deferens, 20, 248*t*, 267
ductus reuniens, 431
ductus venosus, 287, 290*f*
duodenal atresia, 216, 219*f*
duodenal stenosis, 216
duodenum
  congenital anomalies of, 232
  development of, 216, 218*f*
duplex kidney, 256*f*
duplication, chromosomal, 469
dura mater, 384
dyshistogenesis, 459
dysplasia, definition of, 459
dysplastic kidney disease, 256, 257*f*

E
ear
  congenital anomalies of, 434–436
  development of, 430–434, 431*f*, 433*f*
  external, 433–434, 433*f*
  internal, 431–433, 431*f*
  middle, 433, 433*f*
    development of, 165*t*
eccrine sweat glands, 441–442
ectoderm, embryonic, 55, 57
  derivatives of, 75, 77*f*
ectodermal dysplasia, congenital, 444
ectopia cordis, 309, 310*f*
ectopic anus, 239, 240*f*
ectopic kidney, 253*f*, 254
ectopic parathyroid gland, 173
ectopic pregnancies, 45–47
ectopic testes, 281, 281*f*
ectopic thyroid gland, 175, 176*f*, 177*f*
ectopic ureter, 255, 256*f*
ectrodactyly-ectodermal dysplasia-clefting syndrome, 444
Edwards, Robert G., 11
efferent ductules, 267
egg. *See* Oocyte(s)
Egyptians, ancient views of embryology in, 8
eighth week, 81–83, 90*f*, 91
ejaculatory duct, 248*t*
elastic cartilage, 339
electrolytes, transplacental transport of, 119*f*, 120
electromagnetic fields, fetal effects of, 483
eleventh week, 100*f*
embryo(s)
  abnormal, and spontaneous abortion, 39
  blighted, 466
  12-day, 45
  14-day, 45
  16-day, 58*f*
  21-day, 63*f*
  definition of, 2
  development of (*See* Embryonic development)
  folding of, 73–75, 74*f*, 75*f*, 147*f*
    and cardiovascular system, 295*f*
embryo(s)—cont'd
  measurement of, 80*t*
  spontaneous abortion of, 48–49
  ultrasound of, 89–90, 92*f*
embryological terminology, 2–7
embryology
  ancient views on, 8
  applied, 8
  definition of, 7
  in Middle Ages, 8–9
  in Renaissance, 9–11
  significance of, 7–8
embryonic age, 83, 85, 86, 90
  estimation of, 80*t*, 86
embryonic development. *See also specific anatomy and processes*
  control of, 75–77
  eighth week, 81–83, 90*f*, 91
  fifth week, 79–80, 87*f*
  fourth week, 79, 81*f*, 84*f*, 85*f*
  phases of, 73
  seventh week, 80–81, 88*f*
  sixth week, 80
  stages of, criteria for estimating, 80*t*
  third week, 59–75, 82*f*
embryonic disc, 58*f*
  bilaminar, 43*f*, 47*f*, 56*f*
    formation of, 43–52
  trilaminar, 56*f*
embryonic tissues, origin of, 48*f*
enamel, tooth, development of, 448
enamel epithelium, 449
enamel hypoplasia, 451
enamel organ, 449
enamel pearls, 454*f*
endocardial cushions, 293, 296*f*–297*f*, 307*f*
  defects of, 312
endocardial heart tubes, 67, 293*f*–295*f*
endocardium, 292, 293*f*–294*f*
endochondral bone formation, 339–342, 343*f*
endocrine synthesis, in placenta, 121
endocrine system
  pituitary gland
    glandular part of (adenohypophysis), 399, 399*t*, 401*f*, 417
  suprarenal glands, development of, 246*f*, 250*f*, 260
endoderm, embryonic, 55, 57
  derivatives of, 75, 77*f*
endometrial arteries, 44, 115*f*, 116, 116*f*
endometrial veins, 116
endometrium
  compact layer of, 21, 27, 38, 46*f*
  gravid, 111
environmental chemicals, as teratogens, 472*t*, 480
environmental factors, and birth defects, 458, 458*f*, 471–484
epaxial division, of myotomes, 358, 359*f*, 440–441
epiblast, 43*f*
epicardium, 292, 293*f*–294*f*
epidermal ridges, 440
epidermis, development of, 440–441
epididymis, 20, 248*t*, 270
  appendix of, 248*t*, 268*f*, 270
  development of, 267
epigastric hernia, congenital, 155
epiglottis, development of, 198
epiphysial cartilage plates (growth plates), 341
epispadias, 259–260, 276
epithalamic sulcus, 399
epithalamus, 399
epithelial-mesenchymal transformation, 293, 358
eponychium, 448

epoophoron, 248*t*, 270
  duct of, 248*t*
equatorial zone of lens, 427
erythroblastosis fetalis (hemolytic disease of newborn)
  intrauterine fetal transfusion for, 107
erythrocyte mosaicism, 135–136
esophageal atresia, 213
esophageal muscles, formation of, 165*t*
esophageal stenosis, 213
esophagus
  congenital anomalies of, 213
  development of, 212
  dorsal mesentery of, diaphragm development from, 151, 152*f*
  short, 213
ethisterone, avoidance in pregnancy, 477
eventration, of diaphragm, 154*f*, 155
excretory system. *See* Urinary system
exencephaly, 405–407
exocoelomic cavity, 44
exocoelomic membrane, 43*f*, 44
expected date of delivery (EDD), 103
expulsion stage of labor, 123, 124*f*, 125*f*
exstrophy of bladder, 259–260, 260*f*, 261*f*
external acoustic meatus, 80, 88*f*, 169, 179, 433, 433*f*, 434, 434*f*
  absence of, 436, 436*f*
  atresia of, 436
extraembryonic coelom, 44*f*, 45, 46*f*, 47*f*, 50*f*, 74*f*, 222*f*, 224
extraembryonic coelomic space, 45
extraembryonic mesoderm, 44
extraembryonic somatic mesoderm, 45
extraembryonic splanchnic mesoderm, 45
extrahepatic biliary atresia, 220–221
extrauterine implantation, 45–47
extravillous trophoblast, 121
eye(s)
  congenital anomalies of, 422–427
  development of, 78, 420, 421*f*, 426*f*
  movement, fetal, 100
  muscles, 358, 361*f*
eyelid(s)
  coloboma of, 430
  development of, 429–430
  opening of, in fetus, 102
  ptosis of, 430

F
Fabricius, Girolamo (Fabricius of Aquapendente), 9
face
  congenital anomalies of, 185–194
  development of, 179–182, 180*f*–181*f*
facial clefts, 192, 192*f*
facial expression, muscles of, 184
  formation of, 165*t*
facial nerve, formation of, 165, 165*t*, 415
facial primordia, 179
facilitated diffusion, placental transport via, 118
falciform ligament, 220
fallopian tubes. *See* Uterine tubes
fat, fetal
  brown, 101
  white, 101–102, 103
femoral artery, 374*f*
fertilization age, 2, 15, 83
fetal age, estimation of, 96, 98, 103*f*
fetal alcohol syndrome, 476
fetal growth, factors influencing, 103*f*, 104
fetal membranes
  after birth, 111, 123, 126*f*
  development of, 112*f*
  multiple pregnancies and, 134–135
  premature rupture of, 133, 133*f*
fetal period, 6*f*, 100*f*
  definition of, 2
  highlights of, 98–102
  nine to twelve weeks, 98–100
  seventeen to twenty weeks, 100–101
  thirteen to sixteen weeks, 100, 100*f*, 101*f*
  thirty-five to thirty-eight weeks, 102, 103*f*
  thirty to thirty-four weeks, 102
  twenty-one to twenty-five weeks, 101, 102*f*
  twenty-six to twenty-nine weeks, 102, 102*f*
fetal surgery, 8, 108*f*
fetoplacental blood flow
  impaired, and fetal growth, 104
fetoplacental circulation, 117, 117*f*
  impaired, and fetal growth, 104
  umbilical cord Doppler velocimetry of, 128
fetoscopy, 107
fetus
  circulation in, 326–327, 328*f*
  definition of, 2
  measurements and characteristics of, 98, 98*t*, 103*f*
  monitoring of, 107
  status of, assessment of, 104–105
  viability of, 96
fibroblast growth factor(s)
  and digestive system development, 212
fibrocartilage, 339
fibrous joints, 344, 344*f*
fibular artery, 374*f*
fifth week, 79–80, 87*f*
filiform papillae, 177
first arch syndrome, 172, 172*f*
first meiotic division, 15
fistula(s)
  in anal agenesis, 239, 240*f*
  anoperineal, 239, 240*f*
  auricular, 435, 436*f*
  branchial, 170*f*, 171, 171*f*
  lingual, 177
  omphaloenteric, 234, 234*f*
  preauricular, 435
  tracheoesophageal, 198, 202*f*
  urachal, 257, 259*f*
Flemming, Walter, 11
flexures, brain, 385*f*, 392, 396*f*
floating ribs, 347
folding of embryo, 73–75, 74*f*, 75*f*, 147*f*
  and cardiovascular system, 295*f*
foliate papillae, 176
follicles, ovarian. *See* Ovarian follicles
fontanelles, 347, 349*f*
foot
  cleft, 376, 376*f*
  development of, 368*f*, 369*f*
foramen cecum of tongue, 173, 174*f*, 178*f*
foramen of Morgagni, herniation through, 155
foramen ovale. *See* Oval foramen
foramen primum, 295, 298*f*, 299*f*–300*f*
  fate of, 299*f*–300*f*
foramen secundum, 299*f*–300*f*
forebrain, 79, 399–401, 400*f*, 403*f*
foregut, 212
foregut artery, 148*f*, 214*f*
fourth week, 79, 81*f*, 84*f*, 85*f*
fragile X syndrome, 469, 470*f*
frenulum of labia minora, 272*f*, 273
frontal plane, 12*f*, 13
frontal sinuses, 184
frontonasal prominence, 179, 180*f*
fused ribs, 350*f*, 351

G
galactosemia, congenital, 429
Galen, Claudius, 8, 9
gallbladder, development of, 220
gametogenesis, 15
  abnormal, 15, 18*f*
ganglion (ganglia)
  autonomic, 75, 238, 414
gangrene, of intestine, 231
Garbha Upanishad, 8
Garrod, Archibald, 11
Gartner duct, 248*t*, 268*f*
Gartner duct cysts, 268*f*, 270
gases, transplacental transport of, 119*f*, 120
gastroschisis, 155, 229–231, 232*f*
gastrula
  definition of, 2
gastrulation, 55–57
gene(s), inactivation of, 461
gene mutation, 458*f*, 469–470
genetic(s)
  and human development, 11
  and intrauterine growth retardation, 104
genital ducts
  development of, 265–269, 269*f*
  female, 269
  male, 265–269
  vestigial structures derived from, 270
genital glands
  auxiliary, in females, 269
genitalia
  agenesis of, 276, 276*f*
  ambiguous, 273
  development of, 271–273, 272*f*
  female, 272*f*, 273
  male, 271–273
genital system
  congenital anomalies of, 273–277
  development of, 262–273
    indifferent stage of, 262–263
genital tubercle, 271
genotype of embryo, and effects of teratogens, 474–475
germ cells, primordial, 263
germ cell tumors, 281
germ layers
  derivatives of, 75, 77*f*, 161*f*
  formation of, 55–57
gestational age, 15, 96
  definition of, 2
  estimation of, 83
  ultrasound assessment of, 89, 92*f*
gestational choriocarcinoma, 123
gigantism, 354
gingivae (gums), development of, 451
glans clitoris, 248*t*
glans penis, 248*t*, 271
glaucoma, congenital, 428
glial-derived neurotrophic factor, and renal development, 246
glioblasts, histogenesis of, 381
glomerulus, 244, 247*f*
glossopharyngeal nerve, 165, 165*t*, 177, 415
glossoschisis, 179
glottis, primordial, 198
glucose
  in fetal metabolism and growth, 104
gonad(s). *See also* ovaries; testes
  development of, 263–265
  indifferent, 263
    adult derivatives and vestigial remains of, 248*t*
gonadal cords, 263
gonadal dysgenesis, mixed, 275
gonadal ridge, 263, 264*f*
gonadal veins, 289*f*
Graaf, Regnier de, 9
gracile nuclei, 393
gravid endometrium, 111

gravid uterus, 115*f*
gray horns, 383
great arteries, transposition of, 314–315, 315*f*
greater cornu, formation of, 165*t*
greater vestibular glands
  development of, 248*t*
Greece, ancient view on embryology in, 8
Gregg, Norman, 11
growth, 73
  fetal, factors influencing, 104
gubernaculum, 248*t*, 277
gubernaculum testis, 248*t*
gums, development of, 451
gut
  primordial, 212, 212*f* (*See also* Foregut; Hindgut; Midgut)
gynecomastia, 446

H
habitual abortion, definition of, 7
hair
  development of, 442*f*, 447
  lanugo, 101
hair bulb, 447
hand(s)
  development of, 368*f*
hand plates, 80, 366
Hanhart syndrome, 178
haploid nucleus, 20
haploid number, 15
harlequin fetus, 443
Harvey, William, 9
haversian systems, 339
hCG. *See* Human chorionic gonadotropin
head
  congenital anomalies of, 348, 351*f*, 352–353, 352*f*
  fetal
    circumference of, 98, 99*f*, 102
head fold, 73, 75*f*, 76*f*
  and cardiovascular system, 295*f*
heart
  conducting system of, 308*f*, 308–309
  congenital anomalies of, 309–317
  development of, 292–309
    early, 286–292, 286*f*, 290*f*
  position of, head fold and, 295*f*
  primordial
    circulation through, 292, 296*f*–298*f*
    partitioning of, 292–293, 295, 297, 298*f*, 299*f*, 301*f*
  three-chambered, 313
  veins associated with, development of, 286–291, 289*f*–290*f*
heart prominence, 80
heart rate, fetal, monitoring of, 107
heart tubes, 67, 293*f*–295*f*
hematogenesis, 66*f*, 67
hematopoiesis, 220
hematopoietic center, 224
hematopoietic stem cells, 167
hemiazygos vein, 289*f*
hemivertebra, 350*f*, 351
hemolytic disease of newborn, 120
  intrauterine fetal transfusion for, 107
hemopoietic cells, of bone marrow, 339
heparin, use during pregnancy, 477
hepatic cords, 219–220
hepatic diverticulum, 218
hepatic ducts, accessory, 220
hepatic portal system, 287
hepatic segment, of inferior vena cava, 289*f*, 291
hepatic sinusoids, 220, 287
hepatic veins, 289*f*, 326
hepatoduodenal ligament, 220
hepatogastric ligament, 220
hepatopancreatic ampulla, 216
hepatoportoenterostomy, Kasai, 221
hermaphroditism, 273–274, 275*f*
hernia
  diaphragmatic, congenital, 153–155, 155*f*, 156*f*
    and pulmonary hypoplasia, 208
  epigastric, congenital, 155
  hiatal, congenital, 155, 213
  inguinal, congenital, 282
  internal, 232, 233*f*
  parasternal, 155
  retrosternal, 155
  umbilical, 224, 227*f*, 229
herpes simplex virus, as teratogen, 472*t*
hiatal hernia, congenital, 155, 213
hilum of kidney, 249
hindbrain, 393
hindgut, 73
  congenital anomalies of, 238–240
  derivatives of, 235
hippocampal commissure, 402, 404*f*
Hippocrates of Cos, 8
His, Wilhelm, 10
histones, 492
HIV infection, fetal effects of, 481
holoprosencephaly, 409–410, 412*f*, 423, 471
homeobox (HOX) genes, 471
  and skeletal development, 339
homeobox (HOX) proteins, 492–493
homologous chromosomes (homologs), 15, 459
hormones
  masculinizing, 265–266
  transplacental transport of, 119*f*, 120
horseshoe kidney, 255, 255*f*
housekeeping genes, 470
human chorionic gonadotropin (hCG), 43–44
human immunodeficiency virus (HIV) infection, fetal effects of, 481
human parvovirus B19, as teratogen, 472*t*
hyaline cartilage, 339
hyaloid artery, 420, 421*f*, 424*f*
  persistence of, 428
hydatidiform mole, 67
hydatid (of Morgagni), 248*t*, 270
hydranencephaly, 410
hydrocele, 282*f*
  testicular, 282
hydrocephalus, 407–409, 411*f*, 412*f*
hydronephrosis, 250
hygroma, cystic, 335, 444
hymen, 248*t*, 270, 277, 279*f*
hyoid bone, formation of, 165*t*
hypaxial division, of myotomes, 358, 359*f*
hypertrichosis, 443*f*, 447
hypertrophic pyloric stenosis, congenital, 216, 217*f*
hypoblast, 43*f*
hypobranchial eminence, 178*f*
hypogastric vein, 289*f*
hypoglossal nerve, 177, 414
hypoglycemic drugs, fetal effects of, 479
hypoparathyroidism, congenital, 173
hypopharyngeal eminence, 176, 178*f*, 198
hypophysial cartilage, 347, 348*f*
hypophysial diverticulum (pouch), 399, 401*f*
hypopituitarism, 277
hypoplastic left heart syndrome, 317, 319*f*
hypospadias, 275–276, 276*f*
hypotelorism, 410
hypothalamic sulcus, 399
hypothalamus, 399
hypothyroidism, 174

I
ichthyosis, 442–443, 443*f*
ileal diverticulum, 233–234, 234*f*
iliac arteries, 374*f*
  common, 249, 292, 374*f*
  external, 374*f*
  internal, 292, 328*f*, 329*f*
iliac lymph sacs, 334*f*
iliac veins
  common, 289*f*
  external, 289*f*
  internal, 289*f*
immunogobulins, transplacental transport of, 119*f*
immunoprotection, of placenta, 121
imperforate anus, 222, 239, 239*f*, 240*f*
implantation
  of blastocyst, 28, 48
    inhibition of, 51
    sites of, 45–47, 52*f*
  definition of, 2
  extrauterine, 45–47
inactivation, of genes, 461
incisive fossa, 187, 188*f*
incus
  formation of, 160, 165*t*
India, ancient views of embryology in, 9
indifferent gonad, 263
  adult derivatives and vestigial remains of, 248*t*
indifferent stage of sex development, 262–263
indomethacin, and ductus arteriosus closure, 330
induced abortion, definition of, 7
inductions, 78, 78*f*
infancy, 7
infants
  circulation in, 303*f*
infectious agents
  as teratogens, 472*t*, 480
  transplacental transport of, 119*f*, 120–121
inferior colliculi, 398–399
inferior mesenteric artery, 212*f*, 214*f*, 222*f*, 235
inferior vena cava, 302*f*, 303*f*, 310*f*, 311*f*, 329*f*, 330*f*, 331*f*, 332*f*, 334*f*
  development of, 289*f*–290*f*, 291
  double, 291
  hepatic segment of, 289*f*, 291
  postrenal segment of, 289*f*, 291
  prerenal segment of, 289*f*, 291
  renal segment of, 289*f*
  valve of, 304*f*–305*f*
infundibular stem, 400
infundibular stenosis, 316
infundibulum, 399
inguinal canals
  congenital anomalies of, 282
  development of, 277, 280*f*
inguinal hernia, congenital, 282
insulin therapy, fetal effects of, 479
intercalated discs, 360
intercostal arteries, 292, 323*f*, 344
intermediate mesoderm, 65
intermediate zone, 381
intermediolateral cell column, 416
internal capsule, 402
internal hernia, 232, 233*f*
interosseous artery, 374*f*
  common, 374*f*
intersegmental arteries, 292, 321*f*, 324*f*, 326*f*, 344, 345, 374*f*
  dorsal, 67*f*, 287*f*, 344
interstitial cells (of Leydig), 264
interstitial ectopia, 281
interthalamic adhesion, 399
interventricular foramen, 301, 305*f*–307*f*
interventricular septum
  membranous part of, 307*f*–308*f*
  muscular part of, 301, 307*f*
  primordial, 299*f*
intervertebral disc, 344, 345*f*

intervillous space, 114f, 116
interzonal mesenchyme, 342
intestine(s)
  atresia of, 232–233
  congenital anomalies of, 219f
  duplication of, 234–235, 236f
  fixation of, 227, 228f
  gangrene of, 231
  midgut loop of, 224
  rotation of, 226f
  stenosis of, 232–233
intracartilaginous ossification, 339–342, 343f
intracytoplasmic sperm injection, 35
intraembryonic coelom, 65, 76f, 146, 149f, 157, 182f, 222f
intraembryonic mesoderm, 339
intramembranous bone formation, 339
intramembranous ossification, 339
intraretinal space, 420
intrauterine fetal transfusion, 107
intrauterine growth retardation
  cigarette smoking and, 475
inversion, chromosomal, 467f, 468, 469
ionizing radiation, as teratogen, 472t, 482
iris
  coloboma of, 422, 426f
  color of, 426
  development of, 425
ischiadic artery, 374f
isochromosomes, 469
isotretinoin, as teratogen, 472t
IUGR. *See* Intrauterine growth retardation

J
Japanese atomic bomb survivors, birth defect studies in, 482
Jews, ancient views on embryology, 8
joint(s)
  cartilaginous, 344, 344f
  costovertebral, 346–347, 346f
  development of, 342–344
  fibrous, 344, 344f
  synovial, 344, 344f
joint laxity, generalized, 377
jugular lymph sacs, 334f
jugular vein, 289f

K
Kasai hepatoportoenterostomy, 221
keratinization
  disorders of, 442–444
kidney(s)
  blood supply, changes in, 249–250
  congenital anomalies of, 252–256, 254f–257f
  cystic disease of, 255–256, 257f
  development of, 79, 244–250, 247f, 251f
    molecular studies of, 250f
  duplex, 256f
  ectopic, 253f, 254
  hilum of, 249
  horseshoe, 255, 255f
  malrotation of, 253f, 254
  pelvic, 253f, 254
  positional changes of, 249, 251f
  supernumerary, 253f, 255
Klinefelter syndrome, 466f
Klippel-Feil syndrome, 348–350

L
labial commissure, 272f, 273
labia majora, 248t, 272f, 273
labia minora, 248t, 272f, 273
labiogingival groove, 182
labiogingival lamina, 182
labioscrotal swellings
  adult derivatives and vestigial remains of, 248t
labor, 123–133, 124f, 125f
lacrimal glands, development of, 430
lacunae, 44
lacunar network, 45
lamellar ichthyosis, 443–444
lamina terminalis, 402, 403f
lanugo, 101, 447
laryngeal atresia, 198
laryngeal cartilages, 198
  formation of, 165t
laryngeal inlet, 198
laryngeal nerves, 319
  recurrent, 322f
laryngotracheal diverticulum, 198, 199f
laryngotracheal groove, 178f, 198
laryngotracheal tube, 198
laryngotracheoesophageal cleft, 201
larynx
  congenital anomalies of, 201
  development of, 198, 200f
  intrinsic muscles of, formation of, 165t
last normal menstrual period (LNMP), 96
lateral, as descriptive term, 12f, 13
lateral inhibition, 491
lateral mesoderm, 65
lateral palatal process, 186, 188f
lead, as teratogen, 480
Leeuwenhoek, Anton van, 10
legally induced abortion, 7
lens, development of, 427–428
lens capsule, 427
lens epithelium, subcapsular, 427
lens pit, 420
lens placodes, 79, 420
lens vesicle, 420
Lenz, Widukind, 11
leptomeninges, 384
lesser cornu, formation of, 165t
lesser omentum, 220
lesser sac of peritoneum. *See* Omental bursa
Levan, Albert, 11
levator of thyroid gland, 173
levator palpebrae superioris muscle, abnormal development of, 430
levator veli palatini, formation of, 165t
Leydig cells, 264
ligament(s)
  anular, failed differentiation of, 435
  broad, 269, 271f
  falciform, 220
  hepatoduodenal, 220
  hepatogastric, 220
  of malleus, anterior, 165t
  ovarian, 248t, 281
  periodontal, 449
  round
    of liver, 303f, 331
    of uterus, 248t, 281
  sphenomandibular, 165t
  splenorenal, 224
  stylohyoid, formation of, 165t
  umbilical, medial, 303f, 331
  umbilical, median, 62, 257, 258f
ligamentum arteriosum, 321f–322f, 331, 334f
ligamentum teres, 303f
ligamentum venosum, 303f, 331
limb(s)
  blood supply to, 371–372, 374f
  congenital anomalies of, 375–377
  cutaneous innervation of, 368–371
  development of, 80t, 365–372, 367f, 371f
  muscles, 359
limb buds, 365, 365f
  lower, 366
  upper, 366
limb plexuses, 368
lingual cysts and fistulas, congenital, 177
lingual papillae, 176–177
lingual septum, 176
lingual swellings, 176
lingual thyroid tissue, 175
lingual tonsil, 334
lip(s)
  cleft, 188–192, 191f, 192f
lithium carbonate, as teratogen, 472t, 479
liver
  congenital anomalies of, 220–221
  development of, 218–220, 218f, 222f
  primordium of, 219
  round ligament of, 331
  visceral peritoneum of, 220
LNMP. *See* Last normal menstrual period
lobster-claw anomalies, 376, 376f
lobule, 434
low-birth weight, 96, 103
lumbar arteries, 292
lumbar rib, 350
lumbosacral meningomyelocele, 388
lung(s)
  accessory, 208
  agenesis of, 208
  congenital anomalies of, 208, 208f
  cysts of, 208, 208f
  development of, 202–207
    oligohydramnios and, 207
  hypoplasia, 208
  maturation of, 203–207
    alveolar period (late fetal period to childhood) of, 204f, 205f, 206
    canalicular period (16 to 25 weeks) of, 203–204, 204f, 205f
    terminal sac period (24 weeks to birth) of, 204–206, 204f
  neonatal, 207
lymphangioma, cystic, 444
lymphatic nodules, 166
lymphatic system
  congenital anomalies of, 334–335
  development of, 333–334, 334f
lymph ducts
  development of, 333, 334f
  right, 334f
lymphedema, 334–335
lymph nodes, development of, 333
lymphocytes, development of, 167, 333–334
lymph sacs
  development of, 333, 334f
  iliac, 334f
  jugular, 334f
  retroperitoneal, 334f
lymph sinuses, 333

M
macroglossia, 178
macrostomia, 192
magnetic resonance imaging
  for fetal assessment, 107, 107f
major histocompatibility complexes, and placental immunoprotection, 121
malformation, definition of, 459
Mall, Franklin P., 10
malleus
  anterior ligament of, 160, 165t
  formation of, 160, 165t
Malpighi, Marcello, 9–10
mamillary bodies, 399
mammary glands, 444–446
  congenital anomalies of, 446
mammary pit, 445
mandibular prominences, 164f
mandibular teeth, 450
marginal sinus, 371

masculinizing hormones, 265–266
mastication, muscles of, formation of, 162, 165*t*, 166*f*
mastoid antrum, 433
mastoid processes, 433
maternal age
  and chromosomal abnormalities, 20, 105, 461, 465*t*
  dizygotic twins and, 134
  ideal, 21
mature sperm, 20
maxillary prominences, 164*f*
maxillary sinuses, 184
maxillary teeth, 450
McBride, William, 11
meatal plug, 434
mechanical factors as teratogens, 483
Meckel cartilage, 160
meconium, 131, 240
medial, as descriptive term, 12*f*, 13
medial umbilical ligament, 303*f*
median artery, 374*f*
median eminence, 400
median palatal process, 185, 186*f*, 187*f*
median plane, 12*f*, 13
median sulcus of tongue, 178*f*
median tongue bud, 178*f*
median umbilical ligament, 62
mediastinum, primordial, 149
medulla oblongata, development of, 393
medulla of suprarenal glands, 248*t*, 260, 262*f*
medullary cavity, 341
medullary center, 404
medullary cone, 385
megacolon, congenital, 238, 238*f*
megacystis, congenital, 257, 259*f*
meiosis, 15, 17*f*
meiotic division
  first, 15
  second, 15
    in spermatogenesis, 20
melanoblast, 440, 447
melanocytes, 440, 447
membranes. *See also specific membranes*
  fetal
    after birth, 111, 123, 126*f*
    development of, 112*f*
    multiple pregnancies and, 134–135
    premature rupture of, 133, 133*f*
membranous atresia of anus, 239, 239*f*, 240*f*
membranous cochlea, 431, 432*f*
membranous labyrinth of internal ear, 431, 432*f*, 433
membranous neurocranium, 347
membranous viscerocranium, 347
menarche, 8
Mendel, Gregor, 11
meninges, spinal, 384
meningocele, 389–391, 405, 408*f*
meningoencephalocele, 405, 409*f*
meningohydroencephalocele, 405
meningomyelocele, 389–391
meninx, primordial, 384
menopause, 20
menstrual age, 15
menstrual period
  first (menarche), 8
mental retardation, 413
mercury, as teratogen, 472*t*, 480
meroencephaly, 405–407, 410*f*
meromelia, 375, 375*f*, 479
mesencephalon. *See* Midbrain
mesenchymal cells, 57
mesenchyme, 57
  interzonal, 342
  and skeletal development, 339
mesenteric artery
  inferior, 212*f*, 214*f*, 222*f*, 235
  superior, 146, 212*f*, 214*f*, 222*f*, 224
mesentery (mesenteries), 148*f*
  definition of, 146
  development of, 146
  of stomach, 213, 214*f*, 215*f*, 216
mesoblast, 57
mesocardium, 292
  dorsal, 294*f*
mesoderm
  embryonic, 55, 57
    derivatives of, 75, 77*f*
  intermediate, 65
  intraembryonic, 339
  lateral, 65
  paraxial, 65
    derivatives of, 339, 340*f*
mesodermal cells, and skeletal development, 339
mesonephric ducts, 244
  adult derivatives and vestigial remains of, 248*t*
  remnants, 270
mesonephric tubules, 244
  adult derivatives and vestigial remains of, 248*t*
mesonephroi, 244, 246*f*, 247*f*
mesovarium, 265, 270
metabolism, placental, 118
metanephric diverticulum, 244, 248*f*
metanephric tubules, 244
metanephrogenic blastema, 244
metencephalon, 393, 397, 397*f*
methadone, fetal effects of, 480
methotrexate, as teratogen, 472*t*, 478
methylmercury, as teratogen, 472*t*, 480
microcephaly, 353, 407, 410*f*, 476
microdeletions, 467–468, 468*t*
microduplications, 467–468, 468*t*
microglial cells (microglia), histogenesis of, 381
microglossia, 178
micromelia, 479
micropenis, 277
microphthalmia, 423–424
microscopes, and early embryology, 10*f*
microstomia, 192–195
microtia, 435
midbrain, 398–399, 398*f*, 400*f*
midbrain flexure, 392
Middle Ages, embryology in, 8–9
midgut, 73
  congenital anomalies of, 231–235
  derivatives of, 224
  nonrotation of, 231, 233*f*
  return to abdomen, 226*f*, 227
  reversed rotation of, 231
  rotation of, 224, 226*f*
  volvulus of, 231
Miller-Dieker syndrome, 468*t*
Minamata disease, 480
missed abortion, definition of, 7
mitral valve, development of, 308*f*
mobile cecum, 231
molecular biology, of human development, 11
molecular cytogenetics, 468
molecular studies
  of bone development, 339
monozygotic twins, 134, 137–138, 137*t*, 139*f*, 140*f*
  conjoined, 139, 142*f*
mons pubis, 272*f*, 273
morphogenesis, 55, 73
  branching, 206, 246
morphogens, 366, 488–491
morula, 2
mosaicism, 274, 462–465
  erythrocyte, 135–136
motor axons, 368
mouth
  congenital anomalies of (*See* Cleft lip and palate)
multicystic dysplastic kidney disease, 256, 257*f*
multifactorial inheritance, 309, 458*f*, 484, 484*f*
multiple pregnancy. *See also* Twin(s)
  and fetal growth, 104
  spontaneous abortion in, 25
muscle(s). *See also specific muscles*
  accessory, 362
  cardiac, development of, 360, 381
  congenital anomalies of, 361–362
  skeletal, development of, 358–359
  smooth, development of, 360
  variations in, 362
muscular dystrophy, 361
myelencephalon, 393–394, 396*f*
myelination, of spinal nerve fibers, 386, 390*f*
myelin proteins, 386
myeloschisis, 391, 394*f*
mylohoid muscle, formation of, 165*t*
myoblasts, 339, 340*f*, 358
myocardium, 292
  development of, 293*f*–294*f*
myofibrils, 358
myogenic precursor cells, 358
myotomes, 339, 340*f*, 358, 359*f*
myotubes, 358

N

nail(s)
  absence of, 448
  deformed, 448, 448*f*
  development of, 448
nail fields, 448
nail folds, 448
nasal cavities, development of, 182–185, 183*f*
nasal pits, 179, 182, 183*f*
nasal placode, 179
nasal prominences, 179
nasal sacs, primordial, 183, 183*f*
nasolacrimal duct, 169, 180–181
nasolacrimal groove, 179
nasopalatine canal, 187
natal teeth, 451
natural killer cells, killer-inhibitory receptors in, and placental immunoprotection, 121
neck
  congenital anomalies of, 348, 351*f*, 352–353, 352*f*
neocerebellum, 397
neonatal blood flow, 325
  transitional, 327–330
neonatal lungs, 207
neonate
  circulation in, 303*f*
nephrogenic cord, 244, 245*f*
nephron(s), development of, 244, 249*f*
nephron loop, 244
nerve(s)
  abducent, formation of, 414
  accessory, formation of, 415*f*, 416
  chorda tympani, 415, 433
  cochlear, 416
  cranial, 414–415
    formation of, 165*t*
    somatic efferent, 414–415
    special visceral afferent components of, 415
    special visceral efferent (branchial) components of, 162–163
  facial, formation of, 165, 165*t*, 415
  glossopharyngeal, 165, 165*t*, 177, 415
  hypoglossal, 177, 414
  laryngeal, 319
    recurrent, 322*f*

nerve(s)—cont'd
  myelination, 386
  oculomotor, 415, 430
  olfactory, 184, 416
  optic, development of, 416
  pharyngeal arch, 415–416
    derivatives of, 165*t*
  pharyngeal arch, 162–166
  spinal, 414
  trigeminal, 165, 165*t*, 177, 415, 434
  trochlear, formation of, 414
  vagus, 415–416
    formation of, 165, 165*t*
    superior laryngeal branch of, formation of, 165*t*
  vestibular, 416
  vestibulocochlear, formation of, 416
nervous system. *see also* Brain; Spinal cord
  autonomic, 416
  cells in, histogenesis of, 387*f*
  origin of, 381
  parasympathetic, development of, 416
  peripheral, development of, 413–416
neural canal, 381
neural crest
  derivatives of, 389*f*
  formation of, 62–64, 64*f*
neural crest cells, 62
  and cardiovascular development, 305–306
  derivatives of, 75, 77*f*
  and limb development, 368
  and skeletal development, 339
  and spinal development, 383
  and thymic development, 167
neural crest populations, 179
neural folds, 62, 64*f*, 384*f*
neural groove, 62, 64*f*
neural plate, 62
  formation of, 62
  and origin of nervous system, 382*f*
neural retina, 420
neural tube, 382*f*, 383*f*
  development of, 62–64, 64*f*, 381
  nonfusion of, 381 (*See also* Neural tube defects)
neural tube defects, 65, 386–387, 391–392, 394*f*, 395*f*
neuroblasts, 394
neurocranium
  cartilaginous, 347, 348*f*
  membranous, 347
neuroectoderm, 77*f*, 420
neurohypophysial diverticulum, 399
neurohypophysis, 400
neurolemma (Schwann) cells, 386
neuropores, 79, 381, 384*f*
neurula
  definition of, 2
neurulation, 62–64, 381
  abnormal, congenital anomalies resulting from, 65
nevus flammeus, 444
Newton, Isaac, 8
ninth week, 98–100, 98*f*, 99*f*
nipples
  absence of (athelia), 446
  development of, 445–446
  inverted, 447
  supernumerary, 446
nondisjunction of chromosomes, 35, 459, 460*f*
nonrotation, of midgut, 231, 233*f*
norethisterone, avoidance in pregnancy, 477
nose. *See also entries at* Nasal
  bifid, 192
  development of, 182–185, 183*f*
nostril, single, 192
notch-delta pathway, 488, 491, 492*f*
notochord, 59, 62
  development of, 61*f*
  remnant of, and chordoma, 62
notochordal canal, 59
notochordal plate, 59
notochordal process, 59, 60*f*, 62
NTDs. *See* Neural tube defects
nuclear aggregations, 118
nucleus pulposus, 344, 345*f*
numerical chromosomal abnormalities, 459
nutrients
  transfer to embryo, 120
  transplacental transport of, 119*f*

O

oblique vein, 289*f*, 290*f*
obstructive uropathy, 131
ocular muscles, 358, 361*f*
oculomotor nerve, 415, 430
odontoblastic processes, 449
odontoblasts, 449
olfactory bulb, 184, 416
olfactory epithelium, 184
olfactory nerve, 184, 416
oligodendrocytes, 381, 386
oligohydramnios, 130–131, 207
  bilateral renal agenesis and, 252–253
olivary nucleus, 394, 396*f*
omental bursa, 215*f*, 216
omphalocele, 228–229, 230*f*, 231*f*
omphaloenteric duct, 147, 224
omphaloenteric fistula, 234, 234*f*
On the Formation of the Foetus (Galen), 9
oocysts, in toxoplasmosis, 481
oocyte(s)
  prenatal maturation of, 20
  primary, 20, 265
oocyte maturation inhibitor (OMI), 20
oogenesis, 16*f*
  abnormal, 18f
oogonia, 20
optic chiasm, 403
optic cup, 420
optic disc, 420
  edema of, 429
optic groove, 420
optic nerve, development of, 416
optic stalk, 420
optic vesicle, 399, 420
oral contraceptives
  fetal effects of, 477
  and ovulation, 20, 27
oropharyngeal membrane, 59, 73, 75*f*, 212
ossification, 8
  endochondral, 343*f*
  intracartilaginous, 339–342, 343*f*
  intramembranous, 339
  primary centers of, 98, 339
  secondary centers of, 341
osteoblasts, 339
osteoclasts, 339, 451
osteocytes, 339
osteogenesis, 339
  of long bones, 368
osteoid tissue, 339
ostium secundum defect, 312
otic capsules
  cartilaginous, 431, 432*f*, 433, 433*f*
otic pits, 79
otic vesicle, 432*f*
oval foramen, 300*f*, 301*f*, 302*f*, 303*f*, 310, 331
  closure at birth, 303*f*
  patent, 310, 311*f*–313*f*
oval fossa, 310*f*, 331
ovarian cortex, 248*t*, 266*f*
ovarian follicles
  development of, 248*t*
  primordial, 20
  secondary, 20
ovarian ligament, 248*t*, 281
ovarian vein, 289*f*
ovaries
  descent of, 281
  development of, 248*t*, 265, 266*f*, 271*f*
ovulation
  oral contraceptives and, 20, 27
ovum. *See* Oocyte(s)
oxazepam, use during pregnancy, 480
oxygen
  transplacental transport of, 119*f*
oxyphil cells, 169

P

palate
  cleft, 188–192, 191*f*, 192*f*
  development of, 185–187, 186*f*, 187*f*
  primary, 185–186, 186*f*, 187*f*
  secondary, 186, 188*f*
palatine tonsil, 334
paleocerebellum, 397
palpebral conjunctiva, 426*f*, 429
pancreas
  accessory tissue of, 222, 234*f*
  anular, 222–223, 224*f*, 241
  congenital anomalies of, 222–223
  development of, 221–222, 223*f*, 225*f*
  head of, 221
  histogenesis of, 222
pancreatic acini, 222
pancreatic buds, 221
pancreatic ducts, 221–222
pancreatic islets, 222
Pander, Heinrich Christian, 10
papilla (papillae)
  circumvallate, 178*f*
  of tongue, development of, 178*f*
papillary muscles, 301, 308*f*
papilledema of optic disc, 429
parachordal cartilage, 347, 348*f*
paradidymis, 248*t*
parafollicular cells, 169
paralingual sulcus, 179
paralysis, sphincter, with spina bifida cystica, 388
paramesonephric duct
  adult derivatives and vestigial remains of, 248*t*
  development of, 265
  and female genital system, 269
  remnants, 270
parametrium, 269
paranasal sinuses, development of, 184–185, 187*f*, 348
  postnatal, 185
paraoophoron, 270
parasitic twin, 142*f*
parasternal hernia, 155
parasympathetic nervous system, development of, 416
parathyroid glands
  abnormal number of, 173
  congenital anomalies of, 173
  development of, 167, 168*f*
  ectopic, 173
  histogenesis of, 167, 169
paraurethral glands, 248*t*, 269
paraxial mesoderm, 65
  derivatives of, 339, 340*f*
parietal pleura, 203
paroophoron, 248*t*
parotid glands, development of, 179
pars distalis, 399

pars intermedia, 400
pars nervosa, 400
pars tuberalis, 399–400
parturition, 123–133, 124f, 125f
parvovirus B19, as teratogen, 472t
patent ductus arteriosus, 315f, 331–333, 334f
patent foramen primum, 312
patent oval foramen, 310, 311f–313f
Pax genes, 493
pectinate line, 236
pelvic kidney, 253f, 254
pelvis, renal
  development of, 248t
penile hypospadias, 275–276
penile raphe, 271
penis
  bifid, 277
  development of, 248t, 261f, 262f, 271–273, 272f
  double, 277
penoscrotal hypospadias, 275–276
percutaneous umbilical cord blood sampling (PUBS), 107
pericardial cavity, 152f, 292
  development of, 293f–295f
pericardial defects, congenital, 147
pericardial sinus, transverse, 292, 294f
pericardioperitoneal canals, 149, 150, 152f
pericardium
  visceral (endocardium), 293f–294f
perichondrium, 339
periderm, 440
perilymphatic space, 433
perinatology, 104
perineal hypospadias, 275–276
periodontal ligament, 449
periosteum, 339
peripheral nervous system, 413–416
peritoneum, lesser sac of. *See* Omental bursa
phallus
  adult derivatives and vestigial remains of, 248t
phallus, primordial, 271
pharyngeal arches, 79, 160–166, 161f
  arteries of, 163f (*See also* Aortic arches)
    double, 324, 324f
    fifth, 319
    first, 318
    fourth, 319
    second, 318
    sixth, 319
    third, 318
  cartilages of, derivatives of, 160–162, 165f, 165t
  components of, 160, 165t
  fate of, 160
  first, 160
    cartilage, derivatives of, 160, 165f, 165t
    muscles, derivatives of, 162, 165t, 166f
  fourth
    cartilage, derivatives of, 162, 165f, 165t, 178f
    muscles, derivatives of, 162, 165t, 166f
  muscles, 358
    derivatives of, 162, 165t, 166f
  nerves, 415–416
    derivatives of, 162–166, 165t
  second, 160
    cartilage, derivatives of, 162, 165f, 165t
    muscles, derivatives of, 162, 165t, 166f
  sixth
    cartilage, derivatives of, 165t, 178f
    muscles, derivatives of, 165t
  third
    cartilage, derivatives of, 162, 165f, 165t
    muscles, derivatives of, 162, 165t, 166f
  and tongue development, 178f
pharyngeal grooves, 169
pharyngeal hypophysis, 401
pharyngeal membranes, 166, 169, 434
pharyngeal pouches, 163f
  derivatives of, 166
  first, derivatives of, 166, 168f
  fourth, derivatives of, 167, 168f
  second, derivatives of, 166, 168f
  third, derivatives of, 166–167, 168f
pharyngeal tonsils, 334
pharyngotympanic tube, 75, 166, 168f, 169f, 195, 433
pharynx
  constrictor muscles of, formation of, 165t
phenylketonuria (PKU), fetal effects of, 483
phenytoin, as teratogen, 472t, 474–475, 478
physiologic umbilical hernation, 224
Pierre Robin syndrome, 172
pigment granules, 441
pili torti, 447–448
pineal gland (body), 399
pinocytosis, placental transport via, 118–119
piriform sinus fistula, 171
pituitary gland, 399, 399t, 401f
  glandular part of (adenohypophysis), 399, 399t, 401f, 417
placenta, 111–122
  abnormalities of, 125, 129f
  accessory, 123–125, 128f
  afterbirth, 111, 123, 126f
  as allograft, 121
  battledore, 125, 127f
  bidiscoid, 123
  development of, 111, 112f, 113f
  endocrine synthesis and secretion in, 121
  fetal part of, 111
  fetal surface of, 125, 126f
  functions and activities of, 118
  immunoprotection of, 121
  as invasive, tumor-like structure, 122
  maternal part of, 111
  maternal surface of, 123–125, 126f
  metabolism of, 118
  shape of, 113
  transport across, 118–121, 119f
    of drugs and drug metabolites, 119f, 120
    of electrolytes, 119f, 120
    by facilitated diffusion, 118
    of gases, 119f, 120
    of hormones, 119f, 120
    of infectious agents, 119f, 120–121
    of maternal antibodies, 119f
    of nutrients, 119f, 120
    by pinocytosis, 118–119
    by simple diffusion, 118
    via red blood cells, 119
    of waste products, 119f, 120
placenta accreta, 125, 129f
placental barrier. *See* Placental membrane
placental circulation
  fetal, 116f, 117, 117f
  maternal, 118
placental membrane, 118, 127f–129f
  transfer across, 119f
placental septa, 115, 116
placental stage, of labor, 123
placenta percreta, 125, 129f
placenta previa, 48, 125, 129f
plagiocephaly, 352
plantar artery, 374f
pleura
  parietal, 203
  visceral, 203
pleural cavities, 152, 152f
pleuropericardial membranes, 147–149, 150f
pleuroperitoneal membranes, 149–150, 151, 151f, 152f, 153–154
pneumocytes, 204
pneumonitis, tracheoesophageal fistula and, 201
Poland syndrome, 361
polychlorinated biphenyls, as teratogens, 472t, 480
polydactyly, 377, 378f
polyhydramnios, 131, 153
  duodenal atresia and, 218
  esophageal atresia/tracheoesophageal fistula and, 201
polyploidy, 461
polysplenia, 224
pons, development of, 393, 397, 397f
pontine flexure, 392
popliteal artery, 374f
portal system, hepatic, 287
portal vein, development of, 290f, 303f
port-wine stain, 444
posterior, as descriptive term, 12f
posterolateral defects of diaphragm, 153–155, 154f, 157f
postmaturity syndrome, 103–104
postnatal period, 7
Prader-Willi syndrome, 468, 468t
preaortic ganglia, 416
preauricular sinuses, 435
prechordal plate, 45, 59
pregnancy
  abdominal, 47, 52f
  cervical, 52
  ectopic, 45–47
  multiple, 134–140 (*See also* Twin(s))
    and fetal growth, 104
    spontaneous abortion in, 25
  prolonged (postmaturity syndrome), 103–104
  symptoms of, 55
  trimesters of, 97–98
  tubal, 45–47
  uterine growth in, 122, 122f
preimplantation genetic diagnosis, 39
prenatal development
  stages of, 2, 3–5
prepubertal growth spurt, 8
primitive groove, 57
primitive node, 57
primitive pit, 57
primitive streak, 57
  fate of, 57
primordial follicles, 20
primordium, definition of, 2
probe patent oval foramen, 310, 311f
processus vaginalis, 277
  persistent, 282, 282f
proctodeum, 212, 212f, 235, 236, 237f, 240f
profunda fermoris artery, 374f
progenitor cells. *See* Stem cells
progestogens/progestins
  as teratogens, 472t, 476–477
pronephroi, 244, 246
prosencephalic organizing center, 179
prosencephalon. *See* Forebrain
prostaglandin(s)
  and labor, 123
prostate gland, 270f
  development of, 248t, 269
prostatic utricle, 248t, 270
proximal, as descriptive term, 12
pseudohermaphroditism, 274
ptosis, congenital, 430, 430f
puberty
  definition of, 7
  oogenesis in, 20
  presumptive, legal age of, 8

puberty—cont'd
  presumptive age of, 496
  stages of, 8
PUBS (percutaneous umbilical cord blood sampling), 107
pulmonary artery
  left, 307*f*, 315*f*, 319, 321*f*, 322*f*
  right, 319, 321*f*
pulmonary atelectasis, 361
pulmonary trunk, 306, 307*f*, 316*f*
pulmonary valve stenosis, 316
pulmonary vein, 301, 302*f*–303*f*
  primordial, 305*f*
pupillary light reflex, 102
pupillary membrane, 427
  persistent, 428
Purkinje fibers, 360
pyloric stenosis, congenital hypertrophic, 216, 217*f*
pyramids, 393

Q
quickening, 100
Quran, 9

R
rachischisis, 351, 351*f*, 405
radial artery, 372, 374*f*
radiation, as teratogen, 472*t*, 482
radius bone, congenital absence of, 377
receptor tyrosine kinases, 488, 493–494, 494*f*
reciprocal induction, 246
rectal artery
  inferior, 238
  superior, 238
rectal atresia, 240–241, 240*f*
rectouterine pouch, 269
rectum
  development of, 236–238, 238*f*
  partitioning of, 237*f*
recurrent laryngeal nerve, 165*t*, 319, 322*f*
red blood cells, placental transport via, 119
Renaissance, embryology in, 9–11
renal agenesis, 130–131
renal arteries, 249, 250, 251*f*
  accessory, 250, 251*f*
renal calices, 244, 248*f*
renal ectopia, crossed, 253*f*, 254, 254*f*
renal pelvis
  development of, 248*t*
renal veins
  accessory, 250, 251*f*
  development of, 289*f*
reproductive system. *See* Genital system
respiratory bronchioles, 203
respiratory bud, 198, 200*f*
respiratory distress syndrome, 207
respiratory primordium, 198
rete ovarii, 248*t*, 265, 266*f*
rete testis, 248*t*, 263, 266*f*
retina
  central artery and vein of, 420, 423*f*, 426*f*
  coloboma of, 422
  development of, 420
retinal fissures, 420, 423*f*
retinoic acid
  endogenous, and embryonic development, 472
  exogenous, as teratogen, 472*t*, 479
retroesophageal right subclavian artery, 324
retroperitoneal lymph sacs, 334*f*
retrosternal hernia, 155
rhombencephalon. *See* Hindbrain
ribs
  accessory, 350
  cervical, 350
ribs—cont'd
  development of, 346–347, 346*f*
  floating, 347
  fused, 350*f*, 351
  lumbar, 350
rickets, 342
rima glottis, 178*f*
ring chromosome, 467, 467*f*
root canal, 449
rostral, as descriptive term, 12, 12*f*
rostral neuropore, 381
round ligament of liver, 303*f*, 331
round ligaments of uterus, 248*t*
Roux, Wilhelm, 11
rubella virus
  congenital infection, 479, 481*f*
  as teratogen, 472*t*, 480
    in ear development, 434
    in eye development, 428–429, 429*f*
  transplacental transport of, 119*f*
Rueff, Jacob, 9*f*

S
sacral arteries, lateral, 292
sacral vein, median, 289*f*
sacrococcygeal teratoma, 57–58, 59*f*
saddle anesthesia, with spina bifida cystica, 388
sagittal plane, 12*f*
Saint Hilaire, Etienne, 10
Saint Hilaire, Isidore, 10
salicylates, fetal effects of, 479
salivary glands, development of, 179
Samuel-el-Yehudi, 9
Sanskrit treatise on embryology, 9
satellite cells, 414
scalp vascular plexus, 81, 89*f*
scaphocephaly, 352, 352*f*
Schleiden, Mattias, 10
Schwann, Theodor, 10
Schwann cells, 386
sclera, development of, 429
sclerotomes, 339, 340*f*
scrotum
  development of, 248*t*, 271–273
sebaceous glands, 441, 442*f*
sebum, 440
secondary sexual characteristics
  development in puberty, 8
second meiotic division, 15
  in spermatogenesis, 20
segmental bronchi, 203
selective serotonin reuptake inhibitors, 480
semicircular ducts, 431
semilunar valves, 306, 308*f*, 317*f*
seminal colliculus, 248*t*
seminal glands, 267–269
seminiferous cords, 263, 267*f*
seminiferous tubules, 248*t*, 264, 266*f*, 267*f*
sensory axons, 368
septate uterus, 278*f*
septum pellucidum, 403
septum primum, 295, 299*f*, 300*f*, 301*f*, 302*f*, 305*f*, 311*f*
septum secundum, 295, 299*f*, 300*f*, 301*f*, 303*f*
septum transversum, 73, 75*f*, 150, 152*f*, 219, 221*f*, 295*f*
Sertoli cells, 20, 264
seventeenth week, 101*f*
seventh week, 80–81, 88*f*
sex chromatin patterns, 106
sex chromosomes
  disorders of, 278–279
sex determination, 263, 273–274
sexual characteristics, secondary
  development in puberty, 8
shaft of bone, formation of, 339
Shickel, Theophilus, 11
Shprintzen syndrome, 468*t*
signaling pathways
  and bone development, 339
  developmental, and birth defects, 471
simple diffusion, placental transport via, 118
single chromatid chromosomes, 15, 17*f*
single ventricle, 313
sinovaginal bulbs, 269
sinuatrial node, 308, 308*f*
sinuatrial valve, 292, 296*f*–298*f*
sinus(es)
  auricular, 169
  branchial, 169.170*f*, 171*f*
    external, 169.170*f*
    internal, 169.170*f*
  coronary, 290*f*, 291*f*, 297, 302*f*, 304*f*–305*f*, 310*f*
    persistent left superior vena cava and, 291
  frontal, 184
  lymph, 333
  marginal, 371
  maxillary, 184
  paranasal, development of, 184–185, 187*f*, 348
  pericardial, transverse, 292, 294*f*
  preauricular, 435
  spinal dermal, 387, 392*f*
  thyroglossal, 174, 175*f*
  urogenital, 256, 258*f*
    adult derivatives and vestigial remains of, 248*t*
sinus tubercle, 265, 269
  adult derivatives and vestigial remains of, 248*t*
sinus venarum, 297, 304*f*–305*f*
sinus venosus, 287, 289*f*–290*f*, 292, 293*f*–294*f*, 296*f*–297*f*, 297, 374*f*
  changes in, 297, 304*f*–305*f*
  circulation in, 296*f*–297*f*
  horns of, 290*f*, 296*f*–297*f*, 304*f*–305*f*
sinus venosus atrial septal defects, 310–312, 310*f*, 311*f*, 312*f*
sixth week, 80
skeletal muscle, development of, 358–359
skeletal system, development of, 340*f*
skeleton
  appendicular, development of, 353–355, 354*f*, 355*f*
  axial
    congenital anomalies of, 348–355
    development of, 344–348, 345*f*
  cardiac, 309
  congenital anomalies of, 353–355
skin
  angiomas of, 444, 455
  congenital anomalies of, 442–444
  development of, 440–442, 440*f*
  glands of, 441–442
skull. *See* Cranium
Smith-Magenis syndrome, 468*t*
smooth chorion, 111, 112*f*, 114*f*, 115*f*, 116
smooth muscle, development of, 360
somatic efferent cranial nerves, 414–415
somatopleure, 65
somites
  cervical, 153, 153*f*, 246*f*
  development of, 63*f*, 65
  myotomes of, 339, 340*f*
  and skeletal development, 339, 340*f*
Sonic hedgehog, 489–490, 490*f*
Spallanzani, Lazaro, 10
spectrophotometric studies, 105
Spemann, Hans, 11
sperm
  acrosome of, 19f, 20, 29, 30*f*
  acrosome reaction of, 29, 30*f*

sperm—cont'd
capacitation of, 29, 30*f*
components of, 20
definition of, 2
head of, 20
mature, 15, 20
neck of, 20
tail of, 20
spermatic cord, hydrocele of, 282, 282*f*
spermatic vein, 289*f*
spermatids, 20
spermatogenesis, 15–20
abnormal, 18*f*
genetic and molecular factors in, 20
spermatogonia, 15
spermatozoon. *See* Sperm
spermiogenesis, 20, 20*f*
sphenomandibular ligament, 165*t*
sphincter paralysis, with spina bifida cystica, 388
sphincter pupillae muscle, 425
spina bifida, 350, 351*f*, 386, 387–388, 388–389, 391*f*, 393*f*, 394*f*
spina bifida cystica
sphincter paralysis with, 388
spinal cord
adult, 385
central canal of, 381, 386*f*, 388*f*, 396*f*
congenital anomalies of, 386–392
development of, 381–387, 385*f*, 386*f*
in newborn, 385
positional changes of, 384–386
spinal dermal sinus, 387, 392*f*
spinal ganglion, development of, 383, 385*f*
spinal meninges, 384, 390*f*
spinal nerves, 414
spiral endometrial arteries, 44, 115*f*, 116, 116*f*
splanchnic mesoderm, extraembryonic, 45
splanchnopleure, 65
spleen
accessory, 224
development of, 223–224, 225*f*, 334
histogenesis of, 224
splenic artery, 224, 225*f*
splenorenal ligament, 224
spongy urethra, 271, 272*f*
spontaneous abortion
abnormal embryos and, 39
early, 49
of embryos, 48–49, 113*f*, 114*f*
in multiple pregnancies, 25
sporadic and recurrent, 48–49
stapedial arteries, 318
stapedius muscle
formation of, 165*t*
stapes
formation of, 165*t*
stem cells
lymphocytes from, 167
Steptoe, Patrick, 11
sternocostal hiatus, herniation through, 155
sternum
congenital anomalies of, 351
development of, 347
stomach
development of, 213–216, 214*f*, 215*f*, 225*f*
mesenteries of, 213, 214*f*, 215*f*, 216
rotation of, 213, 214*f*
stomodeum, 73, 75*f*, 179, 180*f*, 212
stratum germinativum, 440
streptomycin, as teratogen, 477
stylohyoid ligament, formation of, 165*t*
stylohyoid muscle, formation of, 165*t*
styloid process, formation of, 165*t*
stylopharyngeus muscle, formation of, 162, 165*t*, 166*f*
subarachnoid space, 384
subcardinal veins, 288, 289*f*
subclavian arteries, 319, 321*f*, 322*f*, 323*f*, 325*f*
right, 319, 321*f*, 322*f*, 324*f*
anomalous, 324
subclavian veins, 289*f*
sublingual thyroid gland, 175
submandibular duct, 179
submandibular glands, development of, 179
substantia nigra, 399
sudden infant death syndrome (SIDS), 309
sulci, cerebral, 406*f*
sulcus limitans, 383
sulcus terminalis, 301, 304*f*–305*f*
superfecundation, 140
superior, as descriptive term, 12*f*
superior colliculi, 398–399
superior laryngeal branch of vagus nerve, formation of, 165*t*
superior laryngeal nerve
formation of, 165*t*
superior vena cava, 302*f*–303*f*
development of, 288, 290*f*
double, 291, 291*f*
persistent left, 291
superior vesical arteries, 292, 303*f*, 329*f*, 331
supernumerary breasts and nipples, 446
supernumerary digits, 377, 378*f*
supernumerary kidney, 253*f*, 255
supracardinal veins, 289*f*, 291
suprarenal cortex, 262, 264*f*, 266*f*
suprarenal glands, development of, 246*f*, 250*f*, 260, 262*f*
suprarenal veins, development of, 289*f*
surfactant, 204
sustentacular cells, 264
Sutton, Walter, 11
sutures (cranial), 347, 349*f*
sweat glands, 441–442, 443*f*
apocrine, 442
Swiss cheese ventricular septal defects, 313
sympathetic trunk, 416
syncytiotrophoblast, 38, 43, 43*f*
syndactyly, 377, 378*f*
synostosis
cranial, 407
synovial joints, 344, 344*f*
synovial membrane, 344
syphilis
and birth defects, 472*t*
congenital, 482

T
tail fold, 73, 76*f*
talipes equinovarus, 377, 378*f*, 459, 483
Talmud, 8
taste buds, development of, 176–177
tectum, 398
teeth
abnormally sized, 452
congenital anomalies of, 451–454, 455*f*
development of, 448–451, 450*f*, 451*f*
bell stage of, 449–450, 450*f*
bud stage of, 449, 450*f*
cap stage of, 449
discolored, 453–454, 454*f*
eruption of, 448*t*, 450–451
natal, 451
neck of, 449
root of, 449
supernumerary, 452, 455*f*
variations in shape of, 451–452
tegmentum, 399
tela choroidea, 398
telencephalic vesicles, 399
telencephalon, 401–402
temporal bone, styloid process of, formation of, 165*t*
tendinous cords, 301, 305*f*, 308*f*
tensor tympani, 165*t*, 433
tensor veli palatini, formation of, 165*t*
teratogen(s), 472*t*
and critical periods of human development, 473*f*, 474
dose-response relationship for, 474
drugs as, 472*t*, 475–476
environmental chemicals as, 472*t*
infectious agents and, 472*t*
known human, 475–480
maternal factors as, 483
mechanical factors as, 483
teratogenicity, proof of, 475
teratology
definition of, 7, 458
terms in, 459
terminal filum, 386
terminal sac period, of lung maturation, 204–206, 204*f*
terminal sulcus, of tongue, 176, 178*f*
terminology
descriptive, 11–13, 12*f*
embryological, 2–7
testes (testicles)
descent of, 267*f*, 279–281, 280*f*
development of, 248*t*, 263–265, 266*f*
ectopic, 281, 281*f*
rete, 263, 266*f*
undescended, 276, 281, 282*f*
vesicular appendix of, 270
testicular feminization syndrome, 274–275, 275*f*
testicular hydrocele, 282, 282*f*
testosterone, 263, 264
tetracycline, as teratogen, 454, 472*t*, 477
tetralogy of Fallot, 316
tetraploidy, 465–466
tetrasomy, 462–465
thalamus, development of, 399
thalidomide, as teratogen, 372–373, 375*f*, 472*t*, 479
therapeutic abortion, 7
third trimester, 97, 118
third week, 55–69, 82*f*
thirty-seventh week, 103*f*
thirty-sixth week, 103*f*
thoracic duct, development of, 333, 334*f*
threatened abortion, definition of, 7
three-chambered heart, 313
thymic corpuscles, 167
thymus
accessory tissue of, 173, 173*f*
histogenesis of, 167
thyroglossal duct cysts and sinuses, 174, 175*f*
thyroid cartilage, formation of, 165*t*
thyroid follicles, 174
thyroid gland
accessory tissue of, 175, 176*f*
agenesis of, 175
congenital anomalies of, 174
development of, 173–174, 174*f*
ectopic, 175, 176*f*, 177*f*
histogenesis of, 173–174
isthmus of, 173, 174*f*
levator muscle of, 173
lingual tissue of, 175
sublingual, 175
thyroid hypoplasia, 173
tibial artery, 372, 374*f*
Tjio, Joe Hin, 11
toe buds, 369*f*
tongue
arch derivatives of, 178*f*

tongue—cont'd
bifid or cleft, 179
congenital anomalies of, 177, 178, 178*f*
development of, 176–177, 178*f*
distal buds of, 178*f*
median bud of, 178*f*
median sulcus of, 178*f*
muscles of, 359
nerve supply of, 177, 178*f*
papillae of, development of, 178*f*
posterior third (pharyngeal part) of, 178*f*
terminal sulcus of, 176, 178*f*
tongue-tie, 178, 178*f*
tonsil(s)
development of, 334
lingual, 334
palatine, 334
pharyngeal, 334
tubal, 334
tonsillar crypts, 166
tooth. *See* Teeth
torticollis, congenital, 362, 362*f*
Toxoplasma gondii (toxoplasmosis)
as teratogen, 472*t*, 481, 482*f*
transmission across placenta, 119*f*
trabeculae carneae, 301, 308*f*
trachea
congenital anomalies of, 198, 201, 202*f*
development of, 198
tracheal atresia, 201
tracheal diverticulum, 201
tracheal stenosis, 201
tracheoesophageal fistula, 198, 202*f*
tracheoesophageal folds, 198
tracheoesophageal septum, 198, 200*f*, 212
tranquilizers, as teratogens, 479
transcription factors, 488, 491–493
and bone development, 339
and placental development, 115
transfusion, intrauterine fetal, 107
translocation, chromosomal, 461, 466–467, 467*f*
transport, across placenta, 118–121, 119*f*
transposition of great arteries, 314–315, 315*f*
transverse plane, 12*f*, 13
Treacher Collins syndrome, 172
Treponema pallidum
as teratogen, 472*t*
tricuspid valve, development of, 308*f*
trigeminal ganglion, 415
trigeminal nerve, 165, 165*t*, 177, 415, 434
trigone region of bladder, 257, 258*f*
trigonocephaly, 352*f*, 353
trilaminar embryonic disc, 56*f*
trimester, 97–98
definition of, 7
trimethadione, as teratogen, 472*t*, 477
triploidy, 465, 466*f*
trisomy, 466*t*
of autosomes, 461, 463*f*
of sex chromosomes, 461–462
trisomy 13, 463*t*, 465*f*
trisomy 18, 463*t*, 465*f*
trisomy 21. *See* Down syndrome
trochlear nerve, formation of, 414
trophoblast. *See also* Cytotrophoblast; Syncytiotrophoblast
abnormal growth of, 67
extravillous, 121
true knots, in umbilical cord, 125, 127, 130*f*
truncus arteriosus, 290*f*, 292, 293*f*–294*f*, 296*f*
circulation through, 296*f*–298*f*
persistent, 314, 315*f*
transformation and adult derivatives of, 321*f*
unequal division of, 316, 317*f*
tubal pregnancy, 45–47
tubal tonsils, 334
tubotympanic recess, 166, 433
tumor, placenta as, 122
tunica albuginea, 264
tunica vasculosa lentis, 427
Turner syndrome, 461, 463*f*
twentieth week, 130*f*
twenty-fifth week, 101, 102*f*
twin(s)
conjoined, 139, 140*f*, 142*f*, 143*f*
dicephalic conjoined, 143*f*
dizygotic, 136*f*, 137, 137*t*, 141*f*
early death of single, 139
and fetal membranes, 134–135
maternal age and, 134
monozygotic, 134, 137–138, 137*t*, 139*f*, 140*f*
parasitic, 142*f*
zygosity of, 138–139
twin-twin transfusion syndrome, 136–137, 138*f*
tympanic cavity, 166, 433

U

ulnar artery, 374*f*
ultrasonic waves, fetal effects of, 483
ultrasound
for bone age determination, 353
of chorionic sac, 111, 115*f*
of embryos, 89, 92*f*
for estimation of fetal/gestational age, 89, 92*f*
for fetal assessment, 105
of heartbeat, 305, 306*f*
umbilical artery(ies), 116*f*, 135*f*, 302*f*, 374*f*
absence of (SUA), 128, 130*f*
adult derivatives of, 303*f*
Doppler velocimetry of, 127–128, 130*f*
fate of, 292
umbilical cord, 125–128
color flow Doppler ultrasound of, 125, 130*f*
prolapse of, 125
sampling of, 107
true knots in, 127, 130*f*
velamentous insertion of, 129*f*
umbilical hernia, 224, 229
umbilical ligament, medial, 62, 257, 258*f*
umbilical veins, 220, 286, 293*f*, 296*f*–297*f*, 302*f*, 325, 374*f*
adult derivatives of, 303*f*
development of, 289*f*–290*f*
transformation of, 290*f*
umbilical vesicle
fate of, 134
formation of, 133–134
primary, 44
secondary, 45
significance of, 134
uncinate process, 221
undescended testes, 276, 281, 282*f*
unicornuate uterus, 277, 278*f*
uniparental disomy, 470
urachus, 62, 257, 258*f*
congenital anomalies, 257, 259*f*
cysts of, 257, 259*f*
urea, transplacental transport of, 119*f*
ureter(s)
bifid, 253*f*, 255
congenital anomalies of, 252–256, 254*f*–257*f*
development of, 244–250, 248*t*
ectopic, 255, 256*f*
ureteric ectopia, 255
ureterostomies, fetal, 108*f*
urethra
clitoral, 274
development of, 248*t*, 260, 262*f*
spongy, 271, 272*f*
urethral folds, 271, 271*f*
adult derivatives and vestigial remains of, 248*t*
urethral glands, 269
urethral plate, 271
uric acid, transplacental transport of, 119*f*
urinary bladder
congenital anomalies of, 257–260, 259*f*, 260*f*
development of, 248*t*, 256–257, 258*f*
exstrophy of, 259–260, 260*f*, 261*f*
trigone of, 257, 258*f*
urinary system, development of, 244–250
urinary tract, duplications of, 253*f*, 255
urine formation, fetal, 98
uriniferous tubule, 246, 248*f*
urogenital groove, 271
urogenital membrane, 236, 237*f*, 271
urogenital ridge, 245*f*
urogenital sinus, 256, 258*f*
adult derivatives and vestigial remains of, 248*t*
vesical part of, 257, 258*f*
urogenital system
embryonic structures in, adult derivatives and vestigial remains of, 248*t*
uropathy, obstructive, 131
urorectal septum, 235, 237*f*, 238
uterine tubes
ampulla of, 22*f*, 26*f*
fertilization in, 31
development of, 248*t*
uteroplacental circulation
impaired, and fetal growth, 104
primordial, 44
umbilical cord Doppler velocimetry of, 128
uterovaginal primordium, 265, 269
uterus
absence of, 277
bicornuate, 277, 278*f*, 279*f*
with rudimentary horn, 277, 278*f*
congenital anomalies of, 277, 278*f*
development of, 248*t*, 269–270, 271*f*
double, 277, 278*f*
gravid, 115*f*
growth in pregnancy, 122, 122*f*
round ligament of, 281
septate, 278*f*
unicornuate, 277, 278*f*
utricle, 270
uvula, 187
cleft, 190, 191*f*

V

vagina
absence of, 277
adenocarcinoma of, diethylstilbestrol exposure and, 477
congenital anomalies of, 277
development of, 248*t*, 269–270
vaginal atresia, 277
vaginal plate, 269
vagus nerve, 415–416
formation of, 165, 165*t*
superior laryngeal branch of, formation of, 165*t*
vallate papillae, 176
valproic acid, as teratogen, 472*t*, 478
valve(s)
atrioventricular, development of, 305*f*, 308*f*
cardiac, development of, 305*f*, 306–308, 308*f*
of inferior vena cava, 304*f*–305*f*
mitral, development of, 308*f*
of oval foramen, 295, 299*f*–300*f*, 302*f*
semilunar, 306
sinuatrial, 296*f*–298*f*
tricuspid, development of, 308*f*

varicella virus, 481
  as teratogen, 472*t*
vascular structures, fetal, adult derivatives of, 303*f*, 330
vasculogenesis, 66–67, 66*f*
vas deferens. *See* Ductus deferens
vein(s)
  associated with heart, development of, 286–291, 289*f*–290*f*
  azygos, 288, 289*f*, 290*f*
    lobe of, 207
  brachiocephalic, left, 288, 289*f*–290*f*, 297
  cardinal, 296*f*–297*f*, 374*f*
    anterior, 287–288, 289*f*–290*f*, 291, 296*f*, 297, 302*f*
    common, 149*f*, 286, 287–288, 289*f*–290*f*, 291–292, 293*f*, 296*f*
    development of, 287–288, 289*f*–290*f*
    posterior, 67*f*, 247*f*, 287–288, 287*f*, 289*f*–290*f*, 296*f*
  endometrial, 116
  gonadal, 289*f*
  hemiazygos, 289*f*
  hepatic, 289*f*, 291, 326, 328*f*–329*f*, 330*f*, 331*f*
  hypogastric, 289*f*
  iliac
    common, 289*f*
    external, 289*f*
    internal, 289*f*
  jugular, 289*f*
  oblique, 289*f*, 290*f*
  ovarian, 289*f*
  portal, development of, 290*f*, 303*f*
  pulmonary, 301, 302*f*–303*f*
    primordial, 305*f*
  renal
    accessory, 250, 251*f*
    development of, 289*f*
  sacral, median, 289*f*
  spermatic, 289*f*
  subcardinal, 288, 289*f*
  subclavian, 289*f*
  supracardinal, 289*f*, 291
  suprarenal, development of, 289*f*
  umbilical, 220, 286, 293*f*, 296*f*–297*f*, 302*f*, 325, 374*f*
    adult derivatives of, 303*f*
    development of, 289*f*–290*f*
    transformation of, 290*f*
  vena cava (*See* vena cava)
  vitelline, 286, 287, 293*f*, 296*f*–297*f*, 374*f*
    development of, 289*f*–290*f*
velamentous insertion, of umbilical cord, 129*f*
velocardiofacial syndrome, 468*t*
vena cava
  congenital anomalies of, 291
  inferior, 302*f*
    development of, 289*f*–290*f*, 291
    hepatic segment of, 289*f*, 291
vena cava—cont'd
  inferior—cont'd
    postrenal segment of, 289*f*, 291
    prerenal segment of, 289*f*, 291
    renal segment of, 289*f*
  superior, 302*f*
    development of, 288, 290*f*
    double, 291, 291*f*
    persistent left, 291
Venezuelan equine encephalitis virus, as teratogen, 472*t*
ventral, as descriptive term, 12, 12*f*
ventral abdominal wall defects (VWDs), detection of, alpha-fetoprotein assay for, 105
ventral median fissure, 383
ventral median septum, 383
ventral mesentery, 219
ventricles
  cardiac, 292
    development of, 293*f*, 298*f*–299*f*
    primordial, positioning of, 301, 306*f*–308*f*
ventricular foramina, 402
ventricular septal defects, 312–313
ventricular zone, 381
ventriculoperitoneal shunt, for hydranencephaly, 410
vernix caseosa, 100
vertebrae, variation in number of, 346
vertebral artery, 292, 327*f*
vertebral body, 346
vertebral column
  cleft, 351, 351*f*
  congenital anomalies of, 348–351
  development of, 344–346, 345*f*
    bony stage of, 345–346, 346*f*
    cartilaginous stage of, 345, 346*f*
vesical artery, superior, 292, 329*f*, 331
vesicle(s)
  cerebral, 4*f*, 80*t*, 385, 401*f*, 403*f*
  lens, 420
  optic, 399, 420
  otic, 432*f*
  telencephalic, 399
  umbilical
    fate of, 134
vesicouterine pouch, 269
vesicular appendage, 270
vesicular appendix of testis, 270
vestibular nerve, 416
vestibulocochlear nerve, formation of, 416
viability
  of conjoined twins, 139
  of fetuses, 96
villous chorion, 111, 112*f*, 114*f*, 116*f*, 123, 132*f*
viruses, transplacental transport of, 119*f*
visceral peritoneum of liver, 220
visceral pleura, 203
viscerocranium
  cartilaginous, 347, 348*f*
  membranous, 347
vitamin(s), transplacental transport of, 119*f*
vitelline artery, 67*f*, 212*f*, 234*f*, 374*f*
  fate of, 292
vitelline veins, 286, 287, 293*f*, 296*f*–297*f*, 374*f*
  development of, 289*f*–290*f*
vitreous body, 427–428
volvulus, of midgut, 231
vomeronasal organ (VMO), 185
  remnants of, 185
vomeronasal primordia, 185
von Baer, Karl Ernst, 10
von Beneden, Eduard, 11

W

warfarin, as teratogen, 472*t*, 477
waste products, transplacental transport of, 119*f*, 120
water
  transplacental transport of, 119*f*
Watson, James, 11
weight
  birth
    cigarette smoking and, 104, 475
    extremely low, 96
    low, 96, 103
Wharton jelly, 125, 130*f*
white (anocutaneous) line, 236
white fat, fetal, 101–102, 103
white ramus communicans, 416
Williams syndrome, 468*t*
Wilmut, Ian, 11
Winiwarter, Felix von, 11
Wnt signaling pathway, 490–491
Wolff, Caspar Friedrich, 10

Y

Y chromosome
  and spermatogenesis, 20
yolk sac
  fate of, 134
  formation of, 133–134
  primary, 44
  secondary, 45
  significance of, 134

Z

zona fasciculata, 260, 262*f*
zona glomerulosa, 260, 262*f*
zona pellucida, 20
zone of polarizing acitivity (ZPA), 366
zygosity, in twin pregnancies, 138–139
zygote
  cleavage of, 35, 36*f*
    definition of, 2
  definition of, 2